KU-221-902

WITHDRAWN FROM LIBRARY

BRITISH MEDICAL ASSOCIATION
0757924

Oxford Textbook of

Fundamentals
of Surgery

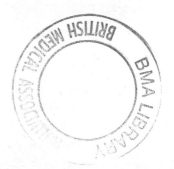

Free personal online access for 12 months

Individual purchasers of this book are also entitled to free personal access to the online edition for 12 months on *Oxford Medicine Online* (www.oxfordmedicine.com). Please refer to the access token card for instructions on token redemption and access.

Online ancillary materials, where available, are noted at the end of the respective chapters in this book. Additionally, *Oxford Medicine Online* allows you to print, save, cite, email, and share content; download high-resolution figures as PowerPoint® slides; save often-used books, chapters, or searches; annotate; and quickly jump to other chapters or related material on a mobile-optimized platform.

We encourage you to take advantage of these features. If you are interested in ongoing access after the 12-month gift period, please consider an individual subscription or consult with your librarian.

Oxford Textbook of
Fundamentals of Surgery

Edited by

Managing Editors

William E. G. Thomas

Malcolm W. R. Reed

Michael G. Wyatt

Section Editors

Mark Fordham

Kevin Sherman

Jonathan Beard

Jeremy Groves

Chris Oliver

James A. Morecroft

Bill Noble

J. Andrew Bradley

Jane M. Blazeby

Sub-section Editors

David A. Adams

Kate Gould

Jonathan D. Spratt

Ian Eardley

Maurice Hawthorne

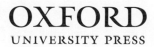

OXFORD
UNIVERSITY PRESS

Great Clarendon Street, Oxford, OX2 6DP,
United Kingdom

Oxford University Press is a department of the University of Oxford.
It furthers the University's objective of excellence in research, scholarship,
and education by publishing worldwide. Oxford is a registered trade mark of
Oxford University Press in the UK and in certain other countries

© Oxford University Press 2016

The moral rights of the authors have been asserted

First Edition Published in 2016

Impression: 1

All rights reserved. No part of this publication may be reproduced, stored in
a retrieval system, or transmitted, in any form or by any means, without the
prior permission in writing of Oxford University Press, or as expressly permitted
by law, by licence or under terms agreed with the appropriate reprographics
rights organization. Enquiries concerning reproduction outside the scope of the
above should be sent to the Rights Department, Oxford University Press, at the
address above

You must not circulate this work in any other form
and you must impose this same condition on any acquirer

Published in the United States of America by Oxford University Press
198 Madison Avenue, New York, NY 10016, United States of America

British Library Cataloguing in Publication Data
Data available

Library of Congress Control Number: 2016939455

ISBN 978–0–19–966554–9

Printed in Great Britain by
Bell & Bain Ltd., Glasgow

Oxford University Press makes no representation, express or implied, that the
drug dosages in this book are correct. Readers must therefore always check
the product information and clinical procedures with the most up-to-date
published product information and data sheets provided by the manufacturers
and the most recent codes of conduct and safety regulations. The authors and
the publishers do not accept responsibility or legal liability for any errors in the
text or for the misuse or misapplication of material in this work. Except where
otherwise stated, drug dosages and recommendations are for the non-pregnant
adult who is not breast-feeding

Links to third party websites are provided by Oxford in good faith and
for information only. Oxford disclaims any responsibility for the materials
contained in any third party website referenced in this work.

Series Preface from Professor Sir Peter J. Morris

This is a new development in surgical publishing; the first two editions of the *Oxford Textbook of Surgery* are to be replaced by a series of specialty-specific textbooks in surgery. This change was precipitated by the ever-increasing size of a single textbook of surgery which embraced all specialties (the second edition of the *Oxford Textbook of Surgery* was three volumes), and a decision to adapt the textbooks to meet the needs of the audience; firstly, to suit the requirements of Higher Surgical trainees and, secondly, to make it available online.

Thus, we have a produced a key book to deal with the Fundamentals of Surgery, such as Anatomy, Physiology, Biochemistry, Evaluation of Evidence, and so forth. Then there are to be separate volumes covering individual specialties, each appearing as an independent textbook and available on *Oxford Medicine Online*.

It is planned that each textbook in each specialty will be independent although there obviously will be an overlap between different specialties and, of course, the core book on *Fundamentals of Surgery* will underpin the required scientific knowledge and practice in each of the other specialties.

This ambitious programme will be spread over several years, and the use of the online platform will allow for regular updates of the different textbooks.

Each textbook will include the proposed requirements for training and learning as defined by the specialist committees (SACs) of surgery recognized by the four Colleges of Surgery in Great Britain and Ireland, and will continue to be applicable to a global audience.

When completed, the *Oxford Textbooks in Surgery* series will set standards for a long time to come.

Professor Sir Peter J. Morris
Nuffield Professor of Surgery Emeritus, and former
Chairman of the Department of Surgery and Director of the
Oxford Transplant Centre, University of Oxford and
Oxford Radcliffe Hospitals, UK

Foreword

A thorough knowledge of the relevant basic sciences and how to manage a patient from presentation to discharge is a prerequisite for all surgeons. Not only does a surgical trainee have to understand the fundamentals of anatomy, physiology, and pathology and acquire the necessary operative expertise, but they must also learn many other skills to be a successful surgeon. These include effective communication with patients, relatives, and colleagues in any circumstance, recognizing the signs of a critically ill surgical patient, dealing with acute trauma and diseases at the extremes of age, and keeping up to date by reading and appraising relevant research publications. These essential skills together with many others are addressed in ten core surgical training modules as part of the Intercollegiate Surgical Curriculum Programme, but to date there has been no single textbook that covers all of these areas. These modules are formally assessed in the Membership of the Royal College of Surgeons (MRCS) examination, which is delivered by the four Surgical Royal Colleges of the United Kingdom and Ireland and managed by the Intercollegiate Committee.

While the MRCS is an entrance requirement for doctors entering higher surgical specialty training in the United Kingdom and Ireland, many overseas doctors also aspire to MRCS, recognizing its value in focusing their learning as well as enhancing their own professional development and reputation.

Mr William Thomas, Professor Malcolm Reed, and Mr Michael Wyatt—three well-respected surgeons, teachers, and educators—have done an outstanding job in editing the *Oxford Textbook of Fundamentals of Surgery* by bringing together the whole core surgical curriculum in one definitive textbook. This is the first such textbook of its kind.

The book, divided into ten main sections, mirrors the ten modules of the core surgical curriculum. The whole curriculum is covered comprehensively in over 800 pages. Starting with the basic sciences, which includes an innovative overview of radiological anatomy for surgeons, the book takes readers through the remaining nine modules covering in detail basic surgical skills, perioperative care, and all aspects of surgical patient management, ending with an informative section on evidence-based surgery, research, and audit.

The editors are to be congratulated on attracting an outstanding group of authors, from established experts, many of whom are MRCS examiners themselves, to more junior colleagues who have passed the examination more recently! In doing so, the book is beautifully balanced, easy to read, and informative throughout. Each chapter is laid out clearly with a summary at the beginning and suggestions for further reading where appropriate. It is clearly illustrated, with over 350 professionally prepared diagrams, figures, and operative photographs to complement the text and assist with learning. In this way, many complex areas that can sometimes be difficult to learn and assimilate become much easier to understand. The text is also pitched at an appropriate level, remaining focused, yet detailed enough to appeal to a variety of readers.

Not only will this book be essential reading for junior doctors embarking on a surgical career, but it also contains a wealth of information which should appeal to more experienced surgeons, examiners, and those wishing to update or widen their knowledge in the basic sciences and 'surgery in general'.

In summary, the editors and publishers have produced a unique textbook that covers in detail the core surgical curriculum and which will be essential reading for trainees preparing for their MRCS examination and beyond. It is informative, easy to read, and its very nature sets it apart from other currently available books. I believe the *Oxford Textbook of Fundamentals of Surgery* will also find its place as a reference book on the bookshelves of many colleagues across surgical specialties as it contains a wealth of up-to-date information and knowledge and advice that underpins our day-to-day practice.

Peter A. Brennan MD FRCS FRCSI FDSRCS

Consultant Maxillofacial/Head and Neck Surgeon
Honorary Professor of Surgery
Queen Alexandra Hospital
Portsmouth, UK
Chairman
Intercollegiate Committee for Basic Surgical Examinations
(MRCS and DOHNS)
Past Chairman
MRCS Court of Examiners
Royal College of Surgeons of England, London, UK

Preface

'Surgery' is an ever changing facet of medical care, and it is crucial that all surgeons, and especially surgical trainees, are fully informed and kept up to date with recent advances as well as with tried and tested methods of diagnosis and management. As a result, surgical examinations have changed over the years to reflect the current needs and demands for a fair and yet objective way of ensuring that all surgeons have a comprehensive understanding of their profession with all its opportunities, advances, dangers, and limitations.

To clearly define a syllabus that would meet these demanding requirements has been a challenging task, but the Intercollegiate Surgical Curriculum was developed in an attempt to provide a clear and logical approach to the fundamentals of surgical training and subsequent practice. The curriculum seeks to provide surgical trainers, trainees, and examiners with a clear basis of what is required in order to have a functional and structured understanding of the fundamentals of surgery, so that the management of the surgical patient is optimal, safe, and compassionate. This has not been a rapid or easy task, but after nearly a decade of refinement, the curriculum is now more mature and robust and is proving a valuable asset to surgical training.

Having achieved a reliable, tried, and tested curriculum, there was a need for a surgical text that would comprehensively reflect, and be accurately mapped to this curriculum. This volume, covering the fundamentals of surgery, was therefore developed to provide such a text and has been closely based upon the surgical curriculum. Each author and section editor is not only an authority on their particular subject, but also an experienced trainer and examiner—many with vast experience of the new MRCS examination. It is the intention of the editors and publisher that this will rapidly be seen as the essential resource for those preparing for the MRCS as well as for any more senior surgeon who wishes to refresh their knowledge of the crucial underpinning evidence base for surgical practice.

The *Oxford Textbook of Fundamentals of Surgery* covers the generic issues that are relevant to all practising and training surgeons. It will form part of a series of reference texts that will make up the Oxford Textbooks in Surgery series with other volumes concentrating on each of the major surgical specialties. Each volume will be published both in print and online with full search functionality and linked references. As editors, we trust that the *Oxford Textbook of Fundamentals of Surgery* will provide the basis and strong foundation for all practising surgeons as well as trainees—after all, if one gets the 'Fundamentals' right, the rest will follow.

William E. G. Thomas, Malcolm W. R. Reed,
and Michael G. Wyatt
Sheffield, Brighton, and Newcastle

Brief contents

Contents

Abbreviations

2,3DPG	2,3-diphosphoglycerate		CEA	carotid endarterectomy or carcinoembryonic antigen
2D	two-dimensional		CES	cauda equina syndrome
3D	three-dimensional		CEUS	contrast-enhanced ultrasound
AAA	abdominal aortic aneurysm		CIN	cervical intraepithelial neoplasia
ABPI	ankle–brachial pressure index		CMM	cutaneous malignant melanoma
ACA	adenocarcinoma		CMV	*Cytomegalovirus*
ACC	American College of Cardiology		CNS	central nervous system
ACTH	adrenocorticotropin hormone		CO	cardiac output
ADH	antidiuretic hormone		CoA	coenzyme A
ADT	androgen deprivation therapy		COX	cyclooxygenase
AES	antiembolic stockings		CPAP	continuous positive airway pressure
AFP	α-fetoprotein		CPET	cardiopulmonary exercise testing
AGE	advanced glycation end product		CPP	cerebral perfusion pressure
AHA	American Heart Association		CPR	cardiopulmonary resuscitation
AI	aromatase inhibitor *or* adrenal insufficiency		CRC	colorectal cancer
AIS	Abbreviated Injury Scale		CRP	C-reactive protein
AKI	acute kidney injury		CSF	cerebrospinal fluid
ALI	acute limb ischaemia		CT	computed tomography
ALT	alanine transaminase		CTPA	computed tomography pulmonary angiography
ANS	autonomic nervous system		CVU	chronic venous ulceration
ANTT	aseptic non-touch technique		DBD	donation after brain death
APC	activated protein C *or* antigen-presenting cell		DBP	diastolic blood pressure
aPPT	activated partial thromboplastin time		DCD	donation after circulatory death
ARDS	acute respiratory distress syndrome		DCIS	ductal carcinoma *in situ*
ARR	absolute risk reduction		DCO	damage control orthopaedics
ASA	American Society of Anesthesiologists		DCR	damage control resuscitation
AST	aspartate transaminase		DCS	damage control surgery
AT	anaerobic threshold		DDAVP	desamino-D-arginine vasopressin
ATLS	Advanced Trauma Life Support		DDU	duplex Doppler ultrasonography
ATP	adenosine triphosphate		DHAP	dihydroxyacetone phosphate
AV	atrioventricular *or* arteriovenous		DHT	dihydrotestosterone
AWS	alcohol withdrawal syndrome		DI	diabetes insipidus
BABT	behind armour blunt trauma		DIC	disseminated intravascular coagulation
BCC	basal cell carcinoma		DNACPR	do not attempt cardiopulmonary resuscitation
BCS	breast-conserving surgery		DTC	differentiated thyroid cancer
BMI	body mass index		DVT	deep vein thrombosis
BP	blood pressure		ECF	extracellular fluid
BUN	blood urea nitrogen		ECG	electrocardiogram
CAI	chronic arterial insufficiency		ECHO	echocardiogram
CAS	carotid artery stenting		EDH	extradural haematoma
CBF	cerebral blood flow		EDV	end-diastolic volume
CDOP	child death overview panel			

eGFR	estimated glomerular filtration rate		ISS	Injury Severity Score
ER	oestrogen receptor		ITT	intention to treat
ERAS	enhanced recovery after surgery		IV	intravenous
ESR	erythrocyte sedimentation rate		IVC	inferior vena cava
ESV	end-systolic volume		IVU	intravenous urogram
ETC	electron transport chain		KG	ketoglutarate
EVAR	endovascular aneurysm repair		LCIS	lobular carcinoma *in situ*
FAA	femoral artery aneurysm		LCSB	local safeguarding children board
FAD	flavin adenine dinucleotide		LH	luteinizing hormone
FAP	familial adenomatous polyposis		LM	lentigo maligna
FAST	focused assessment with sonography for trauma		LMM	lentigo maligna melanoma
FDG	fluorodeoxyglucose		LMN	lower motor neuron
FEV_1	forced expiratory volume in 1 second		LMWH	low-molecular-weight heparin
FGM	female genital mutilation		MAP	mean arterial pressure
FHH	familial hypocalciuric hypercalcaemia		MAS	minimal access surgery
FLAIR	fluid-attenuated inversion recovery		MCC	Merkel cell carcinoma
FLS	Fundamentals of Laparoscopic Surgery		MDT	multidisciplinary team
FNA	fine-needle aspiration		MEA	multiple endocrine adenopathy
FNAC	fine-needle aspiration cytology		MEN	multiple endocrine neoplasia
FRC	functional residual capacity		MET	metabolic equivalent
FSH	follicle-stimulating hormone		MI	myocardial infarction
FTSG	full-thickness skin graft		MODS	multiple organ dysfunction syndrome
FVC	forced vital capacity		MRI	magnetic resonance imaging
G6P	glucose-6-phosphate		MRSA	methicillin-resistant *Staphylococcus aureus*
GABA	gamma-aminobutyric acid		MTC	medullary thyroid cancer
GCS	Glasgow Coma Scale		NAD^+	nicotinamide adenine dinucleotide
GE	gradient echo		NF1	neurofibromatosis type 1
GFR	glomerular filtration rate		NH_3	ammonia
GH	growth hormone		NHL	non-Hodgkin's lymphoma
GI	gastrointestinal		NHS	National Health Service
GIT	gastrointestinal tract		NHSBT	National Health Service Blood and Transplantation
GnRH	gonadotrophin-releasing hormone		NICE	National Institute for Health and Care Excellence
GOJ	gastro-oesophageal junction		NMDA	*N*-methyl-D-aspartate receptor
GORD	gastro-oesophageal reflux disease		NMP	normothermic machine perfusion
HA	hepatic artery		NMSC	non-melanoma skin cancer
Hb	haemoglobin		NOTSS	non-technical skills for surgeons
HbF	fetal haemoglobin		NPC	nasopharyngeal carcinoma
HBsAg	hepatitis B virus surface antigen		NSAID	non-steroidal anti-inflammatory drug
HBV	hepatitis B virus		NSAP	non-specific abdominal pain
HCC	hepatocellular carcinoma		NTS	non-technical skills
HCV	hepatitis C virus		O_2	oxygen
HCW	healthcare worker		OPSCC	oropharyngeal squamous cell carcinoma
HDR	high dose rate		OR	odds ratio
HIV	human immunodeficiency virus		OSA	obstructive sleep apnoea
HLA	human leucocyte antigen		OSATS	Objective Structured Assessment of Technical Skill
HMP	hypothermic machine perfusion		PAA	popliteal artery aneurysm
HPV	human papilloma virus		PACU	post-anaesthetic care unit
IC	intermittent claudication		PAK	pancreas transplant after kidney transplant
ICH	intracerebral haemorrhage		PBA	procedure-based assessment
ICP	intracranial pressure		PBLI	primary blast lung injury
ICU	intensive care unit		PCA	patient-controlled analgesia
IEM	inborn error of metabolism		PDA	patent ductus arteriosus
IGRT	image-guided radiation therapy		PDH	pyruvate dehydrogenase
IM	intramuscular		PDS	polydioxanone suture
IMRT	intensity-modulated radiation therapy		PDSA	plan-do-study-act
INR	international normalized ratio		PE	pulmonary embolism
IOPTH	intraoperative parathyroid hormone		PEEP	positive end-expiratory pressure
IR	inversion recovery *or* interventional radiology		PEP	post-exposure prophylaxis
ISI	International Sensitivity Index		PET	positron emission tomography

PHPT	primary hyperparathyroidism	SPECT	single-photon emission computed tomography
PNS	peripheral nervous system	SPK	simultaneous pancreas and kidney transplant
POSSUM	Physiology and Operative Severity Score for Enumeration of Mortality and Morbidity	SSI	surgical site infection
		SSRI	selective serotonin reuptake inhibitor
PPI	proton pump inhibitor	STM	soft tissue mass
PRL	prolactin	STS	soft tissue sarcoma
PRN	*pro re nata*/prescribed-as-needed	STSG	split-thickness skin graft
PSNS	parasympathetic nervous system	SV	stroke volume
PTA	percutaneous transluminal angioplasty *or* pancreas transplant alone	SVC	superior vena cava
		SVCO	superior vena cava obstruction
PTC	papillary thyroid cancer	T_3	triiodothyronine
PTFE	polytetrafluoroethylene	T_4	tetraiodothyronine (thyroxine)
PTH	parathyroid hormone	TACO	transfusion-related circulatory overload
PTV	planning target volume	TB	tuberculosis
PV	portal vein	TBI	traumatic brain injury
PVC	premature ventricular contraction	TBSA	total body surface area
RAAS	renin–angiotensin–aldosterone system	TCA	tricarboxylic acid
RBF	renal blood flow	TDA	traumatic disruption of the aorta
RCA	root cause analysis	TEVAR	thoracic endovascular aortic repair
RCT	randomized controlled trial	TF	tissue factor
RR	relative risk	TG	thyroglobulin *or* triglyceride
RRR	relative risk reduction	TH	thyroid hormone
RTS	Revised Trauma Score	TIPS	transjugular intrahepatic portosystemic shunt
SA	sinoatrial	TM	tympanic membrane
SAA	serum amyloid A	TNF	tumour necrosis factor
SAH	subarachnoid haemorrhage	TNM	tumour, node, metastasis
SBAR	situation, background, assessment, recognition	TPR	total peripheral resistance
SBO	small bowel obstruction	TRH	thyrotropin-releasing hormone
SBP	systolic blood pressure	TRISS	Trauma Score—Injury Severity Score
SC	subcutaneous	TSH	thyroid-stimulating hormone
SCC	squamous cell carcinoma	UMN	upper motor neuron
ScvO$_2$	central venous oxygen saturation	USS	ultrasound scan
SDH	succinate dehydrogenase *or* subdural haematoma	UV	ultraviolet
SE	spin echo	VATS	video-assisted thoracoscopic surgery
SERM	selective oestrogen receptor modulator	VHL	von Hippel–Lindau disease
SHOT	serious hazards of transfusion	VR	venous return *or* virtual reality
SIADH	syndrome of inappropriate antidiuretic hormone	VRIII	variable rate intravenous insulin infusion
SIRS	systemic inflammatory response syndrome	VTE	venous thromboembolism
SLE	systemic lupus erythematosus	VV	varicose veins
SNB	sentinel node biopsy	vWf	von Willebrand factor
SND	systematic nodal dissection	WBRT	whole-brain radiotherapy
SN-OD	specialist nurse in organ donation	WCC	white cell count
SNS	sympathetic nervous system	WHO	World Health Organization
SOP	standard operating procedure		

Contributors

David A. Adams, Dean of PU-RCSI, Perdana University, Malaysia

Rajesh Aggarwal, Department of Surgery and Cancer, Imperial College and St Mary's Hospital, London, UK; Department of Surgery, University of Pennsylvania, Philadelphia, PA, USA

Nada Al-Hadithy, Plastic Surgery Department, Southmead Hospital, Bristol, UK

William Allum, Department of Surgery, Royal Marsden NHS Foundation Trust, London, UK

Mymoona Alzouebi, Weston Park Hospital, Sheffield, UK

Nicola R. K. Anders, Royal Manchester Children's Hospital, Manchester, UK

Sonal Arora, Department of Surgery and Cancer, Imperial College and St Mary's Hospital, London, UK

Jonathan Beard, Sheffield Vascular Institute, Sheffield Teaching Hospitals NHS Foundation Trust, Northern General Hospital, Sheffield, UK

Timothy A. Beckitt, Vascular Surgery, Bristol Royal Infirmary, Bristol, UK

Mireille Berthoud, Anaesthetics Department, Royal Hallamshire Hospital, Sheffield, UK

Rob Bethune, Royal Devon and Exeter NHS Foundation Trust, Exeter, UK

Jane M. Blazeby, University of Bristol and University Hospitals Bristol NHS Foundation Trust, Bristol, UK

Eleanor M. Bolton, Department of Surgery, University of Cambridge, Cambridge, UK

Laura J. Bowes, Consultant anaesthetist at Birmingham Children's Hospital

Matthew J. Bown, University of Leicester, Leicester, UK

Andrew W. Bradbury, University Department of Vascular Surgery, Solihull Hospital, Birmingham, UK

Aidan Bradford, Department of Physiology and Medical Physics, Royal College of Surgeons in Ireland, Dublin, Ireland

J. Andrew Bradley, University Department of Surgery, Addenbrooke's Hospital, Cambridge, UK

Paul M. Brennan, University of Edinburgh Centre for Clinical Brain Sciences, Western General Hospital, Edinburgh UK

Chris Brearton, Royal Liverpool University Hospital, Liverpool, UK

Daniele Bryden, Department of Critical Care, Sheffield Teaching Hospitals NHS Trust, Sheffield, UK

Neil Burgess, Norfolk and Norwich University Hospital NHS Trust, Colney Lane, Norwich, UK

Dermot Burke, John Goligher Department of Colorectal Surgery, St James's Hospital, Leeds, UK

Katharine Burke, Churchill Hospital, Oxford, UK

Shirelle Burton-Fanning, The Newcastle upon Tyne Hospitals NHS Foundation Trust, Newcastle upon Tyne, UK

Christopher M. Butler, Medway NHS Trust, Medway Maritime Hospital, Gillingham, UK

Christopher J. Callaghan, Renal and Transplant Department, Guy's Hospital, London, UK

Gordon Carlson, The University of Manchester, Manchester Academic Health Science Centre, Manchester; Salford Royal NHS Foundation Trust, Salford, UK

John J. Casey, The Transplant Unit, The Royal Infirmary of Edinburgh, Edinburgh, UK

Helen Cattermole, Hull Royal Infirmary, Hull & East Yorkshire Hospitals NHS Trust, Hull, UK

James Catto, Department of Oncology, The Medical School, University of Sheffield, Sheffield, UK

David Chadwick, Nottingham University Hospitals, Nottingham, UK

Pankaj Chandak, Specialist Registrar in Transplant Surgery, Guy's and St Thomas and Great Ormond Street Hospitals; Research Fellow and Hon. Lecturer King's College London and Royal College of Surgeons of England, UK

Ishmael Chasi, County Durham and Darlington NHS Foundation Trust, Durham, UK

Jon Clasper, Emeritus Defence Professor and Consultant Orthopaedic Surgeon, Visiting Professor in Bioengineering, Imperial College London, Clinical Lead, The Royal British Legion Centre for Blast Injury Studies

Dermot Cox, Molecular and Cellular Therapeutics, Royal College of Surgeons in Ireland, Dublin, Ireland

Ross J. Craigie, Royal Manchester Children's Hospital, Manchester, UK

David M. Cressey, Department of Peri-operative and Intensive Care, Freeman Hospital, The Newcastle upon Tyne Hospitals NHS Foundation Trust, Newcastle upon Tyne, UK

James N. Crinnion, Department of General Surgery, Whipps Cross University Hospital, London, UK

Katy A. L. Darvall, Department of Vascular Surgery, Musgrove Park Hospital, Taunton, UK

Robert Davies, Department of Vascular Surgery, University Hospitals Leicester NHS Trust, Leicester, UK

Marcel Den Dulk, Department of Surgery, Maastricht University Medical Centre, Maastricht, The Netherlands

Kalpesh Dixit, Children's Services, Salford Royal NHS Foundation Trust, Salford, UK

Declan Dunne, Liverpool Hepatobiliary Unit, Department of Surgery, and Liverpool Hepatobiliary Centre, Aintree University Hospital, Liverpool, UK

Ian Eardley, Leeds Teaching Hospitals, Leeds, UK

Stephen Fenwick, Liverpool Hepatobiliary Unit, Aintree University Hospital NHS Foundation Trust, Liverpool, UK

Andrew Fletcher, Chesterfield Royal Hospital, Chesterfield, UK

Mark Fordham, Department of Urology, Royal Liverpool University Hospital, Liverpool UK

Sheila Fraser, Department of Breast and Endocrine Surgery, St. James's University Hospital, Leeds, UK

Peter A. Gaines, The Sheffield Vascular Institute, Sheffield; Sheffield Hallam University, Sheffield, UK

Jeff Garner, The Rotherham Hospital, Rotherham, UK

Mary Garthwaite, James Cook University Hospital, South Tees Hospitals NHS Foundation Trust, Middlesbrough, UK

Vimal J. Gokani, University of Leicester, Leicester, UK

Dhanny Gomez, Liverpool Hepatobiliary Unit, Aintree University Hospital NHS Foundation Trust, Liverpool, UK

Amit Goyal, Department of Surgery, Royal Derby Hospital, Derby, UK

Timothy R. Graham, Department of Cardiac Surgery, Queen Elizabeth Hospital, Birmingham, UK

Jeremy Groves, Department of Anaesthetics, Chesterfield Royal Hospital, Chesterfield, UK

Louise Hall, Infection Prevention and Control, The Newcastle upon Tyne Hospitals NHS Foundation Trust, Newcastle upon Tyne, UK

J. R. Leslie Hamilton, Freeman Hospital, The Newcastle upon Tyne Hospitals NHS Foundation Trust, Newcastle upon Tyne, UK

Anita Hargreaves, Centre for Digestive Diseases, University Hospital Aintree, Liverpool, UK

Judith H. Harmey, Molecular and Cellular Therapeutics, Royal College of Surgeons, Dublin, Ireland; Biochemistry, Perdana University, Malaysia

Simon J. F. Harper, Department of Surgery, Addenbrooke's Hospital, Cambridge, UK

Matthew Q. F. Hatton, Weston Park Hospital, Sheffield, UK

Maurice Hawthorne, Freeman Hospital, The Newcastle upon Tyne Hospitals NHS Foundation Trust, Newcastle upon Tyne, UK

Kenneth B. Hosie, Peninsula School of Surgery, Peninsula Deanery, Plymouth, UK

Benjamin Hughes, Norfolk and Norwich University Hospital NHS Trust, Colney Lane, Norwich, UK

Leanne Hunt, Chesterfield Royal Hospital, Chesterfield Royal Hospital NHS Foundation Trust, Chesterfield, UK

Kamalan Jeevaratnam, Faculty of Health and Medical Sciences, University of Surrey, UK

Robert P. Jones, Department of Surgery, Aintree University Hospital, Liverpool, UK

Mandeep Kang, Department of Plastic and Reconstructive Surgery, Leicester Royal Infirmary, Leicester, UK

John Keating, Department of Orthopaedics, Royal Infirmary of Edinburgh, Edinburgh, UK

Catriona Kelly, Belfast City Hospital, Belfast, UK

Robert D. Kent, University Hospital of North Durham, Durham, UK

Vikas Khanduja, Addenbrooke's Hospital, Cambridge University Hospital NHS Foundation Trust, UK

Adam Kimble, General Surgery, Derriford Hospital, Plymouth, UK

Daniel Kusumawidjaja, The Sheffield Vascular Institute, Old Nurse's Home, Northern General Hospital, Sheffield, UK

Mark Lansdown, Department of Breast and Endocrine Surgery, St. James's University Hospital, Leeds, UK

Chris D. Lee, Clatterbridge Cancer Centre, Bebington, Wirral, UK

Grace Lee, Department of Surgery, University of Pennsylvania, Philadelphia, PA, USA

Olle Ljungqvist, Faculty of Medicine and Health, School of Health and Medical Sciences, Department of Surgery Örebro University, Örebro, Sweden

Dileep N. Lobo, National Institute for Health Research, Nottingham Digestive Diseases Biomedical Research Unit, Nottingham University Hospitals and University of Nottingham, UK

Robbie Lonsdale, Sheffield Vascular Institute, Sheffield Teaching Hospitals NHS Foundation Trust, Northern General Hospital, Sheffield, UK

David Lowe, The London Clinic, London, UK

Rhona M. Maclean, Sheffield Haemophilia and Thrombosis Centre, Royal Hallamshire Hospital, Sheffield, UK

Vishy Mahadevan, The Royal College of Surgeons of England, London, UK

Jehangir Mahaluxmivala, Princess Alexandra Hospital NHS Trust, Harlow, UK

Daoud Makki, Kent Surrey and Sussex Deanery, London, UK

Michael Makris, Sheffield Haemophilia and Thrombosis Centre, Royal Hallamshire Hospital, Sheffield; Department of Cardiovascular Science, University of Sheffield, Sheffield, UK

Hassan Z. Malik, Liverpool Hepatobiliary Unit, Aintree University Hospital NHS Foundation Trust, Liverpool, UK

Michelle Marshall, Academic Unit of Medical Education, University of Sheffield, Sheffield, UK

Peter McCulloch, Nuffield Department of Surgical Sciences, John Radcliffe Hospital, Oxford, UK

Derek McWhirter, Liverpool Hepatobiliary Unit, Department of Surgery, and Liverpool Hepatobiliary Centre, Aintree University Hospital, Liverpool, UK

Pallavi Mehrotra, Department of Radiology, City Hospital Sunderland Foundation Trust, Sunderland, UK

Scott Middleton, Royal Infirmary Edinburgh, Edinburgh, UK

Gary H. Mills, Department of Anaesthesia, Sheffield University, Sheffield, UK

Ian L. Minty, Radiology Department, Sunderland City Hospitals NHS, Foundation Trust, Durham, UK

Amitabh Mishra, Department of Colorectal Surgery, Churchill Hospital, Oxford, UK

Alan A. Montgomery, Nottingham Clinical Trials Unit, School of Medicine, University of Nottingham, Nottingham, UK

Jonathan Moore, Royal Victoria Infirmary, The Newcastle upon Tyne Hospitals NHS Foundation Trust, Newcastle upon Tyne, UK

Matthew Moran, Royal Infirmary Edinburgh, Edinburgh, UK

James A. Morecroft, Royal Manchester Children's Hospital, Manchester, UK

Brian Mullan, Royal Victoria Hospital, Belfast, UK

Arthur Sun Myint, Clatterbridge Cancer Centre, Bebington, Wirral, UK

Lynn Myles, Department of Clinical Neurosciences, Western General Hospital, Edinburgh, UK

Manjusha Narayanan, Royal Victoria Infirmary, The Newcastle upon Tyne Hospitals NHS Foundation Trust, Newcastle upon Tyne, UK

Pierre Nasr, Addenbrooke's Hospital, Cambridge, UK

A. Ross Naylor, Department of Vascular Surgery, Leicester Royal Infirmary, Leicester, UK

Michael Nicholson, University Department of Surgery, Addenbrooke's Hospital, Cambridge, UK

Bill Noble, Medical Director of Marie Curie, London, UK

Simon Noble, Clinical Reader, Cardiff University, Wales

Aidan Noon, Department of Oncology, The Medical School, University of Sheffield, Sheffield, UK

Chris Oliver, Edinburgh Orthopaedic Trauma Unit, Royal Infirmary of Edinburgh, Edinburgh, UK

Alison Pike, Children's Services, Salford Royal NHS Foundation Trust, Salford, UK

Graeme J. Poston, Liverpool Hepatobiliary Unit, Department of Surgery, and Liverpool Hepatobiliary Centre, Aintree University Hospital, Liverpool, UK

Raaj K. Praseedom, Department of Surgery, Addenbrooke's Hospital, Cambridge, UK

Yassar A. Qureshi, The Royal London Hospital Trauma Unit, Barts Health NHS Trust, London, UK

Yujay Ramakrishnan, Freeman Hospital, The Newcastle upon Tyne Hospitals NHS Foundation Trust, Newcastle upon Tyne, UK

Muhammad Raza, Freeman Hospital, The Newcastle upon Tyne Hospitals NHS Foundation Trust, Newcastle upon Tyne, UK

Zahid Raza, Royal Infirmary of Edinburgh, Edinburgh, UK

Malcolm W. R. Reed, Brighton and Sussex Medical School, University of Sussex, Brighton, UK

Rosalind O' Reilly, Intensive Care Unit, Royal Hospitals Belfast, Belfast, UK

Robert Robinson, Chesterfield Royal Hospital, Chesterfield Royal Hospital NHS Foundation Trust, Chesterfield, UK

Timothy Rockall, The Royal Surrey County Hospital NHS Foundation Trust, Guildford, UK

Stephen J. Rooney, Department of Cardiac Surgery, Queen Elizabeth Hospital, Birmingham, UK

Ian Sabin, London Bridge Hospital, London, UK

Robert Sayers, University Hospitals of Leicester NHS Trust, Leicester; Department of Cardiovascular Sciences, University of Leicester, Leicester Royal Infirmary, Leicester, UK

Katie Schwab, Minimal Access Therapy Training Unit, Royal Surrey County Hospital, Guildford, UK

Peter Sedman, Spire Hull and East Riding Hospital, Hull and East Yorkshire NHS Trust, Hull, UK

Eshan L. Senanayake, Department of Cardiac Surgery, Queen Elizabeth Hospital, Birmingham, UK

Hemant Sharma, Hull Royal Infirmary, Hull, UK

David Sharp, The Spinal Unit, Department of Trauma and Orthopaedics, Ipswich Hospital, Ipswich, UK

Kevin Sherman, Spire Hull and East Riding Hospital, Anlaby, UK

Deepak Singh-Ranger, Department of General Surgery and Coloproctology, The Royal Wolverhampton NHS Trust, New Cross Hospital, Wolverhampton, UK

James Singleton, Trauma and Orthopaedics, Frimley Park Hospital, Camberley, UK

Pramudith Sirimanna, Department of Surgery and Cancer, Imperial College and St Mary's Hospital, London, UK; Academic Colorectal Unit, University of Sydney and Concord Hospital, Sydney, Australia

David Smith, Ninewells Hospital and Medical School, Dundee, UK

Frank C. T. Smith, Department of Surgery, Bristol Royal Infirmary, Bristol, UK

Hilary Smith, Solent NHS Trust, Southampton, UK

Mattias Soop, The University of Manchester, Manchester Academic Health Science Centre, Salford Royal NHS Foundation Trust, Manchester, UK

Jonathan D. Spratt, Radiology Department, Sunderland City Hospitals NHS Foundation Trust, Durham, UK

Sasha Stamenkovic, Freeman Hospital, The Newcastle upon Tyne Hospitals NHS Foundation Trust, Newcastle Upon Tyne, UK

Paul Sutton, Center for Digestive Diseases, University Hospital Aintree, Liverpool, UK

Himanshu Swami, ENT Department, James Cook University Hospital, Middlesbrough, UK

Allison Sykes, Infection Prevention and Control, The Newcastle upon Tyne Hospitals NHS Foundation Trust, Newcastle upon Tyne, UK

Nigel R. M. Tai, The Royal London Hospital Trauma Unit, Barts Health NHS Trust, London, UK

William E. G. Thomas, Consultant Surgeon Emeritus and Past Clinical Director of Surgery, Royal Hallamshire Hospital, Sheffield, UK

Andrew Topping, Department of Anaesthetics, Antrim Area Hospital, Antrim, UK

Bruce Tulloh, Royal Infirmary of Edinburgh, Edinburgh, UK

David Ward, Department of Plastic and Reconstructive Surgery, Leicester Royal Infirmary, Leicester, UK

Sheila Waugh, Freeman Hospital, The Newcastle upon Tyne Hospitals NHS Foundation Trust, Newcastle upon Tyne, UK

Bee Wee, Harris Manchester College, University of Oxford, Oxford, UK

Tom Wiggins, Whipps Cross University Hospital and Royal London Hospital, London, UK

Mark Wilson, St Mary's Hospital, London, UK

Stephen Wilson, Department of Critical Care, Sheffield Teaching Hospitals NHS Trust, Sheffield, UK

Caroline Woodley, Department of Medical and Social Care Education, University of Leicester, UK

Michael G. Wyatt, Consultant in Vascular Surgery, Freeman Hospital, Newcastle upon Tyne, UK

Jamie Young, Borders General Hospital, Melrose, UK

SECTION 1

Basic science

Section Editor: Mark Fordham

PART 1.1

Applied surgical anatomy

CHAPTER 1.1.1

Anatomy of the thorax

Vishy Mahadevan

Anatomy of the chest wall

Osseous and cartilaginous elements of the thoracic cage: sternum, thoracic vertebrae, ribs, and costal cartilages

The thoracic cage is approximately conical in shape. Anteriorly it is made up of the sternum which comprises three elements. From above downwards these are the manubrium sterni, body of the sternum (mesosternum), and xiphoid process. Posteriorly the thoracic cage is made up of the entire length of the thoracic part of the vertebral column. The posterior thoracic wall comprises the 12 thoracic vertebrae and intervening intervertebral discs and is thus twice as long as the anterior wall (the sternum). Between the posterior and anterior walls of the thorax, there are, on each side, 12 ribs (with 11 intervening intercostal spaces). The posterior end of each rib is termed the head. The heads of the ribs articulate with the thoracic vertebral bodies. The anterior extremity of each rib is a strip of hyaline cartilage, the costal cartilage. The costal cartilages of the upper seven ribs articulate directly with the sternum. The costal cartilages of the eighth, ninth, and tenth ribs do not reach the sternum directly. Each articulates with the cartilage of the superjacent rib. This arrangement manifests itself as an oblique, somewhat undulant, firm-to-hard palpable ridge running down on either side of the xiphisternum. This is the costal margin.

The costal cartilages of the 11th and 12th ribs neither reach the sternum nor articulate with their neighbours. Consequently they are spoken of as 'free' or 'floating' ribs.

Overlapping the posterolateral part of the thoracic cage is the scapula which extends from the level of the second to seventh intercostal space.

The articulation between the manubrium sterni and mesosternum is a secondary cartilaginous joint. It is an angulated junction (the manubriosternal junction, also known as the *angle of Louis*) and presents as a prominent palpable (often visible) transverse ridge. *It is a clinically useful anatomical landmark, being located invariably at the level of the second costal cartilage.*

Anatomy of the intercostal space

The interval between adjacent ribs is termed the intercostal space. Thus on each side of the midline, the thoracic cage comprises 11 intercostal spaces.

Generally speaking, each intercostal space is wider in front than at the back. The upper intercostal spaces tend to be wider than the lower ones. Typically, it is the anterior part of the third intercostal space which offers the widest intercostal area. Each intercostal space is bridged by a three-ply arrangement of thin muscular sheets. The outer layer is the *external intercostal muscle*. The middle layer is made up of the *internal intercostal muscle*, while the inner layer is made up of thin, discontinuous muscle strips, all in the same plane, and which may be collectively referred to as the *innermost intercostal muscle*.

A similar three-ply arrangement of muscular sheets is to be seen in the anterolateral part of the anterior abdominal wall.

The nerves and vessels of the thoracic wall (anterior and posterior intercostal arteries and veins and intercostal nerves) lie between the middle and innermost layers of intercostal muscles. As they run along the circumference of the intercostal space, the neurovascular structures lie parallel to, and near the lower border of, the rib that forms the upper boundary of the space. *It is important to be mindful of this anatomical feature when performing procedures such as thoracentesis.*

Superficial thoracic muscles

The thoracic cage as described above is overlapped anteriorly, posteriorly, and laterally by powerful muscles. These must be taken into account and dealt with when gaining surgical access to the thoracic cavity through posterolateral, anterolateral, or lateral approaches.

Several of these muscles are attached, in part, to the shoulder girdle or humerus, or both, and thus are functionally related to the upper limb. Overlapping the anterior aspect of the rib cage are the pectoralis muscles, major and minor. The lateral aspect of the rib cage is overlapped by the multiple digitations of serratus anterior, while posteriorly, several muscles, thick and thin, overlap the rib cage. These include trapezius, latissimus dorsi, and the rhomboids, major and minor.

In addition, the very posterior part of the rib cage is overlapped, in part, by the powerful postvertebral muscles which act on the vertebral column.

Surgical access to the thoracic cavity may be gained by dividing the sternum vertically in the midline. This is called a *median sternotomy*. Alternatively, the thoracic cavity may be entered on the right or left sides through an appropriate intercostal space or rib bed, using anterolateral, posterolateral, or lateral skin incisions.

Diaphragm

Structure of the diaphragm

The diaphragm is a dome-shaped, mobile, musculotendinous partition which separates the thoracic cavity from the abdominal cavity. The convex surface of the dome faces the thoracic cavity. The peripheral part of the diaphragm is made up of muscle fibres which arise posteriorly from the upper lumbar vertebral bodies and

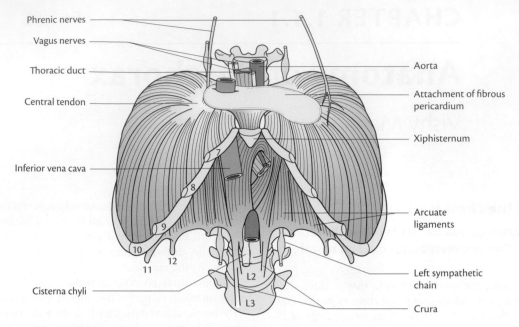

Phrenic nerves
Vagus nerves
Thoracic duct
Central tendon
Inferior vena cava
Cisterna chyli
Aorta
Attachment of fibrous pericardium
Xiphisternum
Arcuate ligaments
Left sympathetic chain
Crura
L2
L3
7
8
9
10
11
12

Fig. 1.1.1.1 The diaphragm and structures passing through it.

elsewhere from the inner aspect of the entire circumference of the inferior aperture of the thoracic cage. From this circumferential, peripheral origin the muscle fibres converge to a *centrally-placed trefoil-shaped tendinous (aponeurotic) part*.

The diaphragm features three large openings, each opening (or hiatus) named for the principal structure which traverses it (Figure 1.1.1.1):

1. The aortic hiatus (at the level of T12 vertebra) transmits the abdominal aorta, the thoracic duct, and often the azygos vein.

2. The oesophageal hiatus (at T10 level) is surrounded by the muscular fibres of the right and left crura of the diaphragm and transmits, in addition to the oesophagus, branches of the left gastric artery and vein and the two vagi.

3. The vena caval hiatus (at T8 level) is situated in the central tendon and transmits, in addition to the inferior vena cava, the right phrenic nerve.

Innervation of the diaphragm

The diaphragm receives its motor innervation exclusively from the right and left phrenic nerves. Each phrenic nerve (root value C3, C4, and C5) arises from the cervical plexus, and is a mixed nerve containing both motor and sensory fibres. The long course of the nerve from the neck to the diaphragm is explained by the embryological derivation of the diaphragmatic muscle from the cervical myotomes.

Injury to the phrenic nerve results in paralysis of the diaphragmatic muscle and consequent elevation of the ipsilateral hemidiaphragm. Two radiological features characterize the paralysed diaphragm: elevation of the diaphragm and paradoxical diaphragmatic movement (in which the diaphragm, instead of descending on inspiration, moves upwards due to upwardly directed pressure from the abdominal viscera).

The sensory nerve fibres from the central part of the diaphragm and from the subjacent peritoneum and superjacent pleura also run in the phrenic nerve; hence, irritation of the diaphragmatic pleura (in pleurisy) or of the peritoneum on the undersurface of the diaphragm by subphrenic collections of pus or blood may present as referred pain to the ipsilateral shoulder-tip area (C4 dermatome).

Function of the diaphragm

The main function of the diaphragm is respiratory. By its descent, the diaphragm greatly increases the vertical dimension of the thoracic cavity, thereby facilitating inspiration Secondarily, the diaphragm, by its contraction and descent, assists other abdominal wall muscles in raising intra-abdominal pressure.

Mediastinum

The mediastinum (Latin for *middle partition*) is the central part of the thoracic cavity, situated between the right and left pleural sacs. It contains numerous mobile and pulsating structures, including the heart, thoracic aorta, and oesophagus.

Boundaries and subdivisions of the mediastinum

The mediastinum is bounded posteriorly by the entire length of the thoracic part of the vertebral column (Figure 1.1.1.2). The inferior boundary of the mediastinum is the upper surface of the diaphragm. The superior limit of the mediastinum is the plane of the superior aperture of the thoracic cage, while anteriorly the mediastinum is bounded by the sternum. As has already been alluded to, the mediastinum is bounded on each side by the medial aspect of the corresponding pleural sac. The mediastinum, thus defined, is customarily and arbitrarily divided into two principal regions: *superior mediastinum* and *inferior mediastinum*.

The plane of demarcation between the two is an imaginary, horizontal plane passing through the mediastinum at the level of the manubriosternal junction.

Situated in its entirety within the inferior mediastinum is the fibrous pericardium, which contains the heart. This feature is availed of to subdivide the inferior mediastinum into three areas: *anterior mediastinum* (anterior to the fibrous pericardium),

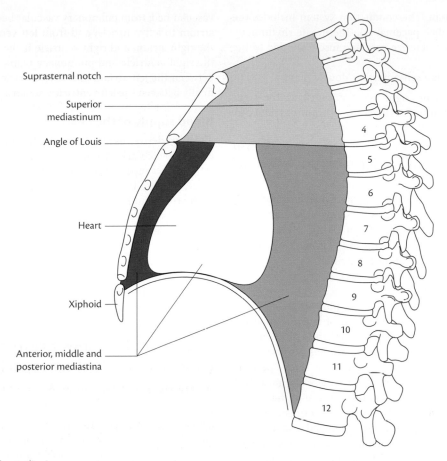

Fig. 1.1.1.2 Subdivisions of the mediastinum.
Reproduced with permission from Ellis H. and Mahadevan V., *Clinical Anatomy*, Thirteenth Edition, Wiley-Blackwell, Oxford, UK, Copyright © 2013.

posterior mediastinum (posterior to the fibrous pericardium), and *middle mediastinum* (the fibrous pericardium itself). Thus the mediastinum may be pictured as being made up of four regions (subdivisions), all of which are in communication with each other. *Knowledge of the contents of each mediastinal subdivision is of utmost importance in the clinical diagnosis and radiological interpretation of mediastinal pathology.*

Principal contents of each subdivision of the mediastinum

Superior mediastinum: by far the most important structure situated in the superior mediastinum is the *arch of the aorta* (which lies in its entirety within the superior mediastinum) and its branches. Other important structures in the superior mediastinum include the oesophagus and trachea (both on their way from the neck to the inferior mediastinum), the right and left vagi and phrenic nerves, lymph nodes, remnants of the thymus, the right and left brachiocephalic veins and their confluence to the right of the midline to form the superior vena cava, and the upper end of the thoracic duct.

The *anterior mediastinum*, the narrowest and smallest of the four subdivision of the mediastinum, occupies the narrow interval between the body of the sternum and the fibrous pericardium. Its contents include thymic remnants, sternal branches of the adjacent internal thoracic arteries, and sternopericardial ligaments (fibrous strands running from the back of the sternum to the fibrous pericardium).

The *posterior mediastinum* contains the descending thoracic aorta and its branches, the oesophagus, the azygos, hemiazygos, and accessory hemiazygos veins, the ganglionated right and left sympathetic trunks and their splanchnic branches, the thoracic duct, and lymph nodes.

The *middle mediastinum* includes the fibrous pericardium and its contents (heart, ascending aorta, pulmonary trunk, the terminations of the superior and inferior venae cavae, and the four pulmonary veins), and the right and left phrenic nerves which are adherent to the outer surface of the fibrous pericardium. (It is conventional to regard the roots of the right and left lungs as contents of the middle mediastinum.)

Cardiac anatomy

Essential functional design of the heart

Situated within the pericardium (and thus *entirely* in the middle mediastinum), the heart is shaped like an irregular cone and lies obliquely with its long axis along a line running from the left midclavicular line anteriorly, to the right mid-scapular line posteriorly. One-third of the heart lies to the right of the median plane of the body and two-thirds to the left of this plane.

The heart is a four-chambered, muscular organ. Cardiac muscle (myocardium) is a highly specialized form of syncytial involuntary muscle, unlike any other in the body. Within the myocardium is a network of specialized myocytes which collectively constitute the cardiac conduction system. The conduction system includes the sinoatrial node (the cardiac pacemaker). The innate rhythmicity and contractility that characterize cardiac muscle are due to the conduction system.

Functionally, the heart is a self-adjusting 'double pump':

- The pulmonary pump, or 'right heart' comprising the right atrium and right ventricle, is a relatively low-pressure system carrying deoxygenated, systemic venous blood.
- The systemic pump, or 'left heart' comprising the left atrium and left ventricle, is a high-pressure system carrying oxygen-saturated blood.

The two pump systems are arranged in series, with the pulmonary vascular bed interposed between the two systems. Topographically, however, the 'right heart' lies largely *in front* of the 'left heart'. The posterior surface of the heart (base of the heart) is made up, almost entirely, of the posterior surface of the left atrium.

Pericardium

The heart is enclosed in the pericardium, a fibroserous sac comprising three concentric layers. The outermost layer, termed the fibrous pericardium, is a strong, fibrous, and inelastic structure which blends inferiorly with the central tendinous portion of the diaphragm. Within the fibrous pericardium is the serous pericardium which consists of two layers. The outer of these two layers (the parietal layer) is firmly applied to the inner surface of the fibrous pericardium while the inner layer, the visceral layer or epicardium, covers the surface of the heart and is firmly applied to it. Between the parietal and visceral layers of the serous pericardium is the pericardial cavity which contains, in health, a thin film of fluid. This film enables the pulsating heart to glide frictionlessly within the pericardium.

The fibrous pericardium fuses with the walls of the great vessels (superior and inferior vena cavae, ascending aorta, pulmonary trunk, and the four pulmonary veins) as these vessels perforate the fibrous pericardium. *Consequently, fluid collections in the pericardial cavity (e.g. haemopericardium) have no natural route of escape, and if sufficiently large, may hinder cardiac expansion and thereby compromise cardiac output. This potentially life-threatening phenomenon is referred to as cardiac tamponade.*

General morphology of the heart

Embryologically, the heart develops from a simple, hollow, endothelium-lined, mesodermal tube which is patent at both ends. As a consequence of a fairly complicated process of simultaneous elongation and folding to which the tube is subjected, and due to the development of internal septation, the heart eventually comes to possess a 'series' of four chambers. Starting at the 'venous end' of the series, the four chambers are, in sequence, the right atrium, right ventricle, left atrium, and left ventricle.

The atria are thin-walled, low-pressure chambers, while the ventricles have thick muscular walls. The wall of the left ventricle is thrice as thick as that of the right ventricle, a reflection of the significantly greater vascular resistance against which the left ventricle has to work. Integrated within the heart are four ingeniously designed valves, each valve being made up of two or more leaflets. These valves ensure unidirectional blood flow during cardiac contraction as follows: from right atrium to right ventricle; from right ventricle to pulmonary artery and thence through the pulmonary

vascular bed; from pulmonary vascular bed to left atrium; from left atrium to left ventricle; and from left ventricle to aorta. Between the right atrium and right ventricle is the tricuspid valve; between the right ventricle and pulmonary trunk is the pulmonary valve; between the left atrium and left ventricle is the mitral valve; and finally between the left ventricle and aorta is the aortic valve.

Blood supply of the heart

The heart derives its arterial supply from the right and left coronary arteries which arise from the aortic root, and are thus the earliest branches of the aorta. Typically the right coronary artery is of greater calibre than the left. Although the terminal ramifications of the right and left coronary arteries do connect with each other, these anastomoses are trivial. The two coronary arteries are thus, effectively, end arteries. *It is both significant and interesting that coronary artery filling takes place principally during ventricular diastole, rather than during systole (as is the case with all systemic arteries).*

The venous drainage of the myocardium is by a number of veins, most of which drain into a venous conduit, the coronary sinus, which in turn opens into the right atrium.

Anatomy of the lower respiratory tract (tracheobronchial tree and lungs)

Anatomy of the tracheobronchial tree

By convention, the nasal passages, pharynx, and larynx are, collectively, referred to as the upper respiratory tract, while the trachea, bronchial tree, and lungs represent the lower respiratory tract. Commencing at the lower border of the cricoid cartilage, the trachea runs down the neck into the superior mediastinum. A short distance below the level of the manubriosternal junction (angle of Louis), it bifurcates into the right and left main (primary) bronchi which enter the right and left lungs respectively. Within the lung, each main bronchus divides into lobar bronchi, which in turn break up into segmental bronchi. These divide repeatedly into smaller and smaller air passages, eventually yielding terminal bronchioles. The latter mark the end of the *conducting portion* of the respiratory tract.

The terminal bronchioles give rise to respiratory bronchioles which, in turn, give rise to alveolar ducts. Coming off the alveolar ducts are clusters of thin-walled sacs, the alveoli. The respiratory bronchioles, alveolar ducts, and alveoli collectively constitute the *respiratory portion* of the tract.

Anatomy of the pleura and lungs

Each lung is enclosed in a thin, double-layered membranous sac, the *pleural sac*.

From the level of the angle of Louis to the level of the fourth costal cartilages, the anterior edges of the two pleural sacs touch each other. Elsewhere the pleural sacs are separated from each other by the fibrous pericardium and other mediastinal structures. Each pleural sac consists of two layers: a *visceral layer* which is intimately related to the surface of the lung and even lines all the natural fissures and crevices of the lung, and a *parietal layer* which lines the inner aspect of the chest wall, the upper surface of the diaphragm, and the sides of the pericardium and other mediastinal structures. The parietal pleura is separated from its overlying structures by a loose, thin layer of connective tissue, the *extrapleural, endothoracic fascia*, which enables the surgeon to strip the parietal pleura from the inner surface of the chest wall with relative ease. Between the two layers of pleura is the pleural cavity, which normally contains no more than a thin film of fluid. The two layers of pleura (visceral and parietal) are continuous with each other around the *hilum* of the lung. The hilum is the well-defined area on the mediastinal surface of the lung through which the bronchus, pulmonary artery, and pulmonary veins enter or leave the lung.

It is important to appreciate that the lung, even at the end of maximal voluntary inspiration, does not obliterate the pleural cavity completely.

Each lung is conical in shape, with a blunt apex superiorly which reaches above the sternal end of the first rib, and a concave base which overlies the diaphragm. The lung also features an extensive, gently convex, costovertebral surface moulded to the inside of the chest wall and a mediastinal surface which is concave and faces the pericardium.

The two lungs are not identical. The right lung is somewhat shorter than the left, owing to the higher position of the right dome of the diaphragm. However, although shorter than the left, the right lung is actually the bulkier and heavier of the two, owing to the greater encroachment of the heart towards the left side.

The right lung is divided into three lobes: the upper, middle, and lower. The oblique fissure divides the upper and middle lobes from the lower lobe while the transverse fissure separates the upper lobe from the middle lobe. The left lung has just two lobes, upper and lower, which are separated from each other by the oblique fissure. The medial (mediastinal surface) of the lung features the hilum through which the bronchus, pulmonary artery, and bronchial arteries enter the lung, and the pulmonary veins emerge from the lung.

Bronchopulmonary segments

Each lobar bronchus and its accompanying lobar branch of the pulmonary artery divide into a constant number of segmental branches. Together, the segmental bronchus and accompanying artery supply a discrete segment of lung within the lobe. Collectively, these three structures constitute a bronchopulmonary segment. Each is an anatomically definable entity that may be resected in isolation. There are typically ten bronchopulmonary segments in each lung.

Anatomy of the breast

General morphology of the breast

In the male, the breast is normally a rudimentary structure comprising just a few ductular elements surrounded by much fibrous tissue. In the adult female, however, the breast is a prominent structure that is located superficial to the pectoralis major muscle. The deep surface of the breast (termed the base of the breast) extends vertically from the level of the second rib to the sixth rib, and transversely from the ipsilateral sternal edge, medially, to beyond the anterior axillary line, laterally. The breast is a modified apocrine gland.

The breast is conventionally described as being made up of 15 or so lobes of glandular tissue embedded in fat; the latter accounting for most of the bulk of the breast. Seventy per cent or more of all the glandular elements in the breast are concentrated in the upper outer quadrant. It is not surprising therefore that cyclical (hormone-dependent), benign conditions of the breast often present as painful nodularity in the upper outer quadrant.

Each lobe of the breast drains by its lactiferous duct on to the summit of the *nipple*.

Blood supply and lymphatic drainage of the breast

The arterial supply of the breast is derived largely from branches of the axillary artery: principally the lateral thoracic and acromiothoracic arteries. The internal thoracic artery (previously known as the internal mammary artery) contributes to the blood supply to the medial part of the breast. The venous drainage is through the veins corresponding to the arteries.

Knowledge of the lymphatic drainage of the breast is of considerable importance in the clinical management of breast cancer. The lymphatic vessels draining the breast are directed to two principal destinations:

1. Along tributaries of the axillary vessels to axillary lymph nodes; this accounts for approximately 75% of the total lymphatic drainage of the breast

2. Along the tributaries of the internal thoracic vessels, to the internal thoracic chain of lymph nodes.

Further reading

Drake RL, Vogl AW, Mitchell AW. *Gray's Anatomy for Students* (2nd ed). Philadelphia, PA: Elsevier; 2010.

Ellis H, Mahadevan V. Anatomy and physiology of the breast. *Surgery* 2013; 31(1):11–14.

Ellis H, Mahadevan V. *Clinical Anatomy: Applied Anatomy for Students and Junior Doctors.* (13th ed). Oxford: Wiley-Blackwell; 2013.

MacKinnon PCB, Morris JF. *Oxford Textbook of Functional Anatomy* (Vol 2, 2nd ed). Oxford: Oxford University Press; 2005.

Mahadevan V. Anatomy of the heart. *Surgery* 2012; 30(1):5–8.

Sadler TW. *Langman's Medical Embryology* (13th ed). Philadelphia, PA: Wolters Kluwer/Lippincott Williams & Wilkins; 2014.

Sinnatamby C. *Last's Anatomy: Regional and Applied* (12th ed). Edinburgh: Elsevier; 2011.

CHAPTER 1.1.2

Anatomy of the abdomen

Vishy Mahadevan

Anterior abdominal wall

An understanding of the design and structure of the anterior abdominal wall is an essential prerequisite to gaining adequate and safe surgical access to the abdominal cavity, and for the safe and satisfactory achievement of procedures such as paracentesis abdominis and suprapubic catheterization of the urinary bladder. The optimal positioning of intestinal stomas (e.g. ileostomies and colostomies) also requires a sound understanding of the architecture of the anterior abdominal wall.

General structure of anterior abdominal wall

The outline of the anterior abdominal wall is approximately hexagonal. It is bounded superiorly by the arched costal margin (with the xiphisternum at the summit of the arch). The lateral boundary on either side is, by convention, taken to be the mid-axillary line (between the costal margin and the summit of the iliac crest). Inferiorly, on each side, the anterior abdominal wall is bounded in continuity, by the anterior half of the iliac crest, inguinal ligament, pubic crest, and pubic symphysis. Situated in the vertical midline of the anterior abdominal wall is the umbilicus, a puckered scar.

The anterior abdominal wall is a multilayered structure, a feature that is readily discernible in a horizontal computed tomography section through the abdominal wall. From the surface inwards, the successive layers are as follows:

1. Skin

2. Superficial fascia comprising two layers—an outer fatty layer which overlies a fibrous layer termed Scarpa's fascia

3. A musculo-aponeurotic plane (which is architecturally complex and is made up of several layers)

4. Transversalis fascia

5. Properitoneal adipose layer

6. Parietal layer of peritoneum.

The transversalis fascia is, in fact, the anterior part of the general endo-abdominal fibrous layer that envelops the parietal peritoneum. The transversalis fascia is closely applied to the deep surface of the rectus sheath medially and to the deep surface of the transversus abdominis muscle laterally.

Musculo-aponeurotic plane of anterior abdominal wall

Anteriorly, on either side of the ventral midline, the musculo-aponeurotic layer is represented by a long, strap-like muscle, the rectus abdominis. Each rectus abdominis muscle arises from the pubic symphysis and adjacent pubic bone. The muscle widens as it runs upwards. The upper attachment of the muscle is to the costal margin alongside the sternum and to a couple of costal cartilages just above the costal margin.

Lateral to each rectus abdominis muscle, the musculo-aponeurotic plane is made up of a three-ply (overlapping) arrangement of flat muscular sheets, termed the anterolateral abdominal muscles. The outermost of these is the external oblique muscle. The intermediate layer is the internal oblique muscle, and the innermost layer is the transversus abdominis muscle. Of these three muscles, only the external oblique has an attachment above the level of the costal margin. Traced anteromedially, each of these muscles becomes aponeurotic. The three aponeuroses enclose the rectus abdominis muscle, the aponeurotic envelope being termed the rectus sheath. Running down the ventral midline of the anterior abdominal wall from the xiphisternum superiorly, to the pubic symphysis inferiorly, and interposed between the two rectus sheaths is a pale, dense, fibro-aponeurotic band termed the linea alba. The linea alba is a midline interlacement of the aponeuroses of the anterolateral abdominal muscles of the two sides. Above the level of the umbilicus it is a prominent, wide, dense, and tough structure, while below the level of the umbilicus it is usually no more than a narrow strip. It is a relatively avascular structure, a feature that is taken advantage of in midline laparotomy incisions.

Innervation and blood supply of the muscles of the anterior abdominal wall

The muscles of the anterior abdominal wall are supplied segmentally by the 7th to 11th intercostal nerves and the subcostal nerve. These nerves (accompanied by their corresponding posterior intercostal vessels) cross the costal margin obliquely to run in the neurovascular plane of the anterior abdominal wall, between the internal oblique and transversus abdominis muscles. The nerves supply the anterolateral abdominal muscles as well as the rectus abdominis segmentally, and eventually emerge as lateral and anterior cutaneous branches. Cutaneous innervation of the anterior abdominal wall by the 7th to 11th intercostal nerves and subcostal nerve is represented by a series of oblique band-shaped dermatomes. The dermatome corresponding to the 10th intercostal nerve is at the level of the umbilicus; that of the 7th intercostal nerve is at the epigastric level. The 11th intercostal and subcostal nerves supply strips of skin below the umbilical level. A strip of skin immediately above the inguinal ligament and pubic symphysis is supplied by the iliohypogastric and ilioinguinal nerves (both L1).

Because there is considerable overlap in the dermal territories of adjacent intercostal nerves, damage to one or two of these nerves will usually not produce any clinically detectable anaesthesia.

The posterior intercostal arteries which accompany the intercostal nerves supply the anterolateral abdominal muscles.

The rectus abdominis muscle, however, has a different blood supply. The upper half of the muscle is supplied by the superior epigastric artery (a branch of the internal thoracic artery). The lower half of the rectus abdominis is supplied by the inferior epigastric artery, a branch of the external iliac artery.

Myocutaneous rotation flaps used in plastic and reconstructive surgery may be fashioned using either the upper or lower halves of the rectus abdominis muscle; the former being based on the superior epigastric vascular pedicle and the latter being based on the inferior epigastric vascular pedicle.

Anatomy of commonly used anterior abdominal wall incisions

Incisions in the anterior/anterolateral abdominal wall may be placed longitudinally, transversely, or obliquely; the choice and site of incision being dictated by a number of factors including the location and nature of the intra-abdominal pathology necessitating the operation.

A vertical midline incision may be supraumbilical, infraumbilical, or full length. The last-named skirts the side of the umbilicus. In adults, a full-length vertical midline laparotomy incision provides the most generous access to the abdominal cavity, and is the preferred incision for open repair of an abdominal aortic aneurysm. Midline incisions are carried through the linea alba and do not traverse muscle.

Vertical incisions placed 2 or 3 cm lateral to the midline are termed paramedian incisions. Paramedian incisions involve incising the anterior and posterior walls of the rectus sheath vertically, but without traversing the rectus abdominis muscle.

A transverse suprapubic incision placed just above and parallel to the pubic crest affords very satisfactory access to the pelvic cavity and lower abdomen. Such incisions generally heal very well leaving a very thin eventual scar, and have a very low incidence of incisional hernia. A Pfannenstiel incision is an example of a suprapubic incision.

An oblique incision through the anterior abdominal wall placed parallel to and 3 or 4 cm below the costal margin is termed a subcostal incision. Access to the peritoneal cavity involves dividing the three-ply arrangement of anterolateral abdominal wall muscles in the lateral part of the wound and dividing the rectus sheath and rectus abdominis muscle in the medial part of the wound. The division of the muscles is performed in the line of the skin incision usually with a diathermy electrode set to cutting mode.

A subcostal incision may be performed on the right or left side. A bilateral subcostal incision is called a rooftop incision and is the preferred incision in some surgical units for such specialized procedures as D2 gastrectomy.

A commonly employed oblique incision is the McBurney incision that is used for open appendicectomy. The incision is placed in the right lower quadrant of the anterior abdominal wall. Following incision of skin and superficial fascia, the anterolateral muscles are incised in the line of their respective fibres (hence, gridiron incision) before the peritoneal cavity is entered.

Groin and inguinal canal

The groin or inguinal region denotes the area adjoining the junctional crease between the front of the thigh and the lower part of the anterior abdominal wall, and includes the inguinal and femoral canals. The inguinal canal is an obliquely orientated, slit-like space within the lower part of the anterior abdominal wall. It may be represented on the surface by a 1.5 cm-wide band, above and parallel to the medial half of the inguinal ligament. The lateral end of the inguinal canal is the deep inguinal ring (a defect in the fascia transversalis). From here the inguinal canal runs inferomedially and anteriorly to open at the superficial inguinal ring (a triangular defect in the external oblique aponeurosis). In adults, the inguinal canal is approximately 5–6 cm long. In males, the inguinal canal contains the spermatic cord and the ilioinguinal nerve, while in females, it contains the round ligament of the uterus and the ilioinguinal nerve. The inguinal canal consists of a floor, a roof, an anterior wall, and a posterior wall. Running obliquely upward and medially behind the fascia transversalis and just medial to the deep inguinal ring is an important artery, the inferior epigastric artery with its companion veins.

Inguinal hernia is an abnormal protrusion of the peritoneal cavity into the inguinal canal. When this protrusion enters the inguinal canal through the deep inguinal ring, it is termed an *indirect inguinal hernia*. Such a hernia has the potential to enlarge and emerge through the superficial inguinal ring, and in men, the hernia may enter the scrotum. The neck of an indirect inguinal hernial sac is lateral to the location of the inferior epigastric artery. By contrast, when the peritoneum protrudes into the inguinal canal, medial to the inferior epigastric artery, through an attenuated and weakened posterior wall, it is termed a *direct inguinal hernia*.

Posterior abdominal wall

The anterior abdominal wall is made up entirely of layers of muscle, aponeuroses, fasciae, and other soft-tissue structures, and is a relatively distensible structure. This is a useful arrangement and allows the abdominal cavity to accommodate large increases in the volume of its contents be that pathological (e.g. ascites, intestinal obstruction, or intra-abdominal tumours) or physiological (e.g. pregnancy).

The posterior abdominal wall, by contrast, is a rigidly constructed structure made up of the sturdy lumbar vertebral column down the middle of its length. This acts as a vertical strut. Inferolateral to the lumbar vertebral column on each side is the iliac wing (ala of the ilium) of the corresponding hip bone. Superolateral to the lumbar vertebral column on each side is the corresponding 12th rib. Collectively, the lumbar vertebral column, the right and left iliac wings, and the 12th ribs make up the bony part of the posterior abdominal wall. Powerful and thick muscles lying on either side of the lumbar vertebral column and on the inner surface of the ala of the ilium make up the muscular part of the posterior abdominal wall (Figure 1.1.2.1).

Lumbar vertebrae

The lumbar vertebrae are five in number. Together with their intervening intervertebral discs they make up the lumbar part of the articulated vertebral column. This forms a prominent vertical ridge on the posterior abdominal wall. The lumbar vertebral column presents a pronounced ventral convexity termed the lumbar lordosis. The lumbar vertebrae are larger and sturdier than any of the individual vertebrae from elsewhere in the vertebral column. Running within the lumbar vertebral column is the lumbar spinal canal. In the adult, the termination of the spinal cord is typically at the level

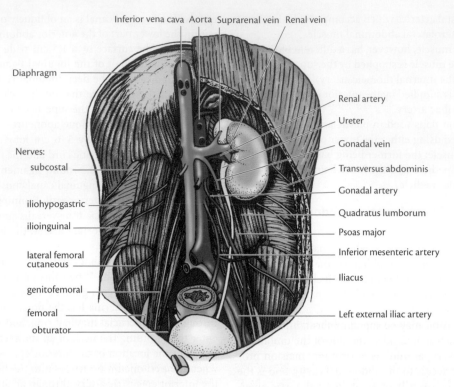

Inferior vena cava | Aorta | Suprarenal vein | Renal vein

Diaphragm

Renal artery
Ureter
Gonadal vein
Transversus abdominis
Gonadal artery
Quadratus lumborum
Psoas major
Inferior mesenteric artery
Iliacus
Left external iliac artery

Nerves:
subcostal
iliohypogastric
ilioinguinal
lateral femoral cutaneous
genitofemoral
femoral
obturator

Fig. 1.1.2.1 Posterior abdominal wall: muscles, nerves, and great vessels.
Reproduced from Sinnatamby C., *Last's Anatomy*, Twelfth Edition, Churchill-Livingstone, UK, Copyright © 2011 with permission from Elsevier.

of the lower border of the first lumbar vertebra. The spinal menin-ges, however, continue distally to mid-sacral level. Contained within the subarachnoid space below the termination of the spinal cord is the cauda equina (the collective name for the roots of the lumbar, sacral, and coccygeal spinal nerves).

Lying behind the vertebral column and providing stability and strong support to the vertebral column from behind, are the post-vertebral muscles. These muscles are arranged in layers and include the large and powerful erector spinae muscle. These muscles are, in the main, innervated by the dorsal rami of spinal nerves.

Muscles of the posterior abdominal wall

When viewed from the ventral aspect, three large muscles on each side of the lumbar vertebral column, symmetrically arranged, are seen to make up most of the muscular part of the posterior abdomi-nal wall. Each of the three muscles is covered on its ventral surface by a dense fascia. The muscles are the psoas major, quadratus lum-borum, and iliacus. In addition, the right and left crura of the dia-phragm which arise from the ventral aspects of the upper lumbar vertebral bodies may also be regarded as muscles of the posterior abdominal wall.

The psoas major muscle arises from the lateral aspect of each of the lumbar vertebral bodies and from the ventral surface of the adjacent transverse process.

The iliacus is a large and powerful muscle that arises from the inner surface of the ala of the ilium. It lies immediately lateral to the lower half of psoas major muscle. Psoas major and iliacus are both covered on their ventral surfaces by dense fasciae. These are the psoas fascia and fascia iliaca, respectively. Distally the tendons of iliacus and psoas major enter the thigh deep to the inguinal liga-ment. Here both iliacus and psoas major (the latter medial to the

former) contribute to the floor of the femoral triangle before they turn inferomedially to gain attachment to the lesser trochanter of the femur. Psoas major and iliacus are powerful flexors of the hip joint. Additionally, psoas major but not iliacus can flex the lumbar vertebral column.

The quadratus lumborum muscle arises from the posterior part of the iliac crest and from the transverse processes of all the lumbar vertebrae. Superiorly, the muscle is attached to the anterior surface of the 12th rib. The fascia which covers the ventral surface of the muscle is the anterior layer of the thoracolumbar fascia.

Peritoneal cavity

The peritoneum is a serous membrane which forms a sac that lines the walls of the abdominal cavity and continues into the upper part of the pelvic cavity. In the male subject the peritoneum forms a completely closed sac. However, in females, owing to the fact that the lateral end of the uterine tube (fallopian tube) opens into the peritoneal sac, the cavity of the latter communicates with the exterior indirectly via the uterine tube, uterus, and vagina (Figure 1.1.2.2).

General disposition of the peritoneum

The peritoneal sac encloses the peritoneal cavity, which, in the nor-mal state, contains no more than a thin film of fluid. The part of the peritoneum which lines the abdominal walls is termed the parietal layer of peritoneum while the part which covers the abdominal and pelvic organs is termed the visceral peritoneum. The two layers are, of course, physically continuous with each other. Thus the perito-neum is very similar in its arrangement to the pleura and serous pericardium.

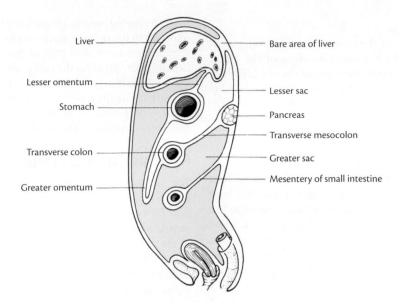

Fig. 1.1.2.2 Schematic sagittal view of peritoneal cavity (female).
Reproduced with permission from Ellis H. and Mahadevan V., *Clinical Anatomy*, Thirteenth Edition, Wiley-Blackwell, Oxford, UK, Copyright © 2013.

In places the parietal peritoneum over the posterior abdominal wall is seen to form ventrally directed infoldings. These double-layered peritoneal infoldings (peritoneal reduplications) are remnants of the dorsal mesentery which, during embryological development, suspended the entire gut from the dorsal body wall.

In reality the peritoneal cavity contains no more than a thin film of serous fluid. This fluid moistens the parietal and visceral layers of the peritoneum, allowing them to glide against each other. Strictly speaking there are no viscera lying *within* the peritoneal cavity: all are extraperitoneal. It is nevertheless useful to make a distinction between (1) those gut-derived structures which are almost completely invested in peritoneum and which invaginate the peritoneal sac from behind and (2) those gut-derived structures which are covered by peritoneum on their anterior aspects only, and are effectively plastered on to the posterior abdominal wall. Viscera which are completely surrounded by visceral peritoneum tend to possess a suspensory mesentery which in turn confers a certain mobility to these viscera.

Principal divisions of the peritoneal cavity

The peritoneal cavity is divided into:

- the greater sac (the term which is used to denote the general peritoneal cavity)
- the lesser sac, which is effectively a diverticulum of the greater sac. The lesser sac also known as the omental bursa, lies behind the stomach and lesser omentum. The long but narrow window through which the greater sac and lesser sac communicate with each other is known as the epiploic foramen. (Other names for the epiploic foramen are *foramen of Winslow* and *aditus to the lesser sac.*)

On first entering the abdominal cavity through the anterior abdominal wall, the most prominent structure that is observed is usually the greater omentum: a long and wide apron of fat which is attached superiorly to the greater curvature of the stomach. The inferior end of the greater omentum is free. Lying posterior to the greater omentum just inferior to the greater curvature of the stomach is the transverse colon. The transverse colon is seen to be fairly mobile, its mobility being due to the presence of a mesentery, the transverse mesocolon, which is attached to the posterior abdominal wall along the lower border of the body of the pancreas.

The transverse mesocolon conveniently divides the peritoneal cavity into two principal compartments: supracolic compartment and infracolic compartment.

The supracolic compartment

The supracolic compartment contains the abdominal oesophagus, stomach, first part of duodenum, lesser omentum and the structures running within its free edge, the liver and biliary tract, and spleen. In addition, there are two spaces within the peritoneal cavity of the supracolic compartment that are of particular surgical significance. These are the lesser sac (omental bursa) and the hepatorenal space (known also as the pouch of Rutherford Morison). The hepatorenal pouch is the most dependent part of the entire peritoneal cavity. Consequently any free fluid in the peritoneal cavity is likely to gravitate to the hepatorenal pouch. The fluid may stagnate in the hepatorenal pouch and become infected, giving rise to a subphrenic abscess.

The infracolic compartment

The infracolic compartment contains the jejunum and ileum in their entirety and also the small intestinal mesentery which suspends all of the jejunum and ileum. The caecum, appendix, sigmoid colon, and transverse colon are additional structures in the infracolic compartment. Since the ascending and descending segments of the colon do not possess a mesentery they may be regarded as retroperitoneal structures lying in the floor of the infracolic compartment. Within the infracolic compartment are the right and left paracolic gutters, respectively lateral to the ascending and descending colons. The paracolic gutters are fairly deep recesses of the peritoneal cavity lying lateral and parallel to the vertical segments of the colon.

Blood supply to the gut

A preliminary consideration of the embryological development of the alimentary tract facilitates understanding of the blood supply (arterial supply and venous drainage) of the tract. The alimentary tract develops in its entirety from the primitive gut tube, which in turn is formed by the infolding of the endodermal germ sheet. Initially the gut tube is closed at either end by the buccopharyngeal membrane at the cephalic end and by the cloacal membrane at the caudal end. Rupture of these membranes, early in the course of embryonic development, results in the gut being open at both ends. Concomitantly, the gut tube differentiates into foregut, midgut, and hindgut. The primitive gut derives its blood supply from a number of vitelline arteries which arise from the ventral aspect of the aorta. All but three of the vitelline arteries disappear during further development. The ones that persist are the coeliac artery, superior mesenteric artery, and inferior mesenteric artery. These supply, respectively, the foregut, midgut, and hindgut.

Developing in concert with the vitelline arteries and their branches are corresponding vitelline veins. These veins eventually come to accompany the coeliac, superior mesenteric and inferior mesenteric arteries, and their branches. Proximally, however, these veins do not drain directly into the inferior vena cava. Instead they empty into the portal vein which in turn is formed by a coalescence of the centrally located vitelline veins.

Arterial supply of alimentary tract

The alimentary tract within the abdominal cavity receives its blood supply entirely from the three visceral branches which arise from the anterior aspect of the abdominal aorta. These are, in succession, the coeliac artery, the superior mesenteric artery, and the inferior mesenteric artery.

Each artery has its fairly well-delineated territory, and these are as follows:

- Coeliac artery: distal oesophagus, stomach, first and second parts of the duodenum, liver, gall bladder, pancreas, and spleen

- Superior mesenteric artery: the duodenum distal to the opening of the ampulla of Vater, the entire jejunum and ileum, caecum, appendix, ascending colon, hepatic flexure of colon, and proximal two-thirds of the transverse colon

- Inferior mesenteric artery: distal third of the transverse colon, splenic flexure of colon, descending colon, sigmoid colon, and rectum.

Venous drainage of the alimentary tract and associated structures

The superior mesenteric vein which drains the territory of the superior mesenteric artery joins the splenic vein behind the neck of the pancreas to form the portal vein. The splenic vein drains most of the territory of the coeliac artery. It also receives, as a direct tributary, the inferior mesenteric vein which carries venous blood from the territory of the inferior mesenteric artery. The portal vein ascends to reach the hilum of the liver (porta hepatis) where it branches to supply the entire liver. The portal vein is thus the final common pathway for venous blood from the distal oesophagus, the full length of the abdominal part of the alimentary tract, the spleen, and pancreas. Portal venous blood is carried to the liver where following passage through the hepatic sinusoids, the blood is returned to the inferior vena cava by the hepatic veins. The portal vein delivers more than 70% of the blood supply to the liver. The hepatic artery provides the remainder. Quite apart from the volume of blood that it supplies, the portal vein is also important for oxygen delivery to the liver. Unlike systemic venous blood, portal venous blood is only partially deoxygenated, and in the preprandial state may possess an oxygen saturation of 92–93%.

Retroperitoneal region

The retroperitoneal region (or retroperitoneum) refers to the region that lies outside the parietal peritoneum, behind the peritoneal cavity and in front of the posterior abdominal wall. Thus the ventral boundary of the retroperitoneal region is the posterior part of the parietal peritoneum, while the dorsal boundary is made up of the lumbar vertebrae and the muscles and fasciae of the posterior abdominal wall. Inferiorly, the retroperitoneum is continuous with the extraperitoneal space of the pelvic cavity.

The retroperitoneum is a relatively large space and its contents include the abdominal aorta and the inferior vena cava. These large vessels, lying side by side, run vertically in front of the lumbar vertebral column. The retroperitoneal region also contains the common iliac vessels, neural structures such as the right and left ganglionated lumbar sympathetic trunks, branches of the lumbar plexi, various autonomic nerve plexi, the cisterna chyli (a large lymphatic sac which continues into the posterior mediastinum as the thoracic duct), a number of lymph nodes, and various retroperitoneal viscera. Some of the retroperitoneal lymph nodes are arranged as clusters in front of the abdominal aorta around the origins of the three gut arteries. These are the pre-aortic lymph nodes. Other lymph nodes lie to either side of the aorta. These are the para-aortic lymph nodes and are situated near the origins of the paired visceral arteries.

Retroperitoneal viscera

The viscera in the retroperitoneal region may be conveniently classified into two broad groups:

1. Those viscera that are derived embryologically from the primitive gut

2. Those viscera that have their embryological derivation from the intermediate mesodermal mass (the embryonic tissue which gives rise to the genitourinary ridge).

The retroperitoneal abdominal viscera derived from the embryonic gut are the duodenum (second, third, and fourth parts; the first part of the duodenum is intraperitoneal), the pancreas, and the ascending and descending segments of the colon including the hepatic and splenic flexures of the colon.

The viscera derived from the genitourinary ridge are the kidneys, ureters, and suprarenal glands (or, to be more precise, the suprarenal cortices).

Abdominal aorta

The abdominal aorta commences at the level of the lower border of the 12th thoracic vertebra, and is the direct continuation of the descending thoracic aorta. The change of name from thoracic to abdominal occurs when the aorta passes through the aortic hiatus of the diaphragm, between the two diaphragmatic crura. The abdominal aorta descends vertically lying immediately in front of the lumbar vertebral bodies.

In front of the fourth lumbar vertebra the aorta divides into its two terminal branches: the right and left common iliac arteries.

The branches of the abdominal aorta may be conveniently classified into four groups as follows:

1. Unpaired visceral branches arising from the ventral wall of the aorta

2. Paired visceral branches arising from the lateral or anterolateral aspect of the aorta

3. Parietal branches arising from the dorsal wall of the aorta and which supply the body wall

4. Terminal branches.

The unpaired visceral branches which arise from the ventral aspect of the aorta are three in number: coeliac artery, superior mesenteric artery, and inferior mesenteric artery. Collectively these branches supply the entire length of the alimentary tract located in the abdominal cavity including all the related viscera derived from the embryonic gut.

The paired (right and left) visceral branches are the renal arteries, gonadal arteries, suprarenal arteries, and inferior phrenic arteries. The inferior phrenic arteries are important sources of blood supply to the diaphragm, but may nevertheless be regarded as visceral since they contribute to the blood supply of the suprarenal glands and the abdominal oesophagus.

The parietal branches arising from the dorsal aspect of the aorta are the four pairs of lumbar arteries and the single median sacral artery. The lumbar arteries supply the lumbar vertebral column and the muscles of the posterior abdominal wall. Through their spinal branches the lumbar arteries also contribute to the blood supply of the terminal part of the spinal cord and the cauda equina.

The terminal branches are the right and left common iliac arteries, each of which bifurcates above the pelvic brim into the external and internal iliac arteries.

The normal abdominal aorta measures approximately 2 cm in diameter. In the elderly, it is frequently thickened and dilated. An aneurysmal dilatation is considered to be present if the aortic diameter reaches 4 cm.

Running across the front of the abdominal aorta and overlapping the origin of the superior mesenteric artery is the body of the pancreas, while crossing the front of the aorta and overlapping the origin of the inferior mesenteric artery is the third part of the duodenum.

A large tumour of the pancreas or stomach, a mass of enlarged pre-aortic lymph nodes or a large ovarian cyst may each be palpable through the anterior abdominal wall. Such masses may transmit the pulsations of the aorta to the anterior abdominal wall and be mistaken for an aortic aneurysm.

Inferior vena cava

The inferior vena cava is the widest and largest vein in the body. It is formed in front of the body of the fifth lumbar vertebra by the confluence of the right and left common iliac veins. It ascends in front of the lumbar vertebral column lying parallel to and immediately to the right of the abdominal aorta, and ends by traversing the central tendinous portion of the diaphragm before opening into the right atrium of the heart. In the upper part of its course, the inferior vena cava lies in a groove on the posterior aspect of the liver. The inferior vena cava carries venous blood from all structures below the level of the diaphragm.

In addition to the right and left common iliac veins, the *direct* tributaries of the inferior vena cava include the right and left renal veins, the lumbar veins of both sides, the right gonadal vein, right suprarenal vein, and the hepatic veins.

Together the two common iliac veins carry all the venous blood from the lower limbs including the gluteal region, and most of the venous drainage from the pelvic walls and pelvic viscera. From the foregoing account it may be readily inferred that the inferior vena cava is the final common pathway for venous thromboemboli originating in the lower limbs, perineum, or pelvic cavity. These emboli may be carried successively through the right atrium, right ventricle, pulmonary trunk, and pulmonary arterial tree before being lodged in the pulmonary vascular bed, causing embolic occlusion of the latter, a potentially fatal condition. In individuals with a high risk of thromboembolism and evidence of proximal extension of a venous thrombus in the lower limb or pelvis, an umbrella filter may be placed in the inferior vena cava to prevent such thromboemboli from being carried proximally. When placing such an occlusive filter, it is important to ensure that the filter is placed below the level at which the renal veins join the inferior vena cava, lest renal venous return be compromised.

Surface anatomy

To facilitate description of the topography of abdominal viscera, and to enable the clinician to convey with precision the location of abdominal lumps and abdominal pain, it is conventional to divide the abdominal cavity into regions by plotting a number of imaginary lines or planes on the anterior abdominal wall. The most commonly employed convention divides the abdomen into nine regions by means of a pair of vertical lines and a pair of horizontal lines. The vertical lines are the right and left mid-clavicular lines. The two horizontal lines are the transpyloric line and the supracristal line. The former is plotted halfway between the sternal notch and pubic symphysis, while the supracristal line lies level with the highest points on the iliac crests. The nine regions thus defined are arranged in three horizontal, parallel rows, with three regions in each row. The upper row includes the right and left hypochondrial regions and the centrally located epigastrium. The middle row consists of the right and left lumbar regions and the centrally located umbilical region, while the lower row consists of the right and left inguinal regions and the centrally located hypogastric region.

The transpyloric line (plane) corresponds to the level of the lower border of the first lumbar vertebra while the supracristal line or plane corresponds to the level of the body of the fourth lumbar vertebra. These lines are of considerable clinical usefulness in the surface representation of deeply placed intra-abdominal structures.

Further reading

Drake RL, Vogl AW, Mitchell AW. *Gray's Anatomy for Students* (2nd ed). Philadelphia, PA: Elsevier; 2010.

Ellis H, Mahadevan V. *Clinical Anatomy: Applied Anatomy for Students and Junior Doctors.* (13th ed). Oxford: Wiley-Blackwell; 2013.

Ellis H. Anatomy of the caecum, appendix and colon. *Surgery* 2011; 29(1):1–4.

Mahadevan V. Anatomy of the anterior abdominal wall and groin. *Surgery* 2012; 30(6):257–60.

Sadler TW. *Langman's Medical Embryology* (13th ed). Philadelphia, PA: Wolters Kluwer/Lippincott Williams & Wilkins; 2014.

Sinnatamby C. *Last's Anatomy: Regional and Applied* (12th ed). Edinburgh: Elsevier; 2011.

CHAPTER 1.1.3

Anatomy of the pelvis and perineum

Vishy Mahadevan

Structure of the bony pelvis and design of the pelvic cavity

The term pelvis is often used interchangeably (and somewhat imprecisely and confusingly) to mean (a) the bony ring formed by the two hip (innominate) bones and the sacrococcygeal part of the vertebral column, (b) the cavity enclosed by the above-mentioned bony ring, and (c) the entire region where the lower part of the trunk meets the lower limbs.

This author favours precision in the use of terminology and recommends strongly, that the term 'pelvis' be reserved for the bony ring and its associated stabilizing ligaments, and the term 'pelvic cavity' be used to denote the space within the bony ring, above the pelvic floor and below the level of the pelvic brim.

The bony pelvis (pelvic wall)

The bony pelvis refers to the irregular but complete bony ring formed by the right and left hip bones at the front and sides, and by the entire sacrococcygeal part of the vertebral column, posteriorly. Externally, on either side, the bony pelvis articulates with the corresponding femoral head to form the hip joint. Superiorly, through the lumbosacral articulation the bony pelvis supports the remainder of the vertebral column. The bony pelvis, as just described, incorporates four articulations, as follows. The two hip bones are held together anteriorly at the pubic symphysis—an extremely strong and virtually unbreachable bond. Posterolaterally, on either side, the medial aspect of the hip bone articulates with the corresponding lateral aspect of the sacrum to form a synovial joint, the sacroiliac joint. Finally, the inferior end of the sacrum articulates with the upper surface of the coccyx to form the sacrococcygeal joint. The pubic symphysis and the sacrococcygeal articulation are both examples of *secondary cartilaginous joints*.

The inner aspect of the bony pelvis features an undulant (wavy), more-or-less complete bony ridge termed the pelvic brim. By convention the plane of the pelvic brim is used to divide the bony pelvis into two parts: the part below the level of the pelvic brim is the lesser pelvis (or true pelvis) and the part above the pelvic brim is the greater pelvis (or false pelvis). The area enclosed by the lesser pelvis is the pelvic cavity, whereas the area enclosed by the greater pelvis (i.e. above the pelvic brim) is in fact the lower part of the abdominal cavity and consists of the right and left iliac fossae.

The pelvic brim, which defines the upper limit of the pelvic cavity, is made up of the sacral promontory (the prominent anterior lip of the upper surface of the body of the sacrum), posteriorly, and is formed on either side by the arcuate line of the ilium and superior ramus of the pubis, while anteriorly it is made up of the pubic crest and the upper edge of the pubic symphysis.

On each side of the midline, the bony pelvis below the level of the pelvic brim, presents three 'gateways'—namely the greater sciatic foramen, lesser sciatic foramen, and obturator foramen. Through these gateways the interior of the bony pelvis connects with areas outside the pelvic ring. Located posterolaterally are the greater sciatic foramen and lesser sciatic foramen which allow the interior of the bony pelvis to communicate with the ipsilateral gluteal region. Located anterolaterally is the obturator foramen, through which the interior of the pelvis communicates with the adductor region of the thigh. The obturator foramen is a large opening in the anterior part of the hip bone, and has a complete bony boundary. In life it is almost completely closed by a dense and fairly strong fibrous sheet termed the obturator membrane.

The bony pelvis serves multiple functions:

1. It transmits the weight of the upper part of the body to the lower limbs through the hip joints, and transmits to the vertebral column the upward thrust generated by the lower limbs during walking, running, and jumping

2. The bony pelvis offers considerable protection to the delicate viscera and vessels contained within it

3. Its external surface provides anchorage to several extremely powerful muscles such as the gluteal muscles and muscles of the thigh including the adductors and hamstrings.

Intrapelvic muscles

The muscles lying within the pelvic cavity are the piriformis, obturator internus, coccygeus, and levator ani. Each of these muscles is complementarily paired (i.e. present bilaterally). Of these, the coccygeus and levator ani muscles shall be considered in the following subsection on the pelvic floor. Piriformis and obturator internus are for the most part intrapelvic structures. Piriformis arises from the front of the sacrum and thus from the posterior wall of the pelvic cavity. Obturator internus arises from the inner surface of the obturator membrane and contiguous bone, and thus from the inner surface of the lateral wall of the pelvic cavity. However, the tendon of each of these muscles leaves the interior of the bony pelvis (the piriformis tendon through the greater sciatic foramen and the obturator internus tendon through the lesser sciatic foramen) to enter the gluteal region. Here the two tendons run immediately behind the capsule of the hip joint capsule before attaching to the greater trochanter of the femur. Functionally the obturator internus and piriformis muscles are external rotators (lateral rotators) of the hip joint.

Pelvic floor

The pelvic floor, also known as the pelvic diaphragm, comprises the right and left coccygeus muscles and the right and left levator ani muscles. The coccygeus is a small, thin muscle that is functionally unimportant and contributes to the posterolateral part of the pelvic floor. It extends from the tip of the ischial spine medially to the side of the sacrococcygeal junction. The levator ani muscle is a larger and wider muscle than coccygeus. Arising from a linear thickening in the obturator fascia (the fascia that covers the *inner* surface of the obturator internus muscle) the levator ani muscle runs inwards, backwards, and downwards and interdigitates with the contralateral levator ani to form a mobile, thin, gutter-shaped muscular sheet, slung like a hammock from the obturator fascia of one side to that of the other. Anteriorly, between the medial edges of the two levator ani muscles is a natural gap termed the *levator hiatus*. The levator hiatus transmits the rectum and urethra in both sexes, and in the female transmits, additionally, the vagina. (Note that the upper quarter of the vagina lies above the level of the pelvic floor and thus within the pelvic cavity, while the lower three-quarters lies in the perineum.) It is the two levator ani muscles that make up the mobile and functionally important part of the pelvic floor. The levator ani is a voluntary muscle. Weakness of the pelvic floor, whether due to physical injury of the muscle (as may be caused by a prolonged and difficult labour) or due to neurological causes, may result in prolapse of intrapelvic viscera and this may, in turn, manifest itself clinically, as faecal and/or urinary incontinence of varying degree. The levator ani muscle acts principally as a support. It also has a sphincteric action on the rectum and vagina and by its contraction, assists in increasing intra-abdominal pressure during defaecation, micturition, and parturition.

Pelvic viscera

Intrapelvic viscera common to both sexes

Those viscera in the pelvic cavity that are present in both sexes include the distal third of sigmoid colon, the entire rectum, the urinary bladder, and the intrapelvic segments of the right and left ureters. In both sexes, the urinary bladder is the most anterior viscus in the pelvic cavity while the terminal portion of the sigmoid colon and rectum are the most posteriorly located of the intrapelvic viscera.

Intrapelvic male genital organs

These include the prostate and prostatic urethra, the right and left seminal vesicles, the intrapelvic segment of each (right and left) vas deferens, and the right and left common ejaculatory ducts (Figure 1.1.3.1).

Intrapelvic female genital organs

These include the uterus, the right and left uterine tubes (Fallopian tubes), the right and left ovaries, and the intrapelvic portion of the vagina (Figure 1.1.3.2).

Pelvic peritoneum and peritoneal recesses

The peritoneum of the abdominal cavity extends into the pelvic cavity as the pelvic peritoneum and partially invests some of the pelvic viscera. Between adjacent viscera it tends to form shallow folds or recesses. The deepest of these peritoneal recesses is the one that lies between the posterior vaginal fornix in front, and the anterior wall of the rectum, posteriorly. This is the rectouterine pouch or pouch of Douglas.

The peritoneum drapes the front and back of the uterus and extends laterally on either side as a double-layered sheet called the broad ligament, whose upper border encloses the uterine tube.

Pelvic blood vessels and lymphatics

The main arteries supplying the walls and contents of the pelvic cavity are the right and left internal iliac arteries. Additionally,

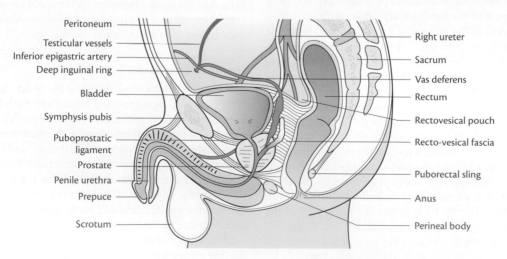

Fig. 1.1.3.1 Sagittal section of male pelvic cavity.

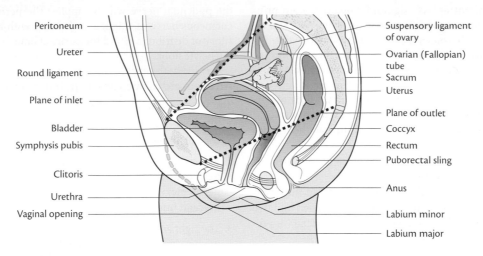

Fig. 1.1.3.2 Sagittal section of female pelvic cavity.

however, are (1) *the superior rectal artery* which is the direct continuation of the inferior mesenteric artery and which is the principal source of blood supply to the rectum; (2) *the median sacral artery*, an unpaired branch of the abdominal aorta which arises from the posterior aspect of the aorta just proximal to the aortic bifurcation and runs inferiorly to lie in front of the sacrum. It is usually an insignificant vessel which supplies the anterior sacral periosteum; and (3) the all-important right and left ovarian arteries. (Note: the male gonadal arteries do not enter the pelvic cavity.) The median sacral artery, the ovarian arteries, and the superior rectal artery (being merely the inferior mesenteric artery by another name) are all direct branches of the abdominal aorta.

Internal iliac artery and its branches

The major arteries of the pelvic cavity are the right and left internal iliac arteries. Together, these two arteries supply the pelvic walls, pelvic musculature, and the pelvic viscera. Indeed all of the pelvic viscera (with the exception of the ovaries and the rectum) rely principally on the internal iliac arteries for their blood supply. Each internal iliac artery is one of two terminal branches of the corresponding common iliac artery; the other terminal branch being the external iliac artery.

Originating at the pelvic brim as the smaller of the two terminal branches of the common iliac artery, the internal iliac artery crosses the pelvic brim and runs just inside the lateral wall of the pelvic cavity with the ureter in front, and the internal iliac vein behind.

Shortly after its origin, the internal iliac artery divides into anterior and posterior divisions, the former being the larger of the two.

The posterior division gives rise to the following arteries: superior gluteal, iliolumbar, and lateral sacral. All three are parietal branches (i.e. they supply the *parietes* or body wall structures) and do not supply viscera. The superior gluteal artery leaves the pelvic cavity through the greater sciatic foramen, enters the gluteal region, and supplies the gluteal muscles.

The anterior division gives rise to two sets of branches: visceral and parietal.

Visceral branches of the anterior division are the superior vesical, inferior vesical, middle rectal, and internal pudendal arteries. The last mentioned supply viscera in the perineum. Additionally, arising from the anterior division of the internal iliac artery in the female is the all-important uterine artery and sometimes a separate vaginal artery for the intrapelvic vagina. Besides supplying the urinary bladder as implied in their names, the superior and inferior vesical arteries supply the intrapelvic segment of the ureter. In the male they also supply the prostate, seminal vesicles, and vas deferens, and in the female, the part of the vagina which lies in the pelvic cavity.

Parietal branches of the anterior division of the internal iliac artery are the obturator artery and inferior gluteal artery. The inferior gluteal artery, like the superior gluteal, crosses the greater sciatic foramen to enter the gluteal region where it supplies the gluteal muscles and contributes to the blood supply of the hip joint. Selective progressive occlusion of the internal iliac artery may result in a significant reduction of blood flow to the gluteal muscles and this in turn may manifest itself in the patient as intermittent gluteal claudication.

Pelvic veins

In the interior of the pelvic cavity the veins tend to be thin walled and plexiform around the pelvic viscera, forming the so-called peri-prostatic venous plexus (the equivalent structure in the female being the uterine plexus and vaginal plexus), the vesical plexus around the urinary bladder, and the rectal venous plexus in relation to the rectum. These plexuses are valveless and communicate fairly freely with each other. Posteriorly this venous plexus communicates through the anterior sacral foramina with the internal vertebral venous plexus. This anatomical pathway is thought to be the route taken by malignant cells from pelvic visceral neoplasms which metastasize to the vertebral column (e.g. prostatic malignancy).

From the venous plexuses lying adjacent to the pelvic viscera emerge small veins which become progressively larger as they are traced laterally. At this stage the veins run alongside the named branches of the internal iliac artery and are named correspondingly. These veins eventually drain into the ipsilateral internal iliac vein.

The rectum and the intrapelvic sigmoid, however, drain principally into the superior rectal vein which runs upwards and on crossing the pelvic brim becomes the inferior mesenteric vein. The latter eventually drains into the splenic vein and thereby into the portal vein. Within the wall of the rectum there are natural venous anastomoses between tributaries of the superior rectal vein and tributaries of the internal iliac vein. In other words, a natural portosystemic anastomosis exists within the wall of the rectum.

The right and left ovarian veins of course drain into the inferior vena cava and left renal vein respectively.

Pelvic lymphatics and lymph nodes

The lymph nodes in the pelvic cavity lie embedded in the extraperitoneal tissue of the pelvic cavity and may be classified into two broad groups: (1) internal iliac lymph nodes and (2) sacral (or presacral) lymph nodes.

The internal iliac nodes are associated with the internal iliac artery and its branches, while the sacral nodes (far less numerous than the internal iliac nodes) lie in the presacral space alongside the median sacral artery and accompanying veins. Much of the pelvic visceral lymph, notably from the urinary bladder, prostate, uterus including uterine cervix, vagina, seminal vesicles, intrapelvic ureters, and part of the rectum drains into the internal iliac nodes bilaterally. Some pelvic lymphatic vessels do cross the pelvic brim from below and drain into lymph nodes associated with the external iliac artery and common iliac artery, while most of the lymph from the rectum and all of the lymph from the intrapelvic sigmoid colon is drained by lymphatic vessels which run alongside the superior rectal artery and eventually empty into the inferior mesenteric lymph nodes situated in front of the abdominal aorta around the origin of the inferior mesenteric artery.

Ovarian lymph is carried in lymphatic vessels which run alongside the ovarian arteries and eventually empty into the para-aortic lymph nodes situated near the origins of the ovarian arteries.

Nerves within the pelvic cavity

Situated in the posterolateral part of the pelvic cavity on either side, and lying in front of the anterior sacral foramina and covered anteriorly by a layer of pelvic fascia is a prominent neural structure—the sacral plexus. Branches of the sacral plexus are distributed to the lower limb, gluteal region, intrapelvic structures, pelvic floor, and perineum. Also within the pelvic cavity are the ganglionated right and left sacral sympathetic trunks, and the inferior hypogastric plexuses. Several branches of the sacral plexus leave the pelvic cavity through the greater sciatic to supply the gluteal region, lower limb, and perineum.

Lumbosacral plexus and its branches

The lumbosacral plexus is formed by the union of the lumbosacral trunk (containing fibres from the ventral rami of the fourth and fifth lumbar spinal nerves) with the ventral rami of the sacral spinal nerves S1 to S4. The sacral ventral rami enter the pelvic cavity through the anterior sacral foramina. The lumbosacral (sacral) plexus thus formed gives rise to a number of branches. Among the more important branches are the superior and inferior gluteal nerves which supply the gluteal region; the sciatic nerve which is

the largest peripheral nerve in the body and which supplies all the muscles in the leg and foot and the hamstring muscles in the thigh; the pudendal nerve which supplies the perineum; the posterior cutaneous nerve of thigh, a large nerve with a fairly extensive territory of distribution; and the perineal branch of S4 which supplies the pelvic floor.

Autonomic nerves in the pelvic cavity

The autonomic nerves in the pelvic cavity comprise:

1. The right and left ganglionated sympathetic trunks which are continuations of the lumbar sympathetic trunks

2. The right and left superior hypogastric nerves which are plexiform branches of the superior hypogastric plexus (a sympathetic nerve plexus situated in front of the aortic bifurcation) that descend into the pelvic cavity

3. The right and left parasympathetic pelvic nerves (pelvic splanchnic nerves) whose fibres originate in the sacral segments of the spinal cord and travel initially in the ventral rami of the sacral nerves S2, S3, and S4 before leaving these nerves to enter the ipsilateral inferior hypogastric plexus

4. The right and left inferior hypogastric plexuses which are elongated nerve plexuses in the pelvic cavity made up of sympathetic fibres (derived from the superior hypogastric nerve) and parasympathetic fibres (derived from the pelvic splanchnic nerves). The inferior hypogastric plexuses are of great functional significance. The parasympathetic fibres in these plexuses innervate the detrusor muscle in the bladder wall, and also mediate penile erection. Significant injury to the inferior hypogastric plexuses, as may occur in the course of surgery for rectal or other pelvic cancers, often results in much postoperative morbidity in the form of bladder hypotonia and sexual dysfunction.

The perineum

The perineum refers to the lowest part of the trunk. It lies immediately below the pelvic floor (levator ani) and is bordered laterally by the inner aspect of the very proximal ends of the thighs and also by the inferior parts of the buttocks. The perineum is subdivided into two regions: (1) the anal region (or anal triangle) and (2) the urogenital region (or urogenital triangle) (Figure 1.1.3.3).

Boundaries of the perineum and subdivisions of the perineum

When the thighs and buttocks are parted, the perineum may be pictured as lying within the osseo-ligamentous framework of the inferior pelvic aperture. This framework has a diamond-shaped outline (Figure 1.1.3.4): the four angles of the *diamond* being the subpubic angle anteriorly, the coccyx posteriorly, and the right and left ischial tuberosities on either side. The four sides of the diamond are the right and left ischiopubic rami, anterolaterally, and the inferior edges of the right and left sacrotuberous ligaments, posterolaterally. A transverse line drawn between the anterior ends of the right and left ischial tuberosities is seen to divide the perineum into two triangular areas. The anterior triangular division is the smaller of the two and is known as the urogenital triangle (urogenital region) of the perineum, while the larger posterior division is the anal triangle (anal region) of the perineum. The anal triangle of the perineum is

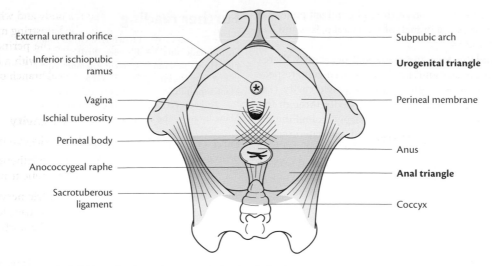

External urethral orifice

Inferior ischiopubic ramus

Vagina

Ischial tuberosity

Perineal body

Anococcygeal raphe

Sacrotuberous ligament

Subpubic arch

Urogenital triangle

Perineal membrane

Anus

Anal triangle

Coccyx

Fig. 1.1.3.3 Outline of perineum and subdivision of perineum into urogenital and anal triangles.

similar in design in the two sexes, and contains the centrally located anal canal flanked by the right and left ischioanal (ischiorectal) fossae. The urogenital triangle, in both sexes, contains the corresponding external genitalia and the distal urethra.

Anal triangle (region) of the perineum

Located in the centre of the anal triangle of the perineum is the anal canal with its integral sphincteric mechanism. On either side of the anal canal is a potentially large, fat-filled space called the ischioanal fossa (formerly known as ischiorectal fossa). Not infrequently, the ischioanal fossa is the site of abscess formation. The right and left ischioanal fossae may communicate with each other posterior to the anal canal. This explains the occasional phenomenon of a horse-shoe abscess (an ischioanal abscess on one side spreading to, and presenting on the other side).

The anal canal is the very terminal segment of the alimentary tract, and lies entirely below the level of the pelvic floor. In the adult it is about 4–5 cm in length; its anterior wall being somewhat shorter than the posterior wall. From its commencement in the levator hiatus as the direct continuation of the rectum, the anal canal passes downwards and backwards. The consequent bend at

the anorectal junction (acute angle directed posteriorly) is termed the perineal flexure, and is produced by the forward pull of the sling-like puborectalis muscle, which is of course derived from both levator ani muscles.

Urogenital triangle (region) of the perineum

Stretching across the width of the urogenital triangle of the perineum from the inner surface of one ischiopubic ramus to the other is a distinct fascial layer termed the perineal membrane. The perineal membrane is quadrangular in outline and is confined to the urogenital triangle of the perineum. It serves to demarcate the two principal subdivisions of the urogenital triangle: the deep perineal pouch and superficial perineal pouch. The former lies deep to (i.e. above) the perineal membrane and contains the membranous urethra, external urethral sphincter (the voluntary, striated muscle sphincter), and the deep transverse perineal muscles. Additionally, in the male, the bulbourethral glands (Cowper's glands) are situated in the deep perineal pouch, posterolateral to the membranous urethra.

The superficial perineal pouch lies superficial to (i.e. below) the perineal membrane. This demarcation into the superficial and deep perineal pouches is more apparent in the male than in the female (owing to the perineal membrane being a more readily demonstrable entity in the male). The external genitalia both in the male and in the female are situated entirely in the superficial perineal pouch. The male external genital organs comprise the penis and spongiose urethra, muscles associated with the root of the penis, scrotum, and scrotal contents. The female external genital organs (collectively known as the vulva) comprise the mons pubis, labia majora and minora, clitoris, vaginal vestibule, and associated structures.

The blood supply and innervation of the perineum

The blood supply to the perineum is derived from the right and left internal pudendal arteries, each being a terminal branch of the corresponding internal iliac artery's anterior division. Venous drainage is to the ipsilateral internal pudendal vein which in turn drains to the internal iliac vein. The motor innervation of all the *voluntary* muscles in the perineum as well as the cutaneous innervation of

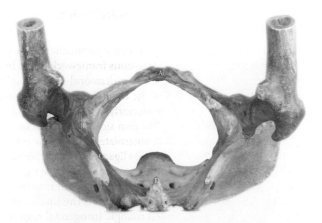

Fig. 1.1.3.4 Articulated pelvis seen from below to show diamond-shaped outline of perineum.

much of the perineum is a function of the right and left pudendal nerves. The pudendal nerve is a branch of the sacral plexus and has a root value of S2, S3, and S4.

The internal pudendal artery and pudendal nerve may therefore be spoken of as the artery and nerve of the perineum, respectively. Both these structures originate in the pelvic cavity (i.e. above the pelvic floor). They leave the pelvic cavity through the ipsilateral greater sciatic foramen. Turning sharply around the tip of the ischial spine, the nerve and artery (and companion vein) run forwards *below* the pelvic floor to enter a fascial sleeve (the pudendal canal) within the obturator fascia in the lateral wall of the perineum.

Further reading

Drake RL, Vogl AW, Mitchell AW. *Gray's Anatomy for Students* (2nd ed). Philadelphia, PA: Elsevier; 2010.

Ellis H, Mahadevan V. *Clinical Anatomy: Applied Anatomy for Students and Junior Doctors.* (13th ed). Oxford: Wiley-Blackwell; 2013.

MacKinnon PCB, Morris JF. *Oxford Textbook of Functional Anatomy* (Vol 2, 2nd ed). Oxford: Oxford University Press; 2005.

Mahadevan V. The anatomy of the rectum and anal canal. *Surgery* 2011; 29(1):5–10.

Sadler TW. *Langman's Medical Embryology* (13th ed). Philadelphia, PA: Wolters Kluwer/Lippincott Williams & Wilkins; 2014.

Sinnatamby C. *Last's Anatomy: Regional and Applied* (12th ed). Edinburgh: Elsevier; 2011.

CHAPTER 1.1.4

Anatomy of the limbs and spine

Vishy Mahadevan

Muscle compartments in the upper and lower limbs

In each of the limbs, the skeletal muscles are collectively ensleeved in a circumferential layer of deep fascia. From the inner surface of this stocking-like deep fascial envelope, fibrous septa project inwards and attach to the bone(s) lying within a given segment of the limb, thereby separating the muscles of that segment of the limb into functional groups. Thus, the muscles within each segment of the upper and lower limbs may be pictured as being located in discrete, osseofascial compartments (Figure 1.1.4.1). As a general rule, it may be stated that each compartment possesses a nerve which supplies all the muscles of the compartment. In addition, each compartment generally carries a principal vessel which supplies the contents of the compartment.

Muscle compartments in the upper limb

The upper limb comprises three segments: arm, forearm, and hand.

Arm

The arm contains two compartments, anterior and posterior, which are separated from each other by the humerus and the medial and lateral intermuscular septa:

- The anterior (flexor) compartment of the arm contains biceps brachii, brachialis, and coracobrachialis; all innervated by the musculocutaneous nerve
- The posterior (extensor) compartment contains the three-headed triceps brachii which is innervated by the radial nerve.

Forearm

The forearm contains two compartments: the anterior (flexor) compartment and the posterior (extensor) compartment, which are separated from each other by the radius, ulna, and interosseous membrane and the medial and lateral intermuscular septa.

The muscles of the anterior compartment of the forearm are arranged in two groups:

- A superficial group comprising pronator teres, flexor carpi radialis, palmaris longus, flexor digitorum superficialis, and flexor carpi ulnaris
- A deep group comprising flexor pollicis longus, flexor digitorum profundus, and pronator quadratus.

In the superficial group, all but flexor carpi ulnaris are innervated by the median nerve. Flexor carpi ulnaris is innervated by the ulnar nerve. In the deep group, the median nerve innervates flexor pollicis longus, pronator quadratus, and the radial half of flexor digitorum profundus.

The medial half of flexor digitorum profundus is innervated by the ulnar nerve.

The muscles of the posterior compartment of forearm (comprising the radial and ulnar extensors of the wrist, the long and short extensors of the thumb, the long abductor of the thumb, the extensors of the digits, and supinator) are innervated by the radial nerve (chiefly through the posterior interosseous nerve).

Hand

The hand contains two regions: a volar (or flexor) region and a dorsal (or extensor) region.

The all-important intrinsic muscles of the hand are located exclusively in the volar region and are arranged in layers, with *most* of the muscles being innervated by the ulnar nerve.

The extensor region of the hand is occupied by the tendons of the so-called *long extensor muscles*.

Muscle compartments in the lower limb

The lower limb comprises three segments: thigh, leg, and foot. Compartments in the segments of the lower limb are as follows:

Thigh

The thigh contains two distinct and physically separate compartments, anterior and posterior, which are separated from each other by the femur and the medial and lateral intermuscular septa:

- The anterior (extensor) compartment comprising quadriceps femoris and sartorius. The nerve of this compartment is the femoral nerve
- The posterior compartment contains two groups of muscles that are functionally distinct—the hamstrings, which are innervated by the sciatic nerve, and the adductors, which are innervated by the obturator nerve.

Leg

In the leg there is a very definite fascial separation into anterior (extensor), posterior (flexor), and lateral (evertor) compartments. Furthermore, the posterior compartment is divided by a distinct fascial layer into superficial and deep subdivisions. Thus, the leg contains four defined compartments.

- The anterior compartment contains tibialis anterior, extensor digitorum longus, extensor hallucis longus, and peroneus tertius, all of which are innervated by the deep peroneal nerve and supplied by the anterior tibial artery

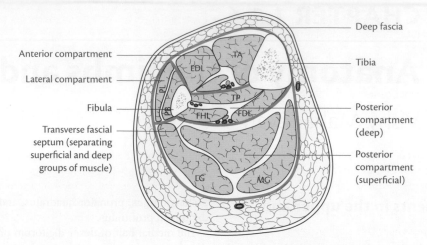

Fig. 1.1.4.1 Cross-section of muscle compartments of the right leg.
Reproduced with permission from Ellis H. and Mahadevan V., *Clinical Anatomy*, Thirteenth Edition, Wiley-Blackwell, Oxford, UK, Copyright © 2013.

- The lateral compartment contains the peroneus longus and brevis muscles, which are innervated by the superficial peroneal nerve

- The superficial group of posterior compartment muscles comprises gastrocnemius, soleus, and plantaris

- The deep group is made up of flexor digitorum longus, flexor hallucis longus, tibialis posterior, and popliteus. All the muscles of the posterior compartment (superficial and deep groups) are innervated by the tibial nerve. (In the view of some authorities, the posterior compartment of the leg has three, rather than two, subdivisions. According to this view, tibialis posterior occupies a compartment of its own.)

Foot

The foot has two regions: a plantar (or flexor) region and a dorsal (or extensor) region. As in the hand, the intrinsic muscles are arranged in layers in the plantar region of the foot, and these plantar intrinsic muscles are innervated by the lateral and medial plantar nerves which are terminal branches of the tibial nerve. The dorsal region of the foot is, generally speaking, similar to the corresponding region in the hand in that it contains the tendons of the extensor muscles. However, it differs from the corresponding region of the hand in that it contains an intrinsic muscle, the extensor digitorum brevis. This muscle, being an occupant of the dorsal region of the foot, is innervated by the deep peroneal nerve.

Compartment syndrome

The fascial boundaries that limit the osseofascial compartments are inelastic sheets. Any condition that leads to an increase in the volume of the compartmental contents is therefore likely to result in a rise in intracompartmental pressure. Such conditions include haemorrhage following closed fractures, muscle swelling caused by trauma or unaccustomed overuse, and local infection. If unrelieved, the increased pressure leads to compression of the vessels in the compartment and secondary ischaemic damage to the nerves and muscles of the compartment. This phenomenon is known as *compartment syndrome*, and involves, most commonly, the compartments of the leg (especially, the anterior compartment of leg).

Compartment syndrome is a surgical emergency and is treated by performing a fasciotomy, a procedure in which a generous incision is made in the deep fascia overlying the compartment in order to decompress the compartment.

Junctional zones in the upper and lower limbs

The axilla, cubital fossa, and carpal tunnel

The axilla (or armpit as it is known colloquially) is a zone of transition between the neck and the upper limb. It is a space which is in the shape of an irregular and somewhat tilted pyramid, and is located between the medial aspect of the upper part of the arm and the lateral aspect of the upper part of the chest.

The apex of the axilla (the upper limit of the axilla) is, in fact, the gap between the middle third of the clavicle and the outer edge of the first rib. This gap, known as the cervicoaxillary opening, transmits the subclavian artery and brachial plexus from the neck into the axilla, and the axillary vein from the axilla into the neck. The cervicoaxillary opening is also traversed by numerous lymphatic channels.

The important contents of the axilla are the axillary artery and its branches, the axillary vein and its tributaries, the cords of the brachial plexus and their branches, and axillary lymph nodes all embedded in the axillary fat, which is usually quite substantial. The axillary lymph nodes are particularly important in the context of cancer of the breast.

The cubital fossa is a zone of transition between the arm and forearm. Situated in front of the elbow joint, the cubital fossa may be described as a triangular intermuscular space between the brachioradialis muscle laterally and the pronator teres medially. The arbitrary proximal limit of the fossa is an imaginary line between the lateral and medial epicondyles of the humerus.

The fossa transmits the median nerve, the brachial artery (flanked by its venae comitantes), and the tendon of biceps brachii. If the brachioradialis muscle is undermined and retracted radially, the radial nerve can be brought into view. Of these contents of the cubital fossa, the brachial artery and the tendon of biceps brachii are readily palpable.

In the distal part of the cubital fossa, the brachial artery divides into its two terminal branches—the radial and ulnar arteries (the latter usually being the larger one).

The contents of the cubital fossa (particularly the brachial artery and median nerve) are vulnerable in supracondylar fractures of the humerus.

The carpal tunnel is an osseofibrous space, bounded dorsally by the concave palmar surface of the articulated carpus. The ventral boundary (i.e. *roof*) of the carpal tunnel is the flexor retinaculum (also known as the transverse carpal ligament), a quadrangular sheet of dense fibrous tissue that attaches by its four corners to four different carpal bones.

The carpal tunnel is traversed longitudinally by the tendons of flexor digitorum superficialis and flexor digitorum profundus, the tendon of flexor pollicis longus. Running within the carpal tunnel, adhering to the deep surface of the flexor retinaculum, is the median nerve. *Carpal tunnel syndrome* denotes a sustained, pathological, symptomatic compression of the median nerve in the carpal tunnel. It is an example (in fact, the commonest example) of a group of conditions termed *entrapment neuropathies*.

The femoral triangle, gluteal region, popliteal fossa, and tarsal tunnel

The femoral triangle is an intermuscular space situated in the anteromedial aspect of the proximal thigh within a triangular outline marked by the sartorius laterally, adductor longus medially, and the inguinal ligament proximally. The latter forms the base of the triangle. The gutter-shaped floor of the femoral triangle, made up of various muscles, lies immediately in front of the capsule of the hip joint. Distally the femoral triangle is continuous with the adductor canal, a narrow intermuscular cleft in the medial aspect of the thigh.

The contents of the triangle are the femoral nerve and its branches, and medial to the femoral nerve, the femoral sheath containing the femoral artery, femoral vein, and femoral canal in that order from lateral to medial. Distally the femoral artery and vein leave the femoral triangle to enter the adductor canal.

The gluteal region lies behind the hip joint and is an important junctional area between the pelvic cavity and the posterior compartment (hamstring compartment) of the thigh. Besides the three gluteal muscles (gluteus maximus, medius, and minimus) the gluteal region also includes several smaller muscles known collectively as the short lateral rotators of the hip joint. A large opening, the greater sciatic foramen, in the posterolateral part of the pelvic wall transmits numerous important neurovascular structures (including the sciatic nerve) from the pelvic cavity to the gluteal region.

The popliteal fossa is a diamond-shaped intermuscular space which spans the posterior aspect of the knee joint, lying successively in the distal part of the hamstring compartment, behind the knee joint and in the proximal part of the posterior compartment of leg.

Through the adductor hiatus, a natural opening in the tendon of adductor magnus, the popliteal fossa communicates proximally with the adductor canal. Indeed it is through this opening that the femoral artery and vein cross over from the adductor canal to the popliteal fossa.

The popliteal fossa contains the popliteal artery and vein which are, respectively, the distal continuations of the femoral artery and vein. The popliteal fossa also contains the terminal branches of the sciatic nerve: the tibial and common peroneal nerves.

The tarsal tunnel is a transitional zone between the posterior compartment of the leg and the sole of the foot. It is situated posteromedial to the medial malleolus and is roofed by the flexor retinaculum of the foot. It is traversed by the posterior tibial artery and its companion veins, the tibial nerve, and the tendons of the muscles of the deep posterior compartment of the leg (namely tibialis posterior, flexor digitorum longus, and flexor hallucis longus).

Vascular arrangement in the upper and lower limbs

The vascular (arterial and venous) arrangements in the upper and lower limbs show many similarities.

Both in the upper and lower limb, a major axial artery enters the proximal segment of the limb (arm/thigh) and supplies the muscle compartments and bone(s) within that segment. On entering the next segment of the limb (forearm/leg) the artery bifurcates into two terminal branches. These terminal branches supply the remainder of the limb through their many branches and in the distal part of the limb form anastomoses with each other. The veins of the upper and lower limbs may be classified into two groups: superficial veins which are superficial to the deep fascia and deep veins which lie deep to the deep fascia of the limb. Communicating veins connect the two systems at various points. Both in the upper and lower limbs, the deep and superficial veins, as well as the communicating veins, contain multiple valves which ensure (a) that blood flows in a proximal direction and (b) that blood flows from the superficial system to the deep veins.

Arterial and venous arrangement in the upper limb

The principal artery in the upper limb is the *axillary artery*, the direct continuation of the subclavian artery beyond the outer border of the first rib. Having traversed the length of the axilla, the axillary artery enters the anterior compartment of the arm as the brachial artery. The latter runs down the medial aspect of the anterior compartment of arm and so enters the cubital fossa. In the distal part of the cubital fossa, the brachial artery divides into its two terminal branches: the radial and ulnar arteries. The latter is usually the larger of the two. The radial and ulnar arteries course distally within the flexor compartment of the forearm, on the radial and ulnar sides respectively. They form a number of anastomoses with each other in the distal part of the limb, two of which are especially significant: the superficial and deep palmar arterial arches.

The veins of the upper limb may be classified into those that are deep to the deep fascia (deep veins) and those that are superficial to the deep fascia (superficial veins). The deep veins of the upper limb are the *venae comitantes* (companion veins) of the major arteries—radial, ulnar, brachial, and axillary. The principal superficial veins in the upper limb are the cephalic and basilic veins which run on the lateral and medial aspects of the limb, respectively. The former eventually drains into the axillary vein while the latter joins the brachial vein. A variable arrangement of superficial veins overlies the cubital fossa. It is these veins that are most commonly used for venepuncture. Both in the upper and lower limbs, the superficial and deep veins contain valves which ensure unidirectional, centripetal blood flow.

Arterial and venous arrangement in the lower limb

The principal artery of the lower limb is the *femoral artery*, the direct continuation of the external iliac artery beyond the inguinal ligament. It traverses successively, the femoral triangle and adductor canal before entering the popliteal fossa through the adductor hiatus. On crossing the adductor hiatus the artery changes its name to the popliteal artery. Throughout its course, the femoral artery is accompanied by its vein, which lies first on the medial side of the artery and then passes posterior to it within the adductor canal.

A major branch of the femoral artery in the femoral triangle is the *profunda femoris artery*. It is the principal vessel supplying the compartments of the thigh. In view of the great functional importance of the profunda femoris, it is the convention among vascular surgeons to refer to the femoral artery proximal to the origin of the profunda femoris as the common femoral artery and distal to the profunda's origin as the superficial femoral artery.

The popliteal artery commences at the adductor hiatus, runs down the popliteal fossa, and distal to the line of the knee joint in the distal part of the popliteal fossa it divides into its two terminal branches, the anterior and posterior tibial arteries.

The posterior tibial artery is the larger of the two terminal branches of the popliteal artery. Initially in the depths of the posterior compartment of the leg, it becomes relatively superficial in the distal third of the leg and passes behind the medial malleolus with its companion vein and the tibial nerve. At, or just distal to, the level of the medial malleolus, the posterior tibial artery divides into the *medial* and *lateral plantar arteries* which are the principal blood vessels in the sole of the foot.

The anterior tibial artery arises at the bifurcation of the popliteal artery and passes forwards between the tibia and fibula through the interosseous membrane to enter the anterior compartment of the leg. The artery continues over the dorsum of the foot as the *dorsalis pedis artery*. The dorsalis pedis artery plunges between the first and second metatarsals to join the lateral plantar artery in the sole of the foot to form the *plantar arch*, from which branches run forwards to supply the plantar aspects of the toes.

The veins of the lower limb are divided into the deep and superficial groups based on the relationship of the veins to the deep fascia of the limb. The deep veins run within the deep fascial envelope and accompany the corresponding major arteries. The superficial veins are the great and small (or long and short) saphenous veins and their tributaries.

The *small (short)* and *great (long) saphenous veins* commence on the dorsum of the foot as proximal continuations of the lateral and medial limbs, respectively, of the venous arch on the dorsum of the foot. The small saphenous vein runs upwards behind the lateral malleolus of the ankle and eventually perforates the deep fascia over the popliteal fossa to drain into the popliteal vein. The great saphenous vein passes upwards immediately in front of the medial malleolus and then along the medial aspect, successively, of the leg, knee, and thigh to reach the groin where it pierces the deep fascia to join the femoral vein. Except at its termination, the great saphenous vein is superficial to the deep fascia. Venous varicosities most commonly involve the great and short saphenous venous systems, and may be the result either of hereditary weakness of the venous valves or valve impairment secondary to venous thrombophlebitis.

Innervation of the upper and lower limbs

The innervation (sensory and motor) of the limbs is derived from specific networks of nerves termed plexuses. The plexuses are formed from the anterior rami of appropriate spinal nerves. Three plexuses are involved in the innervation of the limbs: the brachial plexus innervates the upper limb while the lumbar plexus and lumbosacral plexus innervate the lower limb.

Brachial plexus

The brachial plexus is formed by the anterior rami of spinal nerves C5 to C8, and T1. These five ventral rami are referred to as the roots of the brachial plexus. The plexus spans the lower half of the neck of its side deep to the prevertebral layer of deep cervical fascia. Emerging through the narrow interval between scalenus anterior and scalenus medius, it crosses above the first rib to enter the axilla where the plexus ends by giving rise to five major nerves—median, musculocutaneous, ulnar, axillary, and radial (Figure 1.1.4.2).

The lumbar plexus and lumbosacral plexus

The lumbar plexus is formed within the psoas major (a large and powerful muscle on the posterior abdominal wall) by the union of the ventral rami of the lumbar spinal nerves L1 to L4 inclusive. The two major branches of the lumbar plexus are the femoral nerve and obturator nerve. The former provides the motor innervation for quadriceps femoris while the latter is the motor nerve of the adductor group of muscles. Branches of the femoral nerve and other branches of the lumbar plexus provide cutaneous innervation to the anterior, anteromedial, and anterolateral aspects of the thigh and the medial aspect of the leg.

The lumbosacral plexus is situated within the pelvic cavity and is formed by the union of the lumbosacral trunk with the anterior rami of the spinal nerves S1 to S4. The lumbosacral trunk is formed just below the transverse process of L5 vertebra by the union of the anterior rami of spinal nerves L4 and L5. The trunk crosses the pelvic brim to run in front of the lateral mass of the sacrum where it is joined by the anterior rami of sacral spinal nerves S1–S4. The sciatic nerve, a branch of the lumbosacral plexus, is the largest peripheral nerve in the body. It is distributed to the hamstring compartment of the thigh, and is the motor nerve supply to *all* the muscles in the leg and foot. It also provides cutaneous innervation to the sole of the foot and shares in the cutaneous innervation of the leg.

The bones and joints of the upper and lower limbs

Definition of synovial joint

A synovial joint is an articulation between two or more bones contained within a fibrous capsule with the inner surface of the capsule being lined by synovial membrane. The function of the synovial membrane is to elaborate synovial fluid which acts as an efficient lubricant. The articular surfaces of the bones within a typical synovial joint are covered by articular hyaline cartilage. Of all joints in the body, synovial joints allow the greatest range of movement.

Functional classification of synovial joints in the upper and lower limbs

From a functional or biomechanical point of view, synovial joints may be classified into six types, all of which are represented in the limbs. The six types are *ball and socket* (e.g. hip joint and glenohumeral joint), *hinge* (e.g. ankle joint, elbow joint, and

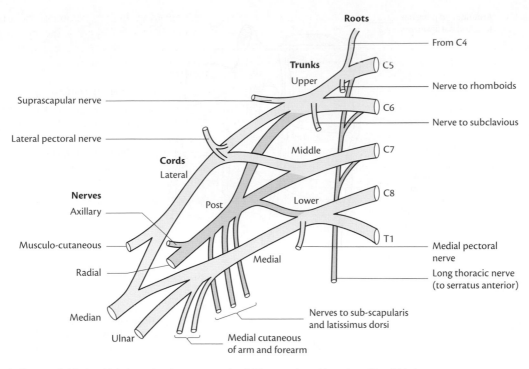

Fig. 1.1.4.2 Schematic diagram of right brachial plexus showing roots, trunks, divisions, cords, and branches of brachial plexus

interphalangeal joints), *pivot* (e.g. superior and inferior radio ulnar joints), *saddle* (e.g. trapeziometacarpal joint in the hand), *condyloid* (e.g. wrist joint), and *plane or gliding* (e.g. calcaneocuboid joint)

Vertebral column

General description of the articulated vertebral column

The adult vertebral column which makes up about two-fifths of the total height of the body, is formed of a vertical sequence of bony elements termed vertebrae. From above downwards these comprise seven cervical vertebrae, twelve thoracic vertebrae, five lumbar vertebrae, the sacrum, and coccyx. The cervical, thoracic, and lumbar vertebrae are termed moveable vertebrae, on account of the fact that the individual vertebrae can move relative to their neighbours. The sacrum and coccyx, by contrast, are each formed by the fusion of vertebrae (five vertebrae fuse to form the sacrum while four fuse to form the coccyx).

Morphology of a typical vertebra

With the exception of the first two cervical vertebrae (atlas and axis respectively), all the moveable vertebrae whether from the cervical, thoracic, or lumbar region share a more-or-less common morphological pattern.

Thus each typical moveable vertebra features a cylindroid *vertebral body* anteriorly. Attached to the back of the body is a bony arch termed the vertebral arch. Between the two is the vertebral foramen. In the articulated vertebral column, all the vertebral foramina 'stacked' one on top of another constitute, collectively, the vertebral canal (spinal canal). Occupying the upper two-thirds of the length of the vertebral canal is the spinal cord.

The most anterior part of the vertebral arch on each side whereby the arch attaches to the back of the body, is termed the *pedicle*. The pedicle bears a notch above and below each of which, with its neighbour, forms an *intervertebral foramen*. The arch bears, on the posterior midline, a spinous process. In addition, the arch possesses, on each side, a laterally directed *transverse process* and upper and lower *articular facets*.

The intervertebral foramina transmit the segmental spinal nerves as follows: nerves C1 to C7 pass over the superior aspect of the pedicles of their numerically corresponding cervical vertebrae, C8 passes through the foramen between the seventh cervical and first thoracic vertebrae, and thereafter each spinal nerve passes inferior to the pedicle of its numerically corresponding vertebra.

On each side of the midline, the part of the vertebral arch medial to the articular processes is termed the lamina. The right and left laminae meet in the posterior midline at the root of the spinous process.

Definition of a spinal motion segment

A spinal motion segment may be defined as any *two successive moveable vertebrae* including the structures and articulations that unite them (Figure 1.1.4.3). Thus, for example, C7 and T1 together constitute a motion segment, as do T9 and T10 and so on.

The principal factor uniting adjacent vertebral bodies is the intervertebral disc: this strong union being reinforced by the anterior and posterior longitudinal ligaments. Uniting adjacent vertebral arches are various strong ligaments (supraspinous and interspinous ligaments and ligamenta flava) and the facet joints on either side between corresponding articular processes.

The spinal motion segment is the functional (biomechanical) unit of the spine.

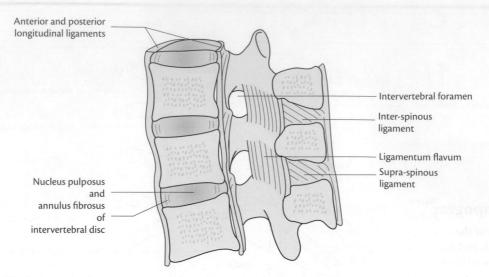

Fig. 1.1.4.3 Sagittal section of lumbar vertebral column showing a spinal motion segment.

Further reading

Drake RL, Vogl AW, Mitchell AW. *Gray's Anatomy for Students* (2nd ed). Philadelphia, PA: Elsevier; 2010.

Ellis H, Mahadevan V. *Clinical Anatomy: Applied Anatomy for Students and Junior Doctors.* (13th ed). Oxford: Wiley-Blackwell; 2013.

MacKinnon PCB, Morris JF. *Oxford Textbook of Functional Anatomy* (Vol 1, 2nd ed). Oxford: Oxford University Press; 2005.

Sadler TW. *Langman's Medical Embryology* (13th ed). Philadelphia, PA: Wolters Kluwer/Lippincott Williams & Wilkins; 2014.

Sinnatamby C. *Last's Anatomy: Regional and Applied* (12th ed). Edinburgh: Elsevier; 2011.

CHAPTER 1.1.5

Head and neck anatomy

Vishy Mahadevan

The general topography of the neck

A sound knowledge of the disposition of the muscles and muscular planes in the neck and a clear understanding of the manner in which the various fascial layers of the neck are arranged are of paramount importance in the surgery of the neck. Equally important is an awareness of the relationship of these muscular planes and fascial layers to the cervical viscera and major vessels and nerves in the neck. An appreciation of such anatomical detail is an essential requisite to safety and precision in all neck operations.

Arrangement of muscles in the neck

It may be stated almost axiomatically, that all the voluntary muscles in the neck are bilaterally represented and symmetrically arranged.

The muscles in the anterior region of the neck may be classified into the following groups:

- *Superficial group* (comprising the right and left platysma muscles).

- *Anterolateral group* (comprising the sternocleidomastoid and trapezius muscles bilaterally).

- *Anterior group* (comprising two subgroups):

  - A *suprahyoid subgroup* made up of mylohyoid, anterior, and posterior bellies of digastric and stylohyoid. Above the level of the hyoid are the suprahyoid anterior cervical muscles. These include the right and left mylohyoid muscles which interdigitate in the anterior midline at the *mylohyoid raphe* which extends from the inner aspect of the symphysis menti to the body of the hyoid. Together the two mylohyoid muscles form a mobile muscular sheet extending between the inner aspects of the right and left halves of the mandible. This mylohyoid 'sheet' is an important surgical landmark as it demarcates the neck below from the oral region above. Lying superficial to the mylohyoid (i.e. on the neck side of mylohyoid) are the stylohyoid and digastric muscles (the latter muscle comprising anterior and posterior bellies).

  - An *infrahyoid subgroup* comprising the strap muscles (i.e. sternohyoid, omohyoid, sternothyroid, and thyrohyoid). Lying immediately deep to the investing layer of deep cervical fascia and running longitudinally on either side of the anterior midline of the neck are the infrahyoid anterior cervical muscles, also known as the strap muscles. On each side of the vertical midline, the strap muscles are disposed in two layers. The superficial layer consists of the sternohyoid and omohyoid muscles lying side by side (sternohyoid medial to omohyoid), and the deep layer consists of the sternothyroid muscle, which

extends vertically from the posterior surface of the manubrium sterni to the oblique line of the thyroid cartilage. Extending upwards from the oblique line of the thyroid cartilage to the greater horn of the hyoid is the thyrohyoid muscle, generally regarded as the upward continuation of the sternothyroid muscle.

- *Prevertebral group* (made up of two subgroups):

  - *Anterior prevertebral subgroup of muscles* exemplified by longus colli, longus capitis, and a couple of other small muscles, all running more or less longitudinally, anterior to the cervical vertebral bodies.

  - *Lateral prevertebral subgroup of muscles* comprising scalenus anterior, medius and posterior, and levator scapulae. All members of this subgroup arise from the transverse processes of cervical vertebrae and run inferolaterally to attach to the upper part of the rib cage or upper border of scapula.

All the muscles in the anterior region of the neck are innervated directly or indirectly by anterior rami of cervical spinal nerves (with the exception of platysma which is, of course, innervated by a branch of the facial nerve).

Arrangement of fascial layers in the neck

The skin of the neck is thinner and generally more mobile over the anterior part of the neck than over the posterior part. Immediately deep to the skin of the neck is the superficial fascia which is essentially a layer of subcutaneous fat arranged circumferentially around the neck. Lying immediately deep to the subcutaneous fat, on either side of the anterior midline is the platysma, a relatively thin but wide sheet of muscle. The platysma is confined to the anterior and anterolateral parts of the neck and is not present at the back of the neck. Superiorly, platysma is loosely adherent to the lower border of the mandible before it crosses over to the face. Inferiorly, platysma crosses superficial to the clavicle and blends with the fascia overlying pectoralis major, just below the level of the clavicle. Above the level of the hyoid, the medial borders of the right and left platysma muscles lie edge to edge, whereas below the hyoid level, they are separated from each other by a narrow interval. Subjacent to the platysma is the *investing layer of deep cervical fascia* which invests the neck like a collar. It is the most superficial of the various layers of the deep cervical fascia: the other layers being the prevertebral fascia, the carotid sheaths, and the pretracheal fascia (Figure 1.1.5.1).

Superiorly, the investing layer of deep cervical fascia is attached to the entire length of the lower border of the mandible, from midline to angle on either side. Traced posteriorly from the angle of

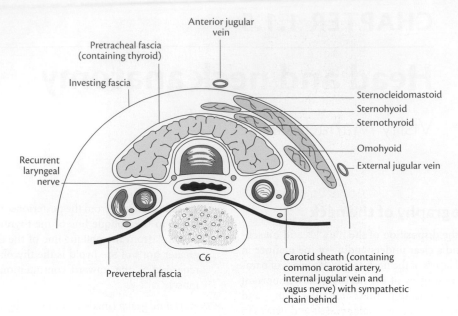

Fig. 1.1.5.1 Cross-section of neck at C6 level showing fascial planes and viscera.
Reproduced with permission from Ellis H. and Mahadevan V., *Clinical Anatomy*, Thirteenth Edition, Wiley-Blackwell, Oxford, UK, Copyright © 2013.

the mandible, it is seen to be attached to the mastoid processes and superior nuchal lines on either side and to the external occipital protuberance in the posterior midline. In the interval between the angle of the mandible and the mastoid process (a distance of nearly 5–6 cm), the investing layer of deep cervical fascia splits to enclose the parotid salivary gland as the parotid fascia or parotid capsule.

Inferiorly, the line of attachment of the investing layer of deep cervical fascia is to the sternal notch (i.e. the notched, thick upper border of the manubrium sterni) anteriorly, and in continuity, on each side, to the upper surface of the clavicle, the acromion, the spine of the scapula, and thus to the posterior midline. Traced laterally from the anterior midline, between its upper and lower attachments, the investing layer of deep cervical fascia splits to enclose, on each side, the sternocleidomastoid initially and then the trapezius muscle. In the interval between the two muscles it forms the roof of the posterior triangle of the neck. The deepest layer of the deep cervical fascia is the prevertebral fascia, a relatively dense layer which runs across from one side to the other in front of the prevertebral musculature and cervical vertebral column. Lying *in front* of the prevertebral fascia along the length of the neck are the right and left carotid sheaths flanking the centrally located visceral column of the neck.

Thus all the cervical viscera, major blood vessels and nerves of the neck, and all the cervical muscles (with the sole exception of the platysma) come to lie within the sweep of the investing layer of deep cervical fascia.

Intermuscular triangles of the neck

For descriptive purposes, the anterior region of the neck is subdivided into the following intermuscular triangular areas:

- Anterior triangle of neck (Figure 1.1.5.2) which is the area between the medial borders of the right and left sternocleidomastoid muscles. The anterior triangle of the neck is limited above by the lower border of the mandible, and inferiorly by the sternal notch.

- Posterior triangle (one on each side of the neck) is bounded anteriorly by the lateral border of sternocleidomastoid muscle, and posteriorly by the anterior border of the trapezius. The base of the posterior triangle is the upper surface of the middle third of the clavicle. The floor of the posterior triangle is the prevertebral fascia overlying the scalene muscles, while the roof is the investing layer of deep cervical fascia stretching from sternocleidomastoid to trapezius.

- Within the upper part of the anterior triangle there lies on each side the corresponding submandibular triangle bounded by the digastric muscle and lower border of mandible. The two bellies of digastric and the lower border of the mandible together form an inverted triangular outline known as the digastric triangle or submandibular triangle. The floor (or deep limit) of this triangular area is the mylohyoid muscle and the roof (or superficial limit) is the investing layer of deep cervical fascia on its way to its attachment along the lower border of the mandible. Situated within the submandibular triangle are the submandibular salivary gland and lymph nodes.

Surface anatomy of clinical and surgical relevance

A number of superficial, palpable landmarks provide useful topographical clues to the precise location of deep structures that are not usually palpable or visualized. Additionally, these landmarks bear a fairly constant relationship to specific vertebral levels, and thus aid the surgeon in siting skin incisions at an appropriate level, when operating on the cervical spine. It is instructive to consider these landmarks in order.

Assuming the subject to be in the anatomical position, with the neck straight, the important landmarks and their corresponding vertebral levels are as follows:

- The *thyroid notch* is readily palpable and often visible. It lies in the midline at the level of the upper border of C4 vertebra (or disc between C3 and C4). The superior borders of the thyroid laminae can be felt on other side of the thyroid notch.

brachiocephalic vein runs obliquely downwards and to the right through the superior mediastinum to meet the much shorter right brachiocephalic vein to form the superior vena cava. Each internal jugular vein receives tributaries corresponding to several of the branches of the ipsilateral external carotid artery. Thus it receives the facial, lingual, superior thyroid, and pharyngeal veins, among others.

The subclavian artery

The right and left subclavian arteries differ from each other in the same way as the two carotid arteries (right and left) do. Thus the left subclavian artery arises directly from the aortic arch behind the origin of the left common carotid, while the right subclavian artery is a terminal branch of the brachiocephalic trunk and commences behind the right sternoclavicular joint. Running laterally in the root of the neck, each subclavian artery crosses above the ipsilateral first rib to become the axillary artery. In the root of the neck each subclavian artery gives off branches, of which the most important is undoubtedly the vertebral artery. Other important branches are the inferior thyroid and internal thoracic arteries.

The vertebral arteries

The vertebral artery is the first (and most important) branch of the subclavian artery. It crosses the dome of the pleura, traverses the transverse foramina of the upper six cervical vertebrae, then turns posteriorly and medially over the posterior arch of the atlas to enter the cranial cavity through the foramen magnum. Here the artery enters the subarachnoid space, and runs in an anteromedial and somewhat superior direction around the medulla oblongata to join its fellow in front of the pons to form the *basilar artery*. The basilar artery runs superiorly in front of the pons and bifurcates just above the level of the pons into the right and left posterior cerebral arteries. The vertebrobasilar system thus formed, supplies all of the brain in the posterior cranial fossa (i.e. brainstem and the entire cerebellum) in addition to a good deal of supratentorial brain. The confluence of the two vertebral arteries forming the basilar artery is the anatomical basis to the *subclavian arterial steal phenomenon*. The two posterior cerebral arteries form the posterior limbs of the circle of Willis.

Cervical lymph nodes

The cervical lymph nodes are of great clinical importance in the context of neoplastic and inflammatory disease involving viscera in the head and neck. The lymph nodes in the neck may be broadly categorized into two sets:

1. Superficial cervical lymph nodes (i.e. those that are superficial to the investing layer of deep cervical fascia)
2. Deep cervical lymph nodes (i.e. those that are deep to the investing layer of deep cervical fascia).

Each of these two categories is further subdivided into groups on the basis of location and territory of drainage.

Scalp and facial skeleton (including oral, nasal, and orbital cavities)

Scalp

The term scalp refers to the layered arrangement of soft tissues which cover the cranial vault. The scalp is made up of five layers. From the surface inwards, these are skin, connective tissue, occipitofrontalis including its aponeurosis, loose areolar tissue, and periosteum.

Each of these layers has features of practical importance.

The *skin* of the scalp possesses the highest concentration of sebaceous glands, and not surprisingly is a very common site for the occurrence of sebaceous cysts. The *subcutaneous connective tissue* consists of loculated fat bound in tough fibrous septa. The blood vessels of the scalp lie in this layer. When the scalp is lacerated, the divided vessels retract between the fibrous septa and cannot be picked up individually by artery forceps in the usual way. The bleeding is stemmed by pressing with the fingers firmly down on to the skull on either side of the wound (thus compressing the vessels), by placing series of artery forceps on the divided aponeurotic layer so that their weight again compresses these vessels and, finally, by suturing the laceration firmly in two layers (aponeurotic and cutaneous).

Facial skeleton (including oral, nasal, and orbital cavities)

The facial skeleton may be regarded as being made up of three horizontally orientated, parallel zones: a lower zone, an upper zone, and a middle zone (Figure 1.1.5.4).

- The lower zone is represented by the mandible
- The upper zone corresponds to the forehead and is made up of the squamous parts of the right and left frontal bones
- The middle zone is the most complex in terms of design and architecture. It may be said to extend from the level of the supraorbital margins above, to the level of the maxillary teeth below. It includes the nasal cavities, the orbital cavities, the maxillary and ethmoidal paranasal sinuses, and the roof of the mouth.

The mandible articulates with the inferior surface of the squamous temporal bone bilaterally at the temporomandibular joints. The oral cavity may, thus, be said to be located between the middle and lower zones of the facial skeleton.

The oral cavity is conventionally described as having an outer part, the vestibule, which lies outside the alveolar processes of the jaws but inside the lips and cheek, and a larger part inside the alveolar processes that is the oral cavity proper. The entire oral cavity is lined by stratified squamous epithelium.

Opening into the oral cavity are the three (complementarily paired) major salivary glands: parotid, submandibular, and sublingual glands.

The nasal cavity which projects anteriorly as the external nose is divided into right and left halves (termed right and left nasal cavities) by a vertically orientated septum which is part bone and part cartilage. The nasal cavity extends from the external nasal aperture (nostril) to the posterior nasal aperture through which it communicates with the nasopharynx. Most of the nasal cavity is lined with respiratory epithelium (ciliated, columnar epithelium alongside numerous mucus-secreting goblet cells). The roof of the nasal cavity, however, is lined with olfactory neuroepithelium. Opening into the lateral wall of each nasal cavity are the four ipsilateral paranasal sinuses: maxillary, ethmoid, frontal, and sphenoid.

The orbital cavities are pyramidal sockets in the facial skeleton in which are located the eyeballs and other elements of the peripheral visual apparatus, all cushioned in orbital fat. The two orbits are separated from each other by the right and left ethmoidal air

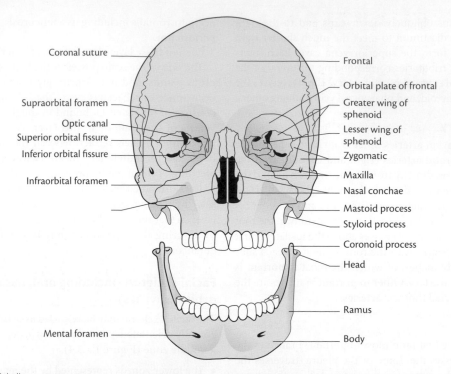

Coronal suture

Supraorbital foramen

Optic canal

Superior orbital fissure

Inferior orbital fissure

Infraorbital foramen

Mental foramen

Frontal

Orbital plate of frontal

Greater wing of
sphenoid

Lesser wing of
sphenoid

Zygomatic

Maxilla

Nasal conchae

Mastoid process

Styloid process

Coronoid process

Head

Ramus

Body

Fig. 1.1.5.4 Anterior view of skull.

Reproduced from M E Atkinson, *Anatomy for Dental Students*, Fourth Edition, Oxford University Press, Oxford, UK, Copyright © 2013, with permission from Oxford University Press.

sinuses and the upper portions of the right and left nasal cavities and nasal septum.

Posteriorly each orbital cavity communicates with the ipsilateral half of the middle cranial fossa through two significant and very important openings: the superior orbital fissure and the optic foramen. The latter transmits the optic nerve and the ophthalmic artery while the superior orbital fissure transmits the cranial nerves III, IV, and VI and the ophthalmic division of cranial nerve V.

Further reading

Drake RL, Vogl AW, Mitchell AW. *Gray's Anatomy for Students* (2nd ed). Philadelphia, PA: Elsevier; 2010.

Ellis H. Anatomy of the salivary glands. *Surgery* 2012; 30(11):569–72.

Ellis H, Mahadevan V. *Clinical Anatomy: Applied Anatomy for Students and Junior Doctors*. (13th ed). Oxford: Wiley-Blackwell; 2013.

MacKinnon PCB, Morris JF. *Oxford Textbook of Functional Anatomy* (Vol 3, 2nd ed). Oxford: Oxford University Press; 2005.

Mahadevan V. Clinical anatomy and developmental aberrations of the thyroid. In Arora A, Tolley NS, Tuttle RM (eds) *A Practical Manual of Thyroid and Parathyroid Disease* (pp. 65–76). Oxford: Wiley-Blackwell; 2010

Mahadevan V. The general topography of the neck. *Surgery* 2012; 30(11):573–7.

Sadler TW. *Langman's Medical Embryology* (13th ed). Philadelphia, PA: Wolters Kluwer/Lippincott Williams & Wilkins; 2014.

Sinnatamby C. *Last's Anatomy: Regional and Applied* (12th ed). Edinburgh: Elsevier; 2011.

Neuroanatomy

Vishy Mahadevan

Central nervous system

Brain

On a functional basis, the brain may be pictured as being made up of four major divisions:

1. Cerebral hemispheres (right and left)

2. Diencephalon (comprising, principally, the thalamus and hypothalamus)

3. Cerebellum

4. Brainstem (comprising, from below upwards, the medulla oblongata, pons, and midbrain).

Each cerebral hemisphere comprises the cerebral cortex and the basal ganglia, and various afferent and efferent neural fibre tracts. Within each cerebral hemisphere lies a cavity, the lateral ventricle, containing cerebrospinal fluid (CSF).

The cortex of the cerebral hemisphere is divided geographically into four major lobes, frontal, parietal, temporal and occipital, each containing discrete areas which subserve specific functions (functional localization).

The frontal lobe harbours the primary motor area which occupies a large part of the precentral gyrus. It receives afferents from the cerebellum and is concerned with the initiation and performance of voluntary movements. The frontal lobe of the dominant hemisphere (the left cerebral hemisphere in the majority of individuals) also includes *Broca's speech area* (the motor speech area).

The parietal lobe features the *primary somatosensory cortex* on the postcentral gyrus. This area receives afferent fibres from the thalamus and is concerned with the recognition of all forms of somatic sensation.

The temporal lobe features *the auditory cortex* whose afferent fibres are derived from the medial geniculate body of the thalamus. It is concerned with the perception of auditory stimuli. The cortical region just above and behind this area on the dominant hemisphere is called *Wernicke's area* and is of considerable importance in the sensory aspects of language comprehension.

The occipital lobe lies behind the parietal and temporal lobes and features on its medial surface *the primary visual cortex*. This area receives afferent fibres from the lateral geniculate body of the thalamus of the same side.

The basal ganglia are compact masses of grey matter which are situated deep in the substance of each cerebral hemisphere and comprise the *corpus striatum* (composed of the caudate nucleus, the putamen, and the globus pallidus) and the *claustrum*. Together with the cerebellum, the basal ganglia are involved in the coordination and control of movement.

The diencephalon

The diencephalon comprises principally the thalamus and hypothalamus, which are coextensive. A median, vertically disposed, cleft-like space between the right and left halves of the diencephalon, is termed the third ventricle. In addition to the thalamus and hypothalamus, the diencephalon includes two small but functionally important regions: the epithalamus and ventral thalamus. The epithalamus is the dorsal portion of the diencephalon and contains the pineal body. The ventral thalamus (also known as subthalamus) contains the subthalamic nucleus, which is one of the basal ganglia.

The thalamus is an ovoid mass of grey matter which forms the upper part of the lateral wall of the third ventricle. The thalamus is the *principal sensory relay station* which projects impulses from the main sensory pathways onto the cerebral cortex. It does this via a number of thalamic radiations in the internal capsule.

The hypothalamus forms the part of the lateral wall and floor of the third ventricle. The hypothalamus performs numerous regulatory functions. As the so-called head ganglion of the autonomic nervous system, it is concerned with the regulation of autonomic (both sympathetic and parasympathetic) activity.

The hypothalamus plays an important role in the control of endocrine secretions by the formation of releasing factors or release-inhibiting factors which act directly on the subjacent pituitary gland. In addition to its major influence on the autonomic nervous system and on pituitary function, the hypothalamus also plays a significant role in temperature regulation, water and electrolyte balance, regulation of appetite, and sleep–wake patterns.

The cerebellum

The cerebellum is the largest part of the hindbrain and occupies most of the posterior cranial fossa. It is made up of the right and left *cerebellar hemispheres* and a median *vermis*.

The cerebellum is connected to the brainstem by way of the paired cerebellar peduncles. Ventrally, the cerebellum is related to the fourth ventricle and to the medulla and pons.

Functions of the cerebellum

The principal function of the cerebellum is to regulate and maintain balance, and to coordinate timing and precision of body movements. The cerebellum has multiple connections with the cerebral cortex, reticular formation in the brainstem, thalamus, and vestibular nuclei. Through these intricate connections, the cerebellum constantly monitors proprioceptive sensory input from joints, muscles, and tendons, and accordingly refines and coordinates the contractions of skeletal muscles. However, unlike the cerebral cortex of the primary motor area, the cerebellum is incapable of *initiating* movement, nor is the cerebellum involved in the conscious perception of somatic or visceral sensations.

The brainstem
Extending from just above the tentorial hiatus to just below the foramen magnum, the brainstem is a stalk-like structure which is continuous superiorly with the diencephalon, and inferiorly with the spinal cord. From above downwards, the brainstem comprises successively the midbrain (mesencephalon), pons, and medulla oblongata. The brainstem and cerebellum are situated in the posterior cranial fossa.

The brainstem serves three major functions:

1. It houses the nuclei of all but two of the 12 pairs of cranial nerves (the exceptions being the cranial nerve pairs I and II which may both be regarded as peripheral extensions of the forebrain)

2. It acts as a 'thoroughfare' for the various ascending and descending nerve tracts running to and from the cerebral cortex, and for other tracts that project to the cerebellum

3. It contains the reticular formation (a fine and diffuse network of nerve cells and nerve fibres) and the reticular activating system. The reticular formation spans the entire length of the brainstem and harbours the 'vital centres'—important reflex centres which regulate respiratory and cardiovascular function. The reticular formation and reticular activating system regulate the individual's level of awareness and wakefulness. Damage to the reticular formation in the upper part of the brainstem may cause the patient to be in a state of prolonged coma.

Spinal cord
The spinal cord in the adult is approximately 45 cm long. It is continuous above with the medulla oblongata at the foramen magnum and ends below at the level of the lower border of the first lumbar vertebra.

The spinal cord bears a fairly deep longitudinal *anterior midline fissure*, and a shallow *posterior midline sulcus*. On either side, is a *posterolateral sulcus* along which the *posterior (sensory) nerve roots* of spinal nerves are arranged serially along the length of the spinal cord. The *anterior (motor) nerve roots* of the spinal nerves emerge serially along the anterolateral aspect of the length of the spinal cord, on either side.

At each intervertebral foramen the anterior and posterior nerve roots unite to form a *spinal nerve* which immediately divides into *anterior* and *posterior rami*, each transmitting both motor and sensory fibres.

Below the termination of the spinal cord, the roots of the lumbar, sacral, and coccygeal nerves continue downwards within the vertebral canal, as the cauda equina, lying in the subarachnoid space, as far as the lower sacral level.

A cross section of the spinal cord (Figure 1.1.6.1) shows the *central canal* around which is the H-shaped *grey matter* packed with nerve cell bodies arranged in a highly orderly manner. Surrounding the grey matter is the *white matter*. The latter contains the long ascending and descending tracts.

On either side of the midline the grey matter presents a somewhat bulbous *anterior (or ventral) horn* packed with motor nerve cells, and a slender *posterior (or dorsal) horn* that extends almost to the periphery of the section. The posterior horn is capped by

the *substantia gelatinosa* in which terminate many of the incoming sensory fibres entering the cord through the posterior nerve roots. In the large *anterior horn* lie the motor cells which give rise to the fibres of the anterior roots.

In that part of the spinal cord that corresponds to the thoracic and upper lumbar segments, and sacral segments, the grey matter features, additionally, a *lateral horn* on each side containing the cells of origin of the sympathetic system in the thoracic and upper lumbar segments, and the cells of origin of the pelvic parasympathetics in the sacral segments.

The white matter of the spinal cord has (a) descending (motor) tracts of which the most important is the lateral corticospinal tract (crossed pyramidal motor tract), and (b) ascending sensory tracts of which the most important are *the lateral and anterior spinothalamic* tracts carrying pain and temperature sensations, and the posterior column fibres which are as yet uncrossed and carry sensations of fine touch, vibration, and proprioception (position sense).

All sensory fibres running up in the spinal cord eventually relay in the thalamus before being projected onto the relevant area of cerebral cortex.

Knowledge of the internal architecture of the spinal cord and the location of various fibre tracts is of immense usefulness in the clinical examination and diagnosis of spinal cord lesions.

Blood supply of the brain and spinal cord
The brain receives its blood supply from the right and left internal carotid arteries (each a terminal branch of the corresponding common carotid artery) and from the right and left vertebral arteries (each a branch of the ipsilateral subclavian artery). Each vertebral artery courses upwards along its side of the neck, through the cervical vertebral transverse processes before entering the posterior cranial fossa through the foramen magnum. The two vertebral arteries then unite in front of the brainstem to form the basilar artery. The latter runs upward and ends by dividing into the right and left posterior cerebral arteries. Each internal carotid artery enters the cranial cavity through the temporal bone of its side and eventually divides into the anterior and middle cerebral arteries. Shortly before its termination the internal carotid artery gives off the all-important ophthalmic artery which enters the orbit through the optic foramen (accompanying the optic nerve) to supply all the

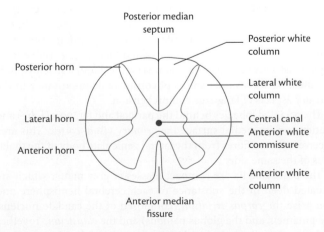

Fig. 1.1.6.1 Cross section of spinal cord at mid-thoracic level.
Reproduced with permission from Ellis H. and Mahadevan V., *Clinical Anatomy*, Thirteenth Edition, Wiley-Blackwell, Oxford, UK, Copyright © 2013.

orbital contents. By means of three narrow communicating arteries, the two internal carotid arteries and the two posterior cerebral arteries form an 'arterial ring' in the middle cranial fossa, termed the *circle of Willis*.

The basilar artery and the two vertebral arteries together supply all of the cerebellum and the brainstem (i.e. the contents of the posterior cranial fossa) and through the two posterior cerebral arteries, a good deal of the medial surface of the cerebral hemispheres including the visual cortex on the occipital lobe. The two internal carotids supply the remainder of the brain. Knowledge of the vascular territories of individual vessels aids in the interpretation of clinical signs caused by occlusion of cerebral vessels.

Venous blood from the brain drains into an interconnected system of *intracranial dural venous sinuses* which are endothelium-lined channels located, in the main, between the dura and the endocranium (the name given to the periosteum that lines the inner surface of the cranial cavity). The intracranial venous sinuses are valveless and eventually drain into the right and left internal jugular veins which leave the cranial cavity through the skull base to run down the neck.

The spinal cord derives its blood supply from the anterior and posterior spinal arteries which are branches of the vertebral arteries. Blood supply to the lower half of the spinal cord is supplemented by the spinal branches of the posterior intercostal arteries which are, in turn, branches of the descending thoracic aorta.

Floor of the cranial cavity

The floor of the cranial cavity is the upper surface of the base of skull. In a dry skeleton it is revealed by removing the cranial vault (skull cap).

The floor of the cranial cavity presents a terraced arrangement of three regions (areas). In anterior to posterior sequence, these are the anterior cranial fossa, middle cranial fossa, and posterior cranial fossa. The anterior fossa is the shallowest and the smallest, whereas the posterior fossa is the deepest and largest of the three areas (Figure 1.1.6.2).

Anterior cranial fossa

The central part of the floor of the anterior cranial fossa is a depressed, perforated plate of bone, the cribriform plate of the ethmoid. This forms the highest part of the roof of the nasal cavity, and is traversed on either side of the midline by the corresponding olfactory nerve filaments, on their way from the roof of the nasal cavity to the olfactory bulb in the anterior cranial fossa. Lateral to the cribriform plate, on either side, the floor of the anterior cranial fossa is somewhat raised and forms the roof of the orbit.

The anterior cranial fossa houses, in addition to the right and left olfactory pathways, the frontal lobes of the cerebral hemispheres and the anterior cerebral arteries as the latter course beneath the frontal lobes. The frontal lobes lie just above the orbital roof.

Middle cranial fossa

The middle cranial fossa floor shows a platform-like elevation in the centre. This is the body of the sphenoid bone. Its upper surface is slightly concave and constitutes the pituitary fossa. Situated immediately above the pituitary fossa is the pituitary gland which is suspended from the hypothalamus by the pituitary stalk. On either side of the central elevation, the floor of the middle cranial fossa accommodates the corresponding temporal lobe of the cerebral hemisphere. Posterolateral to the pituitary fossa on either side lies the corresponding trigeminal ganglion, whereas directly lateral to the pituitary fossa on either side is the cavernous sinus.

Anteriorly, on either side of the midline, the middle cranial fossa communicates with the ipsilateral orbit by means of two openings: the larger, wider, and laterally located one being the superior orbital fissure and the smaller opening being the optic

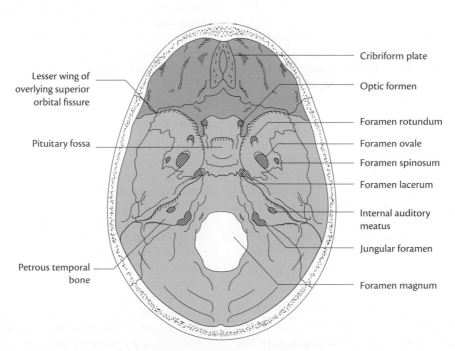

Fig. 1.1.6.2 Floor of cranial cavity showing anterior (blue) middle (light brown), and posterior (green) cranial fossae.
Reproduced with permission from Ellis H. and Mahadevan V., *Clinical Anatomy*, Thirteenth Edition, Wiley-Blackwell, Oxford, UK, Copyright © 2013.

foramen. The latter transmits the optic nerve (ensheathed in the three meningeal layers) and ophthalmic artery, while the superior orbital fissure transmits the oculomotor (IIIrd), trochlear (IVth) and abducens (VIth) nerves, the ophthalmic nerve, and the ophthalmic veins. On each side, the floor of the middle cranial fossa shows three significant foramina. From front to back these are the foramen rotundum, foramen ovale, and foramen spinosum, which transmit respectively the maxillary nerve, mandibular nerve, and the middle meningeal artery.

Posterior cranial fossa

The posterior cranial fossa is the deepest and largest of the three fossae. It houses the entire cerebellum. Lying anterior to the cerebellum in the median part of the posterior cranial fossa is the brainstem comprising, from above downwards, the midbrain, pons, and medulla oblongata. The medulla oblongata leaves the posterior cranial fossa through a large opening in the centre of the fossa's floor, the foramen magnum, to become the spinal cord. The 'slope' of bone which forms the anterior wall of the posterior cranial fossa, and lies in front of the brainstem, is called the *clivus*. The cerebellum is roofed by a large, thick, double-layered sheet of infolded dura mater termed the *tentorium cerebelli*. Above the tentorium cerebelli (and therefore outside the posterior cranial fossa) lie the occipital lobes of the cerebral hemispheres.

Three significant openings, on each side, lead away from the posterior cranial fossa. These are the internal acoustic (auditory) meatus, the jugular foramen, and the hypoglossal canal. The first of these transmits the VIIth (facial) and VIIIth (vestibulocochlear) cranial nerves. The jugular foramen transmits the IXth (glossopharyngeal), Xth (vagus), and XIth (accessory) cranial nerves, and also the sigmoid and inferior petrosal venous sinuses. The hypoglossal canal transmits the XIIth (hypoglossal) cranial nerve.

Peripheral nervous system

Cranial nerves

There are 12 pairs of cranial nerves, all of which leave or enter the cranial cavity through foramina or fissures in its floor or walls. By convention, the cranial nerves are designated in roman numerals. The first and second cranial nerve pairs are unlike the other ten, in that they do not have their 'origins' in the brainstem. For this reason, the first and second cranial nerves are generally regarded by neurophysiologists as fibre tracts of the forebrain, rather than as true nerves.

The numbered cranial nerves (with their corresponding names) are as follows: I (olfactory), II (optic), III (oculomotor), IV (trochlear), V (trigeminal), VI (abducens), VII (facial), VIII (vestibulocochlear), IX (glossopharyngeal), X (vagus), XI (accessory), and XII (hypoglossal).

On a functional basis, cranial nerves may be classified into one or other of three groups:

1. *Wholly sensory cranial nerves*: I (olfactory nerve), II (optic nerve), and VIII (vestibulocochlear nerve)

2. *Wholly motor cranial nerves*: III (oculomotor), IV (trochlear), VI (abducens), XI (accessory), and XII (hypoglossal)

3. *Mixed (motor and sensory) cranial nerves*: V (trigeminal), VII (facial), IX (glossopharyngeal), and X (vagus).

The design of clinical tests undertaken to test the integrity of individual cranial nerves is obviously determined by this classification.

The motor (or efferent) cranial nerves arise from discrete aggregations of neurons in the brainstem, termed *nuclei of origin*.

The sensory (or afferent) cranial nerves arise from neurons situated outside the brain. The central processes of these neurons enter the brain, eventually to join collections of neurons termed *nuclei of termination*. Despite this fundamental distinction, nuclei of origin and nuclei of termination are both commonly referred to as '*origins of cranial nerves*'.

Of the 12 cranial nerve pairs, all but one are confined to the head and neck. The exception is the vagus (Xth cranial nerve) whose distribution extends beyond the head and neck to the thorax and abdomen.

Spinal nerves, spinal cord segments, and dermatomes

The spinal nerves are complementarily paired and symmetrically arranged structures which originate in the central grey matter of the spinal cord. There are 31 pairs of spinal nerves in all (8 cervical, 12 thoracic, 5 lumbar, 5 sacral, and 1 coccygeal). As has already been noted, each spinal nerve is formed by the confluence of a motor (anterior) root with a sensory (posterior) root.

A horizontal section of spinal cord which gives rise to a complementary pair of spinal nerves is termed a *spinal cord segment*. It follows, therefore, that the spinal cord possesses 31 segments.

Each spinal nerve (with the notable exception of the first cervical nerve, which has no cutaneous supply) supplies a specific area of skin. This cutaneous territory of the spinal nerve is termed a *dermatome*.

Autonomic nervous system

The autonomic nervous system is so named because, unlike the somatic nervous system, it is not under voluntary control. The autonomic nervous system consists of three parts: (1) sympathetic nervous system, (2) parasympathetic system, and (3) the enteric nervous system (Figure 1.1.6.3). The autonomic nervous system contains both contain afferent and efferent fibres. These are distributed to the thoracic, abdominal, pelvic, and perineal viscera, and to vascular smooth muscle.

Meningeal coverings of the brain and spinal cord

The brain and spinal cord are surrounded by three layers of protective membranes, arranged concentrically. The outermost layer is the *dura mater*, the middle layer is the *arachnoid mater*, and the innermost layer is the *pia mater*. The pia mater is closely applied to the surface of the brain and spinal cord, and even lines all the major and minor fissures of the brain.

The arachnoid mater is closely applied to the inner surface of the dura mater everywhere, and never normally leaves the dura. In places, the dura in the cranial cavity forms fairly strong, large (double-layered) infoldings. These serve to create compartments within the cranial cavity, and perform the very important function of supporting the delicate brain, and protecting the brain very effectively from the torsional stresses to which it would otherwise be subjected. The most important of these dural reduplications are the falx cerebri and the tentorium cerebelli.

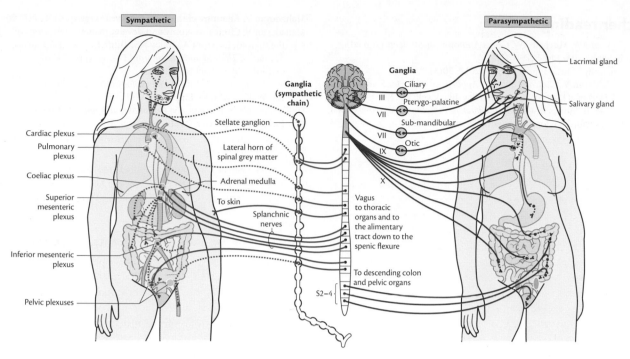

Fig. 1.1.6.3 Organization of the sympathetic (left) and parasympathetic (right) systems.

Between the arachnoid mater and the underlying pia mater is the subarachnoid space in which is contained CSF. Between the arachnoid and the overlying dura is a potential space called the subdural space. Normally, only a thin film of fluid lies in this space which enables the arachnoid to glide on the inner surface of the dura. Abnormally, however, blood may collect in this potential space resulting in a subdural haematoma.

Within the cranial cavity the dura mater is firmly fused to the periosteum that lines the inner surface of the bony walls and floor of the cranial cavity. Within the vertebral canal, however, the dura is free of the wall of the canal. The space between the two is called the epidural (or extradural) space. It contains a thin layer of fat surrounding the dural sheath. Within the fat and arranged circumferentially around the dural sheath is a delicate plexus of (valveless) veins called the internal vertebral venous plexus.

The ventricular system and the cerebrospinal fluid circulation

Developmentally, the entire central nervous system is derived from a simple ectodermal closed but hollow tube. Notwithstanding the eventual transformation of this simple tube into the complex-looking brain and spinal cord, the original lumen is retained in every part of the fully developed central nervous system, and constitutes the ventricular system. It is lined with a specialized epithelium termed ependyma.

Morphology of the ventricular system

The ventricular system comprises the right and left lateral ventricles, the third ventricle, and the fourth ventricle. The right and left *lateral ventricles*, each within the corresponding cerebral hemisphere, are by far the largest components of the system. Each lateral ventricle opens into the third ventricle through an opening

called the interventricular foramen (of Monro) located one on either side in the corresponding lateral wall of the third ventricle. From the third ventricle the CSF passes through a narrow channel in the midbrain, *the cerebral aqueduct (of Sylvius)*, into the fourth ventricle.

The *fourth ventricle* lies between the pons/medulla ventrally and the cerebellum dorsally, separated from the latter by a membrane-like roof. The CSF escapes from the fourth ventricle into the subarachnoid space by way of three natural apertures in the membranous roof of the fourth ventricle, and then flows over the surface of the brain and spinal cord.

Production and circulation of cerebrospinal fluid

CSF is produced mainly in the ventricular system of the brain, whence it enters the subarachnoid space. The production and circulation of CSF are constant, dynamic, and energy-dependent processes.

Besides serving as a 'cushion' for the brain and spinal cord within their respective bony enclosures, CSF plays an important role in the exchange of nutrients and waste metabolites between the blood and neurons of the brain and spinal cord.

CSF is formed by the secretory activity of the choroid plexuses (vascular tufts that are invaginated into parts of the ventricular system) in the lateral, third, and fourth ventricles. CSF is produced constantly at a rate of 0.5 mL/min. It circulates through the ventricular system of the brain and enters the subarachnoid space through three natural openings in the membranous roof of the fourth ventricle. From the subarachnoid space, CSF is extruded into the system of intracranial dural venous sinuses (principally the superior sagittal sinus) by specialized evaginations of arachnoid, termed arachnoid villi.

Any obstruction to the flow and circulation of CSF results in a condition termed *hydrocephalus*.

Further reading

Drake RL, Vogl AW, Mitchell AW. *Gray's Anatomy for Students* (2nd ed). Philadelphia, PA: Elsevier; 2010.

Ellis H. Anatomy of head injury. *Surgery* 2012; 30(3):99–101.

Ellis H, Mahadevan V. *Clinical Anatomy: Applied Anatomy for Students and Junior Doctors.* (13th ed). Oxford: Wiley-Blackwell; 2013.

MacKinnon PCB, Morris JF. *Oxford Textbook of Functional Anatomy* (Vol 3, 2nd ed). Oxford: Oxford University Press; 2005.

Mahadevan V. Anatomy of the cranial nerves *Surgery* 2012; 30(3):95–8.

Mahadevan V. Clinical anatomy and developmental aberrations of the thyroid. In Arora A, Tolley NS, Tuttle RM (eds) *A Practical Manual of Thyroid and Parathyroid Disease* (pp. 65–76). Oxford: Wiley-Blackwell; 2010.

Sadler TW. *Langman's Medical Embryology* (13th ed). Philadelphia, PA: Wolters Kluwer/Lippincott Williams & Wilkins; 2014.

Sinnatamby C. *Last's Anatomy: Regional and Applied* (12th ed). Edinburgh: Elsevier; 2011.

PART 1.2

Applied surgical physiology

Sub-section editor: David A. Adams

CHAPTER 1.2.1

Introduction to Section 1.2: 'Applied surgical physiology'

David A. Adams

Introduction

Knowledge of normal structure and function is essential when trying to understand the consequences of disease. Section 1.2 describes general physiological principles considered to be important in surgical practice.

Chapter 1.2.11 on 'Neurology' describes the functional organization of the nervous system—the sensory, motor, and autonomic pathways together with the specialized functions such as vision, hearing, and reflex arcs.

The various important endocrine glands including thyroid, parathyroids, adrenals, and pancreas are described as well as the controlling hypothalamus and pituitary gland in Chapter 1.2.10 ('Endocrine').

The function of the kidneys in maintaining fluid and electrolyte haemostasis is outlined together with a description of the autoregulation of renal blood flow in Chapters 1.2.4 and 1.2.9 ('Fluid and electrolyte balance and replacement: acid–base balance' and 'Urinary').

Chapter 1.2.8 ('Gastrointestinal') contains a description of the function of the system from salivary glands to colon and includes the processes involved in the digestion of carbohydrates, fats, and proteins. This is augmented by a further chapter dealing with metabolic processes and their regulation (Chapter 1.2.2 'Metabolic pathways, nutrition, and abnormalities').

Fluid and acid–base balance, haemostasis, and thrombosis are important considerations in the surgical patient and are covered in Chapter 1.2.3 ('Blood loss, hypovolaemic shock, and septic shock') and Chapter 1.2.5 ('Haemostasis and thrombosis').

Finally, respiratory and cardiovascular issues are frequently the source of difficult decisions about fitness for surgical intervention. Both are described in detail, in Chapter 1.2.7 ('Respiratory') and in particular in Chapter 1.2.6 ('Cardiovascular'), which gives examples of disordered physiology.

Metabolic pathways, nutrition, and abnormalities

Judith H. Harmey

Overview of metabolism

Humans metabolize nutrients through four interconnected pathways (Figure 1.2.2.1):

1. Oxidative pathways (e.g. tricarboxylic acid (TCA) cycle and oxidative phosphorylation) which use nutrients to generate energy for biosynthesis and mechanical work

2. Fuel storage/mobilization pathways which can be used to generate energy when needed (e.g. glycogen synthesis and breakdown)

3. Detoxification pathways (e.g. urea cycle to remove ammonia (NH_3) generated by amino acid metabolism)

4. Biosynthetic pathways which synthesize macromolecules.

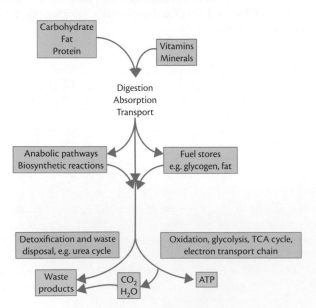

Fig. 1.2.2.1 Overview of metabolic routes for dietary macromolecules. Foods in the diet are digested, absorbed, and transported then converted into energy via oxidative pathways—glycolysis, the TCA cycle, and oxidative phosphorylation—or used as precursors for biosynthesis. The energy generated is used in biosynthetic pathways or for mechanical work such as muscle contraction. Depending on overall energy balance, fuels may be converted into storage molecules such as glycogen and fat which can be used to generate energy when fuels are low. Detoxification and waste disposal pathways remove toxins or by-products of metabolism. The urea cycle, for example, removes ammonia generated from amino acid metabolism.

Through the process of digestion and absorption into the bloodstream, each of the three main nutrients, carbohydrates, protein, and fats, are broken down into smaller molecular units including hexoses (six-carbon sugars, e.g. glucose), amino acids, and fatty acids respectively. These basic building blocks can then be converted to acetyl coenzyme A (CoA) or other intermediates. Pyruvate dehydrogenase (PDH) catalyses the formation of acetyl CoA from CoA and pyruvate generated from oxidation of glucose by glycolysis. Acetyl CoA then enters the energy-generating TCA cycle in the mitochondria. Fatty acids can be used to generate acetyl CoA by β-oxidation. Amino acids can be used to generate acetyl CoA or can enter the TCA cycle after conversion to pyruvate or TCA cycle intermediates. Electrons are transferred to the coenzymes nicotinamide adenine dinucleotide (NAD^+) and flavin adenine dinucleotide (FAD) forming the reduced coenzymes NADH and $FADH_2$ during glycolysis and the TCA cycle and enter the electron transport chain to ultimately produce adenosine triphosphate (ATP) by oxidative phosphorylation.

Carbohydrate metabolism

Almost all carbohydrates can ultimately be digested and converted to glucose which can be broken down further to produce energy and intermediates for other metabolic pathways such as building blocks for glycogen stores or pentoses for nucleotide production. About half of the ingested load of glucose is metabolized to carbon dioxide (CO_2) and water, 5% is stored as glycogen, and 30–40% converted to fat.[1]

Glucose from carbohydrate digestion is absorbed in the small intestine and transported into the plasma (Figure 1.2.2.2), entering most cell types by facilitated diffusion.

Low serum glucose levels stimulate glucagon secretion from the α pancreatic cells which stimulates glycogenolysis and gluconeogenesis. Raised glucose levels stimulate insulin release from the β cells and the insulin stimulates adipose and muscle cell glucose uptake via glucose transporter type 4 (GLUT4) transporters and increases glucose phosphorylation to produce glucose-6-phosphate (G6P) catalysed by hexokinase. In most tissues, hexokinase catalyses the phosphorylation of glucose but in liver parenchyma cells and islet cells of the pancreas, glucose is phosphorylated by glucokinase. G6P is the first step in both glycolysis to produce three-carbon pyruvate for conversion to acetyl CoA which enters the TCA cycle and in the pentose phosphate pathway to produce five-carbon sugars for nucleotide synthesis.

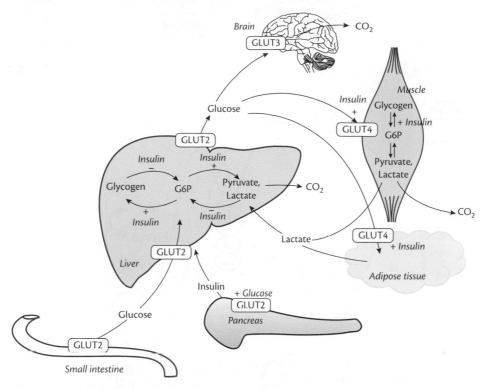

Fig. 1.2.2.2 Overview of carbohydrate metabolism in different tissues. GLUT2 is the high Km non-insulin regulated glucose transporter expressed in liver, kidney and β-cells of the pancreas (i.e. glucose transport is determined by glucose concentration). The GLUT4 transporter expressed in muscle and adipose is insulin regulated (insulin stimulates movement of GLUT4 to the cell surface). GLUT3 is the low Km glucose transporter in the brain (glucose transport is independent of glucose concentration when within normal range).

G6P, glucose-6-phosphate; GLUT, glucose transporter; Km, Michaelis constant (substrate concentration that produces half maximal velocity); + glucose, pathways stimulated by glucose; + insulin, pathways stimulated by insulin; − insulin, pathways inhibited by insulin.

Reproduced from David A. Warrell, Timothy N. Cox and John D. Firth (Eds.), *Oxford Textbook of Medicine*, Fifth Edition, Oxford University Press, Oxford, UK, Copyright © 2010, by permission of Oxford University Press.

Metabolism of glucose in liver cells to G6P is catalysed by glucokinase which creates a concentration gradient facilitating further glucose to enter the cells.

In the fed state when the insulin:glucagon ratio is high, G6P enters glycolysis or glycogenesis in muscle and liver. Excess glucose not required to meet the body's energy demands is transported via GLUT4 into the adipose tissue where it is ultimately converted to triglyceride (TG). In the fasting state when insulin:glucagon ratio is low, glycogen is broken down to provide G6P for glycolysis and gluconeogenesis generates glucose from non-carbohydrate precursors in the liver.

Glycolysis

Glycolysis is the breakdown of six-carbon glucose to three-carbon pyruvate or lactate. Some tissues, including brain and red blood cells, can only generate energy using glucose. Glucose is broken down via glycolysis and the TCA cycle to provide energy in the form of ATP and intermediates for other pathways. In cells that have mitochondria and in the presence of oxygen, pyruvate is the end product of glycolysis which then undergoes reaction with CoA catalysed by pyruvate dehydrogenase (PDH) to form two-carbon acetyl CoA which enters the TCA cycle.

In exercising muscle or cells which lack mitochondria such as erythrocytes, glycolysis is anaerobic and pyruvate is reduced to lactate by lactate dehydrogenase. Although some ATP can be produced from NADH generated during glycolysis, the majority of the cells energy is generated via the TCA cycle and the electron transport chain (ETC). Under anaerobic conditions, the net ATP gain is two ATP molecules per molecule of glucose whereas under aerobic conditions where glucose is completely oxidized via the TCA cycle and the ETC, up to 38 ATP molecules are generated per molecule of glucose (for more detail, see 'Further reading').

Tricarboxylic acid cycle

Each molecule of glucose (six carbon atoms) entering aerobic glycolysis results in two molecules of three-carbon pyruvate which are then converted to the two-carbon acetyl group and linked to CoA by PDH. The TCA cycle starts with synthesis of citrate from acetyl CoA and oxaloacetate and ends with regeneration of oxaloacetate (Figure 1.2.2.3) so the entry of acetyl CoA into the cycle does not result in net production or consumption of TCA cycle intermediates. Each two-carbon acetyl CoA is completely oxidized in the TCA cycle generating two molecules of CO_2 and its electrons are transferred to the electron carriers NAD^+ and FAD. Complete oxidation of one molecule of glucose therefore requires two turns of the TCA cycle.

In addition to its role in energy metabolism, the TCA cycle also acts as a pool of intermediates. It is termed an amphibolic pathway because it is involved in both anabolic and catabolic pathways (Figure 1.2.2.3). For details of the individual enzyme reactions, see 'Further reading'.

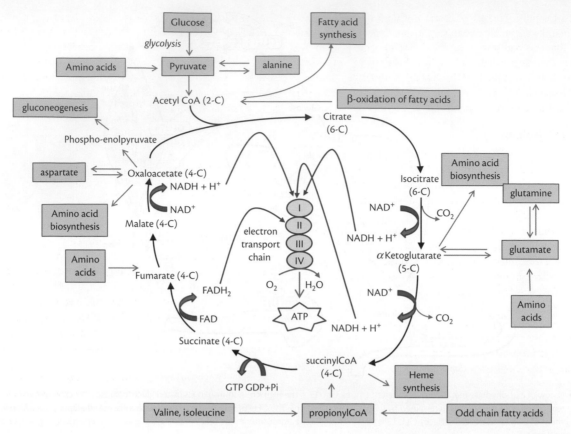

Fig. 1.2.2.3 Integration of carbohydrate, fat, and protein metabolism. Almost all carbohydrates can ultimately enter glycolysis in the form of glucose, a six-carbon (C) sugar, which is oxidized to two three-C pyruvate molecules during aerobic glycolysis. Pyruvate is then converted to acetyl CoA by pyruvate dehydrogenase. Pyruvate can be generated from amino acid metabolism and Acetyl CoA can be generated from TG breakdown. Anaplerotic pathways replenish TCA cycle intermediates and TCA cycle intermediates are also used in anabolic or biosynthetic pathways. The number of carbons in each intermediate is indicated to illustrate that there is no net gain or loss of C during the TCA cycle—two C atoms enter in the form of acetyl CoA and two C leave as CO_2. The reduced electron carriers NADH and $FADH_2$ generated during glycolysis and the TCA cycle are re-oxidized by molecular oxygen in the electron transport chain and ATP is generated by oxidative phosphorylation. Reactions of the TCA cycle are shown in black. Unlike other TCA cycle enzymes which are located in the mitochondrial matrix, succinate dehydrogenase which catalyses the conversion of succinate to fumarate in the TCA cycle is embedded in the inner mitochondrial membrane and also forms part of complex II of the electron transport chain.

Electron transport chain/oxidative phosphorylation

The reduced electron carriers—NADH and $FADH_2$—generated during glycolysis, the TCA cycle, or beta-oxidation of fatty acids—are reoxidized at the electron transfer chain (ETC) to generate ATP by oxidative phosphorylation (Figure 1.2.2.3). NADH and $FADH_2$ pass their electrons to a series of electron carriers (complexes I, II, III, and IV) in the inner mitochondrial membrane. As these electrons are passed along the ETC, protons are pumped into the intermembrane space creating an electrochemical gradient. This proton imbalance—the proton motive force—is used to drive ATP synthesis via oxidative phosphorylation. The movement of protons back into the mitochondrial matrix via a proton channel in the ATP synthase complex drives ATP synthesis from adenosine diphosphate and inorganic phosphate.[2] This ATP is then used to drive enzyme reactions, biosynthesis, and mechanical work such as muscle contraction. Uncoupling proteins or synthetic uncouplers create a proton leak such that electron transport occurs but protons pumped into intermembrane space re-enter the matrix without ATP synthesis and the energy is released as heat. Aspirin overdose results in uncoupling of electron transport and ATP synthesis.

$FADH_2$ is generated during the conversion of succinate to fumarate in the TCA cycle by succinate dehydrogenase. Unlike the other TCA cycle enzymes which are located in the matrix of the mitochondria, succinate dehydrogenase is embedded in inner mitochondrial membrane and also forms part of complex II of the electron transport chain. Electrons from $FADH_2$ therefore enter the ETC at complex II and bypass complex I. Each pair of electrons entering the ETC via $FADH_2$ results in generation of two ATP molecules whereas electrons from NADH which enter at complex I result in formation of three ATP molecules. The final electron acceptor is molecular oxygen. Under anaerobic conditions (e.g. ischaemia, hypoxia) when oxygen is limited, the movement of electrons along the ETC stops and therefore ATP synthesis also stops.

Pentose phosphate pathway

In the pentose phosphate pathway (also known as the hexose monophosphate shunt), part of the energy from G6P is conserved in NADPH (the reduced form of nicotinamide adenine dinucleotide phosphate, $NADP^+$), a biochemical reductant which supplies electrons and hence energy to enzymes involved in fatty acid synthesis, steroid synthesis, and antioxidant reactions. This pathway produces ribose-5-phosphate required for nucleoside biosynthesis (these are five-carbon ribose sugars with purine or pyrimidine) and allows the body to use five-carbon sugars from the diet or from degradation of structural carbohydrates. Insulin increases expression of G6P dehydrogenase, the main regulatory enzyme of pentose phosphate pathway activity, so G6P entry into this pathway is increased when nutrients are plentiful. NADPH is a competitive inhibitor for this enzyme and under most metabolic conditions the NADPH/NADP$^+$ ratio is high enough to inhibit it. The reversible reactions of the pathway are also regulated by supply and demand for pentose phosphate intermediates.

Glycogen metabolism

Glycogen is a rapidly mobilizable storage form of glucose mainly stored in the liver and skeletal muscle. Two key enzymes regulate glycogen synthesis (glycogen synthase) and breakdown (glycogen phosphorylase) in response to levels of metabolites and the energy requirements of the cell.

Glycogen synthase is the key enzyme in glycogen synthesis adding glucose units to form glycogen chains. Glycogen phosphorylase releases glucose-1-phosphate from glycogen which is converted to G6P by phosphoglucomutase.

In the liver, G6P is converted to glucose and released into the bloodstream to maintain blood glucose whereas in muscle, G6P enters glycolysis directly to produce energy for muscle contraction.

High levels of G6P activate glycogen synthase and inhibit glycogen phosphorylase promoting glycogen synthesis. Insulin activates a pathway that activates glycogen synthase and inhibits glycogen phosphorylase.

The net effect is that insulin is anabolic-promoting glycogen synthesis whereas glucagon (liver) and epinephrine (liver and muscle) are catabolic-promoting glycogen breakdown and inhibiting glycogen synthesis.[3]

Gluconeogenesis

Certain tissues such as the brain and erythrocytes require a continuous supply of glucose as a metabolic fuel and blood glucose levels are maintained within a tight range (4.5–5.6 mmol/L in fasting state). In the absence of dietary intake of carbohydrate, liver glycogen can meet the body's glucose requirements for approximately 10–18 hours. However, once glycogen stores are depleted, glucose is formed from non-carbohydrate precursors via gluconeogenesis which is primarily controlled by the levels of circulating glucagon and availability of gluconeogenic substrates. Intermediates of glycolysis and the TCA cycle can act as substrates for gluconeogenesis. For example, oxaloacetate can be converted to phosphoenolpyruvate for gluconeogenesis (Figure 1.2.2.3).

During fasting, initially glycogen stores are adequate, then about 90% of gluconeogenesis occurs within the liver and 10% in the kidney. During prolonged fasting, however, the kidney becomes the major gluconeogenic tissue. Gluconeogenesis is not simply a reversal of glycolysis as four unique enzyme reactions (glucose-6-phosphatase, fructose 1,6-bisphosphatase, and pyruvate carboxylase,/phosphoenolpyruvate carboxylase) are required to bypass the three irreversible reactions of glycolysis (hexokinase, phosphofructokinase, and pyruvate kinase respectively) (see 'Further reading').

Fatty acids stored in the adipose tissue are the body's major fuel reserve. Tri-glycerides (TGs) are hydrolysed to fatty acids and glycerol by hormone-sensitive lipase primarily in response to epinephrine. High insulin and glucose inactivate hormone-sensitive lipase. Glycerol released from TG in the adipose tissue is transported to the liver and used to form dihydroxyacetone phosphate (DHAP), a substrate for gluconeogenesis.

Lactate released into the blood by exercised muscle and by erythrocytes can be converted to glucose in the liver and released back into the circulation to maintain glucose levels.

During prolonged fasting, hydrolysis of tissue protein is the main source of glucose. The α-ketoacids such as α-ketoglutarate (α-KG) and oxaloacetate formed during the metabolism of glucogenic amino acids can enter the TCA cycle (Figure 1.2.2.3).

Fat metabolism

Dietary lipids are digested and absorbed along with fat-soluble vitamins by the enterocytes in the small intestine and then transported in the circulation by chylomicrons assembled within the enterocytes and composed of about 90% TG, cholesterol, cholesteryl esters, fat-soluble vitamins, and apolipoprotein (Apo). Once in the plasma, chylomicrons acquire additional lipoproteins—ApoC and ApoE—by exchange with high-density lipoprotein particles. ApoC-II activates lipoprotein lipase expressed at the surface of endothelial cells lining the capillaries of most tissues (but not liver) which degrades chylomicron TG to fatty acids and glycerol. Adipocytes can re-esterify fatty acids to TG and most cells can oxidize fatty acids for energy. The glycerol released is mainly used by the liver to form glycerol-3-phosphate which can enter either glycolysis or gluconeogenesis.

Following a meal when insulin is high and glucagon low (fed state), most of the fatty acids used for TG synthesis in adipose tissue come from chylomicrons. Following a meal of excess carbohydrate and protein, however, most fatty acids are synthesized in the liver from acetyl CoA. In response to high glucagon and/or high epinephrine (i.e. fasting state), hormone-sensitive lipase hydrolyses TG stored in the adipose tissue to glycerol and free fatty acids. This glycerol is converted to DHAP which can enter glycolysis or gluconeogenesis. Adipocytes lack glycerol kinase and cannot synthesize glucose from glycerol (see 'Further reading').

Beta-oxidation

Fatty acids (saturated) released from TG stored in adipose are transported to various tissues, converted to fatty acid acyl CoA and oxidized to provide energy by beta-oxidation in the mitochondria. Fatty acids cannot be used as a fuel by erythrocytes which lack mitochondria or by the brain due to the blood–brain barrier. Beta-oxidation of fatty acids involves successive removal of two-carbon fragments producing acetyl CoA, NADH, and FADH$_2$ which can be used to generate energy via the TCA cycle and ETC. Acetyl CoA itself is not a gluconeogenic substrate as the PDH reaction is irreversible but it is a positive allosteric regulator of pyruvate carboxylase stimulating production of oxaloacetate as a substrate for gluconeogenesis.

Ketogenesis

Liver mitochondria can convert acetyl CoA from fatty acid oxidation into ketone bodies (there are three: acetoacetate, 3-hydroxybutyrate, and acetone) by ketogenesis. Ketone bodies released into the blood by the liver are a major energy source for other tissues, ultimately metabolized in the TCA cycle via formation of acetyl CoA. Although a normal source of energy, ketone bodies are a particularly important energy source in the heart, adrenal gland, and renal cortex. The brain can also use ketone bodies to meet its energy requirements during prolonged fasting.

Circulating ketone bodies increase in the fasting state or in diabetes mellitus whenever fat breakdown exceeds carbohydrate breakdown and result in increasing acidosis with ketones excreted in the urine and expired breath.

Protein metabolism

Amino acids are not stored in the body and are obtained from the diet, synthesized *de novo*, or obtained by protein degradation. Seventy-five per cent of amino acids obtained from hydrolysis of body protein are recaptured through biosynthesis of new tissue proteins and the balance is metabolized or used as precursors for other compounds. Metabolic loss of amino acids is replaced by dietary protein. Dietary protein is digested in the stomach and by pancreatic enzymes acting in the small intestine. The products of protein digestion—amino acids and di- or tripeptides—are absorbed in the small intestine and released into the portal system as amino acids. Glutamate and aspartate are utilized as energy sources but other amino acids may be released from the liver into the general circulation. The non-essential amino acids can be synthesized from intermediates of metabolism or from the essential amino acids which cannot be synthesized within the body and must be obtained in the diet. Amino acids which can be broken down to pyruvate or TCA cycle intermediates are classified as glucogenic as they can be used as substrates for gluconeogenesis and give rise to net formation of glucose or glycogen. Those that yield acetoacetate (a ketone body) or its precursors, acetyl CoA or acetoacetyl CoA, are termed ketogenic. The ketogenic amino acids cannot give rise to glucose or glycogen (see 'Further reading').

During amino acid catabolism, α-amino groups are removed and the C skeletons enter the pathways of intermediary metabolism (gluconeogenesis, TG synthesis, TCA cycle) (Figure 1.2.2.3). The nitrogen of the amino group can be incorporated into other compounds or excreted via the urea cycle. Aminotransferase enzymes catalyse the transfer of the amino groups from amino acids to an acceptor, usually α- ketoglutarate, forming glutamate. The main aminotransferases are alanine aminotransferase (ALT) which transfers the amino group of alanine to α-KG forming glutamate and pyruvate, and aspartate aminotransferase (AST) which transfers the amino group from glutamate to oxaloacetate forming aspartate and α-KG. As aminotransferases are usually found in the cytosol of cells, especially those of the liver, kidney, intestine, and muscle, the presence of aminotransferases in plasma indicates cell damage. Elevated plasma ALT and AST levels are a feature of most liver diseases.

The second step in amino acid catabolism is oxidative deamination of glutamate by glutamate dehydrogenase using NAD^+ or NADP as a coenzyme regenerating α-KG and releasing the amino group as free ammonia (NH_3). After a high-protein meal, the glutamate dehydrogenase reaction is in the direction of amino acid degradation and formation of NH_3 (oxidative deamination). The α-KG formed can then be used for energy production. However, reductive amination in the opposite direction by glutamate dehydrogenase can synthesize glutamate from α-KG and NH_3 which can be used for amino acid synthesis by aminotransferases. The direction of the glutamate dehydrogenase reaction depends on the concentration of glutamate, α-KG, and the ratio of $NAD(P)^+$ to $NAD(P)H$.

In the majority of tissues, glutamine synthetase forms glutamine from NH_3 and glutamate which acts as a non-toxic storage and transport form of NH_3. Glutamine formed is transported to the liver where it is cleaved to glutamate and NH_3 by glutaminase. NH_3 is disposed of in the urea cycle which takes place in the liver and the urea formed is excreted by the kidneys.

In muscle, alanine is formed from pyruvate by ALT and transported to the liver where it is converted to pyruvate which can be used in gluconeogenesis to synthesize glucose (glucose–alanine cycle; see 'Further reading' for more detail).

Integration of metabolic pathways

Regulation of metabolic pathways

In order for the body to meet its metabolic needs in different conditions, the metabolic pathways are tightly regulated at several levels. In addition to control of the individual pathways and reactions, coordination of metabolism requires interactions between the various tissues and organs of the body. Some individual reactions are controlled by substrate and/or product concentrations which in turn are dependent on enzyme kinetics and transport proteins. Allosteric effects (regulation by the binding of an effector molecule) regulate the activity of individual enzymes.

Two examples of enzymes regulated allosterically are 6-phosphofructo-1-kinase (PFK1) which phosphorylates fructose-6-phosphate to fructose 1,6-bisphosphate in glycolysis, and PDH which converts the end product of glycolysis—pyruvate—to acetyl CoA. PFK1 is inhibited allosterically by high levels of ATP present when the cells energy requirements are adequately met. PDH is inhibited allosterically by its products acetyl CoA and NADH and by high levels of ATP. PDH activity is also regulated by phosphorylation/dephosphorylation as are many enzymes. The availability of intermediates and oxygen influence metabolic activity. Oxygen, as the final electron acceptor of the ETC, regulates rates of glycolysis, the TCA cycle, and oxidative phosphorylation (ATP generation).

The hormonal and nervous systems[4] coordinate and regulate responses involving different tissues. Hormones regulate energy metabolism by phosphorylation/dephosphorylation of an enzyme, changing the rate of enzyme synthesis/degradation, and/or changing the concentration of an activator/inhibitor (see 'Further reading' for more detail).

Plasma glucose is maintained within a narrow range (fasting 4.5–5.6 mmol/L) primarily by the pancreatic hormones insulin and glucagon which are central to control of energy metabolism. Insulin is primarily an anabolic hormone and is countered by the catabolic hormones glucagon, epinephrine, and norepinephrine. At its simplest, the high insulin:glucagon ratio which exists during the 'fed' state promotes glycogen synthesis, glycolysis, and TG synthesis. Conversely, the low insulin:glucagon ratio which exists during the fasting state promotes glycogen breakdown, stimulates gluconeogenesis, suppresses glycolysis, and stimulates fatty acid oxidation and ketogenesis (Table 1.2.2.1).

Insulin affects carbohydrate, lipid, and protein metabolism. Insulin inhibits gluconeogenesis and glycogen breakdown and promotes glycogen synthesis in the liver. In muscle, glucose uptake in response to insulin stimulates glycogen synthesis and carbohydrate use as an energy source for muscle contraction. Insulin activates pyruvate dehydrogenase converting pyruvate to acetyl CoA which can enter the TCA cycle or be used for fatty acid synthesis. In adipose tissue, insulin suppresses breakdown of TGs and promotes fat synthesis. Insulin increases the number of glucose transporters

Table 1.2.2.1 Summary of effects of insulin and glucagon (epinephrine) on metabolic pathways. In the fed state, there is a high insulin:glucagon ratio as a consequence of increased insulin secretion in response to high postprandial glucose levels—overall response is anabolic. Conversely, during the fasting state, the insulin:glucagon ratio (and/or high epinephrine) is low and the overall response is catabolic

System	Fed state—high insulin:glucagon ratio	Fasting state—low insulin:glucagon ratio High epinephrine
Carbohydrate		
Glucose uptake (adipose, muscle)	Stimulates	Inhibits
Glycogen synthesis (muscle, liver)	Stimulates	Inhibits
Glycolysis (liver)	Stimulates	Inhibits
Gluconeogenesis (liver)	Inhibits	Stimulates
Pentose phosphate pathway (liver, adipose)	Stimulates	–
Fats		
Beta-oxidation (liver)	Inhibits	Stimulates
Triglyceride uptake from plasma (adipose)	Stimulates	Inhibits
Triglyceride synthesis (liver, adipose)	Stimulates	–
Triglyceride breakdown (adipose)	Inhibits	Stimulates
Ketogenesis (liver)	Inhibits	Stimulates
Cholesterol synthesis	Stimulates	–
Cholesterol ester breakdown	Inhibits	–
Proteins		
Protein synthesis (liver, muscle)	Stimulates	–
Proteolysis (muscle)	Inhibits	Stimulates
Amino acid degradation (liver)	Stimulates	

in the membrane of adipocytes which increases glucose uptake stimulating glycolysis which produces more DHAP from fructose-1,6-biphosphate which is converted to glycerol-3-phosphate for TG synthesis. Insulin stimulates amino acid uptake into cells and protein synthesis in many tissues and its major effect in protein metabolism is to inhibit protein breakdown.

Glucagon is secreted in response to falling blood glucose and amino acids. Sympathetic adrenergic activation also increases glucagon.[4] Glucagon antagonizes the effects of insulin and prevents hypoglycaemia during fasting. The liver is the primary site of glucagon action where it mobilizes glycogen and stimulates gluconeogenesis. Epinephrine, norepinephrine, and glucagon activate hormone-sensitive lipase promoting TG breakdown. Thus the sympathetic nervous system ensures that TGs are hydrolysed in response to cold, stress, and physical exertion. Glucagon increases proteolysis providing the liver with amino acids for gluconeogenesis.

Glycogen metabolism is controlled by phosphorylation/dephosphorylation of enzymes regulating glycogen synthesis and breakdown particularly glycogen synthase and glycogen phosphorylase (see 'Further reading').

The pathways of gluconeogenesis and glycogen metabolism are highly interconnected. The main source of glucose for glycogen synthesis in the liver is now believed to be gluconeogenic substrates—three-carbon compounds such as lactate, glycerol, alanine, and other glucogenic amino acids—rather than extracellular glucose. Gluconeogenic precursors form G6P which is used for glycogen synthesis.[3] The glycogen formed can then be broken down to provide glucose for release into the bloodstream by the liver or G6P for glycolysis in muscle. In muscle, glycogen metabolism integrates fuel utilization during exercise.[5]

Fed/postprandial state

Following a meal, plasma glucose, amino acids, and TGs (in the form of chylomicrons) are raised. High plasma glucose results in increased insulin secretion. The overall response is anabolic; glycogen synthesis, protein synthesis, and TG synthesis within the liver increase, TG synthesis increases in adipose tissue and protein synthesis increases in muscle. Glucose is used to generate energy via glycolysis, the TCA cycle, and oxidative phosphorylation. In the well-fed state, the high insulin:low glucagon ratio increases the activity of three glycolytic enzymes—glucokinase in the liver, phosphofructokinase, and pyruvate kinase-favouring glucose oxidation to pyruvate. After a high-carbohydrate meal, fatty acid levels are low and glucose is used in glycogen synthesis or fatty acid synthesis.

Fasting state

In the fasting state, several hours after eating a meal, plasma glucose, amino acids, and TGs are low. Insulin secretion falls and glucagon and epinephrine secretion increase. The overall response is catabolic; gluconeogenesis, glycogen breakdown, beta-oxidation of fatty acids, and ketogenesis are increased as well as lipolysis within the adipose tissue. Muscle tissue uses fatty acids and ketone bodies to generate energy and proteolysis supplies amino acids to the liver. The low insulin:high glucagon ratio inhibits the three enzymes glucokinase, phosphofructokinase, and pyruvate kinase reducing glycolysis.

Glycogen stores are depleted within 10–18 hours of fasting and blood glucose is then maintained by gluconeogenesis in the liver using amino acids from proteolysis in the muscle. After 2–3 weeks of fasting, the brain uses ketone bodies as well as glucose. The brain stores minimal TGs and fatty acids cannot cross the blood–brain barrier effectively. Most tissues (but not liver) can use ketone bodies reducing the need for gluconeogenesis from amino acids and therefore reducing proteolysis. Skeletal muscle uses predominantly fatty acids in early stages of fasting but can also use ketone bodies.

Vitamins, trace elements, and metabolic pathways

Vitamins cannot be synthesized by humans and are therefore required in the diet. They play key roles in metabolism and are required as co-factors for many enzymes including those of the metabolic pathways. Vitamins are classed as either water-soluble—folic acid, B_{12}, B_6, B_1, B_2, niacin, biotin, pantothenic acid, vitamin C—or lipid-soluble—vitamins A, D, K, and E. See 'Further reading' for full descriptions of role, signs, and symptoms of vitamin deficiency and treatment.

Trace elements such as iron, magnesium, copper, and selenium are essential nutrients that act as co-factors in enzyme oxidation–reduction reactions. They also function as prosthetic groups of proteins. For example, iron is required for haem biosynthesis and is an electron acceptor in complex I of the ETC. Copper is an electron acceptor in complex III.

Disorders of metabolism

Diabetes mellitus

The myriad complications of diabetes illustrate the critical role of insulin in regulating and coordinating metabolic pathways. Diabetes mellitus is characterized by hyperglycaemia resulting from defects in insulin production or activity (a random venous plasma glucose concentration of > 11.1 mmol/L or a fasting one > 10 mmol/L are diagnostic of diabetes mellitus).

Type 1 diabetes is mainly caused by autoimmune destruction of the insulin-producing β cells of the pancreatic islets whereas type 2 diabetes is caused by impaired insulin secretion or insulin resistance. As type 2 diabetes has a gradual onset, diagnosis is often delayed for years during which time diabetic complications develop. The increased incidence of obesity in society accounts for much of the increase in type 2 diabetes.[6]

Premature mortality in diabetics is usually due to atherosclerotic vascular disease but there is also significant morbidity through microvascular complications which affect the eye, kidney, and nerve tissue (see 'Further reading'). Hyperglycaemia affects a number of processes. Hepatic gluconeogenesis is increased in diabetics despite the high plasma glucose as in the absence of insulin, glucose cannot be transported into cells and the body interprets this as a lack of glucose. Increased gluconeogenesis combined with impaired glucose uptake into cells results in fasting hyperglycaemia. In addition, the absence of insulin results in decreased hepatic glucokinase activity contributing to the inability to regulate blood glucose levels. Chronic hyperglycaemia results in increased formation of advanced glycation end products (AGEs)[7] and glycated haemoglobin (HbA_{1C}) is a clinical marker of glycaemic control in diabetics (see 'Further reading'). AGEs activate monocytes[8] and endothelial cells which play a role in atherosclerotic disease, nephropathy, and retinopathy.[7] AGEs increase susceptibility of low-density lipoprotein to oxidation[9], one of the mechanisms of atherosclerosis,[10] and increased oxidative stress contributes to tissue damage and cell death associated with chronic hyperglycaemia.[7] Hyperglycaemia increases vascular endothelial growth factor in the retina which contributes to macular oedema.[8]

Insulin is not required for glucose entry into cells in the lens, retina, kidney, and Schwann cells so during hyperglycaemia large amounts of glucose can enter these cells and be converted to sorbitol. Osmotic effects of sorbitol accumulation may contribute to diabetic complications such as cataracts, peripheral neuropathy, and vascular problems. (Management of type 1 and type 2 diabetes is covered in the text by Hoogwerf[10] and the 'Further reading' texts.) Diabetic ketoacidosis is the most severe consequence of uncorrected hyperglycaemia. Infections and acute illnesses can precipitate diabetic ketoacidosis; stress may increase insulin requirement

and calorie intake may be reduced at such times. Fatty acids from increased lipolysis of TG in adipose tissue are transported to the liver and oxidized to acidic ketone bodies (e.g. acetoacetate and 3-hydroxybutyrate). These ketone bodies are exported from the liver as an alternative energy source but uptake into peripheral tissues is impaired due to lack of insulin. The build-up of ketone bodies in the circulation leads to severe metabolic acidosis which has a negative ionotropic effect on the heart and increases peripheral vasodilatation. Hyperkalaemia ensues as cells export potassium in exchange for hydrogen ions moving into the cell.

Hypoglycaemia is a common side effect of insulin therapy and more common in type 1 diabetics where there is an absolute insulin deficiency. In normal individuals, as blood glucose falls, insulin secretion falls and glucagon secretion increases. In diabetics, however, these mechanisms are not available. Autonomic symptoms occur due to activation of adrenergic and cholinergic parts of the autonomic system and neurological dysfunction because of inadequate glucose supply to the brain. If plasma glucose is not corrected, hypoglycaemia will ultimately result in coma, seizures, and death.

Obesity

Abdominal obesity is associated with a number of metabolic abnormalities—glucose intolerance, insulin resistance, hyperinsulinaemia, dyslipidaemia, and hypertension—termed metabolic syndrome—which increases the risk of cardiovascular disease and type 2 diabetes in obese individuals.[11] The body mass index (BMI) is calculated using weight in kg divided by height in metres squared. Obesity is defined as a BMI > 30 with 20–25 kg/m² regarded as a normal range.

Inborn errors of metabolism

Most inborn errors of metabolism (IEMs) are due to mutations in the nuclear genome inherited in Mendelian patterns whereas those due to mutations in the mitochondrial genome are maternally transmitted. Mutations which give rise to the IEMs affect primary, secondary, tertiary, or quaternary structure of proteins involved in the metabolic pathways including enzymes, activators, and transport proteins. IEMs affecting carbohydrate, fat, and protein metabolism have been identified (see 'Further reading') and details of individual IEMs can be found in the Online Mendelian Inheritance in Man database.[12] Diagnosis of IEMs can be challenging as symptoms are often vague so a high degree of suspicion and family history are invaluable in reaching a diagnosis. Most IEMs cannot be cured but can often be managed by restricting a substrate that cannot be metabolized or replacing a metabolic product that cannot be synthesized if the specific biochemical abnormality is identified.

Some examples include familial hypercholesterolaemia with an incidence of 1/500; and phenylketonuria (1/10 000). The glycogen storage diseases (all types) only occur in 1/50 000. However, there is considerable variation in the incidence of these conditions in different countries and different ethnic groups.

Further reading

Champe PC, Harvey RA, Ferrier DR. *Lippincott's Illustrated Reviews: Biochemistry* (3rd ed). Philadelphia, PA: Lippincott, Williams & Wilkins; 2005.

or without plasma protein loss.[4] Conditions such as pancreatitis, peritonitis, and burns tend to have high plasma protein loss, while vomiting and diarrhoea, excessive nasogastric and fistula losses, sodium-losing nephropathy, and the use of diuretics tend to be associated with low plasma protein losses.

Physiological responses to hypovolaemia

The physiological response to intravascular depletion is complex and includes immediate and delayed responses.

Immediate response

The immediate response to the loss of intravascular volume occurs within minutes. Reduction in blood volume leads to a fall in venous return, and with it cardiac filling. Atrial pressures fall, causing the activation of low-pressure receptors within the walls of the atria, the pulmonary arteries, great veins, and ventricles. Reduced cardiac preload reduces SV and consequently CO. The reduction in arterial pulse pressure that results produces activation of the high-pressure stretch receptors in the aortic arch and the carotid sinus, that is, these arterial baroreceptors are stretched to a lesser degree.[2] This produces a reduction in parasympathetic stimulation to the heart, with a simultaneous enhanced sympathetic drive to heart and vasculature.[5] Tachycardia and increased myocardial contractility occur, along with widespread vasoconstriction that spares only the vessels of the heart and brain. Vasoconstriction is most marked in the skin, kidneys, and the viscera. In the kidneys, both afferent and efferent arterioles are constricted, with the efferent arterioles to a greater degree. The glomerular filtration rate is reduced, but as the renal plasma flow is decreased to a greater degree, the filtration fraction actually increases.[2] However, very little urine is produced and sodium retention is marked.

There is also an increase in venous tone. This helps to reduce venous capacitance and mobilizes the venous reservoir.

In the event of continuing hypovolaemia, a second paradoxical reflex may be seen that supersedes the baroreceptor reflex.[5] This reflex leads to vagal activation, with consequent bradycardia, and inhibition of sympathetic activity, producing a fall in peripheral resistance and hypotension. This reflex is likely to be protective as it allows for prolonged diastolic filling, prolonged coronary artery perfusion, and a reduction in afterload, thus reducing cardiac work at a time when coronary perfusion is becoming inadequate. This reflex is reversible in the event of restoration of intravascular volume, and may not even be seen in the trauma victim with multiple injuries, as the response to musculoskeletal injury seems to block the increased vagal activity and maintains a high degree of sympathetic activity.[6]

Levels of circulating epinephrine and norepinephrine are elevated in response to adrenal medullary stimulation and as a result of the increased discharge of sympathetic noradrenergic neurons.[2] The increased levels of circulating catecholamines probably contribute relatively little to the ongoing widespread vasoconstriction, but may lead to stimulation of the reticular formation. It may be because of such reticular formation stimulation that some patients are restless and apprehensive.[2]

The chemoreceptors of the carotid and aortic bodies are stimulated in the event of severe hypotension (e.g. MAP of 50 mmHg),[4] but also in response to the reduced oxygen-carrying power of the blood that occurs with the loss of red cells. Stimulation of the chemoreceptors will add to the sympathetic response (via the vasomotor centre in the medulla), and increased activity in chemoreceptor afferents is probably the main cause of respiratory stimulation in shock.[2]

Hypovolaemia will also activate the renin–angiotensin–aldosterone system. Increased levels of angiotensin II contribute to the widespread vasoconstriction and promote thirst. Levels of aldosterone rise, promoting renal retention of sodium and water, although this effect may be delayed by at least 30 minutes.[2]

Delayed response

Capillary pressure drops with hypovolaemia due to the drop in venous pressure, and also with the arteriolar constriction that occurs as part of the immediate response as described earlier. As a result, fluid moves into the capillaries from the interstitium.

There is also a movement of protein, mainly albumin, from the interstitium to the plasma, that increases the colloid oncotic pressure within the capillaries. This further encourages the movement of interstitial fluid into the capillaries.

Glucocorticoid secretion is raised during hypovolaemic shock, producing an elevation in blood glucose.[4] Blood volume may also be replaced in part by the osmotic effect exerted by the elevated blood glucose.

In the long term, there is an increase in the circulating levels of erythropoietin, with a consequent rise in the reticulocyte count that reaches a peak after 10 days.[2]

Clinical presentation

The clinical features of hypovolaemic shock include cold, pale, clammy skin; tachycardia (although bradycardia is also possible, as described earlier); hypotension; tachypnoea; altered levels of mental status (agitation, anxiety, confusion, and even stupor); and reduced urinary output. Hypoperfusion will also be reflected by a rise in lactic acid as aerobic metabolism is overtaken by anaerobic metabolism.

Hypovolaemic shock secondary to blood loss has been classified into four classes, according to the patient's clinical signs, as a tool for estimating the percentage of acute blood loss (Table 1.2.3.2).[1]

These clinical signs are not invariably present. Individual responses to hypovolaemia may vary considerably. This classification of hypovolaemic shock secondary to blood loss is useful as a guide but is not applicable to every patient, and indeed its validity in accurately reflecting clinical reality has been questioned.[7,8]

Management

The treatment goals for hypovolaemic shock are to restore intravascular volume and to prevent further fluid loss.[9]

The choice of fluid used to restore intravascular volume will depend on the cause of the hypovolaemic shock. For example, shock secondary to blood loss should be treated with blood products, while shock resulting from vomiting and diarrhoea should be treated with crystalloid solutions.

Delaying restoration of intravascular volume in severely injured trauma patients until haemostasis has been achieved has been associated with improved outcomes.[10] In these patients, a period of permissive hypovolaemia (or hypotension) is allowable, but it should be kept to an absolute minimum, and if severe hypotension occurs fluid resuscitation may be required before it is possible to achieve haemostasis.

Table 1.2.3.2 Estimated blood loss based on patient's initial presentation

	Class I	Class II	Class III	Class IV
Blood loss (mL)	Up to 750	750–1500	1500–2000	>2000
Blood loss (% blood volume)	Up to 15%	15–30%	30–40%	>40%
Pulse rate (bpm)	<100	100–120	120–140	>140
Blood pressure (mmHg)	Normal	Normal	Decreased	Decreased
Respiratory rate (breaths/min)	14–20	20–30	30–40	>35
Urine output (mL/h)	>30	20–30	5–15	Negligible
Central nervous system/mental status	Slightly anxious	Mildly anxious	Anxious, confused	Confused, lethargic
Fluid replacement	Crystalloid	Crystalloid	Crystalloid and blood	Crystalloid and blood

Reproduced with permission from American College of Surgeons Committee on Trauma, *Advanced Trauma Life Support for Doctors*, Ninth Edition, American College of Surgeons, Chicago, USA, Copyright © 2012.

Septic shock

Definitions

Distributive (or low resistance) shock occurs when the blood volume is normal but the capacity of the circulation increases by vasodilation.[2] This is often caused by the systemic inflammatory response syndrome (SIRS). SIRS is a clinical syndrome characterized by, but not limited to, two or more of the following:[11]

1. Temperature greater than 38°C or less than 36°C

2. Heart rate greater than 90 bpm

3. Respiratory rate greater than 20 breaths/min or $PaCO_2$ less than 4.3 kPa (32 mmHg)

4. White cell count less than 4×10^9/L or greater than 12×10^9/L.

SIRS is caused by widespread inflammation due to infectious and non-infectious processes (e.g. pancreatitis and anaphylaxis).

Sepsis is defined as the presence of infection (probable or documented) together with systemic manifestations of infection, that is, infection plus SIRS.[12] Severe sepsis is defined as sepsis plus sepsis-induced organ dysfunction or tissue hypoperfusion.[12] Sepsis-induced tissue hypoperfusion is defined as infection-induced hypotension, elevated lactic acid, or oliguria, while sepsis-induced hypotension is defined as a systolic of less than 90 mmHg (or a reduction greater than 40 mmHg from baseline), or MAP less than 70 mmHg.[12] Septic shock, then, is sepsis-induced hypotension that persists despite adequate fluid resuscitation. Severe sepsis and septic shock affect millions of people around the world each year and kill at least one in four of these patients.[12]

Pathophysiology

The pathophysiology of sepsis and septic shock is extremely complex, and involves the interaction of cellular and inflammatory mediators (see Figure 1.2.3.1).[13] The inflammatory cascade is triggered by infective pathogens, of which the lipopolysaccharide derived from the cell wall of Gram-negative bacteria, endotoxin, is thought to be particularly important.[11] When bacterial fragments attach to lipopolysaccharide-binding proteins, a complex is formed which stimulates macrophages to release pro-inflammatory

mediators, including the cytokines tumour necrosis factor alpha and interleukin (IL)-1, IL-6, and IL-8, along with platelet activating factor.[13] These mediators then promote the synthesis of prostaglandins from arachidonic acid (via activation of cyclooxygenase), enhance the synthesis of nitric oxide (via both constitutive and inducible forms of nitric oxide synthase), increase the release of lysosomal enzymes from neutrophils, and cause activation of the complement and coagulation cascades.[11]

The overall effects produced include:[2,11,14]

- fever
- vasodilation
- endothelial damage with increased capillary permeability
- platelet aggregation and activation
- disseminated intravascular coagulation
- myocardial depression with coronary vasoconstriction
- defective cellular oxygen utilization.

The sympathoadrenal and neuroendocrine responses that occur in response to hypovolaemic shock will also occur with septic shock. In septic shock, however, these responses are insufficient to overcome the vasodilation that occurs once the inflammatory cascade has been triggered, and can do little to overcome many of the other pathophysiological aspects of septic shock.

Clinical presentation

The clinical features of septic shock include those features characteristic of the underlying disorder (e.g. peritonitis, pyelonephritis, and pneumonia) in addition to the features of SIRS outlined earlier, and other, more specific features.[11]

In the early stages of septic shock, vasodilation and a relative hypovolaemia, due to increased capillary permeability, produce warm peripheries, a rapid capillary refill time, along with tachycardia (often the pulse is bounding) and hypotension. As time progresses, a certain amount of peripheral vasoconstriction may occur, which, in conjunction with myocardial depression and loss of intravascular fluid results in cold peripheries and hypotension,

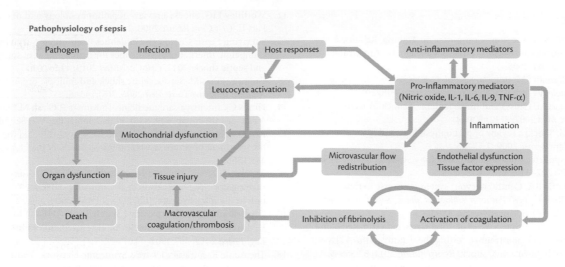

Fig. 1.2.3.1 The pathophysiology of sepsis.

Reprinted from *Anaesthesia and Intensive Care Medicine*, Volume 7, Issue 5, Gupta S, and Jonas M., Sepsis, septic shock and multiple organ failure, pp. 143–146, Copyright © 2006 The Medicine Publishing Company Ltd., with permission from Elsevier, http://www.sciencedirect.com/science/journal/14720299

along with tachycardia, tachypnoea, altered mental status, reduced urinary output, and raised levels of lactic acid.

In addition, patients may present with thrombocytopenia, disordered coagulation, jaundice, reduced serum albumin levels, and, due to defective cellular oxygen utilization, abnormalities in central venous oxygen saturation (ScvO$_2$).[13]

Box 1.2.3.1 Surviving Sepsis Campaign Care Bundles

To be completed within 3 hours

1. Measure lactate level

2. Obtain blood cultures prior to administration of antibiotics

3. Administer broad-spectrum antibiotics

4. Administer 30 mL/kg crystalloid for hypotension or lactate 4 mmol/L.

To be completed within 6 hours

5. Apply vasopressors (for hypotension that does not respond to initial fluid resuscitation) to maintain a mean arterial pressure (MAP) ≥ 65 mmHg

6. In the event of persistent arterial hypotension despite volume resuscitation (septic shock) or initial lactate 4 mmol/L (36 mg/dL):
   • Measure central venous pressure (CVP)*
   • Measure central venous oxygen saturation (ScvO$_2$)*

7. Remeasure lactate if initial lactate was elevated.*

*Targets for quantitative resuscitation included in the guidelines are CVP of ≥8 mm Hg, ScvO$_2$ of 70%, and normalization of lactate.

Reproduced from Dellinger P *et al.*, Surviving Sepsis. Campaign: International Guidelines for Management of Severe Sepsis and Septic Shock, *Critical Care Medicine*, Volume 41, Number 2, pp. 580–637, Copyright © 2012 with permission from Lippincott Williams & Wilkins.

Management

Management priorities in septic shock include:[13]

♦ early recognition and resuscitation

♦ early, appropriate use of antimicrobials (after obtaining specimens for culture)

♦ source control (i.e. searching for and treating a focus of infection)

♦ support for failing organ systems.

The Surviving Sepsis Campaign is an international collaboration that exists to raise awareness of sepsis, to improve diagnosis, and to improve treatment through the development of guidelines of care that are updated regularly. Recent guidelines highlight the importance of early recognition and resuscitation to specific goals (see Box 1.2.3.1),[12] well recognized for some time as a means to reducing mortality and improving outcomes in these patients.[15] Initial resuscitation fluid should be crystalloid,[12] unless large quantities of fluid are required, in which case the colloid of choice should be albumin.[12,16] Starch-based colloids should be avoided.[12,17] Norepinephrine is the initial vasopressor of choice.[12]

Following initial resuscitation and treatment of infection, the focus of management should be on the support of organ systems. A protective ventilation strategy should be employed for lungs affected with sepsis-induced acute respiratory distress syndrome,[12,18] renal replacement therapy may be required for failing kidneys, and red blood cell transfusion may be required to optimize oxygen delivery to tissues.[12] Prophylaxis should be provided against stress ulcers and venous thromboembolism, and blood glucose levels should be maintained at less than 10 mmol/L.[12,19]

Further reading

Guidelines Committee of the European Society of Anaesthesiology.
   Management of severe perioperative bleeding. *Eur J Anaesthesiol* 2013;
   30:270–382.

References

1. American College of Surgeons Committee on Trauma. *Advanced Trauma Life Support for Doctors* (8th ed). Chicago, IL: American College of Surgeons; 2008.
2. Barrett KE, Barman SM, Boitano S, *et al.* (eds). *Ganong's Review of Medical Physiology* (24th ed). New York: McGraw-Hill; 2012.
3. Skinner B, Jonas M. Causes and management of shock. *Anaesth Intensive Care Med* 2007; 8(12):520–4.
4. Worthley LIG. Shock: a review of pathophysiology and management. Part I. *Crit Care Resusc* 2000; 2:55–65.
5. Kirkman E. Applied cardiovascular physiology. *Anaesth Intensive Care Med* 2007; 8(6):227–31.
6. Kirkman E, Little RA. Central nervous system response to trauma. In Schlag G, Redl H (eds) *Pathophysiology of Shock, Sepsis and Organ Failure* (pp. 352–70). Springer-Verlag, 1993.
7. Guly HR, Bouamra O, Spiers M, *et al.* Vital signs and estimated blood loss in patients with major trauma: testing the validity of the ATLS classification of hypovolaemic shock. *Resuscitation* 2011; 82:556–9.
8. Mutschler M, Nienaber U, Brockamp T, *et al.* A critical reappraisal of the ATLS classification of hypovolaemic shock: does it really reflect clinical reality? *Resuscitation* 2013; 84:309–13.
9. Society of Critical Care Medicine. *Fundamental Critical Care Support: A Standardised Curriculum of the Principles of Critical Care* (3rd ed). Des Plaines, IL: Society of Critical Care Medicine; 2001.
10. Harris T, Rhys Thomas GO, Brohi K. Early fluid resuscitation in severe trauma. *BMJ* 2012; 345:e5752.
11. Worthley LIG. Shock: a review of pathophysiology and management. Part II. *Crit Care Resusc* 2000; 2:66–84.
12. Surviving Sepsis Campaign Guidelines Committee. Surviving Sepsis Campaign: international guidelines for management of severe sepsis and septic shock: 2012. *Crit Care Med* 2013; 41:580–637.
13. Gupta S, Jonas M. Sepsis, septic shock and multiple organ failure. *Anaesth Intensive Care Med* 2006; 7(5):143–6.
14. Hinds CJ. Intensive care medicine. In Kumar P, Clark M (eds) *Clinical Medicine* (4th ed, pp. 829–836). Philadelphia, PA: WB Saunders; 2001.
15. Rivers E, Nguyen B, Havstad S, *et al.* Early goal-directed therapy in the treatment of severe sepsis and septic shock. *N Engl J Med* 2001; 345:1368–77.
16. The Saline versus Albumin Fluid Evaluation (SAFE) Study Investigators. A Comparison of albumin and saline for fluid resuscitation in the intensive care unit. *N Engl J Med* 2004; 350:2247–56.
17. Crystalloid versus Hydroxyethyl Starch Trial (CHEST) Investigators. Hydroxyethyl starch or saline for fluid resuscitation in intensive care. *N Engl J Med* 2012; 367:1901–11.
18. The Acute Respiratory Distress Syndrome Network. Ventilation with lower tidal volumes as compared with traditional tidal volumes for acute lung injury and the acute respiratory distress syndrome. *N Engl J Med* 2000; 342:1301–8.
19. The Normoglycaemia in Intensive Care Evaluation-Survival Using Glucose Algorithm Regulation (NICE-SUGAR) Study Investigators. Intensive versus conventional glucose control in critically ill patients. *N Engl J Med* 2009; 360:1283–97.

CHAPTER 1.2.4

Fluid and electrolyte balance and replacement: acid–base balance

Catriona Kelly, Rosalind O' Reilly, and Brian Mullan

Physiology of fluid balance

Fluid homeostasis in the normal adult

Water accounts for 60% of the total adult body weight. In a 70 kg male, the total body water (TBW) is 42 L (NB 1 L of saline weighs ~ 1 kg). Two-thirds is in the intracellular volume (= 28 L) and one-third in the extracellular volume (14 L), of which 11.0 L is in the interstitial fluid and 3.0 L in the plasma.

For normal values see Table 1.2.4.1 and for fluid and electrolyte distribution throughout the compartments see Figure 1.2.4.1.[1–3] Water is present in all compartments and moves freely within these compartments due to changes in the osmotic gradients. Thirst controls the input of fluid and is stimulated by a rising plasma osmolality acting on osmoreceptors in the thirst centre in the hypothalamus and by hypovolaemia via the renin–angiotensin system. In addition, fluid output is hormonally controlled. An increase in serum osmolality or a decrease in circulating blood volume will cause the release of antidiuretic hormone (ADH) from the posterior pituitary, causing water to be reabsorbed from the collecting ducts of the kidney.

The normal daily requirement for water reflects the inevitable losses from the body:

♦ Output:
  • Transpiration is responsible for 500 mL each day but there may be much more with increased perspiration in a hot environment or a pyrexial patient.
  • Expired air accounts for 500 mL. A further 100 mL is lost in faeces. A minimum obligatory 500 mL is lost in urine, though the loss in a normal individual is about 1 L. The normal glomerular filtration rate is 170 L/24 h.

♦ Input:
  • The average person drinks about 1.5 L of fluid each day and gets another 0.5 L from food. There is also a contribution from the metabolic oxidation of food, for example, 100 g of fat will yield 100 g of water and 100 g of starch will give 55 g of water.
  • Large volumes of fluids are secreted and then largely reabsorbed each day, for example, in the gastrointestinal tract: saliva 1.5 L, gastric juice 3.0 L, pancreatic juice 1.0 L, bile 0.5 L, and intestinal juice 3.0 L.

Fluid and electrolyte loss and replacement in the surgical patient

The stress response from surgery or trauma leads to increased levels of circulating catecholamines, aldosterone, cortisol, and ADH. This can lead to sodium and water retention postoperatively and since there is relatively more water retention than sodium retention there is a risk of postoperative hyponatraemia.[4,5]

Postoperative fluid replacement is calculated to replace any specific losses such as drainage from fistulae as well as what is required to replace normal losses (Table 1.2.4.2). In addition, appropriate electrolyte replacement is needed. The average adult patient who is on a 'nil by mouth' regimen after surgery will require about 2.5 L of water each 24 hour (~1.5 mL/kg/h) with suitable electrolyte replacement. Table 1.2.4.3 shows that 1 L normal saline contains 154 mmol of sodium chloride, which is about 6 g, enough for a

Table 1.2.4.1 Normal values

Serum		Arterial blood gases		Urine	
Sodium	135–145 mmol/L	PCO_2	4.5–6.0 kPa	pH	4.6–8.0
Potassium	3.5–5.0 mmol/L	PO_2	11–15 kPa	Osmolality	450–1200 mosmol/L
Chloride	100–108 mmol/L	pH	7.36–7.46		
Osmolality	280–295 mosmol/L	Bicarbonate	22–30 mmol/L		
		Lactate	0.5–2.2 mmol/L		
		Base excess (negative/positive in metabolic acidosis/alkalosis)	−2 to +2		

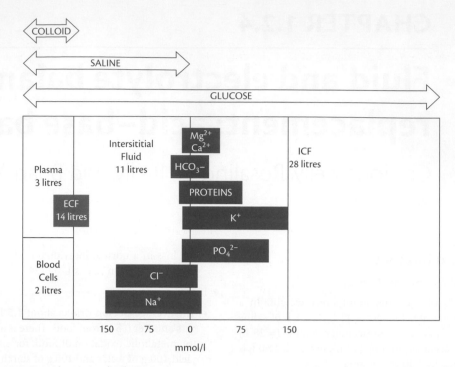

Fig. 1.2.4.1 Body fluid compartments with main ion distribution.

ECF, extracellular fluid; ICF, intracellular fluid.

Reproduced from Doherty M and Buggy DJ, Intraoperative fluids: how much is too much?, *British Journal of Anaesthesia*, Volume 109, Issue 1, pp. 69–79, Copyright © 2012 British Journal of Anaesthesia, with permission from Oxford University Press.

normal daily replacement. A 5% dextrose solution effectively only replaces water loss. If there are electrolyte-containing losses from the gastrointestinal tract then more normal saline together with potassium replacement should be used. Losses due to diarrhoeal illness can cause profound hypokalaemia.

Pyrexia can increase insensible fluid loss by 20% for every degree in Celsius above normal body temperature. An adult can lose 1000 mL per day at normal temperatures through exhalation, which is mainly water vapour, and sweat, which is rich in electrolytes.

In the septic patient or the trauma patient, the purpose of administering fluids in the resuscitation phase is to restore an adequate circulating volume to maintain perfusion pressure, thus ensuring optimum oxygen delivery to end organs. 'Third-space' losses are fluids lost from the intravascular compartment due to trauma or sepsis-induced increased capillary permeability. Large volumes of fluid can be sequestered in the bowel lumen or the peritoneal cavity.[7] See Table 1.2.4.4.

The shocked patient will start to rely on anaerobic metabolism leading to increased production of lactic acid and causing the patient to become acidaemic.

Table 1.2.4.2 Composition of body fluids

Types of fluid	Na (mmol/L)	K (mmol/L)	Protein (g/L)
Serum	135–145	3.5–5.3	70
Nasogastric losses and vomit	60–120	5–10	Minimal
Diarrhoea	80	25–40	Minimal
Third space losses	135–145	3.5–5.3	10–20

Source: data from Wilson WA *et al.*, Peri-operative fluid balance, *Update in Anaesthesia*, Number 20, pp. 11–20, Copyright © 2005.

End points of fluid resuscitation include:

- lactate less than 2.5 mmol/L
- systolic blood pressure greater than 120 mmHg
- mean arterial blood pressure greater than 70 mmHg
- urine output greater than 0.5 mL/kg/h.

Types of fluid for intravenous use

There are three main types of intravenous fluids available to administer: crystalloids, colloids, and blood products. Each will be examined in detail in the following sections. In choosing the appropriate fluid it is important to consider the constituents of the body fluid being lost and try to match the replacement fluid type accordingly.[7] See Table 1.2.4.2.

The different intravenous fluids administered enter the compartments to varying degrees. The electrolyte composition of body fluids is different within each compartment. See Figure 1.2.4.1.

Crystalloid

Crystalloids are aqueous solutions containing dissolved salts or sugars. They distribute evenly throughout the extracellular space. They can be isotonic, hypotonic, or hypertonic.

The most commonly used isotonic crystalloids are normal saline and Hartmann's solution. Being isotonic means they do not cause the loss or gain of water by osmosis. After a rapid infusion of 2000 mL of normal saline (0.9%) or Hartmann's solution, 24% and 18%, respectively, will remain in the intravascular circulation at 1 hour and 22% and 14% at 6 hours.

Crystalloid solutions have the advantage of a long shelf life, they are cheap, and there is no risk of anaphylaxis. Normal saline contains 154 mmol/L sodium and chloride (about 6 g of sodium chloride). If large volumes of normal saline alone are administered, the patient may develop a hyperchloraemic metabolic acidosis. Hartmann's is

Table 1.2.4.3 Electrolyte composition of common crystalloid solutions

Crystalloid solution	Sodium (mmol/L)	Chloride (mmol/L)	Dextrose (mmol/L)	Calcium (mmol/L)	Potassium (mmol/L)	Lactate (mmol/L)
0.9% sodium chloride ('normal saline')	154	154	–	–	–	–
5% dextrose	–	–	278	–	–	–
Dextrose-saline	30	30	222	–	–	–
Hartmann's solution	131	111	–	2.0	5.0	29

a suitable alternative with 131 mmol/L sodium, 110 mmol/L chloride, and 5.0 mmmol/L K^+.

A 5% dextrose solution is a hypotonic crystalloid, once administered it behaves like water and is distributed through all compartments. Its use is limited to correct dehydration, as the administration of water intravenously causes haemolysis.

Hypertonic saline (1.8%, 2.7%, or 30%) is only used in specialized units and its main uses currently are as osmotherapy for patients with cerebral oedema or for the correction of symptomatic hyponatraemia. Specialist advice should be sought in these situations.[6]

Colloid

Colloids are fluids which contain small molecules dispersed in a continuous fluid phase. They exert an osmotic effect as their molecules are too large to cross the endothelium. Gelofusine®, one of the original semisynthetic colloids, was derived from bovine collagen. It was the most commonly used colloid in the United Kingdom but its use was associated with anaphylactoid reactions. The newer colloids are starches derived from maize. They are suspended in carrier solutions with electrolyte compositions similar to plasma. The advantage of these colloids is a lower risk of anaphylactoid reaction; they are relatively inexpensive and have a long shelf life. The incidence of pruritus is higher in this group (13%) and there is evidence to suggest the use of colloids in sepsis may increase the risk of acute kidney injury.[5,6]

Human albumin is a human plasma derivative. The preparation with a concentration of 4.5% is iso-oncotic and the one at 20% is hyperoncotic but salt-poor and so causes movement of water to the intravascular compartment. It is less useful in sepsis where 32% leaves the circulation via leaky capillaries. Anaphylactoid reactions are rare as is pruritus and kidney injury. It is relatively expensive and there is a risk of transmission of new variant Creutzfeldt–Jacob disease.[6]

Blood products

Blood products may be thought of as biological colloids, these include whole blood, red blood cells, fresh frozen plasma (FFP),

and albumin. Whole blood is the ideal resuscitation fluid with the combination of red cells and clotting factors—this is increasingly the fluid of choice in military trauma resuscitation.[5,6]

Blood component transfusion, however, is more widely used in most other settings. This is especially useful when resources are limited allowing specific components to be transfused depending on clinical need.

All red cells preparations in the United Kingdom are leucocyte depleted. The red cells are stored in a SAGM solution (saline, adenine, glucose, and mannitol). These can be stored for up to 35 days. Transfusion indications are decided according to local policy and take into account the co-morbidities and age of the patient as well as their current physiology and stability.

Platelets are usually transfused to a target of 75×10^9/L in the bleeding patient and to a count of 100×10^9/L in the patient with traumatic or haemorrhagic brain injury. Platelets are pooled from several donors and carry a higher risk of transfusion-related lung injury. Each bag transfused should increase the platelet count by 20×10^9/L.

FFP is a volume-expanding resuscitation fluid and its use in the massive transfusion protocol is increasing with many trauma units now adopting a 1:1:1 transfusion of red cells:platelets:FFP policy. FFP is produced from the centrifugation of whole blood. It contains factor VIII and fibrinogen.

Cryoprecipitate is rich in factors VII and VIII as well as von Willebrand factor and fibrinogen. It is predominantly used for correction of coagulopathy associated with disseminated intravascular coagulation.

Acid–base balance

Acid–base balance is regulated within a narrow range by buffer systems. Acid–base disorders are either respiratory or metabolic in origin.

Hydrogen ion concentration

The concentration of hydrogen ions even in very acidic solutions is very low and very small changes result in major shifts between alkali and acid solutions. A logarithmic scale (called pH) allows a simpler numerical representation of this concentration with a tenfold change in concentration for each unit change in pH,[1,9] for example, hydrogen ion concentration [H^+] in mol/L and equivalent pH:

$$10^{-6} \text{ mol/L} = \log_{10}[1/10^{-6}] = \text{pH } 6$$

$$10^{-7} \text{ mol/L} = \log_{10}[1/10^{-7}] = \text{pH } 7$$

$$10^{-8} \text{ mol/L} = \log_{10}[1/10^{-8}] = \text{pH } 8$$

Table 1.2.4.4 Acid–base disturbance demonstrating the primary abnormality and the compensatory mechanism

Disorder	Primary abnormality	Compensation
Metabolic acidosis	↓ [HCO_3^-]	↓ PCO_2
Metabolic alkalosis	↑ [HCO_3^-]	↑ PCO_2
Respiratory acidosis	↑ PCO_2	↑ [HCO_3^-]
Respiratory alkalosis	↓ PCO_2	↓ [HCO_3^-]

Source: data from Corke CF, and Jackson IJB, *Companion to Clinical Anaesthesia Exams*, pp. 171–173, Churchill Livingstone, UK, Copyright © 1994.

The numerical value of pH is a figure expressing the acidity or alkalinity of a solution on a logarithmic scale on which 7 is neutral.

Normal body pH as measured from arterial plasma is 7.40 with an acceptable range[1] of 7.35–7.45. A pH below 7.35 represents acidosis and a pH above 7.45 represents alkalosis. The approximate pH compatible with life is approximately pH 6.8–7.8.[1]

Intracellular pH reflects, but is different from, the extracellular value. Measurement is difficult and rarely undertaken clinically.

Buffers

Normal acid–base balance is regulated by buffer systems, for example, the H^+ concentration is maintained within strict limits by buffering of H^+ ions or elimination of H^+ ions.[9]

A buffer is a substance that is able to bind or release H^+ in solution and can therefore allow a solution to resist any change in acid–base balance.[1,9] A buffer system typically consists of a weak acid, its salt, and its conjugate base and is able to keep the pH of a solution relatively constant despite the addition of considerable quantities of acid or base.[1,9]

There are three main buffer systems: the blood (plasma) buffer system, the respiratory buffer system which excretes CO_2, and the renal buffer system which is responsible for the absorption or excretion of acids, bases, and ions.

Brønsted acid–base model

An acid is a substance that can be a proton donor (H^+) while a base is a substance that can accept protons.[10]

$$HB \text{ (acid)} \leftrightarrow H^+ \text{(proton)} + B^- \text{(base)}$$

A strong acid is one that completely dissociates, for example, hydrochloric acid (HCl) and a weak acid is one that only partly dissociates, for example, carbonic acid (H_2CO_3).[1,10]

Weak acids and their conjugate bases are buffer systems in the body. If H^+ is added to the body it can combine with the base to produce more acid, driving the earlier-given equation to the left, therefore removing H^+ from solution which will limit the increase in H^+ producing less of a pH drop than would have occurred.[1,10]

If H^+ is removed from this system (i.e. if OH^- is added H_2O is formed), the equation will be driven to the right, the acid will dissociate and will release protons (H^+), which will limit the decrease in H^+ concentration thereby limiting the increase in pH.[1,10]

Henderson–Hasselbalch equation

The law of mass action states that the rate of any given chemical reaction is proportional to the product of the concentrations of the reactions.[1,9]

That is, at equilibrium, the earlier-mentioned reaction can be expressed as follows:

$$[H^+]\,[Base^-] = K_a[Acid]$$

where K_a is the dissociation constant for the acid.

Rearranging this equation:

$$[H^+] = K_a[Acid]/[Base^-]$$

Take $\log_{10}$ of this equation and multiply by −1:

$$-\log_{10}[H^+] = -\log_{10}K_a - \log_{10}[Acid] / [Base^-]$$

as by definition $pH = -\log_{10}$ of the $[H^+]$

and $pK_a = -\log_{10}K_a$

This gives the Henderson–Hasselbalch equation:

$$pH = pK_a + \log_{10}[Base^-] / [Acid]$$

which can be applied to the buffer systems in the body.[1,10]

Buffer systems in the blood

The main components of blood buffering are the carbonic acid/bicarbonate system, the plasma protein system, and haemoglobin.

The effectiveness of buffer systems is determined by the pK_a and the closer it is to the physiological pH, the more effective is the system. The pK_a of the bicarbonate system is 6.1 but because of its dual role in kidneys and lungs it accounts for 65% of total buffering capacity. This and the other important blood and extracellular buffer systems are discussed in the following sections.

Carbonic acid—bicarbonate buffer system

$$CO_2 + H_2O \leftrightarrow H_2CO_3 \leftrightarrow H^+ + HCO_3^-$$

The weak acid carbonic acid is only partly dissociated into H^+ and bicarbonate and is an ideal buffer system. The reaction is catalysed by the enzyme carbonic anhydrase, which is absent in plasma, and abundant in red blood cells, gastric acid-secreting cells, and in renal tubular cells.[1,9,10]

Applying the Henderson–Hasselbalch equation for this system, we get:

$$pH = pK_a + \log[HCO_3^-] / [H_2CO_3]$$

In the body, H_2CO_3 is in equilibrium with dissolved CO_2:[1,9,10]

$$H_2CO_3 = K[CO_2] \text{ where } K \text{ is another equilibrium constant.}$$

The amount of dissolved CO_2 is proportional to the partial pressure of CO_2, that is, the PCO_2.[1,9,10]

Therefore the Henderson–Hasselbalch equation for the bicarbonate system can be expressed as:

$$pH = pK' + \log_{10}[HCO_3^-]/[PCO_2]$$

Plasma pH in this setting can therefore be controlled by HCO_3^- and PCO_2, which can be regulated by the respiratory and renal systems:[1,10]

* The amount of dissolved CO_2, that is, the PCO_2, can be controlled by respiration
* The plasma concentration of HCO_3^- can be controlled by the kidneys.

If H^+ is added to a solution the equilibrium shifts to the left and most of the added H^+ is removed from solution:[1,10]

* $H^+ + HCO_3^-$ causes a decline in HCO_3^- and more H_2CO_3 is formed

- The additional H_2CO_3 is converted to H_2O and CO_2, which can be excreted by the lungs

- The rise in H^+ also stimulates respiration, increasing respiratory rate, producing a drop in PCO_2 so some additional H_2CO_3 is removed.

If OH^- is added the equilibrium shifts to the right and:

- H^+ and OH^- combine removing H^+ out of solution

- The decrease in H^+ is countered by more dissociation of H_2CO_3 minimizing the decline in H^+ concentration.

Protein buffer systems

This system is effective because both the acidic and basic residues act as buffers, that is, have a free carboxyl COOH group and a free NH_3^- group that can dissociate.[1,9,10]

For example, for a carboxyl group: $RCOOH \leftrightarrow RCOO^- + H^+$

The pK_a of this system is 7.4 and proteins contribute 5% of total buffering capacity.[9]

Haemoglobin as a buffer system

Haemoglobin can have an intracellular or extracellular effect as protons easily cross the erythrocyte wall. The histidine residues in haemoglobin dissociate and act as buffers. Haemoglobin is abundant with 38 histidine residues and is responsible for 29% of total buffering capacity. The pK_a of the system is 6.8. Deoxyhaemoglobin is a better buffer than oxyhaemoglobin.[1,9,10]

Intracellular buffers

As protons do not readily cross the cell membrane, intracellular buffer systems may take hours to be effective. The intracellular pH is generally lower, around 7.2, and the main intracellular buffers are proteins and organic phosphates.[1,9,10]

Control of pH: renal and respiratory compensatory mechanisms

As shown by the Henderson–Hasselbalch equation, blood pH is dependent on the PCO_2 and the H^+ concentration. Compensatory respiratory and renal control mechanisms are vital to maintain this pH within the narrow range needed for life.

A rise in PCO_2 results in a fall in pH (acidosis) and a fall in PCO_2 leads to a rise in pH (alkalosis).[10]

Arterial PCO_2 varies with the rate of metabolic CO_2 production within the tissues and the ability of the lungs to excrete CO_2. The arterial PCO_2 is detected by respiratory chemoreceptors. This information is sent to the respiratory centre in the medulla oblongata and the respiratory rate is adjusted accordingly. This mechanism requires normal gas exchange in the lungs. The pulmonary removal of CO_2 removes a large acid load. A failure in any part of this mechanism can result in a respiratory acidosis from an increasing PCO_2 or respiratory alkalosis from a decreasing PCO_2.[1,10]

Breathing rate can also be directly affected via chemoreceptors sensitive to H^+ therefore the respiratory system can also compensate for metabolic acid–base disturbances.[10]

The kidneys compensate for changes in pH by the balance of excreting H^+ and absorbing HCO_3^- by the renal tubular apparatus. Under normal metabolic circumstances urine is acidic. The kidneys remove a smaller acid load compared with the respiratory system but the contribution is essential for normal acid–base balance.[1, 10].

Any compensation occurs more slowly taking 24–48 hours to show a response to acute respiratory causes of acid–base imbalance, but chronic respiratory diseases will have established renal compensation mechanisms.

Arterial blood gas analysis

To assess the acid–base status in practice, arterial blood is sampled and the variables are measured either by laboratory testing or point-of-care testing.[10] These variables can be used to determine the degree and cause of the acid–base disturbance (see Table 1.2.4.4).

The following is a suggested method to evaluate an arterial blood gas in clinical practice:

- pH:
  - Normal range 7.35–7.45:
    - Lower than 7.35 = acidosis
    - Higher than 7.45 = alkalosis

- PCO_2:
  - Normal range: 4.5–6.0 kPa
  - At normal pH:
    - Greater than 6.0 kPa suggests mixed respiratory acidosis and metabolic alkalosis
    - Normal range: no acid–base imbalance
    - Less than 4.5 kPa suggests mixed respiratory alkalosis and metabolic acidosis
  - In the acidotic patient, pH lower than 7.35:
    - Greater than 6.0 kPa suggests respiratory acidosis
    - Normal range: a non-respiratory abnormality
    - Less than 4.5 kPa suggests metabolic acidosis
  - In the alkalotic patient, pH higher than 7.45:
    - Greater than 6.0 kPa suggests metabolic alkalosis.
    - Normal range: a non-respiratory abnormality
    - Less than 4.5 kPa suggests respiratory alkalosis

- HCO_3^-:
  - This gives an indication of the metabolic contribution to the acid–base imbalance
  - Normal 22–26 mmol/L
  - Acidosis, pH lower than than 7.35; HCO_3^- less than 22 mmol/L:
    - H^+ increased from a metabolic source
    - Drives buffering reaction to H_2CO_3
    - Removes HCO_3^- from solution
  - Alkalosis, pH higher than 7.45; HCO_3^- greater than 26 mmol/L:
    - H^+ is decreased
    - Drives reaction in opposite direction
    - HCO_3^- released and concentration rises

- Base excess:
  - This gives an indication of the metabolic contribution to the acid–base imbalance

- Its measurement indicates the level of acid–base imbalance when corrected to a normal PCO_2
- Normally −2 to +2
- Positive base excess indicates metabolic contribution to the alkalosis
- Negative base excess indicates metabolic contribution to the acidosis.

When interpreting an ABG result it is helpful to remember that the system never overcompensates, for example, with an acidotic pH of 7.34 with a raised PCO_2 and raised $[HCO_3^-]$ this could be because of respiratory acidosis with metabolic compensation or interpreted as a metabolic alkalosis with respiratory compensation. The primary determining factor is the acidosis as the system cannot overcompensate. Therefore the cause is respiratory acidosis with metabolic compensation increasing the bicarbonate.

Conditions that can give rise to acid–base imbalance

Acidosis
Respiratory acidosis
Caused by accumulation of CO_2 secondary to hypoventilation, resulting in acidosis.
Causes of raised PCO_2:

- Pulmonary disease: chronic obstructive pulmonary disease
- Neuromuscular disorders
  - Guillan–Barré syndrome, myasthenia gravis
  - Flail chest, chest wall deformities
- Drugs:
  - Opiates
  - Residual neuromuscular blockade.

Metabolic acidosis
Caused by either the addition of acid to the system or the loss of base. The causes are divided up on the basis of the anion gap, which represents the unmeasured anions present and is calculated by the following equation.[12–14] The normal anion gap is 10–18 mmol/L.

$$Anion\ gap = (Na^+ + K^+) - (Cl^- + HCO_3^-)$$

Causes of increased anion gap acidosis (addition of acid):[12–14]

- Lactic acidosis:
  - Type A:
    - Strenuous exercise
    - Shock
    - Severe hypoxia
  - Type B:
    - Poisoning (e.g. ethanol paracetamol)
    - Metformin
    - Acute liver failure
- Ketoacidosis:
  - Starvation
  - Diabetes
  - Alcohol

- Uraemic acidosis:
  - Renal failure

Causes of normal anion gap acidosis (base lost):[12–14]

- Loss of alkaline (bicarbonate) GI secretions:
  - Diarrhoea
  - Pancreatic fistula
  - Ureterosigmoidostomy
- Renal tubular acidosis—failure of HCO_3^- re-absorption:
  - Type 1 (distal) and type 2 (proximal)
  - Primary and acquired.

Alkalosis
Respiratory alkalosis
Increased ventilation leading to a reduction in PCO_2 and alkalosis. Causes of increased ventilation:[12–14]

- Psychogenic
- Altitude
- Pulmonary disease
- Salicylate poisoning.

Metabolic alkalosis
Loss of acid or addition of base leading to alkalosis:[12–14]

- Gastrointestinal H^+ loss: vomiting/nasogastric suction
- Intracellular shift of H^+: potassium depletion causes intracellular shift of H^+
- Renal H^+ loss, for example:
  - Mineralocorticoid excess
  - Diuretics
- Addition of base: alkali administration.

The regulation of fluid and acid–base balance are essential for health. In this chapter we have reviewed the mechanisms responsible for maintaining these and have highlighted what happens in disordered function.

Further reading

Loftus I (ed). *Care of the Critically Ill Surgical Patient* (3rd ed). Boca Raton, FL: CRC Press; 2010.
BMJ learning modules (Online learning.bmj.com):

- Fluid management in acutely ill patients.
- Early fluid resuscitation in severe trauma.
- Reducing the risk of hyponatraemia when administering fluids to children.

References

1. Ganong W. *Review of Medical Physiology* (24th ed). New York: McGraw Hill; 2003.
2. Marik P. *Handbook of Evidence-Based Critical Care*. New York: Springer; 2001.
3. Doherty M, Buggy DJ. Intra-operative fluids: how much is too much? *Br J Anaesth* 2012; 109(1)69–79.
4. Grocott M, Mythen MG, Gan TJ. Perioperative fluid management and clinical outcomes in adults. *Anesth Analg* 2005; 100:1093–106.
5. Piper GL, Kaplan LJ. Fluid and electrolyte management for the surgical patient. *Surg Clin N Am* 2012; 92:189–205.

6. Waldmann C, Soni N, Rhodes A. *Oxford Desk Reference Critical Care*. Oxford: Oxford University Press; 2008.

7. English WA, English RE, and Wilson IH. Perioperative fluid balance. *Update Anaesth* 2005; 20:11–20. http://www.wfsahq.org/images/wfsa-documents/updates_in_english/Update_20_2005.pdf

8. Ganong WF. Regulation of extracellular fluid composition and volume. In *Review of Medical Physiology* (pp. 697–704). San Francisco, CA: Appleton & Lange; 1999.

9. Balasubramanian S, Mendonca C, Pinnock C. *The Structured Oral Examination in Anaesthesia*. Cambridge: Cambridge University Press; 2006.

10. McGeown JG. *Physiology: A Core Text of Human Physiology with Self-Assessment*. Edinburgh: Churchill Livingstone; 1999.

11. Corke CF, Jackson IJB. Blood gas analysis. In *Companion to Clinical Anaesthesia Exams* (pp. 171–3). Edinburgh: Churchill Livingstone; 1994.

12. McPherson S. Metabolic medicine. In *Essential Lists for MRCP* (pp. 421–3). Knutsford: PasTest; 2006.

13. Kalra PA. Metabolic acid base disturbances and hypothermia. In *Essential Revision for MRCP* (pp. 421–2). Knutsford: PasTest; 1999.

14. Kumar PJ, Clark ML. Acid-base homeostasis. In *Clinical Medicine* (2nd ed, pp. 502–10). London: Balliére-Tindall; 1990.

CHAPTER 1.2.5

Haemostasis and thrombosis

Dermot Cox

Haemostasis

As blood loss is such a serious threat to life, a complex system has developed to prevent catastrophic loss of blood. To be effective this system must be very responsive to ensure rapid sealing of damaged vessels but not too sensitive to avoid an unwanted thrombosis. This is achieved using three interlinked systems: coagulation, platelets, and thrombolysis.

Coagulation

The coagulation system consists of a cascade of serine proteases that activate other proteins and is accompanied by cofactors that enhance their activity. All of these coagulation factors are synthesized in the liver. The system is designed to generate an insoluble fibrin polymer that plays an important role in preventing blood loss and wound healing. It can be separated into three separate components. The final stage is the generation of the fibrin monomer and this is activated by one of two different pathways: contact (intrinsic) pathway[1] and extrinsic pathway.[2] Associated with this system is an anticoagulation system that acts to control the process (Figure 1.2.5.1).

Clot formation occurs when fibrin polymerizes.[3] To prevent spontaneous clot formation the polymerization sites on fibrin are blocked with short peptides (fibrinopeptides A and B). This inactive fibrin molecule is known as fibrinogen and is a very significant component of plasma with a concentration of 2–3 g/L. Fibrinogen is composed of three chains (α, β, and γ) and the full molecule is composed of two of each of these chains giving it a molecular weight of 340 kDa.[4]

The activation of fibrinogen is achieved by proteolytic cleavage of the fibrinopeptides by the serine protease thrombin.[5] Again, to prevent inappropriate activation of the system, thrombin exists in an inactive form (prothrombin) at a concentration of 100 mcg/mL in plasma. Prothrombin is activated by the serine protease factor (F) Xa that also circulates in an inactive form as FX. Once fibrin polymerizes it is necessary for it to be stabilized by cross-linking the polymers with FXIIIa, which is generated from inactive FXIII by thrombin. This is the common pathway of coagulation.

There are two pathways to the activation of FX. The primary pathway for activation of FX is the tissue factor pathway where FVIIa converts FX to FXa. Tissue factor (TF) is the activator of FVII. Cells within the circulatory system do not express TF on their surface; however, inflammatory cytokines can induce the expression of TF on the surface of endothelial cells which the binds FVII converting it to FVIIa.[2]

The other activation pathway is the contact pathway[1] where FIXa converts FX to FXa. FIXa is generated from FIX by the action of FXIa, which is generated from FXI by FXIIa. It can also be generated by FVIIa–TF complex. FXIIa is generated from FXII when it comes into contact with surfaces hence the name contact pathway.

Coagulation cofactors

Many of the enzymes in the coagulation cascade have very low levels of activity even in their active form. The binding of cofactors serves to greatly increase their activity. One such cofactor is FV which when activated by thrombin binds to FXa and greatly increases its activity. In the contact pathway, FVIII, when activated by FXa or thrombin, binds to FIXa increasing its activity.[6]

Von Willebrand factor (vWF) is a large multimeric protein that primarily mediates the interaction of platelets with subendothelial matrix under high shear.[7] However, FVIII circulates in the plasma in complex with vWF, which has the effect of prolonging the plasma half-life of FVIII.[8]

Vitamin K

Prothrombin, FVII, FIX, and FX are characterized by the presence of a Gla domain. This is a protein domain rich in γ-carboxyglutamate as a result of carboxylation of glutamic acids in the liver in a vitamin K-dependent process.[9] These Gla domains have a high affinity for calcium and are important in binding of the coagulation factors to phospholipid membranes. Phospholipids are essential cofactors for coagulation and typically they are provided by activated platelets. They facilitate the binding of coagulation factors through their Gla domains. This serves to bring the coagulation factors into close proximity thus speeding up the reactions.

Amplification

The coagulation system is arranged as a cascade that serves to amplify the original signal. As the key factors are enzymes, the activation of a single enzyme leads to activation of many substrate molecules. As these are also enzymes they in turn lead to activation of many enzyme molecules. This amplification is further enhanced by feedback mechanisms. Thus, not only does thrombin activate fibrinogen, it also activates other key enzymes such as FV, FVIII, and FXI while FXa also activates FVIII.

Anticoagulant system

There are a number of factors that inhibit coagulation and serve to limit the extent of coagulation. One such inhibitor is activated protein C (APC), which is a vitamin K-dependent serine protease similar to the other coagulation factors.[10] APC is generated from protein C by the actions of thrombin in complex with thrombomodulin, which is an endothelial cell thrombin-binding protein. When thrombin binds to thrombomodulin it loses its ability to activate fibrinogen and platelets and develops an affinity for protein C.

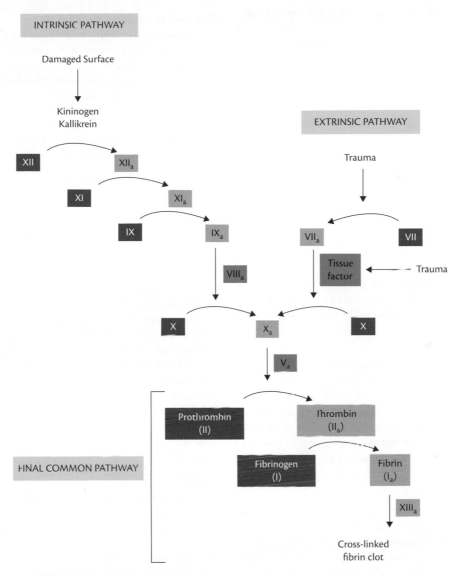

Fig. 1.2.5.1 Coagulation occurs when fibrinogen is activated to fibrin, which polymerizes forming a clot. This is the final common pathway of coagulation. The coagulation cascade can be activated by two distinct methods. The intrinsic pathway is activated by FXII interacting with damaged surfaces while the extrinsic pathway is activated by the exposure of tissue factor on damaged cells.

Reproduced with permission from Anaesthesia UK, *Coagulation-classical model*, Copyright © 2005, available from http://www.frca.co.uk/article.aspx?articleid=100096

Thus, binding to thrombomodulin changes thrombin from being a procoagulant enzyme to being an anticoagulant enzyme. APC cleaves FVa and FVIIIa thereby inactivating them. In a manner similar to that with the procoagulant factors, APC has a low intrinsic activity and it is only upon binding the vitamin K-dependent cofactor protein S that it becomes fully active.

As many of the procoagulant factors are serine proteases they are susceptible to inhibition by serine protease inhibitors (serpins).[11] As its name implies, antithrombin III (AT) inhibits the activity of thrombin but it also inhibits the activity of FXa and to a lesser extent the other serine proteases in the coagulation system. As is frequently the case in the coagulation system, the activity of AT is under the influence of a cofactor, which in this case is heparin. The inhibitory activity of AT is increased around 1000-fold upon binding to heparin. Another inhibitory serpin is protein Z-dependent protease inhibitor; in the presence of protein Z this serpin inhibits FXa and FXIa.

The tissue factor pathway inhibitor (TFPI) inhibits FXa and FVIIa–TF–FXa complex. It is synthesized in endothelial cells and much of it remains bound to the cell surface.

Laboratory testing

There are three basic tests that are used to assess the functional state of the coagulation system and are used for diagnosis and management of pharmacotherapy:[12,13]

- *Prothrombin time* (PT). This test measures the time to clot formation of plasma after the addition of calcium and thromboplastin (TF and phospholipid). Thus, it measures the ability of FVII to activate FX and produce a clot. The typical PT for normal plasma is around 12–15 seconds and depends on the source of thromboplastin. The International Sensitivity Index (ISI) is a comparison of each batch of thromboplastin with an international standard.

- *Activated partial thromboplastin time* (aPTT). This test activates the contact pathway by adding in phospholipid, calcium, and kaolin and thus measures the ability FIX to activate FX and produce a clot. Clot formation occurs between 30–50 seconds in an aPTT test in normal plasma.

- *International normalized ratio* (INR). There can be considerable variation in the PT due to the instrument used and the source of TF. The INR controls for this and is often used to monitor anticoagulant therapy:

$$INR = (PT_{test}/PT_{normal})^{ISI}$$

(where the ISI is a numerical value reflecting the results obtained by different commercial systems and which allows results to be compared between centres).

Coagulation and disease

Disorders of the coagulations system can either be prothrombotic or haemorrhagic and they can either be acquired or hereditary. The hereditary bleeding disorders are probably the major category here especially from a surgical perspective.

Inherited haemorrhagic disorders

Haemophilias are probably the best known bleeding disorders and are due to mutations in one of the coagulation factors: FVIII (type A), FIX (type B),[14] and FXI (type C).[15] Haemophilia A accounts for around 80% of all cases. These hereditary disorders are characterized by bleeding into the joints (haemarthroses) or the muscle (haematoma). However, these are not the only inherited coagulation disorders and mutations in vWF and the other key enzymes also occur.[16]

Acquired haemorrhagic disorders

As well as the inherited disorders patients can also have an acquired disorder. An example of this is vitamin K deficiency as this vitamin is essential for the proper function of a number of coagulation factors. While this is more common in infants it can occur at any age. As most of the coagulation factors are synthesized in the liver, anything that impairs liver function such as cirrhosis can lead to a serious decrease in plasma levels of these coagulation factors. Some patients produce antibodies to coagulation factors that inhibit their activity. This is often seen in haemophilic patients on coagulation factor replacement therapy although it can also occur in patients as a result of a blood transfusion.[17] Sepsis can lead to a condition known as disseminated intravascular coagulation (DIC) where bacteria trigger the formation of microthrombi throughout the circulatory system. This ongoing coagulation leads to a consumption of coagulation factors which, as the sepsis progresses, leads to increased bleeding due to the reduced levels of coagulation factors in the blood.[18]

Inherited procoagulant disorders

Mutations in the genes for coagulation factors can lead to them becoming constitutively active leading to an increased rate of coagulation. FV_{Leiden} has a single point mutation that makes FVa resistant to cleavage by APC, which is the major path for inactivation of FVa. Patients that are homozygous for this mutation have a 50-fold increased risk of venous thromboembolism. Inherited deficiencies in the anticoagulant factors such as anti-thrombin, protein S, and protein C can also lead to an increase in clot formation.[19]

Acquired procoagulant disorders

Hyperhomocysteinaemia is associated with an increase in venous thrombosis[20] and acquired APC resistance is associated with fetal loss during pregnancy.[21] The contraceptive pill is also associated with an increase in venous thromboembolism in part due to increasing levels of procoagulant factors and decreasing levels of anticoagulant factors. Prolonged immobility can also predispose patients to venous thromboembolism such as seen in long-haul flights. Other conditions that predispose to thrombosis formation are polycythaemia vera and antiphospholipid syndrome.

Pharmacology of coagulation

Vitamin K antagonists

The death of cattle from internal haemorrhage in the 1920s after eating spoiled sweet clover led to the discovery of the anticoagulant dicoumarol and subsequently (1954) its derivative warfarin became a widely used as an oral anticoagulant. Warfarin inhibits vitamin K epoxide reductase reducing vitamin K levels. As synthesis of prothrombin, FVII, FIX, and FX are vitamin K-dependent, this results in a reduction in their levels and thus in the ability of blood to coagulate. As expected from its mechanism of action the clinical effects of warfarin take a few days to reach their maximum as it only affects the synthesis of new coagulation factors. Equally, its effects can be overcome by administration of vitamin K but this will also take a few days to act. A more rapid reversal of warfarin requires administration of fresh frozen plasma. As warfarin is highly bound to serum albumin and is metabolized by cytochrome P450 enzymes there is significant potential for interactions with other drugs, which requires constant monitoring of warfarin levels using the INR.[22]

Heparin

As heparin acts to increase the affinity of antithrombin III for both thrombin and FXa it can also be used as an anticoagulant. Unfractionated heparin is a mixture of high-molecular-weight glycosaminoglycans extracted from pig intestines[23] and is administered by either intravenous or subcutaneous injection. Its main advantage over warfarin is its immediate action. More recently low-molecular-weight preparations of heparin such as enoxaparin have become more common. While these have the same mechanism of action as heparin, they have greater inhibition of FXa than thrombin. The minimum active component of heparin was identified as a pentasaccharide, which has been synthesized as fondaparinux.[24] This also binds antithrombin but the complex only inhibits FXa and not thrombin and is administered by subcutaneous injection. The major adverse effect of heparins is an immune-based thrombocytopenia (heparin-induced thrombocytopenia (HIT)) and its occurrence appears to be related to molecular weight of the preparation.[25]

Direct inhibitors

Recently, inhibitors of coagulation factors (FXa and thrombin) that directly inhibit their respective coagulation factors have come to the market. The original thrombin inhibitors were not orally active and most were based on the leech anticoagulant hirudin, along with argatroban. Dabigatran is an oral thrombin inhibitor first approved in 2008. Direct inhibitors of FXa such as rivaroxaban[24] and apixaban have also been approved.[26] These direct-acting agents appear to be more effective than warfarin and the main adverse effect is bleeding. Direct FX inhibitors may have a better profile with respect to bleeding problems. Reversal of excessive inhibition is difficult although some specific reversal agents are under development[27] such as idarucizumab which has been shown to reverse the effects of dabigatran in PIII studies and a decision on its approval by FDA is expected by the end of 2015.

Blood coagulation factors

While pharmacotherapy has focused on inhibitors of coagulation there is also a need to treat patients with bleeding disorders due to deficiency in coagulation factors. There are two approaches to this: fresh frozen plasma and factor concentrates/recombinant coagulation factors. The problem with using plasma is that it contains a large amount of unnecessary proteins. However, it is useful when there is a deficiency in multiple coagulation factors or the deficient factor is unknown such as after warfarin therapy or as a result of DIC. For patients with hereditary deficiencies in specific factors, it is more appropriate to use fractionated plasma that has been enriched for the coagulation factor or where possible to use a recombinant coagulation factor such as FVIII used to treat haemophilia.[28]

Fibrinolysis

To provide effective control over coagulation and to remove clots after healing has occurred it is necessary to have a system for clot removal, that is, fibrinolysis. The heart of this system is the serine protease plasmin, which digests fibrinogen and fibrin into fragments D and E. As fibrin is polymerized, the D fragments are linked and thus D-dimers are produced while D-monomers are produced from the digestion of fibrinogen[29] (Figure 1.2.5.2).

Like the other serine proteases, plasmin exists in an inactive form known as plasminogen, which is activated when plasminogen activators (PAs) convert it from a single-chain to a double-chain complex. The primary PA is a serine protease synthesized by endothelial cells and is known as tissue-type PA (tPA). Urinary-type PA (uPA; urokinase) is produced in the kidney and can also activate plasminogen.

The primary inhibitor of this system is plasminogen activator inhibitor-1 (PAI-1), which is a serine protease inhibitor that exists in complex with tPA.[30] Thus, PAI-1 levels are associated with haemorrhage/thrombotic risk. Plasmin itself is inhibited by α_2-antiplasmin.

Laboratory testing

The important test for detecting activation of the thrombolytic system is measurement of D-dimer levels. This is used to detect deep vein thrombosis. Technically it does not measure clot formation, rather it measures clot breakdown which indicates that clot formation must have occurred.[31]

Pharmacology of thrombolysis

Activation of the thrombolytic pathway is an important way of removing occlusive clots in patients with myocardial infarction. The first such compound was streptokinase, an enzyme isolated from haemolytic streptococci. This binds to plasminogen and activates it. Its main limitation is that it is antigenic and that anti-streptokinase antibodies can limit its activity. This limitation has been overcome with the use of recombinant human tPA.[32,33] The other possibility

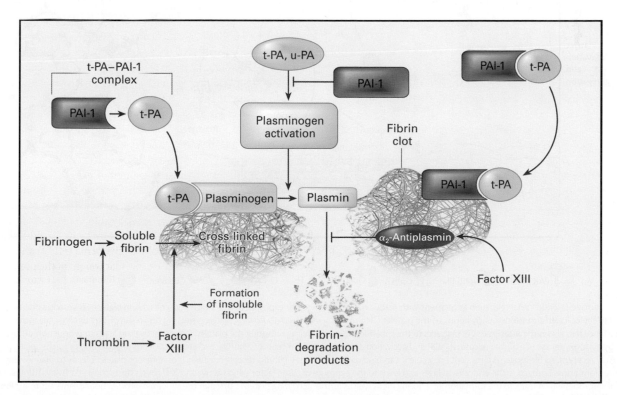

Fig. 1.2.5.2 The coagulation cascade which generates a clot is balanced by the fibrinolytic cascade which breaks down the clot. This is mediated by plasmin which forms fibrin degradation products. Plasmin is formed by the activation of plasminogen by tissue plasminogen activator.

From *The New England Journal of Medicine*, Hans P. Kohler and Peter J. Grant, 'Plasminogen Activator Inhibitor Type 1 and Coronary Artery Disease', Volume 342, Number 24, p. 1792
Copyright © 2000 Massachusetts Medical Society. Reprinted with permission from Massachusetts Medical Society.

for pharmacological intervention is to inhibit the fibrinolytic system thus stabilizing the clots and thereby preventing blood loss. Tranexamic acid is a lysine derivative that inhibits the conversion of plasminogen to plasmin and can be used to prevent blood loss during surgery.[34]

Platelets

Platelets are anucleate fragments of megakaryocytes and are one of the most numerous cell-like particles in the blood at a concentration of 150 000–400 000 platelets/μL.[35] As platelets are anucleate, they are incapable of replication or protein synthesis although there is some synthesis of protein from stable mRNA in the platelet.[36] Platelets are critical elements of both the haemostatic and innate immune systems.[37] This is achieved through three distinct functions: adhesion, activation, and secretion.

Platelet function

Platelet adhesion

When a blood vessel is damaged, the subendothelial matrix is exposed which facilitates platelet adhesion by a number of different surface adhesion receptors.[38,39] The exposed matrix is rich in collagen and thus the two-collagen receptors (integrin $\alpha_2\beta_1$ and glycoprotein (GP)VI) are important in mediating platelet adhesion. The integrin $\alpha_{IIb}\beta_3$ (GPIIb/IIIa) is also important in supporting adhesion to immobilized fibrinogen. In the arterial system, platelets are exposed to high shear, which makes it difficult for these receptors to bind to their ligand. GPIb/IX/V is a receptor for vWF (a component of exposed matrix) but only recognizes vWF under high-shear conditions. Thus, under arterial shear, GPIb binds immobilized vWF allowing platelets to bind transiently. This causes the platelets to roll along the surface, which serves to slow them down sufficiently to allow firm adhesion through collagen receptors or GPIIb/IIIa (Figure 1.2.5.3).

Platelet activation

Adhesion to collagen leads to activation of the platelets. Platelet activation can also be achieved through soluble mediators such as thrombin (protease-activated receptor-1; PAR-1) and ADP (P2Y$_{12}$).[39] Bacteria and viruses can also trigger platelet activation.[40,41] Platelet activation occurs through two complex pathways. Weak platelet agonists mediate activation through phospholipase

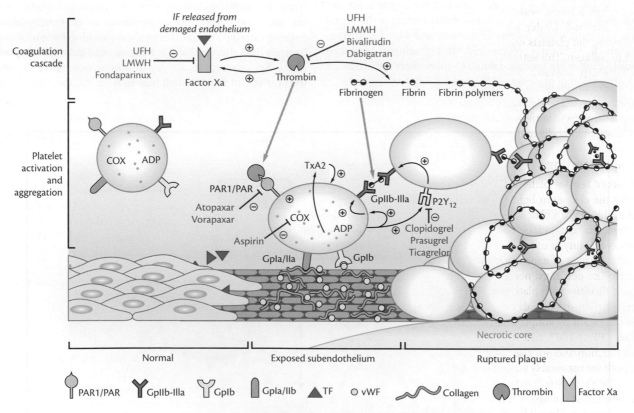

Fig. 1.2.5.3 Damage to endothelial cells, such as happens with plaque rupture, leads to the exposure of subendothelial collagen. In high-shear vessels, von Willebrand factor binds to the collagen and subsequently bonds to the platelet GPIb resulting in the rapidly flowing platelets slowing down sufficiently to allow collagen receptor (GPIa/IIa) to bind. This allows the attachment of platelets to the subendothelium as well as activating the platelet. Platelet activation leads to production of thromboxane A2 (TxA2) by cyclooxygenase (COX), the release of ADP, and activation of the fibrinogen receptor GPIIb/IIIa. Secreted ADP leads to activation of further platelets via P2Y$_{12}$, the ADP receptor. As fibrinogen is a bivalent molecule it can bind to two different GPIIb/IIIa receptors which, if on different platelets, leads to platelet aggregation and thrombus formation. Damage to the endothelial layer also leads to the exposure of tissue factor which activates FX through the extrinsic pathway. This results in the activation of thrombin which leads to the formation of a fibrin clot as well as further activating platelets through the PAR1 receptor. Anticoagulants act to inhibit either FXa (unfractionated heparin UFH), low-molecular-weight heparin (LMWH), or fondaparinux or thrombin (UFH, LMWH, bivalirudin, or dabigatran). Antiplatelet agents act to prevent platelet activation by blocking P2Y$_{12}$ (clopidogrel, prasugrel, or ticagrelor), COX (aspirin), or PAR1 (atopaxar or vorapaxar).

Reproduced with permission from Scott M. Lilly and Robert L. Wilensky, Emerging therapies for acute coronary syndromes, *Frontiers in Pharmacology*, Volume 2, Article 61, Copyright © 2011 Lilly and Wilensky, DOI: 10.3389/fphar.2011.00061, under Creative Commons Attribution 4.0 International (CC BY 4.0).

A2, which cleaves arachidonic from the platelet membrane. This is in turn converted to the potent platelet agonist thromboxane A2 by cyclooxygenase (COX)-1, and thromboxane A synthase. Strong platelet agonists activate platelets through a phospholipase C-dependent pathway. No matter how the platelet is activated the result is activation of GPIIb/IIIa, which allows this receptor to bind soluble fibrinogen (resting GPIIb/IIIa only binds immobilized fibrinogen).[42] Fibrinogen binding to GPIIb/IIIa is mediated by the Arg–Gly–Asp (RGD)-sequence or the γ-chain terminal dodecapeptide. As fibrinogen is a dimer this allows for the possibility of it binding to two different GPIIb/IIIa molecules. If these are on different platelets this leads to platelet aggregation as platelets are cross-linked by fibrinogen binding which acts to seal the damaged vessel preventing further blood loss.

Platelet secretion

Once activated, a platelet secretes the contents of its granules. Platelets contain three types of granules: α-granules, dense granules, and lysosomes. Between them these granules contain over 300 bioactive proteins and numerous small molecules. The platelet secretome contains a diverse array of molecules including ADP, serotonin, chemokines, cytokines, antimicrobial peptides, and adhesion molecules.[43]

Thus, when a blood vessel is damaged, the subendothelial cell matrix is exposed. Under high-shear conditions, GPIb binds to vWF slowing the platelets down sufficiently for collagen receptors to bind to collagen. This activates the platelets triggering the release of ADP, which activates other platelets. Once activated, these platelets bind fibrinogen which cross-links them together to form a platelet aggregate which seals the blood vessel.[44] The activated platelets also secrete antimicrobial peptides and chemokines that attract white blood cells to the area to sterilize the wound.

Laboratory testing

The standard test for platelet function is platelet aggregation. This measures the change in light transmission of platelet-rich plasma after the addition of a platelet agonist. As this test requires specialist equipment, the manipulation of a fresh blood sample, and trained staff, its availability is usually confined to specialist centres. When used with a range of agonists it can be used to diagnose platelet disorders. The perceived need for monitoring antiplatelet therapy and the difficulties with platelet aggregometry has led to the development of point-of-care devices for measuring platelet function and its inhibition by antiplatelet agents. Both the Platelet Function Analyzer (PFA)-100® and Multiplate® systems measure general platelet function and are also used to monitor antiplatelet therapy. While both are reasonably automated, neither are true point-of-care devices. The VerifyNow® system is a point-of-care system for monitoring antiplatelet therapy. The major problem with these systems is lack of agreement. Thus, it is not unusual for a patient to show poor response to therapy with one device but not with the others. This means that it is difficult to interpret the results from these assays.[45,46]

Platelet disorders

Similar to the situation with coagulation disorders, there are both acquired and hereditary disorders of platelet function. Unlike disorders of coagulation, which are associated with haemarthroses and haematoma, platelet defects are associated with bruising and excessive bleeding from a cut.

Inherited platelet disorders

There are a number of hereditary deficits in platelet receptors; however, these are all rare disorders and are often associated with consanguineous marriages. The two most common are Glanzmann's thrombaesthenia and Bernard–Soulier disease, which are due to deficiencies in GPIIb/IIIa and GPIb respectively. There are also defects in platelet secretion known as storage pool deficiency.[47]

Acquired platelet disorders

This is mainly due to thrombocytopenia although severe bleeding does not usually arise until the platelet count drops below 10 000 platelets/μL. This usually presents as idiopathic thrombocytopenia purpura (ITP) and is usually immune mediated.[48] Some cases of ITP can be drug mediated and many drugs have been shown to cause thrombocytopenia. The best-characterized example is heparin-induced thrombocytopenia (HIT)[25] where heparin can bind to platelet factor 4 (PF4) on the surface of platelets and this heparin–PF4 complex is antigenic leading to the formation of antiplatelet antibodies. As well as defects in platelet numbers there can also be acquired defects in platelet function. This is primarily associated with the use of antiplatelet agents.

Prothrombotic disorders

There is also the concept of prothrombotic states where patients have hyperactive platelets.[49] This can be due to the presence of plaque in the coronary arteries, infection, or polymorphisms in platelet receptors that make them more reactive or even the presence of drugs such as selective COX-2 inhibitors.[25]

Platelet pharmacology

Since myocardial infarction is ultimately due to the formation of a platelet thrombus, there has been extensive research on antiplatelet agents.

Cyclooxygenase (COX) inhibitors

Aspirin is one of the oldest drugs in current use with a history of over 2000 years of use (at least as a herbal extract). However, the antiplatelet properties of aspirin have only recently been identified. Aspirin acts to irreversibly inhibit COX, which plays an important role in platelet activation.[50,51] The major drawback with aspirin is its effects on the gastric mucosa where COX-1 plays an important role in production of the mucus that protects the stomach from the surrounding acid environment and as a result some patients are prone to gastric ulceration. Two strategies were developed to minimize this. Firstly low-dose (75 mg or 81 mg) preparations can be used, as platelets lacking a nucleus cannot synthesize fresh COX. Since aspirin is an irreversible inhibitor, the inhibition rapidly accumulates in the absence of fresh COX being synthesized. This is further enhanced by the use of enteric-coated aspirin where aspirin absorption takes place in the small intestine rather than the stomach. A lot has been made of the existence of aspirin-resistance; however, recent studies would suggest that this is a very rare phenomenon and that it is primarily due to poor compliance.[52] There is also evidence that poor bioavailability of enteric-coated aspirin, especially in patients weighing over 90 kg, also contributes to the problem.[53]

P2Y$_{12}$ antagonists

The discovery that ADP secreted from activated platelets is important in triggering further platelets led to the development of antagonists of the platelet ADP receptor P2Y$_{12}$. The original member of this group is clopidogrel and more recently prasugrel.[24,50] Both are orally active irreversible inhibitors of $P2Y_{12}$. More recently, new reversible $P2Y_{12}$ antagonists such as cangrelor and ticagrelor have been developed.[54]

GPIIb/IIIa antagonists

As fibrinogen binding to GPIIb/IIIa is critical for the formation of platelet thrombi, it has been the target for antiplatelet agents.[55] Abciximab is a monoclonal antibody to GPIIb/IIIa and was the first in this class of drug. Based on the idea that the amino acid sequence RGD in fibrinogen mediates the binding, potent analogues were developed that can inhibit GPIIb/IIIa. Two of these—tirofiban and eptifibatide—were ultimately approved. All three GPIIb/IIIa antagonists are intravenous only and are primarily used for acute coronary syndromes and during stent placement.[24,50]

Thrombopoietin receptor agonists

Thrombopoietin is the hormone that regulates platelet production. Recently synthetic agonists of its receptor such as romiplostim and eltrombopag have been developed for the treatment of ITP.[56]

Conclusion

In conclusion, an understanding of the interplay between coagulation, fibrinolysis, and platelet activation is necessary to prevent haemorrhagic and thrombotic complications of surgery.[57] It is also important to appreciate the significance of individual factors in response to pharmacological intervention which can result in patients developing excessive bleeding for the dose of drug used.[58]

References

1. Gailani D, Renné T. The intrinsic pathway of coagulation: a target for treating thromboembolic disease? *J Thromb Haemost* 2007; 5:1106–12.
2. Mackman N, Tilley RE, Key NS. Role of the extrinsic pathway of blood coagulation in hemostasis and thrombosis. *Arterioscler Thromb Vasc Biol* 2007; 27:1687–93.
3. Weisel JW, Litvinov RI. Mechanisms of fibrin polymerization and clinical implications. *Blood* 2013; 121:1712–19.
4. Mosesson MW. Fibrinogen and fibrin structure and functions. *J Thromb Haemost* 2005; 3:1894–904.
5. Cera ED. Thrombin as procoagulant and anticoagulant. *J Thromb Haemost* 2007; 5:196–202.
6. Fang H, Wang L, Wang H. The protein structure and effect of factor VIII. *Thromb Res* 2007; 119:1–13.
7. Springer TA. Biology and physics of von Willebrand factor concatamers. *J Thromb Haemost* 2011; 9:130–43.
8. Schneppenheim R, Budde U. Von Willebrand factor: the complex molecular genetics of a multidomain and multifunctional protein. *J Thromb Haemost* 2011; 9:209–15.
9. Stafford DW. The vitamin K cycle. *J Thromb Haemost* 2005; 3:1873–8.
10. Wildhagen K, Lutgens E, Loubele S, *et al.* The structure-function relationship of activated protein C. Lessons from natural and engineered mutations. *Thromb Haemost* 2011; 106:1034–45.
11. Huntington JA. Serpin structure, function and dysfunction. *J Thromb Haemost* 2011; 9:26–34.
12. Perry DJ, Fitzmaurice DA, Kitchen S, *et al.* Point-of-care testing in haemostasis. *Br J Haematol* 2010; 150:501–14.
13. Chitlur M. Challenges in the laboratory analyses of bleeding disorders. *Thromb Res* 2012; 130:1–6.
14. Fijnvandraat K, Cnossen MH, Leebeek FWG, *et al.* Diagnosis and management of haemophilia. *BMJ* 2012; 344:e2707.
15. Peyvandi F, Bolton-Maggs PH, Batorova A, *et al.* Rare bleeding disorders. *Haemophilia* 2012; 18:148–53.
16. James PD, Lillicrap D. The molecular characterization of von Willebrand disease: good in parts. *Br J Haematol* 2013; 161:166–76.
17. Kruse-Jarres R. Current controversies in the formation and treatment of alloantibodies to factor VIII in congenital hemophilia A. *Hematology Am Soc Hematol Educ Program* 2011; 2011:407–12.
18. Semeraro N, Ammollo CT, Semeraro F, *et al.* Sepsis, thrombosis and organ dysfunction. *Thromb Res* 2012; 129:290–5.
19. Varga EA, Kujovich JL. Management of inherited thrombophilia: guide for genetics professionals. *Clin Genet* 2012; 81:7–17.
20. Di Minno M, Tremoli E, Coppola A, *et al.* Homocysteine and arterial thrombosis: challenge and opportunity. *Thromb Haemost* 2010; 103:942–61.
21. Benedetto C, Marozio L, Tavella AM, *et al.* Coagulation disorders in pregnancy: acquired and inherited thrombophilias. *Ann N Y Acad Sci* 2010; 1205:106–17.
22. Lee A, Crowther M. Practical issues with vitamin K antagonists: elevated INRs, low time-in-therapeutic range, and warfarin failure. *J Thromb Thrombolysis* 2011; 31:249–58.
23. Gray E, Mulloy B, Barrowcliffe T. Heparin and low-molecular-weight heparin. *Thromb Haemost* 2008; 99:807–18.
24. Showkathali R, Natarajan A. Antiplatelet and antithrombin strategies in acute coronary syndrome: state-of-the-art review. *Curr Cardiol Rev* 2012; 8:239–49.
25. Warkentin TE. HIT paradigms and paradoxes. *J Thromb Haemost* 2011; 9:105–17.
26. Yeh CH, Hogg K, Weitz JI. Overview of the new oral anticoagulants: opportunities and challenges. *Arterioscler Thromb Vasc Biol* 2015; 35:1056–65.
27. Daniels PR. Peri-procedural management of patients taking oral anticoagulants. *BMJ* 2015; 351.
28. Ofosu FA, Santagostino E, Grancha S, *et al.* Management of bleeding disorders: basic science. *Haemophilia* 2012; 18:8–14.
29. Castellino F, Ploplis V. Structure and function of the plasminogen/plasmin system. *Thromb Haemost* 2005; 93:647–54.
30. Van De Craen B, Declerck PJ, *et al.* The biochemistry, physiology and pathological roles of PAI-1 and the requirements for PAI-1 inhibition in vivo. *Thromb Res* 2012; 130:576–85.
31. Lapner ST, Kearon C. Diagnosis and management of pulmonary embolism. *BMJ* 2013; 346:f757.
32. Collen D, Lijnen H. Thrombolytic agents. *Thromb Haemost* 2005; 93:627–30.
33. Flemmig M, Melzig MF. Serine-proteases as plasminogen activators in terms of fibrinolysis. *J Pharm Pharmacol* 2012; 64:1025–39.
34. Georgiou C, Neofytou K, Demetriades D. Local and systemic hemostatics as an adjunct to control bleeding in trauma. *Am Surg* 2013; 79:180–7.
35. Hartwig JH. The platelet: form and function. *Semin Hematol* 2006; 43:S94–100.
36. Weyrich AS, Schwertz H, Kraiss LW, *et al.* Protein synthesis by platelets: historical and new perspectives. *J Thromb Haemost* 2009; 7:241–6.
37. Cox D, Kerrigan SW, Watson SP. Platelets and the innate immune system: mechanisms of bacterial-induced platelet activation. *J Thromb Haemost* 2011; 9:1097–107.
38. Kiefer TL, Becker RC. Inhibitors of platelet adhesion. *Circulation* 2009; 120:2488–95.
39. Nieswandt B, Pleines I, Bender M. Platelet adhesion and activation mechanisms in arterial thrombosis and ischaemic stroke. *J Thromb Haemost* 2011; 9:92–104.
40. Fitzgerald JR, Foster TJ, Cox D. The interaction of bacterial pathogens with platelets. *Nat Rev Microbiol* 2006; 4:445–57.
41. Alonso AL, Cox D. Platelet interactions with viruses and parasites. *Platelets* 2015; 26:317–23.
42. Shattil SJ, Newman PJ. Integrins: dynamic scaffolds for adhesion and signaling in platelets. *Blood* 2004; 104:1606–15.

43. Blair P, Flaumenhaft R. Platelet α-granules: basic biology and clinical correlates. *Blood Rev* 2009; 23:177–89.

44. Furie B. Pathogenesis of thrombosis. *Hematology* 2009; 2009:255–8.

45. Rechner A. Platelet function testing in clinical diagnostics. *Hamostaseologie* 2011; 31:79–87.

46. Paniccia R, Priora R, Liotta A, Abbate R. Platelet function tests: a comparative review. *Vasc Health Risk Manag* 2015; 11:133–48.

47. Handin RI. Inherited platelet disorders. *Hematology Am Soc Hematol Educ Program* 2005; 2005:396–402.

48. Cuker A, Cines DB. Immune thrombocytopenia. *Hematology Am Soc Hematol Educ Program* 2010; 2010:377–84.

49. Martin JF, Kristensen SD, Mathur A, *et al.* The causal role of megakaryocyte-platelet hyperactivity in acute coronary syndromes. *Nat Rev Cardiol* 2012; 9:658–70.

50. Eikelboom JW, Hirsh J, Spencer FA, *et al.* Antiplatelet drugs: Antithrombotic therapy and prevention of thrombosis, 9th ed: American College of Chest Physicians evidence-based clinical practice guidelines. *Chest* 2012; 141:e89S–119S.

51. Fuster V, Sweeny JM. Aspirin: a historical and contemporary therapeutic overview. *Circulation* 2011; 123:768–78.

52. Cox D. Aspirin resistance: a nebulous concept. *J Clin Pharmacol Pharmacoepidemiol* 2008; 1:39–47.

53. Peace A, McCall M, Tedesco T, *et al.* The role of weight and enteric coating on aspirin response in cardiovascular patients. *J Thromb Haemost* 2010; 8:2323–5.

54. Damman P, Woudstra P, Kuijt W, *et al.* P2Y12 platelet inhibition in clinical practice. *J Thromb Thrombolysis* 2012; 33:143–53.

55. Armstrong P, Peter K. GPIIb/IIIa inhibitors: from bench to bedside and back to bench again. *Thromb Haemost* 2012; 107:808–14.

56. Lakshmanan S, Cuker A. Contemporary management of primary immune thrombocytopenia in adults. *J Thromb Haemost* 2012; 10:1988–98.

57. Marietta M, Facchini L, Pedrazzi P, *et al.* Pathophysiology of bleeding in surgery. *Transplant Proc* 2006; 38:812–14.

58. Kluft C, Burggraaf J. Introduction to haemostasis from a pharmacodynamic perspective. *Br J Clin Pharmacol* 2011; 72:538–46.

CHAPTER 1.2.6

Cardiovascular

Aidan Bradford

The heart cycle

An example of the heart cycle is shown in Figure 1.2.6.1.

Parameters of normal cardiac function

Systemic arterial blood pressure is 120/80 mmHg.

Pulse pressure is systolic pressure minus diastolic pressure: 120 − 80 = 40 mmHg.

Mean pressure is diastolic + 1/3 pulse pressure: $80 + 1/3 \times 40 = 93.3$ mmHg.

Cardiac output (CO) equals the volume of blood pumped by each ventricle per minute:

$$CO = \text{stroke volume (SV)} \times \text{heart rate (HR)}$$

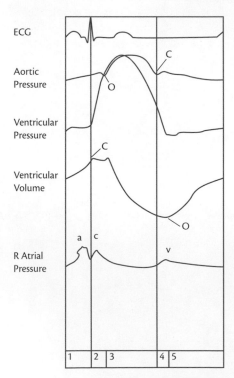

Fig. 1.2.6.1 Electrocardiogram, pressure, and volume changes in the atrium, ventricle, and aorta during the heart cycle. 1 is atrial systole, 2 is isovolumetric or isometric contraction, 3 is ventricular ejection, 4 is isovolumetric relaxation, and 5 is ventricular filling.

Reproduced from Matthew Barnard and Bruce Martin, *Cardiac Anaesthesia*, Oxford Specialist Handbooks in Anaesthesia, Figure 2.4, p. 23, Oxford University Press, Oxford, UK, Copyright © 2010, by permission of Oxford University Press.

$$5 \text{ L/min} = 70 \text{ mL} \times 70$$

$$SV = \text{end-diastolic volume (EDV)} - \text{end-systolic volume (ESV)}$$

$$70 \text{ mL} = 120 \text{ mL} - 50 \text{ mL}$$

$$\text{Ejection fraction} = SV/EDV \times 100$$

$$60 = 70/120 \times 100$$

At a HR of 70/min, the heart cycle duration is 0.8 seconds of which 0.3 seconds is systole and 0.5 seconds is diastole. When HR increases, systolic and diastolic time decrease but there is a greater decrease in diastolic time.

Heart cycle electrical and pressure/valve correlations

The QRS complex of the electrocardiogram (ECG) indicates depolarization of the ventricle and this is followed by contraction and a rise in ventricular pressure. This causes closure of the atrioventricular (AV) valves and the first heart sound.

The ventricular pressure causes bulging of the AV valves and a rise in atrial pressure called the 'c' wave. The aortic and pulmonary valves are also closed and this period of isovolumetric contraction ends when ventricular pressure exceeds aortic/pulmonary pressure.

The semilunar valves open and blood is ejected, rapidly and then more slowly. The descent of the AV ring increases atrial volume and decreases its pressure, that is, the 'x' descent.

The T wave of the ECG indicates ventricular repolarization and relaxation of the ventricle and a fall in pressure. The semilunar valves close causing the second heart sound and the incisura[1] of the aortic pressure pulse (erroneously referred to as the dicrotic notch in many texts). This is the onset of the isometric relaxation period because the AV valves are also shut.

During ventricular systole, atrial pressure rises because the AV valves are shut and blood is entering the atria. The pressure rises to a peak called the 'v' wave which is followed by the 'y' descent when the recoiling ventricle and the rapid fall in ventricular pressure results in the pressure being greater in the atrium than in the ventricle and so the valves open.

For the remainder of diastole, atrial and ventricular pressure is approximately zero. There is rapid followed by slow filling of the ventricle and then the P wave occurs indicating atrial depolarization, contraction of the atria, and the 'a' wave of atrial pressure.

Diastolic murmurs are due to AV valve stenosis and aortic/pulmonary valve incompetence (regurgitation) and systolic murmurs are due to AV valve incompetence (regurgitation) and aortic/pulmonary valve stenosis.

Electrophysiology

The cell

The ventricular cell action potential (Figure 1.2.6.2) consists of five phases:

1. Phase 0, caused by activation of fast Na^+ channels that then become inactivated

2. Phase 1 due to activation of a transient outward current

3. Phase 2 due to activation of L-type Ca^{2+} channels and reduced K^+ channel conductance

4. Phase 3 due to decreased Ca^{2+} and increased K^+ conductance and K^+ exit

5. Phase 4 (−90 mV) when the Na^+/K^+ pump, the Na^+/Ca^{2+} exchanger and a Ca^{2+} pump restore cell ion levels.

The long plateau or phase 2 means that the refractory period is longer than the contraction time so that summation and tetanus cannot occur.

Ca^{2+} channel blockers are used to treat heart failure. This is because they dilate blood vessels and therefore reduce afterload. This increases CO despite the reduction in heart muscle force caused directly by the blocker.

In the sinoatrial (SA) node, the resting membrane potential is −55 mV. Depolarization and repolarization are slower and there is no phase 1 or 2. Phase 4 is unstable (pacemaker potential, diastolic depolarization, prepotential) and it is caused by the 'funny' current[2] which is activated by hyperpolarization and allows Na^+ to enter the cell. The depolarization activates slow L-type Ca^{2+} channels that cause phase 0. Repolarization is caused by activation of K^+ channels and K^+ exit. The intrinsic rate of the SA node is approximately 100/min. This is slowed to a resting HR of 70/min by the vagus.

Cardiac muscle is a functional syncytium with cells electrically connected via intercalated discs. More specifically, it is two syncytia, the atria and ventricles, divided by a fibrous AV ring and linked by the AV node. Current flows from depolarized to non-depolarized muscle. The cardiac impulse spreads from SA to AV node through internodal pathways. There is a delay at the AV node and then the impulse spreads rapidly through the bundle of His and Purkinje system.

The ECG

There are three standard bipolar limb leads (Figure 1.2.6.3): lead I is arm to arm, lead II is left leg to right arm, and lead III is left leg to left arm.

There are three augmented unipolar limb leads (aVR, aVL, and aVF) where one limb is connected to positive and the other two limbs are connected together.

There are six unipolar chest leads, V1–V6 (the indifferent electrode is the three limb leads connected together to give 0 volts—Einthoven's triangle).

Deflections in the ECG occur when current flows between depolarizing and non-depolarizing muscle. The wave of depolarization moving towards a + electrode causes a positive deflection.

The atria depolarize causing the P wave.

The inner wall of the ventricle depolarizes before the outer wall during the QRS complex.

The outer wall of the ventricle repolarizes first, so that the repolarization wave is in the opposite direction to depolarization and so the T wave is in the same direction. During the QRS, the resultant vector is about 60° from horizontal, that is, the electrical axis of the heart.

Left and right ventricular hypertrophy causes left and right axis deviation respectively.

The PR interval is from the beginning of P to the beginning of QRS. In first-degree heart block, the PR interval is prolonged (>0.20 seconds). In second-degree heart block, there are missed beats (e.g. P:QRS of 2:1 or 3:2). In third-degree or complete heart block, ventricular escape occurs and the ventricle beats at 40/min independently of the SA node. There is no relation between P and QRS. In Stokes–Adams syndrome, there is intermittent complete block with fainting followed by ventricular escape.

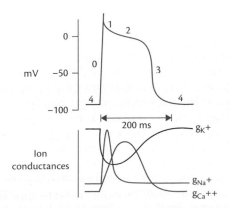

Fig. 1.2.6.2 Ventricular action potential (above) and ionic conductances (below). Phase 4 is the resting membrane potential, phase 0 is the rapid upstroke of depolarization, phase 2 is the plateau, and phase 3 is repolarization.

Reproduced from Matthew Barnard and Bruce Martin, *Cardiac Anaesthesia*, Oxford Specialist Handbooks in Anaesthesia, Figure 2.1, p. 16, Oxford University Press, Oxford, UK, Copyright © 2010, by permission of Oxford University Press.

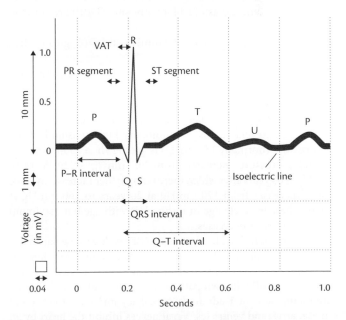

Fig. 1.2.6.3 Electrocardiogram showing the P wave (atrial depolarization), QRS complex (ventricular depolarization, T wave (ventricular repolarization), and various intervals and segments.

Reproduced from Goldschlager N and Goldman MJ, *Principles of Clinical Electrocardiography*, Thirteenth Edition, Appleton and Lange, Connecticut, USA, Copyright © 1989, with permission from McGraw-Hill Education.

The QT interval is from the beginning of QRS to the end of T. In long QT syndrome, the prolonged QT is associated with arrhythmias. The RR interval is the duration of one heart cycle. A prolonged QRS can be due to prolonged conduction through the ventricle (hypertrophy/dilation or Purkinje block) or to a premature ventricular contraction (PVC). An elevated ST segment can occur with acute myocardial infarction.

Sinus arrhythmia is an increase in HR during inspiration.

Ectopic beats are premature contractions due to abnormal impulses from ectopic foci. These can arise from ischaemia, calcified plaques, drugs, and so on. Premature atrial contractions occur in healthy people. There is a pulse deficit, that is, a weak pulse. With PVCs, there is a prolonged QRS, the QRS voltage is larger (one side of heart depolarizes before the other so no cancelling of waves occurs) and there is an inverted T wave (repolarization is in the same direction as depolarization). There is a compensatory pause because the next SA node impulse arrives during the PVC and has no effect. In Wolff–Parkinson–White syndrome, anomalous pathways between atria and ventricles result in re-entrant activity and multiple PVCs. In atrial flutter, the rate is 200–350 beats/min. There is no atrial pumping, there are P waves, and usually 2:1 or 3:1 block. In atrial fibrillation, there is no pumping and no P waves, but CO is adequate at rest. In ventricular fibrillation, multiple ectopic foci or re-entrant activity cause desynchronized contractions, no ejection of blood, and eventually death occurs unless reversed with a defibrillator.

Control of blood pressure and cardiac output

Introduction to control of blood pressure and cardiac output

Grade I hypertension is a systolic blood pressure (SBP) greater than 140 mmHg and a diastolic blood pressure (DBP) greater than 90 mmHg.

Grade II is SBP greater than 160 mmHg and DBP greater than 100 mmHg.

The problem of 'white coat hypertension' can be circumvented with Holter 24-hour recording.

Morbidity and mortality from hypertension arises due to excessive work load on the heart, heart failure, coronary and cerebrovascular events, and renal damage. Pulmonary hypertension is when mean pressure (normally 15 mmHg) is greater than 25 mmHg.

Diastolic pressure increases from 70 mmHg at 20 years to 85 mmHg at 60 years after which there is no further increase. Systolic pressure increases from 120 mmHg at 20 years to 160 mmHg at 70 years. There is no change in resting HR with age but maximum HR during exercise decreases.

Short-term control of blood pressure (BP) is due to the baroreflex but long-term control is the renal mechanism of pressure diuresis. An increase in BP will cause natriuresis and diuresis so that blood volume falls so BP falls. Sympathetic nerves stimulate the heart by acting mainly at beta-1-adrenoceptors. They innervate the SA and AV node, atria, and ventricles. Vagal nerves inhibit the heart by an action at M_2 muscarinic receptors. They act on the SA and AV node and atria but have only a small effect on the ventricles. Sympathetic stimulation opens SA node cation channels so Na^+ enters the cell ('funny inward current') causing rapid depolarization so threshold

is reached earlier so HR increases (positive chronotropic effect). Ivabradine[3] blocks the 'funny' current and so decreases HR (useful in angina, heart failure, and heart transplantation). The sympathetic nerves also increase Ca^{2+} entry into atrial and ventricular cells which increases contractility (positive inotropic effect). Vagal stimulation decreases 'funny inward current'. This reduces phase 4 depolarization so that it takes longer to reach threshold so HR is decreased. In maximal exercise, sympathetic stimulation and vagal withdrawal increases HR to 200/min. Beta blockers (e.g. propranolol) decrease HR to about 60/min. Strong vagal stimulation can cause complete heart block and then 'vagal escape'—an idioventricular beat of 40/min. Atropine will increase HR at rest to about 120/min. Sympathetic and vagal blockade results in a HR of 100/min—the intrinsic pacemaker rate.

Baroreceptors

Baroreceptors are stretch receptors in the aortic arch (vagal afferents) and carotid sinus (glossopharyngeal afferents). A rise in pressure stimulates them and this causes inhibition of the medullary sympathetic outflow, arteriolar vasodilation, venodilation, and decreased HR, SV, CO, venous return (VR), and total peripheral resistance (TPR). Therefore, since BP = CO × TPR, the BP decreases. There is also activation of vagal efferents to the heart to decrease HR. Since CO = SV × HR, CO can be controlled by altering HR and SV. SV is determined by intrinsic and extrinsic factors. Intrinsic control is the Frank–Starling mechanism. If more blood enters the ventricle in diastole, the ventricular muscle fibres are stretched to a greater length (increased preload). The actin and myosin filaments are at a more optimal sarcomere length so the force of ventricular contraction increases and SV increases, that is, the heart ejects what it receives. Extrinsic control is by nervous control and circulating factors that alter contractility. The SV and CO are usually unaffected by the afterload or aortic pressure, except at very high BP or in heart failure. This is partly because of Starling's law, that is, the increased afterload causes a temporary decrease in SV, an increase in EDV and restoration of SV. Thus, hypertensive patients usually have an apparently normal CO.[4]

Haemodynamics

There is a relationship between flow (Q), pressure head (ΔP), and resistance (R), that is, $Q = \Delta P/R$. According to Poiseuille's law, $R = 8\eta L/\pi r^4$. Therefore $Q = \Delta P\, \pi r^4/8\eta L$ where η (eta) = viscosity, L = length of vessel, and r = vessel radius.

Flow depends directly on pressure difference and radius (4th power or r^4). Flow depends inversely on viscosity and length. Blood flow is normally laminar or streamlined when Reynold's number (Re) is less than 2000. Re = ρ (rho). D. v/η (eta) where ρ = density, D = diameter, η = viscosity, and v = velocity.

Beyond a critical velocity, for a given vessel diameter, turbulent flow occurs. Turbulence causes murmurs and Korotkoff sounds. Increased viscosity decreases flow and increases heart work. Factors that alter viscosity are haematocrit and temperature (hypothermia increases viscosity). Small vessels have anomalous viscosity due to axial streaming of red blood cells (RBCs). RBCs travel faster than the plasma so the haematocrit is less in small vessels.

Transmural pressure (P_{TM}) = inside pressure − outside pressure. Pressure inside must be greater or the vessel collapses. But $P_{TM} = T/r$

where T = wall tension and r = radius (Laplace's law). A small radius means that less wall tension is required to balance the distending pressure so thin-walled capillaries do not rupture. A dilated aneurysm is more likely to rupture and a dilated heart must generate more tension. The arterioles have a thick wall of smooth muscle with a rich sympathetic but no parasympathetic innervation. They have high resistance so the blood pressure falls steeply in the arterioles from 80 mmHg at the beginning, to 30 mmHg at the end of the arteriole. Arterioles offer 50% of TPR and they control BP and flow into capillaries.

Tissue blood flow is also controlled by autoregulation. Tissue metabolism produces vasodilator metabolites such as K^+, H^+, CO_2, adenosine, and so on which ensure that the blood flow is adequate to meet the metabolic requirements. If metabolism increases, more metabolites accumulate so the vessels dilate and blood flow increases. If metabolism decreases, there are less metabolites so the vessels constrict and blood flow decreases.

Starling forces

Capillary BP (hydrostatic pressure) forces fluid out of the capillary (30 mmHg at the start and 10 mmHg at the end of the capillary). Interstitial fluid pressure is the pressure of the fluid in the tissue spaces. Interstitial pressure is about −3 mmHg, probably due to lymphatic pumping. The plasma colloid osmotic pressure (25 mmHg) is generated by the plasma proteins (mainly albumin) which cannot pass through the wall. This causes fluid uptake into capillaries. Interstitial fluid colloid osmotic pressure is 8 mmHg because some protein enters the interstitium.

During haemorrhage, the decrease in BP and the arteriolar constriction causes a decrease in capillary hydrostatic pressure that causes fluid uptake by capillaries, hence the pinched appearance of patients.

In congestive heart failure, the decreased VR increases capillary hydrostatic pressure causing oedema. Portal hypertension causes ascites (abdominal oedema) because of increased hydrostatic pressure in gut wall capillaries. A decrease in plasma proteins (e.g. starvation, liver disease, nephrotic syndrome, and burns) causes oedema. Increased capillary permeability (e.g. histamine, bacterial infection, prolonged ischaemia, and burns) also causes oedema as well as lymphatic blockage or removal.

Venous return

The venules and veins carry blood back to the right atrium. They are capacitance vessels with low pressure and thin walls. The veins contain two-thirds of the blood volume. They have a rich sympathetic innervation that causes venoconstriction that mobilizes blood to increase VR and CO. VR is determined by the pressure gradient (10 mmHg in the venules and 0 mmHg in the right atrium). Therefore, VR is increased in exercise and decreased in right heart failure. Contractions of skeletal muscles compress deep veins and push blood back to the heart (muscle pump). The negative intrathoracic pressure during inspiration pulls blood towards the right atrium (respiratory pump).

Gravity causes venous pooling below the heart and decreases VR. Orthostatic hypotension occurs on standing when the decreased VR causes a decrease in CO and BP. Pressure in the sagittal sinus above the heart is negative, hence the danger of air embolism during brain surgery.

Cerebral blood flow

Cerebral blood flow (CBF) is held constant despite large changes in mean arterial blood pressure (MAP). Between a MAP of 60–140 mmHg, CBF is relatively constant at 750 mL/min (15% of resting CO).

The metabolic theory of autoregulation is that if BP increases, blood flow will increase and wash away local vasodilator metabolites such as CO_2, H^+, K^+, adenosine, and so on. This will cause vasoconstriction so that the blood flow does not increase. Cerebral vessels are especially sensitive to CO_2. Hyperventilation can be used to reduce intracranial pressure since the fall in CO_2 will cause cerebral vasoconstriction.

The myogenic theory of autoregulation is that if BP increases, the stretch of the vascular smooth muscle causes it to contract so the vasoconstriction prevents an increase in blood flow. In general, sympathetic nerves are thought to have a minor role in normal control of CBF. The CNS ischaemic response protects CBF when MAP falls. When MAP falls during haemorrhage, the resulting brain ischaemia causes hypoxia/hypercapnia in the brainstem evoking powerful stimulation of sympathetic nerve activity to increase MAP and restore CBF.[5] The brain is enclosed in a rigid structure. An increase in intracranial pressure (e.g. due to a tumour, head injury, or oedema) will compress the blood vessels, decrease CBF and evoke a CNS ischaemic response called the Cushing reflex. The BP will be elevated but HR will be low (presumably because the baroreflex can lower HR but not BP due to vagal slowing of HR). This combination of high BP and low HR is an ominous clinical sign.

Coronary blood flow

Two coronary arteries arise behind the cusps of the aortic valves. Most blood returns to the right atrium via the coronary sinus/anterior cardiac veins. Coronary blood flow is 250 mL/min (5% of CO at rest).

During systole, the contracting ventricle compresses its blood vessels. A systolic pressure of 120 mmHg in the left ventricle means that there is zero flow to subendocardial regions of left ventricle. There is little effect on flow in the right ventricle where systolic pressure is only 25 mmHg. Eighty per cent of coronary blood flow in the left ventricle occurs in diastole. This can be a problem at high HR because diastole is shortened to a greater extent than systole. Most tissues extract 25% of the arterial blood O_2 but the coronary extraction is 75% so that the venous O_2 content is 5 rather than 15 mL/100 mL of blood. This means that increased O_2 consumption must be through increased blood flow since the heart cannot extract much more O_2 from the arterial blood. Coronary flow is closely related to O_2 consumption. Vasodilator metabolites include hypoxia, high CO_2, H^+, K^+, lactate, adenosine, and so on.

Coronary arteries have a sympathetic innervation but control by local metabolites predominates.

Further reading

Barrett KE, Boitano S, Barman SM, *et al. Ganong's Review of Medical Physiology* (24th ed). New York: McGraw-Hill Education; 2012.
Koeppen BM, Stanton BA. *Berne & Levy's Physiology* (6th ed). Philadelphia, PA: Elsevier Health Sciences; 2009.

References

1. O'Rourke MF, Yaginuma T. Wave reflections and the arterial pulse. *Arch Intern Med* 1984; 144:366–71.
2. DiFranesco D, Borer JS. The funny current: cellular basis for the control of heart rate. *Drugs* 2007; 67 (2):15–24.
3. Sulfi S, Timmis AD. Ivabradine—the first selective sinus node If channel inhibitor in the treatment of stable angina. *Int J Clin Pract* 2006; 60(2):222–8.
4. Mayet J, Hughes A. Cardiac and vascular pathophysiology in hypertension. *Heart* 2003; 89(9):1104–9.
5. Dickinson CJ. Reappraisal of the Cushing reflex: the most powerful neural blood pressure stabilizing mechanism. *Clin Sci* 1990; 79:543–50.

CHAPTER 1.2.7

Respiratory

Aidan Bradford

Respiratory muscles

There are three groups of inspiratory muscles: primary, accessory, and airway. The primary muscles are the diaphragm (innervated by the phrenic nerves from C3, C4, and C5, hence spinal transection above C3 is fatal without intervention) and the external intercostal muscles. Accessory muscles such as the scalenes and sternomastoids are used in exercise or respiratory disease. Airway muscles such as the genioglossus and pharyngeal muscles dilate and stabilize the compliant upper airway.

Obstructive sleep apnoea is a common condition caused by decreased upper airway muscle activity during sleep.[1] The pharynx collapses due to the negative pressure in the airway during inspiration so the patient cannot breath (apnoea) for periods of up to 1 minute in severe cases. Arousal from sleep activates the upper airway muscles and the airway opens. The cycle repeats itself during the night (hundreds of times in severe cases).

Expiration in eupnoea (normal quiet breathing) is passive, due to lung recoil but during forced expiration, the internal intercostals and abdominal muscles are recruited.

Alveolar pressure

Alveolar pressure (P_A) is the pressure in the alveolar space. This space is connected to the atmosphere which has a pressure (P_B) of 760 mmHg (P_B, is designated as a baseline at zero pressure) so P_A is about 760 mmHg or 0.

During inspiration, P_A falls to −1 mmHg as the lung expands and air enters the lung and P_A returns to 0. During expiration, P_A increases to +1 mmHg and air leaves the lung.

In artificial respiration, air is pushed into the lungs under positive pressure so P_A is positive during inspiration. Greater P_A changes are seen with forced inspiration and expiration and in airway obstruction.

Intrapleural pressure

The lungs are separated from the chest wall by a potential space called the pleural cavity. The pressure is −5 cmH$_2$O at functional residual capacity (FRC) due to lung and chest wall recoil.

If air enters the pleural space (pneumothorax) the lung collapses and the chest expands and intrapleural pressure (P_{PL}) becomes 0 (i.e. atmospheric pressure P_B). In a tension pneumothorax, a flap of tissue forms a one-way valve so that air enters with each inspiration but cannot leave so pressure becomes greater than P_B.

During inspiration P_{PL} falls to −10 cmH$_2$O. During forced inspiration and expiration against a closed glottis (Muller and Valsalva manoeuvre respectively), large negative and positive pressures are generated. The P_{PL} becomes positive with forced expiration. At FRC, it is −8 cmH$_2$O at the top and −2 cmH$_2$O at the bottom of the lung in the upright position.

Lung volumes and capacities

- The lung volumes and capacities are measured with a spirometer except for residual volume (RV), FRC, and total lung capacity (TLC) (Figure 1.2.7.1).

- FRC can be measured using the helium dilution technique or body plethysmography.

- Tidal volume (V_T), respiratory frequency or rate (f), are used to calculate the minute ventilation (also called minute volume):

  Minute volume = V_T × f = 500 mL × 12 breaths/min = 6 L/min

- FRC is the volume in the lungs after a quiet expiration (2.5 L).

- Inspiratory reserve volume (IRV) is the maximum volume that can be inspired after a quiet inspiration (3 L).

- Inspiratory capacity (IC) is the maximum volume that can be inspired after a quiet expiration (3.5 L). This is equal to IRV + V_T.

- Expiratory reserve volume (ERV) is the maximum volume that can be expired after a quiet expiration (1 L).

- RV is the volume in the lungs after a maximum expiration (1.5 L).

- TLC is the volume in the lungs at maximum inspiration (6 L) and is the sum of RV + ERV + V_T + IRV.

- Vital capacity (VC) is the maximum volume expired after a maximum inspiration (4.5 L) and is the sum of ERV + V_T + IRV.

- FEV_1 is the forced expiratory volume in 1 second and the ratio FEV_1/forced vital capacity (FVC) equals 80% in the normal adult.

- In obstructive disease (asthma, chronic obstructive pulmonary disease), FEV_1 is reduced more than the FVC so that the ratio of FEV_1/FVC is less than 80%.

- In restrictive disease (lung fibrosis, scoliosis), both FEV_1 and FVC are reduced but the ratio of FEV_1/FVC is either normal or greater than 80%.

- Peak expiratory flow rate can be obtained from a peak flow meter or from the flow–volume curve. It is the highest flow rate achieved during a maximal expiration and occurs at the beginning of expiration near TLC.

- Dead space (V_D) air is air that does not take part in exchange with the blood. Of the 500 mL inspired, only 350 mL enters the alveoli for gas exchange. The rest (150 mL) occupies the dead

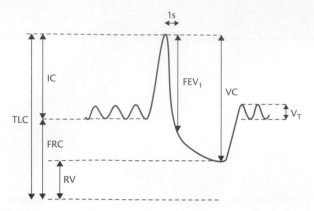

Fig. 1.2.7.1 Spirometer recording showing the lung volumes and capacities. Reproduced from G. J. Gibson, 'Respiratory function tests' in David A. Warrell, Timothy N. Cox and John D. Firth (Eds.), *Oxford Textbook of Medicine*, Fifth Edition, Oxford University Press, Oxford, UK, Copyright © 2010, by permission of Oxford University Press.

space in the mouth, nose, pharynx, trachea, and so on and does not exchange with the blood. Anatomical V_D is the volume of the conducting airways and physiological V_D is this plus air in alveoli that does not exchange with blood. Normally, the volumes are almost the same. Anatomical V_D is decreased by a tracheostomy and increased by breathing through a tube. In respiratory disease, physiological V_D may be much larger than normal. Minute ventilation = $V_T \times f$ but alveolar ventilation is the amount of air that actually reaches the alveoli per minute, that is:

$$(V_T - V_D) \times f = (500 - 150) \times 12 = 4.2 \text{ L/min}$$

Compliance

This is a measure of the ease with which the respiratory system is inflated. It is the change in volume/change in pressure measured in L/cmH_2O.

Compliance is increased when elastic tissue is lost such as in early emphysema and ageing and can be decreased in obstructive and restrictive diseases. Alveoli are lined with liquid creating an air–liquid interface which develops surface tension favouring alveolar collapse. About 50% of lung recoil is due to surface tension. The force is reduced by surfactant secreted by type II alveolar cells. Surfactant increases lung compliance and reduces work, stabilizes alveoli, that is, it counteracts Laplace's law, and reduces lung capillary filtration. Laplace's law states that P is proportional to T/R where P is the distending pressure, T is the wall tension, and R is the radius. If R is small, P is large so small alveoli should empty into large ones and collapse. However, smaller alveoli have more surfactant per unit area than large so when R is small, T is small and P is the same for large and small alveoli so alveoli remain stable.

Surfactant is formed late in gestation so premature infants develop respiratory distress syndrome (RDS). In RDS, there is increased work of breathing, collapse of alveoli (atelectasis), and lung oedema.

Airway resistance

About 50% of airway resistance is in the upper airway above the larynx. Of the 50% in the lower airway, 40% is in the trachea and bronchi and only 10% is in the small airways (<2 mm

diameter). The small diameter is offset by the huge increase in cross-sectional area.

These small airways are most affected in obstructive diseases so that damage in this 'silent zone' may go undetected.[2] Blocking vagal parasympathetic nerve activity with atropine decreases airway resistance by 30%. Sympathetic nerves slightly bronchodilate through beta-2 receptors. Most beta-2 receptors are not associated with these nerves but are stimulated by blood epinephrine (adrenaline) and norepinephrine (noradrenaline) and by drugs like salbutamol.

The airways are held open by radial traction of elastic tissue which increases during inspiration so airway resistance falls. Radial traction is reduced in emphysema so resistance increases as the diameter narrows. During forced expiration, the positive P_{PL} compresses the airways and increases resistance. In obstructive diseases, expiration is difficult and patients will breathe slowly and through partially closed (pursed) lips to maintain pressure to reduce airway resistance.

Ventilation/perfusion ratio

The alveolar–capillary membrane is normally very thin (0.5 μm) and so there is rapid, complete equilibration of O_2 and CO_2 between alveolar gas and blood (perfusion rather than diffusion being the limiting factor). Exchange is by simple diffusion which is directly proportional to pressure difference and the surface area and inversely proportional to distance (i.e. the thickness of the alveolar wall). Exchange is reduced in emphysema (reduced surface area) and in lung oedema and fibrosis (increased distance for diffusion).

The ability of the alveolar–capillary membrane to exchanges gases is measured from the diffusing capacity. Normally, arterial blood PO_2 is slightly less (95 mmHg) than alveolar PO_2 (100 mmHg) (arterial/alveolar PO_2 gradient) because of venous admixture which consists of an anatomical shunt (bronchial veins draining the bronchi directly into the azygous and hemi-azygous systems and the Thebesian veins which drain directly into the cardiac chambers) and ventilation/perfusion (V/Q) mismatch.

In the upright position, P_{PL} is more negative at the apex of the lung. Therefore alveoli are more expanded and therefore less compliant than at the base so more air goes to the base during inspiration. Blood flow is greatest at the base and least at the apex (Figure 1.2.7.2). Because the apex is relatively overventilated, tuberculosis is more likely in the apex where there is a higher PO_2.

In respiratory disease, the V/Q ratio may be increased (overventilation/underperfusion) or decreased (underventilation/overperfusion). An increased V/Q ratio means an increase in alveolar V_D and 'wasted ventilation'. A decreased V/Q ratio means 'shunting' where deoxygenated venous blood bypasses the exchange area and enters the left heart causing arterial hypoxaemia. This is a common cause of hypoxaemia. A 'true shunt' is where blood flows through a region with zero ventilation. Examples would be abnormal right–left shunts in the heart, atelectasis, and consolidation. Oxygen therapy will improve PaO_2 with a low V/Q ratio but not with 'true shunt'. A high V/Q ratio increases alveolar PO_2 (P_AO_2) and decreases P_ACO_2 and vice versa with a low V/Q ratio.

A decrease in P_AO_2 and an increase in P_ACO_2 cause relaxation of airway smooth muscle but contraction of pulmonary arterioles (hypoxic pulmonary vasoconstriction). Hypoxic pulmonary vasoconstriction causes diversion of blood away from poorly

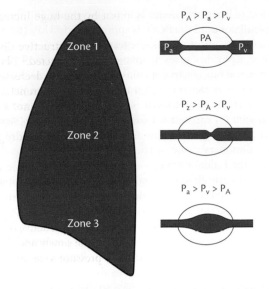

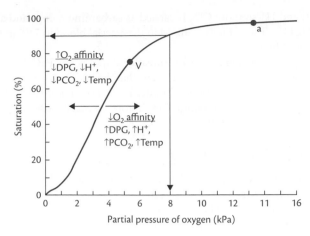

Fig. 1.2.7.2 Diagrammatic representation of the three lung zones of West where PA = alveolar pressure, Pa = pulmonary arterial pressure, and Pv = pulmonary venous pressure.

Reproduced from Catherine Spoors and Kevin Kiff (Eds.), *Training in Anaesthesia*, Figure 13.40, p. 359, Oxford University Press, Oxford, UK, Copyright © 2010, by permission of Oxford University Press.

Fig. 1.2.7.3 The oxyhaemoglobin dissociation curve. Point a is representative of arterial blood and point v is representative of venous blood. The curve can move to the right or left, caused by changes in PCO_2, H^+, temperature, or 2,3-DPG levels.

Reproduced from Nick Maskell and Ann Millar (Eds.), *Oxford Desk Reference: Respiratory Medicine*, Figure 2.1.4, p. 14, Oxford University Press, Oxford, UK, Copyright © 2009, by permission of Oxford University Press.

ventilated/overperfused alveoli and therefore limits 'shunting'. However, generalized alveolar hypoxia (altitude, some respiratory diseases) will cause pulmonary hypertension. Pulmonary hypertension can cause right ventricular hypertrophy and failure (cor pulmonale).[3]

Oxygen and carbon dioxide transport in the blood

Oxygen transport in the blood

Oxygen is carried in the blood physically dissolved in plasma and combined with haemoglobin. Only 0.3 mL/dL is physically dissolved. Haemoglobin consists of four haem groups attached to four protein chains (two alpha and two beta chains). Each haem contains an atom of ferrous (Fe^{2+}) iron. O_2 binds loosely and reversibly with the iron to form oxyhaemoglobin. The percentage saturation (O_2 content/O_2 capacity ratio) is measured non-invasively using a pulse oximeter. O_2 capacity is the volume of O_2 carried when the PO_2 is very high (so the Hb is 100% saturated). There are 15 g of Hb/dL and since every g maximally combines with 1.34 mL O_2, the O_2 capacity is 20 mL/dL.

The 'S' or sigmoid shape of the oxyhaemoglobin dissociation curve (Figure 1.2.7.3) means that at the plateau, where the percentage saturation is almost 100%, the inspired PO_2 can fall without much of a fall in percentage saturation. This is a protection against altitude and respiratory disease. However, it reduces the usefulness of hyperventilation and O_2 therapy. The steep portion allows for O_2 unloading in the tissues.

In the tissues, the increase in PCO_2 and H^+ causes the Hb to release more O_2, that is, the Bohr effect. A similar effect is also caused by an increase in temperature and 2,3-diphosphoglycerate. 2,3-DPG is formed in the red blood cell (RBC) by hypoxia and acidosis and binds to the beta chains of Hb causing O_2 release.

2,3-DPG is increased in exercise, altitude, anaemia, and respiratory disease and is reduced in stored blood. The P_{50} is the PO_2 at which the Hb is 50% saturated.

Examples of states with altered oxygen saturation

Fetal Hb (HbF) binds O_2 better than adult Hb because 2,3-DPG binds poorly to the gamma chains of HbF. This improves O_2 transfer across the placenta.

Myoglobin is found in skeletal and cardiac muscle. It has a higher O_2 affinity than Hb and acts as a tissue store of O_2.

In anaemia, the Hb concentration is reduced so the PaO_2 is normal but the O_2 content is reduced.

The Fe^{2+} of Hb can be oxidized to Fe^{3+} (ferric iron) by chemicals and drugs (e.g. nitrates, nitrites, sulphonamides, local anaesthetics, and cocaine) to form methaemoglobin which does not bind O_2 (methaemoglobinaemia). This can be treated with methylene blue, a reducing agent.

Cyanosis is a blue colouration of the skin and mucous membranes, especially the tongue, mouth, lips, and nail beds. It occurs when the arterial blood is less than 85% saturated ($PO_2 = 6.7$ kPa or 50 mmHg) or when the capillary blood is 70% saturated (5 kPa or 37.5 mmHg). Central cyanosis is due to arterial blood desaturation. Peripheral cyanosis is due to reduced tissue blood flow due to vasoconstriction (exposure to cold, Raynaud's disease, etc.), vascular obstruction or decreased cardiac output (heart failure, shock, etc.).

Hb binds carbon monoxide 240 times more avidly than O_2 forming carboxyhaemoglobin which does not bind O_2 (carboxyhaemoglobinaemia, carbon monoxide poisoning[4]).

In sickle cell anaemia, the abnormal Hb causes deformation of the RBC (sickling) so blood flow is impaired.

Carbon dioxide transport in the blood

Carbon dioxide is carried physically dissolved (3 mL % as molecular CO_2), as carbamino compounds (3 mL % combined with haemoglobin and plasma proteins) and as bicarbonate (42 mL %) due to the reaction $CO_2 + H_2O \leftrightarrow H_2CO_3 \leftrightarrow H^+ + HCO_3^-$.

The deoxygenation of blood increases its ability to carry CO_2, that is, the Haldane effect. The loss of O_2 allows Hb to bind more

CO_2 and H^+ so more CO_2 is carried as carbamino compound and as HCO_3^-. The pH falls from 7.4 in the arterial blood to 7.35 in the venous blood.

Hyperventilation means 'overbreathing', that is, the $PaCO_2$ is less than normal. Hypoventilation means that the $PaCO_2$ is greater than normal. Hyperventilation (altitude, hysteria) causes respiratory alkalosis and hypoventilation (respiratory disease) causes respiratory acidosis.

Control of breathing

Breathing is driven by both a rhythm generator called the pre-Botzinger complex and an inspiratory and expiratory centre all found within the medulla as well as the pontine apneustic and its antagonist, the pneumotaxic centres both within the pons.

Nerve endings in the airway smooth muscle are stimulated by stretch during inspiration. The nerve impulses travel in the vagus nerve to inhibit inspiration. This is the called the Hering–Breuer inflation reflex.

Other nerve endings near the airway epithelial cells are stimulated by noxious gases, cigarette smoke, dust, and cold air. These nerve impulses also travel in the vagus causing reflex bronchoconstriction, mucus secretion, hyperpnoea, sneeze, and cough and may be involved in asthma attacks.

Nerve endings near the capillaries in the alveoli called juxtacapillary (J) receptors are stimulated by pulmonary congestion and oedema. The nerve impulses travel in the vagus causing reflex apnoea or rapid shallow breathing. They may be involved in the rapid shallow breathing and dyspnoea of pulmonary congestion and oedema.

Breathing is also controlled by the pH and gas pressures of the blood and extra cellular fluid. These chemoreceptors consist of peripheral and central chemoreceptors.

The peripheral chemoreceptors (carotid and aortic bodies, supplied by the glossopharyngeal (IX) and vagus nerve (X) respectively) are stimulated by a decrease in PaO_2 and an increase in $PaCO_2$ and H^+. This stimulates the respiratory centre causing an increase in breathing. This causes an increase in PaO_2 and a decrease in $PaCO_2$ and H^+ so there is 'negative feedback' control of blood gases.

The central chemoreceptors in the medulla are stimulated by an increase in brain extracellular fluid PCO_2 and H^+ but not by a decrease in PO_2. They are responsible for 80% of the ventilatory response to increased $PaCO_2$. They have a poor response to arterial blood H^+ because of the blood–brain barrier.

Therefore all of the ventilatory response to decreased PaO_2 is due to the peripheral chemoreceptors, most of the ventilatory response to increased arterial blood H^+ is due to the peripheral chemoreceptors and most of the ventilatory response to increased $PaCO_2$ is due to the central chemoreceptors.

Ventilation is very sensitive to small changes in $PaCO_2$ but there is little response to hypoxia until the PaO_2 falls below 60 mmHg. Hypocapnia causes increased neuromuscular excitability and tetany and hypercapnia causes depression of the nervous system and coma.

One test of brainstem death is to pre-oxygenate and then switch off the ventilator until the PCO_2 is approximately 8 kPa (60 mmHg). If no respiratory effort occurs, the test is positive.

Chronic asphyxia causes adaptation of the ventilatory response to hypercapnia but not to hypoxia. Therefore chronically asphyxic patients are more dependent on their hypoxic drive through the peripheral chemoreceptors in order to breathe. Treatment of asphyxia with O_2 can cause a dangerous rise in $PaCO_2$ due to the elimination of this drive. The CO_2 also rises because of loss of hypoxic pulmonary vasoconstriction and thus V/Q inequality and because of the Haldane effect.

A form of periodic breathing called Cheyne–Stokes breathing[5] where the V_T increases and decreases is associated with heart disease, brain trauma, sleep at altitude, sleep in the newborn, and so on.

Acute altitude exposure does not affect the composition of the air, that is, 21% O_2 in N_2 but the fall in P_B causes a decrease in air PO_2 and in PaO_2. This stimulates the peripheral chemoreceptors and ventilation increases by 65% so that $PaCO_2$ decreases and there is respiratory alkalosis. There is pulmonary hypertension, increased heart rate and cardiac output, and, in the nervous system, drowsiness, decreased manual dexterity, judgement and memory, euphoria, and coma at higher than 23 000 feet. Chronic exposure causes acclimatization where ventilation increases further to 300–500% and $PaCO_2$ decreases further. There is increased erythropoietin, haematocrit (to 60–65%), Hb (to 22 g%), blood volume (by 20–30%), 2,3-DPG, P_{50}, and diffusing capacity. There is renal compensation for the respiratory alkalosis, that is, increased renal HCO_3^- excretion. Acute mountain sickness is associated with dyspnoea, palpitations, fatigue, muscular weakness, drowsiness, sleeplessness, dizziness, headache, nausea, anorexia, decreased visual acuity, high-altitude cerebral oedema, pulmonary hypertension, and high-altitude pulmonary oedema. Treatment consists of descent, acetazolamide, or a Gamov bag. In chronic mountain sickness, there is an excessive increase in haematocrit, severe pulmonary hypertension, and right heart failure.

Further reading

Barrett KE, Boitano S, Barman SM, *et al. Ganong's Review of Medical Physiology* (24th ed). New York: McGraw-Hill Education; 2012.

Koeppen BM, Stanton BA. *Berne & Levy's Physiology* (6th ed). Philadelphia, PA: Elsevier Health Sciences; 2009.

References

1. Dempsey JA, Veasey SC, Morgan BJ, O'Donnell CP. Pathophysiology of sleep apnea. *Physiol Rev* 2010; 90(1):47–112.
2. Kraft M. The distal airways: are they important in asthma? *Eur Respir J* 1999; 14:1403–17.
3. Andrews JL Jr. Cor pulmonale: pathophysiology and management. *Geriatrics* 1976; 31(11):91–9.
4. Prockop LD, Chichkova RI. Carbon monoxide intoxication: an updated review. *J Neurol Sci* 2007; 262(1–2):122–30.
5. Naughton MT. Pathophysiology and treatment of Cheyne-Stokes respiration. *Thorax* 1998; 53(6):514–18.

CHAPTER 1.2.8

Gastrointestinal

Aidan Bradford

Saliva

The parotid glands produce a serous, watery secretion containing amylase, the sublingual glands produce mucus, and the submaxillary glands are mixed serous and mucous. Salivary secretion is approximately 1 L/day and contains mucins (glycoproteins), alpha-amylase (ptyalin), lingual lipase, immunoglobulin A, and lysozyme. It is hypotonic with low Na^+ and Cl^- and high K^+ and HCO_3^- relative to plasma. The pH is 6.0–8.0 (pH optimum for amylase is 7.0). Parasympathetic (cranial nerves VII and IX) stimulation increases the secretion of amylase and mucus, blood flow, and growth of the salivary glands. Sympathetic stimulation increases the secretion of amylase and mucus and decreases blood flow. Stress causes xerostomia or dry mouth.

Swallowing

There are three phases to swallowing: oral (voluntary), pharyngeal (reflex), and oesophageal (reflex). Afferents in cranial nerves V, IX, and X, especially from the pharynx relay to the swallowing centre in the pons and medulla. Efferents run in cranial nerves V, VII, IX, X, and XII. The soft palate is raised, the vocal folds approximate, the larynx is raised, the epiglottis swings back, the upper oesophageal sphincter relaxes, and the superior pharyngeal constrictor contracts initiating a peristaltic wave in the pharynx and breathing is inhibited. Because of the amount of striated muscle involved in swallowing, it can be impaired in conditions which affect striated muscle such as stroke, myasthenia gravis, Parkinson's disease, and multiple sclerosis. In the oesophageal phase, the upper oesophageal sphincter contracts and a primary peristaltic wave (4 cm/s) moves to the lower oesophageal sphincter. Secondary waves clear the oesophagus of food. Peristalsis is controlled by vagal and intrinsic reflexes. The wall in the first third of the oesophagus is striated muscle, the middle third is striated and smooth, and the last third is smooth. The lower oesophageal sphincter smooth muscle is tonically active (pressure approximately 20 mmHg) due to vagal cholinergic activity which prevents reflux. It relaxes ahead of the peristalsis, caused by vagal nerves which inhibit the smooth muscle by releasing vasoactive intestinal peptide and nitric oxide. In achalasia,[1] swallowing is impaired due to excess lower oesophageal sphincter tone and weak oesophageal peristalsis and sphincter relaxation.

Vomiting (emesis)

The causes of vomiting are distension of the stomach and duodenum or emetics acting on receptors in the stomach/duodenum and on the chemoreceptor trigger zone in the medulla, that is, the area postrema, part of the circumventricular organ system. Emetics include cytotoxic drugs, morphine, uraemia, and endogenous substances released from radiotherapy, infection, or disease. Other causes include motion, psychic stimuli, pain, increased intracranial pressure, tactile stimulation of the back of the throat, pregnancy, and so on. Vomiting is preceded by nausea, salivation, sweating, pallor, mydriasis, and irregular heart rate. Afferents from the stomach and duodenum run in sympathetic nerves and the vagus to the vomiting centre in the medulla. Efferents run in cranial nerves V, VII, IX, X, and XII. There is antiperistalsis in the small intestine, relaxation of the pylorus and stomach, elevation of the larynx, elevation of the soft palate, contraction of abdominal muscles, and relaxation of the lower and upper oesophageal sphincter and oesophagus.

Stomach

When a bolus of food enters the stomach, there is receptive relaxation, that is, active relaxation where distension causes reflex (vagovagal) relaxation. The stomach can accommodate 1.5 L with little change in pressure. There is a rapid rise in pressure above 1.5 L. Contractions (peristalsis) spread towards the pylorus (3/min) which mix and propel food towards the duodenum. The narrow pyloric sphincter means that a small amount of food enters the duodenum with each wave of contraction but most pushes back into the stomach to aid mixing.

Gastric juice is secreted at a rate of 2–3 L/day. It contains HCl (pH 2.0) secreted by the parietal (oxyntic) cell (Figure 1.2.8.1), pepsinogen from the chief (peptic) cell, intrinsic factor also from the parietal cell, mucus, water, HCO_3^-, K^+, and Na^+. Salivary amylase gets inactivated eventually by the low pH. Pepsinogen for protein digestion gets activated to pepsin by the low pH. Vagal stimulation causes release of HCl, pepsinogen, water, mucus, and gastrin and increases motility.

Gastrin stimulates acid secretion, increases gastric motility, and relaxes the pyloric sphincter. It relaxes the ileocaecal sphincter. Acid inhibits acid secretion by acting directly on parietal cells, D cells and G cells. In Zollinger–Ellison syndrome, there is excessive acid secretion and ulceration due to a gastrinoma of the pancreas or elsewhere.

Gastric secretion and motility are controlled by a cephalic, gastric, and intestinal phase. In the cephalic phase, the sight, smell, or thought of food activates gastric motility and secretion through the vagus. In the gastric phase, the stomach is activated by local and vagovagal reflexes and by gastrin. During the intestinal phase, chemical stimulation (carbohydrate, fat, and protein digestion products, high osmolarity, acid) and distension of the duodenum causes inhibition of gastric secretion and motility by means of the

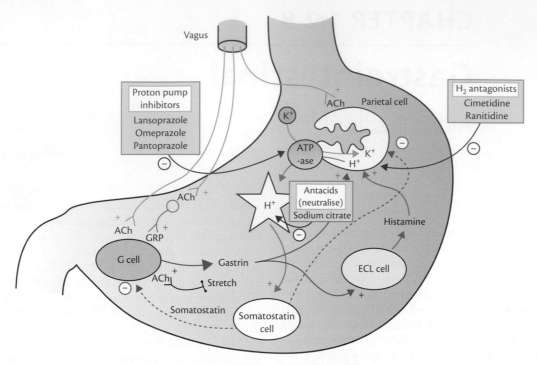

Fig. 1.2.8.1 Diagrammatic representation of the mechanisms involved in the control of gastric acid secretion.
Reproduced from Spoors and Kiff (Eds), *OST Training In Anaesthesia*, Oxford University Press, Oxford, UK, Copyright © 2010, with permission from Oxford University Press.

enterogastric reflex and enterogastrones. The enterogastric reflex is both a local and vagovagal reflex.

Enterogastrones are secretin, cholecystokinin (CCK), and gastric inhibitory peptide. Cholecystokinin may act mainly by activating CCKa receptors on D cells of the pancreas and stomach that release somatostatin that inhibits acid secretion. Peptic ulcers are either gastric or duodenal. They are caused by excess acid secretion or mucosal barrier breakdown. Non-steroidal anti-inflammatory drugs and steroids inhibit prostaglandin synthesis and prostaglandins inhibit acid and stimulate mucus and bicarbonate secretion. Barrier breakdown is caused by *Helicobacter pylori*, the main cause of gastritis and ulcers.[2] This is treated with antibiotics and proton pump inhibitors.

Intestinal motility

The autonomic nerves are not essential for motility. There is a dense vagal innervation to the oesophagus and stomach, a sparser innervation to the small intestine and colon as far as the splenic flexure, and a rich S2, S3, and S4 innervation to the distal colon and rectum. Parasympathetic stimulation increases motility and relaxes sphincters. The sympathetic supply is from T8 to L2 to the entire gut, mainly from prevertebral ganglia (coeliac and superior and inferior mesenteric) and from the hypogastric plexus. Sympathetic stimulation decreases motility and contracts sphincters. The autonomic nerves end mainly on the intramural plexuses which consist of the submucosal (Meissner's) plexus and the myenteric (Auerbach's) plexus (Figure 1.2.8.2). The plexuses consist of cell bodies receiving inputs from extrinsic nerves, other cell bodies, and from gut wall receptors. The output from the cell bodies is to muscle and gland cells. The plexuses are necessary for motility. The basic electrical rhythm or slow waves originate in pacemakers in the muscularis

externa called interstitial cells of Cajal.[3] The pacemaker activity may be caused by an oscillation in calcium conductance. The electrical activity propagates through nexi or gap junctions from one cell to another. The wave amplitude and frequency is determined by extrinsic nerves and hormones and this determines the number of action potentials and therefore the degree of contraction. The pacemaker rate is 3/min in the stomach, 12/min in the duodenum decreasing to 9/min in the ileum. In the large intestine, the frequency is 2/min in the caecum increasing to 6/min in the sigmoid colon. In Hirschsprung's disease, there is a congenital lack of ganglion cells in plexuses of the distal colon and rectum and severe constipation and megacolon. Similar symptoms are seen in Chagas' disease in its megacolon manifestation where *Trypanosome* infestation destroys the colonic plexuses. The migrating motor complex is a 5–10-minute phase of intense contractions which migrates from stomach to ileum in 1.5 hours during fasting. It clears the stomach and small intestine and keeps bacterial counts low in the small intestine. Ileus is a lack of intestinal motility which can occur, especially after abdominal surgery. The gastroileal reflex is a vagovagal reflex which opens the ileocaecal sphincter. Gastrin also relaxes the sphincter. Transit time from pylorus to sphincter is about 5 hours but this is variable. The sphincter allows time for absorption in the small intestine and prevents reflux from the caecum. With obstruction of the colon, gas from bacteria builds up in the caecum and may not be able to pass the ileocaecal sphincter to dissipate in the ileum and this leads to so-called pistol-shot perforation of the caecum. Segmentation contractions in the colon are called haustrations and they almost occlude the lumen. They occur at 2/min in the caecum and increase progressively to 6/min in the sigmoid colon. Peristalsis is weak and slow. Mass movements occur one to three times per day, typically after meals with a duration of approximately 15 minutes but this is highly variable. They are triggered

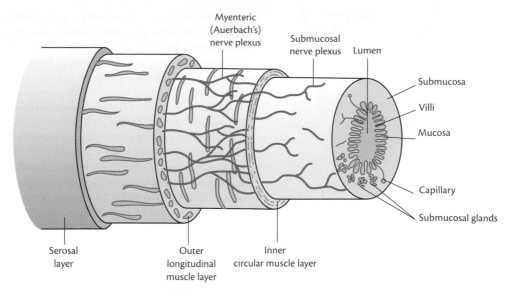

Myenteric (Auerbach's) nerve plexus

Submucosal nerve plexus   Lumen

Submucosa

Villi

Mucosa

Capillary

Submucosal glands

Serosal layer

Outer longitudinal muscle layer

Inner circular muscle layer

Fig. 1.2.8.2 Diagrammatic representation of the structural characteristics of the intestinal wall.
Reproduced from Spoors and Kiff (Eds), *OST Training In Anaesthesia*, Oxford University Press, Oxford, UK, Copyright © 2010, with permission from Oxford University Press.

by gastrocolic and duodenocolic reflexes. This propels faeces into the rectum. Colon transit is slow (18–24 hours approximately) by comparison with the small intestine. Rectal distension causes the defaecation reflex by causing peristalsis in the descending and sigmoid colon and in the rectum and relaxation of the internal anal sphincter. This is controlled by the intramural plexuses. Therefore, with lesions of the extrinsic nerves or spinal cord, defaecation is still possible. However, there is also an extrinsic reflex whereby distension activates stretch receptors running in the sacral parasympathetic nerves. This reflexly activates parasympathetic efferents causing reflex peristalsis in the colon and rectum and relaxation of the internal anal sphincter. The sympathetics do the opposite. Conscious control is through the pudendal nerves to the external anal sphincter which consists of striated muscle. During defaecation, there is voluntary relaxation of the sphincter and a Valsalva manoeuvre. Rectal stretch receptors convey the sense of fullness to the brain. Conscious control is absent in infants, cord and nerve injuries, and mental retardation.

Water and electrolyte absorption

The lumen of the small intestine will have a total volume of fluid of 10 L/day composed of ingested fluid (2 L), saliva (1 L), gastric juice (3 L), bile (1 L), pancreatic juice (1 L), and intestinal juice (2 L). Failure to absorb this fluid would result in diarrhoea, rapid dehydration, and electrolyte imbalance. Normally, 8.5 L is absorbed in the small intestine and 1.4 L in the large intestine leaving 100 mL in the faeces. Excessive secretion can also cause diarrhoea. In the crypts of Lieberkuhn, chloride is secreted by the cystic fibrosis transmembrane regulator (CFTR). Cholera toxin from the bacterium *Vibrio cholerae* activates the CFTR causing excessive sodium chloride and water secretion,[4] producing as much as 20 L/day of watery stool. There is a Na^+/K^+ pump in the basolateral membrane of the intestinal epithelial cell. This lowers the cell Na^+ concentration so that Na^+ enters with amino acids and sugars. This is a major route for salt absorption and is unaffected by bacterial toxins. This is why oral rehydration therapy with solutions containing salt and

glucose is so effective. In the large intestine, HCO_3^- is secreted up to a luminal concentration of 45 mM/L by means of a HCO_3^-/HCl^- exchanger. The Na^+/K^+ pump creates a luminal negative charge of −30 mV which causes K^+ secretion up to a luminal concentration of 25 mM/L. This is why diarrhoea can cause hypokalaemia and metabolic acidosis.

Digestion/absorption

There are two types of digestion, central or luminal and epithelial or membrane digestion.

Carbohydrate digestion begins with salivary amylase (ptyalin) and is completed in the small intestine by pancreatic alpha-amylase and epithelial enzymes. Monosaccharides are absorbed by means of carrier proteins in the epithelial cell membrane. The carriers are closely associated with enzymes.

Glucose is absorbed by secondary active transport requiring luminal Na^+. The glucose carrier is unaffected by insulin.

A deficiency of the lactase enzyme causes intolerance to milk products.

Protein digestion begins in the stomach but gastrectomy has minimal effects on protein digestion. Pepsins are inactivated at a pH greater than 5.0, that is, in the duodenum. In the duodenum, luminal digestion occurs due to pancreatic proteases (trypsinogens, chymotrypsinogens, procarboxypeptidases, and proelastases). Enterokinase from the duodenal wall activates trypsinogens to trypsins which in turn activate other proteases. Digestion is completed by epithelial digestion by dipeptidases, aminopeptidases, and so on. There are at least five different amino acid carriers and the mechanism of absorption is secondary active transport requiring luminal Na^+.

Fat digestion (Figure 1.2.8.3) begins in the duodenum by the action of pancreatic lipase, cholesterol ester hydrolase, and phospholipase. These enzymes are water-soluble and immiscible in fat. However, the fat is emulsified by bile salts. Bile salts are amphipathic with a polar part facing the lumen and a sterol part facing the interior of a fat droplet. This decreases surface tension causing the

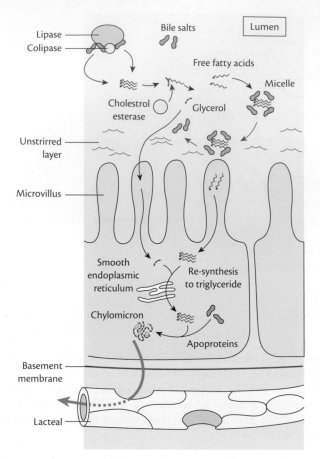

Fig. 1.2.8.3 Diagrammatic representation of the process of fat digestion/absorption in the small intestine.

Reproduced from Spoors and Kiff (Eds), *OST Training In Anaesthesia*, Oxford University Press, Oxford, UK, Copyright © 2010, with permission from Oxford University Press.

droplet to break up into emulsion droplets which increase the surface area exposed to enzyme attack. Lipase converts triglycerides to monoglycerides and fatty acids. These, along with cholesterol, bile salts, and fat-soluble vitamins form micelles which migrate to the brush border and their contents are absorbed by simple diffusion. Bile salts are left in the lumen and absorbed by active transport in the terminal ileum. These return to the liver in the portal circulation for re-secretion (enterohepatic circulation). In the mucosal cells, fatty acids of greater than ten carbon atoms reform triglycerides which, along with phospholipids and cholesterol, form chylomicrons coated with lipoproteins and then enter the lacteals. Fatty acids of less than 10 carbon atoms pass directly into the blood.

Lipid malabsorption is more common than carbohydrate or protein malabsorption. Excess fat in faeces is called steatorrhoea.

Bile consists of bile salts, bile pigments, cholesterol, HCO_3^-, and other electrolytes. Bilirubin is formed from the breakdown of haemoglobin. It is carried to the liver bound to albumin and conjugated to glucuronic acid to form the bile pigment bilirubin diglucuronide which is water-soluble. This enters the intestine and is excreted. Some is converted to urobilinogen which is partly absorbed and appears in the urine and is partly converted to stercobilinogen. Yellowing of the skin is caused by hyperbilirubinaemia which can be prehepatic, hepatic, or posthepatic.[5] In prehepatic hyperbilirubinaemia, there is excessive haemolysis, in hepatic (such as hepatitis) there are problems with uptake, conjugation, or secretion, and in posthepatic (such as gallstones or obstructive jaundice), there is impaired excretion of bile.

Further reading

Barrett KE, Boitano S, Barman SM, *et al. Ganong's Review of Medical Physiology* (24th ed). New York: McGraw-Hill Education; 2012.

Koeppen BM, Stanton BA. *Berne & Levy's Physiology* (6th ed). Philadelphia, PA: Elsevier Health Sciences; 2009.

References

1. Park W, Vaezi MF. Etiology and pathogenesis of achalasia: the current understanding. *Am J Gastroenterol* 2005; 100:1404–14.
2. Marshall BJ, Warren JR. Unidentified curved bacilli in the stomach of patients with gastritis and peptic ulceration. *Lancet* 1984; 1(8390):1311–15.
3. Sanders KM, Koh SD, Ward SM. Interstitial cells of Cajal as pacemakers in the gastrointestinal tract. *Annu Rev Physiol* 2006; 68:307–43.
4. Goodman BE, Percy WH. CFTR in cystic fibrosis and cholera: from membrane transport to clinical practice. *Adv Physiol Edu* 2005; 29(2):75–82.
5. Roche SP, Kobos R. Jaundice in the adult patient. *AAFP* 2004; 69(2):299–304.

CHAPTER 1.2.9

Urinary

Aidan Bradford

Introduction

The functions of the kidney are to regulate the volume and composition of the extracellular fluid (ECF). The kidneys actually regulate the volume and composition of the plasma, maintaining a narrow plasma osmolality between 285 and 295 mosmol/L which results in regulation of the volume and composition of the entire ECF. They therefore play a crucial role in long-term control of blood pressure (BP). The kidneys eliminate potentially toxic metabolic wastes and foreign compounds (urea, uric acid, drugs, etc.). They also release renin, activate vitamin D, and secrete erythropoietin.

The total body water is about 50–60% of body mass (females and males respectively): two-thirds is intracellular fluid (ICF) and one-third is ECF.

In a 70 kg body mass male:

- Total body water (TBW) = 42 L = 0.6 × body mass
- ICF = 28 L = 0.4 × body mass
- ECF = 14 L = 0.2 × body mass.

Na^+ and Cl^- are the main ions in ECF and K^+ and PO_4^- are the main ions in ICF.

In 24 hours, fluid gain is by salt and water intake (~2 L) and metabolic water (~0.5 L). Fluid loss is through urine (~1.5 L), insensible loss (skin ~0.5 L and lung ~0.5 L), sweat, and faeces (~0.1 L).

The nephron (Figure 1.2.9.1) is the functional unit of the kidney. Each nephron consists of a renal corpuscle and a tubular system. The renal corpuscle consists of a tuft of capillaries or glomerulus and Bowman's capsule. The tubular system consists of the proximal tubule (PT), loop of Henle, distal tubule (DT), and collecting duct (CD). The tubular system 'loops down' into the medulla and then returns to the cortex to join a CD. The CD runs from the cortex to the inner medulla. Final urine forms in the CD. The process of urine formation consists of filtration of blood at the glomerulus, tubular reabsorption, and secretion. Blood reaches each nephron via an afferent arteriole. As blood flows through the glomerulus, a fraction of the solutes and water is filtered across the capillary walls into Bowman's capsule. This forms the tubular filtrate. As the filtrate flows through the PT and loop of Henle, most of it is reabsorbed back into the blood. The small volume which remains flows on to the DT and CD. Here, salt and water excretion is regulated so that it matches salt and water intake and the final urine is formed.

Blood flow

Blood flow to the two kidneys is approximately 1.2 L/min or one-quarter of cardiac output. In health, renal blood flow (RBF) is held constant. Blood flow to the cortex is about 90% and blood flow to the medulla is about 10% of total flow. Glomerular capillaries recombine to leave Bowman's capsule as efferent arterioles. Efferent arterioles give rise to peritubular capillaries which surround the tubular system of each nephron. These then recombine to form venules and the renal vein. These capillaries deliver nutrients and oxygen to the epithelial cells lining the tubules and take up fluid from the interstitium that has been reabsorbed from the filtrate.

Over a range of 90–180 mmHg, RBF and hence glomerular filtration rate (GFR) is autoregulated, that is, changes in mean BP

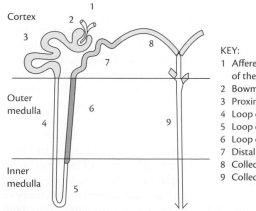

Fig. 1.2.9.1 Structural characteristics of the renal nephron.

KEY:
1 Afferent and efferent arterioles of the glomerulus
2 Bowman's capsule
3 Proximal convoluted tubule
4 Loop of Henle (thin descending limb)
5 Loop of Henle (thin ascending limb)
6 Loop of Henle (thick ascending limb)
7 Distal convoluted tubule
8 Collecting tubule
9 Collecting duct

Reproduced from Reynard et al. (Eds), Oxford Handbook of Urology, Second Edition, Oxford University Press, Oxford, UK, Copyright © 2009, with permission from Oxford University Press.

have little effect on RBF or GFR. This is by two mechanisms: (1) a myogenic mechanism and (2) by tubuloglomerular feedback. The myogenic mechanism is due to the increase in BP causing stretch of afferent arteriolar smooth muscle which then contracts, increasing afferent arteriole resistance and preventing an increase in RBF. The tubuloglomerular feedback mechanism is due to an increase in BP causing an increase in RBF, GFR, and the rate of fluid flow through the tubules so that more Na^+ reaches the macula densa of the ascending limb of the loop of Henle[1] and this causes constriction of the afferent arteriole and a decrease in RBF. However, RBF can be altered by sympathetic nerve activity, hormones, drugs, and so on.

GFR is the volume of plasma filtered per minute, that is, 120 mL/min. Filtration occurs due to a high glomerular capillary hydrostatic pressure of 50 mmHg that is opposed by a lesser plasma colloid osmotic pressure of 25 mmHg and a Bowman's capsule hydrostatic pressure of 10 mmHg, leaving a net filtration pressure of 15 mmHg (the oncotic pressure in Bowman's capsule is 0 mmHg since no protein is filtered normally). Filtration occurs through three layers: the fenestrated endothelium of glomerular capillaries, the basement membrane, and the foot processes of epithelial cells (podocytes). The three layers contain negatively charged glycoproteins. Proteins and cells are not filtered. In nephrotic syndrome, there is an increase in the permeability of the glomerular capillaries to protein and there is protein loss in urine (proteinuria), hypoproteinaemia, and oedema.

Clearance

Clearance is the volume of plasma cleared of a substance per minute or U × V/P (mL/min) where U and P are the concentrations of a substance in the urine and the plasma respectively and V is the volume of urine excreted in mL/min. It is used to measure GFR and GFR is an excellent measure of renal function. A decrease in GFR is often the first sign of renal disease.

The clearance of a substance which meets the following criteria will give a measure of GFR: freely filtered at the glomerulus, not reabsorbed from the filtrate, not secreted into the filtrate, not metabolized by the tubular cells, and does not interfere with kidney function. Creatinine does not fully meet these criteria but is used extensively to measure GFR and hence renal function. The Cockcroft and Gault formula[2] allows calculation of creatinine clearance by measuring plasma creatinine concentration, that is:

Creatinine clearance (mL / min)

= (140 − age)

× mass (kg) / (814 × plasma creatinine concentration)

For example, in a 40-year-old, 70 kg male with a normal creatinine concentration of 0.6mmol/L:

Creatinine clearance = (140 − 40) × 70 / (814 × 60)

= 0.143 mL / min

(For females, the result must be multiplied by 0.85.)

Para-aminohippuric acid (PAH) is freely filtered but not absorbed. All of the PAH that escapes filtration is secreted actively into the tubular fluid. Therefore PAH is completely removed from all of the plasma that flows through the kidneys. Therefore, the clearance of PAH equals the renal plasma flow (RPF) = 700 mL/min, therefore RBF = 700 mL/min × 1/0.58 (assuming a haematocrit of 0.42) = 1.2 L/min.

Control of extracellular fluid volume and electrolytes

Approximately 70% of the filtrate is reabsorbed in the PT and this is not regulated. In the loop of Henle, a further 20% is reabsorbed and only 10% is left to enter the DT and CD. Here, salt and water reabsorption is varied so that salt and water excretion is matched to intake. Sodium reabsorption is regulated by aldosterone and water reabsorption is regulated by antidiuretic hormone (ADH, vasopressin). Normally urine output is 1 mL/min or 1.5 L/day with urine osmolality depending on fluid intake ranging from very dilute at 50 mosmol/L to very concentrated at 1200 mosmol/L. The minimum normal urine output is 0.5 mL/min or 700 mL/day. ADH acts on a V_2 receptor to incorporate aquaporin or water channels[3] that make the CD epithelium permeable to water. In its absence, the CD is impermeable to water. The hypertonic interstitium generated by the loop of Henle and the countercurrent multiplier (Figure 1.2.9.2) allows water to move from the tubular lumen into the interstitium. The thick ascending limb of the loop is impermeable to water but has a $Na^+/K^+/2$ Cl^- pump (that is inhibited by loop diuretics) which moves these three ions into the interstitium and creates an osmotic pressure of 1200 mosmol/L at the base of the loop. Urea absorption also contributes to the high osmolarity. The vasa recta prevent loss of the osmotic gradient by countercurrent exchange. Osmoreceptors located in the hypothalamus control thirst and ADH release from the posterior pituitary. Loss of water causes an increase in plasma osmolarity resulting in ADH release and thirst. In the syndrome of inappropriate ADH secretion (SIADH), for example, lung or brain tumours, there is overhydration and decreased plasma osmolarity falling to as low as 260 mosmol/L. In central diabetes insipidus, there is inadequate release of ADH from the posterior pituitary (e.g. head injury or brain infection). In nephrogenic diabetes insipidus, the CD does not respond to ADH (e.g. lithium treatment). These conditions cause polyuria and polydipsia and, when untreated, serum osmolality rises to higher than 320 mosmol/L and coma can develop.

When the ECF and, therefore, the blood volume falls, BP at the afferent arteriole falls and this causes renin release. Circulating angiotensinogen is acted on by renin to produce angiotensin I which is changed to angiotensin II in the lungs which causes aldosterone release from the adrenal cortex which increases Na^+ absorption from the CD. The increase in plasma Na^+ causes increased osmolarity and increased ADH release so blood volume and BP rise. There are atrial receptors that are stimulated by increased blood volume and cause reduced ADH release and inhibition of sympathetic nerve activity to the kidney. This reduces renin release and also favours salt and water loss by dilating the afferent arteriole and increasing GFR.

The atria also release atrial natriuretic peptide[4] which causes natriuresis and a decrease in blood volume and pressure. In the normal plasma, sodium concentration is 135–148 mM/L. Sodium depletion can be caused by severe diarrhoea, severe vomiting, haemorrhage, and adrenal insufficiency and Na^+ retention can be caused by chronic renal failure, heart failure, and excess adrenocortical hormones. Potassium homeostasis (normal plasma value is 3.5–5.0 mM/L) is controlled by the N^+/K^+ pump in the CD cells. When

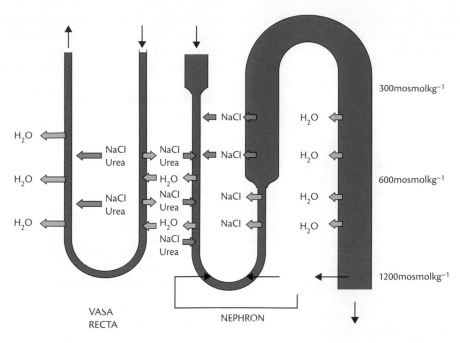

Fig. 1.2.9.2 Diagrammatic representation of the countercurrent multiplier of the nephron and the countercurrent exchanger of the vasa recta.
Reproduced from Pocock and Richards (Eds), *Human Physiology: The Basis of Medicine*, Third Edition, Oxford University Press, Oxford, UK, Copyright © 2006, with permission from Oxford University Press.

plasma K+ increases, this causes aldosterone release which stimulates the pump, increasing CD cell K+, and this K+ is then secreted into the tubule for excretion. The pump is also directly stimulated by the increased ECF potassium concentration. Hypokalaemia is caused by some diuretics, excess aldosterone secretion, metabolic alkalosis, severe diarrhoea, and severe vomiting. Hyperkalaemia is caused by acute kidney injury, adrenal insufficiency, acute acidosis, tissue destruction (burns, rhabdomyolysis, crush injury) and haemolysis. To treat hyperkalaemia, Ca^{2+} is given to prevent arrhythmias, insulin and glucose are given to pump K+ into cells, and ion exchange resins are given to remove K+ from the body through the GIT.

Acid–base balance

The kidneys play a major role in acid–base balance by regulating the HCO$_3^-$ concentration of the plasma which is normally 24 mM. HCO$_3^-$ regulates pH by buffering H+ as follows:

$$H^+ + HCO_3^- \leftrightarrow H_2CO_3 \leftrightarrow H_2O + CO_2$$

The tubule cells synthesize HCO$_3^-$ and replenish that used up by buffering, and add it to the blood (Figure 1.2.9.3). The cells make HCO$_3^-$ and H+ from CO$_2$ and H$_2$O. H+ is secreted into the tubular lumen for excretion and HCO$_3^-$ enters the blood. The secreted H+ ion reacts with a HCO$_3^-$ ion in the filtrate and 'destroys' it. For each HCO$_3^-$ ion 'destroyed', a HCO$_3^-$ ion enters the blood so that the net effect is as though the HCO$_3^-$ in the filtrate has passed through the cell into the blood. In this way, with a normal mixed diet, all of the filtered HCO$_3^-$ is 'reabsorbed' and 'new bicarbonate' is then added to the blood to replenish HCO$_3^-$ 'used up' by buffering the acids generated by the mixed diet. This new HCO$_3^-$ is accompanied

by H+ secretion which lowers the pH of the urine. These H+ ions are buffered by filtered phosphate to form titratable acid and by ammonia (NH$_3$) made from glutamine in the tubular cell,[5] to form ammonium (NH$_4^+$).

In metabolic acidosis, since the plasma, and therefore the filtered load of HCO$_3^-$ is low, more 'new bicarbonate' is added to the blood and the urine pH will be low.

In metabolic alkalosis, the plasma and filtered load of HCO$_3^-$ is high so that not all of it is reabsorbed so HCO$_3^-$ is lost in the urine and the urine pH is high.

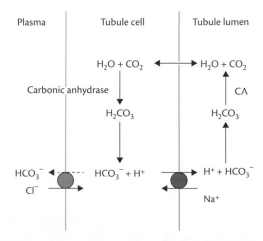

Fig. 1.2.9.3 Diagrammatic representation of the mechanism of bicarbonate absorption from the tubule lumen. For each H+ secreted by the tubule cell that 'destroys' a bicarbonate ion in the filtrate, there is an associated bicarbonate ion that enters the plasma.
Reproduced from Reynard *et al.* (Eds), *Oxford Handbook of Urology*, Second Edition, Oxford University Press, Oxford, UK, Copyright © 2009, with permission from Oxford University Press.

In respiratory acidosis, the blood PCO_2 and tubular cell PCO_2 is high so the cell makes more H^+ and HCO_3^- so that the urine pH is low and 'new bicarbonate' is formed.

In respiratory alkalosis, tubular cell PCO_2 is low so insufficient H^+ is formed and secreted in order to absorb all the filtered HCO_3^- so that HCO_3^- is excreted in the urine.

Renal failure

In acute kidney injury, there is a rapid, sudden decrease in renal function and GFR. In pre-renal failure, the cause is cardiovascular such as heart failure, hypotension, or haemorrhage whereby RBF is inadequate. In intrarenal failure, the cause is some abnormality within the kidney itself such as glomerulonephritis, tubular necrosis, pyelonephritis, and so on. In post-renal failure, there is obstruction of the urinary tract such as stones or high pressure urine retention. The effects of acute kidney injury are hyperkalaemia, metabolic acidosis, hypertension, oedema, increased plasma urea and creatinine, and uraemia. The causes of chronic renal failure are vascular (atherosclerosis), infections (pyelonephritis), immunological (glomerulonephritis), diabetes mellitus, obstruction, polycystic kidney disease, and so on. The effects are similar to acute kidney injury but they occur more gradually. There is also anaemia due to the inability of the kidney to produce erythropoietin and osteomalacia and hyperparathyroidism due to the inability to activate vitamin D to 1,25-dihydoxycholecalciferol. Therefore plasma calcium falls due to reduced calcium absorption from the gut.

Further reading

Barrett KE, Boitano S, Barman SM, *et al*. *Ganong's Review of Medical Physiology* (24th ed). New York: McGraw-Hill Education; 2012.
Koeppen BM, Stanton BA. *Berne & Levy Physiology* (6th ed). St. Louis, MD: Elsevier Health Sciences; 2009.

References

1. Peti-Peterdi J, Harris RC. Macula densa sensing and signalling mechanisms of renin release. *J Am Soc Nephrol* 2010; 21(7):1093–6.
2. Shoker A, Hossain MA, Koru-Sengul T, *et al*. Performance of creatinine clearance equations on the original Cockroft–Gault population. *Clin Nephrol* 2006; 66(2):89–97.
3. Verkman AS. Aquaporins in clinical medicine. *Annu Rev Med* 2012; 63:303–16.
4. Baxter JD, Lewicki JA, Gardner DG. Atrial natriuretic peptide. *Nat Biotechnol* 1988; 6:529–46.
5. Schoolwerth AC, Nazar BL, LaNoue KF. Glutamate dehydrogenase activation and ammonia formation by rat kidney mitochondria. *J Biol Chem* 1978; 253(17):6177–83.

CHAPTER 1.2.10

Endocrine

Kamalan Jeevaratnam

Introduction

The endocrine system uses chemical signals that are released by a group of specialized cells to regulate and coordinate many of the body's physiological function. The main difference between an endocrine gland when compared to the exocrine glands is that they do not have ducts. Chemicals from the endocrine glands are directly secreted into the blood and circulated to the target cells. These chemical signals called hormones exert a cellular response specific to the target cells.[1] Target cells have specific receptors which allow the binding of specific hormones. The synthesis, secretion, and storage of the hormones are dependent on complex pathways that involve a feedback mechanism. Feedback mechanisms can either be a positive feedback in which case the information received promotes further synthesis and secretion of a hormone or a negative feedback in which case the information inhibits the synthesis and secretion of a hormone.[1]

Hypothalamus and pituitary gland

The hypothalamus is situated at the base of the thalamus on each side of the third ventricle. Its anatomical position places it directly above the pituitary gland and it represents less than 1% of brain mass. The hypothalamus indirectly controls a majority of the endocrine glands by regulating secretion and release of several hypophysiotropic hormones (Figure 1.2.10.1) that exert its effect on the

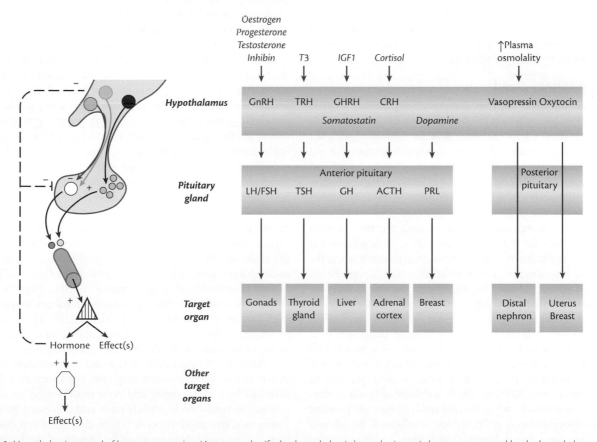

Fig. 1.2.10.1 Hypothalamic control of hormone secretion. Hormones classified as hypothalamic hypophysiotropic hormones secreted by the hypothalamus are gonadotropin-releasing hormone (GnRH), thyrotropin-releasing hormone (TRH), growth hormone-releasing hormone (GHRH), corticotropin-releasing hormone (CRH), and dopamine. Vasopressin and oxytocin are not tropic hormones and are produced in the hypothalamus.

Reproduced from Warrell D. et al. (Eds), Oxford Textbook of Medicine, Fifth Edition, Oxford University Press, Oxford, UK, Copyright © 2010, with permission from Oxford University Press.

pituitary gland. It has neural projections that allow it to maintain connections with several parts of the brain such as the sensory pathways, autonomic nervous system, and the limbic system. This allows the hypothalamus to receive input from both the external environment (sensory pathways providing information about the surrounding environment) and internal environment (information gathered from receptors controlling body temperature, pressure, blood volume, and others). Input from both external and internal environment helps the hypothalamus respond appropriately to maintain homeostasis.

The pituitary gland is a small pea-sized gland which is situated below the hypothalamus and optic chiasm. It is protected inferiorly, anteriorly, and posteriorly by a saddle-shaped bony structure called the sella turcica.[1,2] Physiologically, the pituitary gland can be divided into the anterior pituitary (adenohypophysis) and posterior pituitary (neurohypophysis). Histologically, these two structures have a distinctly different cellular pattern that correspond to their function and hormones released. The anterior pituitary is made up of cuboidal cells which are granular in nature compared to the posterior pituitary which is made up of predominantly unmyelinated axons and glial cells. The histological patterns are directly related to the embryological origin in which the anterior pituitary arises from the epithelium of the pharynx (Rathke's pouch) whereas the posterior pituitary arises from the outgrowth of neural tissues of the hypothalamus. The synthesis and secretion of hormones from both the anterior and posterior pituitary is controlled by the hypothalamus. This is maintained due to the anatomical proximity of the pituitary gland to the hypothalamus which allows for a direct connection. The posterior pituitary is connected by neural projections from the hypothalamus whereas the anterior pituitary is connected by a vascular link to the hypothalamus.[1,2]

Posterior pituitary gland

Together with the hypothalamus the posterior pituitary forms a neuroendocrine system which consists of neurosecretory neurons. The cell bodies in the hypothalamus that are associated with the posterior pituitary are situated in the supraoptic nucleus (SN) and the paraventricular nucleus (PVN). Neuronal cell bodies of SN produce vasopressin (antidiuretic hormone (ADH)) and the cell bodies of the PVN produce oxytocin. These hormones are initially synthesized as prohormones at the SN and PVN and then transported down the nerve endings in combination with a carrier protein called neurophysin. These hormones are stored in vesicles in the posterior pituitary and are released through exocytosis when the nerve impulse stimulates release of these hormones. Upon release, the hormones are immediately absorbed by the capillaries that supply the posterior pituitary and are circulated to the entire body.

The primary effect of ADH is to regulate the body's water retention capacity by the kidney. This is done through the insertion of aquaporin channels in the collecting ducts of the nephron that allow water movement out of the nephron and back into the blood. In a situation where there is an increase in osmotic pressure or reduced blood volume, ADH secretion is enhanced to aid in conserving water. Conversely, when there is reduced osmotic pressure or increased blood volume, ADH section is inhibited. Insufficient ADH secretion can cause polyuria, dehydration, and is associated with diabetes insipidus. ADH also has vasoconstrictive effects which aids in increasing systemic blood pressure through increase in total peripheral resistance.

Oxytocin, on the other hand, is important for lactation and uterine contraction for childbirth. It stimulates the contraction of the uterine wall and promotes cervical dilation during childbirth. Secretion of oxytocin is increased in response to reflexes. As such, when an infant suckles, this serves as a positive feedback for oxytocin release that further promotes milk production thus allowing mothers to continuously breastfeed. The presence of the fetus within the birth canal also promotes oxytocin release which helps with the expulsion of the fetus by uterine contractions.

Anterior pituitary gland

Unlike the posterior pituitary gland, the anterior pituitary synthesizes its own hormones: growth hormone (GH), thyroid-stimulating hormone (TSH), luteinizing hormone (LH), adrenocorticotropin hormone (ACTH), prolactin (PRL), and follicle-stimulating hormone (FSH). As the anterior pituitary produces a variety of hormones, naturally a variety of different cells make up this gland as well. Secretion of hormones from the anterior pituitary is regulated by two primary factors. Firstly, the hypothalamic hypophysiotropic hormone produced by the hypothalamus which is directly delivered to the anterior pituitary gland. These hypophysiotropic hormones have both releasing and inhibitory effect and are transported to the anterior pituitary gland by the hypothalamic hypophyseal portal system. This portal system provides capillary linkages which pass down the stalk of the pituitary gland to form the anterior pituitary gland. The portal system is particularly important as it delivers the hypophysiotropic hormones at a relatively high level direct to the gland bypassing the systemic circulation. The feedback mechanism the anterior pituitary gland receives from the target glands hormones serves as the second factor that regulates the secretion of hormones.

Of all the hormones produced by the anterior pituitary, GH is the most abundantly produced from the somatotroph cells of the gland. GH is particularly important in promoting skeletal growth and bone thickness and length. It also plays a major role in several metabolic pathways such as increasing protein synthesis, mobilization of fatty acids from body fat storage, and reduction in the utilization of glucose by the body. Owing to its primary function of promoting growth, GH is highest in the young and is continuously secreted as we age because GH is also involved in other key metabolic functions. Despite this, the amount of GH secreted steadily declines after middle age. GH does not exert its effects directly as its growth-promoting actions are mediated through somatomedins that are structurally and functionally similar to insulin. Secretion of GH is controlled by several factors, namely the balance between growth hormone-releasing hormone (GHRH) and growth hormone-inhibiting hormone (GHIH), negative feedback loops from somatomedins, and negative feedback loops from GH itself that inhibit GHRH and stimulate GHIH. Reduction of GH secretion can lead to a variety of conditions and is often caused by either a hypothalamic dysfunction, defects in the anterior pituitary, or failure of GH target cells to respond appropriately. Deficiency in GH in the young is commonly associated with dwarfism characterized by a short stature and poor muscle mass. In adults, this can lead to reduction in muscle mass and decreased bone density. Conversely, overproduction of GH in childhood can cause gigantism due to rapid disproportionate growth of the body whereas overproduction in adolescents and adulthood will lead to acromegaly and insulin resistance. Acromegaly is characterized by bone thickening, particularly in the face and extremities.

PRL is secreted by the lactotroph cells in the anterior pituitary and is involved in mammary gland development and milk production in women. It is also particularly important in the immune modulation of the uterus. PRL secretion is controlled by two hypophysiotropic hormones, namely prolactin-inhibiting hormone (PIH) and prolactin-releasing hormone (PRH). High levels of PRL also serve as a negative feedback to reduce the amount of PRL being secreted by the anterior pituitary. Over-secretion of PRL can occur in cases of pituitary tumours and this can cause infertility and decreased libido in both men and women.

Thyroid gland

The thyroid gland is a bow-shaped structure weighing approximately 20 g and is located in the neck below the larynx. It consists of two lobes that lie on either side of the trachea, connected by a band of connective tissue called the isthmus. The thyroid gland primarily secretes thyroxine (T_4) and triiodothyronine (T_3) that come from the follicular cells and calcitonin from the parafollicular cells. Almost all T_4 secreted by the thyroid gland is converted to T_3 in the target tissues which is five times more potent than the T_4. Thyroid hormone (TH) is not essential for life but is an essential hormone for both physical and mental development. It plays a role in nuclear transcription and is involved in the synthesis of several key proteins required by the body. In addition, TH is involved in the regulation of metabolic rate through the regulation of oxygen consumption and energy expenditure. It is also required for the myelination and development of the central nervous system as well as regulation of cardiac output, flow, and rate. Secretion of TH is regulated by TSH which is secreted by the anterior pituitary. Regulation of TSH secretion is in turn controlled by the hypothalamus hypophysiotropic hormone TRH. Increased levels of TRH and TSH promote the production of TH. Increased levels of TH serve as a negative feedback on TSH secretion from the anterior pituitary thus allowing for stable levels of TH to be released throughout the day whereas regulation of TH by the hypothalamus is more long-term modulation. Iodine and tyrosine are the two key ingredients required for the synthesis of TH and deficiency in these can lead to hypothyroidism.

Hypothyroidism can be caused by inadequate dietary intake of iodine, autoimmune conditions affecting the gland, primary pathology of the thyroid gland, or secondary pathology associated with TRH or TSH levels. Decreased TH secretion will primarily affect the body's ability to perform normal metabolic activity. This is associated with a reduction in basal metabolic rate (BMR) which can lead to weight gain. In addition, hypothyroid patients experience frequent bouts of fatigue, weak pulse due to reduction in myocardial contractile strength, with reduced cardiac output as well as depressed reflexes. In cases of prolonged hypothyroidism, myxoedema can occur. This is characterized by a generalized oedematous appearance associated with increased water-retaining carbohydrate molecules. This typically appears as puffiness around the face, feet, and hand as well as pronounced eye bags. Similar to GH, TH is also essential for normal skeletal growth and central nervous system development. If secretion of TH is insufficient from birth, this leads to cretinism which is characterized as dwarfism, delayed mental development or retardation, as well as symptoms directly associated with TH insufficiency.

Hyperthyroidism is characterized by persistent elevation of TH caused typically by an autoimmune condition stimulating TSH receptors in the thyroid cell (Graves' disease), increased TRH or TSH secretion, or a TH-producing tumour, although the last two are less frequent. In the autoimmune condition, long-acting thyroid stimulators stimulate the growth and production of TH and they do not respond to the negative feedback of increased TH thus promoting continued production of TH. Increased circulation of TH leads to an exaggeration of normal metabolic activity associated with TH. There will be elevated BMR, increased sweating due to increased heat production, and reduction in body weight despite increased appetite and food intake. In addition, there will be increased degradation of fat, carbohydrate, and protein as well as episodes of palpitation due to increased contractile strength and rate. A particular feature of hyperthyroidism is exophthalmos caused by the deposition of water-retaining carbohydrates behind the eyes causing protrusion of the eyeball and incidences of corneal ulceration.[1-3]

Goitre is a condition whereby the thyroid gland is so significantly enlarged that it is highly visible. It can occur both in hypothyroidism as well as hyperthyroidism. In cases of hypothyroidism, there are low levels of TH which provide little or no negative feedback to the anterior pituitary. This leads to continuous production of TSH to help further develop the follicular cells. If TH remains low, TSH continuous stimulation of the thyroid gland causes glandular hypertrophy and hyperplasia leading to an enlarged gland. Goitre in hyperthyroidism is related to overstimulation of the thyroid gland and can be related to defects in either the hypothalamus, anterior pituitary, or an immune-mediated condition such as Graves' disease.

In addition to TH, the thyroid gland also produces calcitonin, a polypeptide hormone that is involved in the regulation of calcium in the body. Calcitonin is produced by the parafollicular cells of the thyroid gland and is secreted in response to high blood calcium levels. Calcitonin works to decrease calcium levels in the body by inhibiting reabsorption of calcium from intestines and renal as well as inhibiting osteoclastic activity. Together with parathyroid hormone (PTH), calcitonin plays an important role in the body's calcium homeostasis.

Parathyroid gland

The four parathyroid glands are two paired glands situated on the surface of each lobe of the thyroid gland. The glands are made up of chief cells that secrete PTH and exert their effect on type 1 and type 2 PTH receptors. The primary function of PTH is to increase serum calcium levels. This is done by enhancing release of calcium storage from bones through increased osteoclastic activity, increasing uptake of calcium and magnesium from renal tubules, and inhibiting phosphate reabsorption and increasing calcium uptake from the intestines by enhancing formation of vitamin D. Adenomas or carcinomas of the parathyroid gland can lead to excessive secretion of PTH which can cause increased demineralization of the bone leading to fractures, stones in the kidney and bladder due to increased calcium reabsorption, and several other metabolic disturbances. A parathyroid tumour that keeps producing PTH and does not respond to the negative feedback from PTH causes the condition known as primary hyperparathyroidism. Secondary hyperparathyroidism is related to physiological disturbances associated with hypocalcaemia where there are excessive calcium losses in cases of renal failure or decreased absorption due to vitamin D insufficiency.[1-3] Tertiary hyperparathyroidism occurs after long-standing secondary hyperparathyroidism and is most commonly seen following correction of renal impairment by transplantation or after long-term dialysis. High levels of PTH continue to be secreted producing hypercalcaemia.

Adrenal glands

The adrenal glands are paired glands situated on the upper pole of each kidney. They are pyramidal in shape consisting of two separate endocrine glands embedded in a single organ. The adrenal gland thus can be divided into the outer adrenal cortex which makes up the majority of the gland and the inner adrenal medulla. Each of these structures secretes different hormones that are involved in the body's homeostatic balance.

Adrenal cortex

The adrenal cortex is divided into three distinct layers called the zona glomerulosa (ZG), zona fasciculata (ZF), and zona reticularis (ZR). These three layers produce steroid hormones derived from cholesterol. The adrenal cortex does not typically store these hormones but rather produces them on demand when there is a requirement.

Aldosterone is a mineralocorticoid produced by the ZG layer of the adrenal cortex. It acts on both the collecting and distal tubes of the nephron to aid in the retention of sodium (Na^+) ions thus indirectly retaining water. It is important in the long-term regulation of blood pressure through expansion of extracellular fluid volume. Aldosterone secretion for the adrenal cortex is stimulated by the renin–angiotensin–aldosterone system (RAAS) as well as by direct stimulation due to a rise in plasma potassium (K^+). Maintenance of blood pressure at an optimum level and normal Na^+ and K^+ plasma values provide negative feedback to the adrenal cortex to reduce production of aldosterone thus maintaining balance.

Cortisol is the primary glucocorticoid produced by the ZF and ZR layers of the adrenal cortex. Most of the cortisol is produced in the ZF layer and plays a major role the body's metabolic activity. Cortisol is particular important for the body's adaptation to stress. It increases glucoses levels in the blood through hepatic gluconeogenesis and inhibits glucose uptake by most tissues thus allowing for glucose to be freely available to the brain. It facilitates protein degradation and lipolysis as an alternate source of energy and has strong anti-inflammatory and immunosuppressive effects. Cortisol secretion is regulated by a negative feedback system that involves the hypothalamus and anterior pituitary. ACTH from the anterior pituitary promotes the growth and secretory function of the adrenal cortex which is in turn regulated by corticotropin-releasing hormone (CRH) from the hypothalamus. Increased levels of cortisol then provide a negative feedback to both ACTH and CRH thus regulating its own secretion. In addition to the hormonal influences from the hypothalamus and anterior pituitary, cortisol secretion is also influenced by stress and a diurnal rhythm whereby highest levels are attained in the morning and lowest at night.

The predominant adrenal sex hormone produced by the ZR and ZF is dehydroepiandrosterone (DHEA). In general, several adrenal sex hormones are produced but DHEA is the only androgen hormone that has biological significance. Despite this, most androgen hormone levels are not sufficiently high to exert powerful androgenic effects in most circumstances. In males, DHEA effects are overtaken by testosterone levels whilst in females, DHEA governs androgen-dependent processes. ACTH regulates secretion of DHEA through promoting growth and secretory effects of the adrenal cortex similar to its effect on the cortisol feedback pathway. However, unlike cortisol, increased levels of DHEA do not provide a negative feedback to the hypothalamus and the pituitary gland but negatively feedbacks onto gonadotropin-releasing hormone.[1-3]

Disorders of the adrenal cortex can either be hypersecretion or hyposecretion and is typically uncommon. Over-secretion of aldosterone can lead to excessive Na^+ retention, K^+ depletion, and hypertension due to increased blood volume. This can be caused by an aldosterone-secreting adrenal tumour (e.g. Conn' syndrome) or inappropriate activation of the RAAS in situations such as renal artery stenosis or tumours specifically within the RAAS system. Hyperadrenocorticism, also known as Cushing's syndrome, is characterized by elevation of cortisol levels. This can be caused by a cortisol-secreting adrenal tumour causing suppression of ACTH secretion. Cushing's disease, usually pituitary or hypothalamic in origin, is seen when high levels of cortisol result from overstimulation of the adrenal cortex by excessive CRH or ACTH secretion. In some cases, non-pituitary tumours secreting ACTH can also lead to hyperadrenocorticism. Symptoms of Cushing's syndrome are typically related to excessive levels of glucocorticoid resulting in hyperglycaemia and glycosuria. Excessive circulating glucose leads to deposition of body fat in specific locations such as the abdomen, face, back, and neck. The limbs typically appear thin due to increased muscle breakdown due to protein degradation. Loss of muscle protein leads to fatigue, depressed wound healing, and weakened skeletal muscles. Characteristic reddish linear streaks on the abdominal skin (striae) are suggestive of Cushing's syndrome.

Adrenocortical insufficiency occurs when both of the adrenal glands are affected. If only one gland is affected the other gland undergoes hypertrophy and hyperplasia to compensate, thus there is no insufficiency. Hypoadrenocorticism can either be primary or secondary depending on the cause. In primary hypoadrenocorticism, also known as Addison's disease, the entire adrenal cortex (ZG, ZF, and ZF layers) are under-secreting due to destruction of the adrenal cortex and is typically immune related and less commonly now is associated with tuberculous disease. In Addison's disease, there is both aldosterone and cortisol insufficiency. Aldosterone insufficiency leads to retention of K^+ which can cause disturbances to cardiac rhythm and Na^+ deficiency. There will also be reduction in circulating blood volume and hypotension as aldosterone is involved in water retention and regulation of blood pressure. Together with this, the reduction in cortisol levels will cause hypoglycaemia and the body loses its ability to respond to stress. Excessive ACTH is produced due to insufficient negative feedback from cortisol and this leads to hyperpigmentation of the skin associated with alpha-melanocyte-stimulating hormone receptors. Secondary hypoadrenocorticism is characterized by cortisol insufficiency only, due to reduced ACTH secretion. This is often related to abnormalities in the pituitary or hypothalamus.

Adrenal androgen hypersecretion or hyperandrogenism is typically caused by a defective cortisol pathway and its symptoms are dependent on the age and sex of the individual when onset of hypersecretory activity begins. If onset occurs during adulthood, males are not affected by it as testosterone is the dominant androgen hormone. In adult females, however, this can cause development of male secondary characteristics such as excessive facial hair growth, androgenic alopecia, and adult acne. Hirsutism is a common manifestation of hyperandrogenism in adult females. Hyperandrogenism in newborns can also occur and is manifested as male-type external genitalia in females and precocious pseudopuberty in prepubertal males.[1,3]

Adrenal medulla

The adrenal medulla is the innermost layer of the adrenal gland and is made up of modified postganglionic sympathetic neurons called chromaffin cells. These cells produce two catecholamines derived from tyrosine, namely adrenaline and noradrenaline, with the latter making up the most abundantly produced catecholamine. Unlike the typical sympathetic nervous system innervation, the adrenal medulla does not innervate effector organs. It releases the catecholamines directly into the circulation when stimulated by preganglionic fibres. Release of catecholamines is regulated by sympathetic input such as pain, cold, anxiety, stress, anger, and fear. Metabolic alterations associated with strenuous exercise and hypoglycaemia also stimulate the adrenal medulla. These hormones are important in mounting a stress response, regulating arterial blood pressure, and controlling metabolism. Epinephrine (adrenaline) is the major hormone involved in the 'flight or fight' response in which it increases cardiac contractile strength and rate, and re-channels blood to vital organs and skeletal muscles. It also helps dilate respiratory airways and reduces resistance thus maximizing airway capacity in stressful or demanding situations. It also inhibits digestive function and the micturition reflex but promotes arousal and alertness. As digestive activity is inhibited, adrenaline increases the mobilization of stored fat and glucose through increasing hepatic gluconeogenesis as well as muscle and hepatic glycogenolysis in addition to increased lipolytic activity.

Pancreas

The pancreas functions both as an endocrine and an exocrine gland; the endocrine function of the pancreas will be focused on in this chapter. The endocrine component of the pancreas is made of a cluster of cells called the islets of Langerhans located predominantly in the tail of the pancreas. These islets are made up of five cell types each producing a different hormone. The α-cells secrete glucagon, β-cells secrete insulin, δ-cells secrete somatostatin, pancreatic polypeptide (PP) cells (originally called F-cells) secrete PP, and the more recently discovered ε-cells produce ghrelin. The β-cell of the islets is the most abundant and thus insulin is the major hormone produced by these islets. Collectively these hormones also regulate the secretion of one another. Insulin release is stimulated by increasing glucose levels in the body and by glucagon but is negatively inhibited by somatostatin and catecholamines. Glucagon, on the other hand, is stimulated in hypoglycaemic conditions but is inhibited by insulin and somatostatins. Insulin promotes the uptake and storage of glucose into insulin-sensitive cells; it stimulates glycolysis by activating the enzyme glucokinase in the liver as well increasing glycogen synthesis. It further promotes protein synthesis by increasing amino acid uptake in target cells and delays its degradation. In addition, insulin promotes lipogenesis activity and inhibits lipolytic activity in adipocytes. Glucagon, in contrast, is involved in the metabolism of carbohydrate, protein, and fat in the liver. It promotes glycogenolysis, gluconeogenesis, lipolysis, and ketogenesis primarily in the liver.[1,3]

Further reading

Moini J. *Anatomy and Physiology for Health Professionals*. Sudbury, MA: Jones & Bartlett Learning; 2012.

References

1. Rhodes RA, Bell DR. *Medical Physiology: Principles for Clinical Medicine* (4th ed). Philadelphia, PA: Lippincott, William and Wilkins; 2013.
2. Raff H, Levitzky M. *Medical Physiology: A Systems Approach*. New York: McGraw Hill/Lange; 2011.
3. Marieb EN, Hoehn K. *Human Anatomy and Physiology* (8th ed). Redwood City, CA: Pearson; 2010.

CHAPTER 1.2.11

Neurology

Kamalan Jeevaratnam

Introduction

The nervous system is the central processing centre for the human body. It receives input from both the internal and external environment and responds to allow the body to maintain homeostasis. The nervous system is embryologically derived from the ectoderm which develops to form the neuroectoderm followed by the neural plate and subsequently the neural tube in the first few weeks of gestation. With the aid of the apoptotic process and other developmental processes, the neural tube will give rise to the brain, spinal cord, and the associated neural structures. These structures remain connected as a single unit with the brain being the primary command and control centre, thus allowing for a functional nervous system.

Functional organization of the nervous system

The nervous system is divided into the central nervous system (CNS) which is made up of the brain and the spinal cord and the peripheral nervous system (PNS) which is made up of the nerves that extend beyond the spinal cord and innervate the various structures of the body.[1] These extensive nerve branches are made up of structures called neurons. Neurons are the functional units of the nervous system and are interconnected to one another allowing for two-way transmission of information from the various regions of the body to the CNS. Supporting these neuronal structures are the equally important non-neuronal structures called the glial cells. Glial cells can be divided into macroglia and microglia cells. Macroglia cells are larger in size and consist of astrocytes, oligodendrocytes, and Schwann cells. Astrocytes are the most abundant non-neuronal cells and provide a wide variety of functions including structural support, regulation of blood flow, as well as metabolic homeostasis. The oligodendrocyte cells and Schwann cells are vital in the development of myelin sheaths, facilitation of neurotransmission and some metabolic support. Microglial cells, on the other hand, play largely an immune-supportive role and are typically related to macrophages in the nervous system.

Somatic nervous system

The somatic nervous system is a collection of nerves that control the musculoskeletal system and skin. They are made up of the 12 cranial nerves and the 31 spinal nerves. The somatic nervous system is also a voluntary nervous system in that we are able to exert conscious control over this system. The skin functions as a receptor organ and receives inputs which are then transmitted via the various sensory pathways to the brain. Information is then relayed back to the muscles via motor pathways which are the effector organs.

Sensory pathways

The sensory or ascending pathways carry sensory information from the peripheral receptors to the brain. Receptors such as mechanoreceptors (mechanical input), thermoreceptors (heat and cold input), nociceptors (pain), and proprioceptors (positioning) receive information from the surrounding environment and transmit this information to the brain. Damage to specific areas of the brain and spinal cord will lead to loss of sensory perception. The spinothalamic pathway which decussate at the level of the spinal cord (it ascends a few spinal columns up the Lissauer's tract before decussation contralaterally) is divided into the ventral and lateral tracts which carry sensory information on crude touch and pain and temperature respectively. The dorsal column–medial lemniscal system transmits information such as proprioception, fine touch, and vibration via the medial lemniscus. This pathway crosses over contralaterally at the point of the medulla. The spinocerebellar pathway carries information about the body's positioning and this tract travels all the way to the cerebellum ipsilaterally without any crossover.

Motor pathways

The motor or descending pathways carry motor information from the brain to the muscles. These pathways encompass the upper motor neurons (UMNs) and lower motor neurons (LMNs). The UMNs are neurons that transmit information from the brain to the LMNs. Damage to the UMNs will result in the loss of control of the LMNs leading to exaggerated LMN influence characterized by muscle spasticity. The LMNs are neurons which synapse with the effector organs (muscles) to exert a muscle contraction. They are found in the ventral horn of the spinal cord and also in the brainstem (for cranial nerves). Damage to the LMNs will result in an exaggerated UMN influence which is manifested as flaccid paresis or paralysis. Motor pathways derive their name from the site of origin and their location of distribution. In principle, they can be divided into the pyramidal pathways (pathways that originate at the medullary pyramids) and the extrapyramidal pathways (pathways that do not traverse through the medullary pyramids). The corticospinal and corticobulbar tracts are examples of the pyramidal pathways with the former tract crossing over at the medulla. The corticospinal tract concerns with skilled movements of the trunk, upper limb, and lower limb whereas the corticobulbar tract controls muscles supplied by the cranial nerves (Figure 1.2.11.1).

Autonomic nervous system

Large parts of the body's homeostatic mechanisms are regulated below the level of consciousness under the control of the autonomic nervous system (ANS) which forms part of the PNS. The ANS uses a two-neuron pathway that transmits information from the CNS to the target site and thus involves a preganglionic

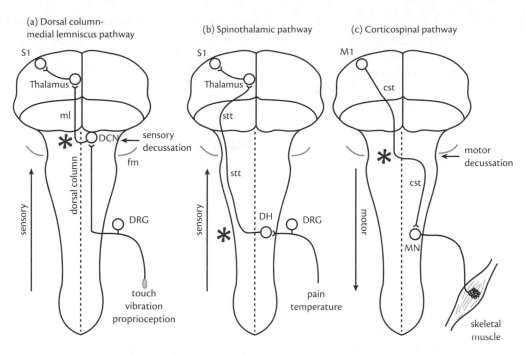

(a) Dorsal column–
medial lemniscus pathway

(b) Spinothalamic pathway

(c) Corticospinal pathway

Fig. 1.2.11.1 Note that the schematics are stretched horizontally for illustrative purposes. The dotted line in the spinal cord and caudal medulla marks the midline. The foramen magnum (fm) separating the spinal cord, below, from the brain, above, is indicated by the blue arcs.
(a) The dorsal column–medial lemniscus pathway carries information about fine touch, vibration, and proprioception from the body to the contralateral cerebral cortex. Primary afferents, often with encapsulated ends, located in dorsal root ganglia (DRG) transmit tactile information from the periphery all the way to the dorsal column nuclei (DCN) in the medulla. Within the spinal cord, these primary afferents travel in the ipsilateral dorsal column of the spinal cord. Cells in the dorsal column nuclei, located in the medulla, receive input from primary afferents and in turn project to the contralateral thalamus. To reach the thalamus, dorsal column nuclear cells send their axons across the midline. The crossing of dorsal column nuclear axons marks the sensory decussation. When the dorsal column nuclear axons reach the contralateral side, they take a turn to travel rostrally through the brainstem as the medial lemniscus (ml). Thalamic cells project to primary somatosensory cortex (S1).
(b) The lateral spinothalamic pathway carries information about pain and temperature from the body to the contralateral cerebral cortex. Primary afferents that innervate the periphery as free nerve endings have cell bodies located in the dorsal root ganglia. They transmit information from the periphery to the dorsal horn (DH) of the spinal cord. Cells in the dorsal horn send an axon across the midline to travel rostrally in the spinothalamic tract (stt) all the way to the contralateral thalamus. Thalamic cells receiving input from the spinothalamic tract project to primary somatosensory cortex.
(c) The corticospinal pathway originates in the primary motor cortex (M1). Cells in primary motor cortex send an axon through the corticospinal tract (cst) to contralateral motoneurons (MN) in the spinal cord. At the spinomedullary junction, corticospinal tract fibres cross the midline, marking the motor decussation. Motoneurons that receive input from the corticospinal tract innervate skeletal muscle, required for voluntary movement. All three pathways cross the midline, at sites marked by the red asterisks. As a result, the cerebral cortex on one side is responsible for both voluntary movement and somatosensory perception of the other side of the body. The dorsal column–medial lemniscus pathway crosses the midline in the caudal medulla. The corticospinal pathway crosses at the spinomedullary junction, and the spinothalamic pathway crosses within the spinal cord at the level of the primary afferent input.
Reproduced from Mason P, *Medical Neurobiology*, Figure 9.1, p. 158, Oxford University Press, Oxford, UK, Copyright © 2011, by permission of Oxford University Press.

neuron and a postganglionic neuron. The common neurotransmitters involved are norepinephrine (adrenergic nerve fibres) and acetylcholine (cholinergic nerve fibres). It is divided into two anatomically and functionally different systems called the sympathetic nervous system (SNS) and the parasympathetic nervous system (PSNS). Both these systems have opposing effects and work together to create a homeostatic balance. These systems are tonically active, meaning that the activity of the SNS and PSNS can either increase or decrease depending on the body's homeostatic requirement. The activity of the SNS often involves a full body response whereas the PSNS involves selected organs in isolation mostly. The SNS, also termed the *flight or fight* system, tends to predominate in stressful and high-energy demand situations such as in emergencies. It has a thoracolumbar outflow (T1 to L2) and its cell body is located in the lateral horn of the grey matter in the spinal cord. The preganglionic neurons exit their respective spinal segments and synapse with the postganglionic neurons within the sympathetic ganglion which is situated along the side of the spinal

cord. These long postganglionic neurons then innervate the various organs where when activated will release neurotransmitters to exert an effect. Among the effects of SNS activation are the redistribution of blood to muscles (skeletal and cardiac), dilation of airway, increased heart rate and contractility, inhibition of digestion peristalsis, and mydriasis. The PSNS, also known as the *rest and digest* system, tends to predominate during quiet and resting periods. It has a craniosacral outflow (cranial nerves III, VII, IX, X, and S1 to S4) with its cell bodies located in the brain stem and sacral spinal cord respectively. The preganglionic neurons exit the CNS and synapse with the postganglionic neurons within the PSNS ganglia situated close to the target organ. As such, the postganglionic neuron of the PSNS is shorter than that of the SNS whereas the preganglionic neuron of the PSNS is longer than that of the SNS. Increased activity of the PSNS will lead to redistribution of blood to the gastrointestinal tract, constriction of the airways when oxygen demand has reduced, and miosis, accelerating digestion and peristalsis among others.

Spinal reflexes

Reflexes are precisely coordinated responses that occur rapidly without conscious effort and occur through neural connections known as reflex arcs. These are autonomic reflexes which we are rarely aware of as they are mediated through the ANS. Such autonomic reflexes occur in the cardiac muscles, endocrine glands, smooth muscles of the stomach, and intestine. The somatic reflexes are more obvious as they involve the somatic system, in particular the skeletal muscles. Although the skeletal muscles receive descending input from the brain, they can contract without conscious control and much of this occurs at the level of the spinal cord, thus the name spinal reflexes. The complexity of spinal reflexes can vary from monosynaptic reflexes (e.g. patellar reflex and Achilles reflex) to polysynaptic reflexes (e.g. withdrawal reflex and cross-extensor reflex) depending on the response required. Spinal reflexes are clinically important as they provide clinicians with valuable information about the integrity of the nervous system. Five main components are necessary for a coordinated spinal reflex. These are (1) the sensory receptors (afferent input), (2) afferent nerve, (3) the integrating centre in the CNS, (4) efferent nerve, and (5) the effecter organ (efferent output). Sensory receptors for reflexes of the somatic nervous system are the muscle spindles and the Golgi tendon organ (GTO). The muscle spindles provide information about muscle length and rate of change in length whereas the GTO provides information about the muscle tension and the rate of change in tension. The muscle spindles, through afferent nerves from the intrafusal fibres, send input to the brain and help regulate muscle tone via the motor neurons (efferent pathway). The GTO encapsulated within the muscles tendon sends input to the brain when muscles tension rises to avoid further increase in muscle tension. When there is damage to this control of reflexes, there is disruption in muscle tone. Clinically this can be characterized as either decreased muscle tone (e.g. flaccid paralysis and muscle hypotonia) or increased muscle tone (e.g. spastic rigidity, lead pipe rigidity, and paratonia).

Synaptic transmission

Neurons in the nervous system communicate with each other through a chemical signalling process called synaptic transmission. Axon terminals from the transmitting neurons communicate with dendrites of the receiving neurons passing through a synaptic cleft.[2] When an action potential travels down the axon it reaches the presynaptic terminal at the axon terminal where depolarization occurs. Depolarization activates voltage-gated presynaptic calcium channels causing localized calcium entry which elicits the release of neurotransmitters (NTs) from the vesicles at the presynaptic terminal. These NTs diffuse out into the synaptic cleft and bind to and activate the receptors on the dendrites of the receiving neurons or postsynaptic neuron. Activation of the receptors at the postsynaptic membrane causes a postsynaptic potential which can either be an excitatory postsynaptic potential (EPSP) or inhibitory postsynaptic potential (IPSP). EPSPs are generated when sodium channels are activated causing depolarization, whereas IPSPs occur when there is increase in potassium or chloride permeability into cells leading to hyperpolarization. Most of the postsynaptic potentials are typically transient and therefore will require a process called summation to actually cause the postsynaptic neuron to reach action potential threshold. As such, an action potential in the postsynaptic neuron is the result of multiple synaptic events from many presynaptic terminals. Temporal summation is when postsynaptic potentials are delivered over a period of time before the preceding potential has ended thus allowing sufficient potential to generate an action potential. Spatial summation is when there is activation of multiple presynaptic terminals in unison to generate an action potential.

Visual pathway

In humans, the visual system plays an important role in daily activity. It is made up of complex pathways that connect the eye to the brain via the optic nerve. The eye itself serves as a receiving device for light input that is than converted to electrochemical signals and transported to the brain for interpretation. This process is called phototransduction and occurs in the retinal layer of the eye. The retina is composed of photosensitive cells called rods which are long, slender cells used for scotopic (night-time) vision and cones which are used for photopic (day-time) vision including colour.[2] Rods are mainly found in the retinal periphery whereas cones are typically found in abundance in the macula region of the retina. Depending on intensity, the photoreceptors cells are activated and an electrochemical signal is generated which passes on to the optic nerve. The fibres from both the left and right optic nerve then enter the optic chiasm where the medial (nasal) fibres decussate on to the contralateral side whereas the temporal fibres travel to the brain on the same side. Input from the right visual field of each eye is sent to the left side of the brain and vice versa. These tracts then travel further to synapse in the lateral geniculate nucleus in the thalamus, and optic radiations from the thalamus project this information to the visual cortex in the occipital lobe.

Auditory pathway

The auditory system uses hair cells which are located in the cochlea to transmit information to the brain. Information from the cochlea is transmitted via the vestibular nerve to the CNS. The input that is interpreted by these hair cells is sound waves that travel from the external ear into the inner ear via the middle ear. Sound waves that enter the ear cause the tympanic membrane to vibrate. These vibrations are then transmitted via the three ossicles of the ear to the oval window which is connected to the stapes. The vibration of the oval window causes fluid within the scala vestibuli to be displaced and this in turn leads to movement of the basilar membrane. Movement of the basilar membrane causes the excitation of the inner hair cells.[2] Hair cell excitation causes serial depolarization due to interconnected channels and an action potential is transmitted to the auditory cortex. There is also an efferent pathway to the cochlea which provides innervation to the outer hair cells. This is thought to prolong the vibration of the basilar membrane and is important in the ability to hear speech in background noises.[1]

Cerebral spinal fluid

The brain is suspended within the skull to avoid it having direct contact with the bony skull internally. This is achieved by having several protective meningeal layers around it. In addition to this, the cerebral spinal fluid (CSF) that lies in the subarachnoid space of the meningeal layer and in the ventricles of the brain provides mechanical cushioning to the brain. This allows the brain to move slightly within the skull in instances of minor head trauma or daily movements without causing it to have direct contact with the internal walls of the skull. The CSF is produced by a group of specialized capillaries known as the choroid plexus (CP) which are made up of endothelial and epithelial cells arranged in tight continuous junctions. The selective permeability capability of this cellular arrangement allows for the production of CSF and provides the blood–CSF barrier. The CP is typically found in the lateral as well as the third and fourth ventricles. CSF flows from the lateral ventricle via the foramen of Monro into the third ventricle. From here it enters the aqueduct of Sylvius and flows into the fourth ventricle of the brain. It exits the ventricles via the foramen of Luschka (lateral openings) and foramen of Magendie (median opening) to fill the subarachnoid space covering the brain and spinal cord.

Regulation of intracranial pressure

The cranium is a rigid box and is filled with the brain, CSF, and its associated structures. A constant ambient intracranial pressure (ICP) is necessary so that these vital structures can maintain their function. ICP is directly proportional to the contents of the cranium, thus if the contents increase, so does the ICP. ICP is typically maintained around 10 mmHg and can be measured when a lumbar puncture or non-invasive techniques such as transcranial Doppler ultrasound. A rise in ICP is potentially life-threatening. This can be caused by an intracranial bleed, a tumour, or a compressive skull fracture. When ICP rises, the vessels that supply the brain are also compressed and this leads to reduction of blood flow to the brain causing ischaemia. This rise is initially characterized as headaches and nausea, and with a continuous rise can lead to confusion, neural dysfunction, abnormal cranial nerve function, and subsequently coma. Continued increase in ICP leads to the compensatory mechanism known as Cushing's reflex. This reflex is activated when the perfusion to the brain is significantly reduced and it has become hypercapnic and hypoxic. This stimulates the vasomotor centre of the medulla which leads to intense peripheral vasoconstriction causing an increase in arterial blood pressure that will eventually help improve blood perfusion to the brain. However, the increased arterial blood pressure will activate the baroreceptors and inhibit the cardio centres. This causes reflex bradycardia. As such, patients with a large increase in ICP have elevated arterial blood pressure that is accompanied by bradycardia.

Regulation of pain by the nervous system

Pain involves both a physiological and psychological response towards an offending stimulus that causes an objectionable sensory and emotional experience. The perception of pain requires pain receptors (nociceptors). Typically, the free endings of these nociceptors receive the input and when threshold is reached an action potential is generated and the impulse is propagated. Different nociceptors respond differently to different stimuli (e.g. thermal nociceptors respond to extreme temperature, mechanoreceptors respond to pressure, and mechanical changes and chemical nociceptors respond to chemical stimuli). Such inputs are converted to electrical impulses which propagate to the spinal cord and brain via pain fibres. There are two types of pain fibres, A-delta fibres which are myelinated fibres and thus conduct the impulse rapidly and C fibres which are unmyelinated fibres which conduct impulse slowly. Both fibres not only differ in their speed of conduction but also in the type of pain information carried. The A-delta fibres carry acute, sharp, and localized pain which aids in the immediate response to remove or withdraw from the noxious stimuli via input from the thalamus. Conversely, C fibres carry dull, aching, and poorly localized pain information which relays via the limbic system thus generating an emotional response and memory to pain. Once the impulse is propagated to the spinal cord and brain, the responses typically will involve the conscious perception of pain in addition to an emotional response, a withdrawal reflex, and ANS-associated change. Pain that comes from within (organs/visceral structures) is typically difficult to distinguish and this is attributed to the fact that many of the structures share similar spinal segments, thus the pain input tends to converge. Referred pain, on the other hand, is pain felt in other locations of the body other than the site of the noxious stimuli. This is frequently seen in cases of cardiac ischaemia where patients complain of pain in the left arm which radiates to the back, or in cases of appendicitis where the pain tends to be periumbilical initially and then spreads to the right iliac fossa.

Consciousness and sleep

The nervous system plays an important role in maintaining a state of consciousness. This is also related to the sleep–wake cycle for humans. Consciousness is typically defined as a state of self-awareness with the ability to perceive stimuli and be able to respond by making a judgement. Sleep is a physiological state of altered consciousness from which an individual can be aroused and which follows a circadian rhythm. There are also cases of severely impaired levels of consciousness such as coma, persistent vegetative state, and brain death. Coma is a state of unconsciousness where the individual is unable to perceive and respond to stimuli with a loss in the circadian rhythm. In cases of persistent vegetative state, the individual has some level of wakefulness with eyes open but is still unaware and unresponsive to stimuli. Brain death, however, is a total lack of any brain activity which will require the individual to be mechanically ventilated. Determination of an individual state of consciousness can be assessed using several physiological measures such as an electroencephalogram, electro-oculograph, and an electromyograph. The electroencephalogram is frequently used to assess brain activity in cases of seizures, altered consciousness, and cerebral disturbances (focal or diffuse).

In humans, the sleep–wake cycle is regulated by genes and can be altered by changing the entrainment (e.g. sunrise and sunset). Melatonin, a hormone released by the pineal gland, is secreted at night and helps induce sleep. There are two main cycles in the sleep process, known as non-rapid eye movement (NREM) and rapid eye movement (REM) sleep. NREM sleep is divided into stages I, II, III, and IV whereas REM sleep is a single stage. During NREM, there is autonomic stability and heart rate, blood pressure, and temperature fall. The opposite occurs in REM sleep. During night-time there are alternating cycles of NREM and REM sleep with REM sleep becoming more prolonged until waking up. Stage IV of NREM sleep is the deepest stage before REM sleep occurs. Wakefulness is maintained by activation of the cerebral cortex by two ascending systems that contribute to the reticular activating system. One synthesizes acetylcholine and the other synthesizes monoamines. During NREM sleep, neuronal activity in both cholinergic and monoaminergic pathways are slowed whereas during REM sleep, cholinergic neurons are active and monoamines are inactive.

Further reading

Marieb EN, Hoehn K. *Human Anatomy and Physiology* (8th ed). Redwood City, CA: Pearson; 2010.

Moini J. *Anatomy and Physiology for Health Professionals*. Sudbury, MA: Jones & Bartlett Learning; 2012.

Raff H, Levitzky M. *Medical Physiology: A Systems Approach*. New York: McGraw Hill/Lange; 2011.

References

1. Purves D, Augustine GJ, Fitzpatrick D, *et al.* (eds). *Neuroscience* (2nd ed). Sunderland, MA: Sinauer Associates; 2001.

2. Rhodes RA, Bell DR. *Medical Physiology: Principles for Clinical Medicine* (4th ed). Philadelphia, PA: Lippincott, William and Wilkins; 2013.

PART 1.3

Applied surgical pharmacology

CHAPTER 1.3.1

Essential pharmacology for surgeons

Chris Brearton

Introduction

The legal ability to prescribe any medication is still one of the major differences between the medically qualified practitioner and other providers of healthcare within the multidisciplinary team. Lack of knowledge of the basic science behind drug action will not prevent drugs from working, but lack of basic knowledge can increase the risk to our patients and does not fit with the duty of care which we owe to them.

No one person is alone in the responsibility for safe prescribing, and no one person can remember all possible medicines. Basic pharmacological science and drug types commonly used in the perioperative period are discussed in detail in this chapter with an overview of important pharmacological aspects of their use.

Principles of pharmacology

The underlying basic science behind pharmacology helps in understanding how our bodies interact with drugs, and how drugs interact with our bodies. This basic knowledge is required for understanding drugs and their safe prescribing.

Pharmacokinetics

This branch of pharmacology deals with what happens to a drug when it enters the body, and is usually divided into four separate stages: absorption and distribution describe drug delivery to the site of action, metabolism and excretion deal with removal of drugs from the body.

Absorption

Absorption describes the way in which a drug enters the body. Most, but not all drugs reach their target via the systemic circulation, the exceptions being drugs administered topically. These are administered at their site of action, although some systemic absorption occurs, and can cause systemic side effects. In order to reach their intended target almost all drugs must diffuse across at least one physiological cell membrane. The physiological membrane is a phospholipid bilayer, which presents a variable barrier to a molecule's passage into or through a cell. A number of factors determine the ability and rate of a molecule to pass through a physiological membrane:

- *Molecular size*: smaller molecules will diffuse at faster rates than very large molecules.

- *Concentration gradient*: with a larger concentration gradient to drive diffusion it will be more rapid.

- *Surface area*: with a larger area available for absorption, it will be more rapid. The gastrointestinal tract (GIT) has evolved to have a huge surface area to absorb dietary intake and so it also presents a large surface area for drug absorption.

- *Blood flow*: absorption is faster in tissues with high blood flow rates; those with limited or variable blood flow will have limited or variable absorption.

- *Time*: with a longer time spent at the absorption site, more absorption will take place.

- *Lipid solubility*: this is probably the most important factor, as molecules that are more lipid-soluble pass through the lipid bilayer much more easily than water-soluble molecules. Lipid solubility is a physical property of a particular drug; however, a drug's lipid solubility will vary depending upon its degree of ionization in solution. All drugs in solution will be present in both ionized and un-ionized forms. The ionized form is electrically charged and therefore water-soluble, and the un-ionized form is not charged and therefore much more lipid-soluble. This physicochemical property of the drug is determined by its pK_a.

- The pK_a is the pH at which there is an equal amount of ionized and un-ionized drug (see Figure 1.3.1.1).

The behaviour of a drug at different pH levels depends upon whether it acts as an acid or a base. In simple terms—does it accept hydrogen ions and become charged, or does it donate hydrogen ions to become charged?

Acids become less charged at low pH as there are more hydrogen ions and dissociation is less favourable so they are more lipid-soluble.

Bases behave in the opposite manner and become more charged at low pH as there are more hydrogen ions and association is more favourable so they are less lipid-soluble.

The further away from the pK_a value the greater the proportion change from 50%. In practice, pH is not a linear scale, it is a logarithmic scale and so small changes imply large differences in hydrogen ion concentration which cause large changes in the proportions of ionized to un-ionized drug. All of these factors combine to affect a drug's absorption, which will in turn affect which route of administration is more optimal.

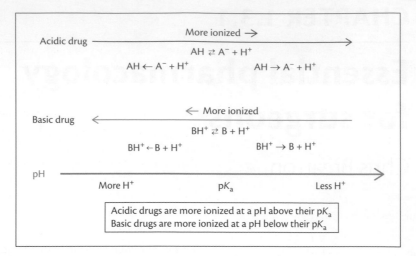

Fig. 1.3.1.1 Changes in drug ionization with altered pH.

• *Routes*: the oral route is by far the most common route of drug administration. Drugs are taken orally and absorbed in the gut, and the small bowel provides such a large surface area that it is the major site of absorption, even in drugs which pass across its membrane poorly.

Changes in diet can affect the amount and speed of absorption as some foods will prevent, or increase drug uptake. The perioperative period often consists of forced changes to diets.

• *First-pass metabolism*: not all of the absorbed drug manages to reach the systemic circulation however, some may be metabolized in the gut wall, and due to the portal circulation almost all blood flow away from the gut passes through the liver. This is the

major site of drug metabolism and so even more drugs are subjected to metabolism before they can reach the systemic circulation. This is termed 'first-pass' metabolism as all gastrointestinal (GI) absorbed drugs must undergo a first pass through the liver (see Figure 1.3.1.2).

Those drugs with extensive or unpredictable first-pass metabolism are not suitable for the oral route as they do not reliably reach sufficient concentrations to be therapeutic.

Bioavailability describes the proportion of an oral dose which reaches the systemic circulation when compared against an intravenous (IV) dose, in which, by definition, the full dose reaches the systemic circulation. Expressed as a ratio or as a percentage it

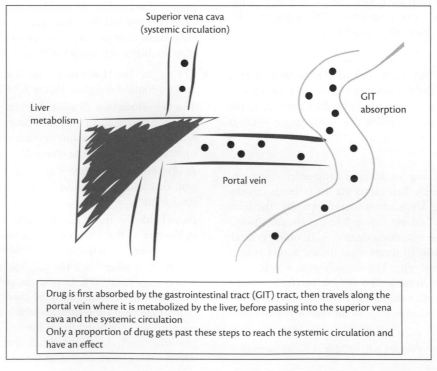

Fig. 1.3.1.2 First-pass metabolism.

gives an indication as to the extent of enteral absorption combined with first-pass metabolism. Highly bioavailable drugs approach a fraction of 1 or 100% whilst those with a very low bioavailability require much higher doses when given orally. Indeed, some drugs have such low bioavailability that they are not suitable at all for this route.

Surgery can present a problem when the oral route is considered; there is always a period of starvation, but medicines are usually an accepted exception. It is the unreliability of the oral route in the postoperative period which causes more issues. Nausea and vomiting are common after anaesthesia and altered GI transit times or prolonged starvation periods can affect the oral route.

Other common routes of administration in surgical patients are:

- *IV*: by definition, this route obtains 100% absorption into the systemic circulation. It is therefore a very reliable route for the administration of many drugs, especially perioperatively. Doses may need to be adjusted and side effects are likely to occur more rapidly. It does require reliable access to the venous system which presents its own problems, but must be reliable as extravasation of some drugs can be limb-threatening. If the IV route is not required then the IV cannula should be removed, as it presents a significant risk of infection.

- *Intramuscular* (IM): this route is popular in surgical patients because it does not require a patent oral route or reliable GI absorption. The proportion of the dose which reaches the systemic circulation is close to 100% in most situations. This route can also be used for some drugs which do not have an oral

preparation. It does, however, require painful injections which may need to be repeated, and each injection carries a risk of injury which can include permanent nerve injury, or significant bleeding in those with a coagulopathy.

Absorption from the IM site is dependent upon blood flow to the muscle, making it less useful and more erratic in those with reduced cardiac output or poor local perfusion.

- *Subcutaneous* (SC): again this route is often used when the oral route is unavailable or there is no viable oral preparation. Insulin and low-molecular-weight heparins (LMWHs) are common drugs given by this route. It requires injection, but tends to be less painful, and absorption is usually good, but is still very dependent on local blood flow.

Other potential routes of administration are shown in Table 1.3.1.1.

Distribution

Distribution describes delivery of a drug to the tissues once it has reached the systemic circulation. There are a number of factors which determine drug distribution to tissues, both drug properties and the physiological properties of tissues are important.

Again, for a drug to cross from the systemic circulation to tissues it must cross cell membranes. The proportion able to cross is a major determinant of distribution. Molecular size and lipid solubility are important factors in this. Drugs which are highly ionized and therefore non-lipid-soluble will cross membranes poorly. Very large molecules will be confined to the plasma because they are too large to pass through membranes—the osmotic diuretic mannitol is a good example of this.

Table 1.3.1.1 Other potential routes of administration

Route	Description	Benefit	Drawback	Example
Buccal	Drug is absorbed via the oral mucus membranes directly into the systemic circulation	Avoids first-pass metabolism. Can have rapid onset	Only suitable for some drugs. Often takes time for absorption. May be variable absorption, especially if swallowed	GTN spray. Buccal nitrates
Rectal	Drug is absorbed from rectum into systemic circulation	Avoids first-pass metabolism. May be used for topical administration	Low patient acceptability, therefore seek consent. Variable absorption, including high absorption levels	Topical steroids in inflammatory bowel disease. Paracetamol and diclofenac are commonly used via this route
Transdermal	Drug is absorbed across the skin into the systemic circulation	Avoids first-pass metabolism. Preparations available with slow release meaning less frequent dosing	Only possible with very lipid-soluble drugs. Absorption may continue after drug removed from outer skin layer	Fentanyl patches for analgesia
Intrathecal	Drug injected into intrathecal space via needle for local effect	Therapeutic concentration reached in cerebrospinal fluid without passing through systemic circulation	Access to space has risks and can be technically challenging. Usually only possible as a single injection. Systemic absorption does occur	Local anaesthetics used for 'spinal' anaesthetic
Epidural	Drug injected into epidural space via needle for local effect	Therapeutic concentration reached without passing though systemic circulation. Avoids direct dural puncture. Often able to use a catheter to allow continuous infusions	Access to space has risks and can be technically challenging. Systemic absorption does occur	Local anaesthetics for epidural analgesia

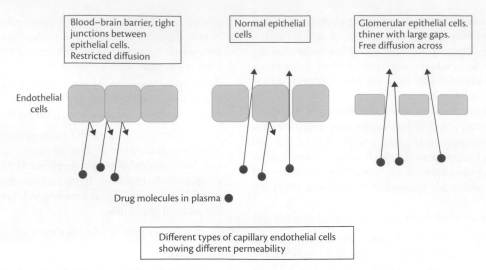

Blood–brain barrier, tight junctions between epithelial cells. Restricted diffusion

Normal epithelial cells

Glomerular epithelial cells. thiner with large gaps. Free diffusion across

Endothelial cells

Drug molecules in plasma ●

Different types of capillary endothelial cells showing different permeability

Fig. 1.3.1.3 Different permeability in specialized endothelia.

However, tissue capillary endothelia have differing permeabilities and therefore allow drugs to cross at different rates. Examples of the wide differences in capillary endothelial permeability are the capillaries of the central nervous system (CNS) and the kidneys.

The blood–brain barrier is a physiological adaptation which protects the brain from exposure to many potential toxins in the plasma. The endothelial cell junctions are tight and the degree of permeability is very low, meaning only very lipid-soluble molecules or those of a small size may pass into the CNS. Active transport mechanisms exist for some molecules important to CNS function, but in general, exogenous molecules will have to pass this relatively impermeable barrier.

The glomerulus of the kidneys is adapted to allow passage of substances across it and into the renal tubule to be excreted. Here not only are the endothelial cells thin, but there are discrete gaps between them—fenestrae—which allow passage of even large molecules out of the plasma (see Figure 1.3.1.3).

Most tissues lie in-between these two extremes and so for normal tissues the determinant of distribution for a drug is organ blood flow. Those with a high blood flow rate will be presented with more drug per unit time than organs with lower blood flow.

A further factor affecting tissue distribution is plasma protein binding (see Figure 1.3.1.4). Many drugs in addition to being carried in solution in the plasma have some degree of binding to plasma proteins. Only free drug is available to act on tissues, and so the degree of plasma protein binding can have a major effect on drug kinetics. The same number of drug molecules in a highly protein-bound drug will lead to far less free active drug available than the amount of free drug available with limited protein binding. States with very low plasma protein levels can occur in the malnourished, after major procedures, and in the critically ill. In these

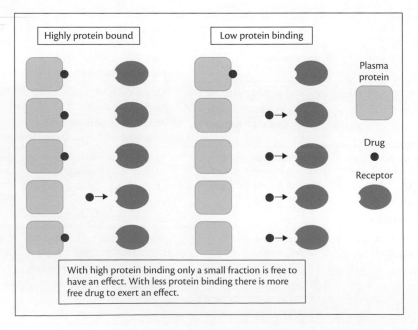

Highly protein bound

Low protein binding

Plasma protein

Drug

Receptor

With high protein binding only a small fraction is free to have an effect. With less protein binding there is more free drug to exert an effect.

Fig. 1.3.1.4 Plasma protein binding.

patients, highly protein-bound drugs have less protein to bind to and this may alter their activity.

Because of varying drug distribution not all of an administered drug is always free in the plasma and available to then have an effect at its target site. Volume of distribution is a calculated theoretical volume that the drug appears to be dissolved in. It is calculated by measuring the initial plasma concentration and then dividing the initial dose by this value. This gives an apparent volume in which the drug appears to be dissolved.

For drugs confined to plasma with minimal distribution the value will be similar to plasma volume. In extensively distributed drugs, it may seem to be very large and may be a value higher than the water content of the body.

Ion trapping is an example of altered distribution which occurs because of body fluids with different pH values. A drug crossing a membrane to a fluid with a different pH will change its proportion of ionization, which may then affect its distribution. This is important to consider in pregnancy, where large, ionized drugs will not cross the placental membrane easily, but any drug which does easily cross membranes will be transferred to the fetus. Because the fetal pH is less than that of the mother, the degree of ionization of drugs will change; basic drug will become more ionized and so less able to cross back over the placenta to the maternal circulation. This ion trapping happens across membranes when the pH is different but is especially important when considering drugs which cross the placenta and may become ion trapped—such as pethidine.

Metabolism

Metabolism describes the way the body changes a drug in order to allow its removal from the body. The overall aim is to alter a molecule to render it more water-soluble so that it is more easily excreted—usually in the urine, but also in bile, and less frequently across the lungs.

Not all drugs require metabolism to be excreted, and whilst the majority of drug metabolism occurs in the liver this is by no means the only site where metabolism takes place. Ideally metabolism would produce, in a single step, a pharmacologically inert substance which is non-toxic and easily excreted in the urine. However, metabolism is often complex, with multiple metabolites produced, some of which may retain active properties, and some of which may be directly toxic.

Many metabolites retain some activity, and some may be more active after metabolism. Indeed, some drugs are given in an inactive state and require metabolism to an active drug in order to exert their effects, and are called pro-drugs. Others, though not inactive on administration, require metabolic conversion to exert most of their effect. A common example is codeine, which undergoes metabolic conversion to morphine in order to produce its analgesic effect.

Wherever metabolism takes place, the reactions involved are classified into phase I and phase II reactions. Many, but not all drugs undergo both types of reaction.

Phase I

These reactions involve reduction, oxidation, or hydrolysis and usually result in an increased availability of reactive sites. The majority of these reactions occur in the liver and are carried out by the system of enzymes called cytochrome P450. There are a wide number of different enzymes within this family, and many forms will metabolize more than one drug. This can lead to potential drug interactions due to altered metabolism.

The cytochrome p450 enzymes are not the only enzymes which catalyse phase 1 reactions, and the liver is not the only organ to take part in drug metabolism. Metabolism of angiotensin-converting enzyme inhibitors occurs in the lungs, and the plasma contains a large number of esterases, which metabolize drugs including the muscle relaxant suxamethonium.

Phase II

These reactions are generally conjugation reactions, whereby the addition of another group to a drug molecule—often at a site rendered functional by a phase I reaction—can increase its solubility. They rely on an enzyme to aid conjugation, and a supply of substrate to conjugate with the drug. This is important as the supply of endogenous substrate is not always enough to keep up with metabolic demand.

Paracetamol is the most common example of a drug which can outstrip its supply of conjugation substrate. In usual dose, multiple metabolites are produced, but only a very small amount of the toxic N-acetyl-p-amino-benzoquinone imine which is conjugated with glutathione. In overdose, much more of this toxic metabolite is produced which uses up the hepatic glutathione allowing the toxic N-acetyl-p-amino-benzoquinone imine to cause direct hepatotoxicity. Early treatment is aimed at maintaining glutathione by administration of precursors. Late treatment is difficult as the hepatic damage has already taken place.

Metabolic enzymes can also be induced or inhibited by other drugs, with many anticonvulsant drugs being potentially potent enzyme inducers. This can be important when a new drug is added which may increase the metabolism of others, or when a new drug is added to an already induced system.

Excretion

Excretion is the final removal of drug from the body. The major organs of excretion are the kidneys, although some drugs will be excreted in exhaled air, sweat, breast milk, and bile. Drugs may be excreted unchanged by the kidneys but the majority undergo at least some metabolism prior to excretion.

Drugs may be filtered at the glomerulus if in solution in the plasma, but highly protein-bound drugs are not free in the plasma to be filtered.

Active secretion takes place in the proximal tubule via nonspecific carriers. These will also remove protein-bound drugs as they will leave the protein to replace drug being lost to the tubule.

Through the tubule, water is reabsorbed to give concentrated urine. This effectively increases the concentration of drugs within the tubule and those that are lipid-soluble may pass back into the plasma and slow their excretion. Ionized drug is more likely to stay in the tubule as it crosses the tubule less easily.

Proportions of ionized to un-ionized drug can be changed with knowledge of their pK_a and manipulation of pH. Acidic drugs will become more ionized in an alkaline environment and this is used to speed excretion of aspirin in overdose by alkalinization of urine. It is a method of inducing ion trapping.

Renal function therefore plays a vital role in the handling of drugs by the body. Those drugs which are largely excreted unchanged by the kidneys may have significantly prolonged action in the presence of renal failure.

Pharmacokinetic modelling

Pharmacokinetic modelling helps describe what happens to drugs when each aspect of its pharmacokinetics is taken into account.

The processes can be described using some mathematical functions:

- Volume of distribution: an apparent volume in which the drug appears to be dissolved at time zero.

- Elimination: describes removal of active drug from the body and includes both metabolism and excretion of the drug.

- Clearance: the volume of plasma cleared of drug in a unit of time. It can be shown with repeated measurement over time that the rate of clearance is proportional to the concentration of the drug. This means that with higher concentrations, clearance rate is also higher.

- Half-life: the time taken for drug plasma concentration to fall by half.

The pharmacokinetic modelling uses these values and specific constants for each drug.

The complex pharmacokinetic interactions can be described using the simple analogy of a bathtub (see Figure 1.3.1.5), where absorption is similar to the tap flow rate, clearance is due to plughole size, and volume of distribution is the size of the bathtub. The pharmacokinetic modelling uses these values and specific constants for each drug.

For a single oral dose, all four stages of its pharmacokinetics are shown in Figure 1.3.1.6.

If a drug is given by IV infusion it will gradually reach a steady-state plasma concentration. As clearance is proportional to plasma concentration, the clearance builds up until it equals the infusion rate and the plasma concentration is static at steady state. This takes five half-lives for the process to be (almost) at steady state. Bolus administration by any other route mimics this and drug concentration also approaches steady-state concentration by this method.

The concentration of drug required in order to produce a clinical effect is not a specific value, rather a range of values. The range of concentrations able to produce the desired effect is called the therapeutic window, or therapeutic index (see Figure 1.3.1.7).

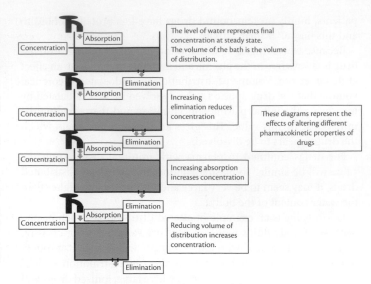

Fig. 1.3.1.5 The bathtub as a pharmacokinetic model.

Levels below this are unlikely to produce the desired clinical effect, whilst levels above this range are more likely to produce either excessive clinical results, overt side effects causing harm, or toxicity. Side effects can occur at normal doses, however, and the level at which excessive clinical effect is produced will vary in individuals.

If the therapeutic range is narrow, then only small concentration changes may change the drug from effective to toxic. Drugs are dosed in order to maximize time in the therapeutic window, whilst minimizing time spent in either the non-effective or toxic range. Usually the lowest dose required to produce an effective response is used to try to prevent potential problems.

Therapeutic drug monitoring describes the need in some drugs to directly measure either their concentration or their effect. The commonest example is probably treatment of hypertension. The blood pressure is sequentially measured over prolonged periods after introduction or titration and when a desired clinical change is measured the dose is maintained. More difficult are drugs with a narrow therapeutic index where toxic effects are more likely to

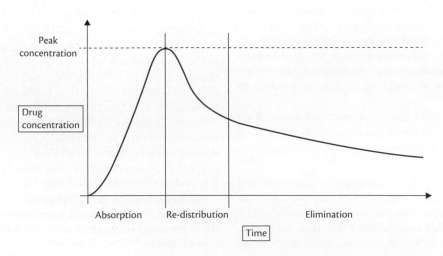

Fig. 1.3.1.6 Oral drug concentration over time.

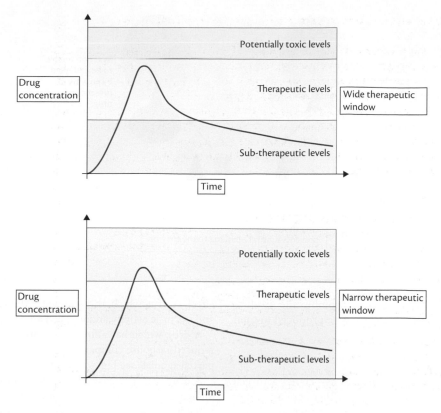

Fig. 1.3.1.7 Therapeutic window.

occur, or for drugs in which the toxic effects are extremely severe and so are monitored to avoid their occurrence.

In some, there is a measurable end point—such as loss of consciousness with anaesthetic induction agents. For others, there is no measurable end point. The aminoglycoside antimicrobial drug gentamicin has a narrow therapeutic index and can cause significant nephrotoxicity. Blood levels should be checked in continued therapy and doses adjusted with advice from the pharmacy team in order to avoid toxic effects.

Pharmacodynamics

This branch of pharmacology deals with the actions of the drug on the body, and so describes how drugs work, or how we think they work. Many drugs will have multiple modes of action, many of which are poorly understood. In most cases, the body is too complex to easily describe all actions of all drugs and their metabolites in such simple terms; however, we try.

Mechanisms of drug action
Chemical interaction
Some drugs work by a simple chemical reaction with either one, or a number of target molecules. A common example is sodium bicarbonate, often given to patients with renal impairment. This simply reacts with hydrogen ions, buffering the pH and maintaining the acid–base balance lost in renal impairment.

Physical action
Mannitol is an osmotic diuretic; it works because the molecule, confined to the plasma, exerts an osmotic effect due to the size of the molecule, drawing fluid into the plasma.

Target protein interaction
This is the major mechanism of action of most drugs. The two major types of active protein within the body which can be targets for drug action are enzymes and receptors. Both have specific physiological roles dependent on their action, which can be manipulated by drugs.

Enzyme interaction
Enzymes within biological systems work as catalysts; they speed up, or reduce the energy required for reactions to take place. They are almost exclusively proteins and are highly selective, allowing specific reactions to take place within the body at the speeds needed to sustain complex life (see Figure 1.3.1.8).

Though separate from true receptor interaction, the concepts are similar and some terms are used in both contexts. An enzyme's selective activity is due to binding sites which are three-dimensionally arranged to allow binding of only specific substrates, or rather to only allow binding of other specific three-dimensional shapes. Drugs with a similar three-dimensional shape to the substrate may also interact with the binding site and therefore interfere with the speed of the biological reaction.

The action of drugs on receptors is usually to reduce the action of the enzyme, and this inhibition can be reversible or non-reversible. Binding to the active site for a short period reduces the effect of the enzyme by temporarily blocking the active site, preventing binding and reaction of the intended substrate. Non-steroidal anti-inflammatory drugs (NSAIDs) bind reversibly to the enzyme cyclooxygenase (COX), preventing prostaglandin synthesis. Irreversible bonding to the enzyme will stop its activity, usually until more enzyme is produced. Aspirin binds

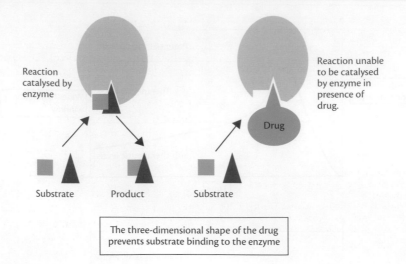

Reaction catalysed by enzyme

Reaction unable to be catalysed by enzyme in presence of drug.

Drug

Substrate   Product   Substrate

The three-dimensional shape of the drug prevents substrate binding to the enzyme

Fig. 1.3.1.8 Enzyme inhibition.

irreversibly to platelet COX, preventing thromboxane production. This reaction requires new platelets to be produced to then be offset.

Receptors

Receptors are large, endogenous molecules associated with cell function and signalling (see Figure 1.3.1.9). There are a number of different types, and multitudes of subtypes, but they share some similar characteristics which can be exploited. A multicelled organism is able to coordinate and regulate many of its functions by the use of signals and receptors. When activated, the receptor usually changes some type of process within the cell, by a number of potential different mechanisms.

The binding of a molecule and subsequent activation of a receptor is specific. This is due to a three-dimensional binding site which can only be accessed by a molecule of a specific shape, and in all cases a molecule exists in the body that activates the receptor, which usually has no activity unless it is activated. This process explains the receptor's susceptibility to external manipulation.

A molecule which binds to a receptor is called a ligand.

The ease of binding by a ligand is termed its affinity.

The ability of a ligand to produce a response in a receptor is called its intrinsic activity.

The endogenous ligand for the receptor will display both affinity and intrinsic activity. It binds to the receptor and produces an effect. A drug which also stimulates the receptor will have affinity and intrinsic activity and is called an agonist.

A drug which has affinity and intrinsic activity but produces a reduced response compared to the endogenous ligand is termed a partial agonist (see Figure 1.3.1.10).

A drug may also have affinity but no intrinsic activity and is an antagonist as it will prevent endogenous activation of the receptor when it occupies the binding site.

Antagonism can be competitive or non-competitive.

Competitive antagonists bind to receptors in a temporary way similar to the endogenous ligand. They are termed competitive because their effect is based on occupying more receptors than the endogenous ligand, and this is more likely at increased concentrations. If the endogenous ligand concentration rises, it can outcompete the antagonist for binding sites.

Non-competitive antagonists form more permanent bonds with the receptor, and their effects cannot be overcome by increasing doses of ligand, only by production of new receptor. Therefore, there is no competition in the production of its effect.

Efficacy is the term used to describe the maximal response able to be produced by an agonist. A drug that cannot produce a maximal response has less efficacy than one which can. Potency describes the drug concentration needed to produce a response. Agonists can be less efficacious as their maximal response is less, but more potent as the response is produced at lower concentrations.

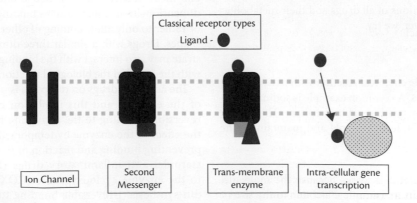

Classical receptor types

Ligand -

Ion Channel   Second Messenger   Trans-membrane enzyme   Intra-cellular gene transcription

Fig. 1.3.1.9 Classical receptor types.

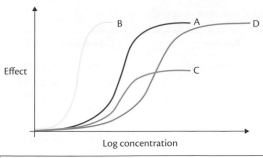

A describes a full agonist drug with maximal effect.
B shows a full effect, so with similar efficacy, but this effect is produced at low concentrations, so it is more potent.
C shows a partial agonist, it cannot produce a maximal effect even at high dose. It may also be drug A in the presence of a non-competitive antagonist.
D shows drug A in the presence of a competitive antagonist. Increased concentration can still give a full effect.

Fig. 1.3.1.10 Drugs as agonists.

Drug interactions

Drug interactions are important instances where the use of multiple drugs changes some aspect of one or more of the concurrent medications. It is important to be aware of drug interactions; many do not present a significant clinical problem, some are beneficial, but others may be fatal.

- *Chemical interactions*: some drugs are chemically incompatible, and cannot be administered together as they undergo a simple chemical reaction with each other, such as sodium bicarbonate and calcium—they will precipitate as calcium carbonate (chalk) if given in the same line.

- *Pharmacokinetic interactions*: this type of interaction occurs because of changes in absorption, distribution, metabolism, or excretion. Epinephrine (adrenaline) added to local anaesthetics causes vasoconstriction, reducing absorption and allowing more drug to be used. This is a beneficial interaction. Warfarin is highly protein bound, and if another highly protein-bound drug is given, it may displace warfarin, causing more free drug and an increase in its action. This could be a potentially fatal reaction due to uncontrolled anticoagulation and is one reason why monitoring of warfarin therapy is important. Metabolism can be induced by certain drugs and alcohol which can then mean more rapid metabolism of other drugs, reducing their effect.

- *Pharmacodynamic interactions*: indirect interactions occur when a drug with different mechanisms of action causes a change, which affects mechanism of action of another. Direct interactions are because of interaction at active sites, such as naloxone antagonizing opioid drugs at the opioid receptors, which is a beneficial reaction.

Analgesics

It is currently impossible to separate surgery and pain; analgesia is an important aspect of surgical practice, and it should be a priority for the whole of the surgical team. A commonly used definition of pain is 'an unpleasant sensory or emotional experience associated with actual or potential tissue damage, or described in terms of such damage'.

Analgesics are the groups of drugs used in the treatment of pain, their modes of action are diverse and they are commonly used in combination.

Paracetamol

Paracetamol is one of the most commonly used drugs. Available to buy from a multitude of outlets it is used for self-medication by a wide range of the population. In standard doses, side effects are remarkably rare, although in overdose it remains a significant problem. Although paracetamol is widely available this does not mean that it is not effective, and it is presented at the start of this section because it should be a baseline analgesic for a majority of our practice.

This drug, though widely used, is not thoroughly understood. In basic terms, it is likely to work by central inhibition of prostaglandin synthesis. It has multiple preparations, and is well absorbed by the oral route. Rectal and IV routes are also used. Its metabolism in the liver is by conjugation prior to urinary excretion.

The main side effects generally only occur when taken in overdose, but are severe, including irreversible liver failure. It is important to understand that in patients with chronic malnutrition and/or liver disease, the dose may need to be reduced to take into account the relative lack of hepatic glutathione. This may well include a number of surgical patients.

Non-steroidal anti-inflammatory drugs

This class of drugs are powerful analgesics, some of which are freely available to buy by the public, but all have potentially significant side effects even at standard doses.

Arachidonic acid is a product of the breakdown of cell membrane phospholipids and is produced during cell damage. It is converted by an enzyme called COX into prostaglandins. Prostaglandins are known to play many roles within the body, and these include the ability to induce and amplify pain, and as an initiator of the inflammatory response (see Figure 1.3.1.11).

NSAIDs work by inhibition of COX enzymes, reducing the availability of prostaglandins to induce pain. As they work both centrally and peripherally, they cause analgesia, reduce inflammation, and have antipyretic effect. Prostaglandins are not just mediators in pain pathways, however.

Other important actions include the generation of a physical barrier in the stomach to protect gastric mucosa from the low pH of gastric secretions, and regulation of renal blood flow by dilatation of afferent arterioles. This explains the two most common serious side effects associated with NSAIDs: gastric ulceration and renal impairment.

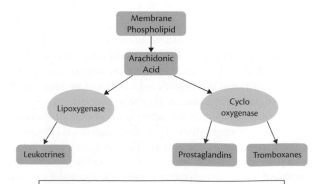

The enzyme cyclooxygenase is essential in the production of prostaglandins which produce pain and inflammation, as well as mediating other physiological processes

Fig. 1.3.1.11 Arachidonic acid pathway.

NSAIDs may also precipitate bronchospasm in those with reactive airways by the production of leukotrienes in an alternative metabolic pathway for arachidonic acid when COX is inhibited.

Most NSAIDs are well absorbed by the oral route, although there are rectal and IV preparations. Metabolism in the liver is followed by urinary or biliary excretion.

Cyclooxygenase isoforms

There are at least two subtypes of COX, COX-1 and COX-2, and it is thought that COX-1 is the form responsible for the production of prostaglandins with functional roles, such as in the GIT and in renal regulation. COX-2 is thought to be expressed in response to tissue damage and has a greater role in the mediation of pain and inflammation. For this reason, COX-2-selective NSAIDs were developed, with the hope of reducing side effects including peptic ulceration, which could be fatal.

The COX-2 inhibitors, however, were found to have potential for increased cardiovascular events including myocardial infarction, and so manufacturers have withdrawn a number of these.

Opioids

Opiate is a term used to describe a naturally occurring substance which works in a similar way to morphine. Opioid is a better term and describes any substance including synthetic substances that display affinity at opioid receptors.

Opioid receptors are presynaptic receptors, which work via second messenger pathways to cause hyperpolarization of the cell membrane, making it more difficult to cause stimulation by depolarization, and play an inhibitory role in the sensation of pain.

Opioid receptors are found throughout the CNS, spinal cord, and in some peripheral tissues including the GIT. There are multiple subtypes with different actions, but opioids cause analgesia, sedation, respiratory depression, meiosis, reduced GIT motility, and euphoria.

Tolerance to opioids describes the situation whereby exposure to a drug results in reduced effect, or the need for a higher dose to produce an effect. It is common in those taking chronic opioid analgesics or those who abuse opioids. The process is complicated, and occurs due to a number of mechanisms. These patients need a tailored dose as they have different requirements; an accurate history is needed to avoid giving high-dose opioids to an opioid-naïve patient.

Morphine is the standard opioid, and is a widely used drug in surgical practice.

Orally, it is less than 30% bioavailable as it undergoes first-pass metabolism, but is well tolerated by this route. IV and IM routes are common in surgical patients. Its duration of action is 2–4 hours and is metabolized in the liver and kidneys to active metabolites, which are excreted in the urine. Significant care must be taken in those with renal impairment as accumulation may occur.

Side effects with opioids are common and include nausea and vomiting which is almost inevitable when high doses of opioids are used. Itching can be a severe side effect and may even be worse than the pain which is being treated. Constipation can be a significant problem in the postoperative period and should be proactively treated.

Sedation and respiratory depression are potentially the most severe side effects. They are in general dose dependent, but not always, as opioid-naïve patients or those with altered clearance will

Table 1.3.1.2 Alternative opioids

Drug	Benefits	Problems
Fentanyl	Rapid acting Very potent High lipid solubility allows for multiple routes of administration, including IV, buccal, and transdermal	Poor oral bioavailability May still cause respiratory depression after removal of trans-dermal 'patch' Can accumulate with continued high doses
Pethidine	Can be given IM or IV	Low potency Toxic metabolite may cause seizures
Methadone	Used to treat opioid dependency Analgesic, with some action at NMDA receptor Long half-life with once-daily dosing	Tolerance may still occur Does not replace the need for increased perioperative analgesia

be at higher risk. Regular observation of the patient's condition is vital in detecting these adverse effects.

Naloxone is an antagonist at the opioid receptors. It will reverse the opioid side effect of respiratory depression rapidly. It can be given via the IV or IM route, and should be used if there is potential for significant respiratory depression. Two problems occur with naloxone use; firstly, it reverses the analgesic effects of opioids, possibly leaving patients with significant pain. Secondly, its half-life is significantly shorter than that of morphine, so its effects will wear off more rapidly than morphine. Repeated doses or an infusion may be required.

Codeine is a weak opioid that is commonly used orally for postoperative analgesia. It can be given via the IM route, but more often orally. It requires hepatic conversion to morphine for its effect. This is via the cytochrome P450 enzyme system, and there is a genetic variation in the activity of the enzyme responsible for this conversion. Some ultra-fast metabolizers will have a higher peak level of the active drug, causing more side effects. This has possibly led to deaths in paediatric patients using codeine after tonsillectomy, and the US Food and Drug Administration has issued a safety announcement stating that codeine should not be used for this indication in children. Alternately, some poor metabolizers will receive little benefit from codeine, as they cannot metabolize it to an active drug rapidly enough. After metabolism, it is excreted via the kidneys.

Multiple other alternative opioids are available with slightly different pharmacological profiles; in general, they share many characteristics (see Table 1.3.1.2).

Antimicrobials

An antibiotic is a substance excreted by an organism that impairs growth of another, but in medicine, this definition is not always adhered to. Antimicrobial is the term better suited to describe the classes of drugs that are used to treat infection by microorganisms. Their use is a common aspect of surgical practice.

They are initially classified according to the type of organism they target, with antibacterials, along with antifungal and antiviral drugs. Further classification is often by the mechanism and/or mode of action.

In pharmacological terms, it is important to understand their mode of action, and the differing pharmacokinetic parameters which may affect choice of agent and side effects. Microbiological sensitivity and its effect upon agent choice are discussed elsewhere.

The aim of these drugs is to damage the pathogen without damaging the host. This gives a number of different potential mechanisms of action based on important cellular differences.

Antibacterial drugs

The aim of these drugs is to damage the pathogen without damaging the host. This gives a number of different potential mechanisms of action based on important cellular differences.

Bacteria are prokaryotic, without a nucleus and with specific other cellular differences to the eukaryote human cells (see Figure 1.3.1.12).

Inhibition of bacterial cell wall synthesis

Many of these drugs contain a molecular component called a beta-lactam ring. This group allows the drugs to bind to and irreversibly inhibit an enzyme necessary in the final steps of bacterial cell wall synthesis. This weakens the cell wall to an extent that cell lysis occurs.

Penicillins and cephalosporins work in this way, and the main problem with their use is production by bacteria of a beta-lactamase which breaks down the beta-lactam ring, a form of resistance.

Beta-lactam antibiotics may be co-administered with a substance to reduce activity of beta-lactamases. Clavulanic acid is combined with amoxicillin as it irreversibly binds to beta-lactamases, reducing their effects on the active portion of the preparation.

There are multiple preparations of penicillin, and absorption varies in these preparations. They are poorly lipid-soluble and so cross membranes poorly. This also includes the blood–brain barrier, and yet they are effective in meningitis. This is because inflammation disrupts the blood–brain barrier and allows better penetration. Penicillins are actively excreted unchanged in the renal tubule.

They can cause GI upset and diarrhoea, and alter the normal flora of the GIT. This can allow infection as other flora become pathological, such as Candida causing oral thrush. There is a significant incidence of allergic reactions.

Cephalosporins are available in multiple 'generations' of development. They have very widely varying pharmacokinetics, tend to be well distributed, and are usually excreted by the kidney, although some undergo metabolism.

Cephalosporins may also allow infection with commensals due to alteration of normal flora. There is also potential for allergic reactions, which may also be because of cross-reactivity in people sensitive to other beta-lactams.

The carbapenems imipenem and meropenem are also beta-lactams, and are used in surgical practice. Imipenem undergoes renal metabolism and excretion, and so will accumulate in renal failure. It may rarely cause seizures and, more commonly, GIT upset.

Glycopeptides such as vancomycin and teicoplanin are not beta-lactam-containing molecules. They inhibit bacterial cell wall formation by inhibition of the enzyme glycopeptide synthetase. They are both excreted unchanged in the urine, and may also cause renal toxicity. Vancomycin is usually dose adjusted according to measured plasma levels.

Inhibition of protein synthesis

A number of antimicrobials target differences in bacterial protein synthesis.

Essentially, prokaryote RNA has different subunits to eukaryote RNA. Some drugs bind to these subunits, blocking transcription and therefore subsequent protein synthesis. A number of antimicrobials work in this way.

Tetracyclines have variable oral absorption, and most have mainly renal excretion. Because they bind to and chelate metals including calcium they can be deposited in bones and teeth and so are contraindicated in young children and in pregnancy.

The aminoglycosides also work this way and the commonest example is gentamicin. It has dose-related toxicity and so is usually monitored with plasma level assay and dose adjustment. It is ototoxic, causing permanent damage to the VIIIth nerve. It is also nephrotoxic, which may not be permanent, but is more likely in those with pre-existing renal disease or use of other nephrotoxic drugs. This is important as aminoglycosides are eliminated almost entirely by the kidneys. This makes renal impairment even more important as it may cause accumulation of the drug.

The macrolides include erythromycin and clarithromycin. They are commonly used in patients with penicillin allergy. Some hepatic metabolism occurs before excretion in the bile.

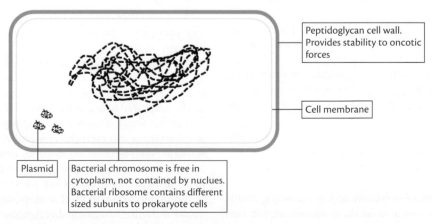

Fig. 1.3.1.12 Bacterial cell structure.

Fusidic acid inhibits bacterial protein synthesis also, but is less commonly used. It is absorbed orally and penetrates well into bone, making it useful in osteomyelitis.

Inhibition of folate

Folate in humans is an essential amino acid and we must obtain it from our diet. Bacteria synthesize folate and the sulphonamides competitively inhibit an enzyme essential in the production of folate, which is then not available for DNA synthesis.

Trimethoprim also works to reduce bacterial use of folate, by inhibiting a different enzyme used in the pathway of folate metabolism, again preventing its use in DNA synthesis.

Interference with DNA replication

The quinolones, including ciprofloxacin, prevent supercoiling of bacterial DNA by inhibiting the enzyme necessary for this—DNA gyrase. This prevents correct replication of DNA, and they are specific for the bacterial version of this enzyme. Elimination is by a combination of hepatic metabolism and renal excretion. There are some important specific side effects, which affect the use of quinolones. They may reduce the seizure threshold, making seizures more likely in all patients, but possibly more so in those with epilepsy. They cause tendon damage, including rupture, and should be stopped if there is suspicion of developing tendonitis.

Rifampicin inhibits RNA polymerase and is well absorbed into most tissues. It can be given orally as well as IV and induces hepatic enzymes. It may also rarely cause liver damage and liver function may need to be monitored.

Metronidazole is thought to work by prevention of DNA replication. It is well absorbed orally and excreted in the urine with little metabolism. Its side effects are few, but it interferes with alcohol metabolism and so alcohol should be avoided during its use.

Antibiotic resistance

This phenomenon occurs because, like any organism, bacteria will adapt to survive. Their generations of replication are many times faster than those of humans and so adaptations are expressed more rapidly. It is a complex area, but occurs because of a number of mechanisms.

Mutations in chromosomes occur at random, and some will confer survival benefit. Most bacteria exposed to drugs will not have these mutations, but some will, and some will survive.

Plasmids are small portions of DNA that are separate, in the cytoplasm. These plasmids may code for a type of resistance, and these are called R plasmids.

Transfer of these resistance genes, usually on R plasmids, can occur within bacteria and between bacteria. This allows for spread of resistance across bacteria even of different species.

Mechanisms of resistance include the production of enzymes, which inactivate the drug being used. The most obvious is that of beta-lactamase which inactivates the functional portion of the beta-lactam antimicrobials.

Other resistance mechanisms include inactivation by enzymatic metabolism and alteration of active binding sites.

Antifungals

Fungi usually cause superficial infection and only rarely systemic infection, but this is more common in the immunocompromised or the critically ill patient.

Fungi have a different plasma membrane, which incorporates a sterol called ergosterol (as opposed to cholesterol) which is the target of many antifungals.

Amphotericin binds to the plasma membrane and forms a pore in the membrane, altering permeability, especially allowing efflux of potassium. It has poor oral absorption, but can still be used orally for treatment of GIT fungal infections. It is heavily protein bound, excreted by the kidneys, and has a very prolonged elimination time. It also causes renal impairment in a significant number of patients undergoing therapy.

Nystatin works in a similar way and is used topically or orally for GIT infection as it has minimal absorption.

The azoles including fluconazole inhibit the bacterial metabolism responsible for production of ergosterol and so inhibit replication of the fungi. Side effects can occur, including hepatic impairment and skin reactions.

Antivirals

Viruses lack the ability to self-replicate and require a host cell to do so. They contain their genetic material and little else. By binding to a cell, they release their genetic material and the host cell's own mechanisms replicate it producing more virus. Antiviral drugs target these points in the life cycle of a virus. There are many new and emerging antiviral drugs (e.g. aciclovir and ganciclovir) which have minimal impact on general surgical patients, but are important in those medical patients with acute or chronic viral infection, in particular immunosuppressed organ transplant patients.

Anticoagulant drugs

Drugs that affect coagulation are invaluable in the prevention and treatment of many conditions. They also cause significant problems in the perioperative period. Knowledge of the clotting cascade is useful, but not always practically clinically relevant as it does not contain platelets, which are a vital part of this physiological process (see Figure 1.3.1.13).

Warfarin

Warfarin is a coumarin and works by antagonizing vitamin K use in the production of a number of clotting factors. Vitamin K is required for the correct functioning of certain enzymes involved in the production of active factors II, VII, IX, and X. These are often termed the vitamin K-dependent clotting factors, and their depletion occurs over 2–3 days.

However, other regulatory proteins C and S are depleted and this may cause an initial prothrombotic effect during the initiation of warfarin therapy.

The anticoagulant effect is measured by the prothrombin time, for which the reagents may vary in laboratories, and so it is standardized as the international normalized ratio (INR). This is routinely monitored to assess the level of anticoagulation.

Warfarin is well absorbed and highly protein bound; the addition of other drugs and even changes in diet may change the effects of warfarin either by reducing absorption or by affecting protein binding or metabolism. It is metabolized in the liver prior to excretion in the urine and bile, and its half-life is around 35–40 hours.

The major side effect is haemorrhage, which may be spontaneous if the anticoagulant effect is overly high. Management of warfarin in the perioperative phase requires planning for elective

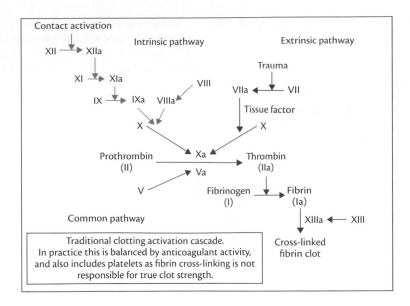

Fig. 1.3.1.13 Clotting cascade.

patients, and is difficult in emergency cases. Reversal of the effects of warfarin is possible. Direct administration of re-constituted vitamin K-dependent factors is possible, and very rapid, but reserved for life-threatening bleeding or emergency surgery that cannot wait. This is due to a risk of the patient becoming prothrombotic. Vitamin K can be given, either orally or IV, and will antagonize the effect of warfarin, but takes time to produce an effect. If warfarin is stopped, its effects will reduce over 3–5 days and can be confirmed by reduction of INR.

Heparin

Heparin is an endogenous molecule produced by the liver and is involved in the normal balance of pro- and antithrombosis. It is a polymer with variable sulphation, and unfractionated heparins are made up of different-sized molecules, usually in the range of 12 000–15 000 Da.

Its mechanism of action involves binding to and increasing the activity of antithrombin. This heparin–antithrombin complex is much more active than antithrombin in isolation and causes significant inactivation of thrombin as the three molecules combine. This method of action is dependent on the size of the heparin molecule being large enough to allow formation of the three-molecule complex.

Other regulatory substances are inactivated by the heparin–antithrombin complex including factor Xa. This activity requires only binding of the molecule to antithrombin and is not size dependent.

LMWHs are not large enough to form the three-molecule combination required for significant thrombin inactivation, but do cause a significant increase in the anti-Xa activity and this is how they exert their effect.

Heparin is given by either the IV or SC route. Dosing should be titrated to the individual by monitoring of the activated partial thromboplastin time (aPTT). A loading dose followed by infusion is according to a standard protocol with aPTT monitoring usual in most units. Its onset is rapid, as is its offset via hepatic and renal metabolism. There is some excretion of unchanged drug via the kidneys.

Because of its rapid offset, usually within 2–3 hours, heparin is used perioperatively where there is a requirement for anticoagulation, but also a risk of haemorrhage. If more rapid offset is required in life-threatening situations, it may also be reversed with protamine sulphate which is manufactured from fish sperm, and essentially chelates heparin molecules forming a salt because of ionic interaction. It is difficult to accurately dose as the time since heparin use needs to be taken into account. It also has significant side effects including anaphylaxis, hypotension, and acts as an anticoagulant in its own right at high doses.

Side effects of heparin are in general related to bleeding, making it vital to adequately monitor therapy. Other side effects may include hyperkalaemia and osteoporosis.

Thrombocytopenia also occurs, including the heparin-induced thrombocytopaenia and thrombosis (HITT) syndrome, which is caused by formation of antibodies to heparin in complex with an antiplatelet protein. Despite the thrombocytopenia, HITT is a prothrombotic state that causes arterial and venous thrombosis. Diagnosis is clinical, aided by laboratory tests to detect the antibodies.

Low-molecular-weight heparins

LMWHs contain only molecules of heparin with a molecular weight of less than 8000 Da. They combine with antithrombin, but lack the size required to significantly affect thrombin. They do, however, have an anti-Xa activity, which produces their anticoagulant effect. Their effect cannot be measured with the APTT, but anti-Xa levels are measurable in certain laboratories and can help guide treatment, but this is usually not needed.

They have a dose-dependent effect and are given via the SC route in a standard dose range based on weight. Their main benefit is once- or twice-daily administration without the need for infusion. They are mainly excreted unchanged in the urine, and so may accumulate in renal impairment. The half-life is prolonged relative to heparin, and the effects are only partially reversed by protamine, making the management of bleeding during administration more complex.

The incidence of HITT syndrome seems to be lower, but is still possible.

Other anticoagulants

Other anticoagulants are also used, but much less frequently in usual practice.

Danaparoid is a heparinoid, which is different from heparin and is used commonly in HITT syndrome. It increases the action of antithrombin and so inhibits activated factor Xa. The half-life is long and it is excreted by the kidneys. There is no reversal agent, but its effects can be monitored by the anti-Xa assay.

Lepirudin is a direct thrombin inhibitor and binds irreversibly to thrombin preventing fibrin binding and clot formation. It is a recombinant hirudin, a class of drug initially isolated from leeches. Lepirudin is excreted via the kidneys and due to its irreversible binding, its actions cannot be reversed.

Fondaparinux is a synthetic drug that mimics heparin's activity on antithrombin and increases its anti-Xa activity; it does not have a direct effect on thrombin. It is excreted by the kidneys and cannot currently reliably be reversed.

Dabigatran is an oral direct thrombin inhibitor. It is used in prophylaxis of thromboembolic events in a similar way to warfarin, but without monitoring. It is contraindicated in treatment of patients with mechanical heart valves due to an increased risk of thromboembolic and bleeding events in these patients.

Antiplatelets

These drugs affect the functioning of platelets, which despite their absence from the traditional clotting cascade play a pivotal role in the formation of stable, functional clot.

Aspirin

Aspirin is widely used in the primary and secondary prevention of thrombotic events in ischaemic heart disease, cerebrovascular disease, and in those with prothrombotic conditions.

It works by inhibition of the enzyme COX. In platelets, this enzyme produces thromboxane, and inhibition of thromboxane production reduces its action in platelet activation and aggregation. COX inhibition in other tissues also accounts for aspirin's analgesic and antipyretic effects.

Aspirin (unlike the other NSAIDs) binds irreversibly to the enzyme, this means its effects persist for the lifespan of the platelet, around 7 days. Aspirin has significant potential side effects, especially peptic ulceration due to its effects on prostaglandins and antiplatelet effect. This is in addition to the potential increase in other bleeding problems. It is also contraindicated in the paediatric populations because of its association with Reye's syndrome, a rare but severe disorder including fatty liver and encephalopathy.

Clopidogrel

This drug also binds irreversibly to platelets, at an ADP receptor. It reduces platelet activation and prevents the binding of fibrin to platelets. It is a pro-drug, which requires metabolism by cytochrome P450 enzymes to be converted to an active molecule. Because of genetic variation in these enzymes, a proportion of people will not metabolize the drug and have a poor response. After metabolism it is excreted in the urine.

Side effects are generally related to haemorrhage, but multiple very rare complications are documented including severe blood dyscrasias.

Dual antiplatelet therapy is common after cardiac intervention, to prevent thrombosis. Bleeding risk is thought to be higher; however, stopping antiplatelets in the perioperative period is likely to increase the cardiac risks associated with procedures.

Others

Dipyridamole is an oral antiplatelet agent with multiple mechanisms of action. It is used in the secondary prevention of cerebrovascular disease—usually in combination with another antiplatelet.

Tirofiban is a glycoprotein IIb/IIIa inhibitor. This is a receptor on the platelet which is involved in platelet activation and aggregation. It is usually only used in the acute phase of a coronary event and this situation poses significant surgical risk itself. It is given IV and has a duration of action of about 6 hours.

Anaesthesia

General anaesthesia

Availability of the safe provision of general anaesthesia is a true advance in surgical practice, and this section will touch on some aspects of the pharmacology of general anaesthesia.

General anaesthesia describes the state of being 'without feeling' but more accurately implies the reversible, induced state of unconsciousness with lack of sensation, pain, and recall. It is a difficult at times to achieve this state and maintain life with otherwise normal physiology. A balanced technique of anaesthesia is often utilized which involves the use of multiple drugs with different actions, in order to produce anaesthesia, whilst minimizing side effects associated with high doses of individual drugs.

During the induction phase of anaesthesia, the patient begins awake and alert with full protective airway reflexes, but induction ends with the unconscious state, absent airway reflexes, and apnoea. The induction phase requires reasonably rapid onset of deep anaesthesia so that the airway can be secured and surgery can begin. Then the maintenance phase where anaesthesia must be maintained whilst allowing the surgical procedure to be performed. The emergence phase is the opposite, offset of multiple drugs must be timed to allow adequate wake up and return of protective airway reflexes prior to removal of airway support.

Induction drugs

An ideal induction drug would produce rapid, dose-dependent depths of anaesthesia, with analgesia and no cardiorespiratory side effects such as respiratory depression or hypotension. It should rapidly lose its effect following a bolus dose, independent of liver or hepatic function, but be able to be used as an infusion to maintain anaesthesia. It should be rapidly eliminated without production of active metabolites to prolong its action, or toxic metabolites to cause side effects.

In reality, no drug is perfect and there is always a balance between intended effects and side effects, and duration of action; most drugs best suited to induction are administered by the IV route.

Propofol is the most commonly used induction drug. It produces dose-dependent sedation, progressing at higher doses to surgical anaesthesia. After a bolus dose, its onset time is around 30 seconds. Offset is due to reduction of peak concentration, not by metabolism, but by re-distribution to other tissues. This is dependent upon the cardiac output redistributing the drug to well perfused tissues. This will occur within 5 minutes and the patient will regain consciousness. Metabolism is in the liver by conjugation with glucuronide and subsequent excretion in the urine.

The mechanism of action of propofol is not completely understood. It seems to have multiple mechanisms of producing anaesthesia including gamma-aminobutyric acid receptor interaction, sodium channel blockade, and some N-methyl-D-aspartate receptor (NMDA) receptor antagonism.

It is a very versatile drug, with minimal residual effect even though its terminal elimination may take up to 24 hours. It does, however, possess significant potential side effects.

The profound anaesthesia produced by propofol is also accompanied by loss of airway reflexes making it a very useful drug at induction where manipulation of the airway is required. Along with unconsciousness, propofol causes respiratory depression and apnoea, which is more significant if opioids are used concurrently. This combination of airway effects necessitates personnel trained in advanced airway techniques to be dedicated to the care of patients receiving propofol, even for sedation only.

The cardiovascular system is also affected by propofol, with significant blood pressure reduction, mainly due to vasodilatation, but also because of direct myocardial depression. This makes propofol potentially very prone to cardiac instability in those with poor cardiovascular reserve or acute hypovolaemia.

Thiopentone is a barbiturate, and is used far less since the introduction of propofol, but is still used in the 'rapid sequence' technique of induction of anaesthesia where speed of induction and subsequent securing of the threatened airway is paramount. This is due to its very rapid onset time, around 10 seconds. Again, offset is due to redistribution long before its hepatic metabolism. Thiopentone metabolism can, however, become saturated with multiple doses or infusion, making it unsuitable for use in infusion as it accumulates.

Due to the profound CNS depression caused by thiopentone, it remains a treatment for status epilepticus and intractable raised intracranial pressure—both of which necessitate intubation and ventilation when thiopentone is used.

Side effects include respiratory depression and cardiovascular instability in a similar manner to propofol.

A specific potential problem with thiopentone is its ability to cause an acute porphyric crisis and so it is contraindicated in those with porphyria, fortunately a rare condition.

Ketamine is infrequently used in the United Kingdom. It produces 'dissociative anaesthesia' with analgesia and amnesia. Its end point can be difficult to determine, it causes hallucinations after use, and is a drug of abuse. These problems, easy availability of alternatives, and so a lack of experience are the main reason for limited ketamine use.

It does have many beneficial aspects relative to other induction drugs, including some cardiovascular stimulation, maintenance of laryngeal reflexes and bronchodilatation. These effects have made it particularly useful in those with acute hypovolaemia or where there is a requirement for a maintained airway without the requirement of endotracheal intubation, such as trauma, and in particular, pre-hospital management. It can also be given IM although with a more prolonged onset time.

Ketamine works by antagonism of glutamate at the NMDA receptor, and is metabolized in the liver by phase I metabolism, including to an active metabolite. These then undergo phase II metabolism prior to urinary excretion.

Volatile anaesthetics

Volatile anaesthetics were the first anaesthetics developed, and include ether and chloroform. They are liquid at room temperature but give off a vapour that induces unconsciousness when inhaled. Modern volatile anaesthetics include isoflurane, sevoflurane, and desflurane, and require highly engineered administration devices (vaporizers) which, in combination with an anaesthetic machine, allow accurate dose administration as a percentage of inspired gas, and titration of the fraction of oxygen in the inspired gas.

Volatile anaesthetics produce a dose-dependent reduction in level of consciousness which is reversible upon elimination of the drug.

The onset of anaesthesia is slower than IV drugs, taking minutes, with an excitation phase at light planes of anaesthesia and a delay in the ability to secure the airway. Inhalational induction is therefore usually reserved for those in whom these risks are acceptable, children who will not cooperate with awake IV access, and in those in whom maintenance of spontaneous respiration is paramount, such as those with potential airway obstruction.

Volatile anaesthetics are mainly used for the maintenance of general anaesthesia as the initial IV induction drug wears off. The organ of both absorption and excretion of the volatile anaesthetics is the lungs. This is a highly unusual situation in drug delivery for systemic effect. However, due to the ability to couple delivery of anaesthetic to the delivery of oxygen it has remained the most widely used method of maintaining anaesthesia. Gas monitoring is mandatory in anaesthesia as it proves adequate oxygen supply, and carbon dioxide output, which confirms ventilation of the lungs.

Measurement of volatile anaesthetic concentration is also possible, allowing both confirmation of delivery and knowledge of sufficient dose. If there is an interruption of anaesthetic due to disconnection of breathing system then an alarm will sound because this also means interruption of oxygen delivery.

Measurement of expired volatile anaesthetic levels allows knowledge of sufficient depth of anaesthetic. The minimum alveolar concentration of each volatile anaesthetic is a value of expired gas known to be a minimum required to keep experimental volunteers asleep to a standard stimulus.

There is minimal metabolic conversion of the modern volatile anaesthetics, unlike older drugs such as halothane, which does undergo hepatic metabolism, and had an incidence of fatal hepatitis linked to metabolites. This is still possible with newer agents, but their hepatic metabolism is minimal and so this is very rare.

Offset is related to reduction in alveolar concentration of the drug, which drops as it is exhaled by the lungs into expired gas. The time taken for offset is related to their blood solubility, the less soluble drugs being given up into the lungs more easily, but is dependent on an adequate ventilation to remove them from the body.

There is no 'reversal agent' for anaesthetic drugs, they have to wear off, and the patient must be awake enough to maintain their own airway before they no longer require direct anaesthetic supervision. Residual volatile anaesthetic will still be evident for a period after the anaesthetic, and after prolonged anaesthesia with deposition into adipose tissue, this residual effect may be prolonged.

Nitrous oxide, or laughing gas, was one of the first gasses used to produce analgesia, and it is still used today. Its use has declined because of the awareness of its limitations and potential adverse effects.

In order to work as an anaesthetic in its own right, nitrous oxide must be given at a partial pressure of around 105 kPa or 105% of the inspired gas mixture. This is not possible at sea level especially as some oxygen must also be involved in the gas mixture and so it is limited to being an addition to other agents. It is used in combination with oxygen, as a carrier gas for other volatile agents. The benefit of additional analgesia, with cardiostability, and the ability to reduce doses of other anaesthetic drugs needs to be balanced against its side effects.

Risks involve accidental hypoxic gas mixture—causing death or hypoxic brain injury; this risk is reduced by engineering solutions within the anaesthetic machine, but is still possible. It expands gas-filled cavities within the body such as in bowel, or a pneumothorax. It also impairs folate synthesis and with prolonged exposure can cause depression of the bone marrow. It is a potent cause of postoperative nausea and vomiting.

The most common use is as a 50:50 mixture with oxygen, 'gas and air', used extensively during labour due to the rapid onset and offset of its analgesic properties.

Neuromuscular blocking drugs

Often called muscle relaxants, these drugs are given at induction in order to allow profound muscle relaxation, which is required for direct laryngoscopy and insertion of an endotracheal tube.

This class of drug is only used in anaesthesia as they cause profound blockade of motor nerve transmission to muscles. This results in complete loss of skeletal muscle power, including the diaphragm. The lungs must therefore be manually or mechanically ventilated to provide oxygen and sustain life until the effects wear off. Inability to ventilate the lungs by any means after administration of these lungs is an anaesthetic emergency that is often unpredictable and called 'can't intubate, can't ventilate' and will rapidly render the patient hypoxic.

The mechanism of action is competitive antagonism of acetylcholine at the neuromuscular junction by blockade of the postsynaptic receptor. Therefore, nerve transmission is unable to stimulate a muscular contraction until the drug has worn off leaving sufficient empty receptors for acetylcholine to stimulate a muscular contraction. Smooth muscle is unaffected.

Offset is due to metabolism reducing the drug concentration available at the neuromuscular junction. This allows acetylcholine to out-compete the drug for its binding site. The offset process can be helped by increasing the concentration of acetylcholine available to compete. This is done by inhibition of the enzyme acetylcholine esterase, but can only be successful if the muscle relaxant is already reducing in concentration, allowing free receptors for the acetylcholine to bind to. In this way, the action of muscle relaxants which are already starting to wear off can be fully reversed at the end of anaesthesia allowing the patient to breathe reliably for themselves.

A novel agent called sugammadex is now available which reverses the action of specific muscle relaxants by chelation within the plasma. It is very specific, but works rapidly enough that it can be used in the emergency 'can't intubate, can't ventilate' scenario—a life-threatening emergency without return of neuromuscular function and spontaneous respiration.

Suxamethonium is the only drug in use which activates the postsynaptic receptor prior to antagonizing it by more prolonged binding than the endogenous ligand—acetylcholine. This is why suxamethonium causes muscular fasciculation as it works, a good end point. It works rapidly, within 90 seconds, and is offset by rapid metabolism within the plasma by esterases. Side effects are

common. It causes postoperative muscular pain, a slight rise in potassium, which can be fatal in some conditions, such as acute kidney injury or after severe burns due to an abnormal receptor proliferation. It is a common cause of anaphylaxis during anaesthesia, and it is a trigger agent for malignant hyperthermia.

Atracurium is a common neuromuscular blocker, of the benzylisoquinolinium type. It causes competitive inhibition of neuromuscular transmission by binding to, but not activating, the acetylcholine receptor. Its duration of action is around 30 minutes and offset is due to diffusion away from the neuromuscular junction down a concentration gradient as the drug is metabolized. In part, this is in the liver, but the molecule also degrades at higher temperatures and with pH changes making its offset of action reliable even in patients with hepatic and renal impairment.

Rocuronium is an amino-steroid muscle relaxant, working by competitive inhibition of acetylcholine at the postsynaptic membrane without activation. It has a rapid onset of action and in high doses can be used for rapid sequence induction as its onset is within 60–90 seconds; however, under normal circumstances its action will last at least 45 minutes, over 40 minutes longer than the brain will be able to survive hypoxaemia in failed intubation. The new reversal/chelation drug sugammadex will, however, reverse its effects, even in high doses, in minutes.

All neuromuscular blocking drugs are common causes of anaphylactic reactions, which can be difficult to recognize during the complex changes at the point of induction.

Total intravenous anesthesia

Total intravenous anaesthesia (TIVA) is a technique of maintenance of anaesthesia without use of volatile anaesthetics. It can be used for many reasons, including anaesthetic preference, where volatile anaesthetics are contraindicated, or in procedures in which there is a 'shared airway' with the surgical team and ventilation may be interrupted.

An infusion of IV anaesthetic agent is given, usually with an infusion of opioids via an IV cannula. Many IV drugs will accumulate if given via infusion, either because their metabolic pathway cannot keep up such as thiopentone, or because they accumulate in tissues to an extent which delays their offset of action. This is called a prolonged 'context-sensitive half-time' and describes the delay in elimination of a drug when it is infused over a period of time.

Therefore, drugs with 'context-insensitive' half-lives are used. The best example of this is the opioid remifentanil which has a rapid offset of action irrespective of duration of infusion because it is rapidly metabolized by esterases in the plasma, with a capacity far larger than required for standard doses. Propofol is also commonly a used drug for TIVA, but does accumulate to some extent in adipose tissue.

Two major issues complicate TIVA use compared with volatile anaesthetics. There is a wide individual variation in dose requirements, and even complex mathematical models used to guide dosing have a range of error. Also unlike volatile anaesthetics carried with inspired gas that is measured, there is no feedback to ensure a presumed dose is reaching the patient. IV access must be accessible at all time to check, which can be difficult in a positioned patient in theatre, and unlike with the airway there is no disconnection alarm. The incidence of awareness is presumed to be higher, but only limited studies of this are available at the time of writing.

In summary, multiple drugs are given during general anaesthesia that have the ability to cause severe morbidity and mortality without close monitoring and the ability to provide advanced airway and cardiovascular support. Some knowledge of this is important in the team approach needed for successful surgical care.

Local anaesthetics

Local anaesthetics are drugs which produce reversible blockage of nerve impulses in the area to which they are applied, without affecting consciousness.

The use of local anaesthetics is an integral part of modern surgical practice. They are versatile drugs that may be used in isolation to allow surgical procedures, or used in combination with analgesics or general anaesthetics as part of a balanced anaesthetic technique. Knowledge of local anaesthetics is therefore important, not least because their use can allow procedures to benefit patients in whom general anaesthesia is of unacceptably high risk or even contraindicated. There are multiple methods of producing anaesthesia, including local infiltration, individual nerve blockade, nerve plexus blockade, and, neuraxial blockade via the epidural and intrathecal spaces.

All local anaesthetics share a common structure, with a lipid-soluble aromatic group and a water-soluble amine group (see Figure 1.3.1.14). They are divided into two classes based upon the chemical link between these two standard groups. Either an ester or amide group joins the two other major groups, and this link provides some of the main differences between the groups.

The ester link is more easily broken down making it less stable in solution with a shorter shelf-life. However, *in vivo*, the major issue is the metabolite produced—para-aminobenzoate is implicated in a significant rate of allergic or hypersensitivity reactions. The amide group, however, causes much less hypersensitivity, and coupled with their stability in solution means it is the main agent used in the United Kingdom.

Mechanism of action

Local anaesthetics prevent transmission of the neuronal action potential by blockade of sodium channels. All excitable cells have a resting potential across their insulating phospholipid membrane, which is created because of different concentrations of charged ions accumulating on opposite sides of the membrane.

The action potential is the mechanism by which electrical potential is transmitted along a nerve. It occurs due to propagation of a wave of depolarization along the nerve as rapid changes in membrane permeability to charged ions occur. A stimulus to depolarization occurs at a point on the nerve. If this reaches a threshold potential then voltage-gated sodium channels open. This rapidly and dramatically increases the permeability of the membrane to sodium ions, which then travel through the open sodium channel into the cell, causing depolarization. Local anaesthetics work by blocking these voltage-gated sodium channels, preventing propagation of a wave of depolarization (see Figure 1.3.1.15). They work from within the cell and on 'open' or active sodium channels, which cannot be 'reset' until the local anaesthetic drug is no longer associated with the sodium channel.

In order to gain access to the intracellular aspect of the sodium channel, the drug must cross the cell membrane. To do this it must be un-ionized as the ionized form is charged and much less lipid-soluble. All local anaesthetics are weak bases—this means they are proton acceptors, and so become ionized when bound to hydrogen ions (protons). As previously stated, it is the pK_a of a drug that determines the proportion of a drug which is ionized or un-ionized in any solution.

As the local anaesthetics are bases, if they are in a solution which is more acidic (lower pH) than their pK_a they will accept more protons and so be more ionized. This explains why local anaesthetics work poorly in infected tissue because it tends to have a lower pH so more hydrogen ions than normal bind with the drug, making

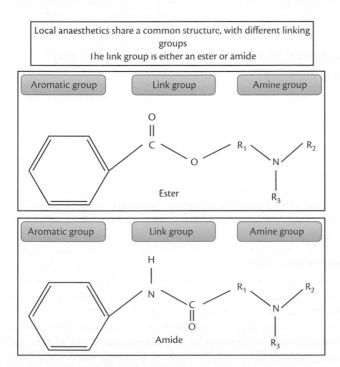

Fig. 1.3.1.14 Local anaesthetic structure.

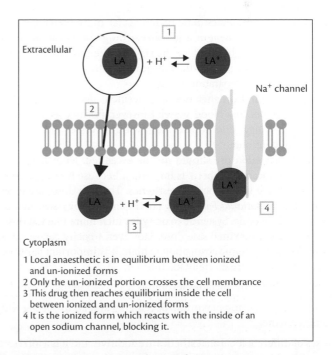

Fig. 1.3.1.15 Local anaesthetic mechanism of action.

the drug more likely to be ionized, and so unable to cross the membrane into the cell.

The absorption of local anaesthetics depends upon their site of administration; direct intravascular injection will obviously give complete absorption, but also poor effect as the drug is carried away from its intended site of action. Local infiltration has a low absorption, but absorption rises if injection is close to major vessels as is often the case for nerve plexus blocks. Most local anaesthetics cause vasodilatation in high doses and so may encourage systemic uptake.

It is the pK_a of a local anaesthetic that determines its onset of action, but the duration of action is linked to the degree of protein binding. More highly protein-bound local anaesthetics have a more prolonged duration of action. Metabolism will depend upon the class of drug: esters are metabolized by hydrolysis in the plasma, with the exception of cocaine, which is hydrolysed in the liver. Amides all undergo hepatic metabolism and so can accumulate in hepatic failure.

In order to manipulate the properties of local anaesthetics multiple additives are used.

Epinephrine is commonly added in low doses to local anaesthetic solutions. This causes local vasoconstriction, reducing systemic absorption of the drug, prolonging its effects, and allowing a higher safe dose to be used. It is important not to use epinephrine-containing solutions in digits or appendages such as the penis, which have an end-arterial supply. Vasoconstriction may result in ischaemia and necrosis in these areas.

Sodium bicarbonate is sometimes added to local anaesthetic solutions in order to manipulate the pH into producing a higher proportion of un-ionized drug. However, although this sounds attractive these solutions are not stable and may precipitate.

Addition of substances to standard solutions is not encouraged, it can be dangerous and is usually outside the product licence and indication. Only products approved and supplied by a pharmacy team should be used as this involves a process for determining safety.

Safe doses

Prevention of local anaesthetic toxicity is far more preferable than emergency management of a life-threatening complication. Some basic measures will help reduce the risk of systemic toxicity.

An awareness of the potential for local anaesthetic toxicity should always be part of preparation for use.

Negative aspiration after needle placement *does not* prove that the needle is not in a blood vessel; however, positive aspiration of blood is very suggestive of placement within a vessel and injection should not continue.

A maximal safe dose should not be exceeded. Knowledge of a safe dose of local anaesthetic is important because it is a prerequisite for the safe use of local anaesthetics. The safe doses are given in the *British National Formulary* (BNF) and can be calculated on a dose per kilo basis. Systemic toxicity is much more likely at doses at or above the maximal safe dose. However, toxicity can occur at lower doses if systemic absorption is high. It is important to obtain an accurate weight, especially in children:

- Bupivacaine—this includes levobupivacaine—150 mg or 2 mg/kg
- Lidocaine—200 mg maximum or 3 mg/kg and up to 500 mg with epinephrine.

Doses of different local anaesthetics are additive, and it is a total safe dose. Reaching the maximal dose of bupivacaine does not mean

that lidocaine can then also be used up to its safe dose. Use of 50% of a safe dose of bupivacaine means that only 50% of the safe dose of lidocaine is then safe to use. It is also therefore important to understand what dose of drug is in an ampoule: 1% solutions contain 10 mg/mL so 100 mg in 10mL; 0.5% solutions contain 5 mg/mL.

Local anaesthetic toxicity

This section describes toxic side effects due to high systemic levels of local anaesthetic. It can occur because of use of an excessive dose or because of inadvertent administration of a standard dose directly IV, or even because of increased systemic absorption.

Systemic side effects can be observed in the two major organ systems with excitable tissue, the CNS and the cardiovascular system. Many of the early signs will be difficult to identify if the patient has an ongoing concurrent general anaesthetic.

In the CNS, peri-oral tingling and paraesthesia is an early sign due to the combination of highly vascular tissue with high nerve density. CNS excitation occurs first, leading to seizures, then global CNS depression with unconsciousness. In the cardiovascular system, outward signs are few, QRS abnormalities occur with QRS widening, prolonged QT interval and progression to ventricular arrhythmias including ventricular fibrillation and death. Cardiac arrest due to local anaesthetic toxicity has been difficult to treat with conventional methods; prevention is ideal, but in extremis, treatment has always been supportive. Standard cardiac arrest protocols with an ABC approach are used, with the need to continue resuscitation if possible until the local anaesthetic has worn off. Outcomes were poor, and worse with the longer-acting highly protein-bound drugs.

A recent advance has been the introduction of high doses of IV lipid emulsions in the treatment of severe local anaesthetic toxicity. They appear to drastically reduce the amount of free local anaesthetic in the systemic circulation in a non-specific form of chelation. This is now incorporated into national treatment guidelines and a supply of lipid with instructions should be available in all areas where significant doses of local anaesthetics are used.

Impact of concurrent medical therapy on surgical practice

The surgical patient will often require some medicines to be prescribed and many will have pre-existing drug regimens or conditions which may affect drugs prescribed. The surgical pathway has its own specific issues which also need to be taken into account. There is often interruption of the oral route, due to preoperative starvation, sedation, nausea, and reduced GIT function. For many drugs, a short interruption in therapy is acceptable, or even desired in the perioperative period. For other drugs, this can cause significant problems and alternatives or alternative routes may be required.

Safe prescribing

It is essential to be able to prescribe drugs safely in the perioperative period, it is also essential to be able to manage existing medicines safely whenever patients are under our care.

As with many aspects of medicine, a multidisciplinary approach to medicines management in surgical patients is key to their safe care. Primary care, preoperative assessment, ward staff, surgical team, anaesthetists, and especially pharmacists play key roles.

The specialist advice given by pharmacists is invaluable, and combined with the BNF and hospital guidelines no prescriber should feel alone in making decisions about drugs in the perioperative period.

Drug history

It is a vital part of safe prescribing practice that an assessment of full drug history is undertaken. In many cases, the medication being taken will be due to pathology separate from the surgical pathology. Some patients will be on few or no medicines, but some will be on multiple medications which may cause issues in the perioperative phase.

A complete medical history will allow a thorough assessment, improving patient safety by knowledge of potential problems and smooth out the patient's surgical journey by dealing with potential problems in advance.

The drug history should be reviewed, ideally at the time of planning a surgical procedure (see Table 1.3.1.3).

Allergy history

Many drugs used in the perioperative period have potential for allergic reactions, commonly antimicrobials and neuromuscular blocking drugs. It is insufficient to merely state a list of drugs, a positive response should prompt further enquiry. This should include name of drug, description of reaction, reactions to related drugs and any investigations of allergy such as skin prick testing in an allergy clinic. Historical allergy from childhood is difficult to disprove, but a clinical history may help denote intolerance of a drug as opposed to true allergic reaction. If allergy history is unclear, it is better to be cautious as anaphylaxis carries a significant mortality.

General anaesthetic exposure history

This must also include family history of exposure. This is worthwhile at the earliest opportunity; a history of repeated exposure to anaesthetic agents without any problems is common. However, there are a number of significant and potentially fatal problems that may be identified early.

Table 1.3.1.3 Drug history

Current drugs	All drugs—generic names. Always check correct drug names
	Indications for drugs
	Routes, doses, and dose timings, confirm doses or timings that are outside the norm
	Duration of current treatment
Recent drugs	Drugs recently stopped, when and why? Ask specifically about steroid treatment
	Confirm reasons for stopping: complete course, condition improved, or intolerance?
Non-prescribed drugs	Over-the-counter drugs, herbal remedies
	Illicit drugs—which? How often? Is there an infection risk?
Absent drugs	With knowledge of medical and medication history there may be drugs which are obviously omitted. This may be intentional, but may not be
Check history	In conjunction with pharmacy and primary care all aspects of medication should be re-checked to ensure completeness and accuracy

Postoperative nausea and vomiting is the most common anaesthetic drug-related adverse event, it is multifactorial, but can be reduced by adjusting the anaesthetic technique and including prophylactic antiemetics.

Anaphylaxis is common to neuromuscular blocking agents, which is difficult to recognize as it tends to occur at induction and has significant mortality. Patients with anaphylaxis during anaesthesia are usually followed up with aggressive investigation so that an alternative plan for drug use can be made.

Suxamethonium apnoea occurs due to a genetic deficit in its metabolizing enzyme. Suxamethonium has a very prolonged duration of action and a period of ventilation in critical care is often needed until return of neuromuscular function. It is familial and so potential problems may be identified even in those not exposed previously to suxamethonium.

Malignant hyperpyrexia is a rare condition which is genetic in origin. An abnormal receptor within skeletal muscle causes muscle contraction and a hypermetabolic state when exposed to either suxamethonium or volatile anaesthetics and stress. Avoidance of these drugs is mandatory if the condition is suspected. In theatres where volatile agents are used extensively, adequate notice is essential. The condition is associated with pyrexia due to excessive muscle contraction and requires a specific muscle relaxant—dantrolene. It still carries a significant mortality; families of suspected cases are investigated in a national unit to help confirm diagnosis in advance.

Drugs commonly prescribed to surgical patients

Cardiac drugs

Cardiac disease is common, and it is common in the surgical population. A wide variety of drugs are used in the treatment of cardiovascular disease, and many can have an impact in the perioperative management of patients.

Antihypertensive drugs are generally prescribed to reduce the long-term risk of cerebrovascular events associated with hypertension. During the perioperative period, there is potential for large swings in blood pressure and so a reasonable control of hypertension is expected prior to elective surgery. In general, they should be continued but with some exceptions, local guidelines may well help. After significant surgery, blood pressure may be lower than normal and so caution may be required in the reintroduction of these drugs.

Beta blockers should be continued but may cause some decrease in blood pressure with general anaesthesia. They are potentially of benefit in reducing cardiac events in high-risk patients. However, the potential risk of stroke means this should be individual decision.

Angiotensin-converting enzyme inhibiters are usually omitted on the day of surgery as they may cause significant hypotension in conjunction with general anaesthesia. This may be exaggerated in the hypovolaemic patient. This also applies to direct angiotensin II antagonists.

Diuretics should usually be continued, they have a potential hypotensive effect and may cause electrolyte imbalance.

Antianginal drugs are prescribed as treatment or prophylaxis of angina, and so aim to reduce myocardial oxygen demand, by reduction of force or rate of contractility, or by reduction in afterload due to vasodilatation. They include beta blockers, calcium and potassium channel blockers, and nitrates. Though usually continued preoperatively they may need to be carefully monitored postoperatively to ensure adequate perfusion pressure in the face of the surgical insult. Suddenly stopping some of these medications may potentially precipitate angina and so caution and specialist advice may be needed.

Antiplatelets are very common drugs, used in primary or secondary prevention of cardiovascular disease. They are discussed in detail elsewhere, but in general, single-agent therapy is usually continued. Dual-agent therapy, however, may have an increased bleeding risk, which may be offset by increased cardiovascular risk if stopped—specialist advice may be required. It is worth noting that both aspirin and clopidogrel bind irreversibly at their site of action and so offset is dependent upon the turnover of new platelets—about a week. If significant bleeding occurs in these patients, discussion with haematology around transfusion of platelets irrespective of platelet count should be considered. Transfused platelets will not have been exposed to the drugs and so will not be inhibited.

Specific antiarrhythmic drugs are used less commonly. In surgical patients, the important drugs include digoxin, amiodarone, and beta blockers. These drugs may cause significant side effects, but in general should be continued due to the risk of perioperative arrhythmia, and if the oral route is unavailable then IV dosing may be required.

Diabetic drugs

Type 1 diabetes describes loss of secretion of insulin due to autoimmune destruction of secretory cells in the pancreas. It is universally treated with injectable insulin. Type 2 diabetes is a condition that involves impaired glucose handling due to reduced insulin secretion, or insulin resistance, or both. It is commonly treated with diet adjustment, oral hypoglycaemic drugs, and insulin in those difficult to manage. The aim of treatment is to ideally maintain a normal blood sugar level, but at least reduce the amount of time with significantly high blood glucose as this is related to end organ damage such as retinopathy, nephropathy, and cardiac disease. The need to avoid potentially fatal high or low glucose levels makes diabetic management a challenge during normal life, more so in the perioperative period.

In the perioperative period, the aim is to maintain normal blood sugar levels despite erratic oral intake and potentially abnormal absorption of diet. Usually an established protocol developed with the diabetic team will exist. There are two major risks: hypoglycaemia due to therapy and lack of oral intake, and hyperglycaemia due to inadequate therapy and surgical stress.

Metformin is a biguanide which inhibits hepatic glucose production and increases insulin sensitivity which improves glucose uptake into cells. It is excreted in the urine and is generally continued when oral diet is re-established. Metformin has the potential to cause severe lactic acidaemia, especially in renal failure.

The sulphonylureas include gliclazide and glimepiride and work by increasing pancreatic release of insulin. They are usually stopped if diet is interrupted as they may precipitate hypoglycaemia in the absence of normal diet.

Pioglitazone is a thiazolidinedione which increases insulin sensitivity and reduces insulin resistance. It is usually used in combination with other diabetic medications. This is usually withheld at surgery until diet is restored.

The administration of the hormone insulin is the major treatment for type 1 diabetes, and is also used in type 2 diabetes. Exogenous insulin is usually recombinant and mimics endogenous insulin function. It is given either SC or IV. Multiple preparations of insulin are available whereby the molecules are adapted—for example, with the addition of zinc—to delay absorption or prolong lifespan. This aims to smooth out the insulin levels allowing multiple dosing with different lengths of action depending upon the time of day and amount of dietary intake. The safe management of insulin therapy is difficult.

Perioperative management of those on insulin essentially requires a titratable method of administration with regular testing of blood sugar to avoid hypoglycaemia and significant hyperglycaemia, which even without ketoacidosis may worsen outcome. Adequate management is intensive and repeated changes to regimens are likely until the patient is back to a normal diet. Local policies and the specialist diabetic teams will help provide care for these patients.

Respiratory disease

Commonly asthma and chronic obstructive pulmonary disease patients often use inhaled medication which should be taken as normal in the perioperative period together with any systemic treatment.

Beta agonists work locally in the lung to cause relaxation of bronchial smooth muscle via beta adrenoreceptors. The aim is for inhaled administration for local effect, although some systemic absorption occurs, causing tachycardia.

Ipratropium bromide is often given via inhaler for local effect as an anticholinergic. This reduces bronchoconstriction and is relatively free of systemic side effects.

Steroids are often given via the inhaled route to reduce local inflammation and improve airflow. This is normally a long-term treatment and should be continued.

Theophyllines are sometimes given as chronic therapy, and are safe when patients are stable. They may produce arrhythmias and cause electrolyte imbalance. Patients on established oral therapy who require IV theophylline should not have a loading dose, as this is more likely to cause side effects.

Leukotriene antagonists such as montelukast are also sometimes used and should be continued where possible in the perioperative phase.

Oral contraceptive pill

This may be either the combined oestrogen and progesterone pill, or the progesterone-only pill. There is a potential increased risk of thrombosis. In some patients with a history or family history of thromboembolism it may be necessary to stop. However, in most cases, the risk of unplanned pregnancy from altered medication schedule is high, and if the pill is to be stopped patients must be advised of this risk. In addition, perioperative antibiotics can alter the dynamics of absorption and directed contraceptive advice is needed.

Proton pump inhibitors and H$_2$ receptor antagonists

These drugs are used to reduce gastric acid secretion in those with peptic ulcer disease, reflux, or increased risk of developing these conditions, such as those patients on aspirin. They should be continued preoperatively to maintain their effect on gastric pH if there is a risk of acid aspiration, and also because of the risk of stress ulceration after major surgery.

Opioid use

These may be legally prescribed, but illicit use is also possible, or they may be used for replacement therapy in long-term drug abusers. In general, baseline doses should be maintained with additional analgesia prescribed in addition for treatment of the surgical pain. The surgical episode is not the correct time to try to reduce or stop chronic opioid use, as there is usually a requirement for additional analgesia and psychological stress. Acute and chronic pain teams will be valuable sources of advice in these patients.

Uncommon drugs

Antiepileptics include sodium valproate, carbamazepine, and phenytoin. Where possible these drugs should be continued perioperatively due to the risk of seizures. If there is interruption in the usual oral route, an alternative should be considered. They are often enzyme inducers and so can affect the metabolism of other drugs introduced.

Antidepressants are generally divided into four categories:

1. Tricyclic antidepressants, such as amitriptyline

2. Selective serotonin reuptake inhibitors such as paroxetine

3. Monoamine oxidase inhibitors (MAOIs) such as isocarboxazid

4. Atypical drugs such as lithium.

MAOI drugs are used far less often, but have significant interactions with drugs used in the perioperative period, causing significant cardiovascular instability. They should be stopped and an alternative added under specialist advice in the weeks prior to theatre. The other agents are generally continued although it is usual to check lithium levels as it has a narrow therapeutic range.

Hormone replacement such as thyroxine is generally continued, and if possible, recent biochemical assessment of therapy should be checked.

Systemic steroids are used for a number of conditions, some of which such as rheumatoid arthritis or inflammatory bowel disease may be reasons for patients to present for surgery. Other indications include autoimmune conditions and chronic chest disease such as asthma or chronic obstructive airways disease.

Steroids reduce immune function and inflammation, but also cause significant side effects including increased risk of gastric ulceration, hyperglycaemia, fluid retention, and suppression of adrenal function. This effect can continue after the drug is stopped and so it is important to elicit any prior steroid use and duration.

Replacement therapy in the perioperative period is required, and depends upon the level of surgical stress and the amount of adrenal suppression. It is important, however, as some patients who cannot mount a response to surgical stress with endogenous steroidal hormones may suffer cardiovascular collapse.

Immunosuppressants are generally prescribed to patients after organ transplant, or those undergoing chemotherapy. They are at increased risk of infection, and decisions regarding timing of surgery and ongoing therapy should be made with a specialist multidisciplinary approach.

Medical conditions with important implications for drugs in the perioperative period

There are a large number of medical conditions which affect surgical patients, but most do not directly affect perioperative prescribing. These conditions involve a component of their disease or disease management that causes potentially significant problems with drugs in the perioperative period. It is impossible to mention all of these conditions, but some, which regularly cause problems, are discussed here.

Obstructive sleep apnoea is a condition that causes apnoea during sleep with periods of airway obstruction. Patients seem to have sensitivity to the sedative effects of opioids and so these drugs should be used with caution in this population.

Parkinson's disease is a disorder of dopamine within the CNS. Patients have multiple symptoms including motor dysfunction with bulbar involvement. Medications are available, but some can only be given enterally. It is therefore important to continue medication up to the point of theatre and then re-establish an enteral route early to facilitate adequate medication. Poor respiratory function without adequate medication may increase risk.

Myasthenia gravis is an autoimmune disease, which affects acetylcholine receptors at the neuromuscular junction. It is characterized by fatigue of skeletal muscle that may progress to respiratory failure. It is important because of the exaggerated response to neuromuscular blockers, and to any drug with a usually modest effect at the neuromuscular junction. Reduced respiratory effort may lead to complications including the need for ventilation. Oral medication with acetylcholine esterase inhibitors should be continued and if not possible, then an IV alternative given.

Phaeochromocytoma is a surgical condition that is well known to require pharmacological intervention prior to surgery. Secretion of vasoactive substances can make handling of the tumour cause significant cardiovascular instability. Alpha adrenoreceptor blockade with or without beta blockade is instituted preoperatively to reduce the effects of excess circulating catecholamines.

Porphyria is a condition, which involves abnormal enzymes that normally handle the haem pigment. Certain drugs which further interfere in these pathways can exacerbate types of porphyria. Because of this, the anaesthetic thiopentone is contraindicated in acute intermittent porphyria which is usually familial.

Applied surgical pathology

CHAPTER 1.4.1

Surgical pathology

David Lowe

Introduction

Surgery and pathology are indivisible. The study of the causes and effects of a disease affects the management and prognosis of it. Many of the processes in pathology are generic and apply in many circumstances, and the common ones of these are included here.

Cell processes

There are two principal ontological imperatives that define living organisms: the imperative for survival and the imperative for procreation. The simplest living organisms such as viruses have defence mechanisms and a genetic impetus to multiply; complicated biochemical structures, such as prions, freely multiply by a cascade effect but have no imperative to do so, and no defined defensive or aggressive capacity to ensure their continued existence.

The cell processes of life as we now recognize it began as:

◆ vegetative growth of single-celled organisms, permitted by the availability of an energy source such as sunlight or thermal energy from crustal fractures, and from simple endocytosis and breakdown of particles that provided energy

◆ differentiation permitting alimentation of inanimate material and of competitors and predators

◆ diversification through chromosomal modifications and sexual division.

Growth mechanisms and the cell cycle

The parts of the cell cycle

Figure 1.4.1.1 shows a cell cycle with checkpoints. G1 and G2 are the gap phases. About 98% of the variation in the duration of the cell cycle is accounted for the time spent in G1, the other 2% variation occurring in G2 phase. The length of both gap phases varies in different cell types and among species. Growth promoter and growth inhibitor products act principally in G1, in which synthesis of RNA leads to translation of cell wall and cytoplasmic proteins. If the cell cycle is permitted to advance beyond the restriction point in G1, the cell will probably complete the other phases of the cycle and undergo mitosis.

S is the synthesis phase in which DNA and other nuclear components are formed. In G2 phase there is more protein synthesis. M is the phase of mitosis. The duration of these phases is relatively constant for a cell type. G0 phase is the so-called resting phase before the cell re-enters the cycle. This phase is variable and also depends on growth-modifying gene products.[1]

Factors that control progression around the cycle

Cyclins are a series of enzymes that act during the different phases of the cycle to ensure their smooth progression. They are controlled by cyclin-dependent kinases (CDKs), another series of enzymes which in turn are affected by growth modifiers.

Growth inhibitor gene products that suppress the actions of CDKs include p53, p27, and p21 proteins. Retinoblastoma gene product and related genes hold the cell in G1 by acting at the restriction point. Once the cell has passed the restriction point it is very likely to undergo mitosis.

Growth-promoting agents include those that are:

◆ circulating:

  • hormones: human growth hormone (hGH), triiodothyronine and tetraiodothyronine (T_3 and T_4), cortisol, testosterone, and oestrogen

  • growth factors: platelet-derived growth factor from α granules, fibroblast-derived growth factor, macrophage-derived growth factors, and insulin-like growth factor 1

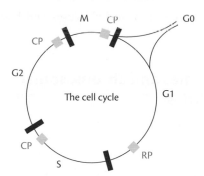

Fig. 1.4.1.1 Cell cycle with checkpoints.

G0 The 'resting phase' in which the cell is active in synthesis, secretion, and other functions but is not undergoing the process of division.

G1 Gap phase 1, in which there is synthesis of cell components necessary for division into daughter cells, except for synthesis of DNA. The checkpoint in G1, at which progress further through the cycle is controlled, is called the restriction point, RP. It is the point at which growth inhibitor factors such as retinoblastoma gene product and *p21* gene product act.

S Synthesis phase, in which DNA is synthesized. The checkpoint (CP) in this phase is towards its end, and also responds to growth inhibitor gene products.

G2 Gap phase 2, in which there is protein synthesis and condensation of chromosomes begins. There is a checkpoint towards the end, at which DNA integrity is examined before the cell is permitted to undergo mitosis.

M Mitosis phase, in which the cell passes through prophase, metaphase, anaphase, and telophase to form two separate daughter cells. The checkpoint is in metaphase, at which the spindle assemblies are examined for competence.

Adapted from David Lowe, *Surgical Pathology Revision*, Second Edition, Cambridge University Press, Cambridge, UK, Copyright © 2006. Reprinted with permission.

- cell membrane bound:
  - protein receptors such as epidermal growth factor receptor (EGFR), homologous with *c-erbB-2* gene product
  - intracytoplasmic: steroid receptors
  - intranuclear: c-myc, c-ras.

Growth-suppressing agents include:

- circulating hormones such as progesterone
- intracellular agents: p53 protein, retinoblastoma gene product, *APC* gene product in familial adenomatous polyposis, *BRCA1* and *BRCA2* gene products in breast and ovarian cancer, and Wilms' tumour gene product. It is abnormalities of these genes and their protein products that permit the development of neoplasia in some cases, not the presence of the genes themselves in the genome.

DNA damage in a cell results in activation of the *p53* gene to make p53 protein. This arrests the cell cycle by increasing the concentration of the CDK inhibitor p21 protein and so prevents the damaged DNA being replicated. The cell will be forced into apoptosis by p53 protein if the DNA defect is not remedied within a time-span that varies among cells.[2]

Abnormalities of the *p53* gene prevent this protective mechanism—*p53* is the commonest growth inhibitor gene found to be abnormal in human neoplasms. Decreased *p53* activity may be by:

- deletion of the *p53* gene or mutation of it into an inactive form
- overactivity of the *mdm-2* gene, the regulator of *p53*, which results in excess protein product which binds with and inactivates p53 protein
- abnormal handling of p53 protein
- metabolism of p53 protein by viruses which stimulate cell division.

Chromosomes and chromosomal abnormalities

Chromosomes in normal cells

Most human cells have 46 chromosomes, 22 pairs of autosomes and one set of sex chromosomes. These can be a pair of X chromosomes or an unmatched set of an X and a Y. When chromosomes developed over 30 million years ago, the X and Y chromosomes were identical in size and composition and would have been at the position of chromosome pair 7 in the modern terminology, in which position 1 represents the largest chromosome and position 21 the smallest (chromosome 22 is in fact larger than 21—this was a labelling mistake). Primates other than human beings have 48 chromosomes; two small non-human primate autosomes fused together resulting in human chromosome 2.

About 10% of tissue cells are in process of mitosis and have built up 96 chromosomes. These coalesce in *prophase*, line up in a bar in *metaphase*, are separated in *prophase* by spindle contraction, and as new sets of 46 chromosomes, are ready to repeat the cell cycle when the daughter cells pull apart in *telophase*.

Cells with 23 chromosomes are haploid. They are found in the testes as late spermatocytes, spermatids, and spermatozoa, and in the ovary as oocytes. When a spermatozoon fertilizes an oocyte they become an ovum, which has 46 chromosomes. Other possible numbers of chromosomes in normal cells include zero, in erythrocytes and reticulocytes which are anucleate, and multiples of 46, such as 92 in cells about to divide, and higher multiples of 46 in multinucleate cells such as osteoclasts and myocytes.

Chromosome abnormalities are classified as those of autosome quality and number, and of sex chromosome quality and number. The two principal types of abnormality of chromosome quality or structure are:

- translocations, in which parts of chromosomes are transposed onto others. Translocations may be balanced, when material is reciprocally transferred and so the total chromosomal material is unaffected, or unbalanced when material is gained or lost
- deletions, in which there is loss of chromosomal material of an amount or type that is compatible with development of a living embryo. Deletion of material from both ends of a chromosome with fusion of the ends results in ring chromosome formation.

DNA ploidy and chromosome numbers

Ploidy is the amount of DNA in a cell, which in a normal cell correlates directly with the number of chromosomes present. A normal cell which has one or more nuclei is haploid, diploid, tetraploid, or polyploid. An abnormal cell may be triploid or aneuploid, either by gaining or losing chromosomal material in odd amounts or by gaining or losing entire chromosomes. A triploid gestation, in which the cells of the embryo have 69 chromosomes, is compatible with a life of only a few weeks. Ploidy is measured by a variety of methods, most commonly flow cytometry; DNA densitometry is less widely used.

Monosomy refers to cells which have one of a pair of autosomes or sex chromosomes missing. The cells have 45 chromosomes, such as in Turner's syndrome, X0 (X zero). Absence of one of a pair of autosomes is almost always lethal, but absence of a Y or one X chromosome is compatible with life. In each cell of a normal woman one of the X chromosomes is inactivated at random, though only partially (the Lyon hypothesis).

Trisomy refers to cells with one extra chromosome in a set, and so 47 chromosomes in a typical cell. In Down's syndrome, there is either an extra chromosome 21 or an extra amount of chromosome 21 genetic material translocated onto another chromosome. Another example is XYY males—as the Y chromosome carries so little genetic material, these men are normal.

In very rare cases, multiple X chromosomes may be present in a viable cell, such as XXX and XXXX, which are examples of trisomy and tetrasomy. As there is at least partial inactivation of the redundant copies this is compatible with life, but the patients are usually infertile and have other developmental abnormalities.

Abnormalities of chromosome quality
Autosomal dominant conditions

If a single copy of an abnormal autosome confers a phenotypic abnormality it is called an autosomal dominant disease. The prevalence is the same in both sexes. At least one parent must be affected, assuming that the patient does not have a spontaneous mutation: if only one, the patient will be heterozygous; if both, the patient may be heterozygous or homozygous. If the patient is heterozygous and has a normal partner, half of their children would be expected to have the condition.[3]

Examples of surgical importance include:

- familial adenomatous polyposis: several chromosomal abnormalities affect mucosal cells in the large bowel and elsewhere in sequence to result in adenomatous polyps and, in almost all cases, adenocarcinoma

- some forms of polycystic disease, which may present in a young adult with the complications of a berry aneurysm such as subarachnoid haemorrhage, and in older adults with hepatic, splenic, pancreatic, and bilateral renal cysts and chronic renal failure. Less commonly, polycystic disease is associated with aneurysm of the aorta, diverticula of the intestines, and ovarian cysts

- Marfan's syndrome, a connective tissue defect in which there are heart valve abnormalities leading to cardiac failure, and an increased risk of aortic dissection and of subluxation of the lens

- spherocytosis, in which there is haemolytic anaemia which may be episodic and an increased risk of gallstones as a consequence.

Autosomal co-dominant conditions

There is random inactivation of one copy of most paired genes (as with the paired X chromosomes in female cells). The other copy contributes all of the body's requirement for the gene product. A small number of genes are unusual in that they provide only about half of the requirement for the gene product and so both copies must be active for normal production; these are called co-dominant genes. Examples include genes for some blood groups, enzymes, red cell constituents, and some antigens such as human leucocyte antigen. The principal condition of surgical interest in which a co-dominant gene is defective is sickle cell disease.

Autosomal recessive conditions

An autosomal recessive disease is one in which both copies of the causative abnormal gene must be present. Both parents must have at least one copy of the abnormal gene. They could be:

- both heterozygous carriers and so asymptomatic

- one a carrier and one homozygous showing symptoms and signs of disease

- very rarely, both homozygous especially if the disease causes little risk of infertility or death before puberty.

When a heterozygous carrier has a normal partner, half of the children would be expected to be carriers. When two carriers have children, one in four would be expected to have the disease, half of them expected to be carriers, and one in four normal.

Autosomal recessive conditions of surgical importance include:

- cystic fibrosis, in which patients have susceptibility to infections and risk of developing intestinal obstruction from meconium ileus, bronchiectasis, pancreatitis, and cirrhosis

- alpha-1 antitrypsin deficiency (better called protease inhibitor deficiency, as the inhibitor is non-specific), in which patients develop hepatitis and cirrhosis, and early-onset emphysema without the usual risk factors.

X-linked (or sex-linked) conditions

These are disorders caused by an abnormality on the X chromosome. The Y chromosome carries little genetic message: the *SRY* gene, genes for immunological functions, and genes which lay down calcium in male animals' teeth. Sex-linked diseases affect males almost exclusively as they have no extra X to compensate; heterozygous females are normal, while homozygous females are affected.

If a woman who is a carrier has children with a normal man actuarially half of all sons would be affected and half of the daughters would be carriers. All of the daughters of a father who is affected must be carriers. Sons who do not have the disease cannot be carriers.

Examples of X-linked diseases include:

- haemophilia and Christmas disease as the result of deficiency or abnormality of factor VIII and factor IX respectively. Affected men suffer from intramuscular bleeding, haemarthrosis, and intracranial bleeding. Undiagnosed, there is a risk of severe intraoperative haemorrhage. Until relatively recently a common cause of death was hepatitis C and human immunodeficiency virus (HIV) infections from contaminated blood transfusions

- glucose-6-phosphate dehydrogenase deficiency, in which there is haemolysis caused by drugs such as antimalarials, sulphonamides, aspirin, and dapsone

- fragile X syndrome, a rare condition but the commonest reason for inherited severe learning disability. Of surgical importance is that these patients have very large testes that could present a diagnostic problem unless the condition is recognized.

- red-green colour blindness, which can be of surgical importance when a surgeon is colour blind and is unaware of the fact (red-green colour blindness is statistically commoner in consultant histopathologists than would be expected by chance. This is unexplained).

Abnormalities of chromosome number

Trisomy 21, Down's syndrome

People with Down's syndrome have three copies of chromosome 21 material, rather than the normal two, in all or some cells. This may be as three distinct chromosomes identifiable as 21, or by translocation of the 21 genetic material onto another chromosome. Chromosome banding and other techniques can be used to clarify this. They can develop many diseases of surgical importance. The commonest include:

- increased susceptibility to infections

- increased risk of glue ear

- congenital heart defects: patent ductus arteriosus, ventricular septal defect, and atrial septal defect

- increased risk of neoplasia.

The three main mechanisms in the development of Down's syndrome are non-disjunction, translocation, and mosaicism. Almost all people with Down's syndrome have the syndrome because of non-disjunction. Their cells all have trisomy 21 with three identifiable chromosomes. The extra copy is the result of non-disjunction (failure of separation) of a pair of chromosomes during anaphase. This occurs during a meiotic division in the formation of oocytes or spermatozoa. One daughter cell receives both copies of chromosome 21 and the other none. The gamete with the extra copy therefore has 24 chromosomes rather than the normal 23 and is viable because 21 is very small. The gamete without a copy of chromosome 21 is non-viable. When the gamete with the extra chromosome 21 is fertilized by a normal gamete from the other parent, three copies are present in the resulting ovum. Non-disjunction is commoner in women but may occur in both sexes: the prevalence of children with Down's syndrome is higher when the father as well as the mother is older.

Translocation of chromosome 21 material onto another autosome, such as chromosome 14, accounts for a small proportion of cases (Figure 1.4.1.2). A normal parent can have absence of one chromosome 21 but one elongated chromosome 14 carrying the missing translocated genes. This is called a *balanced translocation*. The gametes of this parent will be of four types:

♦ one normal chromosome 14 and one normal chromosome 21—23 chromosomes altogether and entirely normal

♦ one normal chromosome 14 and no chromosome 21 material—22 chromosomes altogether and non-viable

♦ one abnormal chromosome 14 with 21 translocation and one normal chromosome 21—23 chromosomes but carrying twice the normal amount of chromosome 21 material

♦ one abnormal chromosome 14 with 21 translocation and no chromosome 21— 22 chromosomes altogether but with the normal amount of chromosome 21 material.

One-quarter of the affected parent's gametes will have two copies of the genetic material of chromosome 21 (the third bullet point in the previous list). When this oocyte or spermatozoon joins with a normal complementary gamete from the other parent, an ovum with three copies of chromosome 21 will result. One in three of the surviving gestations will therefore be normal, one will have Down's syndrome, and one a balanced translocation that can transmit Down's syndrome.

About 1 in 100 cases of Down's syndrome are due to mosaicism. The ovum has a normal complement of chromosomes but there is non-disjunction of chromosome 21 after the blastocyst starts to develop. Only a proportion of cells will be affected by the changes caused by mosaicism.

Abnormalities of sex chromosomes

In Turner's syndrome, the genotype is X0 (X zero). The phenotypic effects are numerous but only some are of surgically importance. Those which are include:

♦ coarctation of the aorta

♦ short stature, important in the differential diagnosis of dwarfism syndromes

♦ germ cell tumours in streak ovaries—the malformed ovaries may contain germ cells.

In Kleinfelter's syndrome the genotype is XXY. The Y chromosome with its *SRY* sex determining region induces testicular development and a male phenotype. Very rarely men with Kleinfelter's syndrome are XXXY or XXXXY. Surgically important features include small external genitalia and infertility, and bilateral gynaecomastia with the risk of breast cancer that is the same as that of a woman.

Hermaphroditism and pseudohermaphroditism

True hermaphroditism is when a person has both ovarian and testicular tissue. This may be either together in the same gonad or as a testis and a contralateral ovary. The karyotype is usually XX though a Y chromosome or translocated Y chromosomal material may be found in some patients. When either of these is present there is a higher risk of the patient developing teratoma, dysgerminoma, and other neoplasms.

Pseudohermaphroditism is when the gonads reflect the genotype but the phenotype is mismatched. For example, a boy may have normal chromosomes and testes but ambiguous genitalia because of androgen insensitivity or deficiency in conversion of testosterone to dihydrotestosterone; a chromosomally normal girl may develop ambiguous genitalia from congenital adrenal hyperplasia.

Inflammation

The immune functions of inflammatory cells, related cytokines, and inflammatory mediators are given in the later section on 'Surgical immunology'. The general pathology aspects of acute and chronic inflammation are dealt with here with specific examples.

Acute inflammation

Acute inflammation has the time-honoured Celsian features of pain, heat, redness, and swelling and the addition by Galen of variable loss of function. Some of these may be honoured in the breach rather than the observance. An acutely inflamed appendix is at core temperature and so cannot become hotter, and loss of function of the appendix would be very difficult to determine. Indeed, whether

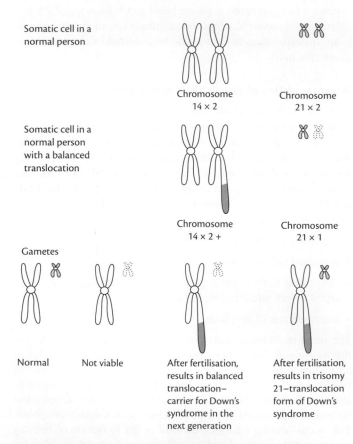

Somatic cell in a normal person

Chromosome 14 × 2   Chromosome 21 × 2

Somatic cell in a normal person with a balanced translocation

Chromosome 14 × 2 +   Chromosome 21 × 1

Gametes

Normal   Not viable   After fertilisation, results in balanced translocation–carrier for Down's syndrome in the next generation   After fertilisation, results in trisomy 21–translocation form of Down's syndrome

Fig. 1.4.1.2 Translocation of chromosome 21.
Reproduced from David Lowe, *Surgical Pathology Revision*, Second Edition, Cambridge University Press, Cambridge, UK, Copyright © 2006. Reprinted with permission.

Galen really did contribute 'functio laesa' or variable loss of function has been questioned.[4] Descriptive terms such as fibrinous, catarrhal, serous, and ulcerative acute inflammation are seldom used nowadays.

In acute inflammation there is a fluid component and a cellular component. The fluid component is characteristically an exudate, but in some specific acute inflammatory conditions such as lobar pneumonia there is an outpouring of fluid from the plasma through endothelial cells that remain intact, a transudate. A transudate characteristically has a protein content of less than 30 g/L and a specific gravity of less than 1.020. This usually forms because of an imbalance between hydrostatic pressures, oncotic pressures, and surrounding tissue pressures resulting in a fluid of low protein content, but can be initiated by inflammation. An exudate is typically formed by an inflammatory process resulting in a fluid of high protein content traversing a damaged endothelial surface. An exudate characteristically has a protein content of more than 30 g/L and a specific gravity of more than 1.020.

Both of these processes but particularly exudation are initiated by macrophages already present at the site of damage (such as by infection, burn, mechanical trauma, foreign bodies, or ionizing radiation) which release inflammatory mediators that have chemotactic effects on granulocytes and other macrophages, vasodilator effects, and stimulatory effects on B lymphocytes to produce immunoglobulins. The cardinal feature of many agents that cause acute inflammation is abscess formation though some, like streptococci, cause spreading infection (cellulitis) without pus formation.

An abscess is a localized tissue collection of pus, characteristically bounded by granulation tissue (the term 'pyogenic membrane' is obsolete). If pus forms in a potential body cavity or hollow viscus like the pleura, gall bladder, or subdural space it is an empyema. Pus is the product of both the exudative and cellular processes of acute inflammation. In inflammation, the exudate consists mostly of water which contains albumin, immunoglobulins, complement components, clotting cascade components, and other inflammatory mediators. If the inflammation is caused by an infective organism, the solid phase would be expected to consist of live and dead bacteria or other microorganisms; human cells which might be alive or dead, including inflammatory cells, epithelial cells and connective tissue cells; and fibrin and neutrophil extracellular trap material.

The natural history of an abscess is to discharge itself. The osmotic pressure in pus constantly increases because albumin and other proteins are broken down by enzymes released by granulocytes and macrophages, and fluid is therefore drawn into the abscess. The pressure increase in time results in discharge of the pus through a line of least resistance—through the skin or mucosa, into a body cavity or hollow viscus, or along fascial lines.

Chronic inflammation

Chronic inflammation is defined as inflammation continuing at the same time as attempts at healing. The tissue changes may be non-specific with a diffuse infiltrate of macrophages, lymphocytes, mast cells and other inflammatory cells, with developing fibrosis, or it may be granulomatous. A granuloma in histological terms is a localized, apparently expansile collection of macrophages (in immunological terms, it is a collection of activated macrophages). Lymphocytes and caseous or other necrosis may be present but are not part of the definition, and the macrophages need not be epithelioid or form giant cells. Collections of macrophages are normal in

the sinuses of reactive lymph nodes ('sinus histiocytosis') but are not expansile.

Granulomatous diseases are classified as caused primarily by inflammation, which may be infective or non-infective, or by a neoplastic process as part of the neoplasm or as a reaction to it. Organisms causing infective granulomas include bacteria such as mycobacteria, *Actinomyces*, and *Treponema*; fungi such as *Aspergillus* and *Mucor*; protozoa such as amoebae and *Leishmania*; and metazoa such as schistosomes and ecchinococci. Non-infective inflammatory granulomas may form around particulate material like beryllium and silica and other inorganic indigestible and foreign materials; they are also features of sarcoidosis, rheumatoid arthritis, and Crohn's disease. A granulomatous response can develop directly around tumour cells, as in seminoma of testis, and severe reactive granulomatous lymphadenitis can be found in axillary lymph nodes of patients with breast carcinoma in the absence of metastatic involvement.[5]

Giant cells can be found in many inflammatory conditions. They are usually formed by fusion of macrophages but lymphocytic and epithelial giant cells can occur. Macrophage giant cells include foreign body multinucleate giant cells in granulomatous reactions around stitch, talc, or other foreign material, which have haphazardly arranged nuclei, and Langhans giant cells in tuberculous infection, Crohn's disease, and sarcoidosis. These have nuclei in a ring or horseshoe and are derived from foreign body giant cells, which reorganize their nuclei if they persist for over a month. Viruses can induce giant cell formation by causing lymphocytes to fuse, as in the Warthin–Finkeldey giant cells of measles, or by infecting epithelial cells and causing nuclear damage with multinucleation as seen in herpes simplex virus and *Cytomegalovirus* (CMV) infections.

Destruction and healing

Cell damage by ionizing radiation

Ionizing radiation can be particulate or electromagnetic (which in current subatomic theory are the same). It supplies enough energy to free an electron from an atom, so making it highly reactive. In some cases a proton can be expelled, which also causes ionization. High-energy radiation such as γ-rays and X-rays are ionizing but even lower-energy, lower-frequency radiation such as radio waves, infrared light, and laser visible light when focused at very high intensity have enough energy to free electrons from tissues. Particles such as α-particles (helium nuclei), β-particles (free electrons), and cosmic rays (which are really particles, mostly free protons) are ionizing—in fact, any charged subatomic particle moving near the speed of light is ionizing.

A cell or tissue exposed to ionizing radiation can be:

♦ unharmed

♦ impaired

  • but able to repair and function normally

  • but unable to function and dies, by necrosis or apoptosis.

A total-body instant dose of 100 000 roentgens (R) results in death within minutes; 10 000 R causes death in hours from central nervous system (CNS) effects; 1000 R causes death in weeks from pancytopenia and gastrointestinal tract (GIT) bleeding. Less than 100 R is not fatal but can cause nausea and vomiting.[6]

In general terms, rapidly dividing cells such as those of the bone marrow, mucosa of the alimentary system, testis and skin (the so-called *labile cells*) are particularly radiosensitive, but other tissues which have few mitoses normally, such as the lens of the eye, the thyroid, and the pituitary, are also relatively sensitive. *Stable cells* divide slowly though the rate increases when there is tissue damage; these include cells in the renal tubules, liver, and fibrous connective tissue. They are less sensitive to the direct effects of ionizing radiation but can suffer from ischaemia or infarction if the radiation damages the tissues' endothelial cells and causes thrombosis. *Permanent cells* have very limited capacity to divide after the very early postnatal period, and include muscle cells and neurons in the CNS and retina. They are the least radiosensitive but can also suffer because of radiation-induced thrombosis.

Diagnostic and therapeutic radiation in surgical practice

The *absorbed dose* is a measure of the likelihood that biochemical changes will be induced in different tissues by ionizing radiation. It is expressed in milligrays (mGy), which is the energy absorbed by a given mass of tissue. One Gy equals 100 rads.

The *equivalent dose*, expressed in millisieverts (mSv), is a measurement of the extent of tissue and cell damage predicted from the absorbed dose, and so considers the type of ionizing radiation used—for a given absorbed dose, different types and frequencies of ionizing radiation have different effects and so are given a different weighting factor. For diagnostic procedures the radiation used has only a small chance of harming the tissues, and the absorbed dose is numerically identical to the equivalent dose. One Sv equals 100 rem.

The *effective dose* is a measure of long-term effects that might arise, and is also expressed in mSv. It is calculated from data on the tissue type, the absorbed dose, and the sensitivity of each tissue to the effects of the radiation.

Free radicals

Free radicals are induced by the energy contributed by ionizing radiation and heat. A free radical is an atom, ion, or molecule that has unpaired electrons or an open electron shell. They are highly reactive, able to damage normal cell components, and also react with each other to form polymers or modified monomers. Free radicals mostly comprise the reactive oxygen species, reactive nitrogen species, hydrogen free radicals, and carbon free radicals which may be alkyl or aryl. They occur normally inside mitochondria and other cellular organelles.[7]

Oxygen free radicals include superoxide $O_2\bullet$ (an O_2 molecule with a missing electron) and peroxides. They are a product of normal cellular metabolism and have an essential function in cell-to-cell signalling, apoptosis, and in the killing of microorganisms. Macrophages in particular make large amounts of superoxide with NADPH oxidase, used internally to kill bacteria and fungi in phagosomes. Superoxide reacts physiologically with nitric oxide in blood vessels and elsewhere to limit its effects on smooth muscle tone and blood pressure. In animal species, free radicals are used for defence and procreation. The bombardier beetle uses the energy from the peroxide reaction to fire boiling liquid at its attacker. In the firefly, a similar reaction provides energy for photoluminescence which in firefly larvae is a defence mechanism and in firefly adults attracts a mate.

Overproduction of free radicals results in damage to:

◆ DNA and RNA: there is abnormal cross-linking of DNA with formation of thymidine–thymidine (TT) dimers, there may be base deletions that make nonsense or harmful sequences, and there may be chain breaks that can be misrepaired to form translocations. If the damage is relatively mild and non-fatal these errors may be replicated in daughter cells and exacerbated by further radiation exposure. Damage to RNA is less harmful as messenger RNA is evanescent but there may be sufficient damage to microsomes to cause cell death

◆ proteins

◆ lipids

◆ enzymes.

Because of this damage, aerobic organisms including human beings require scavenging mechanisms to destroy excess free radicals. These mechanisms may be intrinsic or extrinsic. Intrinsic protection against free radicals is important in plasma and includes molecules of superoxide dismutase, catalase, glutathione peroxidase, and uric acid. Extrinsic factors include vitamins C and E.

Embolus

An embolus is an abnormal mass of undissolved material that is carried in the bloodstream from one place to another. There is no requirement for an embolus to have the capacity to impact: impaction is usual but not essential to the definition.[8]

Most emboli, about 95%, consist of thrombus, clot, or a mixture of both. When a thrombus occludes a vein such as a deep vein of the leg, the blood flow stops and a clot forms in the column of blood proximal to the thrombus, as far as the next communicating vein (the *propagated clot*). Clot retraction (because of platelet contractile filaments) occurs with shrinkage from the endothelium of the vein, so that dislodgement can result in separation. Some of the thrombus would be attached to the clot and so the resulting embolus would be of mixed thrombus and clot.[8]

Others materials that can embolize include:

◆ fat usually from fractured long bones in adults; rare causes of fat embolus include severe burns or soft tissue injuries

◆ bone marrow from fractured long bones in children

◆ malignant tumour cells[9]

◆ lipid material from aortic atheroma

◆ gas, which might be:
  • air from intravenous cannulae, neck veins disrupted by trauma or operative surgery, or dialysis
  • carbon dioxide from fallopian tube or peritoneal insufflation
  • nitrogen in caisson disease

◆ amniotic fluid usually during parturition, which can cause disseminated intravascular coagulopathy (DIC)

◆ microorganisms such as thrombus containing bacteria in infective endocarditis, and metazoa such as schistosomes. In cadavers, diatoms can be found in the bone marrow which have embolized from the lungs to the marrow, evidence of death by inhalation of water from streams and other natural water masses

◆ foreign materials such as talc or chalk in intravenous drug abusers and plastics from medical interventions

- normal cells: adrenal cortical cells pass through the wall of the adrenal vein into the circulation, and trophoblast cells can embolize to the mother's lungs in a normal pregnancy.

The consequences of embolization are dealt with in Chapter 5.7.

Ischaemia and infarction

Ischaemia (Greek *iskaimos*, stanching or stopping blood) is an abnormal reduction of the blood supply to or drainage from an organ or tissue. Infarction (Latin *farcire*, to stuff) is the result of cessation of the blood supply to or drainage from an organ or tissue. Both may have local causes, general causes, or both.

Local causes of ischaemia include:

- arterial obstruction by atheroma, thrombus, embolus, pressure from outside, and spasm
- venous obstruction by thrombus, pressure from mechanical abnormalities (such as strangulation of hernia, torsion, or intussusception), and effective obstruction by stasis from varicose veins
- capillary obstruction
- vasculitis from any cause
- small vessel obstruction in caisson disease with nitrogen bubbles, cryoglobulinaemia, sickle cell disease, and frostbite, and from external pressures such as in decubitus ulcers.

General causes include:

- hypoxaemia: decreased cardiac output as a consequence of myocardial ischaemia, infarction, or heart block
- anaemia.

The extent of ischaemic damage in arterial obstruction depends on the tissues involved and their sensitivity to hypoxia, and is in proportion to the:

- speed of onset
- degree of obstruction of the arterial lumen
- presence of collaterals and of disease in them
- level of oxygenation of the blood supplying the ischaemic tissue
- presence of concomitant heart failure
- state of the microcirculation of the tissue, as in diabetes mellitus.

Infarcts are classified as pale and dark (or white and red, which equate). In venous infarcts, the outflow of blood is obstructed and the reason for the tissues becoming hyperaemic is obvious. If the infarcted tissue is not constrained within a restricted space or by a capsule, the volume can increase to accommodate the inflow of blood. This occurs in the small and large bowel and produces dark or red infarcts. In arterial infarcts, the ischaemia caused by cessation of the incoming blood produces severe tissue hypoxia and vasodilatation of the draining capillaries and veins, permitting backflow of blood into the affected area. If the organ has a fibrous capsule such as the kidney or spleen, the volume cannot change and so the pressure must increase. This local increase in pressure pushes the capsule outwards slightly and forces blood out of the area. The infarct is therefore pale or white with a hyperaemic rim of surviving non-infarcted tissue at the edges; the shape is characteristically triangular on cross-section because of the area of supply of the obstructed artery.

Necrosis

Necrosis is abnormal tissue death during life. It is energy independent, associated with inflammatory changes, and usually results from factors outside the affected cells. The three classical types are coagulative or structured necrosis, colliquative or liquefactive necrosis, and caseous or unstructured necrosis.

In coagulative necrosis, the tissue architecture is preserved, as seen when a tissue is put into boiling water: the proteins coagulate rapidly from the heat, the reticulin framework of the tissue is kept intact, and the architecture is maintained as a consequence. Structured necrosis is seen in kidney, heart, and spleen and can be easily recognized microscopically—the normal tissue components are present but the nuclei of the necrotic cells undergo pyknosis (condensation and shrinkage), karyorrhexis (fragmentation), and karyolysis (dispersal of chromatin) and so disappear.

Colliquative or liquefactive necrosis occurs in the CNS in tissues with cytoplasmic membranes rich in lipid. Enzymes from macrophages and microglia ingest the lipid along with haemosiderin and lipofuscin, and remove it. A cystic space containing liquid derived from plasma results. Colliquative necrosis may also be found in the lung after suppurative inflammation with infection has been overcome by large numbers of polymorphs.

Caseous necrosis is unstructured. It differs histologically from coagulative necrosis as it is impossible to identify the tissue affected by the necrosis because its architecture is destroyed; it differs from colliquative necrosis as necrotic cells and cell debris (from macrophages and mycobacteria, typically) remain. This type of necrosis is classical for mycobacterial infection but may also be found in florid fungal granulomas.

Specific tissue types of necrosis include:

- fat necrosis, which may result from the chemical changes of high plasma concentrations of lipase and amylase on adipose tissue, for example, in the skin. There is no significant inflammatory reaction but because of the change in pH of the tissues, dystrophic calcification can occur. In traumatic fat necrosis, such as in the breast, there is a chronic inflammatory reaction with foreign-body giant cell formation and phagocytosis of extracellular lipid
- dry gangrene is desiccation (mummification) of a tissue without infection, such as can occur in an extremity of a diabetic patient
- wet gangrene is necrosis in which there is infection and digestion by enzymes from the microorganisms and from polymorphs.

Autolysis, homolysis, and heterolysis

Autolysis is the degradation of a cell by activation of enzymes present in the affected cell (self-digestion). Autolysis occurs in the processes of necrosis and apoptosis, and is found at autopsy. Homolysis is degradation of a cell by other cells of the same or similar type: for example, digestion of pancreatic exocrine cells by proteases and lipases from adjacent damaged exocrine cells, or digestion of macrophages by enzymes from other macrophages. Heterolysis is degradation of a cell by enzymes from a different cell line, such as digestion of epithelial cells by enzymes from neutrophils and macrophages in inflammation.

Malnutrition

Malnutrition is the failure to achieve proper nutrition. This failure may be due to undernutrition or overnutrition, obesity being the commonest type of malnutrition in the Western world.

Classification of malnutrition

Undernutrition may be classified as cases that result from inadequate availability of food or from inability to digest and absorb food and its components. Too little food results in starvation, called marasmus (Greek *marasmus*, to wither or waste away) in some parts of the world. Too little protein in food causes protein-energy malnutrition, called kwashiorkor (Ghanaian *kwasioko*, given as 'the jealous one') in parts of Africa—the name derives from malnutrition in a young child who must be weaned from the breast when the next baby arrives.

Vitamin deficiency in starvation manifests as lack of water-soluble vitamins such as the vitamin B series (except vitamin B_{12}), folate, and vitamin C as body stores are small. Large quantities of the fat-soluble vitamins (vitamins A, D, E, and K) and of vitamin B_{12} are stored in the liver and take years to become depleted. Iron, iodine, and trace metals eventually become depleted. All of these have severe implications for wound healing and infection risk.

Food might be available but the patient is unable to utilize it adequately. This might be because of chronic disease of the alimentary system such as malabsorption, increased intestinal transit time, and infections; from chronic renal failure, from malignancy, and other diseases that cause anorexia; and from drug addiction. In a small number of cases food may be plentiful but the lifestyle choice of people not to eat certain components of food leave them open to undernutrition.

Overnutrition may be classified as being from too much food of all kinds, too much specific ingestion of fats or vitamins, too little exercise, and peculiar diets. Vitamins that are toxic in high quantities (such as may be ingested in tablet form by compulsive health-driven people) include vitamin A, niacin (vitamin B_3), pyridoxine (vitamin B_6), and vitamin D. Obesity is defined as a body mass index (BMI) of 30 kg/m^2 or above, and morbid obesity as a BMI of 40 kg/m^2 or above.

Risk of malnutrition

People who are at risk of malnutrition can be classified by age group, the presence of relevant acquired diseases, and people living in certain social conditions. In relation to age groups:

- neonates may have vitamin K deficiency, and vitamin B_{12} deficiency may develop in breastfed babies of vegans

- children on an inadequate diet may develop folate, vitamin A, vitamin C, iron, copper, and zinc deficiencies

- pregnant and lactating women may become folate deficient if not supplemented, and if there is excessive alcohol intake may develop magnesium, zinc, and thiamine (vitamin B_1) deficiencies

- the elderly may develop osteoporosis from relative calcium deficiency and lack of exercise; osteomalacia from lack of sunlight exposure and dietary deficiency of vitamin D; and iron deficiency from an inadequate intake possibly related to poverty.

Patients of any age with chronic diseases:

- patients with potential or chronic diseases from living in areas of famine or extreme poverty

- patients who have had gastrectomy or excision of the terminal ileum and related operations

- patients with AIDS

- patients with drug dependencies including alcohol.

People on unusual diets:

- vegetarians may develop iron deficiency

- vegans may develop vitamin B_{12} deficiency and calcium, iron, and zinc intake tend to be low

- people on very low-calorie diets

- people in societies in which excessive consumption is usual.

Overnutrition is of surgical importance because obese patients may suffer dehiscence of abdominal wounds, ventral herniation, and deep vein thrombosis. They are also at increased risk of impaired respiratory function because of forced elevation of the diaphragm from the upwards force of the abdominal contents.

Undernutrition can lead to poor wound healing, iron and megaloblastic anaemias and impaired immunity with a tendency to pulmonary and other infections. The hypoproteinaemia and risk of infection also contribute to ascites.[10]

Healing by resolution and repair

Resolution is the process of healing by replacement of dead or damaged tissue by the functional tissue normally found at that site. It occurs especially in *partial* thickness loss of an epithelium (an erosion, see 'Erosion and ulceration') and in bone marrow. There is no (or almost no) fibrosis in resolution. Repair is the process of healing by replacement of dead or damaged tissue by collagen or glial fibres which completely or partially fill the defect but have no specialized function. Repair occurs where there is *full* thickness loss of an epithelial surface (an ulcer, see 'Erosion and ulceration'), and in solid organs such as the liver when the capacity for resolution is exceeded.

Fibrosis is the general repair process in the body, in which tropocollagen is secreted by fibroblasts and polymerizes into a linear structure with a repeat offset of three tropocollagen molecules to form collagen. Collagen then contracts to reduce the damaged area. Contraction usually is biologically beneficial but can result in gross scarring, distortion of skin and joints, arthrodesis, and disfigurement.[11]

Gliosis occurs in the CNS. Astrocytes (Greek *astron*, a star) are the principal source of glial fibrillary acidic protein (Greek *glia*, glue) that supports the cytoskeleton of astrocytes as they elongate and complicate their pseudopodia to form a network that fills in the potential space of degenerating neurons. The benefit of gliosis over fibrosis is that gliosis does not contract; fibrosis in the CNS would cause distortion and possibly epileptogenic foci and blockage of cerebrospinal fluid (CSF) flow.

Erosion and ulceration

An erosion is a partial loss of an epithelial surface which heals by resolution. By definition, an erosion can occur only in a stratified epithelium—simple squamous or columnar epithelial can undergo only ulceration. An ulcer is a full-thickness loss of epithelium which heals by repair; there may be resolution as well, or not.

Causes of both include inflammation from an extrinsic agent such as aspirin and other drugs; physical damage from oesophagogastroduodenoscopy, colonoscopy, and radiotherapy; and external pressure as in decubitus ulcers. Intrinsic causes include peptic acid imbalance; infections such as schistosomiasis and amoebiasis; idiopathic inflammatory conditions such as ulcerative colitis and Crohn's disease; ischaemia; and the development of neoplasia.

The rate of healing of an erosion and an ulcer is influenced by the persistence of the causative agent. There may be infection of the ulcerated site secondarily, such as with skin ulcers; complications of ulceration, such as peritonitis and pancreatitis; development of carcinoma in the ulcer, especially in chronic ulcers; immunosuppression from any cause, such as diabetes mellitus, viral infections, and malignancy; and malnutrition.

Organization, granulation tissue, and wound healing

Organization is the process by which material such as clot, thrombus, or pus is transformed into organic, living tissue. Replacement of the inanimate material is characteristically by granulation tissue, which is unspecialized but responsive to the growth control factors of the body. Granulation tissue has three components: proliferating capillary buds, fibroblasts, and macrophages. It is an important part of healing but has little protection against chemical injury or physical damage by trauma or ionizing radiation; it is, though, very resistant to infection. There can be deleterious effects when granulation tissue persists chronically because of the lytic enzymes secreted by macrophages, which can cause joint damage in patients such as those with rheumatoid arthritis. Granulation tissue characteristically lines sinuses and fistulas.

Sinuses and fistulas

A pathological sinus (Latin *sinus*, a hole or bay) is a passage from a focus of inflammation (usually caused by infection, though sometimes by neoplasia or trama) in deep tissues. This is to an epithelial surface. Examples include a skin sinus in chronic osteomyelitis and a pilonidal sinus. Sinuses are usually lined by granulation tissue but can become lined by squamous cell carcinoma (SCC), as in a Marjolin's ulcer in osteomyelitis.

A fistula is an abnormal communication between two epithelial surfaces, also usually lined by granulation tissue. The definition of an epithelial surface in this definition subsumes mesothelial and endothelial surfaces. The length of the fistula is immaterial: there are very short anal fistulas and long gastroenteric fistulas. Examples include anorectal fistulas, enteroenteric fistulas between two parts of the small bowel, enterocolic, enterovesical, enterocutaneous, and gastroenteric fistulas. Fistulas are caused by:

- inflammatory conditions such as Crohn's disease and diverticulitis
- necrosis in a carcinoma that has grown between two epithelial surfaces, such as the vagina and rectum or trachea and oesophagus, or by a sarcoma that has bridged two epithelial surfaces such the pleura and lung
- iatrogenic interventions, such as operative surgery, radiotherapy, and insertion of venous lines. Fistulas are abnormal but not necessarily undesirable—arteriovenous fistula, colostomy, ileostomy, and tracheostomy can be therapeutic.

Factors that determine the rate of healing of a sinus or fistula can be local and systemic. Local factors include:

- continuation of the causative event, such as osteomyelitis or malignancy
- the presence of foreign material
- the presence of infection

- passage of material through the track such as bowel contents or pus
- the width of the track
- reduced local blood supply or drainage
- epithelialization of the track
- malignant change.

Systemic factors that have a bearing on healing include the general state of nutrition of the patient and whether there is immunosuppression, diabetes mellitus, vitamin deficiency, or radiotherapy damage.

Ascites

Ascites (Greek *askos*, a bag) is the accumulation of an abnormal amount of free fluid in the peritoneal cavity. This can be an exudate, which is almost always inflammatory to some extent, or a transudate. Inflammatory causes of protein leakage include peritonitis, pancreatitis, widespread carcinoma, and uraemia. A transudate can be caused by hypoproteinaemia from starvation, nephrotic syndrome, liver failure, and protein-losing enteropathy. It can also be the result of hydrostatic changes from right heart failure, cirrhosis, Budd–Chiari syndrome, and thoracic duct obstruction. Metabolic changes such as secondary hyperaldosteronism in liver failure and hypothyroidism can also contribute.

Investigations helpful in determining the cause of the ascites include microbiology for microscopy for bacteria, and culture and sensitivity; cytology examination for red cells, white cells, and malignant cells that might be carcinoma or lymphoma; and biochemistry for protein content and amylase.

First- and second-intention wound healing

First-intention wound healing refers to the repair process in clean wounds without tissue loss that can be repaired by suturing and heal well classically with only small amounts of fibrosis. Healing by second intention usually involves tissue loss or wounds that have intentionally been left open because of infection. The granulation tissue that forms to fill the defect will heal by fibrosis, but this can be considerable and result in contractures and cosmetic problems.

Taking a skin wound as an example, the stages of healing begin with clot formation. If there is healing by first intention, squamous cells from the wound edges migrate by amoeboid movement to cover the clot. Keratinocytes in damaged skin have surface integrins that are not present in intact skin; these bind to fibronectin, which facilitates migration. In the dermis there is an infiltrate of inflammatory cells, first polymorphs and then macrophages, which secrete chemokines and phagocytose debris. Fibroblasts secrete tropocollagen which polymerizes into collagen and restores tensile strength (in tissues other than skin, this varies from weak to almost normal tissue strength). At the same time there is vascularization of the scar and gradual contraction of myofibroblasts to reduce its size.

There are several cytokine and growth factor systems involved in wound healing. Cytokines include modulators of macrophages and lymphocytes, interferons, and interleukins. Growth factors include:

- epidermal growth factor (EGF) which accelerates the rate of epidermal and dermal regeneration. This family of molecules is found in external secretions such as saliva and tears, internal secretions in the upper GIT, and in platelet granules. Transforming growth factor alpha is part of the EGF family

• platelet-derived growth factor (PDGF) which has a significant role in angiogenesis; vascular endothelial growth factor is part of the PDGF family

• transforming growth factor beta, which controls proliferation and differentiation of most cells and acts as a chemoattractant.

Classification of wounds in relation to surgical site contamination

Clean wounds

Clean surgical wounds have no significant signs of inflammation and do not breach the mucosae of the respiratory, gastrointestinal, or urogenital tracts. Thyroid and breast operations, elective orthopaedic surgery, and vascular surgery operations would be considered clean. This does not mean that prophylactic antibiotics are inappropriate—in the last two cases prophylaxis is important as the consequences of infection would be severe.

Clean contaminated wounds

These are clean wounds that have a greater risk of infection. Wounds that breach the lumen of the respiratory, gastrointestinal, or urogenital tracts (including gynaecological operations) are considered to be clean contaminated. Prophylactic antibiotics are appropriate.

Contaminated wounds

Wounds are considered to be contaminated if there is spillage of GIT contents (especially of the large bowel) into the site; when there are inflamed or infected tissues around the operative site; or when there has been a penetrating injury to the body. Prophylactic antibiotics are inappropriate as therapeutic antibiotics should be given.

Dirty wounds

Dirty surgical wounds are those with pus or faecal material, traumatic wounds when treatment is delayed, and wounds in which a foreign body is present. Therapeutic antibiotics are given.

Scars

A scar results from healing by repair in which there is deposition of fibrous tissue or in the CNS, glial tissue. Scars are generally more florid in young adults; the elderly form scars that have less fibrosis but heal at the same rate as young people. The person's skin type is related to the degree of scarring—those with skin types IV and VI with darker pigmentation tend to have more florid scars. Scarring is often worse over the deltoid and sternal areas, whereas in the conjunctivae and oral tissues can be minimal.

Classification of scars

Typical scar

A typical scar is the type most often encountered after elective abdominal, orthopaedic, thoracic, and skin operations. The healing is by first intention and the scar is clearly visible as a thin red line which fades to white.

Minimal scar

A minimal scar is the result of meticulous apposition of the wound edges, aimed for by reconstructive and aesthetic surgeons. The scar is visible as a faint line which may become unapparent with time.

Wide scar

Widening or sideways stretching of a scar can occur over joints such as the knee and shoulder. It begins about a month after operation, when the scar becomes increasingly pale and thin. Wide scars are usually asymptomatic but are cosmetically undesirable.

Atrophic scar

An atrophic scar is usually small, flat and depressed. They are commonly seen after chicken pox and scarring acne.

Hypertrophic scar

A hypertrophic scar is raised but remains within the boundaries of the scar before the growth excess (which is in fact hyperplasia rather than hypertrophy) occurs. They can be inflamed, itchy, and painful but often regress spontaneously. Intralesional injection of corticosteroid can speed regression.

Keloid scar

A keloid scar (Greek *chele*, like a crab's claw) is raised like a hypertrophic scar but extends beyond the margins of the original scar before the development of keloid change. Keloid scars can affect any site but are found especially on the central sternal area ('necklace area'), over the deltoids, and on the ear lobes after piercings. They continue to grow slowly and rarely regress spontaneously. Treatment is difficult; intralesional cortisone injections are usually ineffective and simple excision is followed by recurrence.

Scar contracture

A distorted or contracted scar classically crosses a skin crease or joint at right angles. They are usually hypertrophic and disabling or dysfunctional. Burns involving joints commonly heal with some degree of contracture.

Predictors of abnormally severe scarring

These include aspects relating to severity, site, and predisposition:

• severe symptoms

• large amount of tissue loss

• large size of scar

• continuing inflammation

• poor response to treatment

• scars in specific anatomical locations, as above

• positive family history of severe scarring

• previous abnormal scarring in the same or other sites.

Complications of skin scars

Scars may be unsightly and be the root of psychosocial problems, and can cause physical symptoms and signs:

• tenderness, pain, and pruritus (with or without formation of a traumatic neuroma)

• physical deformities

• compression of nerves and vessels

• problems of anxiety and depression with sleep disturbance, loss of self-esteem, and post-traumatic stress.

Surgical immunology

Immunology is an essential study for surgeons. Changes in our knowledge of immunology happen weekly. The classical division into humoral and cellular events broadly still holds.[12]

The complement system

The complement cascade starts with cleavage of the C3 component by several mechanisms, including C2b4b complex, antigen/antibody complexes, plasmin, microbial membranes, and polysaccharides. C3 is the most abundant of the complement components in plasma. C3a is an anaphylatoxin and to some extent a chemotactic factor (though not as active as C5a). C3a is further split into more fragments which activate B lymphocytes. C3b is an opsonin and, with C2b4b complex, splits C5 into its components.

Component C5a is an anaphylatoxin, is a strong chemotactic factor, and activates macrophages to secrete interleukin (IL)-5 which is also chemotactic. C5b joins with and anchors C6, C7, C8, and C9 to make the final large component that causes membrane damage; components C7, C8, and C9 have hydrophobic sites that breach the cell membrane, and C9 polymerizes around the hole to keep it open.

Bacterial cells are prokaryotes without a defined nucleus, and so they have very little capacity to repair membrane damage. A single hole results in the death of the bacterium because the osmotic pressure within draws in extracellular fluid which disrupts the bacterial wall. Human cells damaged by complement have much more likelihood of survival as their nuclei can generate more membrane proteins and so they can repair holes quickly.

Immunoglobulins

There are five classes of immunoglobulins: IgG, IgA, IgM, IgD, and IgE in order of abundance in plasma. Each has a basic unit of two light chains and two heavy chains. The two light chain are identical to each other, as are the two heavy chains; both chains have variable regions of the same size and constant regions of different sizes. Two or more of these basic units can be linked to form IgA and IgM molecules. The light chains are lambda and mu chains, shared among all of the five classes, and so are not defining. The heavy chains are specific for the classes. The binding sites are clonal and highly specific for one or more sites on the stimulatory antigen. The heavy chains forming the stem of the Y structure have binding sites for complement, and on IgG have sites for placental transfer. Both of these function only when the antigen-binding sites on the arms of the Y are occupied.

IgG is the most prevalent immunoglobulin, found in the plasma (75–80% of all immunoglobulins) and the tissues. It is composed of one basic Y unit. Its main functions are opsonization and complement activation—macrophages, polymorphs, and some lymphocytes can internalize IgG and so it can act as an opsonin. Cross-linkage of IgG molecules with precipitation is unusual. There is a rise in IgG in all infections in non-compromised patients, in rheumatoid arthritis, and in IgG myeloma.

IgA accounts for about 10% of plasma immunoglobulin. In the plasma, the molecule is a monomer, and only after attachment of the J chain does it dimerize. IgA is produced by plasma cells in the lamina propria of mucosae and elsewhere adjacent to other surfaces. It binds to Ig receptors on the basement membrane aspect of epithelial cells and is taken inside them by endocytosis. The J chain

is also made in plasma cells and links two monomers of IgA to form the typical dimer. The secretory component is synthetized by epithelial cells in the mucosa and it is this extra chain which permits transport through the epithelium. It also confers some resistance to degradation by enzymes in mucus, tears, colostrum, saliva, and other secretions. IgA does not fix complement unless it is aggregated. It can also bind to polymorphs and some lymphocytes, and there are increased plasma concentrations in chronic infection, cirrhosis, rheumatoid arthritis, and IgA myeloma.

The pentamer IgM is the largest immunoglobulin. It is the immunoglobulin that rises quickest after an antigen challenge, and so can be used to monitor the acute phase of a disease. In the fetus, IgM is the first immunoglobulin to be made and also the first synthesized when a B lymphocyte is stimulated by an antigen to become a plasma cell. The five-unit structure cross-links between antigens and between other IgM molecules to form large polymers that do not enter tissues well. The pentamer itself is not a good opsonin, though it is good at fixing complement which acts as an opsonin. IgM increased in infections including malaria, in rheumatoid arthritis, and in Waldenström's macroglobulinaemia. IgM myeloma accounts for only 0.5% of myeloma types.

IgD levels are increased in chronic infections and IgD myeloma, which accounts for 2% of all myeloma types. The precise function of IgD is unknown.

Mast cells carry monomeric IgE molecules on their surfaces attached by their heavy chains. When two or more IgE units are cross-linked by a suitable antigen, the mast cell is triggered to degranulate; attachment to only one IgE does not trigger histamine, bradykinin, and heparin release. Degranulation of mast cells occurs principally in type I hypersensitivity reactions and results in atopy, asthma, and anaphylactic shock. IgE is the rarest type of myeloma.

Lymphocytes

Helper T cells are CD4 positive and bind to major histocompatibility complex (MHC) class II sites principally on macrophages and B cells. They are the most important cells in adaptive immunity. They secrete cytokines that help to change B cells into memory B cells and mature into plasma cells, and they modulate the activity of cytotoxic T cells and macrophages. Helper T cells are activated by antigen-presenting cells like macrophages and dendritic cells.

Cytotoxic T cells are CD8 positive; they bind to MHC class I targets on all nucleated cells, and are able to destroy virus infected cells and some tumour cells. The cytotoxic T cell binds to an infected cell, bores a microscopic hole in the membrane with the enzyme perforin, and injects enzymes from its cytoplasmic granules, the so-called granzymes. These damage mitochondria and other structures in the infected cell and activate that cell's own cytoplasmic enzymes, which then break down DNA and induce apoptosis.

There are three other T cells of particular significance. Memory T cells can be CD4 or CD8 positive and multiply on contact only with recognized antigens. Regulatory T cells, which were called suppressor T cells, are CD4 positive; they inhibit T-cell function at the end of an immune reaction. Natural killer T cells recognize abnormal glycolipid moieties on cells which are seen as antigenic without previous sensitization. They secrete interferon gamma, IL-4, and other interleukins, and tumour necrosis factor alpha (TNF-α), all of which contribute to tumour cell lysis.

Natural killer cells are also part of the innate system but have no T-cell or B-cell markers. They have cytoplasmic granules containing enzymes which make holes in the target cell as do the cytotoxic T cells of the adaptive immune system; natural killer cells can develop adaptive memory in some conditions.

Except for one notable exception, T cells are unable to recognize antigens unless they are presented by another cell type, such as macrophages, dendritic cells, and B lymphocytes. The exception is the so-called superantigen family, produced by viruses, bacteria, and other organisms. Superantigens induce polyclonal T-lymphocyte proliferation and release of large quantities of cytokines which activate macrophages. These produce their own range of cytokines including TNF-α which, at the very high levels involved, can result in shock and multiple organ failure.

Cytokines

Cytokines are signalling molecules that modulate the humoral immune response (such as several of the interleukins) or the cellular immune response (tumour growth factor beta and interferon gamma), or both. They are small proteins soluble in plasma and interstitial fluid. Their effects are to stimulate proliferation of inflammatory cells, to make them secrete their own range of cytokines, They also stimulate growth of epithelial cells (as does insulin-like growth factor 1, which can lead to colonic carcinoma in patients with acromegaly) and cause the liver to secrete acute phase proteins such as C-reactive protein and serum amyloid A (SAA) protein (principally by IL-1 and IL-6 from macrophages). Chemokines are cytokines that are chemotactic.

Acute phase proteins

Acute phase proteins modulate the inflammatory response. C-reactive protein and SAA protein are opsonins; ferritin, haptoglobin, and caeruloplasmin sequestrate iron and prevent its use by microorganisms. C-reactive protein was named for its reaction with the C polysaccharide of the wall of *Streptococcus pneumoniae*.

Macrophages

Macrophage is the generic term for the group of large phagocytic cells that have a part in the innate and adaptive immune systems. The term includes the monocytes in the blood, histiocytes found in almost all tissues, microglia in the CNS, Kupffer cells in the liver, and osteoclasts in bone. Macrophage have several functions, including migration, phagocytosis, digestion, antigen presentation, fusion to form multinucleate giant cells, metabolism of vitamin D, and secretion.

Macrophage functions include:

- migration in response to cytokines
- phagocytosis assisted by opsonization by immunoglobulins, complement, and acute phase proteins
- destruction of microorganisms and digestion by enzymes and peroxides ('respiratory burst')
- multinucleate giant cell formation if the antigen is a particle too large for one macrophage to engulf or if it is indigestible
- antigen presentation to other cells in the immune system, predominantly helper T cells
- secretion of interleukins, prostaglandins, leukotrienes, transforming growth factors, and tumour necrosis factors
- metabolism of vitamin D.

Polymorphonuclear leucocytes or granulocyte

Granulocytes are formed from bone marrow stem cells which differentiate into myeloid-erythroid progenitor cells and common lymphoid progenitor cells. The first differentiate further into myeloblast, megakaryocyte, and erythrocyte precursor cell lines. The myeloblasts mature by two main sequences: granulocyte-precursor maturation into mature neutrophils, basophils, and eosinophils; and monocyte-precursors which mature into macrophages and dendritic cells.

Neutrophils

Neutrophils are found in blood and tissues. They account for about 60% of white cells in the circulation, about 5×10^9 neutrophils/L of whole blood. They have a life of 5–6 days, and once neutrophils leave the circulation they do not return. They are larger than red cells at about 12 μm in diameter (a red cell is 7 μm in diameter) and have polylobate nuclei with three to five segments. The number of lobes increases with the age of the cell and becomes particularly high in vitamin B_{12} deficiency.

Neutrophils are primarily phagocytic, especially of opsonized bacteria and other antigens. They secrete proteins that recruit macrophages and others that kill bacteria by damaging their cell walls directly and by creating free radicals around the organisms. A recently discovered further function is that neutrophils, when they die, release DNA and proteases that trap and kill bacteria in blood vessels without phagocytosis, so-called neutrophil extracellular traps (NETs).

Neutrophils and endothelial cells have been known to interact for some time. Adhesion molecules that bind to neutrophils are present on endothelial cell membranes, and the endothelial filamentous protein actin controls diapedesis. Intercellular adhesion molecules and vascular cell adhesion molecules on endothelium and in vascular smooth muscle have been correlated with the possible damage caused by neutrophils in atheroma and transplant vasculopathy. After margination and attachment, neutrophils take about 30 minutes to push through gaps between endothelial cells, force them apart, and move through the thixotropic basement membrane collagen (a thixotropic material behaves as a solid at rest but as a liquid when moved, like some non-drip paints). They then connect with smooth muscle cells in the vessel wall, move into the extracellular matrix and follow chemotactic signals to the specific site of injury.

Eosinophils

Eosinophils account for about 7% of granulocytes in the blood. Their main function is secretory rather than phagocytic, especially attacking metazoan parasites such as helminths (Greek *helmins*, an intestinal worm). These include nematodes, cestodes, and trematodes such as schistosomes. The secretory granules are strongly eosinophilic, and contain major basic protein, eosinophil cationic protein, and eosinophil-derived neurotoxin. These kill parasites and also induce apoptosis in human cells—there is evidence that malignant tumours with a dense tissue infiltration of eosinophils have a better prognosis than those without. Eosinophils are also antigen-presenting cells and interact with T-helper lymphocytes, B lymphocytes, and other granulocytes; for example, basophils secrete IL-5 which stimulates eosinophil growth and development.

Basophils

Basophils form about 0.1% of circulating granulocytes; the circulating numbers are increased in asthma and other allergies, lymphomas and leukaemias, haemolytic anaemia, Crohn's disease, and hypothyroidism. Activation can be by surface IgE binding to antigen and by complement component C5a. Basophil granules release histamine, heparin, and chondroitin, and proteolytic enzymes such as lipases and elastase. Basophils also secrete lipid mediators like leukotrienes, and several cytokines including IL-4, important in the development of allergies.

Hypersensitivity reactions

Hypersensitivity is generally classified into type I–IV hypersensitivity reactions. Autoimmune interactions against aspects of the cell membrane specifically, such as against hormone and other receptors, have been put into a separate category, type V. These receptors can be stimulated because the antibody mimics the effects of the hormone cognate with the receptor, or they can be blocked because the binding of a ligand is prevented. Examples include Graves' disease and myasthenia gravis respectively. Many people regard this cell membrane effect to be encompassed by type II hypersensitivity rather than being a separate type of its own, though there is no defined cytotoxic effect as in classical type II.

Type I hypersensitivity begins with linkage of two IgE molecules on a mast cell by an antigen, which results in arachidonic acid breakdown products being formed. Prostaglandins and leukotrienes cause release of mast cell contents such as 5-hydroxytryptamine, histamine, heparin, and chemokines from eosinophils. Diseases from this type of hypersensitivity include asthma, allergic rhinitis, atopic eczema, and gastrointestinal effects such as eosinophilic gastroenteropathy in which there is dysphagia, abnormal motility, and abdominal pain.

In a type II hypersensitivity reaction, an abnormal antibody is stimulated to a normal tissue component. This can happen spontaneously or via a hapten. A hapten (Greek *apteo*, to fasten) is a small molecule that is not intrinsically antigenic but that can react with, usually, a larger molecule such as a protein. This protein would not itself normally stimulate antibodies but the attachment to it of a hapten increases its antigenicity several-fold. The enhanced antigenicity is accounted for by activation of B lymphocytes and the production by plasma cells of immunoglobulins against the hapten, and by recognition of the now-abnormal carrier of the hapten by helper T lymphocytes.

The abnormal antibody circulates in the plasma and reacts specifically against a component such as the cell membrane or a cytoplasmic component of the target cell. Cell death is by phagocytosis by macrophages with or without complement activation, or by destruction by natural killer T cells, or both. Diseases related to type II hypersensitivity include complement-mediated haemolysis as in autoimmune haemolysis and blood transfusion reactions, and drug interactions that cause immune reactions against red cells and platelets.

A type III hypersensitivity reaction involves the formation of intermediate-sized immune complexes that activate complement and platelets. These stimulate tissue damage from ischaemia from thrombus formation, membrane attack complexes, and enzyme release from inflammatory cells. The large immune complexes are removed by macrophages and small complexes are filtered out by the glomeruli. Only intermediate ones cause disease and circulate (serum sickness) or are found in tissues and cause disease such as systemic lupus erythematosus (SLE).

A type IV hypersensitivity reaction is characteristically the tissue injury associated with granuloma formation and T-lymphocyte reactions to microorganisms such as mycobacteria, fungi, and other organisms. Organ transplant rejection has a type IV hypersensitivity component. The tissue reaction to stitch material, other implanted surgical objects, beryllium, nickel, and many other chronic irritants is also type IV.

Autoimmune diseases

Autoimmune diseases can be caused by humoral or cell-mediated mechanisms though the prime mover appears to be the helper T lymphocyte, which mediates B-lymphocyte production of antibodies and cytotoxic T-lymphocyte destruction of cells. It may be specific or non-specific. Specific examples include the development of antibodies against:

- thyroid-stimulating hormone (TSH) receptors on thyroid follicle cells in Graves' disease resulting in stimulation
- thyroid peroxidase, thyroglobulin, and TSH receptors with helper T-lymphocyte activation and cytotoxic T lymphocyte destruction of follicle cells in Hashimoto's thyroiditis. Transient hyperthyroidism is caused by release of stored T_4 from thyroglobulin from damaged follicles rather than by TSH receptor stimulation
- intrinsic factor in gastric parietal cells in pernicious anaemia
- acetylcholine receptors at the postsynaptic neuromuscular junction in myasthenia gravis
- mature platelets in idiopathic thrombocytopenic purpura (megakaryocytes in the bone marrow are normal).

Non-specific examples of autoimmune diseases include the development of antibodies against:

- IgG in rheumatoid arthritis, of two types: there are IgM antibodies against IgG, which are large and cannot leave the plasma so are unlikely to cause tissue effects; and IgG antibodies against IgG (they bind to themselves) which do leave the bloodstream and are probably more important in disease
- double-stranded DNA, histones, and other nuclear antigens in SLE, and against single-stranded DNA in some patients with discoid lupus erythematosus
- smooth muscle in chronic active hepatitis: there is an overlap with primary biliary cirrhosis, depending on the class of immunoglobulin—IgG class predominates in chronic active hepatitis and IgM smooth muscle antibodies predominate in primary biliary cirrhosis
- pyruvate dehydrogenase in mitochondria and nuclear components in primary biliary cirrhosis.

Immunization

Immunity can be induced by active and passive means. Each of these can be achieved naturally and by medical intervention. Natural active immunity follows infection by an organism that stimulates a reliable immunological memory. Artificial active immunity is achieved by vaccination. Natural passive immunity is conferred on the fetus by placental transfer of IgG, which lasts for the first few months of life, and artificial passive immunity by injection of preformed antibody from human donors or animals. Artificial passive immunity is used for patients exposed to blood that is positive for hepatitis B surface antigen and in immunocompromised patients with shingles.

Immunization with live attenuated organisms usually results in long-lasting immunity. Examples include the Sabin vaccine for polio, MMR vaccine for measles, mumps, and rubella, and BCG (bacillus Calmette–Guérin) for tuberculosis. Live vaccines can be very dangerous in immunocompromised patients. Killed organisms such as *Bordatella pertussis* for whooping cough result in a less intense immune response. Tetanus toxoid is given not to prevent infection by *Clostridium tetani* but to abolish the lethal effects of the exotoxin that the organism produces.

Immunodeficiency

Patients can be immunocompromised from congenital and acquired conditions. Congenital immunodeficiency may be humoral, such as Bruton type hypogammaglobulinaemia, or cell-mediated as in DiGeorge syndrome. Combined deficiencies with agammaglobulinaemia and stem cell deficiency are rare. A specific deficiency of the capacity of phagocytes to generate oxygen free radicals is present in chronic granulomatous disease, in which patients (usually males as the commonest form is inherited as an X-linked condition) suffer from repeated, severe bacterial infections. Acquired conditions resulting in some degree of immune compromise include HIV infection, long-term steroid therapy, and cytotoxic therapy. Patients with diabetes have deficient neutrophil function which correlates directly with the degree of hyperglycaemia.

Malignant neoplasms of almost any type induce some degree of immunodeficiency, and conversely immune-compromised patients develop malignant disease more frequently than immunocompetent people. A classic example is malignancy in patients with HIV infection (though not necessarily AIDS—only cervical cancer, so-called Kaposi's sarcoma, Burkitt's lymphoma, immunoblastic lymphoma, and primary cerebral lymphoma are on the list of AIDS-defining criteria).

Neoplasms that characteristically arise in patients with HIV infection include:

* lymphoma, most commonly B-cell non-Hodgkin's lymphoma (NHL) but occasionally T-cell NHL or Hodgkin's lymphoma

* squamous cell papilloma and carcinoma of skin

* SCC of cervix, vulva, and anus

* SCC of the larynx

* (Kaposi's sarcoma is now thought to be a non-neoplastic reaction to human herpes simplex virus type 8)

Surgical haematology

Blood transfusion

Surgical use of donated blood accounts for about half of all blood transfusions, so a clear knowledge of the hazards of transfusion is essential. Even simple precautions can save lives—for example, starting a transfusion at night on a general ward should be avoided unless there is a complement of staff trained to identify adverse reactions quickly. Acute transfusion reactions were the leading cause of transfusion morbidity in 2011; the latest Serious Hazards of Transfusion (SHOT) report showed that many incidents were potentially preventable, particularly all adverse events due to human errors, as might be expected.

The National Blood Service in England and North Wales (elsewhere in the United Kingdom there are the Welsh Blood Service in South Wales, the Scottish National Blood Transfusion Service, and the Northern Ireland Blood Transfusion Service) selects and tracks donors, and so excludes donors who can be identified from their medical or social history as unsuitable. Donors must be unpaid volunteers in the United Kingdom. The staff of the Service take blood by a set procedure into a solution of citrate, phosphate, and dextrose for anticoagulation. In the processing laboratory the anticoagulated blood is separated and the packed red cells resuspended in a solution of saline, arginine, glucose, and mannitol (SAGM).

Blood is tested for HIV-1, HIV-2, HTLV-1, HTLV-2, hepatitis B, hepatitis C, and syphilis. In some parts of the world, tests for *Trypanosoma cruzi* (the cause of Chagas disease) and West Nile virus are also performed. Some centres also test for CMV and other viral antibodies but this is not universal. Identification of other organisms with the polymerase chain reaction is being developed. The blood is then typed for ABO, RhD, and Kell blood groups. White cells are removed by specialized centrifugation and filtration to reduce the theoretical possibility of transmitting prion disease.

The transfusion Services prescribe the conditions for storage. When the transfusion blood is used there is a set procedure for checking that it is suitable for the recipient. Adverse reactions must be reported to the relevant blood transfusion laboratory and to the patient's consultant: a report will then be sent to SHOT. All details of the transfused blood and blood products must be recorded in the patient's notes so that they can be traced.

The Services also supply blood components and blood products. A *blood component* is made from one donation (or only a limited number of donations—platelet transfusions are components from pooled blood) to limit antigenicity from blood groups and are wet blood components for transfusion. Examples include packed red cells, platelets, fresh frozen plasma (FFP), and cryoprecipitate. A *blood product* is acellular and produced from thousands of blood donations; these include albumin, coagulation factor concentrates, and immunoglobulins, and are generally produced by industrial processes.

Almost all hospitals in the United Kingdom issue a Maximum Blood Order Schedule. This is an internationally adopted scheme that reduces unnecessary transfusions, reduces clinical requests for excessive amounts of blood for transfusion, and permits better stock control of blood for transfusion. It lists surgical procedures that require cross-match against the number of units that are considered to be required in the experience of the particular hospital. It is reviewed regularly and modified to include new procedures and reassess existing ones. If a procedure does not appear on the list, a 'group and antibody screen' is normally all that is needed. Patients must be judged individually and reasons given to the blood transfusion laboratory if it might be necessary for the listed number of units to be exceeded. In a case of massive haemorrhage, the UK blood transfusion and Tissue Transplantation Services guidelines are clear.[13]

When blood is needed for transfusion, or will probably be needed because of the nature of the surgical operation, a sample of the patient's blood is sent to the blood transfusion laboratory. The sample labelling requirements are stringent.[14]

This may be for 'group and cross-match' or 'group and antibody screen'. Both are automated nowadays. The latter is useful if blood for transfusion might be needed or might not, and permits rapid cross-matching to be done if required at a later date. A sample can usually be stored for up to 3 months, though if the patient is pregnant or has been transfused the sample has to be no more than 3 days before the actual transfusion.

For blood grouping, the patient's red cells are mixed with monoclonal antibodies to determine the ABO and RhD groups. An antibody screen tests the patient's serum against a panel of red cells. Cross-matching tests the bags of donated blood that will be used in this patient's specific case (categorized as being the correct ABO and RhD groups) directly against the patient's serum. This is to pick up antibodies raised by previous transfusions or pregnancy, and antigenicity of minor blood groups. It also acts as a check that the donor blood has been correctly labelled by the Service.

Platelets carry the same blood groups as red cells and so a platelet transfusion must be group-specific for the recipient. Injection of anti-D might be needed in women of child-bearing age who are RhD negative and receive RhD-positive products. Platelets for transfusion are stored at room-temperature.

Albumin transfusion can be indicated in the emergency management of circulatory shock, severe hypoproteinaemia, and burns. Its use nowadays is limited. Crystalloids or colloids are used instead as volume expanders. Crystalloids such as dextrose-saline and Ringer's solutions are not confined by the blood vessel walls and freely diffuse across: colloids have large molecules such as dextran or gelatin. Colloids have more side effects than crystalloids and are more expensive. There is no clinical evidence that colloid solutions are more effective.

Cryoprecipitate contains factors VIII and XIII, von Willebrand factor, fibrinogen, and fibronectin but is usually used as a source of fibrinogen, which might be needed for a patient with DIC after shock, sepsis, or massive blood transfusion.

Indications for blood transfusion

Whether blood is needed for transfusion depends on the patient's haemoglobin concentration and on the estimated blood loss at operation. All efforts should be made preoperatively to optimize the patient's haemoglobin concentration and reduce the risk of bleeding. These might include iron supplements and management of anticoagulant medication such as aspirin and warfarin.

The lowest normal concentration in a man is usually taken as 13 g/dL and in a woman 11.5 g/dL, but people with haemoglobin concentrations well below these can be entirely asymptomatic and managed by investigation with gradual reversal of the anaemia rather than by transfusion. In acute blood loss, crystalloids or colloids are usually better, and in many cases postoperative iron therapy can be used instead of transfusion.

A working scale for perioperative blood loss (expressed as the percentage of total blood volume) is:

- less than 15%, no treatment
- 15–30% loss, crystalloids or colloids
- 30–40% loss, crystalloids or colloids and red cells
- more than 40% loss, rapid replacement by blood transfusion with platelets and clotting factors if indicated.

Alternatives to blood transfusion

Acute normovolaemic haemodilution is a type of autologous transfusion which can be used in patients with normal haemoglobin concentrations. Two or three units of blood are taken from the patient in the anaesthetic room and replaced with an equal volume of colloid or crystalloid solution. The patient's red cell mass is therefore diluted, which reduces the red cell mass lost during the operation. The blood taken at the start is replaced at the end of the procedure when haemostasis has been achieved.

Preoperative autologous deposition of whole blood is no longer practised in the United Kingdom because of the associated risks. In this procedure, blood is taken from patients who have normal haemoglobin concentrations 4 weeks before elective surgery; up to a maximum of four units can be taken, each at intervals of 1 week. The procedure should not be undertaken unless there is a guaranteed date for the operation. In the United States where this procedure is commoner than in the United Kingdom, about half of the deposited blood is discarded unused.

Intraoperative red cell salvage by automated systems may be useful in some instances, when anticipated blood loss is more than two units. Blood from the operative field is collected, filtered, and transfused back. Some systems wash the blood to remove free haemoglobin and cell debris. Side effects include DIC and air embolism. This technique might be acceptable to patients who are Jehovah's Witnesses but might not, and this should be discussed.

Complications of blood transfusion

These can be classified into immediate and delayed. Immediate complications include:

- haemolysis from incompatibility with blood groups, a type II hypersensitivity reaction
- septicaemia from transfusion of infected blood, especially by Gram-negative organisms such as coliforms
- bleeding diathesis: transfusion blood may be deficient in platelets and clotting factors, especially factors V and VIII, though bleeding is usually the result of the underlying condition rather than any deficiency in the contents of the transfused blood
- circulatory changes with hypertension from hypervolaemia and hypotension because of blood group incompatibility; air embolus and other complications of venous access not specific to transfusion can also occur
- metabolic changes, classically hyperkalaemia from damaged red cells releasing potassium; hypocalcaemia is rare nowadays as citrate is generally no longer used as a storage anticoagulant. The patient may also develop acidosis
- temperature changes: hypothermia from rapid transfusion of chilled blood, and hyperthermia from a transfusion reaction.

Delayed complications include:

- septicaemia from deficiency of the aseptic technique of connecting the intravenous lines usually caused by *Staphylococcus aureus* or coliforms
- delayed haemolytic reactions from weak immunoglobulins in the patient's plasma not detected at antibody screening or cross-match
- impaired ability to reject transplanted organs such as renal transplants, especially if repeated transfusions are given. This, of course, might be a good thing
- infection (in unscreened donor blood) from hepatitis B, hepatitis C, HIV, CMV, malaria, and syphilis
- iron overload in patients who have had numerous transfusions, such as patients with thalassaemia.

Indications for platelet transfusion

Platelet transfusion may be indicated in patients with DIC, in patients who have had massive bleeding, and in patients with thrombocytopenia. Patients who have been given aspirin will need a platelet transfusion before a major operation such as aneurysm repair, abdominoperineal excision of rectum, and cardiac bypass.

Indications for transfusion of fresh frozen plasma

These include severe DIC, massive blood transfusion, cardiac bypass surgery, and thrombotic thrombocytopenic purpura. Patients on warfarin who require urgent operative surgery can be treated with FFP to raise clotting factors II, VII, IX, and X to normal.

Anaemia

Anaemia is of great surgical importance. Surgically it is important to understand the significance of the diagnosis of anaemia—surgeons manage patients with anaemia from different causes preoperatively, perioperatively, and postoperatively and surgeons can cause anaemia by many operative procedures.

Iron-deficiency anaemia

Iron-deficiency anaemia is the commonest type of anaemia, related usually to chronic blood loss or a deficient diet. It is commoner in women but not because they menstruate: menstruation is physiological. If a woman develops menorrhagia, excessive menstrual loss, this will overwhelm the capacity of the alimentary system to absorb enough iron compounds and for the bone marrow to convert them into haemoglobin.

The red cell precursors cannot make the proper amount of haemoglobin because of deficiency of iron but have no abnormality in their nuclei and their capacity to multiply is unimpaired. The precursors undergo an extra mitotic division which apportions the deficient cytoplasmic haemoglobin in one parent normocyte between two smaller daughter cells. This increases the mean corpuscular haemoglobin concentration at the expense of the mean corpuscular volume, though the concentration is still low. The blood film shows hypochromic, microcytic anaemia, as would be expected from this sequence.

This blood film picture is not pathognomonic—it is also seen in patients with thalassaemia. Neither is the serum iron particularly helpful: it is low in patients with rheumatoid arthritis and idiopathic inflammatory bowel disease. The serum ferritin concentration is the best measure of iron status, but rises in acute and chronic inflammatory diseases and should be interpreted in context. A low serum ferritin indicates low iron stores.

Macrocytic and megaloblastic anaemia

The red cell maturation sequence in the normal bone marrow is from myeloblasts, myelocytes, early normoblasts, and late normoblasts (all of which are nucleated) to reticulocytes and mature red cells (which are not nucleated—the nuclear remnant has been extruded). Reticulocytes are large red cells that have a 'reticule' (a network or meshwork) of basophilic filaments that are the remnants of RNA in the cell. On a Coulter report, reactive reticulocytosis might speciously appear to be pathological macrocytosis.

Macrocytes are large red cells (without nuclei, and so are like mature normal red cell though too large) which are present in the circulation. Because of the deficiency of absorption of vitamin B_{12} and folate the developing red cells cannot divide efficiently and miss a division. Their progeny are therefore larger than normal, which is reflected on the blood film of a macrocytic anaemia. The film will also show abnormal polymorphs.

Megaloblasts are large, nucleated, abnormal precursors of macrocytes which are never found in normal bone marrow; they are found predominantly in the bone marrow of patients with vitamin B_{12} and folate deficiencies, and very occasionally can be found in a film of peripheral blood. They have abnormal metabolism of DNA precursors into DNA and so can be tetraploid or aneuploid. This nuclear abnormality is present in all cells that have nuclei, so the cytology department will report abnormal nuclear changes on specimens from these patients from, for example, the cervix, bronchus, and bladder. White cell maturation is affected reflected by hypersegmented neutrophils.

Macrocytosis and macrocytic anaemia without megaloblastosis are caused by alcohol ingestion, hypothyroidism, and hepatic and renal failure. The commonest reason for macrocytosis in the United Kingdom is drinking alcohol; most of these people do not develop anaemia. About 3 months of stores of folate are held in the liver, and over 3 years of stores of vitamin B_{12}. This is why pregnant women are given folate supplements but not vitamin B_{12} supplements.

Folate and vitamin B_{12} are used in the cycle of DNA synthesis. The main driver is folate. Vitamin B_{12} acts at a single methylation step which converts homocysteine into methionine and acts as a catalyst rather than a substrate. Vitamin B_{12} is absorbed from meat, predominantly, in the diet. It attaches to intrinsic factor (vitamin B_{12} was originally called extrinsic factor before its nature was known) and they are absorbed by facilitated transport in the terminal ileum. The causes of vitamin B_{12} deficiency include:

- deficiency of intrinsic factor because of:
  - pernicious anaemia from antibodies against parietal cells which secrete intrinsic factor into the gastric lumen
  - partial or total gastrectomy
- absence of vitamin B_{12} absorption because of disease in the terminal ileum such as tuberculosis and Crohn's disease.

Vitamin B_{12} can be absorbed by simple mass action in the jejunum but the patient would have to take several tablets a day rather than one injection of hydroxocobalamin once every few months.

Folate deficiency is cause by dietary deficiency and by pregnancy from increased demands from the fetus. Occasionally folate deficiency is caused by antifolate drugs such as methotrexate but this is almost always closely monitored. Other drugs which interfere with DNA production include zidovudine and hydroxyurea.

Haemolytic anaemia

Haemolytic anaemia is a complex subject, most simply classified into inherited abnormalities and acquired causes of haemolysis. Inherited causes are classified as:

- haemoglobin abnormalities:
  - sickle cell disease, thalassaemia
  - other rarer haemoglobinopathies such as HbC, HbD Punjab, HbE

- red cell membrane abnormalities:
  - spherocytosis is the condition with the most surgical interest, as the symptoms can be cured by splenectomy
  - elliptocytosis is usually asymptomatic
  - enzyme abnormalities such as glucose-6-phosphate dehydrogenase deficiency and pyruvate kinase deficiency.

Acquired haemolytic anaemia can result from many causes. The principal ones of surgical importance are immune mediated and mechanical. Immune-mediated causes can be autoimmune, such as from drug-induced haemolysis, and isoimmune from ABO, RhD, and other blood group incompatibilities. Drugs that stimulate antibodies against red cells with consequent haemolysis by complement include cephalosporins, penicillin, levodopa and methyldopa, and some non-steroidal anti-inflammatory drugs. Mechanical causes include damage to red cells from artificial heart valves, especially metallic ones, and extracorporeal circulation for cardiac surgery.

Haemolytic anaemia is diagnosed when a patient has a low haemoglobin concentration associated with the typical haematological and biochemical changes below. This is characteristically a normochromic normocytic anaemia as there is usually no iron, vitamin B_{12}, or folate deficiency. The raised reticulocyte count in the peripheral blood represents an attempt by the bone marrow urgently to inject mature red cells and reticulocytes into the circulation to compensate for the haemolysis. Reticulocytosis can show on a Coulter result as a specious macrocytic anaemia.

These patients may also have an excess serum concentration of unconjugated bilirubin because the liver's capacity to conjugate is exceeded. There is relative absence of urinary bilirubin and increased serum methaemoglobin concentration.

Sickle cell disease

The clinical features of sickle cell disease are of surgical importance and are protean; the name given used to be sickle cell anaemia, but the patients can suffer severe disease without developing significant anaemia. Sickle cell crises with thrombosis and infarction commonly presents as bone pain but can also cause abdominal and chest pain; splenic infarction causes acute abdominal pain; priapism can be prolonged and becomes a surgical emergency. Sequestration of sickled red cells causes hepatomegaly and splenomegaly, though the spleen can also be small due to infarction. Haemolytic anaemia, especially if longstanding, can cause congestive cardiac failure and pigment gallstones. Unusual infections such as pneumococcal septicaemia and salmonella osteomyelitis can occur.

In sickle cell disease there is a biochemical abnormality of haemoglobin synthesis that results in a less soluble than normal haemoglobin with consequently reduced red cell survival and polymerization of haemoglobin with precipitation under low oxygen tension. There is a single amino acid error in the β-chain at position 6: valine is substituted for the normal glutamic acid which causes polymerization and precipitation of the haemoglobin in its deoxygenated state.

The β-chain genes are on chromosome 11 and act as autosomal co-dominants—each gene contributes about half of the total amount needed for construction of haemoglobin molecules. Patients with sickle cell disease are homozygous and have 90–100% HbS with small amounts of fetal haemoglobin, HbF. People with sickle cell trait are heterozygous, and have only 20–40% HbS with the rest normally being HbA. They are consequently usually asymptomatic.

The blood picture in sickle cell disease is of a normochromic film showing sickled red cells. There is reticulocytosis reflecting compensatory marrow hyperplasia, and features of splenic damage including target cells and fragmented red cells.

Thalassaemia

The intrinsic problem in thalassaemia is defective globin chain synthesis. This results in abnormal haemoglobin molecules and so abnormal red cell production. Alpha-chain thalassaemia affects people in China, Africa, and elsewhere in Asia but can affect their dependants anywhere in the world. Beta-chain thalassaemia is commoner and affects patients especially in Mediterranean countries and the Middle East.

Patients with classical β-thalassaemia have a hypochromic, microcytic anaemia. They have reticulocytosis and other abnormalities on a blood film such as nucleated red cells. There is increased fetal haemoglobin seen on electrophoresis: HbF continues to be produced in patients with thalassaemia as compensation for the production of abnormal HbA. People with the heterozygous β-thalassaemia trait are asymptomatic and have microcytosis without anaemia.

The complications of thalassaemia include marrow hyperplasia to compensate for the anaemia, iron overload from the need for repeated blood transfusions, haemosiderosis with liver damage and endocrine insufficiencies, and pancreatitis.

Splenectomy

Splenectomy is an important surgical procedure, and so it is important that the indication and complications are understood. The most urgent indication is splenic trauma and rupture with haemoperitoneum. Other more predictable indications include those for the treatment of haematological conditions involving the spleen, treatment of some non-haematological conditions, and management of the symptoms of splenomegaly. Splenectomy may be a necessary manoeuvre to permit access in operations in the area of the spleen, such as gastrectomy, adrenalectomy from an anterior approach, left colectomy, and Whipple's operation.

Some haematological diseases respond well to the effects of splenectomy. These include the management of rare haemolytic disorders such as hairy-cell leukaemia and immune idiopathic thrombocytopenic purpura, and the relief of haemolytic problems from hereditary spherocytosis. Splenectomy for the staging of lymphoma has been superseded by computed tomography and positron emission tomography imaging.

Splenic cysts from hydatid disease may need to be excised: congenital splenic cysts are usually asymptomatic. Other than lymphoma, primary and secondary neoplasms of the spleen are rare. Splenectomy may give relief of the symptoms of massive splenomegaly caused by visceral leishmaniasis (kala-azar), myelofibrosis, and chronic myeloid and lymphoid proliferative disorders.

The effects of splenectomy are reflected in red cell changes, platelet changes, and in white cell changes with the immunological consequences of them. Red cell changes are from the incapacity of the spleen to monitor degenerate red cells and abnormal red cell forms. Inclusion bodies in circulating red cells after splenectomy may be Howell–Jolly bodies (which are nuclear remnants) and Heinz bodies (composed of denatured haemoglobin). Abnormal forms include nucleated red cells and acanthocytes, distorted red cells with a spiky shape. Changes in platelet include thrombocytosis, increased adhesiveness, and abnormal cell forms.

White cell changes that characteristically follow splenectomy include a transient neutrophilia followed by permanent lymphocytosis and monocytosis. Immune changes include defective production of antibodies that bind to antigens that have carbohydrate moieties, such as on the cell walls of capsulated bacteria. There is also increased risk of contracting or reactivating malaria.

Splenomegaly

Splenomegaly is an abnormal increase in splenic size and weight, irrespective of function. The causes of splenomegaly are numerous and mostly not of immediate interest to a surgeon but are important to know in its differential diagnosis.

In general, the causes of splenomegaly include:

• inflammation, which may be caused by a large number of infective agents of all sizes from viruses to metazoa, or from non-infective causes of inflammation such as rheumatoid arthritis and sarcoidosis

• congestion of the spleen from complete or partial blockage of the splenic or portal veins by cirrhosis, thrombosis, or involvement by carcinoma of the pancreas

• accumulation of amyloid material, or mucopolysaccharides as in Gaucher's, Hurler's, and Hunter's diseases and other mucopolysaccharide storage diseases

• congenital diseases such as congenital haemolytic anaemia and polycystic disease of the spleen

• neoplastic conditions: any almost any of the leukaemias and lymphomas, and in the myeloproliferative disorders

• drug causes such as antibiotics and psychotropic drugs.

Hypersplenism

Hypersplenism is an abnormal increase in splenic function, almost always linked to size. All of the causes of splenomegaly previously listed can cause hypersplenism. Features of hypersplenism include splenomegaly with removal of red cells, white cells, and platelets whether appropriate or not. It is reversed by removal of the cause of the splenomegaly or by splenectomy.

Polycythaemia

Polycythaemia is classified as primary, secondary, and relative.

Primary polycythaemia is polycythaemia vera (the term has been changed from polycythaemia rubra vera to reflect the fact that white cells and platelets are also raised). It is one of the myeloproliferative diseases, the others being chronic myeloid leukaemia, myelofibrosis, and essential thrombocythaemia. The serum erythropoietin concentration is low in primary polycythaemia. It is characterized by the presence of a mutation in the Janus kinase 2 pathway in 98% of cases, and this is now the diagnostic test for the condition.

In secondary polycythaemia the serum erythropoietin concentration is high. This can be appropriate, stimulated by high altitude, cigarette smoking, lung disease such as emphysema, congestive cardiac failure, and haemoglobinopathies with high-affinity haemoglobins which hold on to oxygen and result in tissue hypoxia.

Secondary polycythaemia due to inappropriate erythropoietin excess is typically caused by excess eutopic secretion from a neoplasm, such as renal parenchymal cell carcinoma and hepatocellular carcinoma, or excess ectopic secretion such as by cerebellar haemangioblastoma, phaeochromocytoma, and prostatic adenocarcinoma. Relative polycythaemia occurs when there is a reduction in plasma volume, in which there is no increase in total red cell mass.

Haemostasis

Platelets

Platelets are of great clinical importance in the control of bleeding, especially from capillaries. Patients with thrombocytopenia present with internal bleeding in the skin (petechiae and ecchymoses) and in the retina. External bleeding, which may be profuse, may come from the alimentary tract, the female genital tract, and the upper respiratory tract as epistaxis. Conversely, patients with thrombocytosis present with coronary thrombosis and digital ischaemia from thrombosis, and with splenomegaly.

Platelets are cytoplasmic fragments of megakaryocytes that are regulated by growth factors such as thrombopoietin. Platelets have no nuclei and no ability to synthesize enzymes, so a continuous supply is needed. The normal concentration in blood is 150–400 $\times 10^9$/L and they have a lifespan of 7–10 days. About two-thirds of platelets stay in the general circulation; the rest are held in the spleen and exchanged with ones from the circulation. In cases of hypersplenism the splenic pool enlarges but the platelet lifespan is unchanged.

Platelets release clotting, vasoactive, and other substances locally to manage a breach in an endothelial cell surface. Platelet cell membranes have proteins that attach to fibrinogen and to von Willebrand factor, which carries factor VIII. The platelet cytoplasm contains:

• storage granules:

  • alpha granules: clotting factors V, VIII, fibrinogen, and von Willebrand factor; platelet factor 4, a heparin antagonist; and platelet-derived growth factor

  • dense granules: 5-hydroxytryptamine (serotonin), ADP, catecholamines, calcium

  • glycogen granules, which provide the energy source for platelet reactions

  • other granules containing thromboxane and prostaglandins

• actin and myosin fibres that cause clot retraction.

When there is a breach in an endothelial surface, collagen is exposed to the bloodstream. Platelets attach to it by membrane proteins and von Willebrand factor, a very large molecule that bridges spaces among platelets and between platelets and collagen. The shape of the platelets changes from discoid to spherical by rearrangement of microtubules. There is release of platelet granules with binding of circulating platelets nearby to fibrinogen which polymerizes to fibrin. Other clotting factors are also bound to the surface of platelets, including factors V and VIII. The platelet plug is stabilized by thromboxane and prostaglandins, and further consolidated when pseudopodia from platelets in the clot link and their actin and myosin fibres contract.

Aspirin blocks the actions of cyclooxygenase (COX) enzymes. These are essential for the formation of thromboxane and prostaglandin in platelets and endothelial cells. The block is permanent in platelets as they have no nuclei to regenerate more COX: in contrast, regeneration is rapidly possible in endothelial cells. New platelets take about a week to repopulate the circulation in adequate numbers.

Blood coagulation

This is achieved by a cascade of pro-enzymes (the clotting factors) and enzymes (the activated clotting factors). Most of the clotting factors are made in the liver (not just factors II, VII, IX, and X, which are the vitamin K-dependent factors). The benefits of the coagulation cascade are that the severity of acute haemorrhage, and to some extent chronic haemorrhage, is limited. The clotting cascade has more effect in venous or capillary haemorrhage rather than arterial. The same factors contribute to localization of acute infection in an abscess.

The cascade was classically divided into the intrinsic and the extrinsic systems but this is no longer considered useful. The intrinsic system has no role *in vivo*. The governing factor is factor VII. With tissue factor this activates factors IX and X. Activated factors IX with activated factor VIII also activate factor X. This, with activated factor V, splits prothrombin to thrombin, which splits fibrinogen to fibrin.

Factors XII and XI are unnecessary—patients with complete absence of factor XII are asymptomatic—but both factors have a small role at sites of major tissue injury. Both are needed for the activated partial thromboplastin time (aPTT test) to be normal. The other main test of clotting is the prothrombin time (PT), which is usually expressed as the international normalized ratio. The PT is prolonged in warfarin treatment, liver disease, DIC, and vitamin K deficiency. The aPTT is prolonged in heparin treatment, haemophilia, DIC, and liver disease. Another test which can be useful is the thrombin time, prolonged in heparin treatment, DIC, and abnormalities of fibrinogen.

Haemophilia syndromes

Men with haemophilia A (and very rarely homozygous women with two abnormal X chromosomes) suffer from repeated haemarthroses, intracranial haemorrhages, and subperiosteal haemorrhages resolving into so-called pseudotumours of bone with new bone formation. The classic form of haemophilia is inherited as an X-linked condition but about one-third are spontaneous mutations. The condition affects 1 in 100 000 men and results in low plasma factor VIII concentrations of variable severity. Patients are classified as severe if their plasma concentration is less than 1% of normal; moderate if they have 1–5% of normal; and mild if they have 6–40% of normal.

Christmas disease or haemophilia B is factor IX deficiency. It is also X-linked but only one-fifth as common as haemophilia A. The clinical picture is the same as haemophilia A. Treatment for both types is replacement of specific clotting factors. Arginine vasopressin (DDAVP) can be used to stimulate secretion of von Willebrand factor with a consequent increase in factor VIII binding and survival in patients with mild haemophilia A but not haemophilia B.

Thrombocytosis

Thrombocytosis (or thrombocythaemia) may be neoplastic in essential thrombocytosis or part of another myeloproliferative disorder such as myelofibrosis, polycythaemia vera, and chronic myeloid leukaemia. Thrombocytosis can also be secondary to:

- inflammation and operative surgery
- iron-deficiency anaemia
- splenic deficiency:
  - splenectomy and congenital absence of the spleen
  - hyposplenism
  - sickle cell disease, thalassaemia, lymphomas, and coeliac disease
  - splenic irradiation before bone marrow transplantation.

Thrombocytopenia and thrombasthenia

Thrombocytopenia is a reduction below normal of the *number* of platelets. Thrombasthenia is a reduction below normal of the *function* of platelets. These conditions are not mutually exclusive. The causes of thrombocytopenia are failure of platelet production, increased platelet consumption, and dilutional or artefactual thrombocytopenia.

Failure of production includes conditions such as:

- aplastic anaemia
  - congenital: Fanconi's anaemia
  - iatrogenic from:
    - drugs: cytotoxics, drugs causing hypersensitivity states
    - radiotherapy
  - autoimmune causes with no known aetiology
  - other: virus infections, pregnancy, accidental radiation exposure
- megaloblastic anaemia
- myelodysplastic syndromes other than idiopathic thrombocythaemia
- bone marrow replacement by metastatic carcinoma
- HIV and other virus infections unrelated to aplastic anaemia
- other congenital causes (rarely):
  - May–Hegglin anomaly
  - Bernard–Soulier syndrome
  - osteopetrosis with obliteration of the marrow.

Increase in consumption in conditions such as:

- thrombotic thrombocytopenic purpura
- splenomegaly and hypersplenism
- DIC
- immunological causes:
  - in a blood transfusion reaction ('post-transfusion purpura')
  - idiopathic thrombocytopenic purpura
  - heparin-induced thrombocytopenia
  - diseases such as SLE and antiphospholipid syndrome
  - drug reactions
- infections: malaria, glandular fever, schistosomiasis.

Relative thrombocytopenia, which may be:

- dilutional from transfusion of stored blood low in platelets, or of large transfusions of fluid such as dextrose saline
- artefactual thrombocytopenia: patients may have antibodies that cause aggregation of platelets in glass.

The causes of thrombasthenia are rare; they can be congenital or acquired. Congenital defects include glycoprotein abnormalities of the platelet membrane, such as Glanzmann's disease and Bernard–Soulier syndrome, or abnormalities of platelet storage granules. Stored platelets have deficient dense granules, alpha granules, or both.

Acquired causes of thrombasthenia include chronic renal and hepatic diseases and drug interactions with platelets. Aspirin blocks the actions of COX enzymes and so inhibits prostaglandin synthetase and prevents release of ADP and thromboxane A2; other drugs causing thrombasthenia include frusemide, sympathetic nerve system blockers, clofibrate, non-steroidal anti-inflammatory drugs, and heparin.

Heparins and warfarin

Unfractionated heparin is a sulphated polysaccharide with a mean molecular weight of 15 kDa that is produced by hepatocytes (hence the name) and by mast cells. It inhibits the actions of thrombin by binding it to naturally occurring antithrombin III, which is also made in the liver. The length of the polysaccharide is important—18 or more saccharide units are essential if the heparin linking chain is to bridge between antithrombin and thrombin. By inhibiting thrombin, heparin prevents conversion of fibrinogen to fibrin, and inhibits thrombin activation of factor V, factor VIII, and platelets. The heparin–antithrombin complex also inhibits activated factor X but does not bind to it. As a consequence the heparin chain length can be as small as five units.

Low-molecular-weight heparin (LMWH) has a mean molecular weight 5 kDa. It has less capacity than unfractionated heparin to inactivate thrombin because of the smaller polysaccharide length, but inhibits activated factor X to the same degree. The advantage of LMWH is that it binds to plasma proteins less than unfractionated heparin and so has a more predictable dose-related half-life, a longer plasma half-life, and a lower risk of heparin-induced osteopenia and thrombocytopenia. The effects of both types of heparin are reversed by protamine sulphate. Heparins do not cross the placenta.

Warfarin antagonizes the effects of vitamin K, which is necessary for the formation of the calcium-binding forms of factors II, VII, IX, and X. Vitamin K in the liver modifies the precursor factor molecules by carboxylating them and this is blocked by warfarin. Protein C and protein S synthesis are also affected. Protein S is a co-factor in the activation of protein C, which acts against activated factors V and VIII to decrease the effects of thrombin. Depletion of all these factors takes several days—warfarin has a half-life of 60 hours—and overlap with heparin should be considered if anticoagulation is urgent. Warfarin crosses the placenta and so cannot be used in pregnancy.

Bridging protocols for patients on anticoagulants have been developed and are regularly scrutinized. When and whether to use bridge anticoagulation will depend on the patient's risk of thromboembolus. This will depend on the indication for long-term warfarin therapy, such as previous deep vein thrombosis with embolus, or heart disease with atrial fibrillation, or a prosthetic valve. Warfarin might not need to be discontinued in patients having minor surgery in which bleeding is likely to be minimal or can easily be staunched. Specific operative risks have been studied—discontinuation of antiplatelet treatment in patients who need to have a coronary artery stent increases the chance of stent thrombosis.[15]

Disseminated intravascular coagulopathy

A surgical knowledge of DIC is clinically important because patients with massive trauma can develop DIC and its complications; patients can present with DIC as a complication of a surgically treatable condition; surgical procedures can cause DIC; and postoperative infections can cause DIC.

Causes of DIC include:

* infections such as Gram-negative septicaemia; Gram-positive septicaemia by meningococci and clostridia; systemic candidiasis and aspergillosis; and malaria
* massive tissue injury from burns, major physical trauma, and extensive surgical procedures
* haematological disorders such as sickle cell disease and other causes of intravascular haemolysis
* vascular and perfusion disorders such as aneurysms, prosthetic grafts, coarctation of the aorta, vasculitis, and occasionally myocardial infarction
* neoplasms such as carcinomas of the bronchus, prostate, ovary, and pancreas
* obstetric complications such as amniotic fluid embolism, eclampsia, and premature separation of the placenta
* other causes including liver failure, acute pancreatitis, hypothermia, amphetamines and other drugs, and snakebites.

The clinical diagnosis of DIC is confirmed by finding a low platelet count, a low plasma fibrinogen concentration, increased PT and aPTT, and fibrin degradation products in urine and serum. Haemolysis and fragmented red cells are usually present to some degree.

Biochemical disorders

Calcium disorders

Hypercalcaemia

The normal serum calcium concentration is in the range of 2.15–2.55 mmol/L with small variations between biochemistry laboratories. Hypercalcaemia is considered to be a corrected serum calcium concentration above 2.60 mmol/L. The commonest cause is recognized or undiagnosed parathyroid disease—about 1% of the population in the United Kingdom has mild primary hyperparathyroidism with consequently raised serum calcium levels.

Hypercalcaemia in relation to malignant disease is also well recognized. Metastatic carcinoma in bone can produce mild or severe hypercalcaemia. Parathyroid hormone-related protein (PTHrP) is secreted by all normal cells as a paracrine communicator, and the plasma concentration of PTHrP increases when there is widespread metastatic carcinoma; this causes generalized demineralization of bone. Carcinomas can also have ectopic secretion of parathyroid-like hormone, such as SCC of bronchus and occasionally oat cell carcinoma. Patients with myeloma, leukaemia, and lymphoma develop hypercalcaemia by several mechanisms including stimulation of osteoclasts by the tumour cells.[16]

Other endocrine diseases associated with hypercalcaemia include phaeochromocytoma, adrenal failure, and severe hyperthyroidism. Phaeochromocytoma that is not part of multiple endocrine adenopathy (MEA) II causes hypercalcaemia by an unknown mechanism; the calcium concentration reverts to normal when the phaeochromocytoma is excised. Iatrogenic causes include prolonged immobilization such as in patients in the intensive care unit and high dependency unit and in patients with Paget's disease of bone. Drugs such as thiazides, lithium, oestrogens, tamoxifen, and overdosage of vitamins A and D also contribute.

Familial causes include hypophosphatasia, idiopathic hypercalcaemia of infancy, and hypocalciuric hypercalcaemia. Other rare causes include severe chronic granulomatous diseases such as sarcoidosis and occasionally tuberculoid leprosy: macrophages hydroxylate vitamin D to its active forms.

The classical and important effects of hypercalcaemia include:

* bone pain, joint pain, and pathological fractures

* depression, confusion, neuroses and psychoses, fatigue, and lethargy

* nausea and vomiting, peptic ulcers, pancreatitis, and constipation

* polyuria and polydipsia, renal calculi, nephrocalcinosis, and renal failure

* in longstanding cases, hypertension, cardiac arrhythmias, and metastatic calcification.

Metastatic calcification

Calcification is classified as normal and abnormal—orthotopic and heterotopic. Orthotopic calcification occurs in bones, teeth, and otoliths. Heterotopic calcification is divided into dystrophic, metastatic, and age-related from no apparent dystrophic or metastatic mechanism.

It is important not to read the word *metastatic* (Greek *metastasis*, change or removal) in this context as referring to involvement by the spread of malignant disease. It means a change in condition from normocalcaemia to hypercalcaemia, calcification secondary to hypercalcaemia rather than dystrophic calcification. Metastatic calcification occurs around the renal tubules as nephrocalcinosis, in alveolar walls in the lungs, around the gastric glands, and in the cornea.

Dystrophic calcification

This is calcification in dead or damaged tissues in the presence of a normal circulating calcium concentration, such as calcification in tissue damage caused by tuberculosis, atheroma, and parasites.

Plasma proteins

Disorders of proteins

Plasma proteins are paradoxically measured in the biochemistry laboratory as serum proteins. Plasma contains all of the constituent proteins in the circulation: serum is plasma depleted of clotting factors. The importance of removing fibrinogen from the plasma before using it for protein electrophoresis is that it forms polymers of itself. There are therefore large numbers of molecules of very many molecular weights and these obscure the bands of the other plasma proteins.

The highest and tightest peaks on electrophoresis are albumin and pre-albumin. The globulin peaks follow: the α-1 band carries α-1-antitrypsin, now called protease inhibitor enzymes, and high-density lipoprotein (HDL); the α-2 band carries α-2 macroglobulin and haptoglobin, a haemoglobin-binding protein important in

haemolytic anaemia; the β-1 and β-2 bands carry low-density lipoprotein (LDL), transferrin, and β-2 microglobulin; and the γ band has the immunoglobulins.

Bilirubin

Bilirubin and jaundice

Bilirubin is derived principally from the haem moiety in red cells, with much smaller amounts derived from myoglobin and cytochrome enzymes. Red cells are degraded in the spleen and the consequent bilirubin is carried in plasma strongly bound to albumin. In the liver, bilirubin is conjugated with glucuronide. Bilirubin glucuronide is excreted in bile. In the colon, conjugated bilirubin is deconjugated by bacterial glucuronidases and reduced to stercobilinogen, which is excreted in the faeces as stercobilin. A small amount of stercobilinogen is absorbed by the colon, recycled by the liver, and excretion in bile. A very small amount of stercobilinogen leaks into the plasma; it is water-soluble and so is excreted in urine as urobilinogen.

Classification of jaundice

Jaundice is classified into haemolytic and other prehepatic causes, hepatocellular causes, and post-hepatic, obstructive causes. In haemolytic diseases the excess of unconjugated bilirubin, which is firmly bound to albumin, is unable to escape through glomerular filtration and so the patient has 'acholuric' jaundice without bile in the urine. In the newborn, the excessive amounts of unconjugated bilirubin such as from RhD incompatibility can attach to lipid-rich areas in the brain such as the basal ganglia and cause kernicterus.

In hepatocellular jaundice there is excess of conjugated and unconjugated bilirubin because the diseased hepatocytes cannot conjugate bilirubin adequately. There may also be failure to excrete in the bile the bilirubin that has been successfully conjugated.

In obstructive jaundice, there is excess of conjugated bilirubin in the plasma because it cannot be excreted in bile and so must be excreted in the urine which is consequently dark. There are less-than-normal amounts of stercobilin production in the colon and so the faeces are pale.

Serological tests for the investigation of a patient with jaundice include full blood count, film, reticulocyte count, erythrocyte sedimentation rate, and C-reactive protein measurement. Other investigations, depending on the clinical picture, may be investigations of clotting function, virological investigations, liver function tests including albumin and total protein measurements, and an autoantibody screen.

Gout

A knowledge of gout is of surgical importance for several reasons. The most important is that gout causes acute and chronic arthritis. It is one of the crystal arthropathies (along with the arthropathies caused by the crystals of calcium pyrophosphate, hydroxyapatite, and oxalate deposition in joints). It is in the differential diagnosis of septic arthropathy and, as in any repeated or chronic joint injury, eventually causes osteoarthritis.

Urological surgeons may diagnose calculi and other diseases caused by urate crystal deposition. Reconstructive surgeons might be asked to treat gouty tophi on visible parts of the body. All surgeons involved with cytotoxic drugs and radiotherapy should know that they can cause or exacerbate hyperuricaemia and clinical gout.

Urate is derived from metabolism of purines (the name was given from the Latin for 'pure urate'). Purines (adenine and guanine) are metabolized to urate; pyrimidines (uracil and thymine in DNA, and uracil and cytosine in RNA) are not, and are eventually degraded to urea, a far simpler molecule than uric acid.

Classification of hyperuricaemia

Primary hyperuricaemia is a congenital abnormality of a phosphoribosyl transferase that causes a defect in the normal recycling of purine breakdown products into new purines. As a consequence, they must be further deconstructed through xanthine and hypoxanthine. The excretory point of their metabolism in human beings is uric acid.

Secondary hyperuricaemia is either from increased cell destruction or decreased urate excretion by the kidneys. The first is caused by increased cell turnover states such as myeloproliferative diseases, leukaemia, psoriasis, and chemotherapy. The second follows decreased excretion of urate as a consequence of chronic renal failure and diuretics such as thiazides and frusemide which modify tubular urate excretion.

Alcohol-related diseases

Ingestion of ethyl alcohol primarily affects the CNS and the stomach, pancreas, larynx, and liver. The CNS is affected the earliest, only minutes after ingestion, by psychological effects such as loss of inhibition and judgement, and physical pharmacological effects of sedation and loss of coordination. The commonest alcohol-related injury in young adults is trauma such as skin lacerations and abrasions, head injuries with intracranial haemorrhage, and long bone fractures. Late complications include cirrhosis, carcinomas of the larynx, stomach, and elsewhere, cerebellar degeneration, encephalopathy, and psychoses. On a practical note, obtaining a clear surgical history from a patient who has ingested alcohol, whether acutely or chronically, may be impossible.

Ethyl alcohol is metabolized principally by the liver and to a lesser extent by the kidney, stomach, and brain. The main pathway is through the microsomal ethanol oxidizing system enzymes, with smaller amounts metabolized by alcohol dehydrogenase and the catalase reaction. All of these have acetic acid as the end result, which is metabolized partly to acetyl-CoA and partly to carbon dioxide in heart, brain, and skeletal muscle cells. Methyl alcohol ingestion is toxic because it is metabolized through formaldehyde to formic acid, both of which have severely deleterious effects on most tissues of the body. Ingestion of as little as 10 mL of methanol can cause blindness and 30 mL can be fatal.

The liver changes on histology as a consequence of long-term alcohol ingestion reflect the degree of hepatocyte damage:

- steatosis with fatty change but no significant inflammation. This usually resolves unless the alcohol challenge continues

- steatohepatitis, which has progressed from steatosis to steatitis with an acute inflammatory cell infiltrate. This can result in fibrosis

- alcoholic hepatitis with demonstrable hepatocyte damage, severe active inflammation, and cholestasis. Some cases are fatal

- progressive hepatic fibrosis with linking fibrosis and early hepatocyte regeneration

- cirrhosis, which is fibrosis of the liver with nodular regeneration. This is classically micronodular unless the patient subsequently gives up drinking, when it can progress to mixed and then macronodular cirrhosis

- in about 5% of cases of alcoholic cirrhosis, hepatocellular carcinoma develops.

Gastric diseases associated with alcohol consumption include acute and chronic gastritis with enhancement of the effects of *Helicobacter pylori* infection if present, gastric erosions and ulcers, and gastric carcinoma.

The pancreas may develop acute pancreatitis, repeated attacks of acute pancreatitis, chronic pancreatitis, and carcinoma of the pancreas. Pancreatic atrophy may occur and sometimes gives no symptoms of abdominal or back pain, only symptoms and signs related to malabsorption.

Alcohol-induced diseases of the larynx are especially associated with consumption of undiluted spirits rather than beer or wine. These patients develop chronic laryngeal inflammation and SCC of the larynx. Other diseases in this group include SCCs of the pharynx and oesophagus.

Surgically important endocrine gland disorders

Thyroid disease

Hyperthyroidism

The three thyroid hormones are T_3, T_4, and calcitonin. Excess of plasma calcitonin, such as in medullary carcinoma of thyroid, has no apparent deleterious effect though the carcinoma itself has a poor prognosis. By convention hyperthyroidism refers only to the iodinated hormones. A patient can be found to have normal thyroid function because it is driven by an elevated TSH concentration, and so in some cases measurement of TSH is important.

Hyperthyroidism and thyrotoxicosis are terms used interchangeably. In mild hyperthyroidism there may be no apparent toxicity. Some of these patients feel full of energy and might become unacceptably lethargic if returned to normal thyroid hormone function. The clinical and biochemical diagnosis of hyperthyroidism gives only a small indication of the underlying disease process.

Biochemically, the synthesis of thyroid hormones requires the coordinated action of several enzyme systems. Iodination of the amino-acid tyrosine provides mono-iodotyrosine and di-iodotyrosine. Coupling of these results in triiodothyronine and tetraiodothyronine, T_3 and T_4 (the name change reflects the fact that tyrosine has one benzene ring and thyronine has two). The reactions depend on the supply of plasma iodine salts, and can be excessive if iodine is in large supply. The tissue causes of hyperthyroidism are varied but all result in excess secretion of T_3 or T_4, or both.

Hyperplasia of the gland is the commonest cause of hyperthyroidism in the United Kingdom. This can be diffuse as in Graves' disease, or focal as in a multinodular goitre in which a hyperactive, toxic nodule develops. In Graves' disease (named for Robert Graves who described the disease in 1835) the gland is diffusely enlarged, dark red, and beefy because of hyperplasia and hypertrophy of the follicular cells and increase in the blood supply. There have been rare reports of Hashimoto's disease developing in patients with treated Graves' disease. It is impossible to identify on routine histopathological sections which of the nodules of a multinodular goitre are oversecreting: there is no relation to size, cellularity, or thyroglobulin content.

Neoplasia of the thyroid can cause hyperthyroidism if the tumour cells are differentiated and hypermetabolic. A follicular adenoma can secrete excess T_3 and T_4. Differentiated carcinomas of the thyroid (papillary and follicular carcinomas) can also secrete T_3 and T_4. Another neoplasm rarely associated with hyperthyroidism is a cystic teratoma (benign dermoid cyst) of the ovary with monophyletic differentiation into thyroid tissue. Surgical removal can cause abrupt hypothyroidism in the patient with hypotension and bradycardia.

Much rarer than all of the neoplasms mentioned above is a TSH-secreting adenoma of pituitary, which occurs with a prevalence of less than 2% of functioning pituitary neoplasms, which they themselves are rare. This can be diagnosed by a raised serum TSH concentration in a patient with an increased serum T_4 concentration.

There are several iatrogenic reasons for hyperthyroidism. There may be overtreatment with thyroxine during replacement after thyroidectomy or treatment of hypothyroidism. Several drugs such as amiodarone contain large amounts of iodine as do radiological investigations using iodine-based contrast media.

Hypothyroidism

Hashimoto's thyroiditis (for Hakaru Hashimoto who described the condition in 1912) is an autoimmune chronic lymphocytic thyroiditis in which the follicular cells are damaged by antibodies and cell-mediated immune reactions. Antibodies are typically against thyroglobulin, thyroid peroxidase, and cell structures including TSH receptors. The cell-mediated damage is by CD4 and CD8 T cells and macrophages, as a type IV hypersensitivity reaction though granulomas are not typical of Hashimoto's disease.

In early Hashimoto's disease there is no hyperplasia but active destruction of the thyroid follicles, which release stored T_3 and T_4 from thyroglobulin and can cause transient hyperthyroidism before the destructive process results in atrophy. Unlike in Graves' disease, in Hashimoto's thyroiditis the gland is enlarged but pale because of the large infiltrate of lymphocytes and developing fibrosis. A rare complication is the development of NHL of B cell type.

Other thyroiditides

Riedel's thyroiditis (first described by Bernard Riedel in 1896) is a rare focal condition characterized by a very dense fibrotic mass that extends beyond the thyroid capsule into surrounding structures such as the strap muscles. The surgical significance is that it closely mimics thyroid carcinoma, and that about one-third of patients with the condition have hypothyroidism. There is no apparent association with the development of fibrosarcoma.

De Quervain's thyroiditis (Fritz de Quervain, 1902) is a rare granulomatous thyroiditis linked with viral infections such as adenovirus and Coxsackie virus. The patient may present with hyperthyroidism in the early stages and hypothyroidism in the later stages. The disease is usually self-limiting but operative surgery may be required to make the diagnosis.

Thyroid neoplasms

The five thyroid neoplasms most commonly seen in general surgical practice are papillary, follicular, medullary, and anaplastic carcinoma, and thyroid lymphoma. The order given for the carcinomas relates to prevalence and prognosis. Other rare neoplasms include thyroid teratoma and lymphangiosarcoma. In view of the high blood supply of the thyroid, metastatic carcinoma to the gland is surprisingly rare.

Papillary carcinoma

Papillary carcinoma accounts for about 80% of thyroid carcinomas and is multifocal in about half of cases (the multifocality can affect both lobes and the isthmus). It is an incidental finding of no significance in about 2% of postmortem examinations in patients with no other malignancy. There is no benign counterpart.

The tumour is related to thyroid irradiation, nowadays more commonly from escape of radioactive iodine from nuclear power plants than from direct radiation used with the intention of therapy. The histological appearance of papillary carcinoma is not directly related to its behaviour in terms of invasiveness except for the tumour size: small tumours of about 0.5 cm diameter are associated with nodal metastases in about half of cases, larger tumours in 80% of cases. It has a prognosis overall of about 90% after 5 years.

Follicular carcinoma

Follicular carcinoma accounts for about 15% of thyroid carcinomas. In contrast to papillary carcinoma it is rarely multifocal, rare as an incidental finding at postmortem, and rarely related to radiation exposure. It metastasizes through the bloodstream to bone marrow and lungs.

The histological appearance is usually of a well or moderately differentiated carcinoma. Diagnosis depends on the behaviour of the tumour cells rather than their appearance—thyroid adenomas can have mitoses and pleomorphic cell forms. Demonstration of capsular or vascular invasion at the periphery of the tumour, or both, is diagnostic. Follicular carcinoma has a prognosis of about 70% after 5 years.

Medullary carcinoma

Medullary carcinoma of thyroid is a malignant neoplasm of C cells; there is no benign counterpart. It has a prevalence of about 5% of thyroid carcinomas overall. When it arises spontaneously, in about three-quarters of cases, it tends to be unilateral. When associated with MEA II syndromes and so genetically determined, it accounts for the other third of cases and is almost always bilateral in the thyroid.

Medullary carcinoma derives from thyroid C cells which make calcitonin. Calcitonin from the tumour cells accumulates within it and has a distinct histological appearance. The deposits of calcitonin among the tumour cells stain with Congo red and have apple-green dichroic birefringence, and so fulfil the simple definition of amyloid material. These amyloid deposits are strongly positive on immunostains for calcitonin.

Metastasis is characteristically to lymph nodes and bone marrow, and is often extensive by the time of diagnosis. Medullary carcinoma has a 5-year prognosis of about 90% if at excision it is completely confined to the thyroid; of about 70% if there are local lymph node metastasis; and about 20% if other tissues are involved. Overall there is a 5-year survival of about 60%.

Anaplastic carcinoma

Anaplastic carcinoma accounts for about 2% of thyroid carcinomas. These characteristically arise in iodine-deficient areas or in a multinodular goitre. Dedifferentiation of a differentiated carcinoma, such as a follicular carcinoma into an anaplastic carcinomas, has almost the same prognosis as the anaplastic type. Metastases of anaplastic carcinoma are early to distant sites through lymphatic and blood vessels. Local, fatal invasive and compressive effects in the neck, especially with retrosternal extension and massive haemorrhage, may preclude the antemortem diagnosis of metastatic spread. It has a 1-year survival rate of almost zero. Young men who develop thyroid carcinoma, which is very rare, almost always develop anaplastic carcinoma.

Diagnosis of thyroid cancer

This depends on clinical examination, fine-needle aspiration cytology (FNAC) and in equivocal cases, diagnostic thyroid lobectomy. Ultrasound of the neck should precede FNAC to exclude vascular and other causes of the neck mass.

All of the five histological types of thyroid cancer can be diagnosed on FNAC except one:

◆ Papillary carcinoma: all papillary neoplasms are malignant: there is no entity of papillary adenoma. They can be diagnosed on FNAC provided that tumour papillae are present on the cytology slide.

◆ Follicular carcinoma: no follicular thyroid lesion can be given a definite diagnosis on FNAC. The differential diagnosis includes normal thyroid parenchyma, follicular adenoma, follicular carcinoma, a dominant nodule in a multinodular gland, and a colloid thyroid nodule. An enlarged parathyroid gland, which also may have follicles and which may be intrathyroid, may also have been sampled.

◆ Medullary carcinoma: this is usually easy to diagnose, with regular polyhedral cells in an amyloid matrix that can be seen on the cytology preparation.

◆ Anaplastic carcinoma: this is usually easy to diagnose; the severe anaplasia is usually very obvious. A possible differential diagnosis is high-grade thyroid lymphoma.

◆ Thyroid lymphoma: this can usually be differentiated from severe lymphocytic thyroiditis because of the monomorphism of the cells of the neoplasm.

The diagnosis of follicular carcinoma depends on the histological demonstration of invasion of the capsule or peripheral vessels. This requires a well-fixed excision specimen of a solitary thyroid mass or of the entire thyroid gland. The concern regarding frozen-section examination is that handling of the fresh tissues can transpose tumour cells artifactually into vessels and outside the capsule. Even on numerous well-orientated sections from fixed tissue this can be a problem. It is resolved by finding an endothelial cell covering of tumour cells in vessels, indicating that this had occurred *in vivo*. This subtlety is very difficult on frozen sections, which are usually at least five times the thickness of a paraffin-wax section.

Lymphomas that involve the thyroid are of NHL type in almost all cases. The development of NHL is associated with Hashimoto's disease and more rarely with Graves' disease. Given a firm diagnosis of NHL, surgery is not indicated: chemotherapy without excision can give a 5-year prognosis of 85%.

Parathyroid disease

Hyperparathyroidism

Almost all cases of excess secretion of parathyroid hormone (PTH) are from eutopic secretion from a parathyroid neoplasm or from parathyroid hyperplasia, which is idiopathic. Frozen section diagnosis has no proper place in the identification of parathyroid disease, only in the confirmation that the tissue sampled is parathyroid. The tissue could be a thyroid nodule, a lymph node, the thymus, a strap muscle, or other tissues. Parathyroid adenocarcinoma is very rare and would usually not be diagnosed on frozen section.

In primary hyperparathyroidism, the disease is an adenoma in 85% of cases, hyperplasia in 15%, and carcinoma in very much less than 1%. Primary hyperparathyroidism is common and often asymptomatic. It causes hyperparathyroid bone disease by generalized stimulation of osteoclasts with bone resorption and of osteoblasts with inadequate mineralization of osteoid, both of which can lead to pathological fractures.

Secondary hyperparathyroidism results from hypocalcaemia, usually from chronic renal failure in which there is abnormal tubular loss of calcium and retention of phosphate, and failure of 1-hydroxylation of vitamin D in the kidney to its active form. Other causes include dietary deficiency of vitamin D, especially aggravated by a long winter with little sunlight. Vitamin D inhibits the transcription of DNA for PTH and so a decrease in plasma vitamin D will result in secondary hyperparathyroidism even without hypocalcaemia. In pregnancy, there are increased demands from the developing fetus which can cause hypocalcaemia. In tertiary hyperparathyroidism, there is adenoma development in one or more of the hyperplastic glands of secondary hyperparathyroidism.

Hypoparathyroidism

Hypoparathyroidism is largely a medical, endocrinological disease but there are important surgical reasons for being aware of the condition. In terms of symptoms, a patient may present surgically with severe abdominal pain or bone pain. The patient may have head injuries because of epileptic fits, bronchospasm causing anaesthetic difficulties, and cardiac arrhythmias, so it is important that hypoparathyroidism is considered.

Operative surgery on the neck for many reasons may result in hypoparathyroidism. In addition to the well-recognized complications of partial parathyroidectomy and bruising or infarction of the remaining gland or glands, there have been cases in which the patient has had hypercalcaemia treated by excision of three glands, and subsequently has needed a partial thyroidectomy for an unrelated reason. About 10% of parathyroid glands are intrathyroid, and so the result can be inadvertent removal of the remaining glands.

Autoimmune destruction in patients who have parathyroiditis, autoantibodies to other endocrine glands such as the thyroid, adrenals, and ovaries can occur. The severe chronic inflammation results in destruction of the parathyroids. Congenital reasons for hypoparathyroidism include T-cell deficiency such as in DiGeorge syndrome, in which the parathyroid glands are hypoplastic or aplastic.

Magnesium is essential for PTH secretion. Deficiency can result from excessive alcohol intake, especially if combined with a poor diet because of vomiting and diarrhoea, and from diabetes mellitus. The hypoparathyroidism is reversed by correction of the hypomagnesaemia.

Adrenal gland disease

Cushing's disease and syndrome

Hypercortisolaemia defines both the disease and the syndrome. Harvey Williams Cushing (1896–1937) was a neurosurgeon in Boston, Massachusetts. He published his widely recognized paper on pituitary adenoma in 1932, though had published before that on the same subject over the previous 15 years. Cushing's disease is a neoplasm of the pituitary gland which is almost always an adenoma. Cushing's syndrome is the collection of symptoms and signs that result from hypercortisolaemia from any cause including, rarely, a pituitary adenoma.

The external and internal features of a patient with severe Cushing's syndrome include:

- cortisol effects such as:
  - change in adipose tissue distribution, such as central obesity which with reduction of muscle tone results in a pendulous abdomen; increase in adipose tissue between the scapulae; and reduction of adipose tissue in the limbs with muscle wasting
  - skin changes such as acne; purple striae and ecchymoses from capillary fragility; furuncles and carbuncles related to the diabetogenic properties of cortisol
  - other changes of diabetes mellitus
  - osteoporosis with the risk of compression fracture
- aldosterone-like effects of cortisol, such as generalized and localized oedema; when this affects the head it gives a rounded face augmented by adipose tissue deposition
- testosterone-like effects of cortisol, responsible for male pattern baldness and hirsutism in women, and amenorrhoea from suppression of ovarian hormone secretion.

The causes of Cushing's syndrome are numerous. The commonest is iatrogenic, usually from treatment with steroids such as prednisolone; adrenocorticotropin hormone (ACTH) is sometimes used instead of steroids in children as it has less effect on growth. Neoplastic causes include eutopic secretion of cortisol from an adrenal adenoma and carcinoma; pituitary adenoma secreting ACTH stimulating the adrenals bilaterally; and ectopic secretion of an ACTH-like substance from atypical carcinoid, oat cell carcinoma, and islet cell tumour of pancreas.

Conn's syndrome

Conn's syndrome is primary hyperaldosteronaemia, whether from bilateral adrenal hyperplasia of the zona glomerulosa cells of the adrenal cortex (in 65% of cases) or an adrenal adenoma which is usually unilateral (in 35% of cases). Other causes, such as adrenal carcinoma and ectopic secretion of aldosterone, are rare. It is named for Jerome W. Conn who described the condition in 1955. Secondary hyperaldosteronism is caused by congestive cardiac failure with a rise in renin secretion from the juxtaglomerular apparatus of the kidney.

The sodium retention by the kidney as a result of the excess mineralocorticoid causes expansion of the plasma volume and hypertension. The latter results in suppression of renin from the juxtaglomerular apparatus. If the patient has Conn's syndrome, the aldosterone:renin activity ratio can be measured to confirm this.

Surgery is usually curative of a solitary adenoma, provided that there is no concomitant hyperplasia of the zona glomerulosa cells adjacent to the neoplasm which might indicate bilaterality. Patients who have bilateral hyperplasia can be treated with spironolactone or other suppressive agents, or by bilateral adrenalectomy and steroid replacement therapy.

Addison's disease

Addison's disease (named for Thomas Addison, who described the disease in 1849 and 1855: his patients had bilateral adrenal tuberculosis) is a rare endocrine disorder in which the adrenal glands are severely damaged. This may be due to infection, inflammation from other causes, or failure of adequate development. The hormone deficiency that results predominantly is from inadequate steroid hormone production rather than inadequate catecholamine production.

The most common symptoms are non-specific and can be difficult to diagnose; President J. F. Kennedy had undiagnosed Addison's disease for some time. Dizziness, muscle pain and weakness, pyrexia, weight loss, postural hypotension, nausea and vomiting, diarrhoea, sweating, and swings in mood and personality are all features and all non-specific. Hyperpigmentation of the skin, especially in sun-exposed sites, skin creases, and the skin of genitalia and nipples can occur as the result of pituitary overproduction of pro-opiomelanocortin, the precursor of ACTH (as a reaction to the hypocortisolaemia) and of melanocyte-stimulating hormone.

Waterhouse–Friderichsen syndrome, in which the adrenal glands are destroyed characteristically in meningococcal septicaemia but also in any severe haemorrhagic diathesis, is not considered to be Addison's disease. Autoimmune endocrine organ destruction of the thyroid and pancreas, such as type 1 diabetes and Hashimoto's thyroiditis, occur more frequently in patients with Addison's disease. Autoimmune adrenalitis is the commonest cause of Addison's disease in the Western world.

Congenital causes of Addison's disease include adrenal agenesis or hypoplasia, and inborn errors of metabolism in terms of steroidogenesis. The commonest form of the rare condition of congenital adrenal hyperplasia (CAH) is 21-hydroxylase deficiency (95% of cases) followed by 11-hydroxylase deficiency (5% of cases). The other enzymes involved in steroidogenesis are much less commonly implicated. The surgical significance of CAH is that the consequent increase in ACTH drive will affect ectopic adrenal cortical gland rests below the capsule of the kidney and below the tunica of the testis. The diagnosis of a testicular mass as a Leydig cell tumour in a young man should raise the question of CAH as the hyperplastic ectopic adrenocortical cells can closely resemble neoplastic Leydig cells (which are also steroidogenic).

Drugs such as ketoconazole and other azole antifungals suppress the enzymes for steroid synthesis. Others stimulate liver enzymes that facilitate its capacity to metabolize steroids, such as phenytoin and some antituberculosis drugs.

Pituitary gland disease

Acromegaly

Acromegaly is the name for the range of clinical effects of excess growth hormone in an adult body, that is, in a patient beyond the age at which bone and other normal growth has ceased.

The cause of acromegaly is almost always hGH excess secreted from a somatotroph adenoma of the anterior pituitary gland. Very rarely there can be ectopic secretion of hGH from a carcinoma of the pancreas, bronchus, or small intestine.

Diseases of surgical importance caused by acromegaly include:

- osteoporosis and pathological fractures
- an increased incidence of neoplastic large bowel polyps and adenocarcinoma of large bowel: hGH acts on the liver to cause it to secrete insulin-like growth factors, which stimulate mucosal cells in the large bowel to divide
- an increased incidence of gallstones and gall bladder disease, hernia, and of the complications of diabetes mellitus
- abnormality of bite from increase in size of the mandible.

Eutopic and ectopic hormone secretion by neoplasms

Eutopic tumour secretion of hormones is from tissues that normally secrete hormones, by neoplasms that are sufficiently differentiated to do so. These include differentiated neoplasms of the:

- adrenal: adrenal adenoma and carcinoma

- thyroid: follicular adenoma (papillary adenoma does not exist) and papillary and follicular carcinoma

- pituitary: adenomas of the cells of the anterior pituitary, many of which are very rare, and carcinomas which are rarer

- liver: hepatocellular carcinoma can secrete erythropoietin (5% of plasma erythropoietin is provided by the normal liver)

- ovary: granulosa cell tumour and thecoma.

Ectopic secretion of hormones is from tumours of tissues that do not normally secrete such hormones:

- the small intestine and respiratory system can develop carcinoid tumours, atypical carcinoids and oat cell carcinoma, all of which are neuroendocrine neoplasms that can secrete 5-hydroxytryptamine, 5-hydroxytryptophane, and polypeptide sequences with the biological activity of antidiuretic hormone and adrenocorticotrophic hormone

- neoplasms of the lung, breast, kidney, pancreas, colon, and adrenal can secrete PTH-like polypeptide sequences with biological activity

- liver neoplasms, especially hepatocellular carcinoma, can secrete beta-human chorionic gonadotrophin

- pancreatic islet cell neoplasms can secrete gastrin, which is not a normal part of the repertoire of the pancreas

- medullary thyroid carcinoma, paragangliomas, prostate cancer, and islet cell neoplasms can secrete ACTH

- breast, bronchial, renal, and prostate tumours can secrete PTHrP, which is a small peptide in which 8 of the first 16 amino acids are homologous with PTH

- lymphomas can produce 1,25-dihydroxycholecalciferol.

Multiple endocrine adenopathy

Multiple endocrine adenopathy is the name for a collection of syndromes involving endocrine organs. The diseases in these organs can be hyperplasia, adenoma, or carcinoma. The syndromes run in families and tend to breed true: a family with MEA I would not be expected to develop phaeochromocytoma more often than chance. In any extended family some members might get one or two aspects of a syndrome, or in severe cases, all.

MEA I

This comprises some or all of:

- adenoma or carcinoma of the pancreatic islet cells

- adenoma (very rarely an aggressive tumour) of the pituitary

- hyperplasia of the parathyroid glands.

MEA IIa

- Medullary carcinoma of thyroid

- Phaeochromocytoma of adrenal, which may be benign or malignant and has a higher prevalence of bilaterality than in phaeochromocytomas not related to MEA II

- Hyperplasia of the parathyroid glands.

MEA IIb

- Medullary carcinoma of thyroid

- Phaeochromocytoma of adrenal, which may be benign or malignant and has a higher prevalence of bilaterality than in phaeochromocytomas not related to MEA II

- Submucosal neurofibromas of the palate

- Hyperplasia of the parathyroid glands.

Vascular diseases of surgical importance

Atheroma

Cholesterol handling

Most cholesterol in the body is made by human cells—only about 1 g/day of preformed cholesterol is absorbed from food. Cholesterol is needed in general for plasma membrane synthesis, for steroid hormone production in the adrenal cortices and gonads, and for vitamin D synthesis in the skin.

The plasma cholesterol concentration is controlled by cytochrome P450-mediated oxidases in the liver; the cholesterol is metabolised into the bile acids cholic acid and chenodeoxycholic acid. These are then conjugated principally with glycine and tauric acid to form bile salts. Normal bile contains cholesterol, bile acids, and bile salts. Almost all of the cholesterol metabolites are reabsorbed in the small intestine linked to lipids from the diet, with which they form micelles necessary for lipid digestion.

Bacterial enzymes in the large bowel dehydroxylate the small proportion of cholesterol metabolites that are not absorbed into secondary bile acids, deoxycholic acid and lithocholic acid; cholic acid becomes deoxycholic acid, chenodeoxycholic acid becomes lithocholic acid. All four bile acids can be reabsorbed and resecreted by the liver.

Low-density lipoprotein

An LDL particle is formed of an apolipoprotein molecule linked with phospholipids synthesized in the liver. This has a hydrophobic layer which wraps around over 1000 cholesterol molecules. Because LDL particles can also transport cholesterol into the artery wall, increased levels are associated with atheroma. The lipid is fixed in the intima by macrophages that engulf the LDL particles and start the formation of plaques.

High-density lipoprotein

HDL particles are smaller than LDL particles—they contain the highest ratio of apolipoprotein to cholesterol. They internalize cholesterol from cell cytoplasm and from other lipoproteins and transport it to the liver and steroid-producing organs. They can remove cholesterol from an atheromatous plaque and carry it to the liver for excretion. Patients with high levels of HDL have relatively low rates of cardiovascular disease, those with low levels of HDL have higher.

HDLs and their contents have antioxidant properties, mediate anti-inflammatory effects, and inhibit platelet aggregation. The acute phase apolipoprotein serum amyloid A (SAA) protein is produced by the liver in response to stress in response to interleukins released from macrophages at an inflamed site. It carries glucocorticoids from the adrenal to sites of inflammation, where it is chemotactic and stimulatory for leucocytes. In its usual low and temporary plasma concentrations, SAA protein is soluble and harmless, but in severe unremitting chronic inflammatory conditions such as rheumatoid arthritis and bronchiectasis, the prolonged exposure causes polymerization of SAA protein in the tissues into insoluble amyloid material.

Atheroma/atherosclerosis

Atheroma or atherosclerosis is the term used for arterial-wall deposits of lipid material which may progress to pools of lipid in the intima and sometimes deeper into the media called atheroma. Many people use these two terms interchangeably for the whole disease process. Atheroma is a disease of elastic and medium-sized muscular arteries down to 1 mm in diameter. The abdominal aorta and the left anterior descending coronary artery (LAD) are the commonest sites of atheroma; the LAD is the commonest site to develop complications of atheroma. The changes in sequence classically begin with endothelial cell interactions with leucocytes, platelets, and myofibroblasts. There is endothelial cell injury from free radical formation from several factors: LDL and the cholesterol carried by it impair the ability of the smooth muscle cells in the wall to contract and dilate, and the antioxidant properties of the endothelial cells is exceeded; hyperglycaemia and chemicals from cigarette smoke damage the metabolism of endothelial cells; and inflammatory mediators from leucocytes cause further damage.[17]

Macrophages derived from monocytes in the circulation enter the intima and phagocytose LDL cholesterol to form characteristic cells with intracellular lipid called foam cells. They secrete cytokines which injure the endothelium further and add to inflammation in the affected intima. As well as the build-up of LDL cholesterol and phospholipids, calcium is deposited and there is developing fibrosis leading to plaque formation with a lipid pool under the fibrous plaque. The flow of blood in the artery is increasingly deranged contributing to platelet deposition and surface thrombosis.

The American Heart Association[18] has classified the changes into six stages leading to the development of full-blown atheromatous disease:

Stage I   Scattered foamy macrophages in the arterial intima

Stage II   Fatty streaks in the intima visible to the naked eye, in which there are more closely aggregated foamy macrophages

Stage III Scattered collections of extracellular lipid in the intima

Stage IV   Pools of extracellular lipid that in time coalesce into a single pool

Stage V   Fibroblasts around the lipid pool secrete tropocollagen which trimerizes into fibrous tissue; dystrophic calcification starts to become common

Stage VI   Complicated atheromatous disease develops with endothelial cell loss and surface thrombus formation; embolization of this and of atheromatous lipid from a ruptured plaque can occur; calcification can become severe.

Reproduced from *Stroke*, Volume 43, Issue 12, Karen L. Furie *et al.*, Oral Antithrombotic Agents for the Prevention of Stroke in Nonvalvular Atrial Fibrillation: A Science Advisory for Healthcare Professionals From the American Heart Association/American Stroke Association, pp. 3442–53, 2012. With permission from Wolters Kluwer Health.

Risk factors in general include being a man, having a family history of atheroma or a complication of it (such as a stroke or myocardial infarct), and having one of the high-risk familial hyperlipidaemias. More specific risk factors include a high plasma concentration of LDL and a low concentration of HDL; hypothyroidism, for example, causes plasma LDL and cholesterol concentrations to rise. The effectiveness of drugs intended to lower cholesterol is debated. Hypertension per se increases the risk of atheroma, as do diabetes mellitus and cigarette smoking. Other factors that probably contribute to some extent include lack of exercise, obesity, high dietary saturated fats, and gout.[19]

The serious complications of atheroma include ischaemia from gradual occlusion of the artery from accumulation of lipid in the plaque; haemorrhage into or rupture of a plaque causing rapid thrombus formation; embolus from a plaque, which may be thrombus from the surface or lipid from the lipid pool; and eventually aneurysm formation.

Aneurysms

An aneurysm is an abnormal localized dilatation of a blood vessel including arteries, the heart, arterioles, and veins in descending frequency. Aneurysmal dilatation of lymphatic vessels may rarely occur.

They are classified variously into:

◆ congenital or acquired: congenital causes include full malformation of vessels, such as veins as in a cirsoid aneurysm of scalp; or malformation of part of a vessel wall, such as in a berry aneurysm of the anterior communicating branch of the circle of Willis, in which there is a congenital deficiency in the media of the artery which manifests as an aneurysm only in adult life

◆ true or false: whether all three layers of the wall are present in the aneurysm or only some, respectively

◆ by shape: saccular if only part of the circumference is involved, fusiform if the entire circumference is involved, and dissecting when the arterial media is deficient

◆ by cause, probably the most informative classification

  • atheroma: descending aorta below the renal arteries below the renal arteries, and the LAD

  • syphilis: dissecting aneurysm of the aorta because of thrombosis of the vasa vasorum in which the *Treponema pallidum* organisms live

  • Erdheim's cystic medionecrosis and Marfan's syndrome from damage to the aortic media. Both of these conditions are autosomal dominant

  • mycotic: low-grade bacterial infection or rarely fungal infection

  • inflammatory other than the above listed: polyarteritis nodosa, aortitis in ankylosing spondylitis

  • ischaemic: ventricular aneurysm after myocardial infarction

  • traumatic: from a penetrating injury, deceleration trauma, and subclavian artery damage from a cervical rib

  • hypertension: microaneurysms in the lenticulosriate artery

  • iatrogenic: arteriovenous aneurysm in a dialysis shunt.

The complications of an aneurysm are internal and external. Internal complications include thrombosis with ischaemic effects, and embolism. External complications usually occur later: from pressure effects in the thorax from an aneurysm of the arch of the aorta on the oesophagus, vertebral column, and sternum, or from an abdominal aortic aneurysm compressing the inferior vena cava; and external haemorrhage from rupture with or without dissection.

Compartment syndrome

Compartment syndrome is caused when the pressure in a closed anatomical space exceeds the perfusion pressure of the blood passing through it. The consequent reduction or cessation of circulation may cause temporary or permanent ischaemic damage to muscles, tendons, and nerves. Acute compartment syndrome comprises recurrent pain and disability on exercise which subside when the exercise is stopped. The pain is induced by passive movement and is intense, out of proportion to the physical clinical changes on examination of the affected part. Late changes indicative of permanent damage are pallor and pulselessness. There is a chronic counterpart of the acute syndrome, in which the volume of the compartment is permanently restricted because of thickened fascia and muscle hypertrophy.

Causes of acute compartment syndrome can be divided into those from external restriction and those from internal restriction. The first include direct physical trauma to a compartment; iatrogenic causes, such as tight fascial closure and tight splints or plaster casts; burns with formation of tight eschar; and very tight clothing. Internal causes include acute bleeding after direct trauma, fractures, or operative surgery; bleeding diatheses; crush injuries and deep burns; and any cause of severe rhabdomyolysis such as drug overdose and snake bite.

Sites typically affected by acute compartment syndrome are the limbs. The forearm has two related compartments, the leg four, and the foot several. The abdomen can develop compartment syndrome after repair of an abdominal aortic aneurysm. Affected indirectly are the kidneys, by acute tubular necrosis from myoglobinaemia, and the heart from the related hyperkalaemia.

Ischaemia reperfusion injury

Ischaemia reperfusion injury is the damage that results from sudden re-introduction of oxygenated blood to an area of ischaemia. There is cellular damage from oxygen free radicals, DNA breaks, and enzyme disruption. Activation of prostaglandins and the complement system causes further inflammatory effects including platelet–leucocyte aggregation, leucocyte–endothelial cell adhesion, and increased vascular permeability. These changes can affect any reperfused tissues, such as muscles in compartment syndrome and after prolonged tourniquet use, the heart after cardiopulmonary bypass, and the liver during liver surgery and transplantation.

Treatment is often difficult. Possible approaches include:

* ischaemic preconditioning where appropriate
* controlled reperfusion
* antioxidant therapy
* prostaglandin inhibition by indomethacin.

Injury and mechanical abnormalities

Endogenous

Herniation

A hernia is a protrusion of tissue from the body compartment in which it is anatomically correct into another body compartment. Predisposing factors include increased pressure in the donor compartment coupled with an actual or incipient weakness in the boundary of the compartment. In the abdomen, this can result in inguinal, femoral, and obturator hernias, and diaphragmatic hernias such as hiatus hernia and those of Morgagni and Bochdalek. In the CNS, increased intracranial pressure can result in herniation of the cingulate gyrus underneath the falx, of the uncus through the tentorium, and of parts of the cerebellum through the foramen magnum.

Other predisposing factors are that there might be congenital absence of normal tissue at a site, such as congenital diaphragmatic hernia with aplastic muscle, or weakness of tissues with normal pressure in the donor compartment, as in an incisional hernia. General factors such as nutrition and immunodeficiency are also important.

The complications of herniation are mainly from pressure effects. There may be obstruction of a hollow viscus such as the small and large intestines (including the appendix) in lower abdominal hernias, and with incarceration and ischaemia or infarction. In the upper abdomen, the effects might be on the upper alimentary system, such as reflux or obstruction, or might be on adjacent organs and cause respiratory compromise and cardiac arrhythmias. In the CNS, the complications are not usually the loss of function of the herniated element but of the part of the brain compressed as a consequence: in the list above these would be the corpus callosum, the midbrain, and the brainstem, respectively.

Diverticula

A diverticulum is an abnormal outpouching of a hollow viscus. Diverticula are classified as congenital and acquired, true and false, and pulsion and traction. True diverticula have all of the components of the wall and are usually the result of congenital malformation, for example, Meckel's diverticulum in the ileum and duodenal diverticula. False diverticula have only part of the wall of the viscus present and tend to be acquired, such as sigmoid, bladder, and oesophageal diverticula.

The complications of diverticula are characteristically the consequences of abnormal anatomy and the predisposition to inflammation and infection: haemorrhage, abscess and fistula formation, and perforation. Inflammation may lead to metaplasia, dysplasia, and malignant change, as in a bladder diverticulum. There may be ectopic gastric and pancreatic tissues in a Meckel's diverticulum, with ulceration as a consequence of the former, and a small tendency to torsion because of the abnormal anatomy. Duodenal diverticula may become colonized by bacteria and result in the blind loop syndrome with vitamin deficiencies.

Exogenous

Fractures and fracture healing

Fractures are classified by[20]:

* location: by the name of the fractured bone and the position of the fracture within that bone, such as fracture through the neck of the femur

- fracture line:
  - transverse, when the line is at 90° to the long axis of the bone
  - oblique when the line is at a straight angle
  - spiral when the line curves, usually resulting from a twisting force
  - comminuted, when more than two fragments are present—this might be segmental, in which the bone is fractured at two separate levels
  - impacted, when the ends are driven together
  - compressed, as in vertebral body fracture
  - depressed, by a localized force that moves one aspect of the fracture site inwards or downwards
- displacement: when bone fragments have moved and are not in alignment.

Fracture healing

From the moment of fracture, there are seven typical stages in the healing of a fracture of a long bone. The first is haematoma formation, the size of which is limited by arterial contraction and by the pressure of the periosteum when it is intact. The second, inflammatory phase follows the usual processes of acute inflammation with vasodilatation, exudate formation, and polymorph infiltration. The demolition phase begins when the inflammatory process becomes chronic: local and recruited macrophages digest the haematoma and with osteoclasts remove dead bone fragments. Organization follows with granulation tissue extending from below the periosteum and out of the fractured bone ends.

In the later stages there is first early callus formation, in which osteoid fibres (a form of collagen) are laid down rapidly and randomly and mineralize to form woven bone, so-called because the pattern of fibres resembles felt, with no organized Haversian canals at this stage. There may also be cartilage formation. Late callus formation follows, when the woven bone is slowly and precisely absorbed by osteoclasts, and osteoblasts lay down lamellar bone with Haversian systems. The final stage, which can take months or years, is remodelling during which the normal shapes of the bone and bone marrow are resumed.

Abnormalities of fracture healing are essentially defects in union of the bone. The most severe is *non-union*, usually as a consequence of interposition between the bone ends of connective tissues, such as muscle or fascia, and sometimes a foreign body. *Delayed union* may result from infection, particularly in compound fractures; movement of the fracture site; presence of a foreign body; and ischaemia which especially affects fractures of the neck of the femur, the shaft of the tibia, and the scaphoid bone. *Malunion* refers to healing that has not followed the usual processes; an example is *fibrous union* when there is excessive fibrous tissue between the fracture ends that permits movement, possibly after repeated fractures at the same site. In some of these pseudarthroses can develop. Osteoarthrosis in the joints above and below the fracture site is the commonest long-term outcome of abnormal union.

Pathological fractures

A pathological fracture is one through a previously abnormal bone, irrespective of the force of the physical trauma. The underling bone disease can be anything that weakens the bone. The two commonest diseases associated with pathological fracture are osteoporosis and metastatic carcinoma. Less common are metabolic bone diseases such as vitamin D deficiency causing rickets with greenstick fractures and osteomalacia, and bone diseases seen in chronic renal failure and primary hyperparathyroidism. Primary bone neoplasms, Paget's disease of bone, and radionecrosis after radiotherapy also cause pathological fracture. Probably the rarest cause is congenital bone disease such as osteogenesis imperfecta.

Burns

Many injurious agents can cause some of the tissue changes found in burns of the skin, but the characteristic causes are thermal injury producing cell damage by protein coagulation, chemical damage destroying cell membranes and organelles directly, and ionizing radiation inducing free-radical formation. Thermal injury could be from the effects of excessive heat, for example, from fire, hot solids like kettles, hot liquids such as water or fat, and from severe friction. Electric current of a high voltage also produces thermal burns.

Chemical injury may be from spillage of corrosives such as acids, alkalis and other industrial products, and from naturally-occurring irritants like the sap of *Rhus typhina*, which cause mild burns in some people but severe burns in many people if they are exposed to sunlight at the same time as the sap (photophytodermatosis). Ionizing radiation causes burns by providing the energy for free-radical formation and also DNA damage.

There are classically three zones of overlapping but recognizable histological change in a burn. In the central part is the coagulation zone, of dead tissue in which the proteins have coagulated and the DNA destroyed. Around this and deep to it is the zone of ischaemia, in which the tissues are viable but subject to sufficient vascular damage that they will die after some days if untreated. Around both of the first two zones is the hyperaemic zone, in which the tissues are not fatally injured and develop vasodilatation from the vascular effects of inflammatory mediators.

Classification of burns

Skin burns are classified in terms of the extent of the burn, the depth of tissue destruction, the prognostic outcome, and by the risk to specific people in a population.

The extent of burns is determined by the percentage of body area involved, estimated by the 'rule of 9s':

- head and neck 9%
- upper limb each 9%
- front of thorax and abdomen 18%
- back of thorax and abdomen 18%
- lower limb each 18%
- genitalia 1%.

In young children, the head is proportionately much bigger and the lower limbs smaller than in adults. Their percentages are reversed—the head and neck in children 18%, the lower limbs each 9%. In terms of risk, the high-risk group includes children under 10 years and adults over 50 years and the low-risk group, patients aged 10–50 years.[21]

A first-degree burn involves only the epidermis. It may have the three zones on histology just described but the central necrotic zone can be very small or missing. The burn is hot, erythematous, and oedematous but does not blister. It remains painful for 2–3 days and usually heals within a week without treatment; lasting tissue damage like fibrosis is rare but pigmentation changes can take months to resolve.

A second-degree burn involves the epidermis and the dermis but not the subcutis. The depth of dermal damage has prognostic importance. The burn has a variegated appearance: it is usually dark red with blister formation and shiny from exudate, with areas of pale grey necrotic tissue. Pain lasts for more than a week. The degree of scarring depends on whether the burn involves superficial dermis alone or the deep dermis as well. In general, superficial second-degree burns heal in about 3 weeks, deep second-degree burns take longer than that.

A third-degree burn destroys tissue at least as far as subcutis. The burn is painless as the dermal nerve-endings are necrotic or vaporized, and is usually pale, dry and rough or black with eschar (Latin *eschara*, a hearth, hence the mark left by a burn). These burns do not heal without debridement and skin coverage, and even then are prone to severe scarring.

In terms of risk and prognosis, burns can be assessed by a combination of several variables.

◆ Minor burns include:
  • partial thickness burns involving less than 15% of body surface area (BSA) in low-risk patients
  • partial thickness burns involving 10% of BSA in high-risk patients
  • full thickness burns of less than 2% of BSA with no other injuries.

◆ Moderate burns include:
  • partial thickness burns of 15–25% of BSA in low-risk patients
  • partial thickness burns of 10–20% of BSA in high-risk patients
  • full thickness burns of 3–10% of BSA with no other injuries.

◆ Major burns include:
  • partial thickness burns of more than 25% of BSA in low-risk patients
  • burns involving the face, hands, feet, or perineum
  • burns involving major joints of a limb
  • burns complicated by:
    ▪ severe electrical damage
    ▪ inhalation injury
    ▪ fractures.

Apart from the direct tissue damage, complications of burns include compartment syndrome, renal damage from myoglobinaemia, hypoproteinaemia, and hypovolaemia, and laryngeal oedema.

Nerve injuries

Nerve injuries are classified in general as *neuropraxia*, axonotmesis, and neurotmesis. *Neuropraxia* (Greek *praxis*, acting on) is a relatively minor injury to a nerve that recovers complete function. The damage involves only the myelin sheath while the extent of the axon remains intact and so there is no Wallerian degeneration. *Axontmesis* (Greek *tmesis*, a cut) refers to injury to the myelin sheath

and to the axon but the rest of the nerve remains with an intact endoneurial sheath and Schwann cell continuity. There is Wallerian degeneration distal to the injury but the axon will normally regrow along the sheath. In *neurotmesis* the whole nerve or nerve bundle is cut across and normal axonal regeneration cannot occur—worse, fibrosis occurs within the nerve sheath and forms a barrier to axonal regeneration. Complete recovery is therefore unlikely.

Nerves can be damaged by several mechanisms of surgical importance, the commonest being trauma. This can be from intentional penetrating injuries from knives or bullets and accidental penetrating injuries from car crashes, falling glass, and tin-opener mishaps. Nerve injury from fractures is uncommon but a recognizable complication, especially in the upper limb: radial nerve damage is caused by fracture of the humerus, and fracture-dislocation of the elbow causes ulnar nerve discontinuations. In the compartment syndrome (which may itself be due to trauma) there may be nerve compression and discontinuity. Compression injury to nerves is also caused by scar contraction and nerve trapping, and in stretch injury there is typically axonotmesis with disruption of axons over long segments.

Degenerations and accumulations

Cyst formation

A cyst is an abnormal fluid-filled cavity characteristically lined by epithelial cells. Amoebic cysts of the liver and spleen have no specific epithelial cell lining but are still called cysts. The cysts of cysticercosis are the intermediate stage in the life cycle of *Taenia solium* and consist of the organism itself with no human epithelial covering. The so-called cysts reported radiologically in diseases such as osteoarthritis are usually solid but transradient and have no specific lining.

Cysts can be congenital or acquired and arise from several processes:

◆ congenital cysts are usually from failure of a duct system to develop properly, such as pancreaticobiliary and renal cysts, or in the case of thyroglossal and branchial cysts, failure to regress properly. Less commonly, extraneous tissue can be included in developmental infoldings, as with dermoid cysts of the face and head

◆ inflammatory cysts are also often the result of obstruction of a ductal system by the inflammatory process. Examples include hydrosalpinx and true pancreatic cyst formation in chronic pancreatitis (as opposed to pseudocyst formation in the lesser sac). Specific organisms such as *Echinococcus granulosus* (causing hydatid disease) and *Taenia solium* have cystic forms in human beings

◆ ischaemia can cause cystic degeneration in leiomyomas and cerebral infarcts but these have no specific epithelial lining

◆ traumatic implantation of surface epithelium can result in cyst formation, as in implantation epidermal cyst and dermal cyst of skin

◆ cysts may be found in hyperplastic tissues such as the endometrium and breast

◆ neoplasia especially in the ovary and pancreas. Large parathyroid adenomas are almost always cystic, though there is no specific epithelial lining.

Calculi

A calculus (Latin *calculus*, a pebble or small stone) is an abnormal mass of solid material precipitated in a duct or bladder. They can be primary, from an increase in the concentration of solute in a solution beyond the capacity for the solvent to carry it. This occurs, for example, in the urinary system in gout when urate calculi form, and in the gallbladder with pigment calculi as the result of haemolytic anaemia. Secondary calculi are secondary to decrease in solvent, stasis, change of pH, nidus formation, or any combination of these. For example, in pyelonephritis the nidus might be a necrotic fragment of a renal papilla and the infecting organism (such as *Proteus* spp.) which causes the urinary pH to rise, resulting in a staghorn calculus that exacerbates the condition with stasis.

Given the conditions for primary or secondary calculus formation, in theory they can develop in any ductal system, but the classic sites are the prostatic ducts, the pancreaticobiliary system, the urinary system, and the salivary ducts, especially the submandibular duct. Corpora amylacea in the prostate ducts are almost universal in men over 65 years and are the commonest kind of calculi, formed of inspissated secretions. In the biliary system, calculi are characteristically derived from cholesterol metabolism or bilirubin metabolism, with a small proportion composed of calcium carbonate. In the kidney, secondary calculi of calcium, magnesium, and ammonium salts are the commonest; primary calculi include urate, oxalate, cysteine, and xanthine stones.

Complications of calculi in general include haemorrhage, obstruction, and tendency to infection. There may be physical obstruction in the pancreaticobiliary system, obstructed by fibrous stricture, and in rare cases gallstone ileus from obstruction of the small bowel after fistulation from the gall bladder to the duodenum. In the urinary tract, there can be obstruction by the calculus itself or as a consequence of fibrosis from inflammation caused by the calculus, which leads to hydronephrosis, hydroureter, and a predisposition to ascending infection. Inflammation also causes squamous metaplasia generally, and carcinoma of the bladder if the calculus is present for some time.

Amyloidosis

The term amyloid was first used in 1839 to describe a semigelatinous starch-like thickening in seeds, and first used to describe a substance in human organs of similar appearance by Rokitansky 3 years later. It is not one substance but a collection of disparate proteins, all of which have a beta-pleated sheet structure (cross-beta structure). Most mammalian systems have no enzymes that will denature these proteins. On Congo red stain histologically, most of the proteins in this group have apple-green birefringence (dichroic birefringence) under polarized light; polarization is important as Congo red stains many tissues, but only the amyloids have the green dichroic colour change. Several recently described amyloids do not stain well with Congo red but do have the expected tertiary structure. Amyloid is not only a human product: it is present in spider silk, some *Escherichia coli* bacteria, and some fungi.

Amyloid used to be classified as primary or secondary, but there was a large overlap between these groups and they took no account of localized deposition. Classification is now by the specific protein deposited. AL (previously primary) amyloid and AA (previously secondary) amyloid produce generalized disease. Aβ or AH amyloid is found adjacent to the neurofibrillary tangles in Alzheimer's disease. Tumour amyloid deposits are found in medullary carcinoma of the thyroid, in which the amyloid is calcitonin; in renal cell carcinoma, mesothelioma, Hodgkin's disease, and some other lymphomas the amyloid is AA type. Deposition of amyloid material around invasive lobular carcinoma of breast has been reported but this was not typed.

AL amyloid, also called light-chain amyloid, used to be called primary amyloid. The disease is found in patients with myeloma, especially IgG and IgA myelomas, and is the result of polymerization in the tissues of immunoglobulin light chains, especially lambda chains. AL amyloid deposits predominate in the heart causing restrictive heart muscle disease; in arteriole walls in skin and deeper tissues related to carpal tunnel syndrome; and in nerves generally or with specific involvement at certain sites causing sweating abnormalities and impotence.

AA amyloid is produced as part of chronic inflammation that persists for years. Stimulated macrophages secrete IL-1 and IL-6 which cause hepatocytes to release SAA, the soluble amyloid precursor. This is a normal, soluble acute phase protein (an apoprotein) that has immunomodulatory effects but polymerizes over time into insoluble amyloid AA. Deposits are found predominately in the kidney, in the glomeruli, renal arterioles, and renal tubules causing nephrotic syndrome; in the spleen, where function is rarely affected; and in the liver in the space of Disse where function is also rarely affected.

Chronic inflammatory diseases causing AA amyloidosis continue for many years. These can include tuberculosis, leprosy, chronic osteomyelitis, bronchiectasis, and Whipple's disease. Rheumatoid arthritis is the commonest cause of AA amyloidosis in the United Kingdom. Familial Mediterranean fever is a congenital chronic inflammatory condition in which IL-1 is unsuppressed and so is permanently higher than normal and raises the SAA concentration. The neoplasms associated with amyloidosis were mentioned earlier; it is likely that the amyloid arises from inflammatory mediators with macrophage stimulation in these cases except for medullary carcinoma of the thyroid.

Deposits of amyloid unassociated with neoplasia can be found rarely in the thyroid, where it diffusely surrounds follicles. It is more commonly seen in the pancreatic islets in patients with diabetes mellitus, where it is composed of calcitonin gene-related peptide and other peptides. Rounded masses of amyloid can occur idiopathically anywhere in the urinary and respiratory tracts and can cause obstruction.

Disorders of differentiation and growth

Deficiencies of initial growth

Agenesis, aplasia, hypoplasia, and atresia

Agenesis is complete failure of an organ or tissue to develop. For example, agenesis of one or more branchial pouches can cause absence of the thymus and parathyroid glands; agenesis of part of a lung in a fetus will cause compensatory emphysema of the formed lung in the neonate, but if more severe will be fatal—neonates must have two lungs to survive, unlike adults.

Aplasia is when there is recognizable tissue present but no indication of differentiation. Hypoplasia is the failure of an organ or tissue to reach a proper size or function. Atresia is the failure of the development of a lumen in a normally hollow structure such as the bile ducts, alimentary system, or choanae, and is a type of aplasia.

Changes in growth in formed tissues

Atrophy

Atrophy is the degeneration of a tissue from its normally developed state to one in which there is a decrease in the normal cell size, cell number, or both. Essentially atrophy is the result of the rate of cell death exceeding the rate of cell proliferation. It is classified into physiological and pathological types. Physiological atrophy occurs in the developing fetus and neonate in the ductus arteriosus, hypogastric arteries, thyroglossal duct, branchial clefts, and notochord. In later life, the thymus normally undergoes atrophy, as does lymphoid tissue generally, and after the menopause there is atrophy of the uterus, vagina, and breasts.

Pathological atrophy is caused by starvation of general nutrients and specifics such as proteins and vitamins. Atrophy of localized parts may be due to disuse from neuropathies; immobilization; fracture; obstruction to a drainage system; and pressure effects such as of an aortic aneurysm on vertebral bone. Some tissues may atrophy for unknown reasons, such as the testis and eye.

Hyperplasia and hypertrophy

Hyperplasia is an increase of the size of an organ or tissue because of an increase in the number of its cells. Hypertrophy is an increase in the size of an organ or tissue because of an increase in the size of its cells. They can occur together, as in the thyroid gland in Graves' disease and in the prostate in nodular prostatic enlargement. Both can be caused by physiological and pathological stimuli. In pregnancy, there is hyperplasia of the breasts and hypertrophy of the uterus (and in late pregnancy a small degree of hyperplasia); the thyroid in pregnancy is stimulated by human chorionic thyrotropin from the placenta and develops hyperplasia and hypertrophy, usually only to a small degree; the lactotrophs of the pituitary undergo hyperplasia because of stimulation by placental oestrogen and increased prolactin secretion. Skeletal muscle undergoes hypertrophy from exercise.

Pathological hyperplasia and hypertrophy can be idiopathic or be caused by a known stimulating process. Idiopathic examples of hyperplasia include parathyroid hyperplasia from an unknown cause in primary hyperparathyroidism and hyperaldosteronism from idiopathic adrenal hyperplasia. The smooth muscle hypertrophy that accompanies hyperplasia in nodular prostatic enlargement is also idiopathic. Known causes of hyperplasia include excess hormone drive, inflammation, and drugs. The hormone drive on some of the effector organs includes, for example, excess oestrogen from an ovarian granulosa cell tumour or thecoma causing endometrial hyperplasia, and a pituitary adenoma secreting excess ACTH and very rarely TSH and follicle-stimulating hormone causing adrenal, thyroid and ovarian hyperplasia. Chronic gingivitis can cause gum hyperplasia, as can antiepileptic drugs. Pathological hypertrophy of cardiac muscle occurs as a consequence of hypertension and several congenital diseases affecting blood flow and direction.

Metaplasia

Metaplasia is defined as a change of one fully differentiated cell type into another fully differentiated cell type. The commonest type is epithelial metaplasia—connective tissue metaplasia is much more rarely encountered. Metaplasia is named for the new epithelial type after the change. Squamous metaplasia forms in glandular and transitional cell epithelia; it develops characteristically in the bladder after calculi and schistosoma infection; in the prostate after transurethral resection, and also in men on antiandrogen therapy for carcinoma. Glandular metaplasia can be found in the bladder as cystitis glandularis, and in glandular organs when there is change from one fully differentiated glandular mucosal type into another—intestinal metaplasia is common in the stomach associated with *Helicobacter pylori* infection; and apocrine metaplasia in the breast is true metaplasia as the breast is a modified eccrine sweat gland.

The surgical significance of metaplasia is that dysplastic and neoplastic change can occur in areas of metaplasia. In the bladder, squamous metaplasia from infection by *Schistosoma haematobium* and occasionally *S. mansoni* in the bladder can develop into SCC. Squamous metaplasia in the bronchus is caused by smoking and inhalation of industrial gases, and if the stimulus for the metaplasia persists and is carcinogenic the patient can develop squamous dysplasia and SCC. In the cervix at puberty, the endocervical glandular mucosa everts and becomes exposed to the acidic milieu of the vagina; the squamous metaplasia that results is more prone to infection by human papilloma virus (HPV) infection and to develop cervical intraepithelial neoplasia and SCC.

Patients with Barret's oesophagus are more likely to develop adenocarcinoma of the oesophagus than carcinoma of the oesophagus. In Barrett's oesophagus, there is metaplasia to gastric mucosa or intestinal mucosa with acid mucin demonstrable in goblet cells (the normal stomach has neutral mucin and no goblet cells). The risk of malignant change appears to be less than originally considered; a recent series of 11 000 patients with Barrett's oesophagus found that in those without dysplasia the risk was 1 case in 1000 patient-years rising to 5.1 cases in 1000 patient-years when dysplasia is present.

Another aspect of surgical importance is that metaplasia can be misdiagnosed. Cystitis glandularis can be misdiagnosed clinically and histologically as dysplastic epithelium and sometimes adenocarcinoma if there is significant inflammatory atypia with hyperchromatism of the metaplastic cells. Florid changes in a Barret's oesophagus can be mistaken for carcinoma on endoscopy.

The principal examples of connective tissue metaplasia are osseous, chondroid, and myeloid metaplasias. The first two can form hard nodules in an abdominal scar many years after bowel resection and so be clinically suspected of being metastatic deposits. A focus of osseous metaplasia can arise in the bladder wall in association with previous surgery at that site. Myeloid metaplasia occurs in the liver, spleen, and lymph nodes if the marrow is unable to function because of widespread bone involvement by myelofibrosis.

Hamartoma and choristoma

A hamartoma (Greek *hamartanein* to err), is a non-neoplastic malformation composed of a haphazard arrangement of different amounts of the tissues *normally* found at that site. A choristoma is the same but formed of tissues *not normally* found at that site. In almost all cases, hamartomas and choristomas stop growing when the patient is about 20 years old, and may regress spontaneously. In surgical practice, both of these defects cause the symptoms and signs of benign neoplasms, they can be mistaken for malignancy, and they can develop malignancy.

Hamartomas occur in the alimentary system classically in Peutz–Jeghers syndrome, an autosomal dominant condition in which there is the development of small and large bowel polyps composed of mucosa, lamina propria, and a tree-like pattern of muscularis mucosa. The last element distinguishes these polyps from neoplastic polyps, irrespective of the presence or absence of dysplasia in the epithelium of the polyp. They are associated with patchy pigmentation (lentigines) around the lips, gingiva, and anus. Hamartoma of the bronchus (called chondroadenoma though it is not a neoplasm) is usually symptomless and found incidentally on chest radiography but can sometimes obstruct the bronchus and adjacent airways. Splenic hamartoma is usually asymptomatic but is very vascular and can spontaneously rupture. Rhabdomyoma of the heart is associated with tuberous sclerosis, in which there are multiple hamartomas in the CNS. Hamartoma of the hypothalamus causes epilepsy, pressure features, and precocious puberty. Malignant change in a hamartoma is rare; a Peutz–Jeghers polyp can become adenocarcinoma, neurofibrosarcoma can supervene in a patient with von Recklinghausen's disease, and chondrosarcoma can arise in an osteochondroma (cartilage-capped exostosis) especially when the cartilage does not regress after the patient is 20 years old.

Choristomas most commonly present with pressure effects. They are commonest in the central and peripheral nervous systems, such as on the facial and trigeminal nerves and in the posterior pituitary. The anterior pituitary may develop a neuronal choristoma, which is classically associated with growth hormone secretion and acromegaly. Choristomas composed of salivary gland acini and ducts can be found in the middle ear.

Dysplasia

Dysplasia is failure of maturation of a tissue associated with a tendency to aneuploidy and pleomorphism but without the capacity for invasive spread. Severe dysplasia has all of the characteristics of malignancy but with no stromal invasion. At specific sites, such as the colon and rectum, dysplastic epithelium can become polypoid and form a neoplastic polyp of large bowel. As this part of the gastrointestinal system has few lymphatic channels, even if the dysplastic epithelium appears to invade the lamina propria it will behave in a biologically benign fashion (though follow-up is important).

There is therefore no concept of carcinoma *in situ* of the large bowel. Only when invasion through the muscularis mucosae has occurred will the neoplastic cells meet lymphatics and gain metastatic potential. This situation does not apply to severe gastric dysplasia and gastric carcinoma *in situ*, as the stomach mucosa has extensive lymphatic drainage.

Histological changes characteristic of dysplasia are pleomorphism and hyperchromatism because of aneuploidy, loss of cohesion between cells, and increased numbers of normal mitoses, and abnormal mitoses such as starburst mitoses, tripolar mitoses, and bizarre mitoses. In the squamous epithelium of a flat or elevated epithelium severely infected by HPV the basal levels are indistinguishable from the highest levels, and there is cell shedding because cohesion is lost. A cuboidal epithelium may develop multilayering. By similar virus, irritant and other effects other tissues can be involved.

In some organs, such as the stomach, the severity of these changes might indicate carcinoma *in situ*, but for a diagnosis of dysplasia there must be no invasion into the underlying connective tissues.

Sites in the body of surgical importance at which dysplasia is relatively common include the stomach in patients with *Helicobacter pylori* infection and intestinal metaplasia; the large bowel when it is extensively and unremittingly inflamed with ulcerative colitis; the bronchus in patients who smoke; and in the oesophagus in patients with Barrett's mucosa and glandular dysplasia, or with candidiasis and squamous dysplasia. The cervix is by far the commonest site in the body involved by dysplasia as cervical intraepithelial neoplasia, but this is unlikely to come to general surgical attention (unlike frank carcinoma of the cervix). The causes of dysplasia are essentially those of neoplasia in general.

Neoplasia

'A neoplasm is an abnormal mass of tissue, the growth of which exceeds and is uncoordinated with that of the normal tissues, and persists in the same excessive manner after cessation of the stimuli which evoked the change' (R.A. Willis, 1952). The common word 'tumour' should be used only when the context is clear, such as when it is obvious that a benign or a malignant neoplasm is being referred to. The word is often used when there is no neoplasm at all: nodular prostatic enlargement is sometimes called a 'tumour'. Conversely, some neoplasms such as leukaemia do not form a recognizable mass or tumour. Used without context, 'tumour' simply means a mass or swelling and implies no predictions of behaviour.

Properly used, the terms 'benign' and 'malignant' refer only to neoplasms—if a swelling is not a neoplasm, the terms are meaningless. No one would call a mass malignant if it was not a neoplasm, but many non-neoplastic masses are called benign. In general usage, a corpus luteum cyst of ovary is called a benign ovarian cyst but it is not neoplastic, has no neoplastic potential, and can behave in a very non-benign way if it ruptures. The common enlargement of the prostate is called benign prostatic hyperplasia, though it is not.

Carcinogenesis

Physical carcinogenesis

The relation between ionizing radiation and heat with DNA and RNA damage has been dealt with earlier above.

Chemical carcinogenesis

Chemical carcinogens act through charged molecules that form covalent bonds with DNA, RNA, and proteins. They are classified traditionally into remote, proximate, and ultimate carcinogens. A remote carcinogen is a precursor of a carcinogenic agent that might be found in food, the environment, by exposure to certain chemicals and physical agents, and in infective organisms. A proximate carcinogen is the metabolite or metabolites of a remote carcinogen that have some carcinogenic potential but may be modified further in the body into an ultimate carcinogen. An ultimate carcinogen is the active carcinogen that interacts with DNA and other aspects of the cell, and causes neoplasia.

Carcinogenesis is usually a multistep process through initiation and promotion. Initiators are classically mutagens that alter DNA. They tend to be rapid and dose related. Most initiators are procarcinogenic and require activation, especially by cytochrome P450-dependent oxygenase enzymes. Initiators that are not activated do not cause neoplasia. A promoter affects normal cells and initiated cells and causes changes that lead to altered gene expression. In most cases the activity of the promoter only affects initiated cells with abnormal DNA; only then does the altered gene expression result in a preneoplastic or a neoplastic cell. Promoters cannot usually induce neoplasia alone but only after an initiator has altered a cell and caused permanent DNA damage in that cell and its progeny. Promoters lead to proliferation which exposes cells to further mutations, and more than one promoter event may be necessary to induce neoplasia.

Hormones and neoplasia

Hormones can cause neoplasia by acting as promoters. Most hormones act by stimulating growth and secretion of the target organ. Some are inhibitory: dopamine used to be called prolactin-inhibiting factor, and so may be considered a hypothalamic hormone; progesterone inhibits proliferation in endometrial cells, but it does support secretion.

Tamoxifen is a drug used to treat breast cancers that express oestrogen receptors on the cell surface by blocking. It works by binding firmly to the receptors and so decreasing the rate of proliferation. Tamoxifen is not an antioestrogen but a partial oestrogen agonist; the agonist effect is negligible in the breast but potent in the endometrium, where it stimulates first hyperplasia, then atypical hyperplasia and adenocarcinoma.

Oestrogen stimulates many tissues in the body but especially the female reproductive system and is a known contributor to the development of endometrial and breast carcinoma. Methylated steroid hormones such as molecules in the testosterone family cause liver neoplasms.

Irrespective of being themselves carcinogenic, hormones may support the growth of malignancies that have arisen spontaneously or from other causes. The rate of growth of breast carcinoma is dependent on oestrogen, and that of prostate carcinoma on testosterone. Growth of papillary and follicular carcinomas of the thyroid is stimulated by TSH from the pituitary. The risk of TSH induction of malignancy in thyroid-irradiated rats is high but in human beings with high plasma TSH levels, even if lifelong, there is only a very small risk. Patients with dyshormonogenetic goitre, in whom there is thyroid insensitivity to TSH because of enzyme errors of metabolism, have a lifelong low thyroxine production and so constantly high TSH levels. These patients very rarely develop malignancy. Papillary and follicular carcinomas have been recorded but only as very occasional case reports and it is not known whether statistically the neoplasms could have occurred by chance.

Hormones or their antagonists may be used to treat neoplasms:

- tamoxifen (a partial agonist) and gonadotrophin hormone-releasing hormone (GnRH) partial agonists such as goserelin are used to treat breast adenocarcinoma
- progestogens are used to treat endometrial adenocarcinoma by suppressing mitoses
- antiandrogens such as flutamide, and GnRH partial agonists such as goserelin or leuprolide, are used to treat prostate carcinoma
- thyroxine can be used to manage thyroid carcinoma, particularly papillary and follicular carcinomas, by suppressing pituitary secretion of TSH.

Viruses and neoplasia

As with hormones, viruses have a strong association with neoplasia. This can be by causing a neoplasm directly, by stimulating the growth of an existing neoplasm, by causing a disease such as HIV and so immunosuppression that predisposes to neoplasia, or simply by providing a new population of neoplastic cells that can become vicariously infected by viruses.

Viruses that cause neoplasia include:

- HPV causing SCC of the cervix, vulva, perineum, and skin. Herpes simplex virus type II was originally said to be causative, then thought to be an incidental passenger, and is now considered to be facultative for HPV-induced neoplasia
- Epstein–Barr virus (EBV) causing Burkitt's lymphoma with the cooperation of malarial infection
- EBV causing nasopharyngeal carcinoma
- HTLV1 and HTLV2 causing lymphoma.

Viral infections that contribute to neoplasia but are not considered to be directly causative include:

- HIV which causes an immunodeficiency state that is permissive for HPV and for the development of lymphoma
- hepatitis B virus infection causing chronic active hepatitis which may progress to cirrhosis and hepatocellular carcinoma. Hepatitis D (which is an incomplete virus, called a virusoid) is a co-factor especially in South East Asia.

Asbestos

Asbestos was used extensively in building ships, houses, and institutions such as prisons and hospitals 50–80 years ago, and was still used in the construction of office blocks in the 1950s. Asbestos, especially blue asbestos (crocidolite) but to some extent most of the numerous compounds in the asbestos family, is now known to be related to an increased risk of several malignancies.

A difficulty in taking out asbestos from buildings, especially public buildings, is that the process of removal increases the asbestos fibre concentration in the air inside the buildings by 100-fold or more, and this stays high for decades afterwards. Occupations most at risk include shipworkers, laggers, builders, industrial plumbers, architects, and workers in old hospitals that have insulation that was installed over 50 years ago. A problem with rare diseases such as mesothelioma is that tying the cause of the disease to a chance exposure to asbestos that could have happened 20 or 30 years before (because of the latent period) can be almost impossible except presumptively.

Diseases considered to be caused by asbestos include:

- asbestosis, a fibrosing lung disease that is dose-exposure related
- carcinoma of bronchus, usually SCC, which might be dose related
- malignant mesothelioma of pleura, pericardium, and peritoneum, which is not dose related and can occur after a single chance exposure over 20 years later
- chronic bronchitis as from any dust-related disease, which is dose related
- misdiagnosis of pleural fibrous plaques (which might be the result of a number of pathogens) as pleural malignancy with consequent morbidity.

Genetic causes of neoplasia

General aspects of cancer genetics

Malignant neoplasms can arise spontaneously and sporadically, in families and from specific genetic abnormalities. Sporadic malignancies account for most cases overall. They arise by chance in patients with no identifiable family history and no apparent genetic abnormalities.

Familial cancer is multifactorial, from abnormalities in several genes in members of the family, not all of which would be present in each person. Environmental factors also play a part. The chance of developing a malignancy is determined by the number of inherited genetic abnormalities, the environmental risk factors, and how all of these act together. There is therefore no entirely predictable way of knowing which family members will develop cancer. For example, the risk of developing carcinoma of the lung is doubled if a person has a first-degree relative who has or had lung cancer, and increased by a third if he or she has a second-degree relative with lung cancer.

Cancers can rarely arise as a consequence of a single gene abnormality, irrespective of environmental influences. The mode of inheritance will depend on whether the abnormal gene is dominant or recessive, but in clinical practice this can be an oversimplification. Retinoblastoma is inherited as an autosomal recessive condition—children born with one *RB* retinoblastoma gene are normal. Early in life the normal *RB* gene in retinoblasts can spontaneously mutate, resulting in loss of heterozygosity and development of the neoplasm.

There are two ways in which a genetic predisposition to cancer can be inherited. One is by inheriting one (or sometimes two) copies of an abnormal gene that will result in malignancy developing. The other is by inheriting an abnormal gene which affects the capacity of a cell to multiply (or to be prevented from doing so), or to repair its DNA adequately. Both apply in many tumours.

Abnormal function of the growth inhibitor gene *p53* is important in many neoplasms. Normally DNA damage in a cell causes the *p53* gene to transcribe RNA for p53 protein. This stops the cell cycle by increasing the concentration of p21 protein, which is a CDK inhibitor; this prevents damaged DNA being replicated.

Specific genetic abnormalities in common diseases
Colorectal carcinoma
Adenocarcinoma of the colon and rectum is usually sporadic. The normal to adenoma to carcinoma sequence involves at least seven major molecular aberrations. Chromosomal abnormalities account for most cases, the earliest detectable being deletions in the growth inhibitor *APC* gene which is followed by abnormalities developing in the *p53* gene. Microsatellite instability accounts for about 15%; microsatellites are repeating DNA units which mutate and persist in the cell line because chromosome repair is defective. The *APC* gene on chromosome 5 codes for a protein that regulates cell adhesion and signal transmission; most defects in the gene are insertions, deletions, and nonsense mutations which cause frameshifts and abnormal positioning of stop codons.

Hereditary non-polyposis colonic carcinoma accounts for about 5% of cases; the genetic abnormality is in DNA repair genes and not the *APC* gene. Familial adenomatous polyposis (FAP) accounts for about 1% of cases of large bowel cancer. Much rarer are Lynch II and Li–Fraumeni syndromes which include colonic carcinoma. FAP is inherited as an autosomal dominant condition, though variants have been identified—there is an attenuated form with fewer polyps and a lower incidence of malignant change, and a non-classical form in Western Jewish populations. FAP may sometimes present with abnormalities outside the large bowel including:

- desmoid tumours
- dental abnormalities, such as supernumerary teeth, unerupted teeth, congenital absence of teeth, dentigerous cysts, and odontomas
- congenital hypertrophy of the retinal pigment epithelium
- malignant tumours of the thyroid, liver, bile ducts, and CNS
- metaplasia, adenoma, and adenocarcinoma of the ileum: adenoma and adenocarcinoma have also been reported in ileal pouches in patients with FAP who have had total proctocolectomy.

Breast carcinoma
About 10% of women with breast cancer in Western countries have a genetic predisposition, with a pattern of inheritance of autosomal dominant with limited penetrance; this means that the abnormal gene or genes can be transmitted by an apparently normal family member. Women who have an inherited breast cancer gene tend to develop malignancy at a younger age and to have more affected first-degree relatives than those with spontaneous mutations. They are also more likely to have bilateral disease. Affected families have a higher incidence of carcinoma of the ovary, colon, prostate, and elsewhere, which has been attributed to the same inherited gene mutation.

The total number of genes that predispose to breast cancer is unknown. The two most studied are the abnormalities of *BRCA1* on the long arm of chromosomes 17 and *BRCA2* on the long arm of chromosome 13. One or both of these are present in most high-risk families.

In general terms, a woman is at risk who has:

- one first-degree female blood-relative who has bilateral breast cancer or breast and ovarian cancer
- one first-degree female blood-relative who has breast cancer under 40 years
- one first-degree male blood-relative who has breast cancer diagnosed at any age
- two first- or second-degree blood-relatives who have breast cancer diagnosed under 60 years or ovarian cancer at any age
- three first or second blood-relatives with breast and ovarian cancer.

Mutations in other genes are also associated with familial breast cancer, in particular abnormalities of growth inhibitor genes. In Li–Fraumeni syndrome, there is inheritance of a mutated, defective *p53* gene in an autosomal recessive manner. This appears to be autosomal dominant because there is loss of heterozygosity of *p53* early in the person's life with the development of two abnormal *p53* genes—the same sequence as occurs in retinoblastoma. The normal inherited *p53* gene copy mutates early in perhaps one cell in several organs so that functional p53, the protein product of *p53*, is absent from the cell line. There is then a considerable reduction in the inhibition of replication of abnormal DNA, and so a greatly increased risk of malignancy in the affected tissues. Most often associated with Li–Fraumeni syndrome are breast carcinoma, osteosarcoma, and soft tissue sarcoma. Other cancers in this syndrome include astrocytoma, leukaemia, and adrenocortical carcinoma. In Cowden's syndrome of multiple hamartomas, several genes are abnormal including *PTEN*, which is also a growth inhibitor gene. Patients with this condition have an increased risk of carcinoma of the breast, thyroid, and endometrium and more rarely of the colon and kidney.

Melanoma

Nodular, superficial spreading and acral lentiginous melanomas have a predictable abnormality on chromosome 6. In familial melanoma, chromosome 9 is usually abnormal with deletion of *p16*, a growth inhibitor gene. In many melanomas there are confounding genetic variables such as the *MC1R* gene for red hair and pale skin, and the abnormal nucleotide repair genes in xeroderma pigmentosum, both of which predispose to melanoma.

Diagnosis of neoplasia

Cytology and histology

Cytology often precedes histological examination of the tissues. The commonest type of cytology is exfoliative; its main use is by gynaecologists and screeners for cervical neoplasia. It is also used by plastic surgeons for diagnosis of skin lesions in aesthetically sensitive areas such as the face. Endoscopic brushings from the stomach or bronchi are also exfoliative though more invasive.

Fluid cytology is used extensively for diagnosis in surgery. Natural fluids of diagnostic value include urine for malignant cells and schistosome ova; sputum for malignant cells such as SCC and oat cell carcinoma; and CSF for malignant glial cells. Unnatural fluids can be helpful, such as ascites and pleural effusion fluid for malignant cells, and bronchial lavage fluid recovery for the same. Aspiration of cyst fluid from the pancreas or thyroid, and the ovary by gynaecologists, can permit the diagnosis of benign and malignant tumours with a high degree of certainty.

Handling of the fluid for cytology is important if a diagnosis is to be achieved or relied upon. Pleural and ascitic fluid must be anticoagulated so that the clotting factors in the fluid will not solidify it and make centrifugation difficult. Urine intended for examination for malignant cells should be a random catch during the day and not an early-morning specimen—left overnight, even normal transitional cells decay in the urine and can look alarming.

FNAC is used principally for the diagnosis for breast tumours, thyroid tumours, and lymph nodes. Imprint cytology, where the fresh specimen is dabbed onto a histology slide, is used for rapid examination of a lymph node or spleen suspected of having lymphoma; some pathologists have experience enough to diagnose melanoma this way.

Tissues are sent for histological examination by incisional and other biopsies and by excision specimens, which can be small for a benign skin tumour on the face and very large for a hind-quarter amputation or pelvic exenteration. A biopsy is usually for diagnostic reasons rather than therapeutic, and ranges in size from scraping or shave biopsy of skin diseases through wide-bore needle core biopsy and punch biopsy to diathermy loop and deeper biopsies. Sometimes the object of the biopsy is diagnostic though the hope is therapeutic—a large cone biopsy of the cervix, for example, is primarily to establish the extent of involvement by cervical intraepithelial neoplasia but hopefully is curative of it. Excision specimens are usually by cutting diathermy, loop diathermy, or scalpel excision.

The only essential similarity between the two modalities of tissue sampling, cytology and histology, is that in both, the number of cells sampled is large. In cytology, the field sampled is usually large and poorly defined; in histology, it is small and focused.

The architecture of the tissue is absent from a cytological sample, unless there is evidence of papillary carcinoma or other specific features; in histology, the architecture is preserved and so invasion of local tissues can be assessed. Cytology is for the most part non-invasive and repeatable; histology by definition must be invasive, and when the specimen is removed it cannot be removed again. Both modalities can be used to diagnose most types of malignancy but the reliability is higher on histology. Cost and speed of both are difficult to assess. Cytology can be quick and cheap, but the great volume of specimens tends to make it slow. Histology takes 24 hours, which can be much faster than routine cytology, and permits multiple sections for special chromatic stains and immunostains.

Frozen section diagnosis

The indications for asking for a frozen section (FS—rapid intra-operative section) are limited, and it is important to appreciate the limitations and hazards of FS diagnosis. The indications include:

◆ tissue identification, for example to establish that a parathyroid gland is not a thyroid nodule or a lymph node

◆ as an intraoperative diagnostic tool in very limited circumstances. The patient's immediate management must depend on the result of the FS and the issue in question must be within the remit of the pathologist who examines the FS. (For example, FS can be useful simply in diagnosing whether a neoplasm is benign or malignant but would largely be useless for distinguishing one malignant lymphoma from another.)

◆ examination of excision margins to establish whether a carcinoma has been excised completely, especially when the least amount of excision may be preferable as in laryngectomy and glossectomy.

The limitations of FS examination are that the process is destructive: a small specimen can be destroyed completely by ice-crystal artefact. There will inevitably be sampling problems and so the result may be misleading. There will be false negatives and false positives, more frequently than in routine histopathological practice. The diagnosis will usually be simplified rather than the fine-tuned diagnosis possible from properly processed tissues. FS is expensive as it disrupts the normal work in the laboratory. Worst of all, the diagnosis might be completely wrong because of the artefacts induced by the process—there are examples of tuberculosis in a lung FS being diagnosed as sarcoma. Surgeons must accept that there are four proper responses, in general, on a FS report: 'it is parathyroid (for example)', 'it is benign', 'it is malignant', and 'wait until tomorrow for the diagnosis on paraffin-wax slides'.

Immunohistochemistry

Immunohistochemistry staining (immunostaining) gives an indication not just of what a cell looks like but what it contains. This is of course predicated on proper fixation to prevent cell constituents dissolving during processing, or translocating into misleading parts of the section. Immunostains are an essential part of diagnostic pathology and in use daily all over the developed world. Thirty years ago when techniques were still being formulated, fresh tissue was needed to ensure that the technique was reliable; nowadays all commercially available antibodies work very well on routine formalin-fixed, paraffin-wax processed blocks and slides.

Microwave heating has been established to reveal antigens 'hidden' by processing and is very successful.

The main uses of immunostaining are for distinguishing:

◆ among a carcinoma, sarcoma, and lymphoma

◆ among all of the lymphoma types

◆ among specific carcinomas, such as papillary carcinomas of the thyroid, ovary, and pancreas, all of which as a lymph node metastasis can be very difficult on routine stains

◆ between connective tissue components such as laminin and CD10

◆ the different hormone-containing cells in pituitary, testicular, and other endocrine organs in normality and disease

◆ tumours with a low proliferation index from those with a high index.

Difficulties in interpreting immunostains can be considerable but overcomeable. For example, cytokeratins are positive in epithelial neoplasms but can occasionally be positive in leiomyomas and some lymphomas. There are often so-called edge effects, in which there is peripheral staining of the tissues which can lead to false-positive staining and misinterpretation. Negative immunostaining does not indicate that a tissue is not synthesizing a substance—it might be excreting it rapidly so that none remains for staining.

Formalin and its effects on tissues

A 40% solution of formaldehyde in water, abbreviated to formalin, is used almost universally as the routine fixing agent. It is very cheap, versatile, and effective. Formalin fixes almost all tissues well. All of the commercially available immunostains work on formalin-fixed tissues. It works by cross-linking tissue components in place, so preserving relations. The water content of the solution prevents dehydration, and the formaldehyde component is a potent microbicide. Formalin is compatible with haematoxylin and eosin (H&E) staining, and as both are used in all countries of the world, routinely stained H&E sections from anywhere can be assessed by all histopathologists.

The problem with formalin is its toxicity. It is severely irritant in solution and as a vapour and can cause severe skin rashes. If insufficient formalin is used to fix specimens, especially large specimens, the tissue will decay and gases may be produced. When the specimen pot is opened the formalin may spray into the laboratory assistant's or the pathologist's eyes.

Tumour markers

A tumour marker is a substance reliably found in the circulation of a patient with neoplasia which is directly related to the presence of the neoplasm (though is not stoichiometric), falls away when the neoplasm is treated and rises again when the neoplasm recurs at the primary site or as metastases. The main use of tumour markers is to aid diagnosis rather than make the diagnosis, and they are particularly used to monitor persistence of the tumour after operation or recurrence. The level of a tumour marker does not directly reflect the volume of tumour present, except for the plasma concentration of carcinoembryonic antigen which reliably changes in proportion.

Tumour markers are grouped mostly as hormones, isoenzymes, and oncofetal and other antigens. Hormones may be produced by tumours eutopically or ectopically. Tumours of endocrine organs are often differentiated enough to secrete the appropriate hormone,

such as thyroid hormones secreted by papillary and follicular carcinomas of thyroid. Isoenzymes as tumour markers include placental alkaline phosphatase for neoplasms of germ cells which is sometimes also raised in carcinoma of the pancreas, colon, and bronchus.

Prostatic acid phosphatase analysis was used as a diagnosis for carcinoma of the prostate but has now been largely superseded by prostate-specific antigen (PSA). The danger of PSA is that many normal activities cause a significant rise in PSA. For example, riding a cycle will raise the PSA; ejaculating will raise the PSA. Patients must be advised *not* to have a PSA measurement for several days after a rectal examination, or intercourse, or ejaculation—the result will be high and might be unnecessarily alarming.

Screening

A screening programme is defined as a codified search for unsuspected disease in a population of apparently healthy people. Success depends on two main modalities: the features of the disease and the variables of the screening test.

The disease should be an important health problem and so be common; asymptomatic or with only non-specific symptoms; and one with a reliably long premorbid latent period. It should be detectable at an early stage in the latent period, and it should be treatable, preferably at the time of detection. The screening test should be non-invasive and acceptable to people, with no significant harm in terms of the test and the information that the test provides. It should be sensitive and specific, cost-effective, and auditable.

The longest-established screening test in the modern sense is for cervical carcinoma and its precursor lesions. Screening for breast carcinoma in the general population has also become routine in most countries (women with a strong family history of breast cancer or a mutation in one or both *BRCA* genes undergo surveillance rather than screening). Colorectal carcinoma screening is now being introduced for people over 60 years. Screening for abdominal aortic aneurysm is less widespread.

General types of neoplasm

Benign neoplasms

A benign neoplasm is one that is characteristically slow-growing, has no infiltrative growth or capacity to metastasis, and does not recur after complete excision. Benign neoplasms grow either on a surface, such as from the skin or into the lumen of a duct or anatomical tract, or within solid tissues such as the thyroid or adrenal gland. The commonest growth patterns from surface epithelium are papillomas which may be pedunculated or sessile, and adenomas which may be tubular, villous, or mixed patterns of these (and also pedunculated or sessile). There can be mixed tissue components, as in pleomorphic adenoma of parotid gland. Many benign neoplasms of glandular tissue are cystic, especially ovarian neoplasms such as serous cystadenomas which can present with torsion and acute abdominal pain. A benign neoplasm can have mixed elements of epithelium and connective tissue proliferations, such as fibroadenoma of breast, and adenolymphoma of salivary gland.

A benign neoplasm can cause the death of a patient by many processes, including:

◆ thrombosis and infarction that can lead to severe haemorrhage from a large bowel or endometrial polyp; torsion of a benign ovarian cyst or subserosal leiomyoma can cause haemoperitoneum

◆ infection of an ulcerated large bowel adenoma that can result in septicaemia; biliary tract infection can complicate stasis from an adenoma of the biliary system

◆ obstruction of a ductal system, such as biliary obstruction as above; intussusception can be caused by a benign neoplastic polyp of large bowel. A meningioma in the posterior cerebral fossa can obstruct the flow of CSF, or if in the spinal meninges can obstruct the nerve supply to a tissue. A large retrosternal adenoma of the thyroid can obstruct the venous return from the head and neck

◆ biochemical abnormalities that are life-threatening, such as eutopic hormone and ectopic secretion, and electrolyte and protein loss from polyps in the large bowel

◆ pathological fracture through a benign bone tumour such as an osteoid osteoma or osteoblastoma

◆ malignant change

◆ misdiagnosis with consequent mortality.

Malignant neoplasms

A cancer is the generic term for any malignant neoplasm. It is useful when writing about neoplasms of, say, the thyroid: there are four classical carcinomas but five classical cancers, as this term includes lymphoma. A cancer with both carcinomatous and sarcomatous differentiation is called a carcinosarcoma, as in the uterus, ovary, and lung. A differentiated teratoma can have a malignant element, such as adenocarcinoma of a glandular element or SCC of a skin element, or be malignant ab initio and composed of immature elements.

Neoplasms have abnormal proliferation, differentiation, and relation of their cells to each other and the surrounding tissues. This results in an abnormal growth pattern with distortion of architecture and compression with or without infiltration of adjacent structures. There may be the cardinal histological features of neoplastic cells, especially in malignant tumours, such as hyperchromatism from accumulation of DNA and its precursors in neoplastic nuclei leading to a raised nuclear/cytoplasmic ratio and nuclear pleomorphism. Aneuploidy, an abnormal and usually raised amount of nuclear DNA, contributes to hyperchromatism and to tripolar, tetrapolar, and starburst mitoses as metaphase and telophase cannot proceed normally.

Loss of normal maturation leads to the disruption of a squamous epithelium and multilayering of a glandular epithelium. The development of abnormal ductal systems can cause cyst formation. Disruption of poorly formed new blood vessels in a neoplasm causes haemorrhage or thrombosis which leads to necrosis, as does compression of blood vessels by expansile growth in a confined space, such as in a meningioma.

The rate of growth of a neoplasm is proportional to the rate of cell multiplication measured by the growth fraction of actively proliferating cells, and inversely proportional to the rate of cell death, whether due to spontaneous apoptosis, apoptosis induced by immune mechanisms, or necrosis. The growth rate depends on the blood supply, general nutrition, local and circulating growth factors, the intensity and type of immune response to the neoplasm, and the degree of resistance to invasion by surrounding tissues. The growth fraction

can be increased by debulking tumours with an initially low growth fraction, such as colorectal cancer. Tumours with a high growth fraction usually respond better to treatment with cytotoxic drugs.

Molecular changes in neoplasia

Tumour cell spread by detachment from the parent mass, invasion of and transport through lymphatics or blood vessels, attachment to vessels at distant sites, and passage through the vessel's basement membrane into the extracellular matrix. Malignant cells have laminin and receptor integrins over the whole surface, not just at the basement membrane aspect. Matrix metalloproteinases are secreted by tumour cells and they stimulate stromal cells also to secrete matrix metalloproteinases, which degrade collagen. Tumour cells can escape immune recognition as they have altered MHCs or immunoglobulin superfamily expression on their surfaces. Tumour cells that survive adhere to endothelial cells with integrins and secrete matrix metalloproteinases to move into extravascular tissues by proteolysis.

Angiogenesis begins only when the mass of neoplasm is more than 2 mm in diameter as the cells within begin to become hypoxic and react by secreting vascular endothelial growth factor and other angiogenesis factors. Microvessel density correlates with the potential to metastasize. Another factor that encourages angiogenesis, in normal cells and tumour cells, is the plasma membrane molecule CD44. This also has a role in many other aspects of cell behaviour, such as cell-to-cell adhesion and cell-to-connective tissue matrix adhesion, cell differentiation, proliferation, capacity for motility, and presentation of growth factors and cytokines to their receptors. High expression of CD44 by tumour cells is usually associated with aggressive features but in some cancers the reverse is true, and there is at present no definite correlation with prognosis.[22]

Cardinal variables for all cancers

The four features of prime importance in management and prognosis of cancer are the site, type, grade, and stage of the neoplasm. Irrespective of the other three variables, the site of origin of the tumour is crucial. An SCC of skin, for example, will behave very differently from an SCC of oesophagus or SCC of cervix.

The type of a neoplasm is indicated by its cell line. A carcinoma is a malignant tumour of epithelial cells. A sarcoma is a malignant tumour of connective tissue cells; by this definition lymphomas and leukaemias are sarcomas but are always considered as a separate group. Most carcinomas are classified simply as SCC, adenocarcinomas, and transitional cell carcinomas and undifferentiated (anaplastic) carcinomas, but some cancers have specific appearances and behaviour; melanoma, choriocarcinoma, nasopharyngeal carcinoma, and adenoid cystic carcinoma have specific names as they behave in their own specific ways. Mixed carcinomas such as adenosquamous carcinomas of the uterus and transitional cell/SCC of the bladder are uncommon but likely to be encountered. Mixed malignancies of epithelial and connective elements such as malignant mixed Müllerian tumour are rare.

The grade of the neoplasm is based on its degree of differentiation, or lack of it, which refers to the closeness of resemblance to the non-neoplastic normal tissue at the site. This is graded into well differentiated, moderately differentiated, and poorly differentiated. There is no grade of moderately well differentiated; of course more than one pattern may be present, when the tumour would be called partly well differentiated and partly moderately differentiated. A carcinoma is graded as undifferentiated when there is no differentiation that permits recognition as a poorly differentiated SCC, adenocarcinoma, or transitional cell carcinoma. Anaplastic simply means undifferentiated, though some writers reserve the term for particularly pleomorphic tumours with bizarre tumour giant cells. If a neoplasm cannot be recognized as a carcinoma or sarcoma, it is an undifferentiated cancer. Nowadays some degree of differentiation into epithelial and connective tissue cell lines can usually be demonstrated by immunohistochemistry.

The stage of a cancer refers to the extent of spread, both local and distant. The principles of any staging system are that it should be simple to understand, apply, and reproduce reliably. The system should establish a clear ranking of the distribution through the different stages, and must be valuable in the management and prognosis of the patient. Examples of staging systems are given later (see 'Staging of cancer').

Factors that determine the extent of local spread of a neoplasm include:

+ the tumour site, type and grade: for example, an adenocarcinoma of anus behaves differently from to an SCC of anus of the same grade

+ the capacity of the tumour cells to influence the extracellular matrix through which they spread

+ local factors around the tumour such as the blood supply and the presence of tissue planes of least resistance

+ the presence of tissues resistant to infiltration such as cartilage, because of lack of blood supply and secretion of inhibitors of hyaluronidase

+ the extent and type of the humoral immune response to the tumour by circulating and local immunoglobulins, and the cellular immune response by lymphocytes and macrophages such as in the spleen, in which metastases of carcinoma are rarely found.

Metastatic spread of cancer

As well as expansion locally, cancers spread metastatically. A metastasis is a deposit of malignant tumour cells away from and unconnected with its site of origin.

The six classical routes of metastasis are via lymphatic vessels, blood vessels, through one or more of the coelomic cavities, through perineural spaces (which may in fact be lymphatics), through the CSF, and through iatrogenic intervention. Most carcinomas spread by lymphatics, which have no type IV collagen or laminin in their walls and so are considered to be more susceptible to invasion, but other factors must also be in play. Sarcomas classically spread via the bloodstream.

The routes of blood spread are into the new vessels stimulated by the tumour cells, into native vessels around the tumour, and into the left subclavian vein by way of the thoracic duct. The number of cells released in a given time into the bloodstream does not correlate with the development of metastases—for example, a renal parenchymal cell carcinoma can grow directly into the renal vein and sheds millions of cells per hour, but characteristically forms solitary or only few metastases.

Transcoelomic spread can be through the peritoneal cavity, the pleura, and, rarely, the pericardium. All three are derived from the embryonic coelome (Greek *koilos*, hollow). In the peritoneum, the commonest cancers to spread by this route are colon and stomach, both of which spread throughout the peritoneal serosa but especially affect the ovaries. Bilateral nodular involvement of the ovaries by metastases from anywhere are called Kruckenberg tumours (Kruckenberg, 1896). Lung cancers, especially peripheral ones, can metastasize to the upper surface of the diaphragm transcoelomically, and occasionally spread through the pericardial cavity. Perineural spread is most often seen in adenoid cystic carcinoma of the salivary glands. Aggressive tumours of the CNS such as medulloblastoma can spread through the CSF to involve the spinal cord.

Iatrogenic spread of a cancer may be because a neoplastic cyst, such as in the pancreas or ovary, is ruptured during excision. Chondrosarcoma of the pelvis can be seeded widely at operation; malignant chondroblasts have a very low metabolic requirement and can survive on diffused nutrients in the normal small amount of peritoneal fluid.

Grading systems

Most malignant tumours are graded by eye by the histopathologist, without any basis except experience of conformity, into the four grades discussed earlier. Formalized, structured grading systems have been developed for some common tumours. The two in common use are the Elston–Ellis system for breast carcinoma and the Gleason system for prostate carcinoma.

Breast carcinomas are assessed on tubule formation (a grade of 1 means that there is clear tubule formation, 3 that there is not), mitotic count per high power field (1 is few, 3 many) and nuclear pleomorphism (1 little, 3 severe). A combined score of 3–5 is considered low grade, 6–7 intermediate, and 8–9 high grade. These combined scores correlate well with prognosis.[23]

Adenocarcinoma of the prostate is graded by the Gleason system of patterns of growth[24]:

1. The adenocarcinoma of the prostate closely resembles normal prostate tissue—the glands are small, well formed, and closely packed.

2. The adenocarcinoma has well-formed glands but they are larger and have more connective tissue between them.

3. The adenocarcinoma has recognizable glands but the glandular cells are hyperchromatic and begin to invade the surrounding tissues.

4. The adenocarcinoma has few recognizable glands and many foci of invasion are present.

5. The adenocarcinoma has no recognizable glands and forms sheets of neoplastic cells.

Gleason system reprinted from *Human Pathology*, Volume 36, Issus 4, Henrik Helin *et al.*, Web-based virtual microscopy in teaching and standardizing Gleason grading, pp 381–386, Copyright © 2005, with permission from Elsevier, http://www.sciencedirect.com/science/journal/00468177

In the United Kingdom, Gleason pattern 3 is the commonest reported. The histopathologist examines the biopsy specimen microscopically and gives a score to two patterns: the first is called the primary grade, which is that found in most of the tumour; the secondary grade is based on the appearances of the second most prevalent aspect of the adenocarcinoma. These grades are added together to form the final Gleason score. This cannot be less than 2 or more than 10, and reflects the prognosis.

Staging of cancer
TNM staging

The TNM staging system was developed to indicate the prognosis of a malignant neoplasm, to assist in management of it, and to formalize data collection so that different treatments and clinical trials could be compared. The system is based partly on the anatomical extent of spread and partly on clinical features, such as those found on physical examination, endoscopy, imaging, biopsy, surgical exploration, and other relevant procedures performed before treatment. The latter are called the cTNM data.[25]

The T category indicates the extent of the primary tumour. The N category documents the presence or absence of *regional* lymph node metastases; involvement of nodes other than regional nodes is included in the M category. These do not have to be distant metastases: a carcinoma of the hepatic flexure of the colon that has metastases in the liver only a few centimetres away has an entry in M.

The T category of local involvement by the tumour includes:

- TX: the primary tumour cannot be assessed
- T0: there is no evidence of the primary tumour (such as after radiotherapy)
- Tis: carcinoma *in situ*
- T1–T4: the size and local extent of the tumour

The N category of regional lymph node involvement includes:

- NX: the regional nodes cannot be assessed
- N0: there are no regional node metastases
- N1–N3: the extent of regional node involvement

The M category of metastases other than in regional lymph nodes includes:

- MX: the presence or absence of distant metastases cannot be assessed
- M0: there are no distant metastases
- M1: distant metastases are present (their site is stated here).

Reproduced with permission from Wittekind C, Greene FL, Hutter RVP, Klimpfinger M, Sobin LH, *TNM Atlas: Illustrated Guide to the TNM Classification of Malignant Tumours, Fifth Edition*, Wiley-Liss, Copyright © 2008 Wiley.

Other staging systems
Dukes' staging of colorectal carcinoma. The Dukes' staging system (Cuthbert Esquire Dukes, 1890–1977) for colorectal carcinoma was derived from Dukes' earlier work on staging of rectal carcinoma. The earliest evidence that an adenomatous polyp has become an adenocarcinoma is when neoplastic glands are identified on the submucosal side of the muscularis mucosae. The grade

of the epithelium in the neoplasm is immaterial in terms of Dukes' staging.

Dukes' stage A is when the neoplasm has invaded through the muscularis mucosae but has not reached the outermost aspect of the muscularis propria (Dukes could not use the anatomical level of the serosa as a marker as the lower rectum does not have a serosa). Dukes' stage B is when the carcinoma has extended through the outermost aspect of the muscularis propria. Dukes' stage C is when there are lymph node metastases. The staging system has been modified since it was introduced to refer to proximal and distant lymph node involvement, C1 and C2. The carcinoma can spread by lymphatics from an apparently stage A tumour into lymph nodes and so become stage C without breaching the muscularis propria.[26]

The Dukes' staging has been useful for many years but it does not address several aspects of prognostic importance. These include whether the tumour is completely excised, whether there is invasion of major veins in the specimen, and whether the tumour extends close to excision margins. Subsequent staging systems, such as the Jass system, include data on the growth pattern of the tumour—whether it is infiltrative or growing as blunt extensions—and whether there is an inflammatory cell infiltrate, both of which are prognostic indicators.

Clark's staging system for melanoma and the Breslow thickness. Clark's levels is a system of grading melanoma by the extent to which it has spread into the dermis and subcutis[27]:

Level 1: tumour cells only within the epidermis

Level 2: tumour cells invade the papillary dermis only

Level 3: tumour cells reach the junction between the papillary and the reticular dermis

Level 4: tumour cells invade the reticular dermis

Level 5: tumour cells invade the subcutis.

Adapted with permission. Copyright © Cancer Research UK 2014.

This staging system takes no account of the normal variation of the thickness of the dermis in different parts of the body: on the nose and eyelid the dermis is very thin and would be breached by a small melanoma; on the lower back the dermis is considerably thicker and would be breached only by a sizeable tumour. Clark's levels are still used but the Breslow thickness has been found to correlate better with prognosis.

The Breslow thickness of melanoma is not a staging system. It makes no attempt to identify the extent of spread of the melanoma but instead addresses only its thickness, which is measured in millimetres from the granular layer of the epidermis overlying the melanoma to the deepest identifiable tumour cell—there is no requirement to identify where in the dermis or subcutis this is. The Breslow thickness is modified if the tumour is ulcerated; the measurement is taken from the most superficial aspect of the melanoma to the deepest malignant cell and the presence of ulceration is clearly recorded. An exophytic nodular melanoma might have a large Breslow thickness and a Clark's level of only 2. It will have a poor prognosis.

Prognostic features of melanoma include the:

- type of melanoma—a nodular melanoma has a worse prognosis than the other types
- Breslow thickness

- Clark's level, to some extent
- presence of ulceration, indicating a poor prognosis
- presence or absence of satellite nodules and lymph node metastases
- histological features of the tumour, such as a high mitotic count and large tumour volume
- site of the tumour: for a given Breslow thickness, tumours on the extremities have a worse prognosis
- sex of the patient: men have a worse prognosis
- age of the patient: older patients have a worse prognosis.

Paraneoplastic syndromes

A paraneoplastic syndrome is one in which the patient develops symptoms and signs because of a neoplasm which are *not* due to the direct presence of the neoplasm or its metastases or associated cachexia, and *not* due to secretion of hormones or other substances that the neoplasm would be predicted to secrete.

A thyroid follicular carcinoma secreting T_4 with the symptoms and signs that follow is not considered paraneoplastic but logically neoplastic. Only ectopic secretions and their effects are considered paraneoplastic. A gastrinoma of the pancreas and its effects would be a paraneoplastic syndrome as the pancreatic islets do not normally secrete gastrin: an insulinoma secreting insulin would not be.

These symptoms and signs may be the presenting features of a neoplasm and so it is surgically important to recognize the possibility. Some are vague but can themselves cause morbidity or mortality irrespective of the presence of the causative neoplasm. Some can be misleading, such as hypercalcaemia which might be taken to indicate bone metastases and lead to up-staging of the neoplasm. Paraneoplastic syndromes fall into four classical groups:

- Haematological:
  - a tendency to thrombosis, with or without thrombophlebitis migrans and sterile thrombotic endocarditis
  - thrombocytopenia
  - polycythaemia
  - DIC.
- Endocrine:
  - ectopic hormone secretion—eutopic secretion is excluded by the definition.
- Neuromuscular:
  - demyelinating disorders
  - cerebellar degeneration with myasthenic features (Lambert–Eaton syndrome)
  - myopathies without myasthenic features
  - polymyositis.
- Dermatological:
  - clubbing of fingers and toes
  - related to changes in blood flow and also growth factors secreted from the lungs such as prostaglandins
  - acanthosis nigricans

- dermatomyositis
- erythroderma
- erythema gyratum repens
- pemphigus
- hypertrichosis.

References

1. Vermeulen K, van Bockstaele DR, Berneman ZN. The cell cycle: a review of regulation, deregulation and therapeutic targets in cancer. *Cell Prolif* 2003; 36:131–49.
2. Malumbres M, Barbacid M. To cycle or not to cycle: a critical decision in cancer. *Nat Rev Cancer* 2001; 1:222–31.
3. Müller H. Dominant inheritance in human cancer. *Anticancer Res* 1990; 10(2B):505–11.
4. Rather LJ. Disturbance of function (functio laesa): the legendary fifth cardinal sign of inflammation, added by Galen to the four cardinal signs of Celsus. *Bull N Y Acad Med* 1971; 47:303–22.
5. Williams GT, Williams WJ. Granulomatous inflammation—a review. *J Clin Pathol* 1983; 36:723–33.
6. Little MP. Risks associated with ionizing radiation: environmental pollution and health. *Br Med Bull* 2003; 68:259–75.
7. Valko M, Leibfritz D, Moncol J, *et al.* Free radicals and antioxidants in normal physiological functions and human disease. *Int J Biochem Cell Biol* 2007; 39:44–84.
8. Wood KE. Major pulmonary embolism: review of a pathophysiologic approach to the golden hour of hemodynamically significant pulmonary embolism. *Chest* 2002; 121:877–905.
9. Roberts KE, Hamele-Bena D, Saqi A, *et al.* Pulmonary tumor embolism: a review of the literature. *Am J Med* 2003; 115:228–32.
10. National Institute for Clinical Excellence. *Nutrition Support in Adults: Oral Nutrition Support, Enteral Tube Feeding and Parenteral Nutrition.* Clinical Guideline 32. London: NICE; 2006. http://www.nice.org.uk/CG032
11. Eming SA, Krieg T, Davidson JM. Inflammation in wound repair: molecular and cellular mechanisms. *J Invest Derm* 2007; 127:514–25.
12. Male D, Brostoff J, Roth D, *et al. Immunology* (8th ed). Philadelphia, PA: Saunders; 2013.
13. Mahambrey T, Pendry K, Nee A, *et al.* Critical care in emergency department: massive haemorrhage in trauma. *Emerg Med J* 2013; 39:9–14.
14. http://www.transfusionguidelines.org.uk/docs.pdfs/"www.transfusion-guidelines.org.uk/docs.pdfs
15. Douketis JD, Berger PB, Dunn AS, *et al.* The perioperative management of antithrombotic therapy: American College of Chest Physicians Evidence-Based Clinical Practice Guidelines (8th Edition). *Chest* 2008; 133(suppl 6):299S–339S.
16. Bilezikian JP. Management of acute hypercalcaemia. *N Engl J Med* 1992; 326:1196–203.
17. Epstein PH, Ross R. Mechanisms of disease: atherosclerosis—an inflammatory disease. *N Engl J Med* 1999; 340:115–26.
18. Furie KL, Goldstein LB, Albers GW, *et al.* Oral antithrombotic agents for the prevention of stroke in nonvalvular atrial fibrillation: a science advisory for healthcare professionals from the American Heart Association/American Stroke Association. *Stroke* 2012; 43(12):3442–53.
19. Lusis AJ. Atherosclerosis. *Nature* 2000; 407:233–41.
20. Singh AP. *Classification of Bone Fractures,* Feb 16 2016. http://www.boneandspine.com
21. Jeschke MG, Herndon DN. Burns in children: standard and new treatments. *Lancet* 2014; 383:1168–78.
22. Ponta H, Sherman L, Herrlich PA. CD44: from adhesion molecules to signalling regulators. *Nature Rev Mol Cell Biol* 2003; 4:33–45.

23. Elston CW, Ellis IO. Pathological prognostic factors in breast cancer: I. The value of histological grade in breast cancer: experience from a large study with long-term follow-up. *Histopathology* 1991; 19:403–10.

24. Gleason DF. Histologic grading of prostate cancer: a perspective. *Hum Pathol* 1992; 23(3):273–9.

25. Wittekind C, Greene FL, Hutter RVP, *et al. TNM Atlas: Illustrated Guide to the TNM Classification of Malignant Tumours* (5th ed). New York: Wiley-Liss; 2008.

26. Cserni G. The influence of nodal size on the staging of colorectal carcinomas. *J Clin Pathol 2002;55:386–90.*

27. Cancer Research UK. *Stages of Melanoma.* 2014. [Online] http://www.cancerresearchuk.org/about-cancer/type/melanoma/treatment/stages-of-melanoma#clark

Applied surgical microbiology

Sub-section editor: Kate Gould

Sepsis

Muhammad Raza

Background and definitions

Sepsis occurs in patients in all ages and in all surgical and medical specialties, with an incidence of 240.4/100 000 population in the United States, with 20% mortality, ranking in the top-ten causes of death.[1] The mortality with sepsis is based on 28-day survival compared with most other mortality studies, for example, diabetes, where the survival rate is measured over 5 years, showing the numbers of years of life lost with sepsis.

Agreement on a precise definition of sepsis has been difficult to reach owing to its heterogeneity. Sepsis is caused by a variety of bacteria invading from different ports of entry into the body. Presence of underlying illnesses and other factors, for example, smoking, cytotoxic drugs and diabetes, make an impact on how an individual patient deals with a threat of infection. More importantly, the nature, intensity and outcome of an episode of sepsis are determined by complex pathophysiology dictated by individual genetic makeup. Whichever definitions and diagnostic criteria for sepsis are preferred, proper knowledge of its pathophysiology underlies the understanding of its clinical features and management.

Whereas viruses and fungi can also be involved in sepsis in synergy with bacteria, in surgical practice, bacteria remain the most important class of pathogens.

Colonization and infection

To understand sepsis it is important to be familiar with the terms of association that bacteria can have with the host. Several bacterial species reside on epithelial surfaces, for example, coagulase-negative staphylococci on the skin, or haemolytic streptococci in the mouth, normally without causing harm to the host, defining 'colonization'. In contrast, 'infection' is defined as the presence of bacteria on normally sterile places (e.g. in the peritoneal cavity) or their presence on sites where they are not normally found (e.g. *Salmonella* in the colon). 'Infection' may remain subclinical or may progress to a state of disease although, in common language, 'infection' usually also denotes 'disease due to infection'.

Sepsis

Infections are met by host inflammatory and immune responses, determined by individual polymorphism. The numerous factors in inflammatory response can broadly be categorized as pro-inflammatory and anti-inflammatory. The two types of responses, tightly regulated, working in harmony, normally allow the body to fight bacteria, with minimal damage to the host by the bacteria or by inflammation itself.

A predominant, uncontrolled, non-resolving, and non-corrective pro-inflammatory response itself may become deleterious to the host. In contrast, with an unchecked anti-inflammatory response, microorganisms may escape challenge, resulting in damage to the host in that way. Whether it is the first case scenario or one from heterogeneous combinations of the two, it is the resultant damage to the host, reaching a significant level necessitating careful or critical management, that defines 'sepsis'.

Systemic inflammatory response syndrome and sepsis

Inflammatory conditions similar to sepsis, characterized as systemic inflammatory response syndrome (SIRS), can also result from non-infectious causes, for example, severe injury to the tissue ensuing from multiple trauma, extensive burns, acute pancreatitis, or severe autoimmune diseases. Sepsis thus comprises of SIRS with evidence, or suspicion, of infection.

SIRS is recognized by the presence of tachycardia, tachypnoea, leucocytosis or leucopoenia (mainly affecting neutrophils), and fever or hypothermia. Additional features in sepsis include delirium, unexplained hyperbilirubinaemia, metabolic acidosis and/or respiratory alkalosis, and thrombocytopenia, plus signs of focal infection pertaining to its source.

Severe sepsis

A progressive septic process can jeopardize several organ systems in the body. When accompanied by evidence of involvement of at least one organ/system distant from the site of infection and/or by 'significant hypotension', sepsis becomes 'severe sepsis'.

Septic shock

Hypotension in 'severe sepsis' is responsive to fluid resuscitation in a proportion of cases. The term 'septic shock' is reserved for conditions where 'severe sepsis' is accompanied by hypotension resistant to adequate fluid resuscitation, needing pharmacological intervention (e.g. vasopressors). It becomes 'refractory septic shock' if it cannot be corrected within an hour of onset despite appropriate intervention.

Pathogenic basis of clinical and laboratory findings

From infection to sepsis

Source of infection

The mucocutaneous surfaces in the body provide a barrier to invasion by bacteria. A breach therein letting bacteria invade the body could be fairly obvious (e.g. perforation of the gut) or could result from subtle leaks difficult to locate (e.g. in occult cancer). The lungs and the abdomen are the most commonly identified sites of primary infection in sepsis.

Alternatively, pathogenic bacteria invade otherwise intact surfaces, for example, in spontaneous bacterial peritonitis or salmonella infecting the intact intestinal mucosa. In some cases of sepsis, the source could be trivial (e.g. a thorn-prick or an insect-bite) or else, in a large number of cases, a source may not be apparent, or not found at all. Culture-negative and culture-positive cases bear similar morbidity and mortality rates.[2]

Host local response

Bacteria at the site of infection meet a host response characterized by release of biochemical mediators (c.g. cytokines) and recruitment of inflammatory cells (e.g. macrophages and neutrophils). These responses may lead to local inflammation, defined as cellulitis, which can progress to abscess formation, but mainly aim at resolution of infection and inflammation. However, in a number of cases, the bacteria evade the local responses by invading the blood resulting in bacteraemia.

Bacteraemia and septicaemia

Blood is continuously invaded by bacteria originating from different sites (e.g. the gut) or from daily activities (e.g. brushing teeth and defecation). However, such episodes of bacteraemia largely remain transient and inconsequential owing to blood's efficient bactericidal mechanisms, which can be non-specific (e.g. neutrophils and complement factors) or specific (e.g. armoury of T lymphocytes and antibodies).

Where virulent bacteria from a significant source overcome these mechanisms, or the mechanisms are inadequate in an individual patient, the resultant bacteraemia leads to symptoms of systemic infection and, in severe cases, sepsis. The term 'septicaemia' is a layman's expression of bacteraemia (blood poisoning) associated with sepsis, severe sepsis, or septic shock.

Pathophysiology

Pathophysiology of sepsis constitutes systemic responses to bacteria and impairment of end organs. Whereas sepsis is clinically different from severe sepsis and septic shock, no theory currently proposed adequately accounts for the transition.

Types of bacterial species

Infection and sepsis may involve bacteria in a commensal relationship with the host (e.g. anaerobic and coliform bacteria in the colon) once they have successfully accessed the normally sterile sites (e.g. peritoneum). Opportunistic bacteria (e.g. *Acinetobacter* spp. or *Stenotrophomonas* spp.) can harm individuals with inadequate immunity and breach the integrity of barrier functions. Other groups of potentially pathogenic bacteria that can be carried by some individuals without harm can cause infection in others, especially when newly acquired. Examples in this category include *Neisseria meningitidis*, group A streptococci, *Staphylococcus aureus*, and pneumococci.

Some Gram-positive bacteria, such as group A streptococci and *Staph. aureus*, sometimes do not directly invade the bloodstream but cause symptoms of toxic shock through release of 'super-antigens' from the site of infection in the tissue, which sometimes can be trivial (e.g. paronychia).

Systemic response to sepsis

The systemic inflammatory response to infection is finely balanced with its anti-inflammatory counterparts.[2,3,4] A failure in the control of the inflammatory process in dealing with infection and in its down-regulation once infection has been dealt with may lead to SIRS and organ failure.

In contrast, from a state of exaggerated inflammatory process in sepsis, its drastic down-regulation may sometimes swing the balance to a state dominated by anti-inflammatory process. This may result in impairment of antibacterial activities leading to uncontrolled infection and extensive tissue damage.

Pro-inflammatory process

Numerous bacterial components, lipopolysaccharides, peptidoglycan, and DNA, bind to inflammatory cells, triggering pro-inflammatory mediators, for example, interleukin (IL)-1b, IL-8, IL-12, tumour necrosis factor (TNF)-alpha, and prostaglandins. It results in increased blood flow to the inflamed sites, with increased tension in the swollen tissue, causing pain and loss of function. It also leads to increased capillary permeability, leaking of immunoglobulins, C-reactive protein (CRP), mannose binding proteins, and complement factors into the inflamed site. Neutrophil traffic towards the site is also increased. Together, all these factors present a fight against the invading pathogens.

In a proportion of cases, however, the battle cannot be won or contained, leading to bacteria invading the blood and distant organs, to an upsurge of the inflammatory mediators causing systemic symptoms, or both.

Anti-inflammatory factors

Certain factors released in sepsis are recognized for their anti-inflammatory properties: cytokines (e.g., IL-4, IL-6, and IL-10), soluble TNF receptors, regulatory $CD4^+$-$CD25^+$ T cells, neuroendocrine hormones (e.g. cortisol, adrenocorticotropin hormone, and epinephrine), and protease inhibitors.

Besides bacterial virulence, spread of infection beyond a local site marks systemic immunosuppression and a net anti-inflammatory balance. Down-regulation of immune and inflammatory responses caused by major trauma and critical illness may also result in increased susceptibility to infection and sepsis.

The usual response to a localized challenge (e.g. acute appendicitis) is of a pro-inflammatory nature at the site of infection (e.g. peritoneal fluid) and of an anti-inflammatory nature at distant sites (e.g. in the lymph and blood), a pattern lost in sepsis.

Neutrophil homeostasis

Neutrophils, being the most abundant circulating leucocytes, play key bactericidal and phagocytic roles. Like other blood cells, neutrophils are generated in the bone marrow under the influence of a range of mediators, granulocyte colony-stimulating-factor (G-CSF) being the principal one. With a short half-life of 6–8 hours, neutrophils need continuous replenishment by the bone marrow.

Around 5–10% of the total neutrophils are circulating at any one time and similar proportions are to be found in the 'margination pool'. This pool refers to the slower transit of neutrophils within the vascular compartment, mainly in the spleen, liver, and bone marrow.

Neutrophilia, a state of increase in the circulating pool, can be found in numerous conditions. Glucocorticoids increase the size of both the margination and circulation pools, with a 'left shift' from the bone marrow, while epinephrine and exercise cause a shift from the margination pool to the circulation pool. Asplenia, by depleting the margination pool, has similar effects on neutrophil homeostasis. Bacterial products increase the size of both the pools and, on a similar principle neutrophils are recruited to the site of inflammation in the tissue.

The bactericidal functions of neutrophils are characterized by release of destructive enzymes, phagocytosis, and production of toxic reactive oxygen species. With these potentially toxic products, neutrophils are regularly implicated in tissue injury, for example, in acute respiratory distress syndrome (ARDS); similarly, their unregulated numbers and activity can add to damage of an organ in sepsis.

In contrast, severe sepsis can lead to neutropenia owing to their over-consumption and destruction in the fight against infection, their sequestration in the infected tissue, disproportional margination, and/or bone marrow suppression owing to sepsis.[5] It is important to note that several classes of antibiotics, penicillins, cephalosporins, sulphonamides, and vancomycin, may also result in transient neutropenia. Phenytoin and H_2 blockers can have similar effects on the circulation pool. Neutropenia can also result from the cytotoxic drugs in the treatment of cancers, or as a part of chronic granulomatous disease.

Apart from absolute neutrophil counts, a high blood neutrophil–lymphocyte ratio is reported as a marker of severity of sepsis; however, a low ratio does not exclude sepsis.

Acute phase response

'Acute phase response' to infection or trauma constitutes release mainly from the liver of soluble factors, the acute phase reactants (APRs), for example, CRP and complement factors. APRs are involved in modulation of inflammatory responses in both pro- and anti-inflammatory manners. They are also directed at recruitment and activation of various inflammatory and immune cells, and at enhancing their bactericidal mechanisms.

CRP is an important biochemical indicator of infection in clinical practice. It is a pentameric protein deriving its name from its ability to bind to C-polysaccharide of *Streptococcus pneumoniae*. Its functions are not very well known, but it efficiently binds to cellular chromatin, and probably helps in clearing cellular debris after tissue damage. It can also activate the classical complement pathway, and helps phagocytosis of bacteria by opsonization.[6]

From its acceptable serum level of 5 mg/L or lower, CRP in sepsis may rise by several hundred-fold. Its rapid response to infection proportional to its severity and its relatively short half-life of 18 hours provide a sensitive diagnostic indicator in measuring in timely fashion the severity and progress of the inflammatory process.

However, its rise during inflammation owing to non-infection causes renders it as a non-specific marker. CRP levels are usually normalized within 48 hours after recovery from infection.

Sepsis down-regulates the production of serum albumin from the liver, another useful biochemical marker easy to measure in the laboratory. Together, CRP and serum albumin provide an important set of markers to monitor infection and sepsis.

Thermoregulatory effects

Infection and sepsis are usually associated with an increase in core body temperature. Fever has beneficial effects of inhibiting bacterial growth and increasing efficiency of bactericidal mechanisms.

Studies have linked fever with increased inflammatory mediators, for example, TNF and IL-6, also called pyrogens. However, the pyrogenic effects arising from an inflamed site can also travel along the nociceptive and vagus nerves to the thermoregulatory centre in the hypothalamus.

Acute rise in core body temperature is achieved with strenuous involuntary muscular activity felt as shivering and rigors, accompanied by redistribution of blood flow from peripheral circulation in the skin to the core organs, resulting in feeling of chills.

Hypothermia may accompany systemic inflammation in more severe cases of sepsis. Several mediators have been implicated in the pathogenesis of hypothermia in inflammation, for example, platelet-activating factor and prostaglandins. A rat model of inflammation has shown that a challenge with bacterial endotoxins at a lower dose causes fever, whereas in higher doses they induce early hypothermia that might either persist or is replaced with fever.[7]

Metabolic responses

Increased metabolic demands during the stress of sepsis are met through maintenance of euglycaemia, or even hyperglycaemia, with numerous factors, for example, epinephrine, cortisol, and insulin-resistance by the muscles. Gluconeogenesis in the liver is favoured at the expense of body muscle mass and adipose tissue, releasing proteins and lipids to meet metabolic needs.

Excessive glycogenolysis and glycolysis result in lactate overproduction, not effectively cleared by the impaired liver. Tissue hypoperfusion, shifting aerobic metabolism to anaerobic form, has an added effect on lactate production. Correction of hypotension may or may not correct lactic acidosis, depending on the actual state of tissue perfusion.

Coagulopathy and microcirculation

As a major player in sepsis pathophysiology, the vascular endothelium is involved in vascular tone, coagulation, and vascular permeability.

Inflammation and coagulation are closely linked. Coagulation, characterized by increased synthesis of thrombin and release of fibrinogen, and decreased synthesis of protein C and anti-thrombin III, help in limiting infection by walling it off as an abscess within a case engineered by fibrin deposition.

Evidence from animal models indicates reduced microvascular density in sepsis. Loss of vessels could be due to blockage of microvasculature owing to less deformable erythrocytes in sepsis, too tough for the fine-calibre vessels. More importantly, platelet aggregation in sepsis leads to microthrombosis resulting in vascular injury and blockage. Damage to endothelium leads to extravasation of fluid into the tissue, with further increase in coagulability.

As the inflammatory response intensifies, this process may cascade into disseminated intravascular coagulation (DIC), reaching approximately 30–50% of vessels in severe cases.[2] Platelets and coagulation factors are consumed in the process resulting in haemorrhage, exhibiting as oozing from wounds or gastrointestinal bleeding.

Activated protein C (aPC), an endogenous proteolytic derivative of protein C, demonstrates anticoagulant and cytoprotective activity. It can potentially halt the above-mentioned process through its anticlotting activity. The 'Activated Protein C Worldwide Evaluation in Severe Sepsis (PROWESS)' study on the use of recombinant human aPC showed a 6.1% decrease in 28-day mortality in patients with 'severe sepsis'. Similar benefits were not, however, seen in a follow-up study, PROWESS-SHOCK.[8]

It has been proposed that aPC is beneficial for its cytoprotective effects in the management of sepsis, but not for its anticoagulant effects. Hence, cytoprotective-selective aPC variants have been under development and a subject of recent research.[9]

Organ dysfunction

Widespread endothelial and parenchymal injury results from endotoxins, inflammatory mediators, hypoxia, and/or from apoptosis. Severe sepsis is characterized by involvement of at least one organ in the body, varying from mild derangements to irreversible changes. Multiple organ dysfunction syndrome (MODS) is characterized with involvement of two or more organs.

Lungs

Deranged capillary blood flow and permeability lead to interstitial and alveolar oedema. It is compounded by entrapped neutrophils within the pulmonary microcirculation, resulting in acute lung injury and, when more severe, in ARDS. Diffuse alveolar damage may eventually resolve, or may organize, leaving pulmonary architecture distorted.

Endotoxins and other inflammatory mediators stimulate the medullary ventilatory centre resulting in hyperventilation with respiratory alkalosis, commonly found in sepsis.

Gastrointestinal tract

Septic shock can cause paralytic ileus interfering with enteral feeding and bacterial homeostasis. The gastrointestinal tract (GIT) has various functions besides digestion: production of hormones, immunological functions, and barrier against translocation of bacteria and endotoxins. It hosts a large population of diverse bacterial species, mainly in the colon, which contains approximately 10^{12} bacteria/g of colonic content.

Sepsis leads to failure in several of these functions, but more importantly, disrupts its barrier function. Malfunctioning GIT in sepsis thus drives a vicious cycle, enhancing it by leaking bacteria into the blood. Translocated bacteria, normally successfully dealt with by the Kupffer cells in the liver, may not be so in sepsis with increasing rates of translocation, compounded by a deranged liver. Bacteria from the GIT can also be aspirated into the lungs from their overgrowth in the upper GIT in ileus, causing pneumonia. These mechanisms provide some rationale to using 'selective gut decontamination' in sepsis.

Liver

The liver plays a key role in the systemic response to infection. The liver also seems to play a role in the sensory system that informs the hypothalamus that microbes have invaded.

Damage to hepatocytes in severe sepsis can lead to a leak of enzymes, defects in metabolism of bilirubin and coagulation factors, and failure to excrete toxins such as ammonia leading to encephalopathy. The function of Kupffer cells (found in the hepatic venous sinusoids) of targeting translocated bacteria and of hepatocytes catabolizing endotoxins are also impaired.

Cardiovascular system

'Shock' can be described as warm or cold depending on the state of peripheral circulation. The warm type is characterized by high cardiac output and low peripheral vascular resistance (PR). Of the two factors, it is held that it is principally the low PR which drives increase in cardiac output, particularly seen in volume-resuscitated patients.

Despite showing increased output, the myocardium in sepsis can in fact be depressed. This is supported by studies utilizing radionuclide cineangiography. The clinical spectrum of cardiac derangement is broad, including left ventricular, right ventricular, and diastolic dysfunction, but is usually reversible.

Kidneys

Acute kidney injury (AKI) has now replaced the term 'acute renal failure' as the injury can take place in the absence of marked renal failure (raised creatinine and blood urea nitrogen (BUN)). AKI is not an uncommon event in critically ill patients and usually occurs as a part of MODS.

Brain

The hypothalamus on receiving information of an infective process in the body activates the thermoregulatory centre, and the hypothalamic–pituitary–adrenal axis, with an upsurge of hormones. Since the microcirculation and tissue metabolism are regulated via peripheral nerves and circulating hormones, their dysregulation in sepsis can add to organ dysfunction.

Encephalopathy is a frequent manifestation in severe sepsis but its pathogenesis is not fully understood. Potential mechanisms involve low tissue perfusion resulting from hypotension, neuroinflammation, and disturbance of the blood–brain and blood–cerebral spinal fluid barriers.

Clinical features

Clinical (and laboratory) features in sepsis are determined by how and in what combination the abnormalities contributed by SIRS, MOD, and hypotension, along with damage by infection, develop in an individual patient.

The occurance of toxic appearance, fever, chills, rigors, fatigue and/or malaise, although not pathognomic for sepsis, indicates its presence. Localizing symptoms provide further clues to the aetiology and source of infection.

While fever, measured as core body (rectal) temperature, is common in sepsis, hypothermia when present indicates severe disease and a worse outcome. Hypothermia from prolonged cold exposure or during anaesthesia or certain surgical procedures may predispose to infections.

Brain involvement shows as altered mentation. Hepatic and renal derangement can be detected with abnormal biochemical markers, the latter also with oliguria or altered urinary concentration capacity. Myocardial abnormalities are detected by cardiac studies.

Hyperventilation with respiratory alkalosis is noted with the deranged lungs, the chief and often the only organ affected in severe sepsis. Acute lung injury and ARDS result in deranged oxygenation capacity of the lungs showing in decreased PaO_2:FiO_2 ratio; chest radiography will show bilateral lung infiltrates.

Findings of full bounding pulses, flushed skin, and fever describe warm shock, while cold shock, usually a progression of the warm type, is characterized with low-volume pulses, hypotension, delayed capillary refill, and clammy skin.

Hypotension (systolic blood pressure < 90 mmHg, or > 40 mmHg fall in the usual value) is associated with sepsis. In severe sepsis, the hypotension remains persistently low despite fluid replacement with 0.5 L (in adults), but is normalized with administration of vasopressors, unless the septic shock has progressed to a refractory stage.

Signs of intestinal bleeding may indicate development of a stress ulcer, or DIC if accompanied by blood oozing from other sites.

Differential diagnosis

+ SIRS
+ ARDS
+ Cardiogenic shock
+ Infective endocarditis
+ Distributive shock
+ Haemorrhagic shock
+ Toxic shock syndrome
+ Anaphylactic shock.

Investigation

Microbiology

+ Blood cultures: peripheral and through vascular catheters
+ Urine: for culture, and for *Legionella* and pneumococcal antigens where necessary
+ Sputum, bronchoalveolar lavage
+ Line-site swabs; skin swabs from skin lesions
+ Serum for appropriate testing—discuss with microbiologist
+ EDTA blood for appropriate molecular testing—discuss with microbiologist
+ Cerebral spinal fluid or samples from abscess, or from joint, pleural, or ascitic fluid where available and indicated.

Tests to monitor sepsis

+ Complete and differential blood cell counts show leucocytosis or leucopenia with corresponding neutrophilia or neutropenia; increased neutrophil:lymphocyte ratio; thrombophilia initially, which progresses in severe sepsis to thrombocytopenia with DIC
+ Hb level greater or equal to 8 g/dL necessary to ensure oxygen delivery to tissue
+ CRP and serum albumin to monitor inflammation; serum lactate dehydrogenase to measure tissue damage or red blood cell haemolysis
+ Serum procalcitonin can help differentiate sepsis from SIRS. It can be used to monitor the impact of antibiotics and other management
+ Metabolic assessment: serum glucose and electrolytes, magnesium, calcium, and phosphate
+ Renal function: serum creatinine, BUN. AKI can occur without major changes in these markers
+ Hepatic function: alkaline phosphate, alanine aminotransferase, and serum bilirubin
+ Serum lactate and pH provide an assessment of tissue hypoperfusion and hypermetabolic state. Serum lactate levels point to severity and risk of mortality from sepsis

+ Coagulation status: prothrombin time (PT) and the activated partial thromboplastin time (aPTT) (increased in sepsis)
+ DIC is marked with a rapid drop in the platelet count or a count reaching lower than 100 000/mm^3; D-dimers (plasma fibrin degradation products); PT or aPTT prolongation; and low plasma levels of coagulation inhibitors (e.g. antithrombin III).

Diagnostic imaging

+ X-ray:
  - Chest radiograph to detect pneumonia, embolism, haemorrhage, fluid overload, ARDS, pleural effusion, pneumothorax
  - X-ray imaging to detect free or soft tissue gas from an intra-abdominal source of sepsis
+ Ultrasonography for biliary tract infection
+ Computed tomography/magnetic resonance imaging:
  - Abdomen: for detecting intra-abdominal or retroperitoneal source
  - Head: before performing a lumbar puncture to detect increased intracranial pressure, space-occupying lesion, and encephalitis.

Principles of management of sepsis

'Early clinical suspicion, rigorous diagnostic measures, aggressive initiation of appropriate antimicrobial therapy, comprehensive supportive care, and measures aimed at reversing predisposing causes are the cornerstones of successful management.'[8]

Evidence holds that early-care resuscitative bundles improve patient outcome and facilitate case review.[10]

Critical care monitoring

Management of critically septic patients follows the 'ABC' of critical care applicable in different phases of the disease and patient-care activities (see 'Further reading').

Management of infection

Antibiotic therapy

Culture results guide specific antibiotic therapy but until then, empirical therapy, based on individual risks, suspected source of infection, and on the local bacterial resistance statistics, must be instituted immediately. It must cover major classes of bacteria, Gram positive, and Gram negative, including *Pseudomonas*, and anaerobic, and must be administered parenterally and in high doses within the permissible range.

Various antibiotic combinations satisfying the above-mentioned criteria have been reported in the literature, with no single combination being clearly superior to others.

A list of combinations based on various studies and local experience by the author is given in the following list applicable in different situations—provided there are no contraindications, including drug allergies and the patient is not known to have had a recent infection with bacteria resistant against the agent proposed. Add linezolid when the patient is a known or suspected meticillin-resistant *Staphylococcus aureus* carrier:

+ Meropenem and linezolid, when the source is not clear, or brain infections are suspected

- Chloramphenicol, with or without fosfomycin (not available in most centres), especially useful in the elderly and in most situations, including in atypical pneumonias, and does not particularly promote *C. difficile*
- Pneumonias: meropenem; add ciprofloxacin when atypical pneumonia is suspected
- Piperacillin/tazobactam and clindamycin where skin and soft tissue is involved (e.g. necrotizing fasciitis)
- Meropenem, and gentamicin as a stat dose in cases where abdominal infections, including biliary tract infections, are suspected as a source, and the kidney functions are not compromised. Gentamicin can be repeated 24 hours after the first dose if desirable, provided its pre-dose level is 1 mg/L or lower
- Piperacillin/tazobactam and vancomycin in cases with vascular catheter-associated infections. Vancomycin can be replaced with daptomycin where available
- Meropenem with or without gentamicin in urinary tract infection.

The therapy will need rationalizing later based on microbiology results.

Surgical drainage
Recovery from severe sepsis can be delayed or fail until and unless surgical drainage of abscess/collection and debridement of the infected tissues, where applicable, is carried out in the early stages of the management.

Other therapies
Use of hydrocortisone in sepsis depends on the clinical judgement. The role of more specialized interventions particularly addressing abnormalities in inflammation, such as anti-TNF, or those in clotting, such as aPC, is unclear as the effect is not consistent and can sometimes be harmful.[10] This may be due to a heterogeneous pathophysiology underlying the sepsis.

Prevention
Meticulous application of infection control and hand hygiene practices and line-care bundles are desirable to prevent spread of infection from one site to another and between patients. Judicious use of antibiotics prevents further complications, for example, infection with *Clostridium difficile*. Role of selective gut decontamination, chlorhexidine throat application, and nebulized colistin in prevention of sepsis or of its progress in critically ill patients needs further research.

Further reading
Azzopardi N, Fenech M, Piscopo T. Sepsis, the liver and the gut. In Azevedo L (ed) *Sepsis – An Ongoing and Significant Challenge*. InTech; 2012. [Online] http://www.intechopen.com/books/sepsis-an-ongoing-and-significant-challenge/sepsis-the-liver-and-the-gut

Lever A, Mackenzie I. Sepsis: definition, epidemiology, and diagnosis. *BMJ* 2007; 335(7625):879.

Mandell GL, Cheatham OR, Bennett JE, *et al. Mandell, Douglas, and Bennett's Principles and Practice of Infectious Diseases* (8th ed). Philadelphia, PA: Elsevier; 2013.

Nimmo GR, Singer M. *ABC of Intensive Care* (2nd ed). London: BMJ Books; 2011.

Young LS. Sepsis syndrome. In Mandell GL, Bennett JE, Dolin R (eds) *Principles and Practice of Infectious Diseases* (pp. 806–16). Philadelphia, PA: Churchill Livingstone; 2000.

References
1. Martin GS, Mannino DM, Eaton S, *et al.* The epidemiology of sepsis in the United States from 1979 through 2000. *N Engl J Med* 2003; 348:1546–54.
2. Rangel-Frausto MS, Pittet D, Costigan M, *et al.* The natural history of the systemic inflammatory response syndrome (SIRS). *JAMA* 1995; 273:117–23.
3. Remick DG. Pathophysiology of sepsis. *Am J Pathol* 2007; 170(5):1435–44.
4. Marshall JC. Inflammation, coagulopathy, and the pathogenesis of multiple organ dysfunction syndrome. *Crit Care Med* 2001; 29(Suppl):S99–106.
5. Summers C, Rankin SM, Condliffe AM, *et al.* Neutrophil kinetics in health and disease. *Trends Immunol* 2010; 31(8):318–24.
6. Husain TM, Kim DH. C-reactive protein and erythrocyte sedimentation rate in orthopaedics. *Univ Pa Orthop J* 2002; 15:13–16.
7. Leon LR. Hypothermia in systemic inflammation: role of cytokines. *Front Biosci* 2004; 9(1):877.
8. Kinasewitz GT, Yan SB, Basson B, *et al.* Universal changes in biomarkers of coagulation and inflammation occur in patients with severe sepsis, regardless of causative micro-organism. *Crit Care* 2004; 8(2):R82–90.
9. Holder AL, Huang DT. A dream deferred: the rise and fall of recombinant activated protein C. *Crit Care* 2013; 17(2):309.
10. Simmonds M, Blyth E, Chikane M, *et al.* Quality assurance in severe sepsis: an individualised audit/feedback system results in substantial improvements at a UK teaching hospital. *Crit Care* 2013; 17(Suppl 2):P500.

Skin and soft tissue infections

Jonathan Moore and Manjusha Narayanan

Introduction

Skin, the largest organ in the human body, is complex and vital. It is composed of a thin outermost layer, the epidermis, and an innermost layer, the dermis. Below the dermis lies the fatty subcutaneous layer which is traversed by blood vessels and nerves. The epidermis provides a mechanical protective barrier and the skin's immune function which is regulated mainly by Langerhans cells (antigen-presenting cells) and keratinocytes.

The Langerhans cells migrate to the dermis and into the draining lymph nodes.

Cytokines secreted by keratinocytes play a role in maintaining skin homeostasis (Figure 1.5.2.1).

Glossary of dermatological terms

- Macule: discoloured, circumscribed area of any size characterized by its flatness and usually distinguished from surrounding skin by its colouration
- Papule: elevated or palpable area 5 mm or less across
- Nodule: elevated, palpable area greater than 5 mm across
- Plaque: elevated, flat-topped area, greater than 5 mm across
- Vesicle: fluid-filled, raised area 5 mm or less across
- Bulla: fluid-filled, raised area greater than 5 mm across
- Blister: vesicle/bulla
- Pustule: pus-filled area
- Scale: dry, horny epidermis
- Lichenification: thick/roughened skin
- Excoriation: traumatic lesion characterized by breakage of epidermidis.

Overview

Skin and soft tissue infections are predominantly caused by Gram-positive cocci like *Staphylococcus aureus* and *Streptococcus pyogenes* (group A *Streptococcus*).[1] These infections vary in severity from self-limiting superficial infections such as impetigo to rapidly spreading, life-threatening infections such as necrotizing fasciitis. Both pathogens have the potential to be very virulent due to their ability to produce exotoxins like toxic shock syndrome toxin-1 (TSST-1) in *S. aureus* and streptococcal toxic shock syndrome toxin. Exfoliative toxins produced by some strains of *S. aureus* are associated with staphylococcal scalded skin syndrome. Panton–Valentine leucocidin (PVL)-positive strains of

S. aureus can cause severe infections and are also capable of producing TSST-1.

An overview of commonly encountered skin and soft tissue infections, common causative pathogens and empirical treatment options is provided in Table 1.5.2.1.[1,2]

Cellulitis

Cellulitis is a common, acute, spreading bacterial infection of the skin and subcutaneous tissues. It usually occurs as a result of *Staphylococcus aureus* and/or *Streptococcus pyogenes* breaching the skin barrier to cause infection.[1] Other rarer causes include group B, C, and G *Streptococcus*, Gram-negative bacilli from the Enterobacteriaceae family ('coliforms'), and anaerobes. Cellulitis can affect all age groups with the main predisposing factors being diabetes mellitus, obesity, immunodeficiency, underlying chronic liver and renal disease, and leg ulcers in peripheral vascular disease. Disruption to the skin barrier may be apparent, providing an obvious portal of entry for bacteria. Examples of this would include tinea pedis, insect bites, cuts, or inflammation such as that seen in eczema.[1,3]

Cellulitis manifests as a spreading, warm, erythematous, tender swelling of the affected skin. It may be accompanied by systemic symptoms such as fever and localized blistering, erosions, and ulceration.[4] Cellulitis is a clinical diagnosis with blood cultures rarely (<5%) positive.[5] Upon resolution of the cellulitis, the skin may flake or peel off as it heals.

Empirical treatment is usually with flucloxacillin. Clindamycin, erythromycin, and doxycycline are alternatives in penicillin-allergic patients.[5] Other options for treating more severe cellulitis caused by meticillin-resistant *Staphylococcus aureus* (MRSA) include linezolid, daptomycin, tigecycline, and vancomycin.[6] If Gram-negative infection is suspected, for instance, in the context of a diabetic ulcer, broad-spectrum agents such as cefuroxime or piperacillin/tazobactam may be required, although Gram-negative organisms are often merely colonizers in most cases. Treatment is usually for 5–10 days until the clinical features of cellulitis have subsided.[7] Intravenous antibiotics would be indicated in patients presenting in acute sepsis or toxic shock syndrome.[1]

Impetigo, folliculitis, furuncles, and carbuncles

Impetigo is a contagious, superficial bacterial infection of the skin caused by *Staphylococcus aureus* and/or *Streptococcus pyogenes*.[2] It commonly affects children, especially in the summer months. It primarily affects the face, extremities, and skin folds (particularly

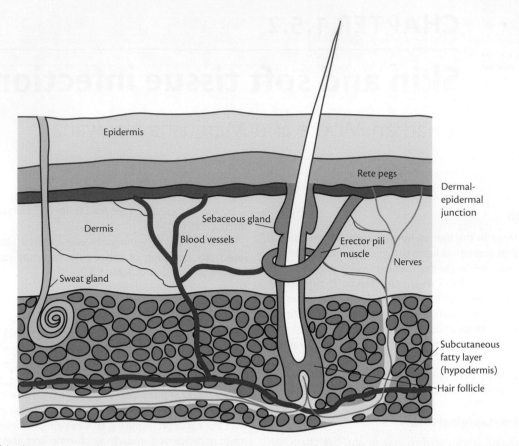

Fig. 1.5.2.1 Layers of the skin.

Table 1.5.2.1 Summary of common pathogens implicated in skin and soft tissue infections along with possible empirical therapies

Condition	Common pathogens	Empirical therapy[a]
Impetigo	*Staphylococcus aureus* *Streptococcus pyogenes*	Topical mupirocin *or* topical fucidic acid
Cellulitis	*Staphylococcus aureus*, Streptococci (groups A–G)	Flucloxacillin *or* clindamycin
Furuncles and carbuncles	*Staphylococcus aureus*	Flucloxacillin *or* clindamycin
Necrotizing fasciitis	Polymicrobial including *Staphylococcus aureus*, *Streptococcus pyogenes*, coliforms, anaerobes	Surgical debridement *plus* piperacillin/tazobactam and clindamycin *or* meropenem and linezolid *or* ciprofloxacin + clindamycin/co-amoxiclav
Pyomyositis	*Staphylococcus aureus* *Streptococcus pyogenes*	Percutaneous or open drainage Flucloxacillin or clindamycin
Gas gangrene	Clostridia species (such as *Clostridium perfringens*)	Surgical debridement Piperacillin/tazobactam, clindamycin and metronidazole
Human bite wound	*Staphylococcus aureus*, *Haemophilus* spp., *Eikenella corrodens*, anaerobes, streptococci, and *Fusobacterium* spp.	Co-amoxiclav *or* clindamycin
Animal bite wound	*Pasteurella multocida*, *Capnocytophaga canimorsus*, *Bacteroides*, *Fusobacterium*, and *Peptostreptococcus*	Co-amoxiclav *or* clindamycin + ciprofloxacin
Burn wound	*Staphylococcus aureus*, 'coliforms', *Pseudomonas aeruginosa*, fungi	Determined by cultures

[a]Antibiotic therapy should always be guided by recent and previous culture results. Infections caused by methicillin-resistant *Staphylococcus aureus* for instance will *not* be covered by flucloxacillin so this will necessitate a change to empirical therapy determined by local sensitivity patterns.[1,2]

Source: data from DiNubile MJ, Lipsky BA, Complicated infections of skin and skin structures: when the infection is more than skin deep, *Journal of Antimicrobial Chemotherapy*, Volume 53, Supplement 2, pp. ii37–50, Copyright © The British Society for Antimicrobial Chemotherapy 2004; and Stevens DL *et al.*, Practice guidelines for the diagnosis and management of skin and soft tissue infections, *Clinical Infectious Disease*, Volume 41, pp. 1373–1406, Copyright © 2005 by the Infectious Diseases Society of America.

the armpits) causing lesions that initially appear as small vesicles and then go on to develop into pustules with golden yellow crusts.[2] Oral antibiotics such as flucloxacillin may be used if the patient is slow to respond to first-line tropical treatment like fusidic acid ointment or chlorhexidine washes.

Folliculitis describes a group of conditions in which there is superficial inflammation of the hair follicles secondary to infection,[2] irritation, or occlusion. It typically presents with small, tender, pruritic erythematous papules, often with a central pustule. It is usually caused by *Staphylococcus aureus*, though *Pseudomonas aeruginosa* is implicated in 'hot-tub' folliculitis.[8] Folliculitis usually resolves spontaneously with or without drainage. If lesions persist, empirical treatment is with flucloxacillin, though other pathogens including Gram-negative bacteria and yeast such as *Malassezia furfur* should be considered if the initial response to therapy is poor. Swabs taken from the pustule can help to guide subsequent therapy.

A *furuncle* (boil) is a deep infection of the hair follicle in which a small abscess forms in the subcutaneous tissue following extension through the dermis. It presents as one or more tender erythematous spots or pustules. A *carbuncle* is a larger deeper abscess, an accumulation of pus extending into the subcutaneous fat with multiple heads. They are usually caused by *Staphylococcus aureus*[2] and may cause surrounding cellulitis, systemic upset, and fever. *Staphylococcus aureus* carriage is often a predisposing factor, with tiny nicks or grazes enabling the bacteria to penetrate the wall of the hair follicle and establish the infection. Treatment is with incision and drainage. The role of antimicrobial therapy is uncertain.[9] Systemic antibiotics such as flucloxacillin or clindamycin should be reserved for cases where there are multiple large (>5 cm) abscesses, surrounding cellulitis, fever, or systemic upset.[2,9] Eradication of *Staphylococcus aureus* carriage may be considered in patients suffering from recurrent abscesses.

Necrotizing fasciitis

Necrotizing fasciitis is a rapidly progressive, life-threatening infection of the fascia that spreads along the fascial plane, with secondary necrosis of the subcutaneous tissues.[2,10] *Fournier's gangrene* is a form of necrotizing fasciitis that is localized to the scrotum and perineal area.

Necrotizing fasciitis usually affects the lower limbs, though any part of the body can be affected. Abdominal surgical wounds are at particular risk. The infected area is excruciatingly painful, tender, and appears red, hot, and swollen.[10] The condition progresses with skin discolouration, bulla formation, and cutaneous gangrene. Alternatively, it may present with a necrotic ulcer with an outer zone of violaceous erythema. Meleney's ulcer presents with multiple fistula tracts surfacing at a distance from the infected wound.[1] In due course, destruction of superficial nerves and thrombosis of small vessels render the area numb. Subcutaneous oedema is seen on imaging, though imaging should never delay surgical exploration due to the rapidly progressive nature of the condition.

The microbiological aetiology of necrotizing fasciitis can be either mono, dual, or polymicrobial and has traditionally been divided into two types [1,2,10] (Table 1.5.2.2). The mainstay of treatment is prompt surgical exploration and debridement.[6,11] Antibiotics are not a sole alternative to surgery but used as an adjunct. Antibiotic coverage should be broad spectrum and include adequate antitoxin and anaerobic cover. Usually piperacillin/tazobactam or

Table 1.5.2.2 Aetiology and classification of necrotizing fasciitis

	Type 1 necrotizing fasciitis	Type 2 necrotizing fasciitis
Frequency	66%	30%
Type of infection	Polymicrobial	Mono or dual microbial
Organisms involved	Anaerobes (e.g. *Bacteroides*, *Peptostreptococcus*, or *Clostridium* spp.) Plus one or more Gram-positive cocci (*Staphylococcus aureus*, *Streptococcus pyogenes*) and/or Gram-negative bacilli ('coliforms')	*Streptococcus pyogenes* on its own or in conjunction with *Staphylococcus aureus*

Source: data from DiNubile MJ, Lipsky BA, Complicated infections of skin and skin structures: when the infection is more than skin deep, *Journal of Antimicrobial Chemotherapy*, Volume 53, Supplement 2, pp. ii37–50, Copyright © The British Society for Antimicrobial Chemotherapy 2004; and Stevens DL *et al.*, Practice guidelines for the diagnosis and management of skin and soft tissue infections, *Clinical Infectious Disease*, Volume 41, pp. 1373–1406, Copyright © 2005 by the Infectious Diseases Society of America; and Bellapianta JM *et al.*, Necrotizing fasciitis, *Journal of the American Academy of Orthopaedic Surgeons*, Volume 17, Number 3, pp. 174–82, Copyright © 2009 by the American Academy of Orthopaedic Surgeons.

meropenem along with clindamycin or linezolid and metronidazole is favoured[1,2,10] or a combination of ciprofloxacin and clindamycin/co-amoxiclav. If infection with *Staphylococcus aureus* or *Streptococcus pyogenes* is suspected, intravenous immunoglobulin may be considered.[2]

Pyomyositis

Pyomyositis describes an acute bacterial infection and abscess formation in the skeletal muscle. It occurs infrequently in Europe, but is more common in the tropics. Predisposing factors include HIV, diabetes mellitus, alcoholic liver disease, and underlying malignancies.[12] *Staphylococcus aureus* and *Streptococcus pyogenes* are responsible for the majority of cases.[2,12] There is often a history of blunt trauma or rigorous exercise to the affected area.

As bacteria invade the muscle, the patient experiences local swelling, erythema, and a subacute onset of fever, though there is mild pain and minimal tenderness. The suppurative stage follows 2–3 weeks later characterized by fever, muscle swelling, and tenderness. This then progresses into a more systemic illness with generalized sepsis and exquisite tenderness. It may be complicated by metastatic abscess formation, shock, and compartment syndrome.

Pyomyositis is usually diagnosed by computed tomography (CT)/magnetic resonance imaging or at surgery. It is managed by either percutaneous or open drainage with or without fasciotomies if compartment syndrome is present. Empirical antibiotic cover should be with IV flucloxacillin or clindamycin.[2]

Gas gangrene (clostridial myonecrosis)

Gas gangrene is caused by *Clostridium* species and is a rapidly progressive skeletal muscle infection that can be life-threatening.[13] There is usually a preceding history of muscle injury and contamination of the wound by soil or material containing clostridial spores. *Clostridium perfringens* is implicated in the majority of cases, with its toxins responsible for the pathological effects after a usual incubation period of 2–3 days although this may be shorter.

Non-traumatic gas gangrene is usually caused by *Clostridium septicum* and is often associated with intestinal pathology such as malignancy or diverticulitis.[2]

Gas gangrene presents with acute onset of excruciating pain and evidence of septic shock and acute kidney injury. Early on, local oedema and foul smelling discharge may be early signs of infection. The diagnosis is clinical, with culture confirming the diagnosis. Initial microscopy (Gram stain) may sometimes help. Plain radiographs and CT imaging may reveal gas in the affected tissues. Prompt surgical exploration and debridement of affected tissues is essential. Antimicrobial therapy is with broad-spectrum agents and should include anaerobic cover using combination treatment such as piperacillin/tazobactam and metronidazole or clindamycin, ciprofloxacin, and metronidazole.[1,2]

Surgical site infection

A *surgical site infection* (SSI) describes an infection that occurs in a wound created by an invasive surgical procedure. By definition, a SSI develops within 30 days of surgery (or up to 1 year if prosthetic material was inserted). They can be superficial, involving just the skin and subcutaneous tissue or deep, involving the muscle, fascia, or even an organ or organ space.[2] One prevalence survey conducted in 2006 found that nearly 5% of patients undergoing a surgical procedure developed a SSI.[14]

The most common organisms implicated in SSI are bacteria found on the skin such as *Staphylococcus aureus* and coagulase-negative staphylococci and organisms found at the site of the operation such as coliforms in lower spinal or bowel surgery.[15] Prosthetic material can provide a protective environment for organisms, meaning relatively few bacteria are required to initiate an infection which can then be extremely difficult to eradicate.

SSIs typically present with erythema, swelling, and purulent discharge with or without fever. They usually appear between 5 days and 2 weeks postoperatively. In obese patients and those with deep, multilayer wounds, the superficial signs of SSIs may take longer to develop. The diagnosis at first is clinical, though cultures of wound swabs and pus can help to obtain a microbiological diagnosis to guide subsequent antibiotic therapy.[16]

The treatment for SSIs is to open the incision, debride infected tissue, consider removal of prosthetic material, and continue dressing changes until the wound heals. Vacuum-assisted wound closure can be considered in wounds with a clean granulating base. Although there is a tendency to try to treat SSIs with antibiotics, there is little evidence to support this practice and often this merely delays surgical intervention.[2,16] This can also be associated with complications of antibiotic use such as *Clostridium difficile* infection and MRSA acquisition. Antibiotics are only really indicated if the patient is unwell with a temperature higher than 38°C on more than two occasions, hypotension, and tachycardia.

SSI can be prevented by thorough preoperative assessment (including screening and eradicating potential pathogens such as MRSA), strict intraoperative asepsis, appropriate timely presurgical intervention (e.g. washouts and debridements), intraoperative prophylactic antibiotics, and good postoperative wound care.[16]

Bite infections

Infections from *human bite wounds* are caused by the oral flora of the assailant and are usually polymicrobial in nature. Typical offending pathogens include staphylococci, *Haemophilus* spp., *Eikenella corrodens*, anaerobes, streptococci, and *Fusobacterium* spp.[17] Patients will often attend with just the bite wound or late presentations of cellulitis or a local abscess. Treatment is with wound irrigation and prophylactic antibiotics such as co-amoxiclav, doxycycline with metronidazole, or in severe cases, piperacillin/tazobactam or meropenem.[2] Prompt surgical debridement may be necessary with wounds left open to enable closure by secondary intention. Human bites have the potential to spread blood-borne viruses such as hepatitis (B and C) and HIV[18] so a risk assessment should be made and post-exposure prophylaxis considered where applicable. Bite wounds may cause tendon and/or nerve damage and be complicated by the development of osteomyelitis or septic arthritis.

Animal bite wound infections are usually polymicrobial[19] and account for 1% of emergency department attendances.[2] Common pathogens include *Pasteurella multocida*, *Capnocytophaga canimorsus*, *Bacteroides* spp., *Fusobacterium* spp., and *Peptostreptococcus* spp.[19] Secondary infections with *Staphylococcus aureus* and *Streptococcus pyogenes* are common. They may present with cellulitis, fever, purulent or non-purulent discharge, and abscesses. Like human bite wounds they can be complicated by osteomyelitis, septic arthritis, and sometimes bacteraemia and systemic sepsis. Wound swabs can be helpful in identifying the aetiology of the infection and targeting subsequent therapy. Treatment is with copious irrigation, removing any debris, debriding devitalized tissue, and steri-stripping the wound (stitching the wound should be avoided).[19] Antibiotics such as co-amoxiclav or ciprofloxacin and clindamycin or piperacillin/tazobactam or meropenem in severe cases can be used both prophylactically to prevent and in the treatment of animal bite infections pending culture results.

Further reading

Bennett JE, Dolin R, Mandell GL (eds). *Mandell, Douglas, and Bennett's Principles and Practice of Infectious Diseases* (8th ed). New York: Churchill Livingstone; 2014.
Finch R, Davey P, Wilcox M, *et al.* (eds). *Antimicrobial Chemotherapy* (6th ed). Oxford: Oxford University Press; 2012.
Greenwood D, Barer M, Slack R, *et al.* (eds). *Medical Microbiology. A Guide to Microbial Infections: Pathogenesis, Immunity, Laboratory Diagnosis and Control* (18th ed). Edinburgh: Churchill Livingstone; 2012.
Williams NS, Bulstrode CJK, O'Connell PR (eds). *Bailey & Love's Short Practice of Surgery* (26th ed). London: Hodder Arnold; 2013.
Wolff K, Johnson RA, Saavedra AP (eds). *Fitzpatrick's Colour Atlas & Synopsis of Clinical Dermatology* (7th ed). New York: McGraw-Hill Medical; 2013.

References

1. DiNubile MJ, Lipsky BA. Complicated infections of skin and skin structures: when the infection is more than skin deep. *J Antimicrob Chemother* 2004; 53,(Suppl 2):ii37–50.
2. Stevens DL, Bisno AL, Chambers HF, *et al.* Practice guidelines for the diagnosis and management of skin and soft tissue infections. *Clin Infect Dis* 2005; 41:1373–406.

3. Björnsdóttir S, Gottfredsson M, Thórisdóttir AS, *et al*. Risk factors for acute cellulitis of the lower limb: a prospective case-control study. *Clin Infect Dis* 2005; 41:1416–22.

4. Phoenix G, Das S, Joshi M. Diagnosis and management of cellulitis. *BMJ* 2012; 345:e4955.

5. Perl B, Gottehrer NP, Ravesh D, *et al*. Cost-effectiveness of blood cultures for adult patients with cellulitis. *Clin Infect Dis* 1999; 29:1483–8.

6. Liu C, Bayer A, Cosgrove SE, *et al*. Clinical practice guidelines by the Infectious Diseases Society of America for the treatment of methicillin-resistant Staphylococcus aureus infections in adults and children. *Clin Infect Dis* 2011; 52:e18–55.

7. Hepburn MJ, Dooley DP, Skidmore PJ, *et al*. Comparison of short-course (5 days) and standard (10 days) treatment for uncomplicated cellulitis. *Arch Intern Med* 2004; 164:1669–74.

8. Ratnam S, Hogan K, March SB, *et al*. Whirlpool-associated folliculitis caused by Pseudomonas aeruginosa: report of an outbreak and review. *J Clin Microbiol* 1986; 23:655–9.

9. Gorwitz RJ. The role of ancillary antimicrobial therapy for treatment of uncomplicated skin infections in the era of community-associated methicillin-resistant Staphylococcus aureus. *Clin Infect Dis* 2007; 44:785–7.

10. Bellapianta JM, Ljungquist K, Tobin E, *et al*. Necrotizing fasciitis. *J Am Acad Orthop Surg* 2009 17(3):174–82.

11. Levine EG, Manders SM. Life-threatening necrotizing fasciitis. *Clin Dermatol* 2005; 23:144–7.

12. Crum NF. Bacterial pyomyositis in the United States. *Am J Med* 2004; 117(6):420–8.

13. MacLennan JD. The histotoxic clostridial infections of man. *Bacteriol Rev* 1962; 26:177–276.

14. Smyth ET, McIlvenny G, Enstone JE, *et al*. Four Country Healthcare Associated Infection Prevalence Survey 2006: overview of the results. *J Hosp Infect* 2008; 69: 230–48.

15. Health Protection Agency. *Surveillance of Surgical Site Infection in England: October 1997–September 2005*. London: Health Protection Agency; 2006. http://www.hpa.nhs.uk/webc/HPAwebFile/HPAweb_C/1194947340094

16. National Institute for Health and Care Excellence. *Surgical Site Infection: Prevention and Treatment of Surgical Site Infection*. Clinical Guideline 74. London: NICE; 2008 (reviewed 2014). http://www.nice.org.uk/guidance/cg74

17. Talan DA, Abrahamian FM, Moran GJ, *et al*. Clinical presentation and bacteriologic analysis of infected human bites in patients presenting to emergency departments. *Clin Infect Dis* 2003; 37:1481–9.

18. Bartholomew CF, Jones AM. Human bites: a rare risk factor for HIV transmission. *AIDS* 2006; 20:631–2.

19. Abraham FM, Goldstein EJC. Microbiology of animal bite wound infections. *Clin Microbiol Rev* 2011; 24:231–46.

CHAPTER 1.5.3

Healthcare-associated infection

Allison Sykes

Surgical site infection

Infections that occur in the wound created by an invasive surgical procedure are generally referred to as surgical site infections (SSIs). These can range from simple wound discharge with no other complications to a life-threatening condition. Nearly 5% of patients who had undergone a surgical procedure were found to have developed an SSI and over one-third of postoperative deaths are related, at least in part, to SSI.[1] However, these figures may be underestimated as many SSIs develop after the patient has been discharged from hospital.

SSIs are usually derived from the patient's own skin flora (endogenous infection). Exogenous infection occurs when microorganisms from instruments or the theatre environment contaminate the site peri- or postoperatively before the skin has sealed. They usually develop within 30 days of an operative procedure and most often between the 5th and 10th postoperative days. On rare occasions, microorganisms from a distant source of infection, principally through haematogenous spread, can cause an SSI by attaching to a prosthesis or other implant. This may occur several months after the operation.

There are three levels of SSI[2]:

- *Superficial incisional* which affects the skin and subcutaneous tissue. Signs of these may be localized (Celsian) redness, pain, heat, or swelling at the site of the incision or the drainage of pus.

- *Deep incisional* which affect the fascial and muscle layers. Signs of these may be the presence of pus or an abscess, fever with tenderness of the wound, or a separation of the edges of the incision, exposing the deeper tissues.

- *Organ or space infection* which involve any part of the anatomy other than the incision, that is opened or manipulated during the surgical procedure, for example, joint or peritoneum. Signs of these infections may be the drainage of pus or the formation of an abscess detected by histopathological or radiological examination or during re-operation.

There may also be microbiological evidence of wound infection from cultures obtained from wound fluid or tissue. However, skin sites are normally colonized by a variety of organisms, therefore positive wound cultures without clinical signs of infection are not usually indicative of SSI.

Risk factors for surgical site infection

The risk of SSI is increased by factors that increase endogenous and exogenous contamination, and diminish the efficacy of the general immune response.[1] These risk factors include:

- age
- diabetes and postoperative hypoglycaemia and the degree of hypoglycaemia

- malnutrition
- low serum albumin
- anticancer treatment and radiotherapy (within 90 days of surgery)
- obesity
- smoking
- wound classification
- complexity of the procedure.

Preventing surgical site infections

Various strategies can be employed to reduce the number of microorganisms introduced into the operative site and optimize the patient's defences to infection. These include the following:

- Maintenance of strict asepsis and removal of microorganisms which normally colonize the skin (as described earlier in this chapter)

- The use of standard precautions during all patient care

- Implementation of the 'Saving Lives' strategies[3]:

  - Meticillin-resistant *Staphylococcus aureus* (MRSA) screening and decolonization

  - Hair removal using clippers

  - Maintaining normothermia

- Use of appropriate prophylactic antibiotics

- Use of appropriate wound dressings to prevent introduction of contaminants.

Saving Lives

The Saving Lives Care Bundle to prevent SSI[3] identified key elements within the clinical process that must be performed consistently for every patient (these are also endorsed by the Association for Perioperative Practice[4]). These elements are discussed in the following sections.

Preoperative actions

MRSA screening

Patients must be screened for MRSA prior to elective surgical procedures or on admission, if an emergency, unless exempt, in accordance with UK Department of Health guidance.[5] This enables risk reduction strategies to be implemented at the pre-, peri-, and postoperative phases. To ensure an adequate risk assessment has been completed, it is essential that the results of these screens are known prior to any surgery, wherever possible.

MRSA decolonization

This must be given to all MRSA-positive patients prior to elective procedures.

Perioperative actions

Hair removal

◆ Use a clipper with a disposable head

◆ Shaving with a razor is not recommended.

The use of electric clippers with a single-use head on the day of surgery is the recommended mode of hair removal. Re-useable heads can be used; however, effective decontamination processes must be implemented to ensure patient safety.

The removal of hair is only necessary if it directly interferes with access to the incision site and if there is a risk that it will contaminate the wound site. If removal is necessary, consent must be obtained from the patient and the method of removal agreed.

Hair should be removed as close to the time of surgery as possible to reduce the risk of bacterial contamination of the skin surface.

Shaving is not a recommended means of removal as it causes micro-abrasions of the skin which may support the multiplication of bacteria within the skin and on the skin's surface.

The use of depilatory creams is an effective method of hair removal, although it can be costly. However, patch testing is recommended prior to use as some patients may experience irritation.[4]

Prophylactic antimicrobial

◆ An appropriate antimicrobial should be administered within 60 minutes prior to incision.

Normothermia

◆ Maintaining a body temperature above 36°C in the perioperative period has been shown to reduce infection rates

Inadvertent hypothermia must be prevented with the use of warming devices during the peri- and postoperative stage, as hypothermia can delay wound healing due to reduced perfusion. However, in some cases, hypothermia can be deliberate for medical or surgical reasons.

Glucose control

◆ Maintaining a glucose level of less than 11 mmol/L has been shown to reduce wound infection in diabetic patients.

Dressings

Where practical, low-adherence, transparent polyurethane dressings should be used to cover all surgical incisions post procedure. This will protect the wound and allow the surgical incision site to be reviewed without having to disturb the dressing. Ideally dressings should be left *in situ* for between 3 and 5 days.

It is recommended that the dressing should have an integral pad of absorbent material. For healing to take place at an optimum rate, all dressing materials used should ensure that the wound remains[1]:

◆ moist with exudate but does not get macerated

◆ free from clinical infection and excessive slough or devitalized/necrotic tissue

◆ free from toxic chemicals, particles, or fibres released from the dressing

◆ at an optimum temperature for healing to take place (around 37°C)

◆ undisturbed by frequent or unnecessary dressing changes

◆ at an optimum pH value.

An aseptic non-touch technique (ANTT) must be used when undertaking dressing changes to reduce the risk of surgical site contamination. The use of a surgical or standard ANTT procedure would be determined by the necessity for wound cleansing or complexity of the procedure.

Standard precautions

Standard precautions are based on the principle that all body fluids are potentially infectious. This requires the identification of high-risk procedures rather than high-risk individuals, to prevent exposure of healthcare workers (HCWs) to potentially pathogenic microorganisms through inoculation, injury, and body fluid splashes to mucous membranes. These precautions also protect patients from the transmission of organisms from other patients and HCWs.

Standard precautions include[6]:

◆ hand hygiene

◆ managing breaks to the skin

◆ use of personal protective equipment (PPE)

◆ body fluid spillage management

◆ sharps management

◆ action following a sharps injury.

Hand hygiene

Hand hygiene is the single most important method to prevent the transmission of organisms and the prevention of healthcare-associated infection. Effective hand hygiene involves several steps including the use of the correct hand cleaning agent and the correct application technique (Figure 1.5.3.1). The correct technique for hand washing and use of alcohol hand rub are detailed in the following paragraphs.

Alcohol hand rub

Alcohol hand rub is only effective on clean, dry skin which is not soiled, sweaty, or greasy as it does not penetrate organic matter. The hand rub must cover all areas of the skin, as for hand washing, and be rubbed in until dry. After several uses the emollients in the hand rub will build-up on the skin, leaving the hands feeling gritty; hands must be washed at this stage.

It must be noted that alcohol hand rub is *not* effective against bacterial spores such as *Clostridium difficile* spores and hands must be washed with soap and water after coming into contact with patients with this organism.

The '5 Moments for Hand Hygiene' defines the key moments when hand hygiene must be performed (Figure 1.5.3.2).[7] These are as follows:

◆ Before touching a patient

◆ Before an aseptic task

◆ After body fluid exposure

HAND CLEANING TECHNIQUES

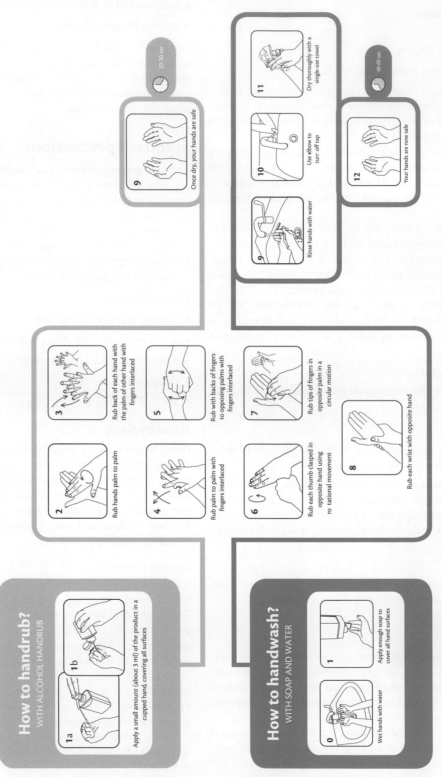

Fig. 1.5.3.1 National Patient Safety Agency hand cleaning techniques. Particular attention must be paid to the finger tips, thumbs, finger webs, and wrists, as these are the areas most commonly missed during this procedure.

Reproduced with permission from National Patient Safety Agency, *Hand Cleaning Techniques*, Copyright © 2011 National Patient Safety Agency, available from www.npsa.nhs.uk/cleanyourhands licensed under the Open Government Licence v3.0; and World Health Organization, *WHO Guidelines on Hand Hygiene in Health Care*, Copyright © 2009, available from http://whql bdoc.who.int/publications/2009/ 9789241597906_eng.pdf

◆ After touching a patient

◆ After touching a patient's surroundings.

Other important points for effective hand hygiene include the following[6]:

◆ Wash hands when gloves are removed rather than using alcohol hand rub

◆ Use emollients regularly to prevent dry and breaking skin

◆ Cover skin breaks with waterproof dressings

◆ Staff with chronic skin lesions to hands or forearms or persistent skin problems must avoid undertaking invasive procedures

◆ Be *bare below the elbow* in clinical settings

◆ Watches, hand or arm jewellery, nail varnish, and artificial nails must not be worn as they harbour microorganisms, prevent effective hand hygiene and can damage the patient.

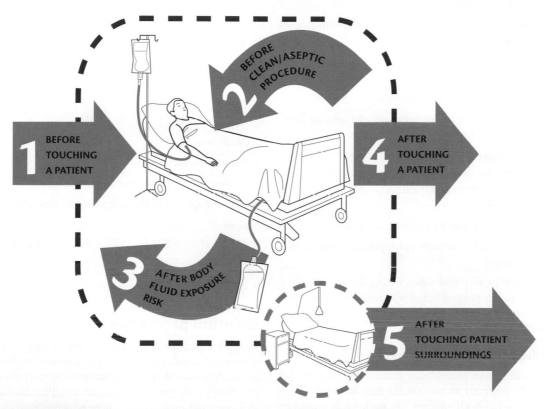

1 BEFORE TOUCHING A PATIENT	WHEN?	Clean your hands before touching a patient when approaching him/her.	
	WHY?	To protect the patient against harmful germs carried on your hands.	
2 BEFORE CLEAN/ ASEPTIC PROCEDURE	WHEN?	Clean your hands immediately before performing a clean/aseptic procedure.	
	WHY?	To protect the patient against harmful germs, including the patient's own, from entering his/her body.	
3 AFTER BODY FLUID EXPOSURE RISK	WHEN?	Clean your hands immediately after an exposure risk to body fluids (and after glove removal).	
	WHY?	To protect yourself and the health-care environment from harmful patient germs.	
4 AFTER TOUCHING A PATIENT	WHEN?	Clean your hands after touching a patient and her/his immediate surroundings, when leaving the patient's side.	
	WHY?	To protect yourself and the health-care environment from harmful patient germs.	
5 AFTER TOUCHING PATIENT SURROUNDINGS	WHEN?	Clean your hands after touching any object or furniture in the patient's immediate surroundings, when leaving – even if the patient has not been touched.	
	WHY?	To protect yourself and the health-care environment from harmful patient germs.	

Fig. 1.5.3.2 National Patient Safety Agency 'Your 5 moments for hand hygiene at the point of care' poster.

Reproduced with permission from SAVE LIVES: Clean Your Hands - WHO's global annual call to action for health workers, *'Your 5 Moments For Hand Hygiene Poster'*, Copyright © 2009, World Health Organization, available from http://www.who.int/gpsc/5may/Your_5_Moments_For_Hand_Hygiene_Poster.pdf

Personal protective equipment

The selection of PPE should be based on an assessment of the risk of transmission of microorganisms to the patient and the risk of contamination of the HCW's clothing and skin by patient's blood/body fluids.

Gloves and aprons/gowns

- Must be worn for invasive procedures, contact with sterile sites, and non-intact skin or mucous membranes and all activities that have been assessed as carrying a risk of exposure to blood, body fluids, secretions, or excretions.
- Must be single use and gloves must *never* be cleaned with alcohol hand rub or washed.
- Must be changed between patients and between different care activities for the same patient.
- Gloves must be non-latex (wherever possible).
- Gowns must be either single use or removed and sent for laundering after each patient contact.

Masks/goggles/face visors

- Face protection must be worn if there is a risk of exposure to the mucous membranes of the face from splashing of blood/body fluids.
- If single use, they must be disposed of once the task is complete.
- If reusable, they must be decontaminated appropriately after each use as per local policy.
- Specific masks may be required when caring for patients with respiratory infections, for example, influenza and *Mycobacterium tuberculosis* (tuberculosis (TB)). Referral to appropriate Trust Policy is essential in these cases.

Blood/body fluid spillage management

When there are spillages of blood/body fluids it is essential that these are dealt with correctly to prevent the risk of transmission of blood-borne viruses to both patients and staff. Spills should be soaked up and the area disinfected as per local policy. Chlorine solutions should not be used on urine as this will cause the release of ammonium gases.

Sharps and splash injury prevention and management

To prevent HCWs sustaining occupational injuries from sharps and potentially acquiring a blood-borne virus or other infection from that injury, it is vital that sharps are used and managed safely. HCWs must always adhere to the following precautions:

- Always dispose of sharps into an appropriate sharps bin
- Never pass sharps from hand to hand
- Never re-sheath needles
- Never remove needles from syringes, they should be disposed of connected
- Never dispose of sharps into domestic or clinical waste bins
- Never leave sharps on beds, lockers, theatre tables, etc.
- Never put anything other than sharps and attached syringes into the sharps bins

- Never place hands into sharps bins to retrieve anything
- Never shake a sharps bin as something may fly out.

If a sharps injury is sustained the following action should be taken:

1. Gently squeeze the puncture site in the attempt to remove any contaminants that may be at the surface.
2. Wash the puncture site with soap and water.
3. Cover with a waterproof dressing.
4. If known, note name of patient the sharp had been used on.
5. Report to the Occupational Health Department (or equivalent) with the patient information.
6. Complete an incident reporting form (as per local policy).

If a splash injury to the eyes or mouth is sustained, the following action should be taken:

Eyes

- Irrigate thoroughly for at least 5 minutes with eyewash or sterile water
- Remove contact lenses
- Report to A&E for assessment of the injury
- Follow steps 4–6 of the sharps injury action list.

Mouth

- Irrigate thoroughly for at least 5 minutes with drinking water
- Do not swallow the water
- Follow steps 4–6 of sharps injury action list.

Isolation precautions

Protective isolation precautions may be required for patients at greater risk of infection due to their medical condition (e.g. neutropenia). Source isolation is required when the patient is a source of potentially pathogenic microorganisms. Patients should be isolated in an en-suite single room where possible; with clearly visible signage identifying the patient is being isolated.

General principles

Protective isolation

- Wash hands and forearms with an antiseptic solution prior to entering room. Don apron and gloves. Masks may be required as per local policy. Gowns often replace aprons in a theatre setting.
- Prior to leaving protective isolation: remove apron and gloves, dispose of into clinical waste, and wash hands.
- It is important that staff or visitors with an infection do not enter a room in which a patient is being nursed in protective isolation.

Source isolation

- Clean hands prior to entering room. Don apron and gloves. In a theatre setting, gowns would be worn rather than aprons.
- Surgical or FFP3 masks will be required for organisms spread via the respiratory route, for example, influenza and multidrug-resistant TB (check local policy). Staff require fit testing for FFP3 masks.

◆ Prior to leaving source isolation: remove apron and gloves dispose of into clinical waste, and wash hands. Remove mask in the ante-room where possible (or as per local policy)

◆ The patient equipment and environment must be disinfected as per local policy after each use / episode.

◆ Although it is not always practical to isolate a patient as per local policy, in the theatre environment, the general principles of isolation can be implemented to reduce the risk of transmission of the organism.

Further reading

Department of Health. *Clean, Safe Care: Reducing MRSA and other Healthcare Associated Infections and Saving Lives*. London: Department of Health; 2008. http://www.dh.gov.uk/en/Publicationsandstatistics/Publications/

Department of Health. *The Health and Social Care Act 2008: Code of Practice for the NHS on the Prevention and Control of Healthcare Associated Infection and Related Guidance*. London: Department of Health; 2009. http://www.dh.gov.uk/en/Publicationsandstatistics/Publications/

Department of Health. *The Health and Social Care Act 2008: Code of Practice for the NHS on the Prevention and Control of Healthcare Associated Infection and Related Guidance*. London: Department of Health. 2015. https://www.gov.uk/government/uploads/system/uploads/attachment_data/file/449049/Code_of_practice_280715_acc.pdf

National Audit Office. *Reducing Healthcare Associated Infections in Hospitals in England*. London: The Stationery Office; 2009. http://www.nao.org.uk/wp-content/uploads/2009/06/0809560.pdf

National Institute for Health and Clinical Excellence. *Prevention and Control of Healthcare-Associated Infections*. NICE Public Health Guidance 36. London: NICE; 2011. http://www.nice.org.uk/guidance/ph36

World Health Organization. *WHO Guidelines for Safe Surgery: Safe Surgery Saves Lives*. Geneva: World Health Organization; 2009. http://www.who.int/patientsafety/safesurgery/tools_resources/9789241598552/en/

References

1. National Institute for Health and Care Excellence. *Surgical Site Infection: Prevention and Treatment of Surgical Site Infection*. Clinical Guideline 74. London: NICE; 2008 (reviewed 2014). http://www.nice.org.uk/guidance/cg74

2. PHE Protocol for the Surveillance of Surgical Site Infection Surgical Site Infection Surveillance Service Version 6. June 2013 [Online]. https://www.gov.uk/government/uploads/system/uploads/attachment_data/file/364412/Protocol_for_surveillance_of_surgical_site_infection_June_2013.pdf

3. Department of Health. *Saving Lives: Reducing Infection, Delivering Clean and Safe Care. High Impact Intervention No 4 Care Bundle to Prevent Surgical Site Infection*. 2007. [Online] http://www.dh.gov.uk/en/Publicationsandstatistics/Publications/PublicationsPolicyAndGuidance/DH_124265

4. Association of Perioperative Practice. *Standards and Recommendations for Safe Perioperative Practice* (3rd ed). Harrogate: Association of Perioperative Practice; 2011

5. Department of Health. *Implementation of Modified Admission MRSA Screening Guidance for NHS (2014). Department of Health Expert Advisory Committee on Antimicrobial Resistance and Healthcare Associated Infection (ARHAI)*. London: Department of Health; 2014. https://www.gov.uk/government/uploads/system/uploads/attachment_data/file/345144/Implementation_of_modified_admission_MRSA_screening_guidance_for_NHS.pdf

6. Fraise A, Bradley C (eds). *Ayliffe's Control of Healthcare-Associated Infection: A Practical Handbook* (5th ed). London: Hodder Arnold; 2009.

7. World Health Organization. Your 5 Moments For Hand Hygiene Poster. 2009. [Online] http://www.who.int/gpsc/5may/Your_5_Moments_For_Hand_Hygiene_Poster.pdf

CHAPTER 1.5.4

Blood-borne viruses

Shirelle Burton-Fanning and Sheila Waugh

Introduction

The principal viruses transmitted via blood are hepatitis B virus (HBV), hepatitis C virus (HCV), and human immunodeficiency virus (HIV). These viruses are of particular importance in surgical practice because of the potential for transmission during invasive procedures.

Patients and healthcare staff are at risk of acquiring these viruses and equally, both patients and staff may act as sources of infection. Adherence to standard infection prevention and control precautions and the safe use of sharps, including surgical instruments, is essential to reduce the risks of infection.

Enormous advances have occurred in recent years in the treatment of viral hepatitis and HIV. Long-term disease-free survival is now possible in the majority of cases. Early diagnosis is important to ensure optimal follow-up and treatment. Infected patients are often seen in a variety of healthcare settings before infection is diagnosed. Although these infections do not classically present in a surgical setting, testing should be considered for patients presenting with suggestive symptoms or signs and should be offered to patients with known risk factors.

Hepatitis B virus

Epidemiology

The World Health Organization (WHO) estimates that 240 million people worldwide are infected with HBV. The majority of these infections have occurred in high-prevalence areas such as sub-Saharan Africa and South East Asia (5–10%), with the prevalence in Western Europe and North America being much lower (less than 1%).[1]

Transmission routes and risk groups

There are three main routes of transmission: vertical, sexual, and parenteral. Vertical transmission occurs perinatally between an infected mother and her child and is the main route of transmission in countries with a high prevalence of infection. Parenteral transmission refers to direct inoculation of infectious blood or body fluids during intravenous drug abuse, tattooing or body piercing, and during medical, surgical, or dental procedures (including needlestick injury).

Clinical features

The incubation period for HBV is between 6 weeks and 6 months following exposure. During the acute infection, many individuals are asymptomatic but may present with acute hepatitis characterized by markedly raised liver transaminases and jaundice. The risk of fulminant hepatitis is less than 0.1%. Clinically HBV infection cannot be distinguished from other causes of viral hepatitis. In many countries, including the United Kingdom, the diagnosis of acute HBV infection requires formal notification to public health authorities.[2]

Following acute infection, the majority of adults will clear the virus and develop immunity. Only 1–5% of immunocompetent adults will progress to chronic infection. In contrast, 90% of those infected perinatally develop chronic infection. Although chronically infected individuals may remain well for many years, eventual sequelae include chronic hepatitis, cirrhosis (20%), and hepatocellular carcinoma (5%).

Diagnosis

HBV should be considered as a potential diagnosis in all cases of hepatitis. Where an asymptomatic patient is known to have risk factors for infection, testing should be offered to enable appropriate follow-up and treatment. Diagnosis in the later stages of chronic infection is associated with a poorer outcome.

HBV infection can be diagnosed by detecting HBV surface antigen (HBsAg) in blood. A number of other markers help ascertain the stage of infection (Table 1.5.4.1). The window period (the interval between infection and the time blood markers are detectable) for HBV is 3–6 months.

Management

Most symptomatic acute infections are self-limiting and require supportive treatment only. Patients are followed up to determine if they clear the infection or become chronically infected.

Specialist management is required for those with chronic HBV infection. Treatment is indicated where there is evidence of ongoing hepatitis to prevent further hepatic sequelae. Clearance of infection is rarely achieved in chronic infection and thus the primary goal of treatment is to suppress viral replication, as monitored by the level of viral DNA in blood. In recent years, potent antiviral drugs have become available which can fully suppress the virus and thus HBV has become a treatable infection associated with long-term disease-free survival.

Hepatitis C virus

Epidemiology

There are 130–150 million people worldwide who are infected with HCV with prevalence varying widely between countries and within individual risk groups.[3] The United Kingdom has a relatively low

Table 1.5.4.1 Serological markers in hepatitis B virus infection

Serological marker	Interpretation of positive result
Hepatitis B virus surface antigen (HBsAg)	Screening test. Presence indicates current HBV infection. Persistence in blood for ≥ 6 months indicates chronic infection
Hepatitis B core Ig G antibody (anti-HBc IgG)	Past HBV infection. In the absence of HBsAg, a marker of past (cleared) infection
Hepatitis B core Ig M antibodies (anti-HBc IgM)	Recent acute infection
Hepatitis B virus e antigen and antibodies (HBeAg and anti-HBe)	Presence of HBeAg in untreated patients indicates high levels of virus in the blood and is often used to denote high infectivity

Many patients who are HBeAg negative and anti-HBe positive have lower levels of virus in the blood, this is not always the case and thus these markers cannot be reliably used to assess infectivity. |
| Hepatitis B surface antibody (anti-HBs) | Produced following clearance of infection and after vaccination. Used to assess vaccine response |

prevalence of under 0.5%; however, up to 50% of intravenous drug users have evidence of infection.[4]

Transmission routes and risk groups

Parenteral transmission through the sharing of contaminated needles and equipment amongst intravenous drug users is the most common route of HCV transmission. Infection can also occur via direct exposure to infectious blood during tattooing, body piercing, and medical, surgical, or dental procedures (including needlestick injury). In the past, HCV was often acquired via blood transfusion; however, screening of blood donors has made this an exceedingly rare occurrence. Vertical and sexual transmission routes are much less common than for HBV.

Clinical features

The incubation period is between 2 weeks and 6 months. Most acute infections are not clinically apparent although jaundice may be reported. Approximately 80% of newly infected individuals fail to clear the virus and develop chronic HCV infection. Patients with chronic infection may complain of fatigue and malaise; however, most remain symptom free for many years. Liver damage will eventually progress to cirrhosis in 5–20% of patients and 1–5% will die of HCV-related cirrhosis or hepatocellular carcinoma. End-stage liver disease due to HCV infection has become the commonest indication for liver transplantation worldwide.

Diagnosis

HCV infection is normally diagnosed by testing for HCV antibodies in blood. This test cannot distinguish active infection from past cleared infection. Detection of hepatitis C RNA (normally using the polymerase chain reaction) or HCV core antigen indicates ongoing active infection. HCV antibodies may not be detectable for up to 3 months after infection (the window period).

Management

Specialist management is required for those with ongoing HCV infection. Historically, treatment consisted of immune modulation with injections of pegylated interferon and oral ribavirin for 6–12 months. Recently, a number of direct-acting antivirals against HCV have been licensed and have resulted in an ability to clear the virus in over 90% of cases. Many more drugs are in development and this figure and the tolerability of treatment regimens is expected to improve.

HIV

Epidemiology

The WHO estimates 30–40 million people worldwide are infected with HIV with 1.5 million deaths per annum. Prevalence varies geographically and in different populations; less than 1% in resource-rich nations to 1 in 20 adults in sub-Saharan Africa.[5] The prevalence is higher amongst men who have sex with men in resource-rich countries although transmissions via the heterosexual route are increasing.[6]

Transmission routes and risk groups

The virus is principally transmitted by direct exposure to infectious blood or body fluids. The three main routes of transmission are vertical, sexual, and parenteral. Vertical transmission occurs perinatally or via breastfeeding from an HIV-infected mother to her child in over 25% of cases; however, this can be reduced to less than 1% with interventions including antiviral treatment. Parenteral transmission can occur as a result of intravenous drug abuse, tattooing or body piercing, and during medical, surgical, or dental procedures (including needlestick injury). HIV is less commonly transmitted via parenteral routes than HBV or HCV.

Clinical features

HIV infects lymphocytes in the blood, and untreated, loss of these cells (measured by CD4 lymphocyte count) results in an increased risk of infection and certain malignancies.

An acute seroconversion illness may occur 2 weeks to 3 months post exposure; this often goes unnoticed, however, but patients may present with non-specific symptoms or a glandular fever-like illness. At this time the patient is highly infectious. A period of asymptomatic chronic infection follows for 5–15 years, although some patients may develop persistent lymphadenopathy. Untreated, eventual loss of immune function results in increasing susceptibility to infections, including opportunistic infections, and this defines the acquired immunodeficiency syndrome (AIDS). Patients at this late stage may present with a wide variety of infections, including recurrent shingles and *Pneumocystis* pneumonia.

Diagnosis

Data from the United Kingdom show that a quarter of HIV-infected individuals remain undiagnosed and that up over 40% are diagnosed at a late stage of infection, when treatment is often less effective.[6] For this reason, national guidelines in the United Kingdom have been developed advising a routine offer of HIV testing for certain clinical presentations.[7]

Current HIV screening tests involve a combined antibody and antigen test and are extremely sensitive. A positive result is expected within 4 weeks of infection, although retesting after the window period (3 months after exposure for HIV) is normally advised.

Management

Patients are managed by specialists. Currently complete clearance of the virus is not possible and treatment is aimed at suppression of viral replication. Over 20 different antiviral drugs are now licensed for the treatment of HIV. Treatment is normally initiated based on CD4 count using a potent combination of three drugs to suppress the virus and prevent the development of viral resistance. Current regimens are relatively non-toxic and in the majority of cases fully suppress the virus to undetectable levels. In those cases where treatment is initiated before later stages of infection, HIV infection is now compatible with a near-normal life expectancy.

Other blood-borne viruses

Human T-lymphotropic viruses

Human T-lymphotropic virus (HTLV)-1 is prevalent in Japan, the Caribbean, Central and South America, and Africa. It is transmitted vertically (principally via breastfeeding), and also via sexual contact, transfusion of infected blood, and intravenous drug use. Infection remains asymptomatic in most individuals. Disease occurs after many years of infection in less than 5%, manifesting as adult T-cell leukaemia/lymphoma or an HTLV-associated myelopathy. HTLV-2 is associated in certain countries with intravenous drug use and currently has no definite disease associations.

Other viruses

Hepatitis D virus is blood-borne, but can only infect individuals also infected with HBV.

A number of recently identified viruses have been linked to the blood-borne transmission route (e.g. GB virus, TT virus, and Parv4); however, no specific disease associations have been identified.

Many other viruses have a viraemic phase during infection; however, this is usually of short duration and is not the principal route of transmission (e.g. cytomegalovirus, Epstein–Barr virus, parvovirus B19, and West Nile virus).

Prevention of infection in the healthcare setting

Infection prevention and control

The key to preventing transmission of blood-borne viruses in the hospital setting is the consistent use of standard infection prevention and control precautions by all staff for all patients.

Many individuals with these infections remain undiagnosed, and even those with negative screening tests may be in the window period of infection. It is also likely that other pathogenic blood-borne viruses exist for which screening tests are not available. For these reasons, standard precautions should be followed in all cases including adherence to hand hygiene, use of appropriate personal protective equipment, and in particular the safe handling of sharps, including needles and surgical instruments. Waste should be appropriately disposed of following appropriate hospital policies. Any spills of blood or body fluid should be immediately dealt with following hospital policies and normally using a bleach (hypochlorite) solution which is effective in the inactivation of blood-borne viruses.

Screening of patients prior to surgical procedures is not recommended, although screening should be offered to patients with compatible signs or symptoms or those in risk groups, to enable early assessment and treatment.

Donated blood and blood products are currently screened to prevent transmission of infections. In the United Kingdom, screening includes HBV, HCV, HIV, and HTLV and involves highly sensitive nucleic acid testing to reduce the window period.

Vaccination

The WHO recommends that all individuals are vaccinated against HBV at birth. In the United Kingdom, only at-risk individuals are currently offered vaccination routinely, including healthcare workers (HCWs).[8] HBV vaccine is not a live virus and consists of purified HBV surface antigen. It is administered as three doses at 0, 1, and 6 months or an accelerated schedule at 0, 1, 2, and 12 months. In HCWs, response should be documented by measurement of antibody levels. Around 10–15% of adults fail to respond to the initial course of vaccine. Many of these individuals may respond to a booster dose or further vaccine course; however, some remain non-responders. Non-responders require the administration of HBV immunoglobulin should significant exposure occur. No effective vaccine is currently available for HCV or HIV.

Needlestick injuries

A needlestick injury is usually defined as an accidental percutaneous injury involving a needle or other sharp instrument contaminated with blood. The vast majority of such incidents are preventable by adherence to standard infection prevention and control procedures and local hospital policies for the handling of sharps. When a potential exposure occurs it should be immediately reported and local policies should be in place to ensure the needlestick recipient obtains appropriate expert advice, risk-assessment, and post-exposure management.

Risk assessment

It has been estimated that the risk of transmission from an infected individual following percutaneous injury from a device visibly contaminated with fresh blood is in the order of 1 in 3 for HBV, 1 in 30 for HCV and 1 in 300 for HIV.[9,10] This risk is lower for other exposure incidents; blood splash onto mucous membranes carries a much lower risk (estimated at 1 in 1000 for HIV).[9,10] Where the source patient is known, consent should be obtained for urgent HBV, HCV, and HIV testing. Experience has shown that most patients are happy to be tested in these circumstances. A risk assessment is required as to the potential for blood-borne virus transmission in a particular incident. This will take into account the mechanism of the injury itself and the likelihood of infection in the source patient, considering viral epidemiology and risk factors. Where the incident is assessed as being high risk for HIV, post-exposure prophylaxis (PEP) should be started immediately and not be delayed while test results are awaited.

Post-exposure management

In all cases, a baseline blood should be taken for storage. This will allow retrospective testing to be carried out should infection occur. Post-exposure management should follow national and local policies.

HBV vaccination status should be ascertained in all cases. This provides effective protection against HBV and responders can be reassured. A booster dose of vaccine is sometimes advised. Known non-responders to vaccine who are exposed to an HBV-positive or unknown source should be offered PEP with HBV-specific immunoglobulin.[8]

Where the source patient is known to be infected with HIV, or where risk assessment suggests it is appropriate, the recipient of the needlestick injury should be started on a course of HIV PEP.[11] This consists of a combination of antiviral drugs and must be started as soon as possible after exposure, ideally within 1 hour. Treatment can be stopped if negative results are subsequently obtained from the source patient.

No PEP is available to prevent the transmission of HCV. Appropriate follow-up is essential, as treatment started soon after infection is associated with a much higher rate of viral clearance than treatment started once chronic infection is established.

All patients with a blood exposure incident should be followed up with screening after the window period to determine if infection has occurred. Most infections will be detectable on testing 3 months after the exposure incident.

Healthcare workers infected with blood-borne viruses

The risk of transmission of a blood-borne virus infection from a HCW to a patient is extremely small and essentially limited to exposure-prone procedures (EPPs). EPPs are defined as invasive procedures where there is a risk of injury to the HCW, which may result in exposure of a patient's open tissues to the HCW's blood. These include procedures where a gloved hand may be in contact with sharp instruments or tissues (spicules of bone and teeth) inside a patient's open body cavity, wound, or confined space where the hand or fingertips may not be completely visible.[12] Guidelines on the screening of HCWs for blood-borne viruses vary between countries. Current guidelines in the United Kingdom[12] require that testing for blood-borne viruses be carried out for HCWs starting in a new post which will involve EPPs; testing should be offered to other staff but is not obligatory.

Regulations regarding employment of infected HCWs in roles which require the employee to perform EPPs vary around the world and exist to limit the risk of transmitting blood-borne viruses to patients. The following relate to the current guidelines in the United Kingdom.[13]

HCWs with HIV, whose viral load is fully suppressed, can perform EPP subject to certain conditions including frequent monitoring. Those with unsuppressed viral load are prohibited from working in positions where they will perform EPPs.[14]

HCWs with active HCV (detectable hepatitis C RNA) are prohibited from performing EPPs; however, those who have cleared the virus naturally or show a sustained response to treatment may undertake EPPs.

EPPs may not be performed by HCWs with HBV if they are hepatitis B e antigen-positive or if the viral load in blood is greater than 10^3 genome equivalents/mL. Under certain circumstances, a HCW on treatment for HBV may be permitted to undertake EPPs.

Infected HCWs who continue to perform EPPs must commit to regular review to ensure criteria for this continue to be met.

Every HCW has a duty of care to be tested if they become concerned that at-risk behaviour or symptoms suggest that they or a colleague may be at risk of blood-borne virus infection.[15] This will result in adequate and timely treatment for the individual as well as protection for their patients. If a HCW carrying out EPPs is subsequently found to be infected with a blood-borne virus, expert advice is required to determine whether notification and testing of patients is required.[13] Although many such look-back exercises have been undertaken, it remains exceedingly rare for a patient to be infected by a HCW.[13]

References

1. World Health Organization. *Fact sheet No. 204: Hepatitis B*. July 2015. [Online] http://www.who.int/mediacentre/factsheets/fs204/en/ WHO http://www.who.int
2. Public Health England. *Notifiable Diseases and Causative Organisms: How to Report*. 2010. [Online] https://www.gov.uk/guidance/notifiable-diseases-and-causative-organisms-how-to-report
3. World Health Organization. *Fact Sheet No. 164: Hepatitis C*. July 2015. [Online] http://www.who.int/mediacentre/factsheets/fs164/en/
4. Public Health England. *Hepatitis C in the UK. 2015 Report*. 2015. [Online] https://www.gov.uk/government/publications/hepatitis-c-in-the-uk
5. World Health Organization. *Global Health Observatory (GHO) Data: HIV/AIDS*. http://www.who.int/gho/hiv/en/
6. Public Health England. *HIV in the United Kingdom: 2014 Report*. 2014. [Online] https://www.gov.uk/government/statistics/hiv-in-the-united-kingdom
7. British HIV Association, British Association of Sexual Health and HIV, British Infection Society. *UK National Guidelines for HIV Testing 2008*. London: British HIV Association; 2008.
8. Joint Committee on Vaccination and Immunisation. *Immunisation Against Infectious Diseases*. London: Stationery Office; 2006. http://immunisation.dh.gov.uk/category/the-green-book/
9. Health Protection Agency. *Eye of the Needle. UK Surveillance of Significant Occupational Exposures to Blood Borne Viruses*. London: Health Protection Agency; 2012.
10. Woode Owusu M, Wellington E, Rice B, et al. *Eye of the Needle. United Kingdom Surveillance of Significant Occupational Exposures to Bloodborne Viruses in Healthcare Workers: Data to End 2013*. Public Health England: London; 2014.
11. Department of Health. *HIV Post-Exposure Prophylaxis: Guidance from the UK Chief Medical Officer's Expert Advisory Group on AIDs*. 2008
12. Department of Health. *Health Clearance for Tuberculosis, Hepatitis B, Hepatitis C and HIV: New Healthcare Workers*. London: Department of Health; 2007.
13. Public Health England. *UK Advisory Panel for Healthcare Workers Infected with Bloodborne Viruses (UKAP)*. [Online] http://www.hpa.org.uk/Topics/InfectiousDiseases/InfectionsAZ/BloodborneVirusesAndOccupationalExposure/UKAP/
14. Public Health England. *The Management of HIV Infected Healthcare Workers Who Perform Exposure Prone Procedures: Updated Guidance*. January 2014. [Online] https://www.gov.uk/government/uploads/system/uploads/attachment_data/file/333018/Management_of_HIV_infected_Healthcare_Workers_guidance_January_2014.pdf
15. General Medical Council. *Confidentiality: Disclosing Information about Serious Communicable Diseases*. London: General Medical Council; 2009.

CHAPTER 1.5.5

Asepsis

Louise Hall

Aseptic technique

Aseptic technique is a specific set of practices and procedures to prevent contamination by microorganisms, thereby protecting the patient from infection. All patients are potentially vulnerable to infection, although the risks are greater for patients undergoing surgical procedures; strict asepsis must be applied in the operating theatre. Failings relating to poor standards of aseptic technique can result in surgical site infection (SSI). For an aseptic technique to be safe and efficient, the staff member must risk assess every procedure for the level of aseptic technique required to maintain asepsis.

Theatre personnel should complete surgical hand antisepsis to remove transient microorganisms; this will also reduce resident microorganisms. Fingernails should be short and not extend beyond the fingertips to prevent the risk of gloves tearing; nails should also be free from polish or false nails. Antiseptic solutions used for hand decontamination should be fast-acting with a residual effect and have a broad spectrum of activity. Theatre personnel with bacterial infections of the upper respiratory tract or infected or exuding skin lesions should not participate in aseptic procedures.

Aseptic non-touch technique

Aseptic non-touch technique (ANTT)[1] is a framework for standardizing aseptic practice across a range of clinical procedures. The principles of ANTT are to protect key-parts and key-sites throughout procedures which require asepsis. When undertaking a procedure requiring asepsis, staff must determine whether standard or surgical ANTT is required.

Standard ANTT

Standard ANTT is the technique required when it is possible to undertake a procedure without directly touching or contaminating key-parts or key-sites. This procedure is short in duration, for example, when preparing intravenous drugs.

Surgical ANTT

Surgical ANTT is the technique required when it is not possible to undertake a procedure without directly touching or contaminating key-parts or key-sites. This form of ANTT will be implemented during surgical procedures.

Key-sites are defined as any breaches in the patient's bodily defences, such as open wounds or the entry point during cannulation. Key-parts are any equipment which comes into contact with other aseptic key-parts or key-sites.

A micro-critical asepsis field is where two key-parts meet and asepsis must be maintained at the point of contact, such as at the tip of syringe and the end of a needle or the tip of a needle and sterile saline being drawn up.

A critical asepsis field is created where a large aseptic working area itself becomes a key-part; this must be protected from contamination at all times. The main asepsis field must be managed as a critical asepsis field (i.e. only sterilized aseptic equipment can come into contact with it). In the operating theatre, during open procedures maintenance of a critical asepsis field is essential.

Surgical hand antisepsis and sterile personal protective equipment must be used as it is not possible to undertake a procedure without directly touching or contaminating key-parts or key sites. To reduce the potential risk of contamination, scrubbed personnel should not leave the immediate area of the critical asepsis field and there should be no contact between scrubbed and non-scrubbed staff.

All equipment necessary to perform the procedure should be gathered in advance and, prior to use, the integrity of the outer packaging of sterilized items must be checked, there must be evidence of sterilization, and the expiry date should be reviewed. Staff must be trained and assessed as competent when opening sterile packs to ensure the contents do not become contaminated; the process should take place in an area where there is enough space to maintain sterility. Non-scrubbed personnel must open the outer wraps of the pack, opening away from the body and towards the critical asepsis field. Scrubbed personnel should initially open the pack towards themselves and then away from their body. Any additional sterile items or solutions must be carefully presented to scrubbed staff.

Skin preparation

The patient's skin is a major source of microorganisms which can cause SSI, therefore appropriate, perioperative skin antisepsis can assist in reducing the risk of postoperative infections. Antiseptic skin preparations should have broad-spectrum activity acting against Gram-negative and Gram-positive bacteria, viruses, and fungi. They should be effective against resident and transient microorganisms. Some examples of skin preparations include:

- 2% chlorhexidine gluconate in 70% isopropyl alcohol
- povidone–iodine alcoholic solution
- povidone–iodine aqueous solution.

Single-use applicators or sachets reduce the risk of contamination in comparison to multiple-use products. However, where they are used, solutions must never be decanted from one container to another as this further increases the risk of contamination. The expiry date must always be checked prior to use.

Skin preparation should be applied by a competent member of the scrub team using ANTT and using appropriate equipment. Cleansing should begin at the incision site in an outward, circular motion, repeating the process with a clean sponge several times. Sufficient solution should be applied to ensure adequate skin coverage; this should extend to the potential location of drain sites and possible extension of the incision. One wipe with an antiseptic solution is not enough to significantly reduce the bacterial load on the skin; however, the solution must not be allowed to pool under the patient.

Decontamination

Reusable medical devices (surgical instruments) can be a vector in the transmission of microorganisms to patients, staff, or the environment if they are not decontaminated effectively; there must be adequate decontamination of these devices to assist in the prevention of SSI.

Definitions

Single-patient use items are any medical devices deemed unsuitable for re-processing as stated by the manufacturers. Equipment labelled as such may be used a number of times by the same patient only.

Single-use/disposable items are any medical devices deemed unsuitable for re-processing as stated by the manufacturers; these items must be disposed of after each use.

Contamination is the soiling or pollution of inanimate objects or living material with harmful, potentially infectious or unwanted material.

Decontamination is the combination of processes (including cleaning, disinfection, and sterilization) used to render re-usable items safe for further use on patients and handling by staff. Effective decontamination is essential in reducing the risk of transmission of infectious agents.

Cleaning is the process that physically reduces the level of contamination (organic matter, dirt, and grease) but does not destroy all organisms. The effectiveness of cleaning is as important as the agent used. It is important to emphasize that thorough physical cleaning must be the first step in decontamination; if items are not appropriately cleaned, subsequent disinfection or sterilization will be ineffective.

Disinfection is the partial removal or destruction of some, but not all organisms present. Heat disinfection is preferable to chemical disinfection and therefore should always be considered in the first instance.

Sterilization is the process used to render an object free from all microorganisms including spores. Routine sterilization of most surgical instruments is achieved in autoclaves using steam under pressure. The duration of the sterilization cycle is dependent on the temperature to which the autoclaves are set; 134–137°C for 3 minutes or 121°C for 15 minutes.

Decontamination life cycle

The decontamination life cycle of surgical instruments highlights the extent to which decontamination affects the whole organization (Figure 1.5.5.1). To achieve adequate decontamination, a surgical instrument must pass through each stage of this cycle.[2]

Effective quality control systems must occur at all stages of the process ensuring:

◆ appropriate automated and centralized decontamination facilities

◆ appropriately trained staff with clear systems of supervision

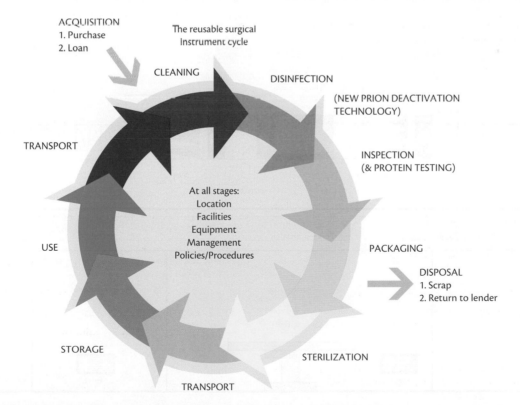

Fig. 1.5.5.1 Decontamination life cycle.

Reproduced with permission from Department of Health, *Choice Framework for Local Policy and Procedures 01-01—Management and Decontamination of Surgical Instruments (Medical Devices) used in Acute Care. Part A: The Formulation of Local Policy and Choices*, © Crown Copyright 2013 licensed under the Open Government Licence v3.0.

- single-use items are not reused

- comprehensive decontamination records are maintained

- an adequate traceability system exists to confirm that instruments are tracked throughout the decontamination process and that they are linked to the patient on which they have been used.

Environmental cleaning

The healthcare environment can also contribute to the transmission of microorganisms; defined cleaning schedules must be in place to ensure regular, high standards of cleaning are achieved. All surfaces should be kept visibly clean and regular audits should be undertaken to demonstrate compliance.

Operating tables and equipment that has direct patient contact are more likely to become contaminated and therefore must be decontaminated in between each case. Daily damp dusting of other surfaces such as shelves and ledges should be sufficient. All equipment must be cleaned at the end of the list and once cleaned, portable equipment removed from the theatre. At the end of each session, the theatre floor should be disinfected. The floor should be scrubbed daily with a floor-scrubbing machine.

Air quality

There are national standards and policies to enable healthcare providers to fulfil their duty of care in relation to engineering governance[3] (Figure 1.5.5.2). These standards ensure ventilation systems in operating departments are appropriately designed, installed, operated, and maintained providing safe environments for both patients and staff. Specialized ventilation is provided in patient treatment areas, for example, operating departments and critical care areas.

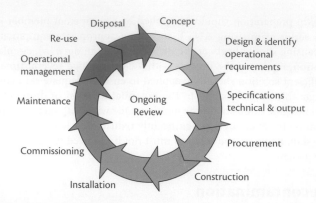

Fig. 1.5.5.2 Healthcare-building life cycle.
Reproduced with permission from Department of Health, *Clean, Safe Care: Reducing MRSA and other Healthcare Associated Infections and Saving Lives*, © Crown Copyright 2005, licensed under the Open Government Licence v3.0.

Types of ventilation

Ventilation is the method of removing and replacing air in a defined space. Mechanical ventilation enables more control of the environment involving fans and collection or distribution ductwork (Figure 1.5.5.3); this may also include the ability to heat and filter the air. A fixed volume of air is supplied within the space ventilated; this is often recorded as the resulting number of air changes per hour. In an operating theatre, the standard is a minimum of 25 air changes per hour.

Ultra-clean ventilation aims to significantly increase the dilution effect of ventilation. It is fitted with a terminal device to supply the working area with a unidirectional, downward air flow; the standard of filtration is capable of delivering air with a very low particle

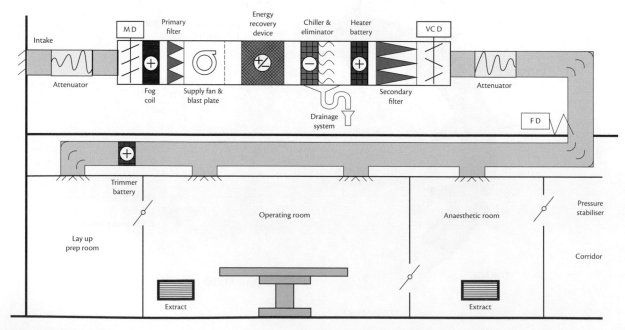

Fig. 1.5.5.3 Example of a typical operating theatre ventilation system. Fire Damper (FD); Motorized Damper (MD); Variable Control Damper (VCD).
Reproduced with permission from Department of Health, *Clean, Safe Care: Reducing MRSA and other Healthcare Associated Infections and Saving Lives*, © Crown Copyright 2005, licensed under the Open Government Licence v3.0.

count. This prevents entry of any contaminants that have originated outside the operating zone and clears the area of any contaminants or particles generated within it. This reduction in contaminants can reduce postoperative SSI and is used most frequently in orthopaedic cases.

Air conditioning enables control of the climate within the space supplied regardless of changes in outside air conditions or the activities within the space; this includes the ability to heat, cool, dehumidify/humidify, and filter air.

Main functions of ventilation

- *Dilute airborne contamination*: airborne contaminants can be shed by operating staff, via the supply air, through surgical activities or transferred from adjacent areas.

- *Control air movement to minimize the transfer of airborne contaminants from less clean to cleaner areas*: transfer grilles and pressure stabilizers should be designed to permit and control the flow of air between spaces to ensure air flow from the clean to less clean areas of the suite is maintained.

- *Control the temperature and where necessary the humidity*: supply flow rates are calculated taking in to account heat and moisture gains and losses, and the temperature differences between the room and supply air.

- *Assist the removal of waste anaesthetic gases*: anaesthetic gases are subject to workplace exposure limits and air extracted from operating theatres should not be re-circulated.

Theatre traffic

Controlling movement within the operating theatre assists in minimizing the movement of microorganisms from the environment, theatre staff, and patients. The doors to the operating theatre should remain closed, with a restriction of movement in and out of the theatre to ensure the ventilation system can work effectively. The number of personnel present during a case should be restricted to numbers essential to safely care for the patient during the procedure.

Commissioning

Prior to a ventilation system becoming fully operational there must be a rigorous and robust commissioning process. This is usually undertaken by specialist commissioning contractors in collaboration with equipment suppliers and Estates personnel. At the final stage of commissioning, a full report detailing the findings should be produced. This report must include a clear statement identifying whether the ventilation system does or does not achieve the required standard. This report must also be distributed to the users of the department, infection prevention and control, and estates department.

Further reading

Association of Perioperative Practice. *Standards and Recommendations for Safe Perioperative Practice* (3rd ed). Harrogate: Association of Perioperative Practice; 2011.

Department of Health. *Clean, Safe Care: Reducing MRSA and Other Healthcare Associated Infections and Saving Lives*. 2008. [Online] http://www.dh.gov.uk/en/Publicationsandstatistics/Publications/

Department of Health. *The Health and Social Care Act 2008: Code of Practice of the Prevention and Control of Infections and Related Guidance*. 2015. [Online] https://www.gov.uk/government/uploads/system/uploads/attachment_data/file/449049/Code_of_practice_280715_acc.pdf

Health and Safety Executive. *COSHH: A Brief Guide to the Regulations: What You Need to Know About the Control of Substances Hazardous to Health Regulations*. London: Health and Safety Executive; 2005.

Loveday HP, Wilson JA, Pratt RJ, *et al.* epic3: National Evidence-Based Guidelines for Preventing Healthcare-Associated Infections in NHS Hospitals in England 2014. *J Hosp Infect* 86S1: S1–S70.

NHS Estates. *Infection Control in the Built Environment—Design and Planning*. Health Facilities Note 30. London: NHS Estates; 2002.

National Collaborating Centre for Women's and Children's Health (Commissioned by the National Institute for Health and Clinical Excellence). *Surgical Site Infection Prevention and Treatment of Surgical Site Infection*. 2008 (reviewed 2014). [Online] http://www.nice.org.uk/CG74

References

1. Rowley S, Clare S, Macqueen S, *et al.* ANTTv2: an updated practice framework for aseptic technique. *Br J Nurs* (Intravenous Supplement) 2010; 19(5):S5–S12.

2. Department of Health, Estates and Facilities Division. *Choice Framework for Local Policy & Procedures (CFPP) 01-01—Management and Decontamination of Surgical Instruments (Medical Devices) Used in Acute Care*. London: Department of Health; 2012.

3. Department of Health, Estates and Facilities Division. *Health Technical Memorandum 03-01: Specialised Ventilation for Healthcare Premises. Part A—Design and Installation*. London: Department of Health; 2007.

Applied surgical radiology

Sub-section editor: Jonathan D. Spratt

CHAPTER 1.6.1

Plain film radiology for surgeons

Jonathan D. Spratt

Introduction

A 'plain film' is a radiograph taken without the use of a barium or iodine-based contrast agent. X-rays were discovered in Germany in 1895 by Wilhelm Röntgen, gaining him the first Nobel Prize in Physics in 1901. In 1896, Major John Hall-Edwards made the first use of X-rays under clinical conditions at Birmingham General Hospital, United Kingdom, when he radiographed a needle stuck in a colleague's hand.[1] A month later he took the first radiograph to direct a surgical operation. Unfortunately his left arm was amputated in 1908 due to X-ray dermatitis.

In an X-ray tube, electrons generated by thermionic emission from a heated cathode accelerate through a kilovoltage potential and collide with a rotating tungsten target creating X-rays that can pass through the body and are captured nowadays usually by a digital detector rather than film. Four densities are demonstrated: gas (black), fat (dark grey), soft tissue/fluid (light grey), and bone/calcification (white).

At diagnostic energies, X-ray photons interact with atomic electrons of tissues either through the photoelectric effect at lower energies with total photonic absorption and the emergence of a highly energetic electron or via Compton scatter at higher X-ray energies resulting in the freeing of a lower-energy outer electron and a deflected less energetic X-ray photon. These emergent electrons create highly reactive ions that alter chemical bonds in tissue, inducing cancer with a latent period of years or decades after exposure.

A comparative list of typical effective absorbed doses from various examinations reveals that the abdominal film results in 35 times the dose of a frontal chest film (Box 1.6.1.1).

The use of medical exams that would expose children to ionizing radiation needs special consideration. Children have a three to five times larger radiation-induced cancer mortality risk than adults.[2,3]

Referral and justification

A referrer is identified as a registered medical or dental practitioner or health professional who is entitled to refer individuals for medical exposure to a practitioner.

The criminal law governing medical ionizing radiation exposure[4] states that the referrer is responsible for the provision of sufficient clinical information to enable justification. This involves consideration of the appropriateness of each and every request, optimization of the imaging strategy, analysis of risk versus benefit, understanding of the immediate and cumulative radiation effects, consideration of age-specific issues (e.g. seeking alternative non-ionizing radiation procedures in children and younger adults), the

---

Box 1.6.1.1 Comparative estimates of effective dose (mSv)

Single radiograph

- Skull (posteroanterior (PA) and lateral) (0.04), limb or joint (0.06)
  - Chest (PA) (0.02), chest (lateral) (0.04)
  - Abdomen (0.7), pelvis (0.7).

Contrast examination, X-ray series, or computed tomography

- Spinal series: cervical (0.27), thoracic (1.4), lumbar (1.8)
  - Barium exam: swallow (1.5), follow through (3.0), enema (7.0)
  - Intravenous urogram (2.5)
  - CT: head (2.0), chest (8.0), abdomen (10), pelvis (10).

---

urgency of the exposure (e.g. in potential or actual pregnancy), the efficacy of imaging in different clinical situations, and appropriate delegation.

The referrer has a legal responsibility to ensure the completeness and accuracy of data relating to the patient's condition and to be kept fully informed about patient history, the presenting complaint and relevant physical signs, past history, and previous imaging. If an inappropriate exposure occurs, legally termed a 'radiation incident', this must be reported by law to the local Radiation Protection Advisor and then to the Department of Health in the United Kingdom.

The diagnostic value of plain films is greatly enhanced with full, legible, and accurate clinical information. It is best practice to record immediate interpretation of plain films in the medical notes, and legally compulsory if there are no arrangements for formal reporting.

Plain abdominal film

Analysis of the abdominal plain film

Despite its partial eclipse by more ready access to latest-generation ultrasound, computed tomography (CT) and magnetic resonance imaging, the abdominal plain film still retains a position in the imaging firmament. Traditional uses have come under critical scrutiny and its efficacy in roles either as a separate examination for the evaluation of abdominal disorders or as a preliminary 'control film' at the start of a contrast series has been questioned.

Analysis starts with a systematic assessment of the size, contour, radiodensity, and position of the liver, kidneys, and spleen then a search for abnormal gas patterns should be undertaken, for example, retrocolic appendix (Figure 1.6.1.1), or intrahepatic, biliary, or portal venous gas (Figure 1.6.1.2). Bowel calibre, wall thickness, and irregularity are assessed (e.g. mural oedema ('thumbprinting') in colitis) and any wall displacement noted (e.g. paracolic abscess).

An absent psoas shadow can be a marker of retroperitoneal haemorrhage or mass. A curvilinear paravertebral calcification may indicate aortic aneurysm; both calcified walls must be inspected for loss of parallelism to exclude simple tortuosity.

Ureteric calculus (Figure 1.6.1.3) along the line of the transverse process tips and medial to the ischial spines may be detected. Diagnostic dilemma may occur with the clinically irrelevant, smooth rounded or oval pelvic phleboliths ('vein stones') that have radiolucent centres and also with calcified mesenteric nodes, which tend to be irregular, clustered, and mobile when compared with previous films.

Surgically relevant bony findings include metastases and sacro-iliitis, the latter associated with Crohn's disease with an increased incidence of gallstones and renal calculi.

Fluid levels within bowel do not appear on supine films. If there is no gas in the bowel, obstruction can be missed, and it is best to seek radiological advice when there is significant clinicoradiological discrepancy as often proceeding to CT examination has a far better diagnostic yield than the decubitus or erect anteroposterior film from yesteryear.[5]

Diagnosis of bowel obstruction and volvulus

Abdominal films and CT have similar overall accuracies in diagnosing small bowel obstruction but where obstructive symptoms are associated with specific medical conditions, such as a history of a previous malignant abdominal tumour, known inflammatory bowel disease, palpable abdominal mass, or sepsis, CT not radiography should be the primary imaging modality of choice.[6]

Large bowel is characterized on plain film by its haustrations and sacculations in the periphery of the film most prominent in

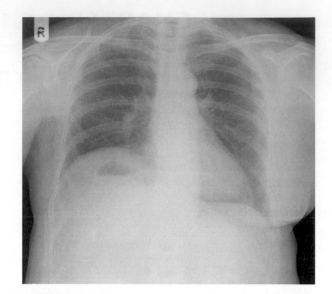

Fig. 1.6.1.2 Intrahepatic abscess.

the ascending and transverse colon. The plicae of the large bowel are more widely spaced than the valvulae conniventes of the small bowel. With moderate distention of the large bowel, the plicae appear to extend entirely across the lumen but this appearance may disappear with further distention.

The addition of an erect film does not significantly increase the accuracy of diagnosis of obstruction or help in the correct identification of its level.[7]

Bowel dilatation occurs when the small bowel exceeds 3 cm in diameter, the colon 6 cm, and the caecum 9 cm (the '3, 6, 9 rule'). In large bowel obstruction, when the caecal diameter exceeds 10 cm, the probability of perforation is high with the caecum always dilating to the largest extent no matter where the obstruction is sited.

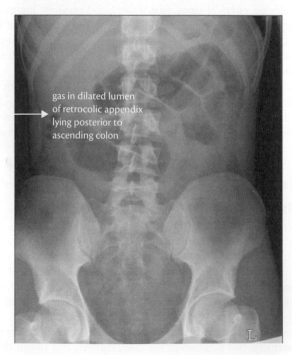

gas in dilated lumen of retrocolic appendix lying posterior to ascending colon

Fig. 1.6.1.1 Retrocolic appendicitis.

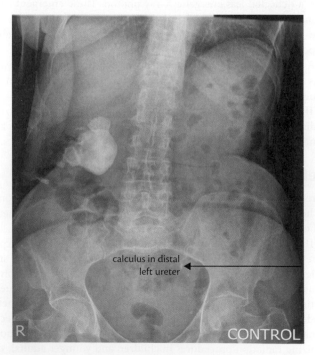

calculus in distal left ureter

Fig. 1.6.1.3 Staghorn calculus (right), uretric calculus (left), and phleboliths.

With an incompetent ileocaecal valve, small bowel obstruction may be mimicked.

A generalized adynamic ileus is quite characteristic with the large and small bowel extensively air-filled, 'looking the same', and minimally dilated.

Caecal volvulus reveals the characteristic relocation of the caecum to the mid-abdomen or left upper quadrant (Figure 1.6.1.4) with accompanying small bowel obstruction and dilated distal colon rarely seen. Sigmoid volvulus extends into the right upper quadrant and the colon proximal to the twist distends and the rectum is usually empty with a coffee-bean sign as with other closed-loop obstructions (Figure 1.6.1.5). The classic triad in gastric volvulus (Figure 1.6.1.6) consists of severe epigastric pain, retching, inability to pass a nasogastric tube (NGT) and occasionally with severe, referred left shoulder pain.

Role of the plain film in the acute abdomen

With the increasing availability of CT, use of the plain abdominal radiograph in the acute abdomen is now restricted to only a small number of suspected diagnoses.[8]

A recent multicentre prospective study evaluating the added value of plain radiographs (supine abdominal and erect chest radiographs) on top of clinical assessment in patients presenting to the emergency department with acute abdominal pain revealed that the diagnosis changed in only 11% of cases. Only sensitivity in detecting bowel obstruction was significantly higher. Their routine use gave no added value.[9]

As little as 1 mL of gas can be detected below the right hemidiaphragm on properly exposed erect chest radiographs taken with correct technique (5–10-minute erect position maintained prior to exposure). Despite being the first line of investigation, the erect chest film is diagnostic in only 50–70% of cases of free gas.[10] A left lateral decubitus film can also be used in the detection of small

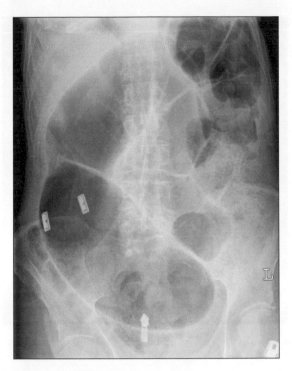

Fig. 1.6.1.5 Sigmoid volvulus.

amounts of free air that may be interposed between the free edge of the liver and the lateral wall of the peritoneal cavity. However, not only is CT superior in detecting small amounts of free intraperitoneal gas, it can accurately determine the exact site of perforation in 86% of cases.[11]

The erect chest film may also reveal a pneumomediastinum and surgical emphysema of Boerhaave's syndrome as a cause of epigastric and chest pain (Figure 1.6.1.7).

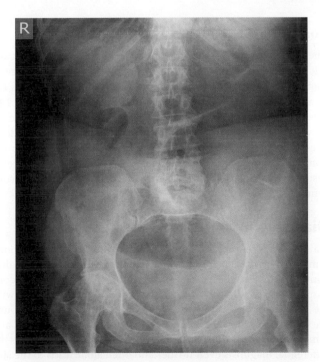

Fig. 1.6.1.4 Caecal volvulus.

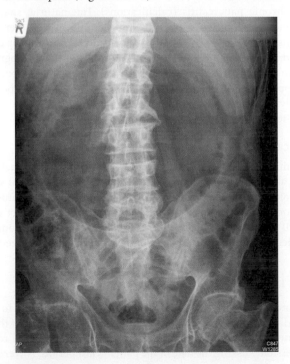

Fig. 1.6.1.6 Gastric volvulus.

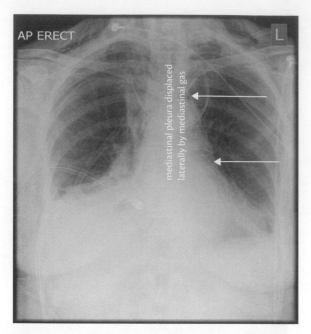

AP ERECT

mediastinal pleura displaced
laterally by mediastinal gas

L

Fig. 1.6.1.7 Pneumomediastinum and surgical emphysema in Boerhaave's syndrome.

Royal College of Radiologists' referral guidelines for abdominal plain films

The Royal College of Radiologists' referral guidelines on requesting plain abdominal film on an adult general surgical admissions unit include acute abdominal pain with suspected obstruction/perforation, acute small bowel obstruction (diagnosis and level assessment), acute large bowel obstruction, exacerbation of inflammatory bowel disease (identifying toxic megacolon), acute pancreatitis (only in excluding other causes in cases of unclear diagnosis), and chronic pancreatitis (calcifications). Haematuria, sharp or poisonous foreign body ingestion and stab injury are other indications.[12] A palpable mass warrants consideration of CT or ultrasound. Constipation may be an indication. Plain film radiography has no role in gastrointestinal haemorrhage, peptic ulceration, classic appendicitis, urinary tract infection, or non-specific abdominopelvic pain. The 28-day rule applies in patients over 12 years of age (Box 1.6.1.2).

Indications for abdominal plain films in children

In children, indications include pain with prior abdominal surgery, abnormal bowel sounds with distention or peritoneal signs, gastrointestinal bleeding (if necrotizing enterocolitis or intussusception suspected), and foreign body ingestion, with erect chest film if perforation is suspected.[14] For suspected renal stones in smaller children, an abdominal film should only be authorized by a

Box 1.6.1.2 28-day rule

Before an examination where the uterus is within or close to the irradiated area, the operator is required to ask the patient if there is any possibility of pregnancy. An unequivocal negative reply necessitates asking the date of the patient's last period. If overdue, the examination must be postponed.

radiologist who has performed an ultrasound. An ingested foreign body requires abdominal and erect chest films.

Role of primary survey plain films in major trauma

Whole-body CT is being used increasingly in the primary survey of major trauma patients. The Advanced Trauma Life Support (ATLS®) version 8 guidance advocates plain film of the chest and pelvis as part of the primary survey prior to transfer to CT or theatre.[15] The Royal College of Radiologists' guidance in severely injured patients states that where definitive imaging such as CT is deemed necessary, less accurate imaging such as plain X-rays should be omitted as they are irrelevant.[16]

Skull and cervical spine trauma films

In the investigation of all patients for suspected brain injury, CT has totally replaced the skull radiographic series,[18] which is only now used as part of a skeletal survey in the investigation of non-accidental injury in children.

In most circumstances of cervical spine injury, three-view cervical spine radiographic series are the initial investigation of choice, required if the patient cannot actively rotate the neck to 45° to left and right.

In patients with a Glasgow Coma Scale (GCS) score less than 13 on initial assessment or in multi-region trauma,[19] CT is mandatory as well as in those patients needing urgent clearance prior to surgery. Continued clinical suspicion of injury despite normal or equivocal plain film series also warrants CT.

Children under 10 years do not need a peg view and CT should be restricted to those with either severe head injury (GCS score ≤ 8) or strong suspicion of injury despite normal or inadequate plain films. CT is superior for depressed and diastatic skull fractures.[20]

Position of catheters and stents

Chest radiography for NGT position positively confirms that the exit holes of the NGT are within the stomach. The importance of confirming the correct position cannot be overstated. Patients fed or administered drugs via a malpositioned NGT (Figure 1.6.1.8) have a high risk of complications. Confirmation of position by drawing back gastric contents and testing with pH paper alone does not rule out the side hole within the oesophagus. The position of stents within the common bile duct (Figure 1.6.1.9), ureter, oesophagus, pylorus, large bowel, and vascular system can be confirmed and monitored.

Diagnosis of bone tumours

Plain film radiographs remain crucial in the diagnosis of bone tumours. The term *bone tumour* encompasses benign and malignant neoplasms, metabolic abnormalities, and miscellaneous 'tumour-like' conditions. The majority arise in the extremities, with the lower limbs affected more frequently. In primary bone tumours, the two most important aspects of evaluation are patient age and tumour location. The specific radiographic appearance narrows the differential diagnosis even further and often alone leads to the single correct diagnosis.[21]

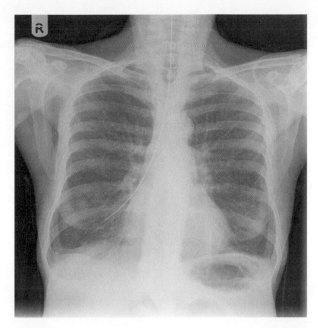

Fig. 1.6.1.8 Malpositioned nasogastric tube down right main bronchus.

Most bone tumours occur in a characteristic location, some at sites of rapid bone growth, usually the metaphysis (e.g. osteosarcoma), while others follow the distribution of red marrow (e.g. Ewing sarcoma). Aggressive features include ill-defined margins, abnormal mineralization, spiculated periosteal reaction, and soft tissue component. Infection and malignancy may appear similarly aggressive.[22]

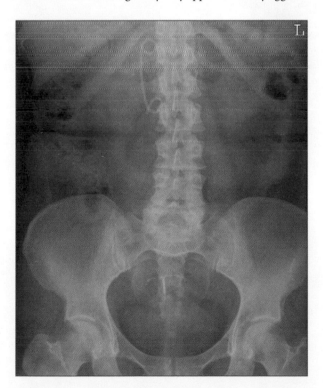

Fig. 1.6.1.9 Stent in common bile duct (and intrauterine contraceptive device).

Further reading

Bregg JD (ed). *Abdominal X-Rays Made Easy* (2nd ed). Edinburgh: Churchill Livingstone; 2006.

Corne J, Pointon K. *Chest X-Ray Made Easy* (3rd ed). Edinburgh: Churchill Livingstone; 2009.

Di Mizio R, Scaglione M (eds). *Small-Bowel Obstruction: CT Features with Plain Film and US Correlations*. Milan: Springer; 2007.

Pettet G, Rodrigues J, Gandhi S (eds). *Basics of Abdominal Radiology* (Kindle ed). Derby: JMD Books; 2012.

Raby N, Berman L, de Lacey G, *et al.* (eds). *Accident and Emergency Radiology: A Survival Guide* (3rd ed). Philadelphia, PA: Saunders/Elsevier; 2015.

References

1. Meggitt G. *Taming the Rays: A History of Radiation and Protection*. Raleigh, NC: Lulu.com; 2008.

2. National Council on Radiation Protection and Measurements. *Sources and Magnitude of Occupational and Public Exposures from Nuclear Medicine Procedures*. NCRP Report 124. Bethesda, MD: National Council on Radiation Protection and Measurements; 1996.

3. United Nations Scientific Committee on the Effects of Atomic Radiation. *Sources and Effects of Ionizing Radiation, Volume 1: Sources*. New York: United Nations Publishing; 2000.

4. Department of Health. *Ionising Radiation (Medical Exposure) Regulations IS 1999/3232*. Norwich: Stationery Office; 2000.

5. Kottler NE, Aguirre DA, Casola G, *et al*. Imaging the obstructed bowel and other intestinal emergencies. *Appl Radiol* 2005; 35(4):20–34.

6. Balthazar E. CT of small-bowel obstruction. *AJR Am J Roentgenol* 1994; 162:255–61.

7. Simpson A, Sandeman D, Nixon SJ, *et al*. The value of an erect abdominal radiograph in the diagnosis of intestinal obstruction. *Clin Radiol* 1985; 36(1):41–2.

8. Hampson F, Shaw A. Assessment of the acute abdomen: role of the plain abdominal radiograph. *Rep Med Imaging* 2010; 3:93–105.

9. van Randen A, Laméris W, Luitse JS, *et al*. The role of plain radiographs in patients with acute abdominal pain at the ED. *Am J Emerg Med* 2011; 29(6):582–9.e2.

10. Miller RE, Nelson SW. The roentgenologic demonstration of tiny amounts of free intraperitoneal gas: experimental and clinical studies. *AJR Am J Roentgenol* 1971; 112:574–85.

11. Hainaux B, Agneessens E, Bertinotti R, *et al*. Accuracy of MDCT in predicting site of gastrointestinal tract perforation. *AJR Am J Roentgenol* 2006; 187(5):1179–83.

12. The Royal College of Radiologists. *Making the Best Use of Clinical Radiology Services: Referral Guidelines*. London: The Royal College of Radiologists; 2007.

13. Loughborough W. Development of a plain radiograph requesting algorithm for patients presenting with acute abdominal pain. *Quant Imaging Med Surg* 2012; 2(4):239–44.

14. Rothrock SG, Green SM, Hummel CB. Plain abdominal radiography in the detection of major disease in children: a prospective analysis. *Ann Emerg Med* 1992; 21(12):1423–9.

15. American College of Surgeons Committee on Trauma. *Advanced Trauma and Life Support for Doctors Student Course Manual* (8th ed). Chicago, IL: Hearthside Publishing Services; 2008.

16. The Royal College of Radiologists. *Standards of Practice and Guidance for Trauma Radiology in Severely Injured Patients*. London: The Royal College of Radiologists; 2011.

17. Hudson S, Boyle A, Wiltshire S, *et al*. Plain radiography may be safely omitted for selected major trauma patients undergoing whole body CT: database study. *Emerg Med Int* 2012; 2012:432537.

18. National Institute for Health and Clinical Excellence. *Head Injury: Triage, Assessment, Investigation and Early Management of Head Injury in Infants, Children and Adults.* London: NICE; 2007.

19. Grogan E, Moore D, Speroff T, *et al.* Cervical plain films should be eliminated in the high risk patient: results from decision analysis using an institutional cost perspective. *J Am Coll Surg* 2004; 199(3 Suppl):77.

20. Young-Im K, Cheong JW, Yoon SH. Clinical comparison of the predictive value of the simple skull X-ray and 3 dimensional computed tomography for skull fractures of children. *J Korean Neurosurg Soc* 2012; 52(6):528–33.

21. Resnick D. *Diagnosis of Bone and Joint Disorders* (4th ed). Philadelphia, PA: Saunders, 2002; 3757:3922–4.

22. Miller TT. Bone tumors and tumorlike conditions: analysis with conventional radiography. *Radiology* 2008; 246:662–74.

23. Robinson PJA. Radiology's Achilles heel: error and variation in the interpretation of the Rontgen image. *Br J Radiol* 1997; 70:1085–98.

Nuclear medicine for surgeons

Ian L. Minty

Introduction to nuclear medicine for surgeons

Nuclear medicine is an established type of molecular imaging that uses small amounts of radioactive tracers to diagnose, determine the severity of, and treat a variety of disorders including many cancers, cardiac disease, gastrointestinal, endocrine, and neurological conditions. Abnormal molecular activity can be pinpointed at very early pathological stages and immediate response to therapy may be assessed.

Depending on exam type, the radiotracer is either injected intravenously, swallowed, or inhaled as a gas. Radioactive emissions from the radiotracer are detected by a special imaging device.

Nuclear medicine encompasses positron emission tomography–computed tomography (PET-CT) which is the subject of a separate chapter (Chapter 1.6.3).

Tumours

Non-PET neoplasm imaging

Nuclear medicine is important in the management of many common malignant tumours. Its strength is to identify abnormal areas of metabolic activity, which can then often be anatomically defined by other imaging. It is used in the protocols of common malignancies to help stage the cancer by determining the presence of local spread or of metastatic disease.

Bone scanning

Bone avid diphosphonates are used which are excreted via the urinary tract which also shows on the scan. Metastatic as well as degenerative bone disease and trauma show increased uptake. A single 'hot spot' represents benign disease in 90% of cases. When two or more adjacent ribs show focal uptake this is most commonly due to trauma. Bony metastases typically manifest as randomly distributed lesions of variable size and activity most commonly in the red marrow-rich axial skeleton (spine, pelvis, rib cage, and skull).

The bone scan is very sensitive at detecting disease and, like PET-CT, images the entire skeleton. Radiographic detection of a lesion requires 30% bone loss and a bone scan can detect lesions unseen on conventional CT.

Osteolytic lesions can fail to take up isotope as they are mainly destructive with no significant new bone formation, the so-called cold lesions. These are often seen in myeloma (without pathological fracture), and sometimes in renal, thyroid, breast, lung, and poorly differentiated tumours. Early avascular necrosis can also be cold.

A pattern of diffuse increased uptake throughout the entire skeleton, the so-called super scan, is typically seen in metastatic prostate cancer,[1,2] but the differential diagnosis includes metabolic disease (e.g. hyperparathyroidism).

Within the first 3 months of chemotherapy, bony metastases may show enhanced isotope uptake, the 'flare phenomenon', which may give a false impression of a deteriorating clinical status.

Biopsy of an osteoid osteoma can be aided with a hand-held gamma probe.

Bone scanning is useful in the follow-up of metastatic primary bone malignancies, in particular osteosarcoma.

Sentinel lymph node imaging

Sentinel lymph node imaging (SLNI) is most commonly used in breast cancer and is also useful in skin, neck, and soft tissue tumours. Radiolabelled tracer particles are injected around the tumour and activity is traced with a hand-held gamma probe in theatre to the first draining 'sentinel' node. The decision to perform a full regional lymphadenectomy is based on the SLN histology. If negative in breast cancer, this obviates the need for an axillary dissection with its risk of lymphoedema. SLNs in patients with breast cancer can be identified in 85–94% of patients.[3–5]

SLNI can also be used in skin or soft tissue tumours preoperatively, for example, in malignant melanoma to demonstrate the pattern of lymphatic nodal drainage (Figure 1.6.2.1).

Neuropeptide receptor imaging

Neuroendocrine tumours such as carcinoid, pancreatic islet cell tumours, medullary carcinoma of the thyroid, phaeochromocytoma, and small cell lung can be imaged by using octreotide, a radiolabelled analogue of the natural neuropeptide somatostatin (Figure 1.6.2.2).

Thyroid cancer

Discrete thyroid cancers are seen as cold nodules on the thyroid scan. Commoner in women, most are papillary or follicular.

Metastatic lesions from well differentiated tumours tend to take up radioiodine, detectable on follow-up whole-body imaging. Postsurgical metastases may be treated with iodine-131 which has a relatively long half-life of 8 days making it also suitable post thyroidectomy to ablate residual thyroid tissue.

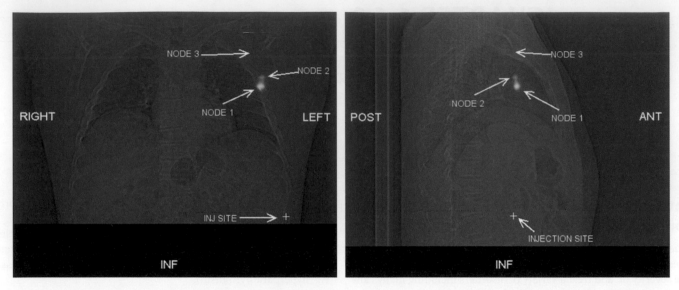

Fig. 1.6.2.1 SPECT-CT of sentinel lymph node imaging in breast cancer. Identification of site of the sentinel nodes in a patient with breast cancer (labelled node 1 and 2). Images using SPECT-CT with the location of the nodes superimposed on the low-dose CT scout to anatomically locate it. A third apical axillary node is identified (node 3).
Courtesy of Jim Phillips, Clinical Scientist, Medical Physics—University Hospitals Birmingham NHS Foundation Trust, UK.

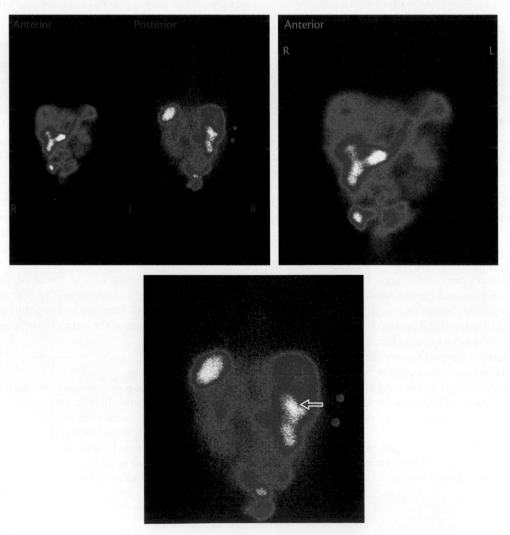

Fig. 1.6.2.2 Octreotide scan of phaeochromocytoma.

Gastrointestinal tract

Assessing biliary function

Radionucleotide studies using hepatobiliary iminodiacetic acid (HIDA) can be used to assess gallbladder function and excretion. This isotope is normally excreted into the biliary tree and then passes along the cystic duct into the gallbladder. In acute cholecystitis, the cystic duct is usually blocked and the gallbladder is not visualized. In normal patients, the isotope is excreted into the small bowel which can be encouraged by a fatty meal or cholecystokinin and the ejection fraction can be calculated as a percentage.[6] These scans can be used postoperatively to assess gallbladder or cystic duct remnants, biliary obstruction, and bile duct leaks.[7]

In biliary obstruction, a magnetic resonance cholangiopancreatogram (MRCP) is often used to look for common duct calculi. HIDA scanning is useful to investigate unexplained biliary type pain in the presence of a normal ultrasound and MRCP (Figure 1.6.2.3).

Diagnosis of Meckel's diverticulum

Ectopic gastric mucosa found in a Meckel's diverticulum takes up technetium-99m pertechnetate within its mucin-secreting cells and accumulates activity synchronously with normal gastric uptake. The sensitivity is less after adolescence with a decreasing incidence of gastric mucosa within Meckel's diverticula. H_2 blockers (e.g. cimetidine) are often used in this test to block the release of pertechnetate by the mucin-secreting cells (Figure 1.6.2.4).

Gastrointestinal bleeding

Technetium-99m is used in the investigation of gastrointestinal (GI) bleeding particularly in the intermittent or slow type from

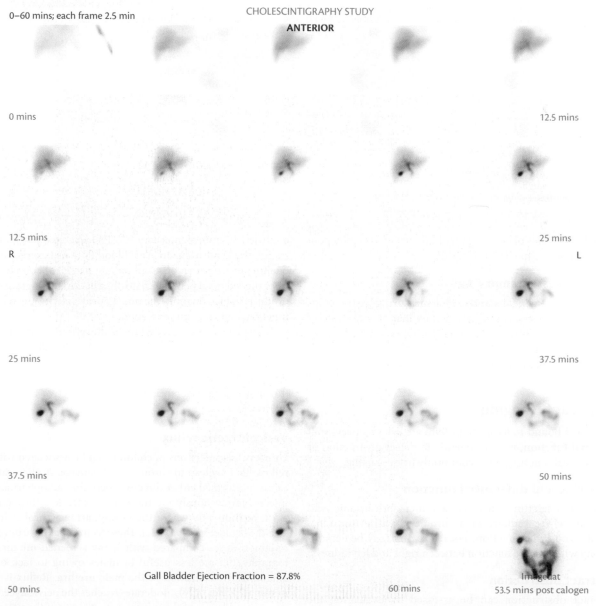

Fig. 1.6.2.3 HIDA scan.

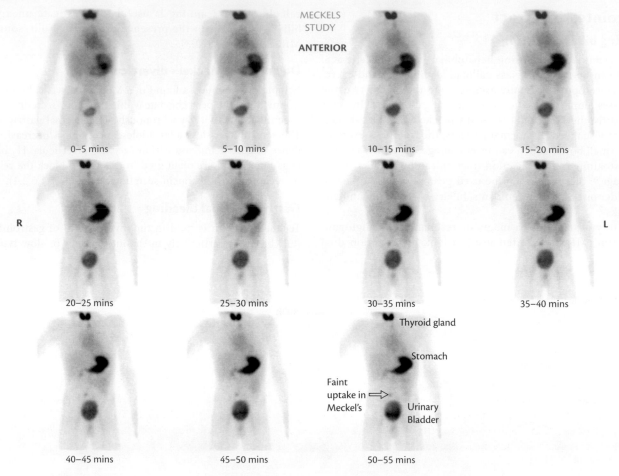

MECKELS STUDY

ANTERIOR

0–5 mins   5–10 mins   10–15 mins   15–20 mins

R   L

20–25 mins   25–30 mins   30–35 mins   35–40 mins

Thyroid gland

Stomach

Faint uptake in ⟹ Meckel's   Urinary Bladder

40–45 mins   45–50 mins   50–55 mins

Fig. 1.6.2.4 Meckel's diverticulum.

the lower GI tract. Sites of bleeding manifest during the blood pool phase changing with time[8] (Figure 1.6.2.5).

Evaluation of gastric emptying

Isotope studies are the gold standard for measuring gastric emptying. In practice, there are multiple factors that alter the rate of emptying of solids and liquids. The patient takes a meal labelled with technetium-99m isotope and is assessed over a 4-hour period. Delay is seen in diabetic gastroparesis, previous surgery, and drug therapy.

Urinary tract imaging

Different agents bound to technetium-99m are used to assess split dynamic renal function, most frequently to detect obstruction or decreased cortical function, most commonly from scarring.

Renal scarring and differential function

Assessment of renal function is via a dimercaptosuccinic acid (DMSA) scan where radiotracer accumulates within the renal tubular cells with little excretion. Focal scarring may be demonstrated along with relative function between right and left kidneys.

Urinary tract obstruction

Urinary tract obstruction can be assessed by evaluating the renal passage of isotopes mercaptoacetyltriglycine (MAG3) or

diethylenetriaminepentacetate (DTPA), excreted by glomerular filtration thus informing on renal blood flow and excretion. This can quantify urinary tract obstruction into partial or complete or identify a dilated renal pelvis with no obstruction. Renogram curves are produced which quantify the time to peak activity, the relative renal function, and half-time excretion.

Diuretic renography is where a diuretic is given in combination with the isotope. The increased urine flow should cause rapid transport of the isotope through the kidney, producing a rapid washout of isotope if unobstructed. Quantified with a half-time, this is useful in differentiating non-obstructive from obstructive hydronephrosis.

Vesicoureteric reflux

Urinary tract infections in children can be associated with urinary reflux that may lead to chronic renal damage. A micturating study can be performed either directly where the radiopharmaceutical is injected intravenously and the activity is tracked through the renal tract, or indirectly where the radiopharmaceutical is introduced into the bladder via a catheter. These techniques have lower gonadal radiation doses compared with X-ray-screened micturating cystography, but are less useful in males owing to lack of detailed anatomical visualization of the male urethra. Reflux is graded as minimal (ureter only), moderate (reaches the pelvicalyceal system), or severe (dilation of the calyces or tortuosity of the ureter).

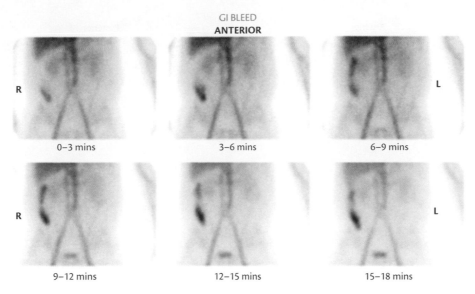

GI BLEED
ANTERIOR

R   L

0–3 mins   3–6 mins   6–9 mins

R   L

9–12 mins   12–15 mins   15–18 mins

Fig. 1.6.2.5 Technetium-99m blood pool of lower GI bleed.

Function in transplanted kidney

Ultrasound is the usual initial investigation. Renal scintigraphy helps monitor perfusion and function and may detect post-surgical complications such as acute tubular necrosis and ciclosporin toxicity. In transplant rejection, there is usually both poor perfusion and excretion. Donors may also be assessed to confirm that they will tolerate nephrectomy.

Skeletal system

The bone scan is the most commonly used, practical, and cost-effective method to evaluate the entire bony skeleton due to its high sensitivity in identifying sites of abnormal bone metabolism. As well as the uses in neoplastic disease described separately, it has non-neoplastic applications.

The most commonly used isotope, methylene diphosphonate (MDP) is preferentially taken up by bone. Technetium-99m is chemically attached to MDP so that radioactivity can be transported and attached to bone via the hydroxyapatite for imaging. An increase in physiological function, such as due to a fracture in the bone, will normally cause an increase in the concentration of the radioisotope.

Infection in prosthetic joints

A conventional bone scan can be difficult to interpret as these scans can show increased uptake even 1–2 years after surgery due to normal healing and bone repair. A loose hip prosthesis usually has delayed focal uptake at the tip of the stem and adjacent to the upper stem near the greater trochanter whilst an infected prosthesis shows increased uptake along the length of the stem.

Labelled leucocyte imaging is time-consuming but is the procedure of choice for diagnosing prosthetic joint infection.

Most of the leucocytes labelled are neutrophils so the test works best on bacterial infections. It is less useful when the cellular response is other than neutropenic, for example, in opportunist infections and spinal osteomyelitis.[9]

Stress fractures

Stress fractures may be difficult to identify on conventional radiographs. Bone scans, if performed early (within 4 weeks of presentation) show increased uptake on the early blood pool images.

A common clinical problem is tibial pain in physically active individuals. Bone scan imaging helps differentiate stress fractures from shin splints (medial tibial stress syndrome). The latter on a bone scan show linear uptake along the posteromedial cortical margin along the site of insertion of the soleus muscle. In older patients, stress fractures can occur in the pelvis through the sacrum, called insufficiency fractures. Bilateral vertical stress fractures passing through the sacral foramina give rise to the H-shaped uptake called the Honda sign.

Osteomyelitis

Conventional radiographs do not show changes early in the disease, and only become positive after 7–10 days. A three-phase bone scan is extremely sensitive and can be positive within 2 days of onset of symptoms with an accuracy of over 90%.[10] Images typically show increased uptake of isotope on both the early blood pool images and the delayed images taken at 3 hours.

Cellulitis shows as increased soft tissue uptake on the blood pool scan but decreased activity on the delayed scans. This has a sensitivity of 80%. In difficult clinical cases, a labelled white blood cell scan has greater sensitivity (95%) and specificity (90%).

Septic arthritis of a joint usually shows increased activity on both sides of the joint. There is no risk in patients with renal impairment which is an advantage over magnetic resonance imaging scanning which usually uses contrast in these cases, for example, when planning possible surgery in osteomyelitis of diabetic feet (Figure 1.6.2.6).

Benign causes of uptake

Paget's disease typically shows increased uptake on a bone scan. This can be mistaken for metastatic disease when it occurs in the pelvis in patients with prostatic carcinoma. If there is doubt,

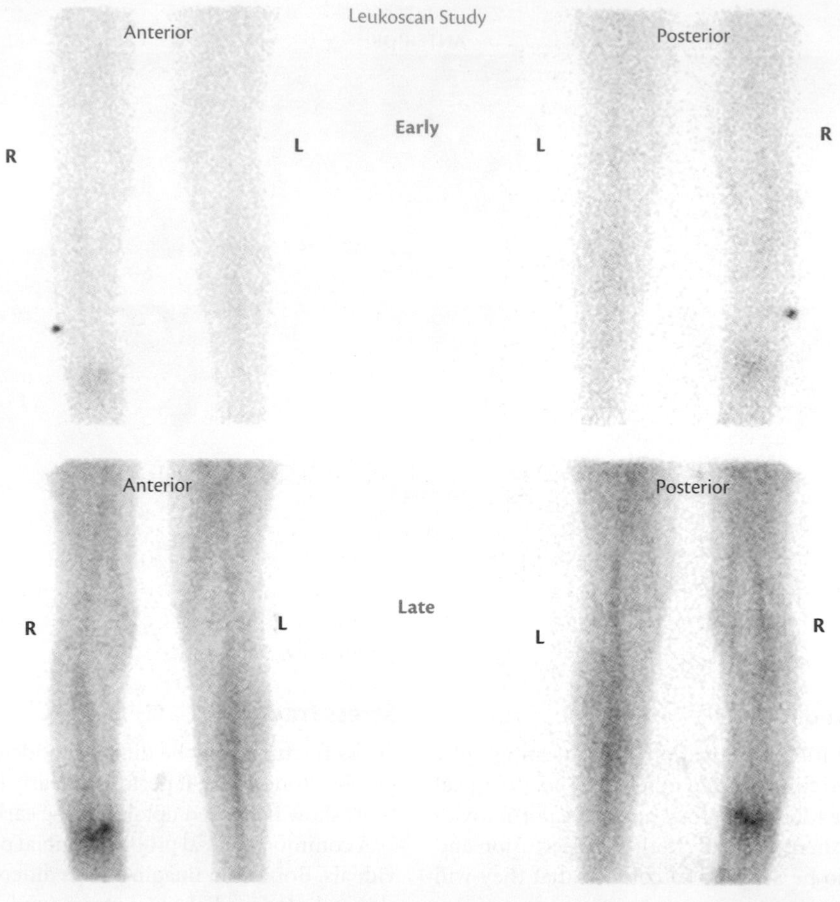

Fig. 1.6.2.6 Bone scan of foot osteomyelitis.

plain X-rays will often show the typical appearances. Paget's disease can affect a single bone or more commonly multiple bones—polyostotic. Sarcomatous change in Paget's disease is quoted at 1%. Other benign causes of uptake include fractures, osteomyelitis, enchondromas, or osteomyelitis.

Multiple sequential cold vertebral bodies is usually due to previous radiotherapy.

Soft tissue uptake

Soft tissue uptake can be seen in bone scans. Free unbound isotope can be seen taken up normally by the stomach and thyroid gland. Soft tissue calcification following trauma or surgery (heterotopic calcification) or around neuropathic joints (dystrophic calcification) all show activity on a bone scan. Degenerative uptake is common in the spine where it is often seen in osteophytes or facet joints. This can usually be correlated with radiographs if clinically suspicious. Tumours that produce metastases with calcification can show activity (e.g. bowel, breast, and osteosarcoma).

Thorax

Lungs: ventilation/perfusion scan

Technetium-99m macro-aggregated albumin is used to image pulmonary perfusion. These particles are trapped in their first pass through the pulmonary capillaries. Aerosols labelled with technetium-99m are commonly used to assess ventilation. The test should be interpreted with a chest X-ray within the last 2 days which can be used to asses pre-existing disease (e.g. bullae or pleural effusions). In a normal individual, the perfusion of the lung and ventilation are matched. This test is less sensitive in patients with chronic obstructive pulmonary disease.

Defects in perfusion that are not matched in the ventilation imaging are suggestive of pulmonary embolus. CT pulmonary angiography is often the first test to diagnose pulmonary emboli. Ventilation/perfusion imaging when performed with single-photon emission computed tomography (SPECT) is diagnostic in 88% of patients in the diagnosis of pulmonary embolism.[11] It has the advantages of a lower dose of radiation and can be used in patients with renal impairment and contrast allergies. In pregnant patients, where radiation dose is important, a perfusion-only scan may be performed. If this is normal, it excludes a pulmonary embolus with a reasonable degree of certainty.

Other uses of lung scans include assessment of lung function in patients considered for pulmonary resection surgery or lung transplant surgery and to detect lung transplant rejection.

Heart: myocardial perfusion scan

A SPECT myocardial perfusion scan is used to visualize heart blood flow and function. Stress and rest images are obtained to distinguish reversible from non-reversible defects. This is valuable in the assessment of hypoxic but viable myocardium that would benefit from revascularization. It can detect coronary artery disease and to evaluate damage to heart muscle after a heart attack. This is useful in assessing treatment options including coronary artery stenting and bypass surgery. It can be used in the preoperative risk assessment of major surgery, particularly in those with a cardiac history.

Cardiac function may be calculated from the ejection fraction in assessing patients before and after cardiotoxic chemotherapy.

Endocrine

Thyroid gland

This gland is now most commonly imaged using technetium-99m pertechnetate. The relative sizes of the right and left glands can be assessed and the overall percentage uptake can be calculated. Congenital ectopic thyroid tissue can be identified. Known nodules can be assessed to see if they have normal uptake or have no uptake (cold). These cold nodules may indicate thyroid cancer and warrant consideration of further investigation (possibly ultrasound with fine-needle aspiration), Hot nodules can be identified which represent hyperactive adenomas. Thyroiditis in the earlier stages of the disease shows a diffuse increase in glandular uptake of isotope.

Parathyroid adenoma

These small tumours can be difficult to detect particularly if in an aberrant location or at re-operation. Usually four in number (range is reported from three to eight) Technetium-99m sestamibi is the radionucleotide primarily used. Approximately 20% of adenomas are ectopic, often in the lower neck adjacent to the carotid sheath or oesophagus or within the superior or anterior part of the inferior mediastinum, sometimes within the thymus gland. Technetium-99m sestamibi is taken up both by parathyroid adenomas and normal thyroid gland, but parathyroid adenomas are best seen in early and delayed images due to avid early uptake and delayed washout. Over 95% of adenomas can be detected (Figure 1.6.2.7).[12]

Adrenal glands

The adrenal medulla can be imaged using meta-iodobenzylguanidine (MIBG) which is taken up by chromaffin cells. It is useful in the imaging of adrenal phaeochromocytomas and it can detect ectopic tumours. It can also be used to detect neuroblastomas and their metastases.

Miscellaneous

Vascular graft infection

Conventional CT imaging can identify late cases of vascular graft infection but labelled leucocyte scans may offer early diagnosis of infections involving arterial bypass and dialysis grafts. False-positive results can occur in graft thrombosis and perigraft haematoma (Figure 1.6.2.8).[9,10]

Lymphoedema

In patients with swollen legs, lymphoscintigraphy can be performed to identify problems with the lymphatic drainage. In particular, delay in drainage can be ascertained.

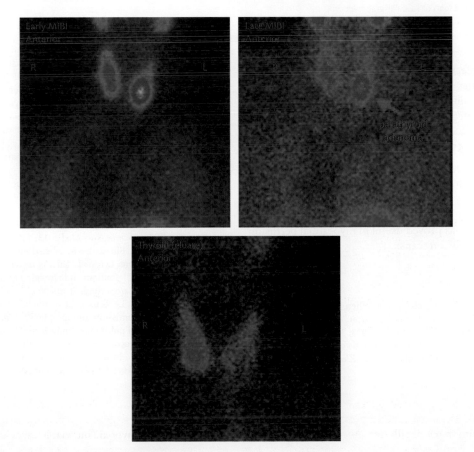

Fig. 1.6.2.7 Technetium-99m sestamibi scan of parathyroid adenoma.

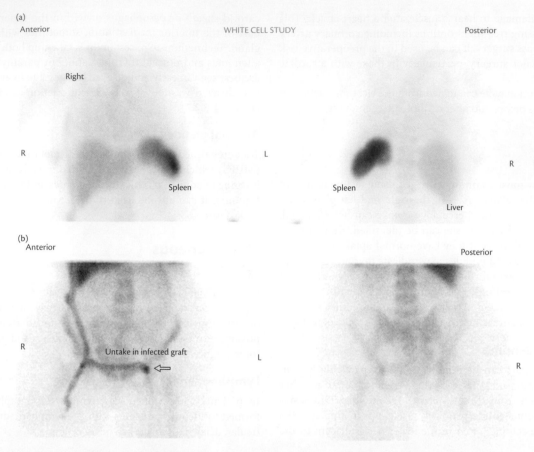

Fig. 1.6.2.8 Labelled leucocyte scan of vascular graft infection.

Infection

The site of an occult infection may be identified using technetium-99m-labelled leucocytes in a patient with a fever of unknown origin. This test can facilitate the differentiation of normal postoperative changes from infection.[9,10]

Planar imaging and SPECT

The mathematical algorithms used successfully in CT imaging have also been applied to radionucleotide techniques where images are acquired in a multiplanar format and displayed cinematically as a three-dimensional image or in the three standard axial, coronal, and sagittal planes. This has proved useful in myocardial perfusion and lung ventilation/perfusion scans.

References

1. De Nunzio C, Leonardo C, Franco G, *et al*. When to perform bone scan in patients with newly diagnosed prostate cancer: external validation of a novel risk stratification tool. *World J Urol* 2013; 31(2):365–9.
2. Zhou JQ, Zhu Y, Yao XD, *et al*. Necessity analysis of bone scan in patients with newly diagnosed prostate cancer. *Zhonghua Yi Xue Za Zhi* 2013; 93(4):248–51.
3. Langer I, Zuber M, Köchli OR, *et al*. Validation study of the sentinel lymph node (SLN) method in invasive breast carcinoma. Personal data and review of the literature. *Swiss Surg* 2000; 6(3):128–36.
4. Borgstein PJ, Pijpers R, Comans EF, *et al*. Sentinel lymph node biopsy in breast cancer: guidelines and pitfalls of lymphoscintigraphy and gamma probe detection. *J Am Coll Surg* 1998; 186(3):275–83.
5. Krag D, Moffat F. Nuclear medicine and the surgeon. *Lancet* 1999; 354(9183):1019–22.
6. Ziessman HA. Nuclear medicine hepatobiliary imaging. *Clin Gastroenterol Hepatol* 2010; 8(2):111–16.
7. Uliel L, Mellnick VM, Menias CO, *et al*. Nuclear medicine in the acute clinical setting: indications, imaging findings, and potential pitfalls. *Radiographics* 2013; 33(2):375–96.
8. Allen TW, Tulchinsky M. Nuclear medicine tests for acute gastrointestinal conditions. *Semin Nucl Med* 2013; 43(2):88–101.
9. Palestro CJ, Love C, Bhargava KK. Labeled leukocyte imaging: current status and future directions. *Q J Nucl Med Mol Imaging* 2009; 53(1):105–23.
10. Love C, Palestro CJ. Radionuclide imaging of inflammation and infection in the acute care setting. *Semin Nucl Med* 2013; 43(2):102–13.
11. Le Duc-Pennec A, Le Roux PY, Cornily JC, *et al*. Diagnostic accuracy of single-photon emission tomography ventilation/perfusion lung scan in the diagnosis of pulmonary embolism. *Chest* 2012; 141(2):381–7.
12. Saengsuda Y. The accuracy of 99m Tc-MIBI scintigraphy for preoperative parathyroid localization in primary and secondary-tertiary hyperparathyroidism. *J Med Assoc Thai* 2012; 95(Suppl 3):S81–91.

CHAPTER 1.6.3

Positron emission tomography–computed tomography for surgeons

Ian L. Minty

Basic principles

Positron emission tomography (PET)[1] is a nuclear medicine, functional, three-dimensional (3D) imaging technique which detects pairs of gamma rays from a matter–antimatter annihilation event between tissue electrons and a positron emitted by a tracer introduced into the body riding on a biologically active molecule. 3D imaging is mapped precisely with the aid of a computed tomography (CT) X-ray scan performed simultaneously by the same machine and images are 'fused'.

The commonest biologically active molecule chosen for PET is fluorodeoxyglucose (FDG), an analogue of glucose, and the concentrations of tracer imaged will indicate tissue metabolic activity as in the resting fasting state many tumours use glucose to a greater degree than normal cells. Ninety per cent of current scans use the FDG tracer to explore the possibility of cancer metastasis.

On a minority basis, many other radioactive tracers are used in PET to image other molecules of interest.

Scanning protocols

Patients fast for 4 hours which ensures that most of their tissues are using fatty acids as their source of energy. The blood glucose level is checked to be normal—if it is high then the FDG may not be taken up well.

The standardized uptake value (SUV) takes into account the amount of activity injected, the patient's weight, and the time from the injection. The value obtained for normal vascular structures and the liver can be compared with focal areas of uptake. It also allows comparative measurements to be made between two scans performed weeks or months apart.

Lung cancer

The role of PETCT in the staging of non-small cell lung cancer is well established. The sensitivity is decreased in tumours smaller than 1 cm. PET-CT scans have replaced bone scans for the detection of bone metastases. FDG PET-positive lesions still require histological confirmation in most cases as FDG uptake can occur in infection and inflammatory diseases such as sarcoid.[1]

Curative lung cancer

Patients with lung cancer in whom curative surgery or radiotherapy is being considered now routinely undergo PET-CT imaging. In the differentiation of benign from malignant disease, PET-CT has an overall sensitivity of 86–100% and specificity of 40–90%.[2] The accurate staging of hilar and mediastinal nodes is a crucial factor in determining operability. PET-CT can detect nodal involvement when CT size criteria are unmet, with a sensitivity of 83% and specificity of 92% which is approximately 15% higher than CT alone[3] (Figure 1.6.3.1). PET-CT can also exclude unexpected distant metastatic disease particularly liver, adrenals, and osseous (Figure 1.6.3.2). The sensitivity is 95% for both nodal and bony metastases.[4] This is most cost-effective in patients who are mediastinal node negative on conventional CT scanning.[5]

Solitary pulmonary nodule

These are commonly indeterminate after CT analysis and may be technically difficult or hazardous to biopsy. The diagnostic accuracy of PET-CT is over 90% with over 85% of metabolically active nodules being malignant. There is increasing likelihood with increasing FDG uptake with a SUV of over 2.5 being a cut-off between benign and malignant. Lesions less than 10 mm in diameter are often indeterminate as they are too small to be accurately resolved. Certain malignant tumours including carcinoid and alveolar cell tumours are associated with low levels of FDG uptake.

Detection of recurrent disease

A year after stereotactic radiotherapy, greater levels of FDG uptake are seen in recurrent disease which can have a sensitivity of up to 100%, certainly better than any other imaging modality to differentiate radiotherapy change from recurrence.[6]

Radiotherapy planning

PET can be used in patients being considered for radical radiotherapy. It can show FDG-avid tumour which lies outside the planning target volume and leads to changes in the volumes used in 25–60% of patients. PET-CT frequently changes planning management and is associated with much improved survival.[2,7,8]

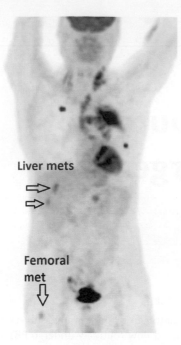

Fig. 1.6.3.1 Lung cancer with lung, liver, and right femoral bone metastases.

Gastro-oesophageal cancer

Oesophageal and gastro-oesophageal cancer

Although endoscopic ultrasound is good at local T and N staging, PET-CT is valuable at detecting tumour in sub-centimetre supraclavicular nodes and occult distant disease with a sensitivity of 67% and specificity of 97%.[2] PET-CT is well established in the evaluation of oesophageal tumours but gastro-oesophageal junction tumours have variable FDG uptake,[9] with some exhibiting low levels similar to normal background.

Gastric cancer

The gastric mucosa has normal physiological FDG uptake which makes the identification of smaller tumours more difficult; this is compounded by the fact that only 60% of gastric tumours take up significant levels of FDG. The detection of recurrent

gastric cancer is better at 77%, including recurrent anastomotic disease.[10]

PET-CT is useful in evaluation of metabolic response to chemoradiotherapy, which has useful prognostic value in helping to identify good responders.[11]

Colorectal cancer

PET-CT is not routinely useful in the preoperative staging and evaluation of primary colorectal cancer. It does, however, have a sensitivity of 91% for recurrent disease.[12] PET-CT is most accurate 6 months after surgery when FDG-avid residual inflammatory change has largely resolved. PET-CT is used in patients with liver or lung metastases being considered for curative resection to exclude other sites of occult metastatic disease, commonly the retroperitoneum, peritoneum, and ovaries. PET-CT is useful in patients suspected of local recurrence on conventional CT/magnetic resonance imaging (MRI) or in those with a rising carcinoembryonic antigen without cause (Figure 1.6.3.3).

Gastrointestinal stromal tumours

Gastrointestinal stromal tumours show high FDG avidity and PET-CT is used for primary evaluation and therapeutic response. The metabolic and clinical responses correlate.

Head and neck

The commonest head and neck tumours involve the tonsils or tongue base. Interpretation is made more difficult in this area by muscular and vocal cord uptake so some centres use a 'silent protocol' or diazepam to reduce FDG uptake in neck musculature. PET-CT is superior at detecting nodal metastases compared to standard cross-sectional imaging and detects hitherto occult metastases in about 10% of patients.

PET-CT is superior at detecting regional nodal metastases in primary head and neck cancer with a sensitivity and specificity of

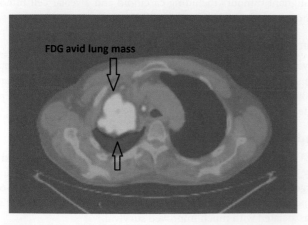

Fig. 1.6.3.2 Lung tumour with small FDG-positive mediastinal node.

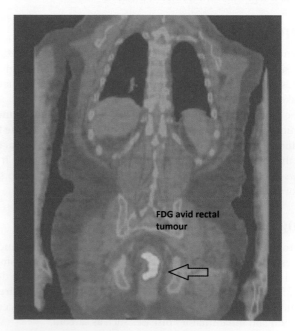

Fig. 1.6.3.3 Rectal cancer localized.

95%.[13] It can also assess treatment response where it is useful in the identification of residual or recurrent disease post therapy with a high negative predictive value.

Lymphoma

This is the second commonest disease after lung cancer to be imaged by PET-CT with profound advantages of whole-body analysis (Figure 1.6.3.3).[14] Treatment response is assessed by metabolic and physical parameters. Reduced accuracy for bone marrow involvement necessitates a continued role for bone biopsy.

Melanoma

PET-CT is used for the initial staging of patients with cutaneous malignant melanoma, particularly in an adjunctive role in those with nodal or distant metastases (stages III and IV). It detects almost all metastases greater than 10 mm and 80% between 6 and 10 mm, and detects deep soft tissue, lymph node, and visceral metastases.[15] There is no evidence that PET is of value in the regional staging of melanoma as it has a lower sensitivity compared to sentinel lymph node biopsy for detecting regional lymph node metastases.[16]

Male/female reproductive organ tumours and breast cancer tumours

Testicular cancer

PET-CT is most helpful in seminoma recurrence, differentiating residual tumour from fibrosis, and in patients with elevated tumour markers. Mature teratoma tumours show poor FDG uptake and can give false-negative results.

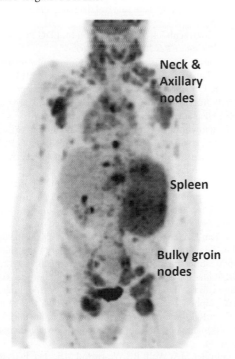

Fig. 1.6.3.4 Lymphoma stage IV disease with FDG-positive marked splenic enlargement.

Cervical cancer

In locally advanced cases, PET-CT is superior to other imaging modalities in assessing lymph node status and distant metastases with high FDG uptake in the primary tumour and in regional lymph nodes predictive of a worse prognosis. Radiation treatment volumes can be tailored according to the PET data.[17]

Ovarian cancer

Normal physiological FDG uptake can be seen in the ovaries in women of reproductive age. However, focal uptake in postmenopausal women is suspicious of malignancy and warrants further evaluation. PET-CT has a role in ovarian cancer patients with indeterminate lymph nodes, in those with rising CA125 levels and those with a clinical suspicion of recurrence in whom conventional CT scanning has been unhelpful.

Breast, thyroid, and pancreatic cancer

Breast cancer

Many types of primary breast cancer are not FDG avid enough to be detected by PET-CT. The accuracy in axillary node staging is better by sentinel node biopsy. PET-CT is most useful in patients with recurrent breast cancer where it can offer improved diagnostic accuracy compared with current standard imaging.[18] It has a role in symptomatic patients with negative tumour markers and asymptomatic patients with positive tumour markers.

The conventional technetium bone scan is the standard method for the detection of bone metastases. PET-CT is better at detecting osteolytic disease.

Thyroid cancer

After thyroidectomy for carcinoma approximately 20% of patients develop local recurrence or metastases which cannot be detected by iodine-131 scanning. PET-CT is used in post-surgical patients with rising serological markers (thyroglobulin serum) with a negative iodine-131 scan. It is suggested that patients with thyroglobulin levels above 10 ng/mL are investigated and PET-CT reveals metastases in up to 90% of these patients.

In post-thyroidectomy patients with medullary cancer and elevated calcitonin levels, FDG-PET-CT has a sensitivity of 70–75% for localizing metastases.[19]

Pancreatic cancer

PET-CT can help distinguish between benign and malignant disease [2] Its value is in the detection of involved lymph nodes, peritoneal disease, and occult lesions, although its sensitivity is low in nodes/nodules below 1 cm in size.

Cancer of unknown primary and sarcoma

Cancer of unknown primary

PET-CT can detect the primary tumour in approximately 33% of cases with lung, oropharyngeal, and pancreatic cancer being the most frequently uncovered.[20]

Sarcoma

These rare tumours have a wide pathology spectrum and PET-CT has difficulty in distinguishing between low-grade malignant sarcomas and benign tumours.

Therapy response

The level of FDG uptake as measured by the SUV can be used to assess response to therapy early and late in the course of treatment. The initial staging scan evaluates the FDG tumour avidity and a second scan early at 2–4 weeks after commencement of treatment predicts histological response and survival.

Incidental findings, FDG-averse tumours, and normal variants

Significant incidental findings

Early use of PET-CT identified many incidental findings and those reported should have reasonable probability of significance. For example, focal large bowel FDG uptake is due to pre-malignant polyps in about 10% of patients and should always be investigated.

Poorly FDG-avid tumours and averse physiology

* Renal tumours are better assessed by helical CT scan.[21]

* Bladder tumours are not reliably detected, as FDG urinary excretion can confuse diagnosis.

* Prostate cancer nodal metastases are not FDG avid (11C choline or acetate may be).

Normal variants in FDG uptake: pitfalls in diagnosis

* Cerebral FDG uptake due to normal glucose metabolism makes it relatively difficult to detect tumours; MRI is more sensitive.

* Cardiac uptake is commonly seen due to normal glucose metabolism.

* Renal activity is seen due to normal excretion of the FDG in urine.

* FDG uptake is seen in normal active muscles.

* Activated brown fat can take up FDG; seen more often in the winter months, usually in the supraclavicular fossa and in the paraspinal distribution within the thorax.

* Vascular FDG uptake is seen in the great vessels and at the site of plaque.

* Gastrointestinal tract: the stomach commonly has physiological uptake. Bowel commonly shows strips of segmental (not localized focal) uptake. Anorectal inflammatory uptake is common, but caution is needed here as this can also be a site for pathology.

* Salivary and thyroid glands commonly show incidental diffuse uptake (focal uptake warrants further investigation, usually by ultrasound).

* The use of granulocyte stimulating factor in oncology can stimulate normal bone marrow FDG uptake which can mimic lymphomatous bone marrow infiltration.

Further reading

Barrington S, Maisey MN, Wahl RL. *Atlas of Clinical Positron Emission Tomography* (2nd ed). London: Hodder; 2005.
Blodgett TM. *PETCT: With Correlative Diagnostic CT*. Philadelphia, PA: Lippincott Williams & Wilkins; 2008.
Lynch TB, Clarke J, Cook G, et al. *PETCT in Clinical Practice*. Berlin: Springer; 2007.
Oehr P, Biersack HJ, Coleman RE (eds). *PET and PETCT in Oncology: Basics and Clinical Applications*. Berlin: Springer; 2003.

References

1. Cuaron J, Dunphy M, Rimner A. Role of FDG-PET scans in staging, response assessment, and follow-up care for non-small cell lung cancer. *Front Oncol* 2012; 2:208.
2. Fletcher JW, Djulbegovic B, Soares HP, et al. Recommendations on the use of 18F-FDG PET in oncology. *J Nucl Med* 2008; 49(3):480–508.
3. Konishi J, Yamazaki K, Tsukamoto E, et al. Mediastinal lymph node staging by FDG-PET in patients with non-small cell lung cancer: analysis of false-positive FDG-PET findings. *Respiration* 2003; 70(5):500–6.
4. Wu Y, Li P, Zhang H, et al. Diagnostic value of fluorine 18 fluorodeoxyglucose positron emission tomography/computed tomography for the detection of metastases in non-small-cell lung cancer patients. *Int J Cancer* 2013; 132(2):E37–47.
5. Facey K, Bradbury I, Laking G, et al. Overview of the clinical effectiveness of positron emission tomography imaging in selected cancers. *Health Technol Assess* 2007; 11(44):iii–iv, xi–267.
6. Nakajima N, Sugawara Y, Kataoka M, et al. Differentiation of tumor recurrence from radiation-induced pulmonary fibrosis after stereotactic ablative radiotherapy for lung cancer: characterization of (18) F-FDG PET/CT findings. *Ann Nucl Med* 2013; 27(3):261–70.
7. Mac Manus MP, Everitt S, Bayne M, et al. The use of fused PET/CT images for patient selection and radical radiotherapy target volume definition in patients with non-small cell lung cancer: results of a prospective study with mature survival data. *Radiother Oncol* 2013; 106(3):292–8.
8. Krause BJ, Schwarzenböck S, Souvatzoglou M. FDG PET and PET/CT. *Recent Results Cancer Res* 2013; 187:351–69.
9. Wu AJ, Goodman KA. Positron emission tomography imaging for gastroesophageal junction tumors. *Semin Radiat Oncol* 2013; 23(1):10–5.
10. Herrmann K, Ott K, Buck AK, et al. Imaging gastric cancer with PET and the radiotracers 18F-FLT and 18F-FDG: a comparative analysis. *J Nucl Med* 2007; 48(12):1945–50.
11. Cuenca X, Hennequin C, Hindié E, et al. Evaluation of early response to concomitant chemoradiotherapy by interim 18F-FDG PET/CT imaging in patients with locally advanced oesophageal carcinomas. *Eur J Nucl Med Mol Imaging* 2013; 40(4):477–85.
12. Brush J, Boyd K, Chappell F, et al. The value of FDG positron emission tomography/computerised tomography (PET/CT) in pre-operative staging of colorectal cancer: a systematic review and economic evaluation. *Health Technol Assess* 2011; 15(35):1–192, iii–iv.
13. Yongkui L, Jian L, Wanghan, et al. 18FDG-PET/CT for the detection of regional nodal metastasis in patients with primary head and neck cancer before treatment: a meta-analysis. *Surg Oncol* 2013; 22(2):e11–16.
14. Kumar R, Maillard I, Schuster SJ, et al. Utility of fluorodeoxyglucose-PET imaging in the management of patients with Hodgkin's and non-Hodgkin's lymphomas. *Radiol Clin North Am* 2004; 42(6):1083–100.
15. Krug B, Crott R, Lonneux M, et al. Role of PET in the initial staging of cutaneous malignant melanoma: systematic review. *Radiology* 2008; 249(3):836–44.
16. Schröer-Günther MA, Wolff RF, Westwood ME, et al. F-18-fluoro-2-deoxyglucose positron emission tomography (PET) and PET/computed tomography imaging in primary staging of patients with malignant melanoma: a systematic review. *Syst Rev* 2012; 1:62.

17. Herrera FG, Prior JO. The role of PET/CT in cervical cancer. *Front Oncol* 2013; 3:34.

18. Pennant M, Takwoingi Y, Pennant L, *et al.* A systematic review of positron emission tomography (PET) and positron emission tomography/computed tomography (PET/CT) for the diagnosis of breast cancer recurrence. *Health Technol Assess* 2010; 14(50):1–103.

19. Schöder H, Yeung HW. Positron emission imaging of head and neck cancer, including thyroid carcinoma. *Semin Nucl Med* 2004; 34(3):180–97.

20. Kwee TC, Kwee RM. Combined FDG-PET/CT for the detection of unknown primary tumors: systematic review and meta-analysis. *Eur Radiol* 2009; 19(3):731–44.

21. Schöder H, Larson SM. Positron emission tomography for prostate, bladder, and renal cancer. *Semin Nucl Med* 2004; 34(4):274–92.

Principles of magnetic resonance scanning and its use in surgical practice

Ishmael Chasi

Basic physical principles

Magnetic resonance imaging (MRI) resonates mobile hydrogen nuclei (solitary protons) in water in the body to create high-contrast images, enabling multiplanar lesion characterization crucial for accurate diagnosis to facilitate curative or palliative surgical procedures. MRI is also integral for detecting complications of surgical intervention or radiotherapy.

Transmitter coils broadcast radio waves into a magnetized patient (0.5–7 Tesla) at circa 46 MHz, the resonant frequency of the proton. Receiver coils then detect the radio 'echo' emitted from the patient as proton resonant energy is released. This sequence is repeated many times per second and complex mathematical calculations generate images. Tissues exhibit varying properties which provide inherent contrast.

There are three main categories of magnetic resonance (MR) sequences: spin echo (SE), inversion recovery (IR), and gradient echo (GE). SE sequences include T1, T2, and proton density weighted. Typical signal characteristics of these are shown in Table 1.6.4.1.

IR sequences are fluid-attenuated inversion recovery (FLAIR) and short T1 inversion recovery (STIR), both exhibiting T2-weighted features with the additional characteristics of fluid signal suppression in FLAIR and fat suppression in STIR sequences.

GE sequences image moving blood and extravasated blood products but are more prone to artefact (magnetic susceptibility).

In practice, a combination of SE, IR, and GE sequences can be used depending on clinicoanatomical context. Other specialized sequences in clinical practice include diffusion-weighted imaging mainly used in stroke imaging, magnetic resonance spectroscopy utilized for assessing metabolic disorders and tumour metabolism, and functional MRI.

Gadolinium is a paramagnetic compound that is the most commonly used MRI contrast agent which can be administered intravenously or into joints to enhance contrast between normal and abnormal tissue.

Magnetic resonance angiography (MRA) can be performed with or without intravenous contrast agents. The latter is achieved by using special sequences such as time-of-flight and phase contrast.

Safety

Exposure to strong magnetic and radiofrequency fields raises safety concerns. Attraction of non-fixed ferromagnetic objects to the main magnetic field can result in dangerous projectiles, and wires in or on the patient can become incandescent. Therefore only MRI-compatible equipment and material should be brought into the scanning room. Thus standard anaesthetic equipment, oxygen tanks, monitors, pillows with steel springs, cutlery, belts, inhalers, and floor buffing machines are strictly excluded. Credit cards will be wiped.

Damage can occur to pacemakers, neurostimulators, insulin pumps, cochlear implants, and physiological monitors. Certain types of heart valves and intracranial aneurysm clips are unsafe; documented evidence of safety of specific devices is mandatory. Six to eight weeks should be allowed to elapse before patients with non-ferromagnetic stents, filters, coils, and staples are scanned.

Metallic foreign bodies may move when the patient is moved in and out of the scanner. This can cause damage in certain areas such as the eye. Plain radiographs should be obtained where there is any doubt or suspected exposure such as in sheet metal workers or welders.

The effects of MRI in pregnancy are as yet unknown, with no good evidence of harm. However, MRI is avoided in the first trimester. The use of gadolinium in pregnancy should only be reserved for cases where the concern for the immediate well-being of the mother is deemed paramount.

Gadolinium contrast has a much lower frequency of adverse reactions than the iodinated contrast agents used in computed tomography (CT). Allergic reactions are extremely rare. The use

Table 1.6.4.1 MRI signal characteristics of tissue in the human body

	Fat	Water	Cortical bone	Air	Muscle
T1	High	Low	Low	Low	Low to intermediate
T2	Intermediate to high	High	Low	Low	Low to intermediate
Proton density	Intermediate	Intermediate	Low	Low	Low to intermediate

of gadolinium in patients with acute kidney injury or chronic renal failure has been known to cause nephrogenic systemic fibrosis.

For claustrophobic patients, alternative imaging methods, sedation, and open magnets should be considered.

Artefacts

Most artefacts are due to patient movement, respiratory motion, vascular flow, signal heterogeneity, metallic implants, or chemical shift. Artefacts are generally greater with higher-strength magnets. Images tend to be more compromised in older unwell patients who may find it difficult to keep still, hold their breath, and who may have had metallic implants. Rapid MRI sequences allow breath-hold imaging to be performed thereby negating or minimizing the effects of respiratory motion artefact. Buscopan® can be administered for imaging bowel to reduce peristalsis and electrocardiogram-gating allows for cardiac imaging to be performed.

Common areas and indications for scanning

Brain

MRI is the modality of choice for stable patients with suspected non-traumatic brain and spine pathology. It is excellent in detecting lesions that may be occult on CT, particularly if they are small or superficial without significant mass effect or oedema. Intravenous contrast medium is invaluable in assessing patients with neoplastic and inflammatory disease. Malignant or inflammatory meningeal disease is also far more readily detected on post-contrast MR scans.

Neoplasms

Tumours can be classified according to histology, age, location, and prevalence. Analysis of tumours on MRI should include the following:

◆ *Age*: metastases are rare in children. In adults, approximately half of central nervous system lesions are metastases. Older patients tend to have more aggressive tumours although they can occur at any age.

◆ *Location*: tumours may be intra-axial (arising from the brain parenchyma) or extra-axial (arising from the meninges, nerve sheaths, or skull), supra- or infratentorial. Gliomas are the largest group of primary intra-axial tumours and include astrocytoma, ependymoma, oligodendroglioma, and choroid plexus tumours. Primary extra-axial neoplasms are typified by meningiomas and schwannomas. Most infratentorial tumours in adults are metastases. Metastases are usually located at grey–white matter junctions.

◆ *Solitary versus multiple*: multiple lesions are much more likely to be metastatic. Primary tumours are typically solitary; however, multiple primary tumours can be seen in the form of gliomas or lymphoma. Fifty per cent of metastases are solitary. The commonest sites of origin outside the cranium include lung, breast, and melanoma.

◆ *Lesion characteristics*: most tumours will appear high signal on T2-weighted imaging and low signal on T1-weighted reflecting an increase in the water content (Figure 1.6.4.1). However, tumour signal can be variable. Tumours which are calcified, haemorrhagic, highly proteinaceous, or secondary to extracranial melanoma and mucinous tumours may exhibit low signal on T2-weighted and high signal on T1-weighted images.

◆ *Contrast enhancement*: extra-axial tumours such as meningioma do not possess a blood–brain barrier so will typically demonstrate prominent enhancement (Figure 1.6.4.2). Intra-axial tumours will show some degree of enhancement once the blood–brain barrier is broken down (Figure 1.6.4.1). Enhancing areas in mid- to high-grade tumours usually correspond to viable tumour, making this a useful aid in targeting biopsies. With low-grade infiltrative tumours, often the blood–brain barrier is intact and there is no enhancement. Metastases characteristically demonstrate ring or nodular enhancement whilst irregular

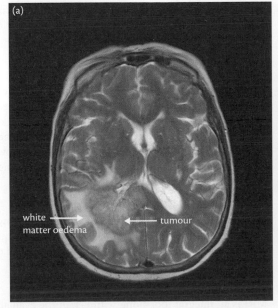
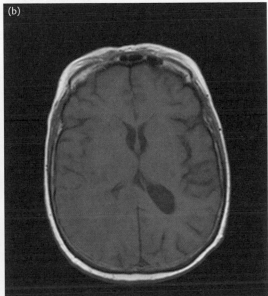

Fig. 1.6.4.1 Brain glioma, axial-, T2-, and T1-weighted post-gadolinium image.

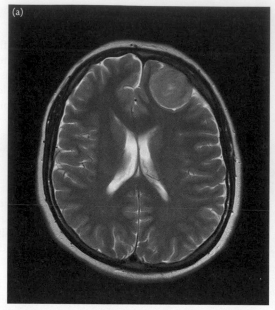
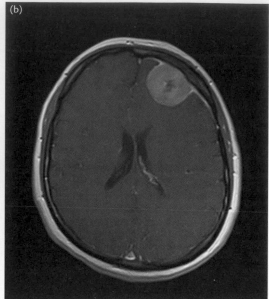

Fig. 1.6.4.2 Meningioma, axial-, T2-, and T1-weighted post-gadolinium image.

enhancement is more a feature of high-grade primary tumours such as glioblastoma multiforme.

◆ *Effect on surrounding structures*: MRI scans should be evaluated for the presence of mass effect, white matter oedema (high T2 and FLAIR signal with no enhancement), midline shift, hydrocephalus, sulcal and ventricular effacement. Metastases tend to have a disproportionately large degree of mass effect compared with larger primary tumours.

Whilst MRI is very good at predicting the nature and grade of tumours based on the above-listed features, ultimately definitive diagnosis can only be obtained by histological examination of material obtained by brain biopsy, open surgery, or metastases inferred from the clinical context.

A solitary lesion on brain CT requires MRI to characterize and determine lesion number in the brain in addition to a body CT to detect any potential primary malignancy elsewhere.

Infections

Herpes simplex encephalitis typically affects the temporal lobes with bilateral, asymmetrical high T2 signal oedema often complicated by limited haemorrhage.

Alongside CT, MRI allows accurate diagnosis of cerebritis and brain abscesses. Abscesses are typically thin walled with rim enhancement and associated extensive white matter oedema, some with restricted diffusion. They may be difficult to differentiate from cystic tumours but the clinical scenario should assist. Local spread from middle ear infections, sinusitis, and mastoiditis may be apparent and should be actively sought. Subdural and epidural empyema may complicate intracerebral, middle ear, or paranasal sinus infection (Figure 1.6.4.3). Venous sinus thrombosis associated with intracranial sepsis can be readily diagnosed using conventional MRI and MR venography.

Trauma

There is no major role for MRI in acute cranial trauma. GE sequences are very sensitive for detecting microscopic foci of blood

products in the non-acute setting to help diagnose and define the extent of diffuse axonal injury for prognostic purposes.

Vascular

MRI and MRA are excellent for diagnosing congenital vascular anomalies. Arteriovenous malformations, dural fistulae, venous malformations, and aneurysms are well characterized (Figure 1.6.4.4).

Intracranial aneurysms appear as signal voids, 'black' on a T2-weighted MRI scan of the brain. Partially thrombosed aneurysms may show variable signal. MRA will readily depict the location and size of aneurysms to aid interventional or surgical planning. Endovascular coils used for embolizing aneurysms are MRI compatible. The ability to assess the secondary brain parenchymal changes after haemorrhage and surgery such as ischaemia, gliosis, and hydrocephalus is self-evident. In practice, a combination of MRI/MRA, CT, and conventional angiography will be employed depending on the condition of the patient (Figure 1.6.4.5).

Head and neck

Congenital

MRI is ideal for evaluating the rare congenital solid and cystic lesions in the head and neck. Ultrasound scan is the initial investigation of choice but MRI will provide greater detail of the contents and surrounding structures. Cysts are easily identified as homogeneous T2-hyperintense structures which do not show any evidence of enhancement. These include branchial cleft and thyroglossal cysts and cystic hygromas.

Inflammatory

Patients with pharyngeal abscesses are usually unwell. Although MRI provides better tissue characterization, the far quicker CT with contrast is preferred to demonstrate any thin-walled rim enhancing fluid collections typical of abscesses.

Neoplasms

MRI is an integral tool along with CT in the evaluation and management of head and neck cancers, assisting in the delineation of

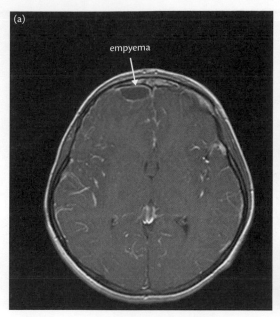
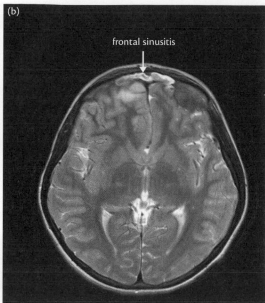

Fig. 1.6.4.3 Subdural empyema from sinusitis.

local disease involvement as well as nodal spread.[1] MRI is crucial for planning initial radiotherapy and surgery as well as the depiction of later disease recurrence. Although MRI is inferior at evaluating bony detail, it is superior for characterization of soft tissues such as muscles, fat, fascial planes, and neural structures. MRI is utilized as a powerful staging tool revealing clear contrast between tumoural and non-tumoural tissue. The relative inaccessibility of the skull base to clinical evaluation means that MRI has a unique role in this region.

MRI has the ability to localize lesions within the deep anatomical compartments subdivided by deep cervical fascia. Thus lesions can be localized to one of seven spaces: mucosal, retropharyngeal,

parapharyngeal, masticator, carotid, parotid, and prevertebral spaces. Differential diagnoses can be formulated based on location, contents of the space, and the MRI signal appearances. MRI is excellent for defining intracranial and intra-orbital extension. Parotid, nasopharyngeal, and sinonasal tumours are best imaged with MRI. Squamous cell carcinoma lymphadenopathy is typically necrotic.

Thorax

Mediastinum

Foregut duplication cysts usually demonstrate high T2 and low T1 signal, but this may be variable with proteinaceous or haemorrhagic fluid. Cysts typically do not enhance post contrast.

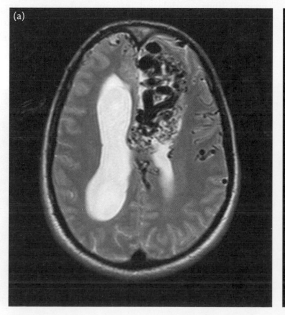
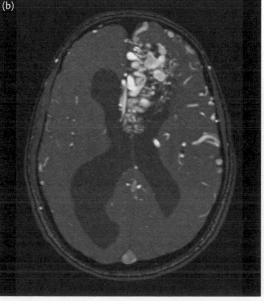

Fig. 1.6.4.4 Brain arteriovenous malformation.

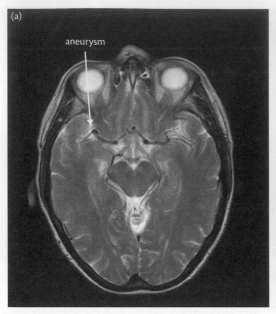
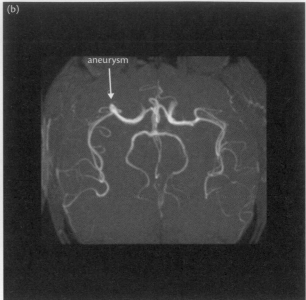

Fig. 1.6.4.5 Brain aneurysm, axial T2 and time-of-flight MRA.

Other more solid posterior mediastinal lesions include mesenchymal tumours, pleural fibromas, neurogenic tumours, sarcomas, and metastases. Neurogenic tumours may extend into the intervertebral foramina and spinal canal.

Cardiac

Pre-surgical cardiac MRI is used where other tests are insufficient, inconsistent, or equivocal, and is ideal for assessment of congenital cardiac conditions such as tetralogy of Fallot, coarctation of the aorta, atrial septal defect, vascular rings, and cardiac masses/tumours such as atrial myxoma. Sedation or general anaesthetic can be used in those children unable to cooperate without assistance.

Hepatobiliary

Benign

The commonest benign liver lesions are cysts, haemangiomas, and focal fatty change, encountered incidentally on ultrasound and CT. Where there is diagnostic doubt, MRI is usually confirmatory. Haemangiomas have typical appearances on ultrasound and CT but MRI is useful for atypical cases. They appearing as lobulated moderate to high T2 signal intensity lesions with discontinuous nodular peripheral enhancement with centripetal contrast in-filling on delayed images (Figure 1.6.4.6).

Chemical shift GE sequence is used to detect fat-containing lesions.[2] Signal loss is identified on out-of-phase images with focal fatty change whilst with fatty sparing, signal loss occurs in the rest of the liver.

Adenomas are usually asymptomatic with a strong link to oral contraceptives. They may contain fat, often difficult to see on pre-contrast MRI but readily visible in the arterial phase of a dynamic post-contrast study. They fade to a similar appearance to background liver on delayed imaging. Adenomas carry a significant risk of spontaneous haemorrhage and are therefore potentially surgically treated. Focal nodular hyperplasia (non-surgical lesion)

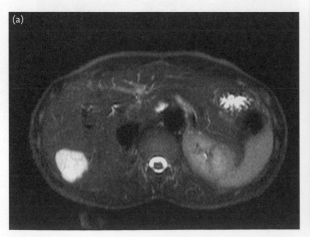
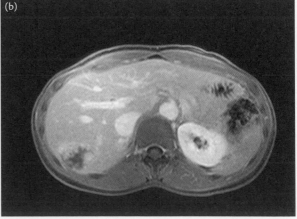

Fig. 1.6.4.6 Hepatic haemangioma.

may be equally hypervascular but may possess a central scar (Figure 1.6.4.7). Special liver-specific contrast agents can be used to differentiate adenomas from focal nodular hyperplasia.[3]

Malignant

Metastases are the commonest malignant liver lesion. Most are relatively hypovascular, appearing low signal on T1-weighted images, mildly high signal on T2, and typically with peripheral enhancement most conspicuous on portal phase images (Figure 1.6.4.8). Lesions can be easily localized within segments providing useful information for guiding surgery and radiofrequency ablation. Hypervascular metastases usually show prominent arterial phase enhancement and are typically due to renal carcinoma, carcinoid or islet cell pancreatic tumours.

Hepatocellular carcinoma (HCC) is the commonest primary malignant liver tumour[4] usually occurring in alcoholic or hepatitic cirrhosis. HCC usually appears low signal on T1, mildly high signal on T2, and hypervascular on post-contrast T1-weighted images with rapid wash-out on delayed images becoming darker than the surrounding liver. Lesions may be solitary or multifocal. Direct invasion of the portal or hepatic veins may result in enhancing tumour thrombus which has a similar appearance to the tumour. Fatty change may be observed in well-differentiated lesions. HCC does occur in patients without cirrhosis or apparent risk factors. This includes a variant in younger patients called fibrolamellar HCC (Figure 1.6.4.9).

Cholangiocarcinoma may appear as a dominant bile duct stricture with prominent duct wall thickening and enhancement.[5] Both intra- and extrahepatic mass lesions can be encountered, usually hypovascular poorly marginated with associated biliary tract dilatation. A Klatskin tumour (hilar cholangiocarcinoma) is a variant that occurs at the liver hilum. MRI is extremely useful for assessing operability and vascular involvement (Figure 1.6.4.10).

Liver transplant

MRI is invaluable for assessing patients being worked up for liver transplant, both recipients and donors in particular for identifying variant anatomy that may affect surgical approach. It is also a non-invasive method for evaluating patients post transplant detecting vascular, biliary, and liver parenchymal complications.

Magnetic resonance cholangiopancreatography

Heavily T2-weighted sequences brighten the bile ducts (and any fluid-containing structures) and calculi will be readily identified as

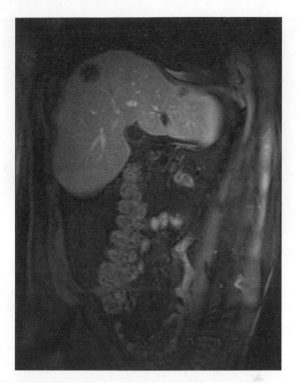

Fig. 1.6.4.8 Hepatic metastasis.

dependent filling defects (Figure 1.6.4.11). Flow artefacts, pneumobilia, and stents may simulate and or hide calculi. Magnetic resonance cholangiopancreatography is highly accurate in determining the cause and level of biliary tract obstruction. This allows selection of patients who need endoscopic retrograde cholangiopancreatography and biliary intervention. Malignant strictures are typically shouldered and abrupt.

Pancreas

Pancreatitis

MRI plays a supporting role in imaging patients with pancreatitis. In young patients who may be at risk of receiving repeated CT scanning and therefore high radiation burden it is a reliable method of detecting complications such as pseudocyst formation.

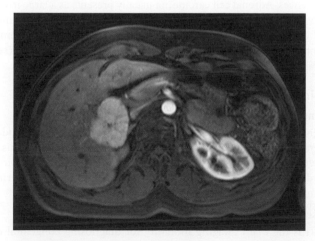

Fig. 1.6.4.7 Focal nodular hyperplasia.

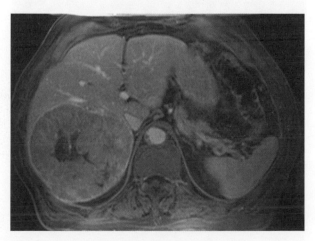

Fig. 1.6.4.9 Hepatocellular carcinoma (fibrolamellar type).

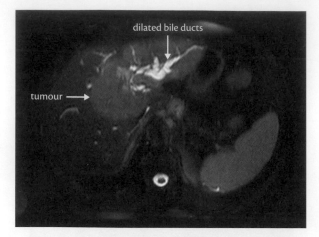

Fig. 1.6.4.10 Cholangiocarcinoma—Klatskin type.

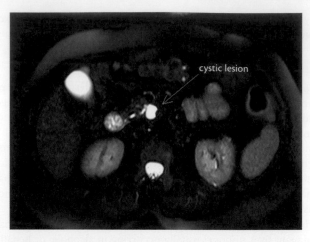

Fig. 1.6.4.12 Pancreatic cystic lesion.

The pancreatic duct appears irregular and dilated in chronic pancreatitis, together with dilated side branches.

Neoplasms

Triple-phase CT is the investigation of choice for suspected pancreatic tumours, particularly ductal adenocarcinomas and evaluating for potential resectability. However, MRI alongside endoscopic ultrasound has a major role to play in preoperative lesion characterization.[6] MRI has the ability to differentiate solid from cystic lesions and assess vascular involvement and nodal disease. Secondary effects such as biliary and pancreatic duct obstruction will be well visualized. Areas of fatty change which may be difficult to interpret on CT are easily recognized with MRI. Cystic lesions seen in the pancreas may represent post-pancreatitis pseudocysts or cystic neoplasms. Epithelial pancreatic cysts are rare. Cystic neoplasms may have a low risk of malignancy (e.g. serous microcystic adenomas) and solid pseudopapillary neoplasm or a higher malignancy risk (e.g. mucinous and intraductal papillary mucinous cystic neoplasms) (Figure 1.6.4.12).

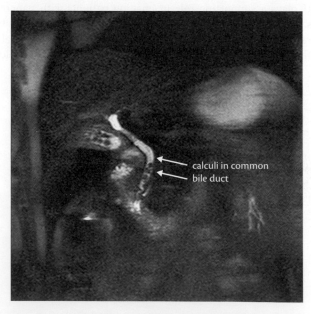

Fig. 1.6.4.11 Magnetic resonance cholangiopancreatogram of ductal calculus.

Islet cell tumours are typically hypervascular and may be cystic.

Kidneys

Focal lesions

Indeterminate lesions on CT or ultrasound are ideal for dynamic contrast-enhanced MRI. Angiomyolipomas and haemorrhagic or proteinaceous cysts may be confirmed. Lesions which do not fall readily into any of these categories should be considered suspicious for renal cell carcinoma.

Magnetic resonance urography

This is a useful technique using heavily T2-weighted sequences to highlight urine as bright and therefore providing contrast with ureteric calculi which will appear as filling defects. This may be performed in pregnant patients.

Magnetic resonance angiography

Renal MRA can identify hypertensive patients with stenosis which may be amenable to endovascular treatment. MRI is also used for assessing vascular anatomy and ureters in patients being evaluated for renal transplant.

Adrenals

Adenomas can be diagnosed on MRI by detecting the presence of fat with suppression on out-of-phase, phase contrast, and STIR sequences. Adrenal cell carcinoma usually presents as a large irregular mass with heterogeneous enhancement. Phaeochromocytomas are bright on T2-weighted images (light bulb sign) with prominent enhancement; 10% are bilateral, 10% extra-adrenal (see Chapter 1.6.2), and 10% malignant.

Spine

Congenital

Spinal anomalies are well characterized with MRI. This includes segmentation anomalies and spinal dysraphism/spina bifida. This is useful for diagnosing associated anomalies such as low lying spinal cord, meningoceles, meningomyeloceles, diastematomyelia, syringomyelia, and Arnold–Chiari malformation.

Disc disease

MRI is the main imaging modality for diagnosing congenital or acquired spinal canal stenosis, disc protrusions, and post-surgical

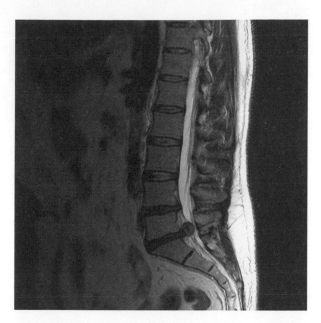

Fig. 1.6.4.13 L5/S1 disc prolapse.

complications such as haematoma, infection, disc recurrence, and post-surgical fibrosis. Abnormalities in disc morphology are reliably characterized with MRI. A disc protrusion has an intact annulus fibrosus, a disc extrusion occurs beyond the annulus, whilst a sequestration results when the disc fragment loses contact with the parent disc. Cervical disc protrusions often at C5/6 and C6/7 may be accompanied by osteophytes to form disc–osteophyte complexes. Lumbar disc protrusions most often at L4/5 and L5/S1 may combine with hypertrophied degenerate facet joints and a hypertrophied ligamentum flavum to cause central canal, lateral recess, and exit foraminal stenosis with compression of the thecal sac, spinal cord, and nerve roots (Figure 1.6.4.13).

Spondylolisthesis occurs when there is slip of one vertebra over another. The commonest causes are congenital or acquired pars defects (spondylolysis) and facet joint degenerative change. Exit foramina and lateral recesses may be severely stenosed, resulting in compression of nerve roots.

Infection

MRI is the most sensitive and specific modality for evaluating spinal infections which may involve the disc (discitis), the vertebral body (spondylitis), or, typically as in pyogenic infections, a combination of the two (spondylodiscitis). MRI findings include high T2 disc signal, loss of disc height with associated subchondral endplate bone marrow oedema (low T1, high STIR), and bony, disc, or paravertebral/epidural soft tissue contrast enhancement on T1-weighted images. Paraspinal abscesses and epidural empyema may complicate spondylodiscitis, appearing as rim-enhancing low T1-weighted fluid collections. An epidural empyema can occur without discitis. Septic arthritis of the facet joints is also readily diagnosed. Contrast is essential for investigation of suspected spinal infection (Figure 1.6.4.14).

Trauma

The challenges posed by the logistics of transferring the sick, major trauma, possibly ventilated patient in and out of the MRI suite mean that it is best used in a targeted manner typically in specialist neuro centres. It is the best method for diagnosing soft tissue injuries, ligamentous disruption, traumatic disc herniations, spinal cord injury, and epidural haematomas. In patients with partial neurological deficits, MRI is crucial for detecting surgical lesions and predicting outcomes. STIR sequence is essential in trauma patients, useful for identifying ligamentous injury and bone marrow oedema.

Neoplastic

Extradural tumours usually arise from the vertebra, typically metastases, myeloma, or lymphoma.

Intradural extramedullary tumours include metastases, meningioma, and nerve sheath tumours.

Intramedullary lesions include ependymoma, astrocytoma, metastases, and haemangioblastoma.

MRI is the prime investigation for suspected spinal cord and cauda equina compression syndromes, excellent for detecting the level and cause of the neurological compromise.

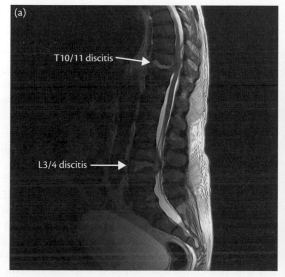

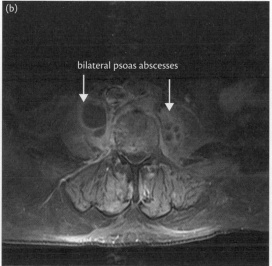

Fig. 1.6.4.14 Discitis.

Gastrointestinal

Inflammatory bowel disease

MRI is now the imaging modality of choice for assessing young patients with inflammatory bowel disease, having the ability to differentiate quiescent from active disease and depict sites of strictures and obstruction without subjecting the patient to ionizing radiation (Figure 1.6.4.15). Active Crohn's disease demonstrates high T2 signal in the wall with prominent contrast enhancement on T1-weighted images.

Fistulae complicating Crohn's disease, particularly in the pelvis, can be classified according to sphincter involvement aiding treatment planning. MRI assists surgical planning in patients with perianal sepsis, being able to reliably demonstrate the course of fistulae and sinuses and the location of abscesses with respect to the sphincters and levator ani.

Rectal cancer staging

Local staging of rectal cancers with MRI is performed by obtaining high-resolution, triplanar T2-weighted images through the tumour. The rectal wall and perirectal anatomy is well depicted. The mesorectal fascia corresponds to the circumferential resection margin in patients undergoing total mesorectal excision. The following need to be accurately determined: site (anorectal, low, mid, or upper rectum), distance from anal verge, length, tumour morphology (annular or polypoidal), axial spread and status of the resection margin, and involvement of adjacent structures including vessels and local nodes. MRI thus helps in deriving a tumour/node/metastasis status that enables appropriate decisions to be made about treatment options and minimizing of local tumour recurrence[7] (Figure 1.6.4.16).

Gynaecology and surgical disorders in pregnancy

General aspects

The excellent contrast resolution of MRI makes it ideal for evaluating pelvic structures where the relatively small amount of fat makes

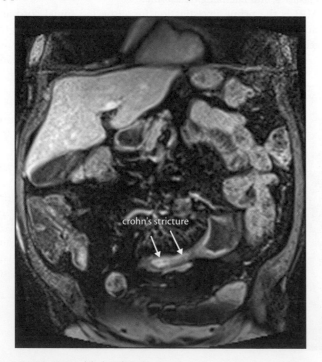

Fig. 1.6.4.15 Terminal ileal Crohn's disease.

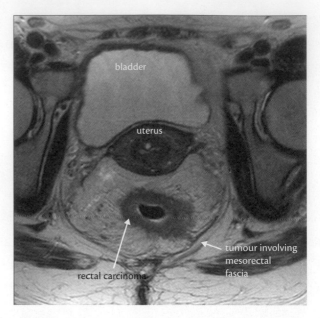

Fig. 1.6.4.16 Rectal cancer.

CT less suited. Whilst transvaginal ultrasound is the easily accessible gold standard modality for investigating pelvic masses, MRI is particularly useful in assessing the young woman with a nonspecific pelvic mass seen on ultrasound.[8]

Uterine fibroids are the commonest uterine mass, usually low signal on T2-weighted images. Specific diagnoses of adenomyosis, endometriosis, functional ovarian cysts, haemorrhagic cysts, dermoids (Figure 1.6.4.17), and ovarian torsion can be readily established.

Where there is doubt on ultrasound, MRI can demonstrate complex features such as septations and mural nodules, and help surgical planning by evaluating surrounding structures.

MRI can assess the depth of invasion and parametrial spread of endometrial and cervical cancers.

Pelvic tubo-ovarian abscesses, hydrosalpinx, adhesions, and other sequelae of pelvic inflammatory disease can be shown in great detail on MRI. Contrast is mandatory for suspected inflammatory disease.

Surgical diagnosis in pregnancy

Where clinical examination and ultrasound are equivocal, MRI has a role to play in investigating pregnant patients with the potential to diagnose conditions such as appendicitis, ureteric calculi, complicated herniae, and complications of pregnancy such as placental accreta.

Musculoskeletal

MRI is extensively utilized in musculoskeletal imaging. The STIR sequence is especially sensitive in detecting bone marrow oedema and therefore diagnosing conditions such as occult fractures, osteonecrosis, transient osteoporosis, and osteoid osteoma.

In patients who have suspected hip fractures and equivocal plain radiographs, MRI is very sensitive in detecting occult femoral neck or scaphoid fractures or stress fractures (Figure 1.6.4.18). Avascular necrosis is detected much sooner than would be possible with plain films and with greater specificity than isotope bone scanning.

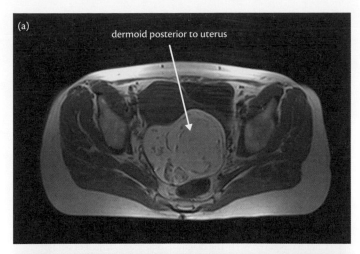

(a) dermoid posterior to uterus

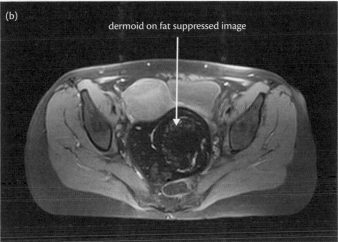

(b) dermoid on fat suppressed image

Fig. 1.6.4.17 Ovarian dermoid.

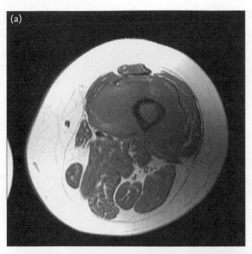

(a)

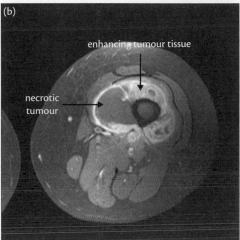

(b) enhancing tumour tissue

necrotic tumour

Fig. 1.6.4.19 Sarcoma.

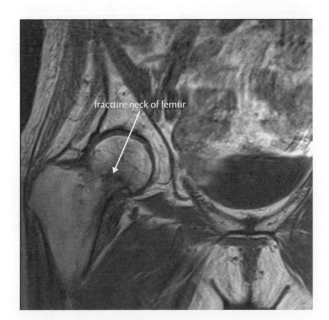

fracture neck of femur

Fig. 1.6.4.18 Hip fracture.

Benign and malignant bone and soft tissue tumours are shown with excellent detail, aiding surgical planning by delineating compartmental and regional nodal spread.[9] MRI may specifically diagnose lipoma, haemangioma, schwannoma, fibromatosis, or sarcoma (Figure 1.6.4.19).

Osteomyelitis and septic arthritis are readily evaluated with MRI, particularly when STIR and fat-suppressed post-contrast T1-weighted images are used. Inflammatory arthropathies are equally easily diagnosed with changes appearing prior to the development of any abnormalities on plain radiographs.

In the shoulder, MRI is used for diagnosing rotator cuff tears, impingement, and bursitis, and with MRI arthrography, labral and bicipitolabral complex tears can be diagnosed. MRI is extensively utilized in knee joint imaging to detect ligamentous injury in addition to meniscal tears (Figure 1.6.4.20) and extensor mechanism abnormalities. Loose bodies in the joint are readily identified as are joint effusions, popliteal (Baker's) cysts, and ganglia.

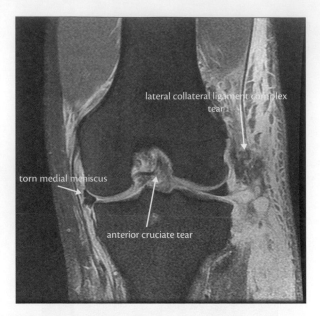

Fig. 1.6.4.20 Anterior cruciate and meniscal tears.

MRI is ideal for investigating children with unexplained hip pain (e.g. preslip/early slip of capital femoral epiphyses), where clinical examination, ultrasound, and plain radiographs are non-diagnostic.

Non-malignant synovial swellings such as pigmented villonodular synovitis and synovial osteochondromatosis have typical appearances on MRI scan.

Further reading

Castillo, M. *Neuroradiology Companion: Methods, Guidelines, and Imaging Fundamentals* (4th ed). Philadelphia, PA: Lippincott Williams and Wilkins; 2011.

Helms CA, Major NM, Anderson MW, *et al. Musculoskeletal MRI* (2nd ed). Philadelphia, PA: WB Saunders; 2008.

Semelka, RC (ed). *Abdominopelvic MRI* (3rd ed). Hoboken, NJ: Wiley-Blackwell; 2010.

References

1. Alberico RA, Husain SH, Sirotkin I. Imaging in head and neck oncology. *Surg Oncol Clin N Am* 2004; 13(1):13–35.
2. Basaran C, Karcaaltincaba M, Akata D, *et al.* Fat-containing lesions in the liver: cross-sectional Imaging findings with emphasis on MRI. *AJR Am J Roentgenol* 2005; 184:1103–10.
3. Choi BY, Nguyen MH. The diagnosis and management of benign hepatic tumours. *J Clin Gastroenterol* 2005; 39(5):401–12.
4. Bolog N, Andreisek G, Oancea I, *et al.* CT and MR imaging of hepatocellular carcinoma. *J Gastrointestin Liver Dis* 2011; 20(2):181–9.
5. Lim JH. Cholangiocarcinoma: morphologic classification according to growth pattern and imaging findings. *AJR Am J Roentgenol* 2003; 181:819–27.
6. Jani N, Bani Hani M, Schulick RD, *et al.* Diagnosis and management of cystic lesions of the pancreas. *Diagn Ther Endosc* 2011; 2011:478913.
7. Klessen C, Rogalla P, Taupitz M. Local staging of rectal cancer: the current role of MRI. *Eur Radiol* 2007; 17(2):379–89.
8. Hubert J, Bergin D. Imaging of the female pelvis. When should MRI be considered? *Appiled Radiol* 2008; 37(1):9–24.
9. Helms CA. *Fundamentals of Skeletal Radiology* (2nd ed). Philadelphia, PA: WB Saunders; 1996.

Principles of computed tomography: advantages and disadvantages

Pallavi Mehrotra

Introduction

The importance of computed tomography (CT) has significantly increased with a rapidly rising clinical demand together with the increased accessibility, speed, and improved image quality, alongside more versatile presentation formats. Modern detectors provide a massive three-dimensional (3D) volume data set acquired in a single breath hold. Standard triplanar reconstructions are sent to a picture archiving and communication system while other important reconstructions such as CT angiography or virtual endoscopy can be manipulated at specialist workstations. The CT image is composed of tiny 3D cubes of data (voxels) represented as two-dimensional (2D) pixels, each having a relative density measured in Hounsfield units (HU). Water is the reference level at zero HU giving values in the range for soft tissues at 70 HU, bone 1000 HU, fat −100 HU, and air −1000 HU. Consequently bone appears white, soft tissue grey, fat very dark grey, and gas jet black on CT images.

Important artefacts which can degrade the image quality include movement and streak artefact, the latter due to dental amalgam, metallic implants, adjacent high concentration of contrast medium, or even the patient's own arms that cannot be elevated.

CT uses ionizing radiation which can cause DNA damage and with repeated use can increase the risk of a radiation-induced malignancy. The most commonly induced malignancies include lung, breast, thyroid, and stomach cancer and leukaemia as these tissues are the most sensitive to radiation exposure.[1] Background radiation in the United Kingdom is approximately 2.7 mSv and the effective dose of a chest X-ray is 0.02 mSv, a head CT 1–2 mSv, and an abdomen and pelvis CT 8–11 mSv.[1] The legally enforceable 'as low as reasonably achievable' (ALARA) principle should be constantly at the forefront of the referring clinician's and radiologist's thoughts during the justification process.

Rapid cellular division in the fetus and in children make them more sensitive to the effects of radiation and at a greater risk of induced cancer than adults, and CT should only be used with extreme caution in pregnant women and in children.

To enhance visualization of different structures and to appreciate tissue vascularity, intravenous (IV) contrast agents are often administered during CT. Non-ionic, low, or iso-osmolar IV agents are preferred for their better safety profile although life-threatening reactions including anaphylaxis can very rarely occur. Patients who are at increased risk of reactions include those with asthma and previous contrast reactions (e.g. bronchospasm and urticaria). Contrast agents are also nephrotoxic and the risk of nephrotoxicity is related to the degree of pre-existing renal impairment, the patient's state of hydration, and presence of diabetes. The risks and benefits of contrast administration should be carefully weighed up for patients in renal failure. Alternative imaging techniques or a non-contrast CT should also be considered. If contrast is to be administered, then the risks should be reduced as far as possible, for example, by ensuring the patient is as well hydrated as possible.[2]

Abdominal imaging

The acute abdomen

Many acute abdominal events can be diagnosed on CT. Free intra-abdominal air can confidently be identified (Figure 1.6.5.1) and the site of hollow viscus perforation can frequently be established which can guide any subsequent surgery. However, for some conditions such as acute cholecystitis or ovarian pathology, an ultrasound scan (USS) often has greater diagnostic accuracy than CT.

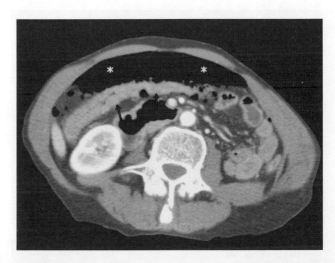

Fig. 1.6.5.1 Axial CT demonstrating intra-abdominal free air (asterisks) anterior to the transverse colon (arrows). Colonic perforation had occurred during colonoscopy.

Acute appendicitis

Whilst USS is an excellent imaging modality, particularly in young, thin patients with right iliac fossa pain, CT can be helpful in older patients with atypical clinical findings. The normal appendix is often identified on CT which is a useful factor in excluding acute appendicitis.

In the early stages, the appendix distends with fluid and later circumferential thickening, wall enhancement, periappendiceal soft tissue stranding, and local lymphadenopathy become evident. The presence of an appendicolith in the presence of an abnormal appendix supports this diagnosis (Figure 1.6.5.2). Secondary inflammation around the caecum and terminal ileum may also develop. Complications of acute appendicitis are well demonstrated on CT, particularly phlegmon or abscess formation, small bowel obstruction (SBO), and appendiceal perforation.

Acute cholecystitis

Gallbladder wall thickening, pericholecystic inflammation, and a target appearance of the gallbladder with an enhancing mucosa and serosa are features of acute cholecystitis on CT. USS is a more accurate technique for diagnosing acute cholecystitis particularly as gallstones and mild gallbladder wall thickening are more readily identified on USS. However, CT has a role particularly with atypical clinical findings.

In gangrenous cholecystitis, the gallbladder may have intraluminal membranes and haemorrhage and its wall appears irregular or disrupted and may enhance poorly. These features are strong indicators of gangrenous cholecystitis but are often not seen on CT in confirmed surgical cases.

Emphysematous cholecystitis is a life-threatening complication of acute cholecystitis, more common in diabetic patients. On CT, gas is seen in the wall of the gallbladder or in the non-dependent part of the gallbladder lumen. Gas may extend out into the pericholecystic soft tissues and abscesses may form in or around the adjacent liver. Diagnostic features may be seen on USS; however, if the gallbladder is poorly seen or findings are equivocal with a strong clinical suspicion, CT is indicated.

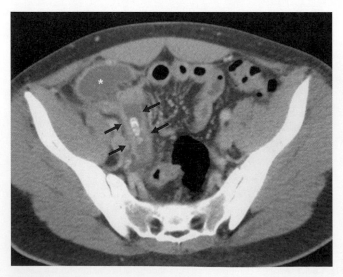

Fig. 1.6.5.2 Axial CT of a patient with appendicitis. The appendix is thick walled and contains appendicoliths (arrows). The caecum is identified by the asterisk.

Pancreatitis

CT is particularly useful in evaluating both acute and chronic pancreatitis. A pre-contrast pancreas CT can provide additional information on the underlying cause of pancreatitis such as pancreatic calcification indicating chronic inflammation or common bile duct calculi. The radiation dose may be an important factor particularly in young patients with severe pancreatitis who may require repeat CTs.

In acute pancreatitis, the gland becomes enlarged and oedematous with a poorly defined contour and adjacent inflammation. Fluid extravasation from the pancreas leads to peripancreatic and intra-abdominal collections with free fluid. When pancreatitis sometimes only involves part of the pancreas, most commonly the head, differentiating pancreatitis from malignancy can be difficult. Patients may require further investigations such as endoscopic USS or a follow-up CT.

In necrotizing pancreatitis, the parenchyma has patchy areas of poor enhancement which correlate well with the presence of pancreatic necrosis at surgery. Furthermore, the presence of air bubbles and debris within a necrotic pancreas suggests superimposed infection. Other complications of pancreatitis such as pseudocysts, abscess, and pseudoaneurysms which can lead to retroperitoneal haemorrhage may be detected on CT. Common sites for pseudoaneurysm formation are the pancreaticoduodenal and the perisplenic regions.

Acute diverticulitis

On CT, colonic wall thickening and pericolic stranding in the presence of diverticula with the appropriate clinical findings suggest acute diverticulitis. Pericolic abscesses can initially develop within the mesocolon and can be walled off by the small bowel and adjacent structures. As the inflammation progresses, abscesses may extend to other parts of the peritoneal cavity.

Differentiating certain cases of diverticulitis from colonic carcinoma can be difficult on CT. In colonic carcinoma, features such as asymmetrical, abrupt margins at the site of colonic thickening and pericolic lymph nodes are seen.

Coloenteric fistulae are a complication of diverticulitis and are difficult to diagnose on CT; however, colovesical fistulae are often well demonstrated. A thickened segment of sigmoid colon with an adjacent thickened bladder wall and air in the bladder indicate this diagnosis. Often a fluid and air filled track between the two structures is present.

Small bowel obstruction

The cause and level of SBO and resultant complications such as bowel ischaemia or perforation may be seen on CT. Demonstrating a transition point between dilated and non-dilated small bowel is the hallmark of obstruction but can be difficult, particularly in the distal small bowel, and here it may be difficult to differentiate SBO from ileus. In addition, the site of obstruction on CT (e.g. left lower quadrant) does not always correlate with the exact surgical findings as the bowel may be quite mobile. Pneumatosis and poor bowel-wall enhancement suggest ischaemia but not necessarily infarction, unlike gas in the portal venous system.

In the Western world, adhesions are the most common cause of SBO and appear as an abrupt transition between dilated and non-dilated small bowel, sometimes with a beak-like morphology with no other obvious abnormality at the transition site. Other pathology may have similar imaging features such as short strictures due to ischaemia or inflammation, small peritoneal metastases, or carcinoid tumours. However, with adhesions there is usually a previous history of abdominal surgery. If SBO occurs due to a hernia, there is dilated bowel proximal and collapsed bowel distal to the hernia with thick-walled bowel within the hernia sac (Figure 1.6.5.3). Peritoneal carcinomatosis particularly from colon, gastric, and ovarian malignancies can cause multifocal SBO due to a widespread desmoplastic response and peritoneal masses. Imaging features include ascites, peritoneal, mesenteric, and omental masses, and tethered small bowel folds.

Crohn's disease

In the active phase of Crohn's disease, the affected bowel has enhancing inner mucosal and outer serosal layers with a low-attenuation thickened submucosal layer (Figure 1.6.5.4). Increased mesenteric vascularity and enhancing mesenteric lymph nodes also suggest active inflammation. In the later fibrostenotic phase, fixed strictures with thickened bowel wall and dilatation of the bowel immediately proximal to the stricture develop. The small bowel is particularly affected in this phase although large bowel strictures also occur. Other complications of Crohn's disease such as fistulation into adjacent bowel vagina, bladder, and perianal/perineal regions may also be identified on CT.

Cancer staging

Colorectal cancer

Incidental colorectal cancers on a normal CT appear as focal areas of bowel wall thickening or focal masses (Figure 1.6.5.5). However, this finding is non-specific as collapsed bowel can sometimes have a similar appearance therefore subsequent endoscopic correlation is usually required. Staging CT for confirmed colorectal cancer includes

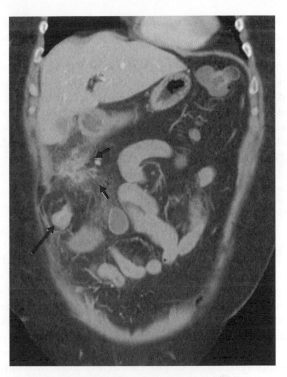

Fig. 1.6.5.4 Coronal CT showing an inflammatory Crohn's mass (short arrows) in the right upper quadrant. Tracts extend between small bowel and the distal stomach. The neo-distal ileum (previous right hemicolectomy) is inflamed (long arrow).

the whole torso to identify lung, liver, bone, and nodal metastases. Tumour extension to adjacent organs and bowel perforation which signify T4 stage can be evaluated on CT. Magnetic resonance imaging (MRI) is also required for local staging of rectal tumours.

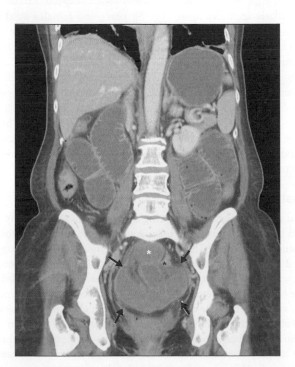

Fig. 1.6.5.3 Coronal CT of a patient with small bowel obstruction due to an internal hernia (arrows) with dilated bowel proximal (white asterisk) and collapsed bowel distal (black asterisk) to hernia sac.

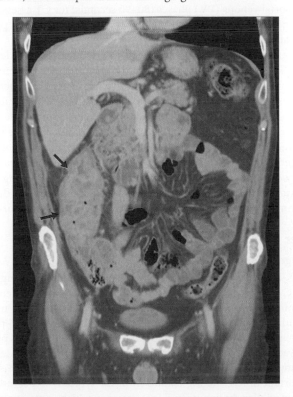

Fig. 1.6.5.5 Coronal CT demonstrating a thick-walled and irregular ascending colon in a patient with colonic malignancy (arrows).

Computed tomography colonography (CTC) is an excellent technique for identifying colorectal polyps and cancers and is more sensitive than barium enema at identifying colorectal cancer and large polyps (> 1 cm).[3] CTC is particularly useful in patients who are unsuitable for conventional colonoscopy as it is usually well tolerated. In this technique, the large bowel is insufflated with carbon dioxide via a rectal catheter. Patients are usually scanned in both prone and supine positions to allow optimal distension of different colonic segments and to allow movement of colonic fluid. Both the 2D and 3D endoluminal views (virtual colonoscopy) are interpreted. Liquid colonic residue can be 'tagged' by prior oral intake of a contrast agent.

Oesophagogastric cancer

Neck, chest, abdomen, and pelvis CT is performed in thin sections to stage oesophagogastric cancers. Patients drink water prior to the CT to ensure distension of the oesophagus and stomach, and spasm is reduced by IV hyoscine butylbromide (Buscopan®) (gastric protocol CT). With a well-distended oesophagus and stomach, the local T stage of the tumour can be determined. Invasion of oesophageal and gastric tumours into adjacent structures such as the pericardium, aorta, diaphragmatic crura, and colon can be identified (T4 disease). Suspected aortic and crural invasion and perioesophageal nodes can be further evaluated by endoscopic USS. Ascites and peritoneal and omental nodularity suggest peritoneal carcinomatosis. Abnormal neck nodes are often further evaluated with neck USS and fine-needle aspiration. All of these factors are important in fully staging these tumours and in guiding the patient's treatment options.

Pancreatic cancer

Two post-contrast phases need acquisition, arterial (40–50 seconds) and portal venous (PV) phases (80–90 seconds) for CT assessment of pancreatic tumours. Many centres include a pre-contrast phase. Ductal adenocarcinoma is the commonest pancreatic tumour, most frequently arising from the pancreatic head, often of lower density than the adjacent normal pancreas with an irregular contour. An ancillary finding of a dilated pancreatic duct distal to a pancreatic mass is a helpful CT feature. Tumours in the pancreatic head can cause dilatation of both the pancreatic duct and common bile duct, termed 'double duct dilatation'. Tumour involvement of the superior mesenteric vein and artery, portal vein and splenic artery are important features to identify on CT as they suggest inoperability. Endoscopic USS can be particularly helpful in locally staging pancreatic tumours by evaluating vessel invasion and also in distinguishing between chronic pancreatitis and pancreatic tumours.

Liver

Benign lesions

Cysts and haemangiomas are common incidental findings on CT. Cysts have a water density with no contrast enhancement. Haemangiomas appear as a hepatic mass with peripheral nodular enhancement on arterial phase which fills in on the PV phase although larger lesions do not always completely fill in by this phase. If an additional delayed CT scan is performed in approximately 4–5 minutes, enhancement in a haemangioma is seen to persist, an important differentiating feature from the typically hypervascular hepatocellular carcinoma and metastases in which contrast quickly washes out.

Hepatocellular carcinoma

Multiphasic CT, MRI, and contrast USS are all used to characterize liver lesions. On unenhanced CT, hepatocellular carcinoma (HCC) often exhibits central tumour necrosis. On the arterial phase, avid enhancement is noted due to dominant supply from the hepatic artery. In later phases, HCC often washes out and exhibits capsular enhancement. HCC has a propensity to invade the portal and hepatic venous systems. An expanded vein which contains enhancing thrombus is more suggestive of tumour rather than bland thrombus. The hepatic artery origin can also be assessed on CT which is important in patients who are potential surgical candidates.

Hepatic metastases

Most metastases to the liver are hypovascular including those from colon, gastric, and lung primaries. They appear hypodense relative to the background liver on the PV phase CT. Hypervascular metastases are less common and include those from carcinoid, melanoma, and breast primaries. These may only be identified on the arterial phase later becoming isodense to the background liver on the PV phase. Some metastases including those from mucinous colon carcinomas can be calcified on CT. Liver metastases can also be cystic, particularly mucinous primary tumours such as colorectal and ovarian tumours and sometimes differentiating these lesions from simple cysts can be difficult on CT. In addition, rim enhancement around some liver metastases may make it difficult to differentiate these lesions from hepatic abscesses.

Uroradiology

Stones

Low dose, non-contrast CT-kidney, ureter, and bladder (KUB) is the investigation of choice in patients with suspected renal colic particularly in males aged over 55 years and females aged over 50 years old with no stone-forming history. In some centres, CT-KUB is performed with the patient prone which is helpful in differentiating vesicoureteric from bladder calculi. It is an accurate technique and useful in identifying important alternative diagnoses such as ruptured aortic aneurysm, pancreatitis, and ovarian pathology. Ureteric calculi as small as 1–2 mm can be detected on CT and secondary effects of ureteric obstruction including hydroureter, hydronephrosis, and perinephric stranding are well demonstrated. Perinephric stranding may remain for several days after an obstructing calculus has passed.

Renal cysts

Renal cysts are a common finding on CT. These were initially classified by their CT characteristics into four groups by the Bosniak classification system.[4] The 2F subcategory was added later. Category 1 and 2 cysts are benign and do not require further follow-up. Category 2F cysts have more complex features but are still thought to be benign and so may be followed up radiologically. Category 3 cysts are indeterminate cystic masses with thickened irregular walls or septae in which enhancement may be seen. They turn out to be malignant in over 50% of cases and hence require urological referral. Category 4 cysts are cystic malignancies with solid enhancing components. Ultrasound can be helpful for assessing some renal cysts particularly if a cyst is hyperdense on CT and suspected to be a benign haemorrhagic cyst.

Urological tumours

Renal masses

Angiomyolipomas are fat-containing vascular tumours that are a common benign finding. Patients with sub-centimetre lesions are usually discharged. On CT, renal cell carcinomas (RCCs) are usually solid masses with heterogeneous enhancement (Figure 1.6.5.6). Lesions may calcify and necrose with a pseudocapsule. RCCs have a propensity to grow along the renal vein and IVC. In this situation, the renal vein becomes expanded and is filled with heterogeneous enhancing tumour. RCC lung metastases are usually well-defined, round 'cannonball' lesions and bony lesions typically large, lytic, and vascular and respond well to spinal embolization if causing neural compromise.

Prostate cancer

Although MRI is routinely used for local staging of prostate cancer, CT has a role in evaluating nodal and distant metastases in patients with advanced prostate disease where skeletal metastases are common, appearing sclerotic. Liver and lung metastases from prostate cancer rarely occur.

Carcinoma of the urinary tract

Triple-phase CT-intravenous urogram (IVU) is becoming the gold standard for investigation of macro- and microscopic haematuria. This typically includes a non-contrast CT-KUB followed by 100-second nephrographic and 8–10-minute urographic phases. CT-IVU is mainly utilized to rule out and evaluate renal and ureteric lesions and to stage bladder cancer. Bladder cancers appear as areas of thickening or protrusions of the bladder wall which enhances to a similar level to the bladder wall. This feature should be interpreted with caution as an underdistended bladder can falsely give the same appearance.

Renal injury

CT is the radiological investigation of choice in assessing stable patients suspected to have renal injury. Indications include frank haematuria and microscopic haematuria following a significant blunt injury. Many renal injuries are not detected on USS. The CT scan technique may include an arterial phase CT to identify active bleeding and a 5–10-minute delayed post-contrast CT to assess collecting system and ureteric integrity.

In minor renal injury, renal contusions (grade 1), superficial lacerations (grade 2), segmental renal infarcts, or subcapsular renal haematomas may be seen. In more severe injuries, deep renal lacerations (grade 3) which may extend into the collecting system (grade 4) can occur. As a result, urine (i.e. contrast) extravasation into the retroperitoneum is seen on CT. In the most severe renal injuries, features such as shattered kidney (grade 5) and renal pedicle disruption (grade 5) may occur with resultant catastrophic haemorrhage. Nowadays, the majority of renal injuries are managed conservatively with the help of CT angiography and embolization of active bleeding vessels.

Adrenal lesions

Adrenal adenomas are common incidental findings on CT and are usually small (<2 cm), low-attenuation lesions which rarely calcify. If an adrenal lesion has been detected incidentally on a post-contrast CT, a subsequent non-contrast adrenal CT may be helpful as adenomas are low attenuation on these scans. MRI also has a role in identifying intralesional fat which is present in adenomas.

Phaeochromocytomas are usually round, avidly enhancing masses with central necrosis. Multiple lesions may be present and extra-adrenal lesions may be seen in the paravertebral region or aortic bifurcation. The adrenal gland is also a common site of metastasis particularly from lung, breast, and renal cancer and melanoma.

Vascular imaging

Aortic dissection

CT has a role in diagnosing acute aortic dissection in stable patients. Thoracic aortic dissections are classified by the Stanford classification into types A and B. Type A are the most common type and involve the ascending aorta and are associated with serious complications such as pericardial tamponade and dissection of the coronary or brachiocephalic arteries. Type B dissections originate distal to the left subclavian artery origin and usually have a more indolent course.

An initial non-contrast CT is helpful as acute mural haematoma can be identified. Following contrast administration, contrast may flow through the dissection flap into the false lumen. If there is no communication between the true and false lumens it can be difficult to differentiate dissection from atheroma. The location of intimal calcification can help in distinguishing these entities.

Abdominal aortic aneurysm rupture

Abdominal aortic aneurysm (AAA) rupture is seen on CT as a retroperitoneal haematoma, periaortic stranding, and extravasation of IV contrast. An initial non-contrast CT is helpful in impending AAA rupture to demonstrate hyperdense haematoma within the aneurysm wall and focal disruption of intimal calcification.

The ischaemic limb

CT peripheral angiography is an excellent non-invasive technique to demonstrate the peripheral arteries. Post-processing with digital removal of adjacent bone and arterial wall calcification can greatly

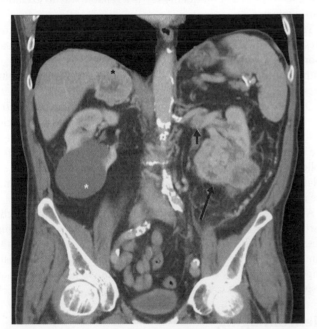

Fig. 1.6.5.6 Coronal CT showing a large RCC arising from the lower pole of the left kidney (long arrow) with tumour thrombus in the left renal vein (short arrow). A right adrenal metastasis (black asterisk) and a simple right renal cyst (white asterisk) are also present.

help vascular visualization. This technique is particularly of value in patients with intermittent ischaemia but is also used in patients with acute ischaemia and to ensure vessel patency following a revascularization procedure.

Thorax

Pulmonary embolus

Pulmonary emboli (PE) are diagnosed by identifying filling defects within the pulmonary arteries on CT pulmonary angiograms (Figure 1.6.5.7). PE can be difficult to diagnose if contrast opacification in the pulmonary arteries is poor. Several factors influence pulmonary artery contrast opacification such as contrast flow rate, concentration of contrast media, timing of CT, and patient factors such as superior vena cava obstruction.

Pulmonary neoplasm

CT has an important role in initial diagnosis and staging of pulmonary malignancies and in guiding biopsies of peripheral tumours. Primary lung malignancy often appears as a solid, lobulated mass which may cavitate. Associated lung collapse or consolidation often occurs, particularly with central tumours. Adverse features of a lung cancer on CT such as hilar/mediastinal nodal involvement and mediastinal/chest wall invasion can help guide subsequent management and appropriateness for surgery. Enlarged mediastinal nodes on CT don't always indicate involvement with tumour and further investigations such as mediastinoscopy and positron emission tomography-CT may be necessary for patients who are otherwise surgical candidates.

Pulmonary metastases

Pulmonary metastases can have a variable shape but are often well-defined, rounded nodules (Figure 1.6.5.8). In adults, breast, kidney, head and neck, and gastrointestinal tract cancers are particular primary sites. Squamous cell carcinomas in particular have a propensity to cavitate. Pulmonary metastases rarely calcify even if the primary tumour is calcified (e.g. breast or colorectal cancers). Some tumours, in particular lung, breast, stomach, and colon cancers, spread within the lungs by the lymphatic system leading

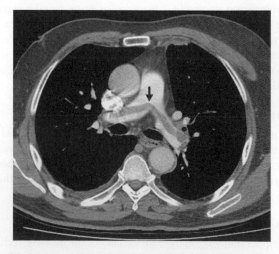

Fig. 1.6.5.7 Axial CT of a saddle pulmonary embolus involving both main pulmonary arteries (arrow).

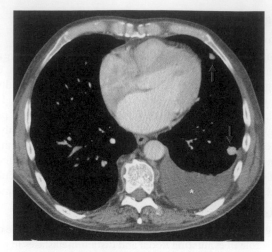

Fig. 1.6.5.8 Axial CT with well-defined, left renal cell carcinoma pulmonary metastases (arrows) and a left pleural effusion (asterisk).

to lymphangitis carcinomatosis which appears as nodular septal thickening and patchy interstitial and ground-glass shadowing. This condition must be differentiated from pulmonary oedema.

Thoracic trauma

Thoracic CT has an important role in trauma and the need for CT is usually guided by the initial chest X-ray, clinical symptoms and signs, and mechanism of injury. Aortic injury usually occurs as a result of rapid deceleration during road traffic accidents and is well demonstrated on CT. Most aortic injuries occur immediately distal to the origin of the left subclavian artery. Frank aortic rupture, intimal flaps, irregularity of the aortic contour, and focal thrombus in the lumen are all features. The complete absence of these features in a good quality CT is a reliable way to exclude an aortic injury.

Tracheobronchial injury can occur as a result of chest compression with a closed glottis. Most cases occur in the mainstem bronchus. In complete tracheobronchial rupture, the lung may fall within the pleural cavity. A pneumothorax which persists despite a chest drain and pneumomediastinum may be a tell-tale sign.

Oesophageal injuries can occur as a result of blunt or penetrating trauma including endoscopy. On CT there may be a clear oesophageal defect but other features include focal thickening of the oesophageal wall with perioesophageal air, mediastinal fluid collections, and pleural effusion/food debris. The CT must be correlated with the level of clinical suspicion as the CT appearances are not specific.

A fracture of the first rib is associated with severe injuries such as aortic injuries, tracheobronchial tears, and subclavian vessel injuries. A flail chest occurs when two or more fractures occur in the same rib or if five or more ribs are fractured in a row. This is an important diagnosis as the flail segment moves paradoxically and respiratory difficulties may rapidly develop.

Neuroimaging

Intracranial haemorrhage

Non-contrast CT has an integral role in imaging patients in head trauma as recommended in the UK guidelines from the National

Institute for Health and Care Excellence.[5] Extradural haematomas occur between the inner surface of the skull and the outer surface of the dura and have a bi-convex (lentiform) shape. An associated fracture is often present and the haematoma will not cross the suture lines of the skull. Subdural haematomas (SDHs) most commonly occur in the frontoparietal region and in the middle cranial fossa. They occur between the dura and arachnoid layers and have a crescentic shape. SDHs are usually larger than extradural haematomas as the blood is unrestricted and can spread over a larger area. The appearance of SDHs further depends on the age of the clot. An acute SDH appears hyperdense relative to the brain and cerebral oedema may be seen. A subacute SDH becomes isodense to the adjacent brain and the window parameters may need to be adjusted to identify the haematoma. A chronic SDH is of low density and in some instances can be difficult to differentiate from a subdural hygroma (accumulation of cerebrospinal fluid).

Subarachnoid haemorrhages (SAHs) occur following head injury or following rupture of a cerebral aneurysm. Blood accumulates between the arachnoid and pia layers. On CT, blood is seen in the basal cisterns and sulci. The sensitivity of CT in identifying SAH reduces as the time of onset of bleed increases and in these circumstances a lumbar puncture may be required. The CT angiogram has a role in identifying cerebral aneurysms in spontaneous SAH.

Cerebral neoplasms

The commonest primary cerebral tumours are gliomas. Their features on CT vary greatly depending upon the tumour type and grade. Cerebral oedema, mass effect with midline shift, hydrocephalus, and enhancement following IV contrast may all be features. Glioblastoma multiforme are aggressive tumours which have central necrosis on CT.

Cerebral metastases appear as round, enhancing, often small lesions usually with marked surrounding oedema. Common primaries include breast, lung, and renal cancers. Meningeal metastases on CT appear as focal or diffuse areas of contrast enhancement and breast cancer is a common primary site. MRI has better sensitivity in identifying meningeal metastases than CT.

Ear, nose, and throat

Rhinosinusitis and nasal polyps

CT particularly with coronal reformats has an important role in the preoperative assessment of patients with rhinosinusitis and nasal polyposis. CT provides an important roadmap to the surgeon. The disease extent, anatomical variations, bone destruction, and complications such as intracranial or orbital abscesses can be assessed. Hyperdense material within a paranasal sinus is often due to inspissated secretions, fungal disease, or blood rather than a tumour. Bone destruction and solid enhancement are more suggestive of tumour rather than benign disease.

Deep neck infections

CT can have a role in diagnosing and assessing the extent of retropharyngeal abscesses in stable patients (Figure 1.6.5.9). In these situations, CT is performed with IV contrast to differentiate cellulitis from abscess. Retropharyngeal abscesses most commonly occur in young children secondary to upper respiratory tract infections. In adults, they develop secondary to trauma or foreign bodies. These abscesses can extend between the base of the skull and the tracheal bifurcation.

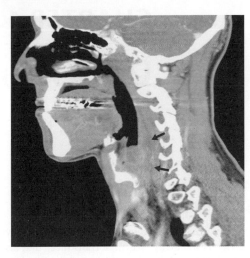

Fig. 1.6.5.9 Sagittal CT of an adult with a retropharyngeal abscess (arrows). The enhancing collection extends proximally towards the skull base. This patient had had a cervical bone graft many years ago which may have been the cause of infection.

Parapharyngeal space (PPS) infections more commonly occur in adults. The PPS is an inverted pyramid lateral to the pharynx which is in contact with the skull base and the greater cornu of the hyoid bone. This space connects with the retropharyngeal, masticator, and submandibular spaces. Infections can reach the PPS from the tonsils, teeth, salivary glands, or the pharynx and the cause can be demonstrated on CT.

Head and neck tumours

CT is important for staging head and neck tumours. A neck CT includes the area between the skull base and the thoracic inlet. Patients are asked not to swallow during the CT to reduce artefact and IV contrast is administered. Dental amalgam can cause quite significant artefact. Close correlation between clinical and CT findings is essential to correctly stage the tumour.

Further reading

Bent C, Lyngkaran T, Power N, et al. Urological injuries following trauma. *Clin Radiol* 2008; 63:1361–71.

Bharwani N, Patel S, Prabhudesai S, et al. Acute pancreatitis: the role of imaging in diagnosis and management. *Clin Radiol* 2011; 66:164–75.

References

1. Furlow B. Radiation dose in computed tomography. *Radiol Technol* 2010; 81(5):437–50.
2. The Royal College of Radiologists. *Standards for Intravascular Contrast Administration to Adult Patients* (2nd ed). London: The Royal College of Radiologists; 2010.
3. Halligan S, Wooldrage K, Dadswell E, et al. Computed tomographic colonography versus barium enema for diagnosis of colorectal cancer or large polyps in symptomatic patients (SIGGAR): a multicentre randomised trial. *Lancet* 2013; 381(9873):1185–93.
4. Bosniak MA. The current radiological approach to renal cysts. *Radiology* 1986; 158:1–10.
5. National Institute for Health and Care Excellence. *Head Injury: Triage, Assessment, Investigation and Early Management of Head Injury in Children, Young People and Adults*. Clinical Guideline 176. London: NICE; 2014.

CHAPTER 1.6.6

Ultrasound for surgeons

Robert D. Kent

Basic physical principles

Ultrasonic waves are produced by electric field-induced vibrations of piezoelectric crystal arrays within a transducer that also vibrate on receiving reflections that coherently generate electricity.

The speed of sound through tissue (around 1540 m/s) is determined by its density and acoustic impedance or stiffness (Z). Echo amplitude is proportional to tissue Z values. The transmission of an ultrasound pulse depends largely on the frequency and whether the medium is gas, liquid, or solid. See Table 1.6.6.1.[1]

As with light, ultrasound energy is attenuated by being scattered, absorbed, or reflected.

Bright echoes are typically produced by gas and calcification, grey echoes from soft tissue propagation, and anechoic black regions due to unimpeded transmission through fluid Therefore ultrasound distinguishes between solid and fluid-filled structures reliably.

The higher the frequency of the ultrasound probe, the better the resolution but with a lower depth of penetration into tissue. The highest frequency transducer that can image the region of interest is used.

Echo characteristics of a lesion may be described as:

- *anechoic/echolucent*: appearing 'black'

- *hypoechoic*: revealing few echoes appearing darker than surrounding tissues

- *echogenic/hyperechoic*: appearing brighter than the surrounding tissues

- *isoechoic*: similar to surrounding tissue, and may not be visualized.

Ultrasound transducers are supplied in a variety of shapes and sizes depending on application. For example, linear, high-frequency probes are used for superficial structures (e.g. testes, breast, thyroid, and musculoskeletal applications), while curved, lower-frequency probes are used for general abdominal imaging.

Specialized probes are available including:

- endovaginal: used primarily for obstetric and gynaecological applications

- transrectal: useful for imaging the prostate with a guide for biopsies

- endoanal: uses a rotating axial transducer for imaging the anal sphincter

- endoscopic: for the distal oesophagus and pancreas

- intravascular: for coronary artery analysis

- endobronchial: to guide mediastinal nodal biopsies

- 'hockey stick': a small probe for joints of the extremities and tendons.

Colour flow Doppler

The Doppler effect is the frequency difference between the transmitted and received wave reflected off a moving object with the frequency shift being proportional to object speed. For example, the direction of blood flow within the portal vein can be identified when assessing portal hypertension, or within the peripheral deep venous system when excluding deep venous thrombosis as velocities are colour coded depending on flow direction and viewed in real time.

Power Doppler

This is more sensitive for detecting low velocities but offers no directional information, and is ideally suited to demonstrate perfusion within a solid mass or a lymph node.

Pulsed Doppler

This enables peak/mean velocities and resistive index calculation. B-mode (brightness mode) and colour Doppler information can be displayed simultaneously as 'duplex scanning'.

Advantages and disadvantages of ultrasound

Advantages

- Relatively low cost compared to other imaging modalities

- Real-time diagnosis

- Portability at the bedside

Table 1.6.6.1 Table of speeds of sound within human tissues

Material	Speed of sound (m/s)
Air	344
Water	1500
Soft tissue (mean value)	1540
Muscle	1570
Fat	1440
Bone	3500

- Readily differentiates fluid-filled structures from solid masses
- Non-ionizing therefore non-cancer inducing or teratogenic
- Guidance for biopsy needles.

Disadvantages

- Difficult to learn and interpret
- Heavily operator dependent
- Limited usefulness in obese or oedematous patients
- Overlying bowel gas may obscure underlying structures
- Artefacts may mimic pathology and it is vital that operators are properly trained to recognize potential pitfalls.

Abdominal applications

Hepatobiliary system

Gallbladder

An ideal first-line investigation for the assessment of hepatobiliary disease, ultrasound has a high sensitivity for the detection of gallbladder pathology, particularly acute cholecystitis, which manifests as a thick-walled, oedematous gallbladder (and gallbladder bed) containing either a single calculus which has obstructed the cystic duct, multiple calculi within the gallbladder lumen, both, or acalculus disease.

Gallbladder polyps, adenomyomatosis of the gallbladder, and gallbladder carcinoma may be readily detected. See Figure 1.6.6.1.

Biliary tract

Biliary obstruction is readily identifiable with ultrasound; indeed, even mild early dilatation of the intrahepatic biliary tree may be identified in most patients. While the presence of biliary obstruction can be confirmed, its cause cannot always be determined sonographically. Ultrasound is useful to determine the level of obstruction with a sensitivity approaching 85%.[2]

In skilled hands, obscuring bowel gas notwithstanding, an obstructing calculus within the distal common bile duct can usually be seen. Other causes of biliary obstruction, for example, by a small ampullary pancreatic cancer, would not be easily visualized.

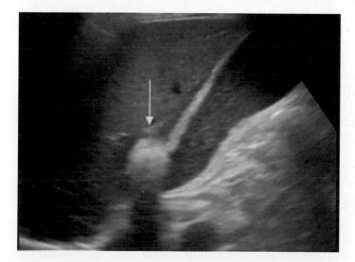

Fig. 1.6.6.1 Calculus impacted in gallbladder neck (arrow). Note the thickened wall and low-level echoes within the gallbladder lumen due to inspissated bile.

Pancreas

There is no role for ultrasound in the diagnosis of acute pancreatitis, similarly with computed tomography (CT) or magnetic resonance imaging (MRI) as it is a clinical diagnosis. Once the acute phase has resolved, ultrasound of the biliary tree is indicated to rule out biliary tract calculi as a cause.

Complications of acute pancreatic disease can often be resolved sonographically, for example, pseudocyst formation. Similarly, pancreatic fibrosis and calcification may also be visualized in the absence of unfavourable body habitus and overlying duodenal gas.

Large masses arising from the pancreatic head and nodal disease within the porta hepatis can usually be resolved. Small ampullary lesions are unlikely to be visualized.

Liver

Ultrasound is an ideal first-line investigation for diffuse hepatocellular disease. It is superior to CT for differentiating cystic from solid parenchymal lesions when smaller than 1 cm diameter. Its sensitivity is greatly enhanced by the use of contrast-enhanced ultrasound (CEUS) agents (e.g. microbubbles).[3]

Focal lesions as small as 0.5 cm can usually be visualized, and cyst versus solid can be differentiated. However, it may not be possible to differentiate benign from malignant disease in the absence of other clinical indicators. For example, giant cavernous haemangioma may be indistinguishable from metastatic disease, hepatocellular carcinoma, or cholangiocarcinoma using greyscale ultrasound in isolation. MRI or CEUS is preferred in doubtful situations.[4]

Ultrasound is frequently used to determine the appropriate route for guided liver biopsy and is the preferred method of localization for percutaneous drainage.

Hepatic fibrosis or cirrhosis is also readily detectable with ultrasound. Steatosis, for example, usually exhibits a uniform increase in parenchymal reflectivity with increased attenuation. A cirrhotic liver parenchyma may have a similar appearance and may also show an irregular edge, best seen with a high-frequency probe.

Portal venous hypertension can be demonstrated by means of colour Doppler, which will show absent or retrograde flow within the portal vein.

Portal venous thrombosis can usually also be demonstrated as a hypoechoic, avascular mass within the lumen.

Abdominal collections

MRI, CT, and ultrasound all have a place in detecting and assessing potential collections within the abdominal cavity and pelvis.

Ultrasound should be the initial investigation of suspected intraperitoneal sepsis being particularly useful delineating the subphrenic, subhepatic spaces. CT or MRI is more sensitive for detecting retroperitoneal or deep pelvic collections which are difficult regions to image sonographically.

Percutaneous drainage of abdominal fluid collections can be achieved by ultrasound or CT depending on the site of the collection.

Ultrasound in trauma: focused assessment with sonography for trauma

Clinical examination of the abdomen in blunt trauma is frequently equivocal.

Focused assessment with sonography for trauma (FAST) is aimed purely at detecting the presence of haemoperitoneum and can be

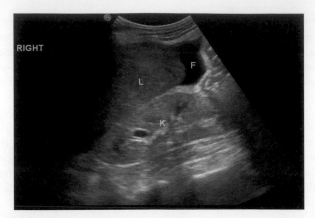

Fig. 1.6.6.2 Free fluid or blood within the hepatorenal space.
F, fluid; K, right kidney; L, liver.
Reproduced by kind permission of Taco Geertsma MD, Radiologist, Hospital Gelderse Vallei,
The Netherlands.

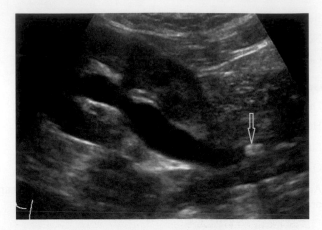

Fig. 1.6.6.3 Calculus impacted within upper third of right ureter. Note proximal dilatation of the renal pelvis.

integrated into the primary clinical pathway, being reproducible and rapidly accessible in the resuscitation room.[5]

Four standard scanning positions are used:

1. Perihepatic: particularly looking for fluid in the hepatorenal space (Rutherford–Morison)

2. Perisplenic: concentrating on identifying fluid around the spleen or left kidney

3. Pelvis: detecting fluid in the pouch of Douglas or rectovesical pouch

4. Pericardial: essentially for detecting fluid or blood within the pericardium.

See Figure 1.6.6.2.

In many centres, the FAST scan is now regarded as being an extension of clinical examination rather than a definitive diagnostic investigation. A standard four-view examination can be completed in less than 2 minutes by a suitably trained operator.

FAST is indicated in any patient who has sustained blunt abdominal trauma who may or may not be haemodynamically unstable, although some authorities have questioned the usefulness of the technique in the stable patient.[6]

Ultrasound at the bedside has been shown to be at least equivalent to plain radiography in the detection of haemothorax in addition to peritoneal injury. Some centres have extended the FAST examination (EFAST), to evaluate the thorax.[7,8]

FAST should not be used to assess the severity of visceral injuries. Such assessments require CT examination.

Genitourinary applications

Kidneys

Ultrasound is a highly sensitive modality for detecting upper renal tract dilatation which may be graded subjectively as mild, moderate, or gross dilatation. It is paramount to note that mild dilatation can be associated with complete obstruction, and marked dilatation may be present without any accompanying obstruction.

Renal tract obstruction

Renal colic secondary to an impacted ureteric calculus is one of the most common presentations of renal tract obstruction. The affected kidney may appear normal initially, but as the obstruction progresses, structures proximal to the obstruction (ureter, renal pelvis, and calyces), will begin to dilate.

Tumours within the ureter or in the region of the vesicoureteric junctions may cause more insidious obstruction, as will extrinsic ureteric compression.

If the obstruction is of long standing, as in benign prostatic hypertrophy, the renal parenchyma may become compressed which will compromise renal function (Figure 1.6.6.3).

Renal cysts

Cortical simple cysts have a characteristic anechoic appearance with a smooth, thin wall and posterior acoustic enhancement; the sonographic hallmarks of benignity. Any complex cyst within the renal cortex should undergo further imaging by means of CT to exclude cystic malignancy.

Solid renal masses

Solid kidney tumours usually appear as heterogeneous, well-defined masses which exhibit increased reflectivity when compared to the adjacent renal cortex: all should be considered malignant until proven otherwise. Eighty-five per cent of solid renal masses represent renal cell carcinoma (RCC), while 10% are due to other malignancies such as sarcoma, lymphoma, transitional cell carcinoma, or metastases. The remaining 5% are benign and include oncocytoma, angiomyolipoma, and fibroma. Of these, only angiomyolipoma is distinguishable from the others sonographically due to the presence of characteristically highly reflective fat within.[9]

Transitional cell carcinoma within the ureter or renal pelvis is poorly visualized with ultrasound, unless seen within a dilated upper tract.

Although not suitable as a staging modality, ultrasound occasionally reveals extension of RCC into the renal vein and inferior vena cava (Figure 1.6.6.4).

Bladder

Ultrasound is excellent for imaging the distended urinary bladder with even a small polypoid bladder tumour well visualized. Bladder wall thickening/trabeculation and mobile calculi may be visualized. Software can be used to calculate bladder volume in the assessment of bladder outflow obstruction.

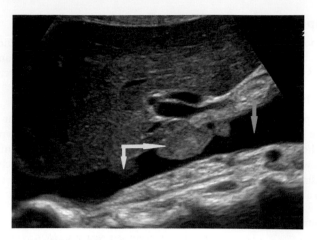

Fig. 1.6.6.4 Sagittal view of right lobe of liver and inferior vena cava. Note tumour seedlings of renal cell carcinoma (yellow arrows) within the lumen of the inferior vena cava (blue arrow).
Reproduced by kind permission of Taco Geertsma MD, Radiologist, Hospital Gelderse Vallei, The Netherlands.

Prostate

Prostate morphology and volume can be easily assessed by using the distended bladder as an acoustic window. Focal prostatic disease, assessment of capsular breach, and nodal involvement in malignancy can be assessed with transrectal probes that are also used to guide prostate biopsy needles.

Scrotal contents

The testis and epididymis are ideally suited to high-frequency, high-definition ultrasound evaluation. Testicular ultrasound is used for:

- determining whether a palpable scrotal mass is within the testis
- assessment of testicular pain
- assessment of scrotal trauma
- assessment of hydrocoele and varicocoele
- undescended testes may be visualized within the inguinal canal

Testicular torsion

Testicular torsion is a urological emergency and early diagnosis is vital. Ultrasound is a valuable tool in detecting torsion, although in the early stages appearances may be subtle. Complete absence of blood flow using colour or power Doppler techniques is diagnostic. However, in the early stages before torsion is complete, or if the torsion is intermittent, there may be some remaining flow in the affected side which may be erroneously reported as normal. It is essential, therefore, that comparison is made with the normal testis.

Greyscale appearances in testicular torsion can be variable, depending upon the duration of the insult. The affected testis may be enlarged and its parenchyma hypoechoic. The parenchyma usually becomes more heterogeneous as the torsion progresses to infarction.

Testicular salvage rates are approximately 100% at 3 hours, 75% at 8 hours, and 50–70% at 10 hours. The salvage rates decrease to 10–20% when torsion persists for more than 10 hours. After 24 hours, salvage of the testicle is rare unless torsion is intermittent.[10]

Acute epididymo-orchitis

Usually presenting with a painful, tender scrotum, pyrexia, and dysuria, ultrasound typically reveals an enlarged, heterogeneous testis and epididymis sometimes with a reactive hydrocoele with colour and power Doppler assessment invariably showing marked hyperaemia of both. See Figure 1.6.6.5.

Scrotal mass disease

High-resolution ultrasound has long been the gold standard for evaluation of scrotal masses, with a sensitivity approaching 100%.[11]

There are no reliable sonographic criteria to distinguish benign from malignant focal intratesticular lesions. Lesions within the epididymis strongly suggest a non-neoplastic or benign process, while all intratesticular masses should be considered malignant until proven otherwise.[12]

Vascular applications

Aneurysmal disease

Aneurysmal disease is discussed in detail in Chapter 2.7.4.

Abdominal aortic aneurysm (AAA) rupture is a vascular catastrophe responsible for 1–3% of deaths in men from the age 65–85 in developed countries.[13]

Patients with leaking AAA frequently present with atypical symptoms, such as suspected renal colic. While ultrasound will exclude AAA in 98% of patients, the modality should not be relied upon for detecting a leaking aneurysm. Fresh blood within the retroperitoneum appears highly reflective or isoechoic on ultrasound and may be indistinguishable from surrounding tissues, with a sensitivity of only 4%. Attempting to detect a leaking AAA with ultrasound will result in potentially catastrophic delay.[14]

Aneurysms of the popliteal and iliac arteries are well visualized.

Other vascular applications

Ultrasound is widely used in the assessment of the following:

- Stenotic carotid artery disease

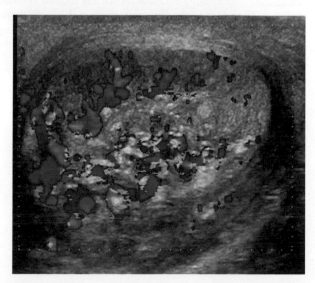

Fig. 1.6.6.5 Acute epididymo-orchitis. Note the marked hyperaemia and heterogeneous testicular parenchyma.
Reproduced by kind permission of Taco Geertsma MD, Radiologist, Hospital Gelderse Vallei, The Netherlands.

- Chronic and acute limb ischaemia (likely performed within vascular lab)
- Varicose vein mapping
- Leg ulceration (diabetic ulceration)
- Venous thromboembolism.

Head and neck applications

The superficial nature of neck structures lends itself readily to high-resolution ultrasound assessment. Ultrasound can provide reliable real-time guidance for fine-needle aspiration cytology (FNAC) or core biopsy. Recognition of its versatility and diagnostic accuracy has led to its routine incorporation in head and neck clinics.

Lymph nodes

Enlarged cervical lymph nodes are the most commonly encountered neck lumps. The role of ultrasound is to differentiate pathological nodes from normal or reactive nodes. While no specific criteria exist to differentiate benign from malignant nodal disease within the neck, any node with a short-axis dimension greater than 8 mm, or one that reveals chaotic or peripheral perfusion or cortical irregularity should be viewed with suspicion. These signs help determine which lymph node to sample using ultrasound-guided FNAC (Figure 1.6.6.6).[15]

Branchial cleft cyst

These are generally found superficial to the common carotid artery and internal jugular vein, posterior to the submandibular gland, and along the anteromedial margin of the sternocleidomastoid muscle.

The ultrasound appearances may be variable, although the anatomical site significantly aids diagnosis. Complex branchial cleft cysts may be indistinguishable from pathological lymph nodes. In such cases, ultrasound-guided FNAC should be performed.

Thyroglossal duct cyst

This congenital abnormality is characteristically located anteriorly slightly off midline deep to the strap muscles just above the thyroid cartilage. It is usually a well-defined, anechoic or hypoechoic, avascular fluid-filled structure[16]

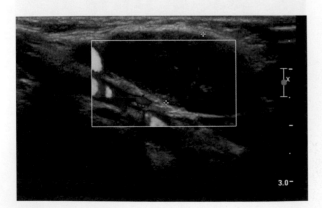

Fig. 1.6.6.6 Enlarged cervical lymph node in lymphoma showing hypoechoic parenchyma and scant perfusion.
Reproduced by kind permission of Taco Geertsma MD, Radiologist, Hospital Gelderse Vallei, The Netherlands.

Lipoma

About 13% occur in the head and neck, typically well-defined, encapsulated compressible hypovascular/hypoechoic subcutaneous mass with linear, echogenic streaks parallel to the transducer.[17]

Venous vascular malformation

Approximately 15% of venous vascular malformations occur in the head and neck, appearing as well-defined heterogeneous hypoechoic masses on ultrasound. Multiple sinusoidal spaces containing slow-flowing internal echoes are also seen. The presence of phleboliths (small echogenic foci with posterior acoustic shadowing) seen in about 20% of cases is pathognomonic.[18]

Lymphangioma

Most present in early childhood and are commonly located in the posterior triangle and cervicothoracic junction. In adults, submental, submandibular, and parotid regions are more commonly affected. Appearances are variable and often present a diagnostic challenge.[19]

Thyroid

Ultrasound contributes little in the diagnosis of thyroid lumps. It is useful to determine whether a nodule is solitary or a component of multinodular disease. It is also of benefit as an aid to FNAC when a nodule or lump is small and difficult to palpate.

Salivary glands

Focal masses within the parotid can usually be targeted for FNAC using ultrasound guidance. Pleomorphic adenoma and Warthin's tumour are the predominant focal lesions seen in the United Kingdom. Other focal masses may be due to intraparotid lymphadenopathy, abscess, or necrotic tumour.[20]

Sialectasis is well seen with ultrasound. Calculi within the parotid or submandibular glands can usually be visualized, although obstructing calculi within the distal ducts may be obscured. Abscess formation within the salivary glands may be aspirated using ultrasound guidance.

Musculoskeletal applications

Most musculoskeletal applications of ultrasound refer to superficial structures where it is ideally suited.

Hip

High-resolution ultrasound is used for the exclusion of infantile developmental hip dysplasia and to accurately detect joint effusions and aid aspiration in paediatric and adult patients. Subclinical subluxation of the infant hip may be demonstrated in real time while the hip is subjected to the standard Ortolani and Barlow clinical examinations.

Shoulder

Ultrasound is ideal at detecting rotator cuff tears and bursitis and guides subacromial steroid injections. Intra-substance and articular surface rotator cuff tears as small as 2–3 mm may be seen in suitable subjects.

Upper and lower limbs

Ultrasound is excellent in the diagnoses of tendon rupture, tendinopathies, locating retained foreign bodies, and the assessment of soft tissue masses and haematomas. Tendon sheaths are particularly well visualized when inflammatory processes manifest as excess fluid within and thickening of the sheath. Colour or power Doppler may show hyperaemia of synovitis. Peripheral neuropathies may be assessed sonographically. The ulnar and median nerves are particularly well seen and in most cases sites of entrapment may be determined.

Specialist applications

Breast

Ultrasound (and MRI) are useful supplements to mammography for detecting breast pathology that is mammographically invisible. While MRI is more sensitive than ultrasound in detecting breast cancers, it is not readily available in all centres.

Ultrasound is the modality of choice for performing guided, free-hand breast biopsies.

Real-time elastography

Real-time elastography is a recent ultrasound application utilizing strain-gauge technology that measures the 'hardness' of tissue which may detect malignancy in lesions thought benign by other methods, thus reducing the number of patients requiring biopsy.[21] See Figure 1.6.6.7.

Endoanal ultrasound

This technique is employed in the investigation of idiopathic or traumatic faecal incontinence and in patients with anal pain, sepsis, or malignancy, as well as in the assessment of sphincter repair following surgery. Endoanal ultrasound probes are specialist implements that have rotating axial transducers.

Gastrointestinal ultrasound

With technical advances, ultrasound used in the initial evaluation of patients with abdominal pain may allow earlier detection of bowel disease.

In specialist centres, its use is many and varied to include:

◆ assessment of inflammatory bowel disease (Crohn's disease, ulcerative colitis, tuberculous ileocolitis, etc.)

◆ detection of infantile hypertrophic pyloric stenosis

◆ neoplastic diseases of the stomach, small bowel, and colon

◆ acute appendicitis and diverticulitis

◆ intussusception and midgut malrotation.

Endoscopic ultrasound may be employed as a screening procedure for oesophageal, gastric, and pancreatic cancer and to target biopsies.[22]

Contrast-enhanced ultrasound

CEUS involves the intravenous administration of micro bubbles in suspension. As the speed of sound within a gas is much lower than within soft tissue, micro bubbles are highly echogenic and they highlight the abnormal vascularity within tumour tissue including the delayed 'wash out' of the suspect region due to abnormal vascular plexi. It is usually possible to differentiate benign from malignant liver disease.

Other uses relate to inflammatory bowel and cardiovascular diseases.[23]

Intravascular ultrasound

Intravascular ultrasound (IVUS) is being used increasingly in the assessment of atherosclerosis within coronary, carotid, and peripheral arteries. Its main advantage is in diagnosing angiographically invisible atheroma hidden by vascular dilatation from 'physiological remodelling' producing non-stenotic disease. A better assessment of plaque burden is possible by assessment by virtual histology IVUS.[24]

The IVUS catheter and probe are, however, expensive which precludes their use other than in specialist centres.

Gynaecological applications

The uterus and ovaries may be visualized by using a distended bladder to displace them superiorly and acting as an acoustic 'window' to enable optimum visualization.

Transvaginal probes use higher more resolute frequency, and their ability to be placed close to the region of interest is a major

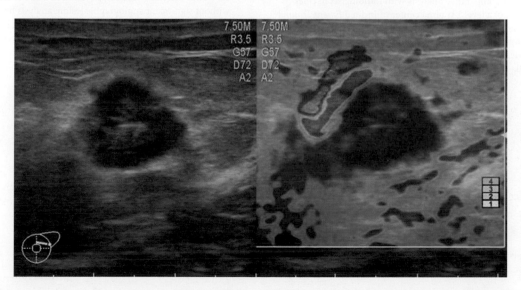

Fig. 1.6.6.7 Breast elastography. Elastography image on the right shows predominantly blue pattern indicative of tissue hardness consistent with scirrhous carcinoma.

advantage. They are used routinely, being especially useful in the detection of ectopic pregnancy.

Ultrasound is excellent for assessing pelvic mass disease. The organ of origin can usually be determined, or a gynaecological cause of the mass excluded.

Differentiation between cystic and solid masses is possible. There are some features of cystic ovarian lesions that suggest malignancy, such as a multiloculated appearance and solid elements within. Transvaginal ultrasound may also be used to guide drainage and biopsy needles.[25]

Further reading

Cardinal E, Chhem RK, Beauregard CG. Ultrasound-guided interventional procedures in the musculoskeletal system. *Radiol Clin North Am* 1998; 36(3):597–604.

Dodds PR, Anderson CO, Dodds JH. Transrectal ultrasound-guided biopsies. *Conn Med* 2013; 77(1):62–3.

Gardner TB. Endoscopic ultrasonography. *Gastrointest Endosc* 2012; 76(3):510–15.

Lee JM, Yoon JH, Kim KW. Diagnosis of hepatocellular carcinoma: newer radiological tools. *Semin Oncol* 2012; 39(4):399–409.

Lehman CD, Lee CI, Loving VA, *et al*. Accuracy and value of breast ultrasound for primary imaging evaluation of symptomatic women 30–39 years of age. *AJR Am J Roentgenol* 2012; 199(5):1169–77.

Kang SK, Chandarana H. Contemporary imaging of the renal mass. *Urol Clin North Am* 2012; 39(2):161–70.

References

1. Shin HC, Prager R, Gomersall H, *et al*. Estimation of average speed of sound using deconvolution of medical ultrasound data. *Ultrasound Med Biol* 2010; 36(4):623–36.
2. Ferrucci JT. Noninvasive imaging of the biliary ducts. *J Gastrointest Surg* 2001; 5(3):232–4.
3. Quaia E. Solid focal liver lesions indeterminate by contrast-enhanced CT or MR imaging: the added diagnostic value of contrast-enhanced ultrasound. *Abdom Imaging* 2012; 37(4):580–90.
4. Sood D, Kumaran V, Buxi TB, *et al*. Liver hemangioma mimicking cholangiocarcinoma—a diagnostic dilemma. *Trop Gastroenterol* 2009; 30(1):44–6.
5. Bhoi S, Sinha TP, Ramchandani R, *et al*. To determine the accuracy of focused assessment with sonography for trauma done by non-radiologists and its comparative analysis with radiologists in emergency department of a level 1 trauma center of India. *J Emerg Trauma Shock* 2013; 6(1):42–6.
6. Natarajan B, Gupta PK, Cemaj S, *et al*. FAST scan: is it worth doing in hemodynamically stable blunt trauma patients? *Surgery* 2010; 148(4):695–700.
7. Dulchavsky SA, Schwarz KL, Kirkpatrick AW, *et al*. Prospective evaluation of thoracic ultrasound in the detection of pneumothorax. *J Trauma* 2001; 50:201–5.
8. Kirkpatrick AW, Sirois M, Laupland KB, *et al*. Hand-held thoracic sonography for detecting post-traumatic pneumothoraces: the extended focused assessment with sonography for trauma (EFAST). *J Trauma* 2004; 57:288–95.
9. Scheible W, Ellenbogen PH, Leopold GR, *et al*. Lipomatous tumors of the kidney and adrenal: apparent echographic specificity. *Radiology* 1978; 129(1):153–6.
10. Kessler CS, Bauml J. Non-traumatic urologic emergencies in men: a clinical review. *West J Emerg Med* 2009; 10(4):281–7.
11. Aganovic L, Cassidy F. Imaging of the scrotum. *Radiol Clin North Am* 2012; 50(6):1145–65.
12. Mirochnik B, Bhargava P, Dighe MK, *et al*. Ultrasound evaluation of scrotal pathology. *Radiol Clin North Am* 2012; 50(2):317–32.
13. Sakalihasan N, Limet R, Defawe OD. Abdominal aortic aneurysm. *Lancet* 2005; 365:1577–89.
14. Eckford SD, Gillatt DA. Abdominal aortic aneurysms presenting as renal colic. *Br J Urol* 1992; 70(5):496–8.
15. Imani Moghaddam M, Davachi B, Mostaan LV, *et al*. Evaluation of the sonographic features of metastatic cervical lymph nodes in patients with head and neck malignancy. *J Craniofac Surg* 2011; 22(6):2179–84.
16. Marsot-Dupuch K, Levret N, Pharaboz C, *et al*. [Congenital neck masses. Embryonic origin and diagnosis. Report of the CIREOL]. *J Radiol* 1995; 76(7):405–15.
17. Fornage BD, Tassin GB. Sonographic appearances of superficial soft tissue lipomas. *J Clin Ultrasound* 1991; 19(4):215–20.
18. Hendrickx S, Hermans R, Wilms G, *et al*. Angiomatosis in the neck and mediastinum: an example of low-flow vascular malformations. *Eur Radiol* 2003; 13(5):981–5.
19. Gritzmann N. Sonography of the neck: current potentials and limitations. *Ultraschall Med* 2005; 26(3):185–96.
20. Musani MA, Sohail Z, Zafar S, *et al*. Morphological pattern of parotid gland tumours. *J Coll Physicians Surg Pak* 2008; 18(5):274–7.
21. Cosgrove DO, Berg WA, Doré CJ, *et al*. Shear wave elastography for breast masses is highly reproducible. *Eur Radiol* 2012; 22(5):1023–32.
22. Rodgers PM, Verma R. Transabdominal ultrasound for bowel evaluation. *Radiol Clin North Am* 2013; 51(1):133–48.
23. Ten Kate GL, van den Oord SC, Sijbrands EJ, *et al*. Current status and future developments of contrast-enhanced ultrasound of carotid atherosclerosis. *J Vasc Surg* 2013; 57(2):539–46.
24. Ouldzein H, Elbaz M, Roncalli J, *et al*. Plaque rupture and morphological characteristics of the culprit lesion in acute coronary syndromes without significant angiographic lesion: analysis by intravascular ultrasound. *Ann Cardiol Angeiol (Paris)* 2012; 61(1):20–6
25. Mohaghegh P, Rockall AG. Imaging strategy for early ovarian cancer: characterization of adnexal masses with conventional and advanced imaging techniques. *Radiographics* 2012; 32(6):1751–73.

Essential interventional radiology for surgeons

Daniel Kusumawidjaja and Peter A. Gaines

Introduction

What is interventional radiology?

Interventional radiology (IR) refers to minimally invasive image-guided procedures that are often therapeutic but can also be diagnostic. Imaging modalities employed include fluoroscopy, computed tomography (CT), magnetic resonance imaging (MRI), and ultrasound, used either singly or in combination. The IR practitioner is frequently but not always a radiologist. He or she will possess the essential skills necessary to carry out 'pin-hole surgery' which includes the manipulation of needles, fine wires, and catheters under image guidance to precisely target intervention (or biopsy in the case of diagnosis).

The benefits of IR procedures include shorter hospital stays, lower costs, reduced risk compared to procedures requiring a general anaesthetic, quicker recovery, and, in general, greater acceptability by the general public compared to open surgery.

Vascular intervention

Trauma

Interventional radiologists play an increasingly important role in the initial management of trauma, especially to stem acute haemorrhage through the use of minimally invasive endovascular techniques. These techniques include blocking bleeding vessels (embolization) or by relining them with covered stents (stent-grafting). IR may also be asked to place a temporary inferior vena cava (IVC) filter in selected patients for the prevention of potential life-threatening pulmonary embolism (PE).

Haemorrhage

Aggressive treatment of haemorrhage saves lives, both acutely and late deaths by preventing trauma-related multi-organ failure. There is evidence that the increased use of IR plays an important role in the management of the severely injured patient and may improve patient outcomes.[1] The United Kingdom National Confidential Enquiry into Patient Outcome and Death (NCEPOD) 2007 report on trauma stipulates that IR services must be available at level 1 trauma centres.[2]

IR techniques are particularly suited to visceral bleeding (spleen, pancreas, liver, kidney, and gastrointestinal tract) and haemorrhage from fractures (particularly pelvic). Following initial stabilization, patients should be considered for urgent CT scanning, particularly if haemorrhage is suspected. Contrast-enhanced CT is a highly sensitive tool to pinpoint sites of active bleeding and can be useful in delineating vascular anatomy before embolization is attempted. It can reveal unexpected retroperitoneal bleeding or occult pelvic fractures.[3]

The spleen is the commonest site of injury in blunt trauma.[4] Embolization preserves the spleen; splenectomy increases the risk of postoperative infection with consequences to long-term immunity.[5] In addition, embolization has been shown to reduce the rate of laparotomy while achieving similar rates of survival (in excess of 85%).[6]

Prophylactic vena cava filter insertion

PE has been shown to be the third major cause of death in trauma patients who survive longer than 24 hours after onset of injury.[7] Patients recovering from trauma have the highest rate of venous thromboembolism (VTE) among all subgroups of hospitalized patients. The likelihood of developing VTE does not appear to correlate with overall severity of trauma but with immobility and prolonged hospital stays.[8] Therefore, IVC filters should be considered in the polytrauma patient with a severe head injury, spinal injury, or pelvic and long-bone fractures. IVC filters are discussed later in this chapter (see 'Inferior vena cava filters').

Embolization

General principles

The aim of embolization is to deliberately occlude flow within blood vessels. Applications include stopping haemorrhage and the treatment of tumours and vascular malformations. Common indications are listed in Box 1.6.7.1.

There are a variety of embolic agents available. Temporary agents provide transient haemostatic control, allowing bleeding vessels a chance to heal, for instance, in pelvic trauma. Autologous blood clot (now rarely used) and absorbable gelatin sponge (Gelfoam®) are examples of temporary agents. Coils are made of stainless steel or platinum and may contain fibres to aid thrombosis. They are used to occlude specific small to medium sized vessels. Particulate embolic agents such as polyvinyl alcohol (PVA) particles can occlude multiple small vessels to elicit ischaemia in target tissue. Tumour embolization is a good example of when particulate embolic agents are used.

Box 1.6.7.1 Indications for embolotherapy

◆ *Haemorrhage*—trauma, visceral, and gastrointestinal bleeding

◆ *Genitourinary*—varicocoele (males), pelvic congestion syndrome (females), prostate (benign prostatic hypertrophy), priapism, angiomyolipoma (reduces risk of haemorrhage), renal cell carcinoma (palliation)

◆ *Gynaecological*—postpartum haemorrhage, uterine fibroids

◆ *Respiratory*—arteriovenous fistulae, thoracic duct (chylothorax), haemoptysis

◆ *Aneurysms*—visceral and intracranial

◆ *Oncology*—chemoembolization and radioembolization

◆ *Vascular malformations*.

Gastrointestinal haemorrhage

The 2008 Scottish Intercollegiate Guidelines Network (SIGN) guidelines on the management of GI haemorrhage have recommended repeat endoscopy, embolization, or surgery for bleeding not controlled by initial endoscopy.[9] Before embolization is considered, patients should undergo urgent imaging evaluation, ideally with CT angiography. This enables the precise localization and confirmation of active bleeding (Figure 1.6.7.1). Scans should be performed during periods of haemodynamic instability in order to give the best chance of demonstrating active contrast extravasation as GI bleeding is by its very nature, intermittent.

If the bleeding point is not demonstrated on CT, it is unlikely to be seen with catheter angiography—embolization cannot proceed without knowing which vessel to target. Nevertheless, in critically ill patients with upper GI bleeding refractory to endoscopic treatment and where no bleeding point is seen on catheter angiography, empiric embolization of the gastroduodenal artery may be effective.[10] Where bleeding is identified on angiography, success rates are very high (typically > 90%).

Poor clinical outcomes are seen in patients who have undergone prolonged resuscitation and received large volumes of blood, consequently developing coagulopathy and multi-organ failure. This highlights that fact that early referrals are crucial to success.[11–14] The risk of bowel infarction in the upper GI tract is low due to its rich collateral blood supply. Beyond the ligament of Treitz, the risk of bowel ischaemia is related to the level of embolization (the more

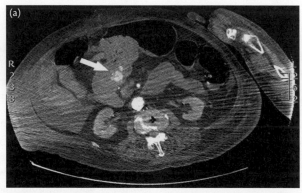

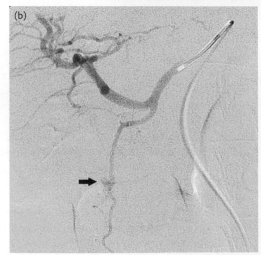
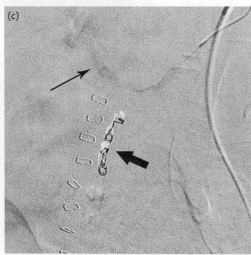

Fig. 1.6.7.1 (a) Upper gastrointestinal haemorrhage—contrast-enhanced abdominal CT scan in arterial phase showing active extravasation of contrast in the duodenum (white arrow). The culprit vessel here is likely to be the gastroduodenal artery;
(b) Digitally subtracted angiogram with the tip of the catheter at the common hepatic artery (a branch of the coeliac artery). Contrast extravasation (black arrow) is demonstrated from the gastroduodenal artery as seen on CT; and
(c) Coils are laid across the bleeding point (thick arrow). Angiogram shows preservation of flow towards the liver (fine arrow).

selective the better) and the length of bowel treated.[15] Selective embolization refers to the use of microcatheters and coils to block off fine vessels as near to the bowel wall as possible, thus reducing the risk of ischaemia to a much smaller area.

Varicocoele embolization

A varicocoele is an abnormal enlargement of the pampiniform venous plexus in the spermatic cord. Percutaneous embolization requires selective catheterization of the testicular vein (via the left renal vein on the left and via the IVC on the right). An example of left testicular vein embolization using coils is shown in Figure 1.6.7.2. Technical success rates are very high (>95%) and recurrence rates low (<2%).[16] Complications are uncommon (<5%) and include thrombophlebitis of the pampiniform plexus if sclerosant is used.[16,17] This minimally invasive outpatient procedure should be offered to all patients considered for treatment as it has similar rates of success and complications to surgery.[18]

Arterial intervention

Angioplasty and stenting

Angioplasty and stenting have revolutionized the treatment of vascular diseases and are the two most common IR techniques performed today.

Percutaneous transluminal angioplasty (PTA) involves the dilatation of vessel stenosis or occlusion with a balloon catheter. PTA causes fractures of the arterial plaque to develop and localized dissections of the arterial wall. The tear may extend into the internal elastic lamina or into the media while the adventitial layer remains intact.

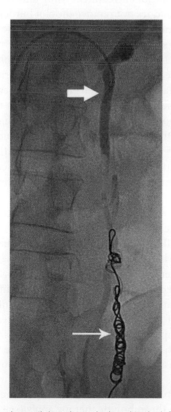

Fig. 1.6.7.2 Varicocoele—coils have been deployed in the left testicular vein (fine arrow). An injection of contrast opacifies the top of the vein (thick arrow). The configuration of the catheter demonstrates the route taken from right femoral vein access—IVC to left renal vein to left testicular vein.

Concentric arterial lesions respond well to angioplasty, as the plaque and the arterial wall layers are dissected uniformly, increasing the vessel luminal diameter. Eccentric arterial lesions may respond less well, as the wall opposite the plaque is stretched by the balloon rather than the plaque itself. Once the balloon is deflated, the normal elastic wall may recoil back to its original size.

During this process, microscopic plaque material may embolize distally. This is usually asymptomatic in the peripheral circulation but can have more serious consequences elsewhere, for instance, during carotid artery intervention.

These difficulties have led to the development of vascular stents, which provide an internal scaffold for the vessel lumen. Advantages include a sustained increase to the luminal diameter, entrapment of vulnerable plaque material that may embolize and elimination of elastic recoil.

In the setting of chronic lower limb ischaemia, guidance on the choice of treatment (endovascular versus open surgery) can be found in recommendations from the Trans-Atlantic Inter-Society Consensus Working Group and the Society of Interventional Radiology.[19] In general, short focal lesions are best treated with endovascular therapy while complex, extensive, and bilateral disease should be considered for surgery.

In general, PTA is used to treat stenosis while stenting is reserved for occlusions (Figure 1.6.7.3) or when results are poor following angioplasty (e.g. residual pressure gradient in the iliac arteries or dissection).[20,21] Endovascular treatment should be performed sequentially from proximal to distal as aorto-iliac intervention has been shown to improve quality of life and compare favourably with surgery for primary and long-term success.[22–25]

Stent grafting and aneurysms

A stent graft is a metal stent covered in fabric or polytetrafluoroethylene (PTFE) and is primarily used in the treatment of aneurysms or for haemorrhage. An interventional radiologist generally performs stent grafting procedures. A discussion on the endovascular repair of abdominal aneurysms (EVAR) is found in Chapter 2.7.4.

Stent-grafts are also used in the treatment of a range of thoracic aortic diseases by a procedure termed 'thoracic endovascular aortic repair' (TEVAR). For instance, TEVAR is the treatment of choice for thoracic aortic aneurysms (TAAs) and has high technical success rates. TAAs are generally treated above a threshold of 6 cm.[26]

Special consideration is given to anatomical suitability for TEVAR, which is assessed by a preoperative CT angiogram. In particular, there must be at least 20 mm of 'landing zone' length to achieve a seal in order to avoid an endoleak. The landing zone refers to the area of normal calibre aorta just proximal or distal to the aneurysm. If there is inadequate length, a surgical de-branching procedure may be required to create a sufficient landing zone (Figure 1.6.7.4). Paraplegia (1–2%) is another serious complication and results from covering the intercostal supply of the spinal cord resulting in ischaemia; prophylactic cerebrospinal fluid drainage may be required.

Thoracic aortic dissections can be complicated by rupture, malperfusion of viscera, persistent pain, refractory hypertension, or false aneurysm formation. TEVAR is the treatment of choice for complicated type B dissections (not involving the ascending

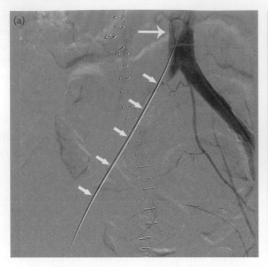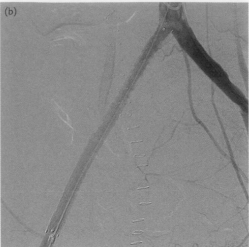

Fig. 1.6.7.3 (a) Right iliac artery stenting—angiogram from a pigtail catheter located in the distal aorta (fine arrow). A guidewire has successfully traversed the occluded right common and external iliac artery (multiple arrows) from a right groin puncture.
(b) A stent has been deployed across the right iliac artery occlusion. A repeat angiogram from the same catheter shows contrast opacifying the right iliac artery, proving that it has reopened.

aorta). The rationale is to cover the entry tear of the dissection in order to depressurize the false lumen and to eventually enable aortic remodelling to take place. Traumatic aortic injuries may also be treated with TEVAR. While uncomplicated type B aortic dissections are often best managed with medical therapy, there is emerging evidence of improved long-term outcomes with TEVAR.[27,28]

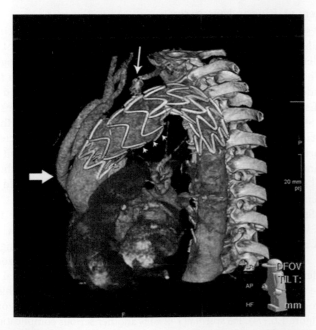

Fig. 1.6.7.4 Thoracic endovascular aortic repair (TEVAR)—stent graft treatment for a thoracic aortic aneurysm (small arrowheads). As there was insufficient landing zone length, the left common carotid artery has been debranched and connected to the right brachiocephalic artery (thick arrow) thereby enabling the proximal stent graft to seal by creating a longer landing zone. The left subclavian artery has been embolized (fine arrow) to prevent flow back into the aneurysm sac (endoleak). The left arm now derives its blood supply from the left vertebral artery.

Venous intervention

Deep vein thrombosis therapies

Lower limb deep venous thrombosis (DVT) carries a risk of clot propagation and PE, which increases the more proximally the clot is located—iliofemoral DVT poses a higher risk than popliteal or calf DVT. The traditional treatment using anticoagulation seeks to lower this risk but does not remove the clot burden nor does it prevent the long-term effects and disabling sequelae of DVT, namely post-thrombotic syndrome (PTS).[29–33]

To prevent PTS, it is likely that the thrombus needs to be removed at an early stage. Iliofemoral DVT rarely recanalizes with anticoagulation alone. Surgical thrombectomy has been superseded by interventional techniques, which include catheter-directed thrombolysis (CDT) or the use of mechanical thrombectomy devices. Of the 208 patients with iliofemoral DVT in the CaVenT study,[34] patients who underwent additional CDT compared to conventional therapy alone had significantly lower rates at PTS at 24 months, corresponding to an absolute risk reduction of 14.4%.

Mechanical thrombectomy may also entail the additional use of a thrombolytic agent and may be performed in a single session whereas CDT will invariably necessitate a short stay on a monitored ward such as the high dependency unit as treatment times may last 24 hours or longer.[35,36]

Additional preprocedural non-invasive imaging in the form of magnetic resonance or CT venography is essential for delineating the extent of thrombus and may reveal a stenosis of the iliac vein due to compression of overlying iliac artery (May–Thurner lesion) for which stenting may be required. The ideal referral for endovenous therapy is a first episode of iliofemoral DVT with an acute clot of less than 2 weeks old, a low risk of bleeding, good performance status, and reasonable life expectancy. The usual contraindications to thrombolytic therapy apply (see Box 1.6.7.2). The American Society for Vascular Surgery has recommended these interventional techniques as first-line therapy for patients meeting the above criteria.[37]

Box 1.6.7.2 Contraindications to thrombolysis

Absolute contraindications

- Active bleeding
- Recent (3 months) ischaemic stroke or transient ischaemic attack
- Recent (2 months) intracranial surgery
- Recent (3 months) major blunt head or facial trauma
- History of haemorrhagic stroke
- History of spontaneous intracranial haemorrhage
- Intracranial neoplasm or vascular malformation
- Suspected aortic dissection
- Bleeding diathesis.

Relative contraindications

- Recent (3 weeks) major thoracic or abdominal surgery
- Recent major trauma
- Recent (1 month) internal bleeding
- Recent (3 months) gastrointestinal haemorrhage
- Uncontrolled hypertension (increased risk of intracranial haemorrhage)
- Prolonged (>10 minutes) or traumatic cardiopulmonary resuscitation
- Pregnancy.

Inferior vena cava filters

IVC filters are principally indicated in patients who have suffered venous thromboembolism (VTE), including PE and DVT, despite adequate anticoagulation or in whom anticoagulation is contraindicated (e.g. active haemorrhage, recent or impending major surgery, brain tumour or haemorrhage, or pregnancy). Softer, but often-used indications include pulmonary hypertension following pulmonary thromboembolic disease, free-floating IVC thrombus, and as prophylaxis in those patients at high risk of PE (e.g. previous history of VTE, trauma, and bariatric surgery).[38,39]

There are a variety of caval filters on the market—the majority are termed 'optional' filters which means they can be removed (typically within 3 months but ideally within 4 weeks) or may be left in permanently. Most filters are used to provide protection against PE for a short defined period of time. The decision on the use of permanent filters depends on the anticipated duration of treatment or risk of PE. Other factors such as poor clinical status, unfavourable life expectancy, poor patient compliance with anticoagulation, filter thrombosis, or other adverse factors that may lead to difficult retrieval should also be considered.[40] Conversely, filters inserted in younger patients should be removed due to the risk of IVC thrombosis in the longer term—reported rates vary depending on the filter type and may be as high as 13%[38] although 5% is a more representative rate.[41]

Factors that preclude filter retrieval include trapped clot within the filter, filter tilt, or adherence to the caval wall. Other complications of filters include caudal migration, strut fracture, and IVC perforation. The latter was seen in all cases in one study after 71 days following removable filter insertion, reinforcing the need to remove caval filters as early as possible.[42]

Superior vena cava obstruction

The majority of superior vena cava (SVC) obstruction (SVCO) is caused by malignant mediastinal disease, typically bronchial carcinoma but may also result from lymphoma and other rarer mediastinal tumours such as thymoma.[43] Non-malignant causes include prolonged transvenous cardiac devices and the prolonged use of indwelling venous access catheters.[44]

Symptoms can be debilitating and include upper body oedema, glottis oedema, hoarseness, and headaches. Surgical treatment has previously consisted of venous bypass following median sternotomy but cannot be justified in cancer patients who have poor prognosis. SVC stenting has emerged as the preferred adjunctive treatment for SVCO as it is the most effective and rapid treatment for the relief of symptoms of malignant SVCO, a conclusion supported by a Cochrane review.[45] Patency rates appear to be similar for patients with complete obstruction and with stenosis.[46] There is currently no evidence supporting the use of stenting in asymptomatic SVCO.

Hepatobiliary (vascular)

Transjugular intrahepatic portosystemic shunt

Transjugular intrahepatic portosystemic shunt (TIPS) is essentially a side to side portacaval shunt created under fluoroscopic guidance to reduce portal venous pressure in patients suffering from the complications of portal hypertension. In recent years, the introduction of PTFE-covered endografts which are able to achieve durable long-term patency, has seen the resurgence of the use of TIPS.

The indications of the use of TIPS are given in Box 1.6.7.3. There is at least a 50% increased risk of re-bleeding following a variceal bleed and is associated with a high mortality rate.[47] The literature suggests that TIPS reduces re-bleeding rates compared to endoscopic therapy but at the risk of new or worsening encephalopathy.[48] New evidence suggests that in high-risk cirrhotic patients with acute variceal bleeding, the early use of TIPS is associated with marked and significant reductions in both treatment failure and mortality.[49,50]

Box 1.6.7.3 Indications for TIPS

- Secondary prevention of variceal bleeding*
- Refractory ascites*
- Refractory acute variceal bleed
- Portal hypertensive gastropathy
- Bleeding gastric/ectopic varices
- Refractory hepatic hydrothorax
- Hepatorenal syndromes (types 1 and 2)
- Budd–Chiari syndrome
- Hepatic veno-occlusive disease
- Hepatopulmonary syndrome.

*Denotes most common indications.

The development of refractory ascites in cirrhotic patients represents close to 50% mortality at 12 months.[51] TIPS is more effective for refractory ascites than paracentesis and is associated with significantly better transplant-free survival at 12 and 24 months.[52]

In the era of bare metal stents, shunt dysfunction (including thrombosis and hyperplastic stenosis) was of significant concern. These have improved with the introduction of PTFE-covered stent grafts. In a study comparing bare metal stents with PTFE stent grafts in 80 patients, primary patency rates at 1 and 2 years were 86% and 80% respectively in the PTFE group, compared with 47% and 19% in the bare metal stent group. Stent thrombosis occurs early; none were seen in the PTFE group compared to three patients with bare metal stents.[53] Encephalopathy is another serious complication, seen in 20–30% of patients, the incidence of which is always higher when compared to other therapies.[54] Patients presenting with refractory encephalopathy or worsening liver failure may require shunt reduction (i.e. reducing the flow through the shunt).[55]

Haemodialysis and venous access

Interventional therapies for haemodialysis fistulae

For patients with chronic renal failure, haemodialysis should ideally be performed via an arteriovenous fistula. Fistulae are the result of the surgical anastomosis of a vein to an artery and must be performed as peripherally in the arm as possible in order to preserve more central access sites for the future. Native fistulae are by far the most durable type of vascular access and the least prone to complications but maturation can take from a few weeks to 3 months before routine cannulation for dialysis is possible.[54] Prosthetic interposition grafts may be used if a suitable superficial vein is unavailable but are prone to infection and much poorer patency rates, usually due to stenosis at the venous anastomosis.[56,57]

A temporary central venous dialysis catheter can be placed while waiting for a fistula to be fashioned or in patients with limited life expectancy but are prone to thrombosis and infection with low-rates of longer-term patency.[58,59]

The majority of fistula-related complications result from stenosis. This may range from 'upstream' anastomotic stenosis leading to a failure of maturation and inadequate blood flow for dialysis to more 'downstream' stenosis of the draining vein or central vein causing prolonged haemostasis following fistula access, oedema, and thrombosis. The nature of the problem can often be elicited non-invasively by ultrasound or a fistulogram, whereby contrast angiogram is performed.

Fistuloplasty refers to balloon dilatation (angioplasty) of fistula-related stenosis and is effective and safe. In most cases, fistuloplasty should be attempted before surgical revision is considered.[60] On the whole, results are better for native fistulae compared to grafts, with reported success rates of 91–95%. Unfortunately, recurrences are common with primary patency rates between 44% and 51% at 1 year[61,62] highlighting the fact that repeat interventions are often necessary.

Thrombosed fistulae may be amenable to percutaneous techniques (thrombolysis or mechanical thrombectomy) if there is adequate venous drainage. Otherwise, surgical revision is necessary.

Central venous access

Central venous access is required for a variety of reasons, including chemotherapy, long-term antibiotics, and total parenteral nutrition. There is also a wide range of catheters and insertion methods—lines can be tunnelled into subcutaneous tissue for medium to long-term access (e.g. Hickman line) and access sites may vary including jugular, subclavian, femoral, or peripheral, the latter applies to peripherally inserted central catheters (PICC). Femoral routes showed a higher incidence of infectious colonization and thrombotic complications, probably because of the higher bacterial density of local skin flora in the groin area.[63] Catheter-related thrombosis also occurs more frequently in lines inserted via the femoral route.[64] Furthermore, it is estimated that a third of all thromboses of the upper extremity are related to intravenous catheters.[65]

While most lines are designed to protrude out of the insertion site for easy access, totally implantable port devices are available that may reduce catheter-related rates of infection.[66,67]

Vascular malformations

General principles

The term 'vascular malformations' encompass a range of vascular abnormalities. Vascular anomalies are categorized into vascular tumours (haemangiomas) and vascular malformations (VMs), a classification adopted by the International Society for the Study of Vascular Anomalies.[68,69]

Haemangiomas usually present 6 weeks after birth and are often self-limiting. VMs are present at birth but are often small and clinically undetectable at the time. As VMs contain embryonic cells from the early stages of development, such as angioblasts, which are mesenchymal cells in origin, proliferation and recurrence is more frequent. Growths of these malformations can be stimulated by hormones (pregnancy, menarche) or by trauma or surgery to the lesions.[70] VMs are further divided by flow dynamics into low- or high-flow malformations, a useful classification as it determines appropriate treatment[71] (Table 1.6.7.1).

Treatment of VMs is most effective in the multidisciplinary setting led by the interventional radiologist and plastic surgeon. The objective of imaging is to delineate the extent of the malformation, as the clinically apparent lesion is often the 'tip of the iceberg'. MRI is generally best at determining this and is helpful in eliciting flow characteristics.[72] Hand-held Doppler is a useful screening tool if a high-flow malformation is suspected and can be used in the outpatient clinic setting. In general, treatment is reserved for when the patient is symptomatic (e.g. pain, bleeding, growth or cosmetic problems).

Arteriovenous malformations—these high-flow malformations are abnormal connections between an artery and vein, bypassing the normal capillary bed. The venous interface between the artery and vein is termed a 'nidus' and it is the aim of treatment to eliminate the nidus. Patients may complain of a pulsatile mass, bleeding, or pain.

Table 1.6.7.1 Classification of vascular malformations

High flow	Low flow
Arteriovenous malformation	Capillary malformation
	Venous malformation
	Lymphatic malformation
	Mixed malformation

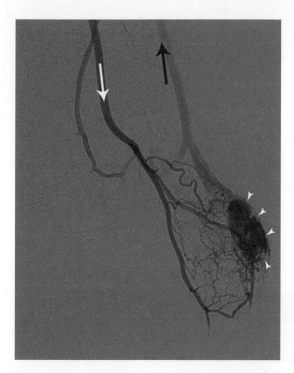

Fig. 1.6.7.5 Arteriovenous (high-flow) malformation (AVM)—high-flow malformation (small arrowheads) on the side of an adolescent's foot. This is fed primarily by the dorsalis pedis artery (white arrow) and drained by the long saphenous vein (black arrow). The digital arteries of the toes are not seen due to the steal effect of the AVM diverting blood away from the toes.

Catheter angiography or venography is almost always performed to determine the exact vascular anatomy of the lesion in order to plan treatment (Figure 1.6.7.5). There are a variety of ways to eliminate the nidus; the approach may be arterial or venous or percutaneous, the latter termed 'direct stick'. There is also a wide variety of embolic agents that may be used.

Low-flow malformations—these lesions may respond to conservative treatment; elastic compression garments (i.e. class 2 compression stockings) should be attempted first.[68] Younger patients concerned about the appearances of the lesion should be referred for a trial of camouflage cosmetics. Often, reassurance about the benign nature of the malformation is all that is required.

The treatment of choice for low-flow malformations is sclerotherapy; this involves the percutaneous injection of a sclerosant (e.g. sodium tetradecyl sulphate, ethanol, or bleomycin) under imaging guidance, often via multiple needles. Complications are rare but patients must be warned of the risk of damage to surrounding muscle, nerve, and skin. The latter may be severe enough to warrant skin grafts. Historically, surgical treatments have resulted in distressing cosmetic consequences and high recurrence rates.[73]

Oncological intervention

The aim of cancer treatment is to deliver therapy effectively to improve patient outcomes while minimizing systemic toxicity. Interventional techniques are increasingly being employed as a weapon in the multidisciplinary armoury available to cancer treatment. The advantage of image-guided oncological treatments is the ability to deliver targeted therapy; these currently fall into two broad categories—catheter-directed techniques and ablative techniques. Other emerging techniques (e.g. high-intensity focused ultrasound) are beyond the scope of this text.

Vascular interventions

Liver embolization

Hepatic arterial embolization may be performed using embolic agents alone (bland embolization) or in combination with chemotherapeutic or radiotherapeutic agents. The last two techniques are termed 'transarterial chemoembolization' (TACE) and 'selective internal radiotherapy treatment' (SIRT) respectively. In the case of hepatocellular carcinoma (HCC), current practice recommendations are given in Figure 1.6.7.6.[74]

Historically, a wide range of embolic agents has been used for bland hepatic tumour embolization demonstrating varying degrees of success.[75,76] The rationale of treatment is that vascular hepatic tumours derive supply from the hepatic artery while the remainder of the (normal) liver derives most of its supply from the portal venous system.[77] Complications related to bland hepatic tumour embolization can include 'post-embolization syndrome' that consists of fever, nausea, fatigue, elevated white cell count, and liver enzyme elevation.[78] Liver necrosis, hepatic abscess or biloma formation, and liver failure are recognized, but less common serious complications of liver embolization.

TACE consists of the intra-arterial delivery of a chemotherapeutic agent mixed with an embolic agent directly to the tumour bed within the liver. The rationale is based on the theory that tumour ischaemia caused by embolization has a synergistic effect with the chemotherapeutic drugs. It has emerged as the first-line therapy for HCCs not amenable to resection or local ablation and has been shown to improve survival compared to supportive care.[79,80] More recently, drug-loaded (typically with doxorubicin) embolization particles have garnered popularity due to their favourable pharmacokinetics, which has been shown to reduce systemic toxicity while maintaining higher intralesion doxorubicin concentration and dwell times.[81] Compared to conventional chemoembolization with doxorubicin in an oil-rich emulsion, treatment with drug-eluting particles has been shown to have higher rates of response, improved tolerability with significantly lower rate of doxorubicin-related side effects, and longer median survival.[82,83]

SIRT involves radioembolization with yttrium-90 microspheres, instilled through a catheter directly into the tumour arterial supply. Yttrium-90 is a beta emitter with a short half-life. As a consequence, a much higher dose of radiation can be delivered to the target lesion, sparing higher doses to the remaining liver. In contrast, external beam radiation delivers an equal dose to both the lesion and non-tumour-bearing liver. In addition to complications involving chemoembolization (discussed earlier), there are three unique complications that may result from radioembolization—radiation pneumonitis (<1%), gastroduodenal ulceration (<5%), and radiation-induced liver disease (<4%). These are eminently preventable through careful preprocedural planning and patient selection.[84,85]

Results of TACE on colorectal metastases to the liver have been disappointing with partial response rates of 2–14%.[86,87] SIRT, on the other hand, is a viable alternative to the treatment of unresectable or unablatable colorectal metastases with improved survival, albeit in the palliative setting.[88–90]

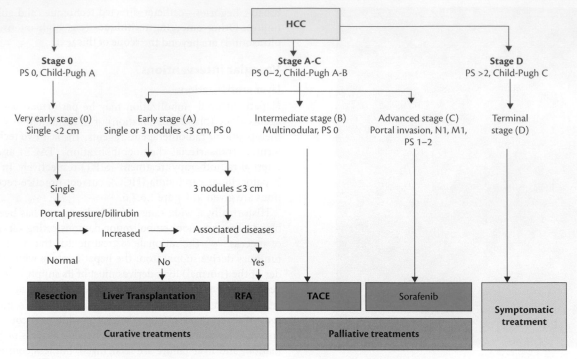

Fig. 1.6.7.6 The Barcelona Clinic Liver Cancer (BCLC) staging system for HCC.

M, metastasis classification; N, node classification; PS, performance status; RFA, radiofrequency ablation; TACE, transarterial chemoembolization.

Reproduced with permission from Forner, A., M.E. Reig, C.R. de Lope, and J. Bruix, Current strategy for staging and treatment: the BCLC update and future prospects, *Seminars in Liver Disease*, Volume 30, Issue 1, pp. 61–74, Copyright © Georg Thieme Verlag KG 2010.

Ablation

General principles

Ablation involves the image-guided insertion of a probe directly into a lesion to precisely deliver a focal area of destruction (most commonly thermal) via radiofrequency (RF) energy. RF ablation induces irreversible cellular injury from focal high-temperature tissue heating that is generated around an RF electrode. Benefits include reduced cost and morbidity compared to standard surgical resection, and the ability to treat patients who are not surgical candidates. However, limitations exist, which include growth of residual tumour at the ablation margin, the inability to effectively treat larger tumours, and variability in complete treatment based upon tumour location.

It has become an accepted treatment option for focal primary and secondary malignancies in a wide range of organs including the liver, lung, kidney, bone, and adrenal glands. In the case of hepatic malignancies, long-term outcomes have been reported to be similar to surgical resection in matched patient populations.[91] RF ablation may be considered for HCCs according to the Barcelona Clinic Liver Cancer (BCLC) liver cancer staging system (Figure 1.6.7.6). In the case of colorectal hepatic metastases, RF ablation may be considered in patients unsuitable for surgical resection, with fewer than five lesions, each less than 3 cm diameter measured in the longest axis.[92]

Early major complications of RF ablation include liver abscess, intestinal perforation, pneumo/haemothorax, intraperitoneal bleeding, and bile duct stenosis (2.2–3.1%). Tumour seeding along the needle track is an uncommon late complication (0.5%). Minor complications include pain, fever, asymptomatic pleural effusion, and asymptomatic self-limiting intraperitoneal bleeding (5–8.9%).[93]

Non-vascular intervention

Biopsy and drainage

These procedures encompass the passage of a biopsy or access needle under image guidance (typically CT or ultrasound) in order to reach the target tissue safely and accurately. In the case of drainage procedures, a locking pigtail catheter may be left *in situ* so that the contents of the target collection may be allowed to drain over a period of time. Prior imaging is usually required (perhaps except for the most superficial lesions) in order to plan for the most appropriate imaging method and route of access.

Patients should have a normal coagulation profile and normal platelet count. Uncooperative patients may require additional support in the form of extra staff or sedation. It is best to plan for these beforehand.

Biopsy techniques include fluid aspiration for cytology, fine-needle aspiration (particularly suited to superficial lesions such as thyroid and breast), and core needle biopsy. Core biopsy devices come in a variety of sizes (usually 14–18 G) and are essential if invasive status of a malignant lesion is sought. Typical sites of core biopsies include liver, breast, lung, intra-abdominal, and nodal.

In patients with diffuse liver disease and consequent coagulopathy or with ascites, transjugular liver biopsy may be performed in which a long vascular sheath is introduced into the right hepatic vein via a right internal jugular approach and a biopsy is obtained using a long cutting biopsy needle. The theory is that as there is no breech of the liver capsule (as occurs with a percutaneous approach), any bleeding is either contained within the liver or flows back into the hepatic vein.[94]

Percutaneous abscess drainage is the treatment of choice for intra-abdominal sepsis and should be attempted before surgical drainage (i.e. laparotomy) if there is a safe route of access in a suitable patient. CT guidance is often necessary, as the presence of bowel gas will obscure ultrasound views. For the majority of cases, access is percutaneous and depending on the site of the collection, may be from the back or flank, which will require the patient to be placed prone in the scanner. Pelvic collections can be tricky and may necessitate a transrectal, transvaginal, or transgluteal approach.

Urological

Percutaneous nephrostomy

Percutaneous nephrostomy denotes the image-guided placement of a draining catheter to the renal pelvis for decompression of obstruction or to act as a portal for future minimally invasive procedures (e.g. ureteric stent insertion, nephrolithotripsy, or ureteric dilatation). The most common indications are ureteric obstruction secondary to calculi, extrinsic compression due to malignancy, or pelvic mass. It also enables healing to take place in cases of ureteric injury or renal fistulae by allowing the diversion of urine. Transplant kidneys are also candidates for nephrostomy. Drainage is particularly urgent if the renal pelvicalyceal system is infected as the consequent loss of renal function and septicaemia can be rapid. Urgent intervention is also indicated in an obstructed solitary kidney or in cases of bilateral obstruction. Coagulopathy is considered a contraindication for nephrostomy and should be corrected beforehand.[95]

Technical success is typically achieved in 96–99% in dilated system but falls in non-dilated systems to approximately 85%.[96,97] Minor complications (1–5%) include catheter misplacement, catheter obstruction due to debris, ileus, urinary tract infection, urinary leakage, access site skin inflammation, and pleural effusion.[98] Transient minor bleeding is common (95%); blood-tinged urine in the nephrostomy bag normally resolves within 24–48 hours.[99] Major haemorrhage occurs in less than 4% and may be associated with pseudoaneurysm formation. Septic shock (< 4%, higher in infected kidneys) is the most serious complication and provides the rationale for preprocedural antibiotics.[100]

Ureteric stenting

Ureteric stents are plastic conduits for urine to flow normally from the renal pelvis into the bladder and while the indications for ureteric stenting are similar to nephrostomy insertion (i.e. obstructed renal collecting systems), stents are generally only considered if longer-term drainage is required. Stents can be placed via the bladder through a cystoscope (retrograde stent) or through an existing nephrostomy (antegrade stent). In most cases, retrograde stenting should be attempted first. They are called 'double-J' stents as both ends of the stent are fashioned into 'pigtails' to prevent migration. Complications and success rates are similar to percutaneous nephrostomy insertion.

Percutaneous nephrolithotomy

Percutaneous nephrolithotomy (PCNL) creates an access tract into the renal collecting system through which nephroscopy can be performed. Percutaneous access is ultrasound guided and typically performed by the interventional radiologist following which the urologist performs nephroscopy. A nephroscope has a working channel through which a lithotripsy device can be introduced and stone fragments removed through a variety of methods (basket extraction, graspers, or suction). The technique enables stones to

be removed so that the patient does not have to pass any fragments, as opposed to shock wave lithotripsy and ureteroscopy. Although more invasive than other treatments, PCNL is safe and effective, and is particularly suited to staghorn, large, multiple, or complex stone disease.[101] Renal stone disease is covered in Chapter 2.9.1.

Hepatobiliary

Percutaneous biliary interventions

Percutaneous biliary techniques have advanced beyond percutaneous transhepatic cholangiography (PTC) as a means of investigating the obstructed biliary tree, especially as CT and magnetic resonance cholangiography are readily available and effective non-invasive tests. The increased use of endoscopy for biliary tract evaluation and intervention (namely endoscopic retrograde cholangiopancreatography) has served to supersede percutaneous techniques, resulting in a decrease in primary percutaneous transhepatic biliary interventions. Therefore, patients requiring percutaneous biliary procedures often have had failed endoscopic procedures or who have altered anatomy (e.g. previous biliary-enteric anastomosis) and often represent a more technically difficult subset of patients.

The purpose of biliary drainage is to decompress an obstructed biliary tree. This is often secondary to malignant disease (e.g. cholangiocarcinoma or pancreatic cancer) but may be due to benign disease (e.g. cholelithiasis, pancreatitis, or injury—traumatic or iatrogenic). An internal–external drainage catheter allows bile to drain both externally into a bag and also internally into the small bowel, thereby preserving the normal enterohepatic circulation of bile, whereas an external drainage catheter is placed when one is unable to advance a catheter through the obstruction and into the duodenum. A stent may also be deployed across the point of stricture, often in cases of malignancy.

Patients requiring biliary drainage have the potential to become ill rapidly, often due to sepsis, which is also the most common complication related to biliary drainage.[102] Other complications include hepatic abscess, haemobilia rarely causing significant haemorrhage, and bile peritonitis which may occur when drainage catheter is blocked.

Percutaneous cholecystostomy

Percutaneous cholecystostomy (placement of a gallbladder drain) represents an alternative treatment in patients with acute cholecystitis who are at high risk for surgery resulting in significantly lower morbidity and mortality compared to cholecystectomy.[103] It is contraindicated in gallbladders packed full of stones and in those with severe coagulopathy. Leakage of bile is the most common complication.

Gastrointestinal

Image-guided gastrostomy

For patients with swallowing disorders, a gastrostomy serves as a lifeline in providing nutritional support. Gastrostomy tubes come in several varieties—the percutaneous endoscopic gastrostomy (PEG) is inserted with the aid of an endoscope; the radiologically inserted gastrostomy (RIG) is inserted percutaneously under fluoroscopic guidance and fixed to the anterior abdominal wall by sutures or anchors; and the peroral image-guided gastrostomy (PIG) is pulled down through the oropharynx and out through a guidewire previously inserted through image-guided gastrostomy. The PIG allows for larger gastrostomy sizes (typically 14–20 Fr), which helps prevent blockage. Complications include inadvertent puncture of adjacent viscera and consequent peritonitis (<5%).[104]

Gastrointestinal stenting

Metallic stenting of the GI tract was initially used in oesophageal obstruction, superseding plastic stents due to their superior ability to relieve dysphagia and safety profile.[105,106] Indications for stenting include malignant or benign strictures, malignant fistulae, and perforation. Metallic stents are available in uncovered or covered versions; the rationale for the latter is to impede tumour in-growth with consequent luminal stenosis. The main complications include stent migration, which may require the insertion of overlapping stents to prevent further migration, and tumour in-growth, which may be treated with endoscopic laser therapy and haemorrhage. Perforation is uncommon.[107] Stenting is also performed in the duodenum, stomach, and colon for similar indications. Consideration should always be given to colonic stenting as a temporizing measure in frail and often dehydrated patients with acute colonic obstruction who are high-risk candidates for emergency surgery. This will allow time to correct electrolyte imbalances caused by colonic obstruction and to allow for accurate tumour staging before surgical resection and primary anastomosis.

Further reading

Trauma

Zealley IA, Chakraverty S. The role of interventional radiology in trauma. *BMJ* 2010; 340:c497.

Embolization of gastrointestinal haemorrhage

Gillespie CJ, Sutherland AD, Mossop PJ, *et al.* Mesenteric embolization for lower gastrointestinal bleeding. *Dis Colon Rectum* 2010; 53(9):1258–64.

Mirsadraee S, Tirukonda P, Nicholson A, *et al.* Embolization for nonvariceal upper gastrointestinal tract haemorrhage: a systematic review. *Clin Radiol* 2011; 66(6):500–9.

Wee E. Management of nonvariceal upper gastrointestinal bleeding. *J Postgrad Med* 2011; 57(2):161–7.

Varicocoele embolization

Beecroft JRD. Percutaneous varicocele embolization. *Can Urol Assoc J* 2007; 1(3):278–80.

Angioplasty and stenting for peripheral vascular disease

Beard JD, Gaines PA (eds). *A companion to Specialist Surgical Practice: Vascular and Endovascular Surgery* (4th ed). Edinburgh: Saunders Elsevier; 2009.

Norgren L, Hiatt WR, Dormandy JA, *et al.* Inter-Society Consensus for the Management of Peripheral Arterial Disease (TASC II). *J Vasc Surg* 2007; 45 Suppl S:S5–67.

Interventional DVT therapies

Mehrzad H, Freedman J, Harvey JJ, *et al.* The role of interventional radiology in the management of deep vein thrombosis. *Postgrad Med J* 2013; 89(1049):157–64.

O'Sullivan GJ. The role of interventional radiology in the management of deep venous thrombosis: advanced therapy. *Cardiovasc Interv Radiol* 2011; 34(3):445–61.

IVC filters

Baglin TP, Brush J, Streiff MB, Guidelines for the use of vena cava filters. *Br J Haematol* 2006; 134: p.590–5.

SVC stenting

Ganeshan A, Hon LQ, Warakaulle DR, *et al.* Superior vena caval stenting for SVC obstruction: current status. *Eur J Radiol* 2009; 71(2):343–9.

TIPS

Fidelman N, Kwan SW, LaBerge JM, *et al.* The transjugular intrahepatic portosystemic shunt: an update. *AJR Am J Roentgenol* 2012; 199(4):746–55.

Haemodialysis fistulae

Surlan M, Popovic P. The role of interventional radiology in management of patients with end-stage renal disease. *Eur J Radiol* 2003; 46(2):96–114.

Central venous access

Mauro MA, Jaques PF. Radiologic placement of long-term central venous catheters: a review. *J Vasc Interv Radiol* 1993; 4(1):127–37.

Zaghal A, Khalife M, Mukherji D, *et al.* Update on totally implantable venous access devices. *Surg Oncol* 2012; 21(3):207–15.

Vascular malformations

McCafferty IJ, Jones RG. Imaging and management of vascular malformations. *Clin Radiol* 2011; 66(12):1208–18.

Interventional oncology

Bruix J, Sherman M. Management of hepatocellular carcinoma: an update. *Hepatology* 2011; 53(3):1020–2.

Memon K, Lewandowski RJ, Riaz A, *et al.* Chemoembolization and radioembolization for metastatic disease to the liver: available data and future studies. *Curr Treat Options Oncol* 2012; 13(3):403–15.

Smith KA, Kim HS. Interventional radiology and image-guided medicine: interventional oncology. *Semin Oncol* 2011; 38(1):151–62.

Percutaneous abscess drainage

vanSonnenberg E, Wittich GR, Goodacre BW, *et al.* Percutaneous abscess drainage: update. *World J Surg* 2001; 25(3):362–9.

Percutaneous urological procedures

Antonelli JA, Pearle MS. Advances in percutaneous nephrolithotomy. *Urol Clin North Am* 2013; 40(1):99–113.

Hausegger KA, Portugaller HR. Percutaneous nephrostomy and antegrade ureteral stenting: technique-indications-complications. *Eur Radiol* 2006; 16(9):2016–30.

Percutaneous gastrostomy

Laasch HU, Wilbraham L, Bullen K, *et al.* Gastrostomy insertion: comparing the options—PEG, RIG or PIG? *Clin Radiol* 2003; 58(5):398–405.

Gastrointestinal stenting

Morgan R, Adam A. Use of metallic stents and balloons in the esophagus and gastrointestinal tract. *J Vasc Interv Radiol* 2001; 12(3):283–97.

References

1. Pryor JP, Braslow B, Reilly PM, *et al.* The evolving role of interventional radiology in trauma care. *J Trauma* 2005; 59(1):102–4.
2. National Confidential Enquiry into Patient Outcome and Death. *Trauma. Who Cares?* London: NCEPOD; 2007. http://www.ncepod.org.uk/2007report2/Downloads/SIP_report.pdf.
3. Frevert S, Dahl B, Lonn L. Update on the roles of angiography and embolisation in pelvic fracture. *Injury* 2008; 39(11):1290–4.

4. Fang JF, Wong YC, Lin BC, *et al*. Usefulness of multidetector computed tomography for the initial assessment of blunt abdominal trauma patients. *World J Surg* 2006; 30(2):176–82.

5. Wiseman J, Brown CV, Weng J, *et al*. Splenectomy for trauma increases the rate of early postoperative infections. *Am Surg* 2006; 72(10):947–50.

6. Gaarder C, Dormagen JB, Eken T, *et al*. Nonoperative management of splenic injuries: improved results with angioembolization. *J Trauma* 2006; 61(1):192–8.

7. Knudson MM, Collins JA, Goodman SB, *et al*. Thromboembolism following multiple trauma. *J Trauma* 1992; 32(1):2–11.

8. Geerts WH, Code KI, Jay RM, *et al*. A prospective study of venous thromboembolism after major trauma. *N Engl J Med* 1994; 331(24):1601–6.

9. Scottish Intercollegiate Guidelines Network. *Management of Upper and Lower Gastrointestinal Bleeding*. Guideline 105. Edinburgh: SIGN; 2008. http://www.sign.ac.uk/guidelines/fulltext/105/index.html

10. Dixon S, Chan V, Shrivastava V, *et al*. Is there a role for empiric gastroduodenal artery embolization in the management of patients with active upper GI hemorrhage? *Cardiovasc Interv Radiol* 2012; 36(4):970–7.

11. Walker TG, Salazar GM, Waltman AC. Angiographic evaluation and management of acute gastrointestinal hemorrhage. *World J Gastroenterol* 2012; 18(11):1191–201.

12. Aina R, Oliva VL, Therasse E, *et al*. Arterial embolotherapy for upper gastrointestinal hemorrhage: outcome assessment. *J Vasc Interv Radiol* 2001; 12(2):195–200.

13. Schenker MP, Duszak R Jr, Soulen MC, *et al*. Upper gastrointestinal hemorrhage and transcatheter embolotherapy: clinical and technical factors impacting success and survival. *J Vasc Interv Radiol* 2001; 12(11):1263–71.

14. Mirsadraee S, Tirukonda P, Nicholson A, *et al*. Embolization for non-variceal upper gastrointestinal tract haemorrhage: a systematic review. *Clin Radiol* 2011; 66(6):500–9.

15. Rossetti A, Buchs NC, Breguet R, *et al*. Transarterial embolization in acute colonic bleeding: review of 11 years of experience and long-term results. *Int J Colorectal Dis* 2013; 28(6):777–82.

16. Nabi G, Asterlings S, Greene DR, *et al*. Percutaneous embolization of varicoceles: outcomes and correlation of semen improvement with pregnancy. *Urology* 2004; 63(2):359–63.

17. Reyes BL, Trerotola SO, Venbrux AC, *et al*. Percutaneous embolotherapy of adolescent varicocele: results and long-term follow-up. *J Vasc Interv Radiol* 1994; 5(1):131–4.

18. Dewire DM, Thomas AJ Jr, Falk RM, *et al*. Clinical outcome and cost comparison of percutaneous embolization and surgical ligation of varicocele. *J Androl* 1994; 15 Suppl:38S–42S.

19. Norgren L, Hiatt WR, Dormandy JA, *et al*. Inter-Society Consensus for the Management of Peripheral Arterial Disease (TASC II). *J Vasc Surg* 2007; 45 Suppl S:S5–67.

20. Bosch JL, Hunink MG. Meta-analysis of the results of percutaneous transluminal angioplasty and stent placement for aortoiliac occlusive disease. *Radiology* 1997; 204(1):87–96.

21. Tetteroo E, van der Graaf Y, Bosch JL, *et al*. Randomised comparison of primary stent placement versus primary angioplasty followed by selective stent placement in patients with iliac-artery occlusive disease. Dutch Iliac Stent Trial Study Group. *Lancet* 1998; 351(9110):1153–9.

22. Chetter IC, Spark JI, Kent PJ, *et al*. Percutaneous transluminal angioplasty for intermittent claudication: evidence on which to base the medicine. *Eur J Vasc Endovasc Surg* 1998; 16(6):477–84.

23. Bosch JL, van der Graaf Y, Hunink MG. Health-related quality of life after angioplasty and stent placement in patients with iliac artery occlusive disease: results of a randomized controlled clinical trial. The Dutch Iliac Stent Trial Study Group. *Circulation* 1999; 99(24):3155–60.

24. Wolf GL, Wilson SE, Cross AP, *et al*. Surgery or balloon angioplasty for peripheral vascular disease: a randomized clinical trial. Principal investigators and their Associates of Veterans Administration Cooperative Study Number 199. *J Vasc Interv Radiol* 1993; 4(5):639–48.

25. Adam DJ, Beard JD, Cleveland T, *et al*. Bypass versus angioplasty in severe ischaemia of the leg (BASIL): multicentre, randomised controlled trial. *Lancet* 2005; 366(9501):1925–34.

26. Elefteriades JA. Natural history of thoracic aortic aneurysms: indications for surgery, and surgical versus nonsurgical risks. *Ann Thorac Surg* 2002; 74(5):S1877–80.

27. Fattori R, Montgomery D, Lovato L, *et al*. Survival after endovascular therapy in patients with type B aortic dissection. A report from the international registry of acute aortic dissection (IRAD). *J Am Coll Cardiol Intv* 2013; 6:876–82.

28. Nienaber C, Kische S, Rousseau H, *et al*. Endovascular repair of type B aortic dissection. Long-term results of the randomized investigation of stent grafts in aortic dissection trial. *Circ Cardiovasc Interv* 2013; 6:407–16.

29. Kahn SR, Ginsberg JS. Relationship between deep venous thrombosis and the postthrombotic syndrome. *Arch Intern Med* 2004; 164(1):17–26.

30. Shbaklo H, Kahn SR. Long-term prognosis after deep venous thrombosis. *Curr Opin Hematol* 2008; 15(5):494–8.

31. Kahn SR, M'Lan CE, Lamping DL, *et al*. The influence of venous thromboembolism on quality of life and severity of chronic venous disease. *J Thromb Haemost* 2004; 2(12):2146–51.

32. Kahn SR, Shbaklo H, Lamping DL, *et al*. Determinants of health-related quality of life during the 2 years following deep vein thrombosis. *J Thromb Haemost* 2008; 6(7):1105–12.

33. Ashrani AA, Heit JA. Incidence and cost burden of post-thrombotic syndrome. *J Thromb Thrombolysis* 2009; 28(4):465–76.

34. Enden T, Haig Y, Klow NE, *et al*. Long-term outcome after additional catheter-directed thrombolysis versus standard treatment for acute iliofemoral deep vein thrombosis (the CaVenT study): a randomised controlled trial. *Lancet* 2012; 379(9810):31–8.

35. Lin PH, Zhou W, Dardik A, *et al*. Catheter-direct thrombolysis versus pharmacomechanical thrombectomy for treatment of symptomatic lower extremity deep venous thrombosis. *Am J Surg* 2006; 192(6):782–8.

36. Kim HS, Patra A, Paxton BE, *et al*. Adjunctive percutaneous mechanical thrombectomy for lower-extremity deep vein thrombosis: clinical and economic outcomes. *J Vasc Interv Radiol* 2006; 17(7):1099–104.

37. Meissner MH, Gloviczki P, Comerota AJ, *et al*. Early thrombus removal strategies for acute deep venous thrombosis: clinical practice guidelines of the Society for Vascular Surgery and the American Venous Forum. *J Vasc Surg* 2012; 55(5):1449–62.

38. Decousus H, Leizorovicz A, Parent F, *et al*. A clinical trial of vena caval filters in the prevention of pulmonary embolism in patients with proximal deep-vein thrombosis. Prevention du Risque d'Embolie Pulmonaire par Interruption Cave Study Group. *N Engl J Med* 1998; 338(7):409–15.

39. Eight-year follow-up of patients with permanent vena cava filters in the prevention of pulmonary embolism: the PREPIC (Prevention du Risque d'Embolie Pulmonaire par Interruption Cave) randomized study. *Circulation* 2005; 112(3):416–22.

40. Eifler AC, Lewandowski RJ, Gupta R, *et al*. Optional or permanent: clinical factors that optimize inferior vena cava filter utilization. *J Vasc Interv Radiol* 2013; 24(1):35–40.

41. Sangwaiya MJ, Marentis TC, Walker TG, *et al*. Safety and effectiveness of the celect inferior vena cava filter: preliminary results. *J Vasc Interv Radiol* 2009; 20(9):1188–92.

42. Durack JC, Westphalen AC, Kekulawela S, *et al*. Perforation of the IVC: rule rather than exception after longer indwelling times for the Gunther Tulip and Celect retrievable filters. *Cardiovasc Interv Radiol* 2012; 35(2):299–308.

43. Ostler PJ, Clarke DP, Watkinson AF, *et al*. Superior vena cava obstruction: a modern management strategy. *Clin Oncol* 1997; 9(2):83–9.

44. Kee ST, Kinoshita L, Razavi MK, *et al*. Superior vena cava syndrome: treatment with catheter-directed thrombolysis and endovascular stent placement. *Radiology* 1998; 206(1):187–93.

45. Rowell NP, Gleeson FV. Steroids, radiotherapy, chemotherapy and stents for superior vena caval obstruction in carcinoma of the bronchus. *Cochrane Database Syst Rev*, 2001; 4:CD001316.

46. Crowe MT, Davies CH, Gaines PA. Percutaneous management of superior vena cava occlusions. *Cardiovasc Interv Radiol* 1995; 18(6):367–72.

47. Sharara AI, Rockey DC. Gastroesophageal variceal hemorrhage. *N Engl J Med* 2001; 345(9):669–81.

48. Papatheodoridis GV, Goulis J, Leandro G, *et al.* Transjugular intrahepatic portosystemic shunt compared with endoscopic treatment for prevention of variceal rebleeding: a meta-analysis. *Hepatology* 1999; 30(3):612–22.

49. Garcia-Pagan JC, Caca K, Bureau C, *et al.* Early use of TIPS in patients with cirrhosis and variceal bleeding. *N Engl J Med* 2010; 362(25):2370–9.

50. Garcia-Pagan JC, Di Pascoli M, Caca K, *et al.* Use of early-TIPS for high-risk variceal bleeding: results of a post-RCT surveillance study. *J Hepatol* 2013; 58(1):45–50.

51. Gines P, Cardenas A, Arroyo V, *et al.* Management of cirrhosis and ascites. *N Engl J Med* 2004; 350(16):1646–54.

52. Salerno F, Camma C, Enea M, *et al.* Transjugular intrahepatic portosystemic shunt for refractory ascites: a meta-analysis of individual patient data. *Gastroenterology* 2007; 133(3):825–34.

53. Bureau C, Garcia-Pagan JC, Otal P, *et al.* Improved clinical outcome using polytetrafluoroethylene-coated stents for TIPS: results of a randomized study. *Gastroenterology* 2004; 126(2):469–75.

54. Zuckerman DA, Darcy MD, Bocchini TP, *et al.* Encephalopathy after transjugular intrahepatic portosystemic shunting: analysis of incidence and potential risk factors. *AJR Am J Roentgenol* 1997; 169(6):1727–31.

55. Riggio O, Nardelli S, Moscucci F, *et al.* Hepatic encephalopathy after transjugular intrahepatic portosystemic shunt. *Clin Liver Dis* 2012; 16(1):133–46.

56. Rodriguez JA, Armadans L, Ferrer E, *et al.* The function of permanent vascular access. *Nephrol Dial Transplant* 2000; 15(3):402–8.

57. Ascher E, Gade P, Hingorani A, *et al.* Changes in the practice of angioaccess surgery: impact of dialysis outcome and quality initiative recommendations. *J Vasc Surg* 2000; 31(1 Pt 1):84–92.

58. Hodges TC, Fillinger MF, Zwolak RM, *et al.* Longitudinal comparison of dialysis access methods: risk factors for failure. *J Vasc Surg* 1997; 26(6):1009–19.

59. Schwab SJ, Oliver MJ, Suhocki P, *et al.* Hemodialysis arteriovenous access: detection of stenosis and response to treatment by vascular access blood flow. *Kidney Int* 2001; 59(1):358–62.

60. NKF-DOQI clinical practice guidelines for vascular access. National Kidney Foundation-Dialysis Outcomes Quality Initiative. *Am J Kidney Dis* 1997; 30(4 Suppl 3):S150–91.

61. Turmel-Rodrigues L, Pengloan J, Baudin S, *et al.* Treatment of stenosis and thrombosis in haemodialysis fistulas and grafts by interventional radiology. *Nephrol Dial Transplant* 2000; 15(12):2029–36.

62. Manninen HI, Kaukanen ET, Ikaheimo R, *et al.* Brachial arterial access: endovascular treatment of failing Brescia-Cimino hemodialysis fistulas—initial success and long-term results. *Radiology* 2001; 218(3):711–8.

63. Lorente L, Henry C, Martin MM, *et al.* Central venous catheter-related infection in a prospective and observational study of 2,595 catheters. *Crit Care* 2005; 9(6):R631–5.

64. Merrer J, De Jonghe B, Golliot F, *et al.* Complications of femoral and subclavian venous catheterization in critically ill patients: a randomized controlled trial. *JAMA* 2001; 286(6):700–7.

65. Ge X, Cavallazzi R, Li C, *et al.* Central venous access sites for the prevention of venous thrombosis, stenosis and infection. *Cochrane Database Syst Rev* 2012; 3:CD004084.

66. Kock HJ, Pietsch M, Krause U, *et al.* Implantable vascular access systems: experience in 1500 patients with totally implanted central venous port systems. *World J Surg* 1998; 22(1):12–6.

67. Bouza E, Burillo A, Munoz P. Catheter-related infections: diagnosis and intravascular treatment. *Clin Microbiol Infect* 2002; 8(5):265–74.

68. Mulliken JB, Glowacki J. Hemangiomas and vascular malformations in infants and children: a classification based on endothelial characteristics. *Plast Reconstr Surg* 1982; 69(3):412–22.

69. Enjolras O, Mulliken JB. Vascular tumors and vascular malformations (new issues). *Adv Dermatol* 1997; 13:375–423.

70. Lee BB, Laredo J, Lee TS, *et al.* Terminology and classification of congenital vascular malformations. *Phlebology* 2007; 22(6):249–52.

71. Jackson IT, Carreno R, Potparic Z, *et al.* Hemangiomas, vascular malformations, and lymphovenous malformations: classification and methods of treatment. *Plast Reconstr Surg* 1993; 91(7):1216–30.

72. Konez O, Burrows PE. Magnetic resonance of vascular anomalies. *Magn Reson Imaging Clin N Am* 2002; 10(2):363–88.

73. Emery PJ, Bailey CM, Evans JN. Cystic hygroma of the head and neck. A review of 37 cases. *J Laryngol Otol* 1984; 98(6):613–19.

74. Forner A, Reig ME, de Lope CR, *et al.* Current strategy for staging and treatment: the BCLC update and future prospects. *Semin Liver Dis* 2010; 30(1):61–74.

75. Chuang VP, Wallace S. Hepatic artery embolization in the treatment of hepatic neoplasms. *Radiology* 1981; 140(1):51–8.

76. Chuang VP, Wallace S, Soo CS, *et al.* Therapeutic Ivalon embolization of hepatic tumors. *AJR Am J Roentgenol* 1982; 138(2):289–94.

77. Taylor I, Bennett R, Sherriff S. The blood supply of colorectal liver metastases. *Br J Cancer* 1978; 38(6):749–56.

78. Hemingway AP, Allison DJ. Complications of embolization: analysis of 410 procedures. *Radiology* 1988; 166(3):669–72.

79. Lo CM, Ngan H, Tso WK, *et al.* Randomized controlled trial of transarterial lipiodol chemoembolization for unresectable hepatocellular carcinoma. *Hepatology* 2002; 35(5):1164–71.

80. Llovet JM, Real MI, Montana X, *et al.* Arterial embolisation or chemoembolisation versus symptomatic treatment in patients with unresectable hepatocellular carcinoma: a randomised controlled trial. *Lancet* 2002; 359(9319):1734–9.

81. Varela M, Real MI, Burrel M, *et al.* Chemoembolization of hepatocellular carcinoma with drug eluting beads: efficacy and doxorubicin pharmacokinetics. *J Hepatol* 2007; 46(3):474–81.

82. Lammer J, Malagari K, Vogl T, *et al.* Prospective randomized study of doxorubicin-eluting-bead embolization in the treatment of hepatocellular carcinoma: results of the PRECISION V study. *Cardiovasc Interv Radiol* 2010; 33(1):41–52.

83. Dhanasekaran R, Kooby DA, Staley CA, *et al.* Comparison of conventional transarterial chemoembolization (TACE) and chemoembolization with doxorubicin drug eluting beads (DEB) for unresectable hepatocelluar carcinoma (HCC). *J Surg Oncol* 2010; 101(6):476–80.

84. Kennedy AS, Dezarn WA, McNeillie P, *et al.* Radioembolization for unresectable neuroendocrine hepatic metastases using resin 90Y-microspheres: early results in 148 patients. *Am J Clin Oncol* 2008; 31(3):271–9.

85. Riaz A, Lewandowski RJ, Kulik LM, *et al.* Complications following radioembolization with yttrium-90 microspheres: a comprehensive literature review. *J Vasc Interv Radiol* 2009; 20(9):1121–30.

86. Albert M, Kiefer MV, Sun W, *et al.* Chemoembolization of colorectal liver metastases with cisplatin, doxorubicin, mitomycin C, ethiodol, and polyvinyl alcohol. *Cancer* 2011; 117(2):343–52.

87. Vogl TJ, Gruber T, Balzer JO, *et al.* Repeated transarterial chemoembolization in the treatment of liver metastases of colorectal cancer: prospective study. *Radiology* 2009; 250(1):281–9.

88. Mulcahy MF, Lewandowski RJ, Ibrahim SM, *et al.* Radioembolization of colorectal hepatic metastases using yttrium-90 microspheres. *Cancer* 2009; 115(9):1849–58.

89. Bester L, Meteling B, Pocock N, *et al.* Radioembolization versus standard care of hepatic metastases: comparative retrospective cohort study of survival outcomes and adverse events in salvage patients. *J Vasc Interv Radiol* 2012; 23(1):96–105.

90. Chua TC, Bester L, Saxena A, *et al.* Radioembolization and systemic chemotherapy improves response and survival for unresectable colorectal liver metastases. *J Cancer Res Clin Oncol* 2011; 137(5):865–73.

91. McWilliams JP, Yamamoto S, Raman SS, *et al*. Percutaneous ablation of hepatocellular carcinoma: current status. *J Vasc Interv Radiol* 2010; 21(8 Suppl):S204–13.

92. Crocetti L, de Baere T, Lencioni R. Quality improvement guidelines for radiofrequency ablation of liver tumours. *Cardiovasc Interv Radiol* 2010; 33(1):11–17.

93. Livraghi T, Solbiati L, Meloni MF, *et al*. Treatment of focal liver tumors with percutaneous radio-frequency ablation: complications encountered in a multicenter study. *Radiology* 2003; 226(2):441–51.

94. Sporea I, Popescu A, Sirli R. Why, who and how should perform liver biopsy in chronic liver diseases. *World J Gastroenterol* 2008; 14(21):3396–402.

95. Stables DP, Ginsberg NJ, Johnson ML. Percutaneous nephrostomy: a series and review of the literature. *AJR Am J Roentgenol* 1978; 130(1):75–82.

96. Farrell TA, Hicks ME. A review of radiologically guided percutaneous nephrostomies in 303 patients. *J Vasc Interv Radiol* 1997; 8(5):769–74.

97. Ramchandani P, Cardella JF, Grassi CJ, *et al*. Quality improvement guidelines for percutaneous nephrostomy. *J Vasc Interv Radiol* 2003; 14(9 Pt 2):S277–81.

98. Lee WJ, Patel U, Patel S, *et al*. Emergency percutaneous nephrostomy: results and complications. *J Vasc Interv Radiol* 1994; 5(1):135–9.

99. Dyer RB, Regan JD, Kavanagh PV, *et al*. Percutaneous nephrostomy with extensions of the technique: step by step. *Radiographics* 2002; 22(3):503–25.

100. Lewis S, Patel U. Major complications after percutaneous nephrostomy-lessons from a department audit. *Clin Radiol* 2004; 59(2):171–9.

101. Preminger GM, Assimos DG, Lingeman JE, *et al*. Chapter 1: AUA guideline on management of staghorn calculi: diagnosis and treatment recommendations. *J Urol* 2005; 173(6):1991–2000.

102. Winick AB, Waybill PN, Venbrux AC. Complications of percutaneous transhepatic biliary interventions. *Tech Vasc Interv Radiol* 2001; 4(3):200–6.

103. Boland GW, Lee MJ, Mueller PR, *et al*. Gallstones in critically ill patients with acute calculous cholecystitis treated by percutaneous cholecystostomy: nonsurgical therapeutic options. *AJR Am J Roentgenol* 1994; 162(5):1101–3.

104. Wollman B, D'Agostino HB. Percutaneous radiologic and endoscopic gastrostomy: a 3-year institutional analysis of procedure performance. *AJR Am J Roentgenol* 1997; 169(6):1551–3.

105. Knyrim K, Wagner HJ, Bethge N, *et al*. A controlled trial of an expansile metal stent for palliation of esophageal obstruction due to inoperable cancer. *N Engl J Med* 1993; 329(18):1302–7.

106. De Palma GD, di Matteo E, Romano G, *et al*. Plastic prosthesis versus expandable metal stents for palliation of inoperable esophageal thoracic carcinoma: a controlled prospective study. *Gastrointest Endosc* 1996; 43(5):478–82.

107. Adam A, Ellul J, Watkinson AF, *et al*. Palliation of inoperable esophageal carcinoma: a prospective randomized trial of laser therapy and stent placement. *Radiology* 1997; 202(2):344–8.

SECTION 2

Common surgical conditions

Section editor: Kevin Sherman

PART 2.1

Assessing the acute abdomen

CHAPTER 2.1.1

Assessing the acute abdomen

Tom Wiggins and James N. Crinnion

Introduction

The primary symptom in most patients presenting with an 'acute abdomen' is severe abdominal pain. Such patients are usually referred to general surgeons, and their management represents a large proportion of the workload of the general surgical team. In 2011, United Kingdom Hospital Episode Statistics revealed that 289 133 patients presented with abdominal symptoms[1] with the vast majority of these suffering with abdominal pain. A focused history, skilled clinical examination, and appropriate investigations will enable the clinician to make a rapid and accurate diagnosis of the cause of the abdominal pain. In recent years, the clinical acumen of the surgeon has been greatly assisted by the widespread availability and rapid access to computed tomography (CT) scanning.

This chapter describes the clinical assessment of patients with acute abdominal pain and includes a discussion of the common acute presentations of peritonitis, abdominal distension, and non-specific abdominal pain.

Pathophysiology of abdominal pain

Abdominal pain may be either visceral or somatic in origin.

Visceral pain

Visceral pain emanates directly from the abdominal, pelvic, and thoracic viscera in response to stretching, ischaemia, or inflammation, which stimulate the organ's nociceptors creating the sensation of visceral pain. The pain felt is usually vague, poorly localized, and often referred to a distant and superficial location.

Pain arising from the stomach and duodenum (foregut) is typically referred to the epigastrium. Similarly, pain arising from the midgut (jejunum to transverse colon) is felt in the periumbilical region, and pain arising from the transverse colon to rectum (hindgut) is felt in the suprapubic area.

Visceral pain is appreciated through stimulation of the autonomic nervous system and can therefore be associated with an alteration of blood pressure, heart rate or temperature, and sweating, flushing, pallor, and nausea.[2]

Somatic pain

Somatic pain arises from stimulation of nociceptors within muscle and fascial structures. Within the abdomen it arises from irritation of nerve fibres within the parietal peritoneum, and is typically sharp and localized to the site of the abdominal pathology.

Peritonitis

Inflammation of the peritoneum results in the clinical syndrome of peritonitis that may be localized to the site of the involved viscus, or become more generalized, typically following visceral perforation. Peritonitis produces the classic triad of Classic triad of severe pain, sharp contraction of the overlying muscles upon palpation (guarding) and eventually rigidity (involuntary contraction of the abdominal muscles).

Differential diagnosis of acute abdominal pain

There are a myriad of potential causes of abdominal pain and therefore the surgeon must adopt a systematic approach when formulating a differential diagnosis. In this regard the surgical sieve is helpful (Table 2.1.1.1). Also, the site of the pain and local tenderness will help to narrow down the differential diagnoses (Figure 2.1.1.1).

Surgical sieve

This may be remembered by using the mnemonic INVITED MD that stands for:

◆ Infection
◆ Neoplasia
◆ Vascular
◆ Inflammatory/autoimmune
◆ Trauma
◆ Endocrine
◆ Degenerative causes
◆ Metabolic causes
◆ Drugs and other causes.

Differential diagnosis by site of pain

Figure 2.1.1.1 shows the potential causes of abdominal pain in relation to the site. This list is by no means exhaustive but provides an outline of common causes of abdominal pain by position.

Clinical history in abdominal pain

On many occasions a careful focused history will provide the clinician with enough information to form a likely diagnosis. This clinical suspicion will then be confirmed by the examination findings and subsequent investigations.

Table 2.1.1.1 A list of the most common diagnoses that may manifest as abdominal pain for each section of the surgical sieve

Infective causes	Appendicitis
	Cholecystitis
	Cholangitis
	Diverticulitis
	Pyelonephritis/urinary tract infection
	Pelvic inflammatory disease
	Infective colitis
	Gastroenteritis
	Hepatitis
	Chest infection
	Meckel's diverticulitis
Neoplastic causes	Colonic carcinoma
	Gastric carcinoma
	Small bowel tumour (e.g. GIST/carcinoid)
	Gynaecological malignancy
	Renal carcinoma
	Lymphoma
Vascular causes	Ruptured abdominal aortic, iliac or rarely other visceral aneurysms
	Aortic dissection
	Ischaemic bowel
	Myocardial infarction
	Ruptured ectopic pregnancy
	Testicular torsion
	Mesenteric arterial or venous thrombosis
	Sickle cell crisis
	Rectus sheath haematoma
Inflammatory/ autoimmune causes	Inflammatory bowel disease (Crohn's disease or ulcerative colitis)
	Pancreatitis
	Peptic ulcer disease
	Mesenteric adenitis
Trauma (haemoperitoneum) causes	Splenic injury
	Hepatic injury
	Renal injury
	Bowel injury
Endocrine causes	Addisonian crisis
	Diabetic ketoacidosis or hyperosmolar non-ketotic state
	Porphyria
Degenerative causes	Radiculopathy from spinal pathology
Metabolic causes	Renal failure with uraemia
Drugs and other causes	Medications
	Adhesional small bowel obstruction
	Incarcerated herniae

History of pain

Of particular importance is to elicit a systematic history of the pain. By using the mnemonic SOCRATES (Box 2.1.1.1) as an aide-memoire, all the features of the pain will be recorded and this will assist greatly in forming a differential diagnosis.

The site of pain is a valuable guide to the likely aetiology (Figure 2.1.1.1). Pain of sudden onset suggests either visceral perforation, aneurysm rupture, mesenteric infarction, or acute pancreatitis. The character of pain is very helpful in elucidating the diagnosis. Pain that is intermittent and of a griping nature is often described as 'colicky', and typically occurs following obstruction of a viscus, for example, intestinal, ureteric, or biliary colic. Some pain radiates in a characteristic pattern, for example, pancreatic pain radiates from the epigastrium to the back and ureteric colic radiates from the loin to the iliac fossa. The pain from diaphragmatic irritation is referred to the shoulder tip and pain that is aggravated by movement suggests peritonitis. The symptoms associated with the abdominal pain often clinch the diagnosis, for example, colicky pain and vomiting, distension and absolute constipation imply bowel obstruction.

Past medical history

Assessment of a patient's past medical history will determine whether they have an underlying systemic condition that may present as abdominal pain such as diabetes, sickle cell disease, or acute porphyria. The medication history is important with steroids and non-steroidal anti-inflammatory drugs predisposing to peptic ulceration. Anticoagulants will predispose to a spontaneous rectus sheath haematoma.

General principles of physical examination

General examination

Initially the clinician should objectively assess the severity of the pain, and then record the pulse, blood pressure, and temperature. The patient is inspected for signs of sepsis (flushed, sweaty) or shock (cold, clammy). The skin turgor and tongue are examined to assess hydration. Inspection of the eyes may reveal evidence of jaundice or anaemia. A cold, clammy patient who is lying still in obvious pain will most likely have advanced peritonitis.

Abdominal examination

The abdomen is adequately exposed and carefully observed to detect distension, visible peristalsis (bowel obstruction), incarcerated herniae, abdominal pulsation (possible leaking aneurysm), or scars from previous surgery. Asking the patient to cough or distend the abdomen exacerbates the pain of peritonitis.

The abdomen should be gently palpated in each quadrant observing the patient's response and recording the sites of tenderness and guarding. Any loin (renal angle) tenderness should be elicited. Without causing undue pain, deeper palpation is performed to detect any masses and to exclude an aortic aneurysm. If gentle percussion over areas of tenderness exacerbates the pain then this is suggestive of peritonitis. A tympanic note on percussion may be a sign of gas-filled bowel loops within the abdomen

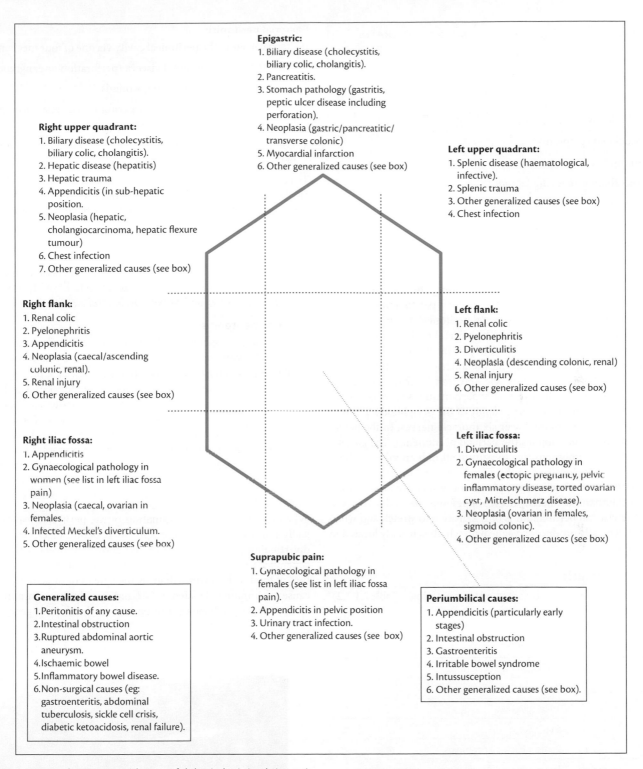

Epigastric:
1. Biliary disease (cholecystitis, biliary colic, cholangitis).
2. Pancreatitis.
3. Stomach pathology (gastritis, peptic ulcer disease including perforation).
4. Neoplasia (gastric/pancreatitic/transverse colonic)
5. Myocardial infarction
6. Other generalized causes (see box)

Right upper quadrant:
1. Biliary disease (cholecystitis, biliary colic, cholangitis).
2. Hepatic disease (hepatitis)
3. Hepatic trauma
4. Appendicitis (in sub-hepatic position.
5. Neoplasia (hepatic, cholangiocarcinoma, hepatic flexure tumour)
6. Chest infection
7. Other generalized causes (see box)

Left upper quadrant:
1. Splenic disease (haematological, infective).
2. Splenic trauma
3. Other generalized causes (see box)
4. Chest infection

Right flank:
1. Renal colic
2. Pyelonephritis
3. Appendicitis
4. Neoplasia (caecal/ascending colonic, renal).
5. Renal injury
6. Other generalized causes (see box)

Left flank:
1. Renal colic
2. Pyelonephritis
3. Diverticulitis
4. Neoplasia (descending colonic, renal)
5. Renal injury
6. Other generalized causes (see box)

Right iliac fossa:
1. Appendicitis
2. Gynaecological pathology in women (see list in left iliac fossa pain)
3. Neoplasia (caecal, ovarian in females.
4. Infected Meckel's diverticulum.
5. Other generalized causes (see box)

Left iliac fossa:
1. Diverticulitis
2. Gynaecological pathology in females (ectopic pregnancy, pelvic inflammatory disease, torted ovarian cyst, Mittelschmerz disease).
3. Neoplasia (ovarian in females, sigmoid colonic).
4. Other generalized causes (see box)

Suprapubic pain:
1. Gynaecological pathology in females (see list in left iliac fossa pain).
2. Appendicitis in pelvic position
3. Urinary tract infection.
4. Other generalized causes (see box)

Generalized causes:
1. Peritonitis of any cause.
2. Intestinal obstruction
3. Ruptured abdominal aortic aneurysm.
4. Ischaemic bowel
5. Inflammatory bowel disease.
6. Non-surgical causes (eg: gastroenteritis, abdominal tuberculosis, sickle cell crisis, diabetic ketoacidosis, renal failure).

Periumbilical causes:
1. Appendicitis (particularly early stages)
2. Intestinal obstruction
3. Gastroenteritis
4. Irritable bowel syndrome
5. Intussusception
6. Other generalized causes (see box).

Fig. 2.1.1.1 Diagram showing potential causes of abdominal pain in relation to site.

and percussion can also be used to elicit shifting dullness indicating the presence of ascites. Normally percussion over the liver produces a dull note but following perforation of a peptic ulcer a large amount of intraperitoneal air may be trapped between the abdominal wall and the liver and a resonant percussion note will be audible.

On auscultation, loud, frequent, and high-pitched (tinkling) bowel sounds will be heard in association with intestinal obstruction whereas in advanced peritonitis the abdomen will be silent.

It is important to examine the heart and lungs as a myocardial infarction and lower lobe pneumonia may present with abdominal pain.

Box 2.1.1.1 Taking a history of abdominal pain—'SOCRATES'

- Site
- Onset
- Character
- Radiation or referred pain
- Associated symptoms
- Timing
- Exacerbating/relieving factors
- Severity.

Peritonitis

The peritoneum

The peritoneum is a serous membrane lining the abdominal cavity. It consists of two parts with the visceral peritoneum covering the abdominal organs and the parietal peritoneum lining the inner surfaces of the abdominal cavity. The parietal peritoneum is richly innervated and extremely sensitive to painful stimuli.

The parietal peritoneum lining the anterior abdominal wall is supplied by the lower six thoracic and first lumbar nerves. The central portion of the diaphragmatic peritoneum is supplied by the phrenic nerves whilst the nerve supply of the peripheral regions of the diaphragm is from the lower six thoracic nerves. In the pelvis, the obturator nerve supplies the parietal peritoneum. The parietal peritoneum is highly sensitive to painful stimuli and the resultant pain is accurately localized to the affected dermatome.

In contrast, the nervous supply of the visceral peritoneum is from the autonomic afferent nerves supplying the underlying viscera. The visceral peritoneum is only sensitive to stretch and when irritated typically produces a vague pain which is usually located in the midline.[3]

Acute peritonitis

Peritonitis can be classified according to its aetiology (Table 2.1.1.2).

Table 2.1.1.2 Causes of peritonitis

Bacterial peritonitis	Perforated diverticulum
	Acute appendicitis
	Tuberculosis
	Salpingitis
	Primary bacterial peritonitis
Chemical peritonitis	Perforated peptic ulcer (usually chemical peritonitis initially then soon progresses to bacterial peritonitis)
	Biliary peritonitis
Ischaemic	Strangulated bowel
	Mesenteric ischaemia
Trauma	Traumatic injury
	Postoperative complications
Allergic reaction	Starch peritonitis

Bacterial peritonitis

Bacteria can enter the peritoneal cavity via one of four mechanisms:

1. From the intra-abdominal viscera (perforation or gangrene)

2. From the outside (penetrating wound)

3. From the bloodstream: primary peritonitis can result from translocation of bacteria following septicaemia

4. From the female genital tract: the uterine tubes provide a portal of entry (acute salpingitis).

The concentration of bacteria within the gastrointestinal tract is usually low until the distal small bowel is reached, and the highest concentrations are found within the colon. The biliary system is usually sterile but becomes contaminated when obstructed leading to cholangitis. Bacteria of gastrointestinal origin include *Escherichia coli, Streptococcus, Bacteriodes, Clostridium, Klebsiella,* and *Staphylococcus.* Primary bacterial peritonitis rarely may arise from organisms outside the gut including *Chlamydia, Gonococcus,* beta-haemolytic streptococci, *Pneumococcus,* and *Mycobacterium tuberculosis.*

Localized peritonitis

The parietal peritoneum produces two potential spaces within the abdominal cavity: the greater and lesser sacs. The greater sac is subdivided into several regions—subphrenic, pelvic, supracolic compartment (above the transverse colon mesentery) and infracolic compartment (below the transverse colon mesentery). These anatomical divisions provide a natural barrier to the spread of infection and help to localize the pathological process.[3] In addition, fibrin produced by the inflamed peritoneum promotes local adhesion of bowel loops and the greater omentum that together reduce the spread of infection (Figure 2.1.1.2).

Generalized peritonitis

When there is rapid contamination of the peritoneal cavity, typically following a perforated appendix, peptic ulcer, or sigmoid diverticulum, the factors described above are overwhelmed and generalized peritonitis occurs. Peristalsis stimulated by the ingestion of food or laxatives enhances the spread of infection, and any cause of immune deficiency (steroid use, human immunodeficiency virus) predisposes the patient to developing generalized peritonitis (Figure 2.1.1.3).

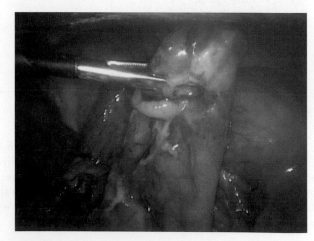

Fig. 2.1.1.2 Localized peritonitis with pus formation around an inflamed appendix.

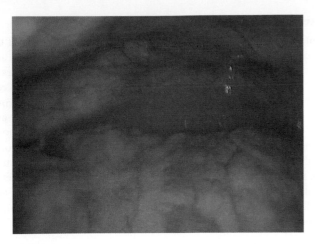

Fig. 2.1.1.3 Diagnostic laparoscopy in a patient with generalized peritonitis reveals free pus within the pelvis.

Clinical features

Severe, constant abdominal pain is the predominant feature of peritonitis and this is sharply aggravated by the slightest movement. Radiation of the pain to the shoulder tip implies irritation of the peritoneum lining the diaphragm. Vomiting frequently occurs as result of a secondary ileus, and the patient will mount a systemic inflammatory response manifest by a high temperature and tachycardia.

Tenderness and guarding occur at the site of peritoneal irritation, which is aggravated by gentle percussion or releasing the examining hand (rebound tenderness). Localized pelvic peritonitis (pelvic appendicitis or salpingitis) produces minimal abdominal signs but severe pain is elicited by rectal or vaginal examination (Figure 2.1.1.4).

Although a patient with generalized peritonitis typically lies still with an exquisitely tender and rigid abdomen, the signs may be attenuated in the elderly or immunosuppressed. With onset of paralytic ileus, the bowel sounds will reduce and eventually disappear. This is a surgical emergency and without rapid intervention septic shock develops. The temperature and pulse initially rise but without treatment the patient eventually decompensates becoming hypotensive, cold (hypothermic), and clammy. This presentation carries a dismal prognosis.

Investigations in peritonitis

Blood tests

A significant leucocytosis is usually present, although in advanced cases a normal leucocyte count or even leucopenia may be evident, which signifies bone marrow suppression, and is a worrying abnormality. Sequestration of fluid and secondary sepsis will impair renal function. A significantly elevated serum amylase (greater than three times times normal) is strongly indicative of pancreatitis, but remember, moderately raised levels are frequently detected in other causes of peritonitis.[4,5] Metabolic acidosis or raised lactate levels are typically found in advanced cases of mesenteric ischaemia or septicaemic shock. However, the lactate level may be normal in bowel strangulation as the venous obstruction prevents the increased lactate from entering the systemic circulation.[6]

Plain chest and abdominal X-rays

An erect chest radiograph often (in around 70% of cases) but not invariably shows free air below the diaphragm following visceral perforation.[7] An abdominal radiograph may show dilated loops of bowel due to paralytic ileus, or may reveal free air trapped between the dilated loops of bowel giving the appearance of gas on both sides of the bowel wall (Rigler's or double-wall sign).

Abdominal CT scan

This is extremely valuable in identifying the cause of peritonitis, being particularly helpful in confirming a perforated viscus. The detailed information provided often enables a decision to be made on the need for surgery and the operative approach. However, unstable patients with obvious peritonitis require immediate surgery and waiting for a CT scan may reduce survival (Figure 2.1.1.5).

Treatment

Initial management of patients with peritonitis

This includes intravenous fluid resuscitation, broad-spectrum antibiotics, adequate analgesia, and patient optimization prior to definitive treatment.

Early administration of broad-spectrum antibiotics against both aerobic and anaerobic organisms has been shown to provide a survival benefit.[8] Insertion of a nasogastric tube will reduce peritoneal

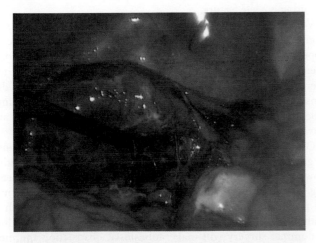

Fig. 2.1.1.4 Acute salpingitis with associated peritonitis and secondary inflammatory adhesions to the small bowel.

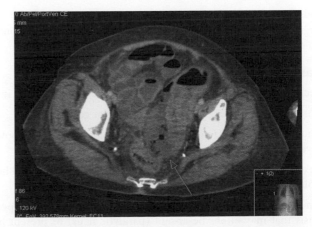

Fig. 2.1.1.5 CT scan of a patient with signs of generalized peritonitis. The arrow show free intraperitoneal air between loops of swollen bowel, confirming the presence of a perforated viscus.

contamination from a perforated peptic ulcer, and help to prevent vomiting and aspiration. Resuscitation should occur rapidly and not delay surgery and definitive control of the septic focus.

Basic principles of surgical treatment

Although a laparotomy remains the mainstay of treatment for generalized peritonitis, localized peritonitis is often managed conservatively, particularly sigmoid diverticulitis or an appendicular mass. Increasingly, interventional radiology is used to drain a septic focus, thus avoiding major surgery.

When performing a laparotomy for peritonitis it is necessary to identify and correct the cause, followed by a very thorough saline lavage of the entire peritoneal cavity, with special attention to paid to the pelvis, sub-phrenic, and sub-hepatic spaces to avoid the development of postoperative collections.

Perforated peptic ulcer

Patients with a perforated peptic ulcer require closure of the defect with an omental patch. This procedure is usually performed via an upper midline laparotomy, but in the stable patient may also be completed laparoscopically. Around 50% of perforated peptic ulcers seal spontaneously[9,10] and it may therefore be possible to treat these patients conservatively, particularly the elderly with significant pre-morbid disease. However, failure to improve will dictate urgent surgical intervention despite the risks.[11]

Perforated diverticular disease

Traditionally this has been treated with a laparotomy and Hartmann's procedure. However, a more minimal approach with an initial laparoscopy is gaining acceptance. If there is gross faecal spillage then the surgeon would proceed to a Hartmann's procedure. However, if there is minimal contamination, a thorough peritoneal washout, local drainage, and intravenous antibiotics may suffice.[12]

Other causes

Perforated acute appendicitis requires prompt appendicectomy. Gangrenous cholecystitis is occasionally encountered, necessitating cholecystectomy. Small bowel infarction following large vessel occlusion or strangulation will require resection of the necrotic segment.

Abdominal distension

Abdominal distension may be a feature in numerous medical and surgical conditions, although when considering the acute abdomen the most common cause is intestinal obstruction.

Classification of bowel obstruction

Mechanical (dynamic) obstruction is conveniently subdivided into:

- intraluminal causes (e.g. impacted faeces or gallstone ileus)
- intramural causes (e.g. malignant pathology within the bowel wall or inflammatory strictures)
- extramural causes (e.g. adhesional obstruction, strangulated herniae, or volvulus).

Functional (adynamic) obstruction is due to impaired peristalsis that may either be absent (paralytic ileus) or present but non-propulsive (e.g. pseudo-obstruction or mesenteric vascular occlusion).[13]

Pathophysiology of bowel obstruction

During dynamic obstruction there is progressive dilatation of the proximal bowel due to swallowed air, overgrowth of bacteria, and fluid secreted from the bowel wall. Increased peristalsis occurs in an attempt to encourage bowel transit and this causes severe colicky pain. In the early stages, increased peristaltic waves beyond the obstruction can cause spurious diarrhoea. Systemic fluid and electrolyte losses occur due to sequestration within the bowel lumen, and stagnant bacteria may translocate through the bowel wall to produce a bacteraemia. This is particularly likely to occur if the natural barrier is impaired due to bowel ischaemia. Unrelieved obstruction results in a progressive increase in wall tension and oedema, which together impair venous drainage and eventually arterial flow. Ischaemia and even perforation may ensue.[14]

Causes of bowel obstruction

The dynamic causes include adhesions, herniae, malignant large bowel obstruction, inflammatory bowel disease, volvulus, gallstone ileus, intussusception, and other rare pathology. In addition, colonic pseudo-obstruction must be considered, especially in the elderly patient with comorbidity. A detailed discussion of these pathological processes is provided in Chapter 2.5.1.

Clinical history in bowel obstruction

The four symptoms experienced are pain, vomiting, distension, and constipation. The preponderance of each symptom at presentation will depend upon the site and duration of the obstruction, the underlying pathology, and the presence of intestinal ischaemia. The pain experienced is often severe but typically colicky in nature. The development of constant pain with features of peritoneal irritation is a worrying event suggesting bowel ischaemia. Most patients describe constipation that can be absolute (with neither faeces nor flatus passed) or relative (where only flatus is passed). In some cases, the onset of constipation is delayed as a result of evacuation of bowel content distal to the obstruction.

Proximal small bowel obstruction will usually present with profuse vomiting, whereas a more distal occlusion will produce initial symptoms of pain and distension, with more delayed vomiting. Large bowel obstruction usually causes significant abdominal distension and absolute constipation, but the pain is less severe, and vomiting is a late feature.

Vomiting occurs early in cases of proximal small bowel obstruction but much later in colonic obstruction. The vomitus changes in appearance as the condition progresses from initial digested food, then bile, and eventually feculent material which is due to the fermentation of bacteria within the dilated bowel. The degree of distension is dependent upon the level of obstruction being minimal when the lesion is in the proximal small bowel, but an early and obvious feature of distal small bowel and colonic obstruction.

Other features in the history are related to the underlying cause. A groin swelling may have been noticed, or the patient with a bowel tumour may describe a change in bowel habit, rectal bleeding, or weight loss. A history of inflammatory bowel disease may be present or prodromal symptoms of Crohn's disease such as cramping pain, diarrhoea, and weight loss. A history of previous abdominal surgery will make adhesional obstruction the most likely diagnosis.

Clinical examination in bowel obstruction

In advanced cases, there may be evidence of dehydration and a compensatory tachycardia. A pyrexia and hypotension are very worrying features that suggest bowel ischaemia or perforation and the need for rapid intervention.

Inspection may reveal abdominal distension and in thin patients the peristaltic waves may be clearly visible. Visible peristalsis is a characteristic feature of mechanical obstruction.

Gentle palpation of the abdomen will often elicit diffuse mild tenderness in simple obstruction, but localized signs of peritonitis suggest bowel ischaemia. A rigid abdomen with obvious peritonitis is indicative of bowel infarction and/or perforation. In left-sided colonic obstruction, the finding of distension and marked tenderness in the right iliac fossa usually indicates caecal wall ischaemia as a result of a closed-loop obstruction (obstruction of the large bowel with a competent ileocaecal valve), with the possibility of imminent caecal perforation.

All hernial orifices must be carefully examined to fully exclude a strangulated hernia (a tense, tender irreducible swelling).

Auscultation will usually reveal high-pitched (tinkling), overactive bowel sounds in distal small bowel and colonic obstruction. In marked contrast, the bowel sounds will be sluggish or absent in cases of paralytic ileus or bowel ischaemia.

Rectal examination may help to differentiate between dynamic or adynamic causes of colonic obstruction. In pseudo-obstruction the rectum is often dilated, whereas it is usually collapsed in the presence of a proximal obstruction.

Investigations in bowel obstruction

Blood tests

All patients require a blood count and full biochemical screen. Iron deficiency anaemia is strongly suggestive of an underlying malignancy, and a leucocytosis may indicate the presence of bowel ischaemia or perforation. In cases of likely pseudo-obstruction it is important to check the serum magnesium, as low levels can be a causative factor. Arterial blood gas analysis may reveal a metabolic acidosis and a raised lactate level indicative of bowel ischaemia.

Plain X-rays

Following an obstruction there is progressive dilatation of large and small bowel that can be easily visualized on an abdominal radiograph. Dilated loops of small bowel are recognized by their valvulae conniventes (radio-opaque bands which traverse the full diameter of the bowel loop). Dilated colon is distinguished from small bowel by anatomical position and typical haustral folds. Small bowel and large bowel loops are considered to be pathological when their diameters exceed 4 cm and 6 cm respectively.

A grossly dilated caecum (> 9 cm) in the absence of small bowel obstruction implies that there may be a closed-loop obstruction that will necessitate emergency intervention to avoid caecal ischaemia. In mechanical obstruction, the rectum is usually empty and not visible, in contrast to a pseudo-obstruction, when the gas-filled rectum can be clearly seen. Both sigmoid and caecal volvulus produce classical X-ray appearances with the former being compared to a 'coffee-bean' (Figure 2.1.1.6).

CT scan

In patients who are clinically stable and have no indication for immediate laparotomy (peritonitis, septic shock, evidence of

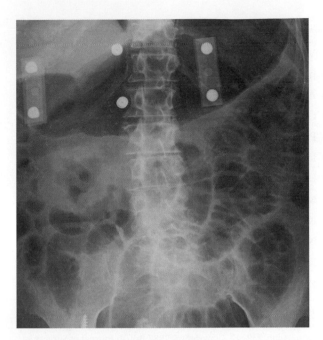

Fig. 2.1.1.6 Plain abdominal X-ray showing marked dilatation of the stomach and small intestine. The valvulae conniventes are easily seen especially in the bowel loops on the right side of the upper abdomen.

intestinal perforation on erect chest X-ray), an urgent CT scan can confirm a mechanical obstruction, usually identify the site, and often the pathological cause. Tumours and inflammatory strictures may be identified allowing an appropriate and planned intervention. CT imaging can also diagnose gallstone ileus (an opacity within the lumen of the small bowel coupled with aerobilia), and intussusception ('target-sign' appearance). An acute 'transition point' without a visible soft tissue mass is diagnostic of obstruction due to adhesions or a congenital band.

Initial management of bowel obstruction

The initial management consists of fluid and electrolyte replacement, and insertion of a wide-bore nasogastric (Ryle's) tube to decompress the distended bowel (so-called drip and suck). Urinary catheterization and hourly measurement of urine output helps guide fluid management, Nasogastric decompression reduces pain, and stable patients may then be investigated. Although some patients will improve and the obstruction will resolve, many will require definitive treatment, which is tailored to the specific aetiology. The indications for surgery and the specific operative management are described in Chapter 2.5.1.

Non-specific abdominal pain

Non-specific abdominal pain (NSAP) is defined as 'pain for which no immediate cause can be found and specifically does not require any surgical intervention'. It is considered a diagnosis of exclusion and has been reported to account for up to 40% of presentations with abdominal pain.[15] However, some patients may be inappropriately labelled as suffering NSAP, and if they are thoroughly investigated (including laparoscopy) the overall incidence of NSAP reduces to around 27%.[16,17]

NSAP is potentially a dangerous diagnosis to make as serious underlying pathology can be missed. It has been documented that

> **Box 2.1.1.2** Causes of non-specific abdominal pain
>
> ◆ Viral or bacterial infections
> ◆ Irritable bowel syndrome
> ◆ Abdominal wall pain
> ◆ Gynaecological causes
> ◆ Psychosomatic pain
> ◆ Iatrogenic peripheral nerve injuries
> ◆ Hernias
> ◆ Myofascial pain syndromes
> ◆ Rib tip syndrome
> ◆ Nerve root pain
> ◆ Rectus sheath haematoma
> ◆ Worm infestations.
>
> Source: data from Gray DWR, Collin J, Non-specific abdominal pain as a cause of acute admission to hospital, *British Journal of Surgery*, Volume 74, Issue 4, pp. 239–42, Copyright © 1987 British Journal of Surgery Society Ltd.

10% of patients over 50 who present to hospital with abdominal pain have an intra-abdominal malignancy.[18] In this series, half of those who were subsequently diagnosed with a malignancy had initially been discharged with a diagnosis of NSAP.

Potential causes of NSAP are shown in Box 2.1.1.2.[15]

Assessment and management of non-specific abdominal pain

A thorough history and physical examination is mandatory. In females, it is important to obtain a full gynaecological history, and a pregnancy test to exclude an ectopic pregnancy. Routine blood investigations and urinalysis must be performed and an ultrasound scan is helpful in excluding obvious pathology. If the diagnosis remains elusive then NSAP is a possible diagnosis.

These patients are difficult to manage as their pain is genuine but there is no particular remedy. The traditional management is to admit and actively observe. A specific diagnosis may become evident, but usually the symptoms either resolve or persist without any clinical deterioration, or change of the inflammatory markers (leucocyte count or C-reactive protein). CT scanning is occasionally helpful in older patients who may have an occult malignancy, but does impart a significant radiation dose, and must therefore be used judiciously, particularly in young women. The mean hospital stay of patients undergoing active observation for NSAP ranges from 2 to 7.3 days.[19]

Some studies have suggested that early laparoscopy in patients with NSAP can increase the proportion of patients in whom a definitive diagnosis is established.[20] This potential benefit was supported by a 2011 systematic review.[19] In a group of patients undergoing early laparoscopy a final diagnosis was established in 79.2–96.9% of patients compared to 28.1–78.1% of patients who only had active observation. Laparoscopy also led to a therapeutic procedure in 10.9–86.5% of patients. Eventual hospital stay was also shorter in the early laparoscopy group (1.3–4.18 days compared to 2–7.3 days in the active observation group). However, the studies assessed were very heterogeneous and it is the authors' view that laparoscopy should only be performed if clinically indicated. In the senior author's experience, diagnostic laparoscopy is rarely of help in a patient with normal inflammatory markers and an unequivocally normal ultrasound examination. Such patients can be discharged with careful advice and early follow-up.

References

1. Health & Social Care Information Centre. *Hospital Episode Statistics, Admitted Patient Care—England 2011-2012.* [Online] http://www.hscic.gov.uk/catalogue/PUB08288
2. Parchment Smith C. Acute abdominal pain. In *Essential Revision Notes for Intercollegiate MRCS Book 2.* Cheshire: PasTest; 2006:232–7.
3. Thompson J. The peritoneum, omentum, mesentery and retroperitoneal space. In Russel RCG, Williams NS, Bulstrode C (eds) *Bailey and Love's Short Practice of Surgery* (24th ed). London: Arnold; 2004:1133–52.
4. Swensson EE, Maull KI. Clinical significance of elevated serum and urine amylase levels in patients with appendicitis. *Am J Surg* 1981; 142:667–70.
5. Wilson C, Imrie CW. Amylase and gut infarction. *Br J Surg* 1986; 73:219–21.
6. Filsoufi F, Rahmanian PB, Castillo JG, *et al.* Predictors and outcome of gastrointestinal complications in patients undergoing cardiac surgery. *Ann Surg* 2007; 246:323–9.
7. Chen CH, Yang CC, Yeh YH. Role of upright chest radiography and ultrasonography in demonstrating free air of perforated peptic ulcers. *Hepatogastroenterology* 2001; 48:1082–4.
8. Dellinger RP, Levy MM, Rhodes A, *et al.* Surviving Sepsis Campaign: International Guidelines for Management of Severe Sepsis and Septic Shock: 2012. *Crit Care Med* 2013; 41(2):580–637.
9. Donovan AJ, Berne TV, Donovan JA. Perforated duodenal ulcer: an alternative therapeutic plan. *Arch Surg* 1998; 133:1166–71.
10. Bucher P, Oulhaci W, Morel P, *et al.* Results of conservative treatment for perforated gastroduodenal ulcers in patients not eligible for surgical repair. *Swiss Med Wkly* 2007; 137:337–40.
11. Ng E. Perforations of the upper gastrointestinal tract. In Paterson-Brown S (ed) *Core Topics in General and Emergency Surgery* (4th ed). Edinburgh: Saunders Elsevier; 2009:97–108.
12. Swank HA, Mulder IM, Hoofwijk AG, *et al.* Early experience with laparoscopic lavage for perforated diverticulitis. *Br J Surg* 2013; 100(5):704–10.
13. Winslet M. Intestinal obstruction. In Russel RCG, Williams NS, Bulstrode C (eds) *Bailey and Love's Short Practice of Surgery* (24th ed). London: Arnold; 2004:1187–202.
14. Paterson-Brown S. Acute conditions of the small bowel and appendix. In Paterson-Brown S (ed) *Core Topics in General and Emergency Surgery* (4th ed). Edinburgh: Saunders Elsevier; 2009:147–66.
15. Gray DWR, Collin J. Non-specific abdominal pain as a cause of acute admission to hospital. *Br J Surg* 1987; 74:239–42.
16. Paterson-Brown S. The acute abdomen: the role of laparoscopy. In Williamson RCN, Thompson JN (eds), *Balliere's Clinical Gastroenterology: Gastrointestinal Emergencies, Part 1.* London: Balliere Tindall; 1991:691–703.
17. Paterson-Brown S. Organisation of emergency general surgical services and the early assessment and investigation of the acute abdomen. In Paterson-Brown S (ed) *Core Topics in General and Emergency Surgery* (4th ed). Edinburgh: Saunders Elsevier; 2009:81–95.
18. de Dombal FT, Matharu SS, Staniland JR, *et al.* Presentation of cancer to hospital as 'acute abdominal pain'. *Br J Surg* 1980; 67:413–16.
19. Dominguez LC, Sanabria A, Vega V, *et al.* Early laparoscopy for the evaluation of nonspecific abdominal pain: a critical appraisal of the evidence. *Surg Endosc* 2011; 25(1):10–18.
20. Morino M, Pellegrino L, Castagna E. Acute nonspecific abdominal pain, a randomized, controlled trial comparing early laparoscopy versus clinical observation. *Ann Surg* 2006; 244(6):881–7.

Abdominal wall and hernias

Abdominal wall and hernias

Peter Sedman

Introduction

Hernia repairs comprise a significant proportion of the general surgeon's workload in both elective and emergency practice and present a variety of challenges in their treatment.

The constant evolution of the methods of hernia repair over the years testifies to the imperfection of the techniques in common use and this evolution will continue for the foreseeable future. Perhaps the two most significant developments in recent years have been the introduction of laparoscopic surgery and the continuing development of mesh materials and, for both, there is an evolving appreciation of the benefits they bring to specific situations.

A hernia is defined as the abnormal protrusion of a viscus or fat through a defect in the surrounding wall. Although they can occur at many sites, most are predictable and the techniques used to repair them vary from site to site; in some, meshes are invaluable, whereas in others they are best avoided. Most herniae are 'reducible', meaning that the contents may be manipulated back into the cavity. They are 'incarcerated' when they cannot be returned and 'strangulated' when the blood supply to the contents of the hernia becomes obstructed, a serious, potentially fatal complication when bowel is involved. Some herniae are more likely to strangulate than others; when there is a narrow and/or indistensible neck, such as occurs in the femoral canal or where the hernias are recurrent and breach scar tissue. Herniae with wide pliable necks, in contrast, rarely strangulate.

Occasionally, just one edge of the bowel may strangulate, a condition known as a Richter hernia, and these may or may not present as bowel obstruction.

Most herniae occur through defects in the full thickness of the abdominal wall and are visible externally, but others pass through the diaphragm (e.g. hiatus hernia) or pelvis (e.g. obturator hernia) or within peritoneal defects (internal herniae), and may be very difficult to diagnose. Occasionally, they pass only part way through the abdominal wall and are termed 'interparietal'.

Approximately 75% of abdominal wall hernias are located in the groin (inguinal and femoral hernias), with umbilical and incisional herniae forming the majority of the remainder.

Inguinal hernia

Inguinal herniae are the commonest herniae to occur and, in England, over 60 000 inguinal hernia repair operations are performed annually (1 per 1000 of the population). Approximately 1 in 20 men will develop an inguinal hernia during their lifetime, 1 in 4 of whom may develop a contralateral defect. Over 95% of groin hernia in men and two-thirds in women are inguinal with the remainder being femoral. Inguinal herniae are approximately 100 times less common in women than men and, overall, are slightly more common on the right compared to the left (perhaps as a result of previous appendicectomies weakening the abdominal wall).

Anatomy

A thorough understanding of the inguinal anatomy is essential to the hernia surgeon.

The groin above the inguinal ligament operates as a shutter mechanism comprising three muscle layers with staggered openings, creating an oblique passage through the anterior abdominal wall (the inguinal canal). This canal runs above and parallel to the inguinal ligament. Through this canal, the testicular vessels and vas deferens pass. These structures exit the abdomen through the superficial inguinal ring, which is an opening in the external oblique aponeurosis located above and medial to the pubic tubercle. They pass collectively into the scrotum. Posteriorly, they enter the abdomen through the deep inguinal ring, an opening in the transversalis fascia immediately lateral to the inferior epigastric artery at the midpoint of the inguinal ligament and here they diverge; the vas deferens passing inferomedially over the pectineal line of the pelvis to join the seminal vesicles, while the testicular vessels pass inferolaterally to their destinations at or near the renal vessels 20–30 cm from the deep ring. In a woman, the inguinal canal transmits the round ligament, which is the embryonic remnant of the gubernaculum (and which may be readily divided during hernia repair).

In a child, the openings of the three layers of muscle overlay each other and it is only with growth that the shutter mechanism evolves. This is relevant because, in a child, it is necessary only to ligate the peritoneal sac of the hernia to repair it and allow natural growth to mature the obliquity and ultimate strength of the inguinal canal.

It is important to appreciate the course of the nerves passing close to the inguinal canal because surgical damage to these can cause chronic groin pain, a very important cause of postoperative morbidity. The nerves, which need to be considered, depend upon whether an anterior approach to repair is used (open surgery) or a posterior approach (laparoscopic surgery).

For the anterior approach, the relevant nerves are the ilioinguinal and iliohypogastric nerves and the genital branch of the genitofemoral nerve. These lie just deep to the internal oblique muscle in the lateral part of the inguinal canal, and more medially in the plane between the internal and external oblique muscles.

The important nerves for laparoscopic repair are the lateral femoral cutaneous nerve and the genitofemoral nerve, which lie in the preperitoneal space lateral to the inferior epigastric artery and below the inguinal ligament. Care should be taken and staples avoided in this area.

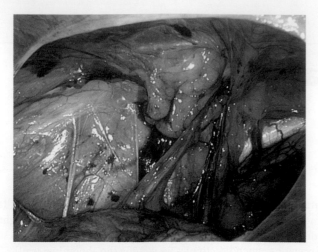

Fig. 2.2.1.1 The laparoscopic appearance of the right groin in a man demonstrating the anatomy and the presence of a direct, an indirect, and a femoral hernia.

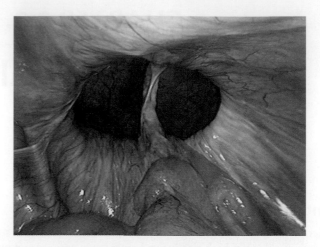

Fig. 2.2.1.2 A 'pantaloon' hernia in the right groin.

Within the inguinal wall, there are two common sites of potential weakness in the transversalis fascia through which two different types of inguinal hernia can occur. These are the indirect and direct type of inguinal hernia (Figure 2.2.1.1).

Indirect herniae are the commonest and account for approximately 80% of inguinal herniae overall. Almost all inguinal herniae in women and, in men under 55 years of age, are indirect, with the weakness lying above the cord structures at the deep inguinal ring causing the peritoneal sac to prolapse along the route of the inguinal canal and testicular vessels. Its deep origin through the transversalis is, therefore, lateral to the inferior epigastric vessels. It exits the inguinal canal through the superficial ring and, when very large, into the scrotum.

'Direct' inguinal herniae (~20%) follow a different route and 'punch' their way directly through the three layers of inguinal muscles. This weakness occurs medial to the epigastric vessels and pushes directly towards the skin.

Sometimes the route may be modified by the external oblique, in which case external examination is unable to confidently distinguish it from an indirect hernia. In addition, a direct and an indirect hernia can coexist in the same groin; this is the 'pantaloon' hernia (Figure 2.2.1.2).

Large inguinal hernia usually contain small bowel, which is usually easily reducible, but on the left side the sigmoid colon may be involved. This is called a 'sliding' hernia, in which the inferior border of the hernia sac is the sigmoid colon and mesentery. Direct and sliding hernias rarely cause obstruction and in elderly men may not need operation where symptoms are minimal.

The Nyhus classification (Box 2.2.1.1) is a common classification of all groin herniae.

Diagnosis

Most inguinal herniae are clinically obvious and present with a palpable or visible swelling in the inguinal canal. Further investigation is usually unnecessary. Demonstration of a cough impulse is usually possible, but a cough impulse in the absence of a palpable, and usually reducible, lump is insufficient to diagnose a hernia. An innocent lipoma of the spermatic cord is enough to cause these findings and does not need treatment.

Where clinical findings are equivocal, ultrasound may be used in addition to clinical examination, but this is controversial with high false-positive rates and definitely not to be interpreted in the absence of careful clinical examination. It is, therefore, recommended that its use be reserved for the secondary care setting. Magnetic resonance imaging may have some additional value in evaluating chronic pain in the absence of clinically apparent hernia, but the decision to operate is ultimately based on clinical judgement alone.

Box 2.2.1.1 The Nyhus classification of groin herniae

Type 1

Indirect inguinal hernia with normal internal ring (e.g. paediatric hernia).

Type 2

Indirect inguinal hernia—internal inguinal ring dilated but posterior inguinal wall intact; inferior epigastric vessels not displaced.

Type 3

Posterior wall defect:

A. Direct inguinal hernia

B. Indirect inguinal hernia—internal inguinal ring dilated, medially encroaching on or destroying the transversalis fascia of Hesselbach's triangle (e.g. scrotal, sliding, or pantaloons hernia)

C. Femoral hernia.

Type 4

Recurrent hernia:

A. Direct

B. Indirect

C. Femoral

D. Combined.

Reprinted from *Surgical Clinics of North America*, Volume 73, Issue 3, Nyhus LM, Iliopubic tract repair of inguinal and femoral hernia: The posterior preperitoneal approach, pp. 487–499, Copyright © 1993, http://www.sciencedirect.com/science/journal/00396109

Who should be offered surgery?

The routine use of a truss is not recommended, but may rarely be useful in highly selected patients. Beyond this, the only decision is to operate or not.

All patients with recurrent hernia should be offered surgery, unless there are prohibitive medical risks, because the strangulation rate may be as high as 50% over 5 years. Up to 80% of patients have attended, primarily because they fear cancer, when the lump is first noticed and initial reassurance is necessary. For patients with symptoms (groin pain or dragging ache), the decision to proceed to surgery is usually obvious, but for the patient with an asymptomatic primary hernia, it is more difficult and judged on the natural history of inguinal herniae.

If untreated, approximately one-third of asymptomatic hernias will become symptomatic over the subsequent 2 years and patients will reconsider the surgical option. Of all inguinal hernia at presentation (both symptomatic and asymptomatic), the cumulative risk of strangulation at 2 years is just under 5%. Strangulation is more likely in women than in men and some priority on the waiting list should be given to higher-risk patients.

Elective repair of inguinal hernia carries a mortality of 0.5% and is ten times higher in emergency repair (5%) and if emergency bowel resection is needed the mortality approaches 20%. These figures present a strong argument for the elective repair for all indirect inguinal hernia and most inguinal hernia overall. Direct hernia may be less likely to strangulate than indirect ones and there is an argument for not operating, especially as these patients are usually elderly, but it can be difficult to confidently distinguish direct from indirect herniae.

Surgical techniques for inguinal hernia repair

There are many inguinal hernia repairs described in the literature, but by far the most important to current practice are the Shouldice and Lichtenstein repairs for open surgery and the transabdominal preperitoneal (TAPP) and totally extraperitoneal (TEP) repairs for laparoscopic surgery. In experienced hands all have low morbidity and low recurrence rates (<1%), but in inexperienced hands morbidity may be significant.

Anterior (open) approach

The Shouldice and Lichtenstein repair are both performed by open surgery under either local or general anaesthesia. There are some advantages to the use of local anaesthesia, especially in the elderly, as these operations are associated with a higher day case and lower urinary retention rate.

The Shouldice repair gives excellent results when performed by appropriately trained high-volume surgeons, but is a difficult technique to learn and very operator dependent. A meticulous approach through the layers of the inguinal canal is required to expose and then reinforce the posterior transversalis muscle layer by dividing it and then repairing and strengthening it by performing a double breasting repair. No mesh is used, and this is the only technique of anterior repair without mesh that gives good long term results (<1% recurrence rates). No other non-mesh open repair of inguinal hernia can be recommended, as recurrence rates for these of over 15% are the historic norm.

The Lichtenstein repair is the commonest mesh repair and reinforces the inguinal canal with prosthetic mesh placed in the plane between the internal and external oblique muscles. It became possible only when mesh technology was sufficiently advanced in the 1980s onward, and replaced all other options except the Shouldice repair. In this repair, the external oblique aponeurosis and the muscle fibres surrounding the cord are dissected to allow the sac to be mobilized, separated from the cord, opened, and transected at the level of the deep ring. A mesh is then placed superficial to the external oblique muscle, with a lateral slit to accommodate the spermatic cord near the deep inguinal ring. Steps are made to ensure that the mesh extends medially to at least 1 cm beyond the pubic tubercle. The mesh is secured to the inguinal ligament and the external oblique muscle is closed superficial to this. The mesh creates a tension-free repair of the posterior inguinal wall.

Posterior/laparoscopic approach

In the laparoscopic approach, the lower abdominal wall is approached from behind and the anterior wall tissues of the inguinal canal are left untouched. By approaching from high behind the anterior abdominal wall, it is possible to utilize the natural plane between the peritoneum and the transversalis fascia without disrupting the muscles. The distal hernia sac may be reduced (always possible in a direct hernia) or simply transected (if the hernia is indirect). A large (15 × 10 cm) mesh is then placed in this newly created preperitoneal plane. This mesh is much larger than that used at open surgery and covers not only the two weak areas of the inguinal canal, but also the femoral canal and the obturator foramen. Providing the defect being covered is a reasonable size and there is at least 3 cm of healthy tissue to support the mesh in all directions from the neck, the mesh will be held in place by the peritoneum once restored and further fixation is unnecessary. Where additional mesh fixation is used, great care must be taken to avoid stapling the vessels passing under the inguinal canal and, more laterally, the lateral cutaneous nerve of thigh and the genitofemoral nerve.

TEP and TAPP merely refer to the slightly different techniques of developing the preperitoneal plane and subsequently restoring the peritoneum. In each, primary access is through the umbilicus. In the TEP repair, the peritoneal cavity is not entered and the secondary trocars are progressively inserted into the preperitoneal plane as it is developed. Consequently, at the completion of the procedure, no peritoneal repair is required as the peritoneum collapses back into its anatomical position naturally. In the TAPP approach, the primary trocar enters the peritoneal cavity directly, secondary trocars are inserted under direct vision and the peritoneum opened again in the groin to access the preperitoneal plane. In this technique the peritoneal opening needs to be closed either by suturing or with staples in order to stabilize the mesh position. It is a matter of surgical preference whether TAPP or TEP repair is used laparoscopically, as there is no consensus data to favour one over the other.

Laparoscopic repairs are technically challenging operations and considered in the spectrum of advanced laparoscopic procedures. Using the laparoscopic approach may have particular advantages in women (where there is a high rate of femoral hernia appearing simultaneously or after inguinal repair), in herniae, which are recurrent after open repair, and in bilateral hernia. Laparoscopic approaches almost always require general anaesthesia.

In the United Kingdom, the commonest means of inguinal hernia repair is the Lichtenstein repair under local anaesthetic. At least 70% of elective inguinal hernia procedures may be performed as day cases.

Femoral hernia

The vast majority of femoral herniae occur in women and comprise approximately 3% of all groin herniae overall. They are uncommon before middle age and are most common in the elderly where they are notorious as an occult cause of small bowel strangulation and primary small bowel obstruction.

The boundaries of the femoral canal through which the hernia passes are the inguinal ligament, the pectineal and lacunar lines of the pelvis, and the femoral vein. These are relatively inflexible tissues and this accounts for the high rates of strangulation seen for femoral hernias (up to 50%).

Clinically, a femoral hernia may be distinguished from an inguinal hernia as it appears below and lateral to the pubic tubercle (the superficial inguinal ring through which an inguinal hernia appears is above and medial to the pubic tubercle). A femoral hernia is usually firm, irreducible, and the size and shape of a walnut. The 6-month survival after emergency femoral hernia repair is approximately 50%, similar to that of fractured neck of femur and reflects that these herniae are often a reflection of senescence. All femoral hernias should be repaired using one of the three techniques described in the following sections.

The high approach

Both the Lothiessen and McEvedy operations approach the femoral canal from above the inguinal ligament and along the preperitoneal plane, allowing easy access into the peritoneal cavity in the event of strangulated bowel needing resection. They are, therefore, usually reserved for emergency femoral hernia repair. The Lothiessen approach involves opening the inguinal canal through all its layers in a transverse plane and the McEvedy approach involves opening the lateral part of the low anterior rectus sheath vertically retracting the rectus abdominis medially to access the preperitioneal plane.

The low approach

Named after Lockwood, this is especially useful in elective surgery and approaches the femoral canal from below the inguinal ligament. The hernia sac is mobilized and opened to inspect the contents. If tissue is incarcerated, a gentle medial splitting of fibres of the lacunar ligament with the finger widens the femoral canal allowing its contents to be inspected and reduced. The sac is transected, the femoral canal closed with either non-absorbable sutures between the pectineal line and the inguinal ligament or by using a mesh rolled up to mimic a 'cigarette stub' and used to plug the femoral canal.

The laparoscopic approach to the femoral canal is possible in experienced hands, but it is unclear whether it conveys significant advantage over the low approach which is generally very well tolerated.

Umbilical hernia

True umbilical herniae (through the umbilical sac) are congenital, present from birth, and the vast majority will heal spontaneously before the age of 6 (although not always in Afro-Caribbean children). All other herniae at the umbilicus are acquired defects and are termed 'para-' umbilical herniae, as they appear immediately above or immediately below the umbilical cicatrix, but not directly through it.

Para-umbilical herniae affect 1–2% of the population, occurring usually in midlife, in women, and the obese. Many are asymptomatic but they may range in size, sometimes becoming very large and containing the transverse colon. Where reducible, the diameter of the neck is the important parameter as those less than 1 cm in diameter will not strangulate and, if asymptomatic, may be left untreated. Those with a neck greater than 2 cm in diameter are prone to strangulation and should be repaired.

Both sutured and tension free mesh repairs are described depending on the size of the defect. For very small defects, a simple suture closure usually suffices, but where the defect is large or recurrent, mesh repair is increasingly preferred. Mesh infection in the umbilicus remains a significant postoperative complication with such repairs and usually the mesh needs removal before the infection settles. The recurrence rate after elective repair should be under 2%.

Parastomal hernia

The incidence of parastomal hernia is very high, and complicate at least 40% of ileostomies and 50% of colostomies. They may be difficult to diagnose in obese patients and are difficult to treat successfully in all patients. Such is the incidence of herniae after stoma formation, that there is a current vogue to pre-emptively use mesh during primary siting of the stoma to reduce this risk.

Both open and laparoscopic approaches are described, but there is a high failure rate and as a last resort the stoma may need to be re-sited.

Primary suture repair is simple, but almost always unsuccessful in the long term and meshes are generally preferred. Even with mesh, the failure rate is high for both open and laparoscopic approaches, the latter of which may also have to contend with abdominal adhesions. Since they rarely strangulate, routine repair of parastomal herniae is not advocated unless they become huge, very symptomatic, or stop the stoma bags from sealing effectively.

Incisional hernia

Collectively these herniae cause the most difficulties to the hernia surgeon and patient. Repair varies from the relatively simple to the incredibly complex and the realm of superspecialization. The incidence of incisional hernia after laparotomy remains stubbornly between 10% and 20% and, whilst more common after surgical site infections, they also occur as a result of patient-related biological problems (drugs, obesity, underlying diseases, etc.), which cause a failure to produce stable scar tissue. Typically these factors can be identified at the time of planned re-repair.

Incisional herniae do tend to progressively enlarge, at varying rates, and may cause pain, incarceration, and occasionally obstruction. However, if they are wide necked and causing few problems, it may be wiser not to reoperate and each hernia must be very carefully judged on its merits.

Surgical techniques

Simple suture repair has a very high recurrence rate of 60% or more and should be reserved for small herniae or in situations where there has clearly been a technical failure of closure (suture fracture etc.). For all other repairs, meshes are strongly recommended as they can halve the recurrence rates. They must, however, be placed such that they produce an overlap of at least 5–6 cm onto healthy tissue in all directions.

Incisional hernia repair is becoming a subspecialty in its own right.

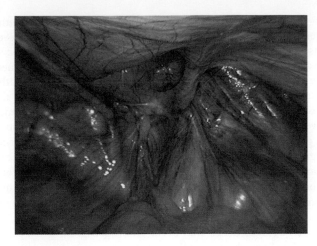

Fig. 2.2.1.3 The dissected left groin demonstrating the nerves relevant to laparoscopic groin hernia repair.

In principle, meshes may be used to either bridge the defect in a tension-free manner, or to reinforce an abdominal wall reconstruction in which the edges of the fascial defect are restored to their normal anatomical position. In this latter approach (which is increasingly favoured), this may involve extensive dissection and a degree of tension on the repair, which must be minimized. Techniques to relieve this tension are various, but the components separation techniques originally described by Ramirez, and variations on this, currently give the best results. These operations are major surgery and may take several hours to perform. Even where laparoscopic surgery is used for incisional hernia surgery, there is a growing appreciation of the need to close the fascial defect wherever possible for, without this, there will remain significant bulging and an increased risk of seroma.

In incisional hernia surgery there are a variety of positions in which the mesh can be placed and the type of mesh that will be used will reflect the position needed (Figure 2.2.1.3). Of the differing mesh placement sites, inlay meshes have very high recurrence rates and are not recommended. Onlay and sublay techniques are the most favoured for open surgery with intraperitoneal onlay mesh being the position usually adopted by laparoscopic surgeons.

Complications after incisional hernia surgery are not uncommon and include recurrence, infection, and seroma.

Ventral hernia

These are small herniae which occur in the anterior abdominal midline between the xiphoid and umbilicus, frequently in younger patients with an athletic build. They usually present with local pain and discomfort and a subcutaneous nodule to palpate. The defect in the linea alba is often tiny and the protrusion is of preperitoneal fat only. They are diagnosed by the palpation of a tiny discreet fatty lump in the midline, usually 1 cm or less in diameter, and they are relatively easy to repair by simple suture closure either under local or general anaesthetic.

They should not be confused with divarication of the rectus abdominis, which is a broad separation of the recti above the umbilicus, producing a diffuse bulge on straining. These are cosmetic changes and there is no risk of strangulation associated with them and no surgery is necessary.

Obturator hernia

These are uncommon herniae, which are difficult to diagnose and usually present as emergencies when a Richter hernia through the obturator foramen causes primary small bowel obstruction. They may occasionally be picked up on preoperative computed tomography (CT) scanning, but for the vigilant, a prodromal history of inner thigh and knee pain may be elicited. These herniae almost always occur in elderly women and lend themselves to laparoscopic mesh repair of the obturator foramen.

Spigelian hernia

These are uncommon herniae, which tend to affect elderly women and may be interparietal rather than transfascial. They occur just lateral to the rectus abdominis muscle at the point where the posterior rectus sheath disappears, one-third of the distance between the umbilicus and the pubic tubercle.

They may be repaired with either open or laparoscopic approaches.

Lumbar hernia

Lumbar herniae and complications from them are very rare. They occur through either the superior or inferior lumbar triangles and usually contain extraperitoneal fat and thus may be mistaken for lipomas. They are frequently bilateral and, if repair is chosen, this involves a mesh repair with either the open or laparoscopic approach.

Mesh technology

Prosthetic meshes are widely used in modern hernia surgery and their use has increased over the last two decades. They facilitate tension-free repairs and undoubtedly reduce the recurrence rates after surgery. Over time, there has been a massive proliferation in the range of meshes available with well over 150 different types currently available. There is very little scientific background to choose one specific mesh over another, but four broad categories may be considered: standard polypropylene, lightweight, composite, and biological.

The first meshes of 40 years ago were prone to the development of chronic infection, and this precluded their routine use. They were superseded by standard polypropylene-based mesh, which had a large pore size of 100 microns. Bacteria, being approximately 8 microns in size, could readily 'hide' in the original meshes which had pore sizes in the order of 50 microns preventing the 80 micron macrophages from effective phagocytosis and only become effective in the newer larger-pore material. Infection is, therefore, less of a problem than previously, but does still occur causing significant problems. Caution and care should still be exercised when using standard prosthetic meshes when contamination is a significant possibility.

Polypropylene incites a fibrotic response in the tissues it touches and this is one of the mechanisms of effectiveness. Over time, however, this scarring will progress and the mesh contracts. In some cases, mesh contraction of as much as 40% may be seen and this may be too much. Lightweight meshes were, therefore, introduced to lessen this effect and these are shown to contract less without significantly compromising strength or repair success rates. They are lighter in part because of their component material (part absorbable, part permanent) and because of the more open weave, which inhibits bridging fibrosis between the filaments and therefore contraction. Lightweight meshes may reduce postoperative pain caused by fibrotic scarring and neuropathic injury, which is a significant complication when it occurs.

The fibrogenic aspect of meshes mean also that they must be placed in environments where this is not a problem. They should not be used in growing tissues (children) or within the peritoneal cavity next to bowel unless absolutely necessary. A specific example is the avoidance of non-absorbable meshes around the oesophagus in hiatus hernia repair wherever possible, because of the risk of erosion into the gullet.

For use near to bowel, composite meshes have been developed. These are coated on one side with a layer designed to inhibit adhesions allowing them to be used within the peritoneum, notably for incisional hernia repair.

The fourth category of mesh is the absorbable mesh, which will slowly dissolve/resorb over time. Their major advantage is in infected or colonized wounds, where short-term strength is needed, but chronic infection will not occur once the mesh has been replaced by fibrotic tissue after 6 months or so. Most of this class of mesh are based on porcine, bovine, or human decellularized collagen and they are often referred to as biological meshes. They are manufactured by a labour-intensive process, which decellularizes pericardial or dermal tissue to leave a collagen lattice into which host fibroblasts can grow, ideally replacing the original scaffold over time. These meshes are extremely expensive and cost prohibits their routine use, but more recently, synthetic materials have been introduced which it is claimed achieve the same effect at a lesser cost. These meshes may also be the materials of choice when next to the bowel (e.g. in hiatal hernia repair).

Internal hernia

These are difficult to diagnose and usually present as intestinal obstruction. The commonest current cause is iatrogenic following laparoscopic Roux-en-Y gastric bypass for obesity. The internal rerouting of the intestinal limbs in this operation leaves two or three internal spaces, which, if not formally closed, may allow small bowel to prolapse, twist, and obstruct. These are potentially dangerous complications and may occur several years after the primary operation. Herniation into abnormal paraduodenal fossa may also be a cause of internal herniae in the virgin abdomen, but these too are very rare and usually diagnosed at acute CT or laparotomy.

Hiatus hernia

Hiatus herniae occur commonly and are of two types. The commoner sliding hiatus hernia may be present in up to 20% of adults. They usually manifest with reflux symptoms or are found incidentally at endoscopy. Treatment is usually based around the severity of the gastrointestinal reflux symptoms. They almost never cause local pain and, when asymptomatic, are treated medically.

Rolling hiatus herniae are much less common than sliding herniae and tend to occur in the elderly. In a rolling hiatus hernia, the gastro-oesophageal junction sits at the level of the crura and the defect lies anterior to this. These are acquired defects, which may be very large. They behave in a similar manner to direct herniae in the groin, in that the peritoneal sac may be readily reduced during surgical repair. Rolling hiatus herniae are important since they can incarcerate and/or cause a gastric volvulus. They should, therefore, all be repaired electively and they are ideally suited to the laparoscopic approach. The recurrence rate following repair is high as the tissues are often flimsy. Mesh repairs are currently discouraged.

Rarely a rolling hernia may occur on the background of a previous sliding hiatus hernia. In this mixed type, surgical repair is also recommended, but crural closure may be even more challenging and there may be a shortened oesophagus.

Further reading

International guidelines for hernia management

British Hernia Society and Association of Surgeons of Great Britain and Ireland. *Groin/Hernia Guidelines*. London: Association of Surgeons of Great Britain and Ireland; 2013. http://www.british-herniasociety.org/wp-content/uploads/2013/04/Groin-Hernia-Guidelines-BHS-2013.pdf; http://www.asgbi.org.uk/download.cfm?docid=21BC920F-290E-4CDE-B415CA77DFF1E0A0

Simons MP, Aufenacker T, Bay-Nielsen M, *et al*. European Hernia Society guidelines on the treatment of inguinal hernia in adult patients. *Hernia* 2009; 13:343–403. http://www.ncbi.nlm.nih.gov/pmc/articles/PMC2719730/

Natural history of hernias

Chung L, Norrie J, O'Dwyer PJ. Long-term follow-up of patients with a painless inguinal hernia from a randomized clinical trial. *Br J Surg* 2011; 98:595–9.

Fitzgibbons RJJr, Giobbie-Hurder A, Gibbs JO, *et al*. Watchful waiting vs repair of inguinal hernia in minimally symptomatic men: a randomized clinical trial. *JAMA* 2006; 295(3):285–92.

Incisional hernia repairs

Ramirez OM, Ruas E, Dellon AL. 'Components separation' method for closure of abdominal-wall defects: an anatomic and clinical study. *Plast Reconstr Surg* 1990; 86(3):519–26. http://education.surgery.ufl.edu/lectures/separationofcomponentsvhr.pdf

Other

Rosenberg J, Bisgaard T, Kehlet H, *et al*. Danish Hernia Database recommendations for the management of inguinal and femoral hernia in adults. *Dan Med Bull* 2011; 58(2):C4243.

Sanders DL, Kingsnorth AN. Prosthetic mesh materials used in hernia surgery. *Expert Rev Med Devices* 2012; 9(2):159–79.

PART 2.3

Upper gastro-oesophageal

CHAPTER 2.3.1

Upper gastro-oesophageal surgery

William Allum

Anatomy and physiology

Anatomy

Oesophagus

Topographical anatomy

The oesophagus is a muscular tube approximately 25 cm long connecting the oropharynx to the stomach. It is in three parts: cervical, thoracic, and abdominal. The cervical oesophagus is a continuation of the pharynx at the lower end of the cricopharyngeus muscle. Its upper limit is level with the sixth cervical vertebra. It enters the thorax at the level of the thoracic inlet lying between the trachea anteriorly and the prevertebral fascia posteriorly. Laterally are the lobes of the thyroid, the inferior thyroid artery, and the carotid sheath. The recurrent laryngeal nerves lie either side in the tracheo-oesophageal groove.

The upper thoracic oesophagus extends from the thoracic inlet to the carina. The middle and lower oesophagus lie in the posterior mediastinum subdivided at the midpoint between the carina and the gastro-oesophageal junction (GOJ). As it descends through the thorax it is closely related to the aortic arch, azygos vein, left main bronchus, right pulmonary artery, and the posterior aspect of the left atrium.

The lower thoracic oesophagus passes through the oesophageal opening in the diaphragm and lies within fibres of the left crus inside a sling passing across from the right crus. The intra-abdominal oesophagus extends to the GOJ. It is covered by peritoneum and lies posterior to the left lobe of the liver.

Blood supply

The oesophagus receives its blood supply segmentally superiorly from the inferior thyroid artery, in the chest via direct branches from the aorta, and inferiorly from ascending branches of the left gastric artery. The venous drainage is similar to the arterial supply. Venous drainage via the left gastric vein creates a portosystemic anastomosis, which results in oesophageal varices in portal hypertension.

Lymphatic drainage

The lymphatic drainage is unique for the gastrointestinal (GI) tract as there are extensive submucosal networks of lymphatic channels throughout the length of the oesophagus. As a result, lymphatic spread of tumours can be extensive. The nodal drainage reflects the arterial supply with cervical, superior, and posterior mediastinal nodes and intra-abdominal nodes.

Nerve supply

The oesophagus receives its nerve supply from parasympathetic vagal branches and the sympathetic innervation originating from the fifth and sixth thoracic spinal cord segments passing to the cervical, thoracic, and coeliac ganglia. In the chest, the vagal trunks lie to the right and left sides. At the diaphragm, the trunks lie respectively anteriorly and posteriorly having emerged from the oesophageal plexuses on its lower surface.

Histology

The oesophageal mucosa is non-keratinizing squamous epithelium with a basement membrane separating it from the underlying lamina propria and muscularis mucosa. Deep to the mucosa is the submucosa which forms the principal layer of the oesophagus. The muscle layer comprises inner circular and outer longitudinal fibres. The oesophagus does not have a serosal surface but is covered with an adventitial layer. The submucosa is clinically important as it is the strongest layer for suturing surgical anastomoses.

Stomach

Topographical anatomy

The stomach is the most dilated part of the digestive tract. It is situated between the end of the oesophagus proximally and the duodenum distally. It lies in the epigastrium, umbilical, and left hypochondrial regions of the abdomen. It occupies a recess bounded by the upper abdominal viscera, the anterior abdominal wall, and the diaphragm. It is divided into four parts: cardia, fundus, body, and antrum. The lesser curve is the right border and measures approximately 10 cm. The junction between the body and antrum is designated by the incisura. The greater curve forms the left border and is approximately 15–20 cm long.

The peritoneal attachment to the lesser curve forms the lesser omentum which extends from the cardia along the undersurface of the liver as far as the porta hepatis. The anterior peritoneal surface of the stomach provides attachment for the greater omentum, which on the proximal upper third gives rise to the gastrosplenic omentum and distally forms the gastrocolic omentum. The proximal third of the greater curve is closely related to the spleen laterally and the body and tail of the pancreas posteriorly. The distal end of the antrum forms the pylorus, which is a circular muscular ring between the stomach and duodenum.

Blood supply

The blood supply of the stomach is from the branches of the coeliac axis: the hepatic, the splenic, and the left gastric arteries. The left gastric artery supplies the lesser curve via ascending and descending branches. The right gastric artery arises from the hepatic artery supplying the antrum and distal lesser curve. The right gastro-epiploic artery arises from the gastroduodenal artery, a branch of the hepatic artery, and supplies the distal half of the greater curve. The left gastro-epiploic artery arises from the splenic artery and with the short gastric arteries supplies the proximal greater curve. Venous drainage reflects the arterial supply.

Lymphatic drainage
Lymphatic drainage is closely related to the arterial supply. It is arranged in tiers as perigastric (right and left cardia, lesser and greater curve, and supra and infra pyloric) and then related to artery of origin of the local vessels (left and right gastric artery, hepatic and splenic artery, and coeliac axis)

Nerve supply
The stomach receives its nerve supply from the anterior and posterior vagus nerves, the former arising from the intra-thoracic left vagus and the latter from the right trunk. The anterior vagus supplies the anterior wall and ends in the hepatic plexus; the posterior vagus supplies the posterior wall and ends in the coeliac and splenic plexuses. The sympathetic supply originates in the coeliac plexus with fibres accompanying the arterial supply.

Histology
The stomach comprises a columnar lined mucosa with a deeper submucosa. The muscularis is an inner oblique layer, with middle circular and outer longitudinal fibres. The outer serosal coat, which is attached to the muscle layer, is formed by the peritoneum. The mucosa is separated from the luminal contents by a layer of mucus.

Physiology
Oesophagus
The oesophagus is a conduit for swallowed food propelled by anti-grade peristaltic contractions from the pharynx to the stomach. Swallowing consists of a partly voluntary oropharyngeal phase and an involuntary oesophageal phase. Functionally the oesophagus has sphincters at the upper and lower end to prevent aspiration of refluxed gastric content.

The upper oesophageal sphincter lies between the pharynx and the upper oesophagus and is created by continuous muscle contractions of the cricopharyngeus and inferior constrictor muscles. Manometric pressure studies show a high pressure zone 2–4 cm long. Relaxation occurs with pharyngeal peristalsis of the food bolus with rebound high pressure once oesophageal peristalsis has started to prevent retrograde reflux.

Oesophageal peristalsis occurs by circular muscle contraction preceded by a wave of muscle inhibition. Once the bolus reaches the lower oesophagus there is a reduction in the resting tone of the circular muscle just above the GOJ. The muscle arrangement differs from the upper end although at rest there is a zone of high pressure 2–4 cm long. This together with the angulation created by the crural muscle sling produces a flap valve to minimize reflux. Failure of the lower oesophageal sphincter to relax is characteristic of achalasia in which there is defect in the myenteric plexus.

At rest, a small volume of reflux occurs at the GOJ as a normal physiological event. This is cleared by spontaneous peristalsis of food or fluid back into the stomach. Refluxed gas usually returns by peristalsis or may be expelled via the pharynx as a belch. Significant reflux is minimized by the lower oesophageal sphincter, the crural diaphragm, and the presence of the intra-abdominal part of the oesophagus, which is compressed by positive intra-abdominal pressure.

Stomach
The principal function of the stomach is to mix food with acid, mucus, and enzymes to prepare it for passage at a controlled rate as chyme into the duodenum and subsequently absorption within the small bowel. Specific physiological function is therefore considered in terms of gastric secretion and gastric motility.

The gastric glands normally secrete approximately 2500 mL of juice daily. Gastric juice contains mucus, acid, and enzymes to protect the stomach mucosa, kill ingested bacteria, provide an acid environment for pepsin to begin protein degradation, and to stimulate the flow of bile and pancreatic juices. Gastric acid is produced by an active secretion of hydrogen ions from the parietal cells of the proximal stomach. This is in exchange for potassium ions via a so-called proton pump.

The stomach also secretes a number of hormones, the most important being gastrin which is involved in acid secretion and gastric motility. In addition, intrinsic factor is secreted by the parietal cells and is responsible for combining with dietary vitamin B_{12} for absorption in the terminal ileum.

Although the stomach absorbs few substances, it does absorb alcohol and lipid-soluble compounds including aspirin and non-steroidal anti-inflammatory drugs (NSAIDs). It also absorbs water readily with half the ingested volume absorbed in 20 minutes.

Gastric secretion of acid is controlled by neural and hormonal processes. The cephalic phase initiated by seeing and smelling food is mediated centrally via the vagi. This stimulation results in the release of gastrin which together with secreted acetyl choline and histamine stimulates gastric parietal cells to secrete acid. The histamine is released by mast cells situated close to the parietal cells and acts to sensitize them to gastrin.

The gastric phase occurs when food enters the stomach and a combination of gastric distension and mucosal irritation creates both further gastric secretion but also increased vagal activity via vasovagal reflexes. Once the mixed food is passed into the duodenum and small bowel, gastric inhibitory factors are released including cholecystokinin (CCK) and secretin as well as gastric inhibitory reflexes in the enteric nervous system, which are sensitive to acid in the duodenum.

Gastric motility is effected by stretch receptors in the gastric wall which induce a wave-like peristalsis by contraction of longitudinal and circular muscle. Once this reaches the antrum there is an initial contraction, which closes the pylorus to allow recirculation of gastric contents to enhance food mixing to create chyme. Following a fall in the duodenal pressure, the pylorus relaxes and chyme is propelled onwards. The effect of vagotomy is directly on the antrum and as a result a gastric drainage procedure is required after vagotomy to enable gastric emptying.

Pathophysiology of oesophageal and gastric disorders
Oesophageal cancer
Incidence
In the United Kingdom, oesophageal cancer is the ninth most common malignancy accounting for 8500 new cases annually.[1] It

predominantly affects men, commonly in the seventh decade. Over the last 20 years there has been an almost exponential rise in the incidence of adenocarcinoma (ACA) in middle-aged men in the United Kingdom: 50% of oesophageal cancers are ACA and 50% are squamous cell carcinoma (SCC).

Predisposing factors
SCC is associated with smoking and alcohol. Worldwide incidence is highest in countries where food and liquid intake includes strong irritants such as hot spices and concentrated alcohol. Predisposing conditions include achalasia in which long exposure to stagnant food residue is likely to be the carcinogenic factor.

ACA is strongly associated with gastro-oesophageal reflux disease (GORD). Significant reflux for a prolonged period of time, particularly nocturnal, raises the risk of developing ACA by a factor of 43.[2] This may be a simple association and give rise to sporadic cases or may be associated with Barrett's columnar lined oesophagus; 10% of patients with GORD develop Barrett's. This reflects the damaging effect of acid on the squamous epithelium causing metaplastic change to glandular epithelium. Although usually symptomatic, Barrett's metaplasia can occur without associated symptoms.

Dysplasia can occur in association with the metaplasia although this may spontaneously reverse. Current research is accumulating evidence of biological markers, which may allow identification of those with Barrett's who are either at high or low risk of malignancy.[3] There is also evidence of a relationship between obesity and oesophageal ACA. This is likely to be related to raised intra-abdominal pressure and thus reflux although there is some evidence of specific tumour-promoting factors being released, particularly from excess retroperitoneal fat.[4]

Pathology
Pathologically, oesophageal cancer develops in the mucosal epithelium and spreads by local infiltration through the wall into surrounding structures. The network of intra-mural lymphatics results in spread both cranially and caudally for considerable distances away from the primary site. Both lymph node spread to local mediastinal and regional cervical and intra-abdominal nodes and blood-borne spread to distant sites including liver, lung, and bone are common.

Grossly, oesophageal cancer can be ulcerating, exophytic, or form strictures which result in the typical presentations of difficulty or pain on swallowing.

Oesophageal cancer is staged according to the tumour, node, and metastasis (TNM) system. The current TNM 7th edition includes any cancer within 5 cm of the GOJ as an oesophageal cancer.[5] Nodal disease is considered according to the number of nodes involved.

The overall prognosis for either SCC or ACA is poor, reflecting the late stage at presentation. Approximately 38% present at a stage when radical therapy can be considered.[6] The 5-year survival is 12% and this has only slightly improved over the last few years. Nevertheless, if diagnosed early, when limited to the mucosa or submucosa, 5-year survival is in excess of 70%.[7]

Gastric cancer
Incidence
Worldwide the incidence of gastric cancer has steadily decreased. This has reflected improvements in hygiene as well as consumption of fresh food and changes in food preservation from salt preservation to refrigeration. In the United Kingdom, gastric cancer

incidence has almost halved in the last 25 years to 8.6/100 000 (age adjusted).[1] It is more common in men and prevalent in the 7th and 8th decades. The increase in the ageing population will continue to produce significant numbers of new cases.

Predisposing factors
The classic aetiological model for gastric cancer comes from the Far East where salt-preserved fish was commonly eaten. This created carcinogenic nitrosamines within the stomach. Fresh fruit and vegetable consumption with intake of vitamin C has removed this risk factor. In 1994,[8] the World Health Organization designated the bacterium *Helicobacter pylori* as a carcinogen for gastric cancer. Evidence from high incidence areas such as Colombia showed a relationship between early exposure to *H. pylori* and development of gastric cancer in later life. Direct causal evidence is not available as *H. pylori* can cause duodenal ulceration and these patients do not develop gastric cancer. Further evidence suggests that a specific type of *H. pylori* is more likely to increase the risk of malignancy.[9]

Pathology
The majority of gastric cancers are ACA. These arise in the mucosa and penetrate the gastric wall to the serosa. Lymphatic spread is common to perigastric nodes and those associated with the principal arterial supply. Haematogenous spread is usually via the portal vein to the liver but widespread metastasis can occur to the lung and bone. An unusual feature of gastric cancer is transperitoneal or coelomic spread, which can give rise to Kruckenberg tumours of the ovary.

Macroscopically, gastric cancer can be polyploidal or ulcerating and can infiltrate submucosally creating the linitus plastica appearance. Although gastric cancer can affect any part of the stomach, in the United Kingdom there has lately been a migration proximally with an increase in the incidence of cardia cancer.

Experience in Japan has defined early gastric cancer (EGC), which is limited to the mucosa and submucosa. This definition of EGC and associated prognostic implications include nodal involvement.[10]

The overall survival for gastric cancer has shown marginal improvement in the last 10 years in the United Kingdom, partly reflecting better case selection and awareness of earlier diagnosis.[7] However, approximately 60% of patients still present with established disease and rarely survive beyond 12 months.[6]

Gastro-oesophageal reflux disease
Oesophageal reflux creates a clinical problem when chronic acid reflux produces persistent symptoms and associated complications. GORD is a very common condition accounting for a significant number of consultations with general practitioners. It is estimated that 25% of the adult population in the United Kingdom experience reflux symptoms on a regular basis.[11]

Although oesophageal sphincter disorders may be congenital, the majority are acquired. They present in the fourth and fifth decades and there may be a familial background.

Environmental and dietary factors, which lower oesophageal tone, include coffee, dietary fat, and GI hormones such as CCK. Obesity aggravates reflux and is related to hiatal herniation, inducing the sphincter to slide into the chest.

Exposure of the oesophageal squamous mucosa to excess acid results in a range of injury from superficial linear erosions to confluent patches of inflammation to circumferential erosions with oedema and friability to extensive ulceration and stricture formation.

In many cases, there is disordered motility caused by the chronicity which aggravates the presentation. Paradoxically, many patients with significant reflux symptoms do not have objective evidence of oesophagitis. It is therefore essential to combine endoscopic assessment with pH and manometric physiology studies.

Peptic ulceration

Although peptic ulceration including gastric and duodenal ulcers is less common, it remains a significant cause of morbidity and mortality, particularly amongst the elderly because of the complications of bleeding and perforation. Annual incidence estimates rates of 19.4–57.0/100 000 for acute bleeding and 3.8–14/100 000 for perforation.[12]

Factors associated with gastric and duodenal ulceration include systemic sepsis, drugs, stress, tobacco, and alcohol, and rarely gastrin-secreting tumours.

The two commonest aetiological factors are NSAIDs and *H. pylori*. The effect of NSAIDs appears to be direct damage to the mucosal barrier. This is mediated by prevention of prostaglandin synthesis, which decreases intragastric mucus production and gastric mucosal blood flow. In addition, the ability of mucosal repair is decreased.

H. pylori damages gastric mucosa by a number of mechanisms. Initial infection leads to reduced gastric acid secretion. The associated acid environment results in a reflex stimulation of parietal cell gastric secretion and hyperacidity. In duodenal ulceration, there is mucosal metaplasia with islands of ectopic gastric mucosa which is colonized by *H. pylori*. As a result there is a decrease in acid-stimulated release of bicarbonate and hence acid-induced ulceration. *H. pylori* also blocks secretin release from the duodenal mucosa, which counteracts the usual effect of secretin on delaying gastric emptying and stimulating bile secretion, all of which increase an abnormal acid environment in the duodenum.

Gastric ulceration tends to occur in the lesser curve of the stomach and duodenal ulceration, which is more common, in the first part of the duodenum. *H. pylori* colonizes the gastric mucosa principally of the pyloric antrum. It secretes a urease enzyme, which converts urea to ammonia and carbon dioxide. These buffer gastric acid to allow the bacteria to survive. This property is used in diagnosis, the urease breath test, whereby exhaled radiolabelled carbon dioxide is measured.

Common clinical presentations

Dysphagia

Dysphagia presents either spontaneously or in the context of previous heartburn. Increasingly, dysphagia is occurring in the context of morbid obesity which is often complicated by diabetes and sleep apnoea. Although in older age groups dysphagia is commonly due to oesophageal carcinoma, in younger age groups GORD and reflux stricture and achalasia need to be excluded.

Investigations

The principal investigation is endoscopy. Contrast radiology is rarely indicated apart from the evaluation of functional disorders.

Endoscopic biopsy is required for histological diagnosis and the position of the primary lesion needs to be carefully documented to aid treatment planning. It is important to differentiate histological types with SCC usually more proximal and ACA more distally located.

Once a diagnosis of cancer is made, further investigations are directed to staging disease spread. Multidetector CT scanning establishes distant metastatic disease. It can also provide information on the extent of local disease although accuracy of tumour and nodal staging is limited. Local disease spread is best assessed by endoluminal ultrasound (EUS) with accuracy for T staging of 61–78% and N stage of 65–75%.[13] Positron emission tomography (PET)-CT scanning provides details of both local and distant spread.

Oesophageal and GOJ cancers have been classified clinically as type I, lower oesophageal, type II, junctional, and type III, cardia cancers.[14]

Treatment

A key component in the treatment planning for a patient with oesophageal cancer is the assessment of comorbidity. This includes pulmonary and cardiac assessment with pulmonary function tests, electrocardiography, and echocardiography. Cardiopulmonary exercise testing allows a predictive score of cardiac and respiratory reserve to be determined, which is useful for risk discussion with the patient.[15]

Selection of treatment for oesophageal and gastric cancer is based on multidisciplinary team discussions taking into consideration all details of the individual presentation and pretreatment staging. Although radical surgery is an option, this is only indicated in early stage disease, which is not suitable for endoscopic therapy. Small T1 cancers usually in association with Barrett's are treated by endoscopic mucosal resection if well or moderately differentiated and limited to the mucosa as the risk of lymph node disease is less than 5%.

Combination chemotherapy with radical surgery is the current approach in the United Kingdom for locally advanced oesophageal cancer. Trials have confirmed a survival benefit for preoperative chemotherapy.[16] European studies have also shown an advantage for preoperative chemoradiotherapy.[17]

Surgery is performed via a combined laparotomy and thoracotomy or via a transthoracic approach. The stomach is fully mobilized and pulled up either into the chest or neck for anastomosis after resection of the oesophagus. Increasingly, stomach mobilization is being undertaken laparoscopically and trials are evaluating totally minimally invasive oesophagectomy.

Principal postoperative complications include anastomotic leak and cardiopulmonary dysfunction.

Dyspepsia and epigastric pain

Dyspepsia and epigastric pain are common and often non-specific symptoms. However, a long history with failure to respond to appropriate medication or recent onset of symptoms over 55 years of age are considered 'alarm' presentations requiring urgent investigation to exclude gastric cancer. The differential diagnosis includes benign gastric ulcer or gastric cancer.

Investigations

Endoscopy and endoscopic biopsy are the principal diagnostic investigations. Careful description of the lesion and its relationship to the GOJ and the pylorus should be carefully recorded.

CT scanning should be done to exclude visceral metastatic disease. It has limited accuracy in establishing T and N stage. Because of the risk of intraperitoneal spread, laparoscopy is undertaken to inspect peritoneal surfaces as well as the outer surface of the stomach.

EUS is used in gastric cancer for staging but there can be difficulties differentiating inflammation associated with ulceration from malignant infiltration.

PET-CT scanning also has a role although in certain histological types may not visualize the tumour,[18] particularly the diffuse subtype. The details from the staging assessment allow selection of treatment based on the extent of disease at presentation. This requires careful discussion by the multidisciplinary team.

Treatment

In gastric cancer, combination chemotherapy with radical surgery is the standard of care with chemotherapy given before and after surgery.[19] The extent of surgical resection is dependent on the position of the tumour in the stomach in order to obtain clear proximal and distal margins. The alternatives are subtotal or total gastrectomy. Adequate nodal dissection to remove possible sites of nodal spread is recommended. The extent of lymphadenectomy is contentious but in a fit patient most recommend excision of the perigastric and the next tier of nodes.[20]

Postoperatively, patients can experience a number of symptoms because of the effect of the gastrectomy. These include early satiety, weight loss, and diarrhoea often with steatorrhoea. Dumping can occur after gastrectomy because of rapid transit of undigested food with high osmolarity. Patients may express pain, dizziness, and nausea reflecting either fluid shifts with hypovolaemia or insulin production. All patients require vitamin B_{12} supplement after total gastrectomy because of loss of intrinsic factor and some may develop anaemia because of impaired iron absorption.

Heartburn and reflux

Heartburn and reflux are common symptoms. Many patients self-medicate and keep symptoms under control. Those who relapse on proton pump inhibitors (PPIs) need intervention. In addition, there is a strong case for endoscopic assessment in those over 55 years presenting with heartburn and reflux before starting PPIs. Some patients can present with features of insidious reflux such as persistent unproductive cough. The differential diagnosis includes GORD, hiatus hernia, oesophageal dysmotility, peptic ulcer, and malignancy.

Investigations

Endoscopy is essential to document mucosal changes, hiatal herniation, and to exclude rare conditions such as eosinophilic oesophagitis. Histology is important to confirm or exclude Barrett's and to document any dysplasia.

Oesophageal physiology studies are required to confirm pathological reflux. Measurement of oesophageal pH confirming regular and/or prolonged exposure to refluxate with a pH lower than 4 is indicative of abnormal physiology. Oesophageal manometry is also required as motility disorders can cause similar symptoms and antireflux surgery is ineffective in such patients.

Treatment

The management of significant GORD is based upon patient wishes with selection of treatment options determined by confirmatory evidence of pathological reflux. Patients whose symptoms recur after discontinuing PPIs or who have breakthrough reflux despite adequate medical therapy have the option of lifelong PPI with dose escalation as appropriate or surgery.

The aim of antireflux surgery is to recreate the mechanisms to minimize gastro-oesophageal reflux. Fundoplication is the preferred procedure as it ensures the GOJ is kept within the abdomen and the angle between the oesophagus and the stomach is re-created. Repair of any associated hiatus hernia completes the procedure.

The common complications of antireflux surgery include initial dysphagia, which normally settles. Occasionally, if persistent, the fundoplication may be too tight and requires revision. Patients may find difficulty with belching and experience bloating which usually settles with time.

Epigastric pain—acute onset

Acute onset of epigastric pain particularly in the elderly usually presents as an emergency when the pain is very severe. The history should consider predisposing factors such as ingestion of NSAIDs but also careful assessment of comorbidity. Common clinical signs include abdominal tenderness with guarding and rigidity and absent bowel sounds. The differential diagnosis includes acute perforated peptic ulcer, acute pancreatitis, ruptured abdominal aortic aneurysm, and acute myocardial infarction.

Management and investigations

After appropriate resuscitation with intravenous access, oxygen supplement, and analgesia, erect chest radiograph and blood investigations including serum amylase are required.

Free subdiaphragmatic gas particularly above the liver is indicative of a perforated viscus. It is, however, visible in just over 50% of cases. Serum amylase may be raised but not to the same level as in acute pancreatitis. If there is any doubt, a CT scan is indicated if the patient is stable and is usually conclusive.

Treatment

Surgical repair of a perforated peptic ulcer is a relatively straightforward procedure. At laparotomy a thorough peritoneal lavage is required to remove any contamination. The ulcer is usually in the anterior wall of the first part of the duodenum and is simply closed with sutures and an omental patch. If a gastric ulcer has perforated, biopsies should be taken to exclude malignancy. Although open procedures are the conventional approach, laparoscopic repair is now increasingly performed. There is no difference in outcome although the laparoscopic repair can take longer and has a slightly greater risk of recurrent leakage.[21]

Despite a straightforward surgical procedure, operative morbidity and mortality are high, reflecting the comorbidity of this patient group. The associated cardiac disease and the use of aspirin will increase postoperative complications. Occasionally a very unwell patient can be treated conservatively with antibiotics and radiological drainage of any collections. The mortality, however, can be more than 50%.

Acute upper gastrointestinal haemorrhage

Acute upper GI haemorrhage commonly presents without warning with haematemesis or melaena or both. There may be a background of insidious bleeding with progressive tiredness reflecting a slowly evolving anaemia. Important features in the history are similar to acute epigastric pain with reference to NSAIDs and comorbidity but also medication, which could promote bleeding such as anticoagulant therapy. The differential diagnosis includes peptic ulcers (60%), mucosal erosions (25%), Mallory–Weiss tears, oesophageal varices, and bleeding from tumours such as cancer, GI stromal tumours and arteriovenous malformations.

Management and investigations

Patients presenting with acute upper GI haemorrhage require appropriate urgent resuscitation with intravenous access and invasive monitoring. In patients with active bleeding, urgent/immediate endoscopy is indicated. In stable patients, endoscopy within 24 hours is required. Few patients require immediate endoscopy but such patients should be managed with airway protection and availability of surgery if endoscopic measures fail. Fortunately, peptic ulcer bleeding stops spontaneously in 70–80% of patients.[22]

Treatment

At endoscopy it is possible to determine high- and low-risk lesions based upon risk of re-bleeding. In low-risk lesions with no evidence of recent bleeding, no endoscopic therapy is required. High-dose infusional PPI therapy is indicated to raise the gastric pH, which improves clot formation and platelet aggregation.

In high-risk lesions, with either active bleeding or visible vessel and adherent clot, endoscopic therapy with a combination of epinephrine (adrenaline) injection and thermal or mechanical treatments with endoscopic clips is indicated. Such patients may require repeat endoscopy if the initial view is poor and there is uncertainty about control of bleeding.

Age, presence of shock, comorbidity, cause of bleeding, and endoscopic features are combined to predict the risk of re-bleed and mortality.[23] The overall 30-day mortality for acute upper GI haemorrhage is approximately 8%, which has changed little from the period when many patients required surgical rather than endoscopic control.[12]

Further reading

Allum WH, Blazeby JM, Griffin SM, et al. Guidelines for the management of oesophageal and gastric cancer. *Gut* 2011; 60:1449–72.

Griffin SM, Raimes SA. *Upper Gastrointestinal Surgery. A Companion to Specialist Surgical Practice* (4th ed). London: WB Saunders Ltd; 2009.

Lamb P (ed). Oesophagus and stomach. *Surgery* 2011; 29(11):537–80.

References

1. Office for National Statistics. *Cancer Statistics Registrations: Registrations of Cancer Diagnosed in 2008, England.* Series MB1 No. 39. London: National Statistics; 2011.
2. Lagergen J, Bergstrom R, Londgren A, et al. Symptomatic gastro-oesophageal reflux as a risk factor for oesophageal adenocarcinoma. *N Engl J Med* 1999; 340:825–31.
3. Fitzgerald RC. Molecular basis of Barrett's oesophagus and oesophageal adenocarcinoma. *Gut* 2006; 55:1810–18.
4. Vaughan TL, Kristal AR, Blount PR, et al. Non-steroidal anti-inflammatory drug use, body mass index and anthropometry in relation to genetic and flow cytometric abnormalities in Barrett's oesophagus. *Cancer Epidemiol Biomark Prev* 2002; 11:745–52.
5. Sobin LH, Gospodarowicz MK, Wittekind C (eds). *TNM Classification of Malignant Tumours* (7th ed). Oxford: Wiley-Blackwell; 2009.
6. The NHS Information Centre. *National Oesophago-Gastric Cancer Audit. Annual Report 2015.* London: The NHS Information Centre; 2008.
7. Coupland VH, Allum WH, Blazeby JM, et al. Incidence and survival of oesophageal and gastric cancer in England between 1998 and 2007, a population-based study. *BMC Cancer* 2012; 12:11–20.
8. International Agency for Research on Cancer Working Group on the Evaluation of Carcinogenic risks to Humans. Infection with Helicobacter pylori. In *Schistosomes, Liver Flukes and Helicobacter pylori.* Lyon: International Agency for Research on Cancer; 1994:177–240.
9. Tomb JF, White O, Kerlavage AR, et al. The complete genome sequence of the gastric pathogen Helicobacter pylori. *Nature* 1997; 388:539–47.
10. Japanese Gastric Cancer Association. Japanese classification of gastric carcinoma: 3rd English Edition. *Gastric Cancer* 2011; 14:101–12.
11. Klauser AG, Scindlbeck NE, Muller Lissner SA. Symptoms in gastro-oesophageal reflux disease. *Lancet* 1990; 335:205–8.
12. Lau JY, Sung J, Hill C, et al. Systematic review of the epidemiology of complicated peptic ulcer disease: incidence, recurrence, risk factors and mortality. *Digestion* 2011; 84:102–13.
13. Kelly S, Harris KM, Berry E, et al. A systematic review of the staging performance of endoscopic ultrasound in gastro-oesophageal carcinoma. *Gut* 2001; 49:534–9.
14. Siewert JR, Stein HJ, Feith M. Adenocarcinoma of the esophago-gastric junction. *Scand J Surg* 2006; 95:260–9.
15. Forshaw MJ, Strauss DC, Davies AR, et al. Is cardiopulmonary testing a useful test before esophagectomy? *Ann Thorac Surg* 2007; 85:294–9.
16. Allum WH, Stenning SP, Bancewicz J, et al. Long-term results of a randomized trial of surgery with or without preoperative chemotherapy in esophageal cancer. *J Clin Oncol* 2009; 27:5062–7.
17. van Hagen P, Hulshof MC, van Lanschot JJB, et al. Pre-operative chemoradiotherapy for esophageal or junctional cancer. *N Engl J Med* 2012; 366:2074–84.
18. Dassen AE, Lips DJ, Hoekstra CJ, et al. FDG-PET has no definite role in preoperative imaging in gastric cancer. *Eur J Surg Oncol* 2009; 35:449–55.
19. Cunningham D, Allum WH, Stenning SP, et al. Perioperative chemotherapy versus surgery alone for resectable gastroesophageal cancer. *N Engl J Med* 2006; 355:11–20.
20. Allum WH. Optimal surgery for gastric cancer: is more always better? *Recent Results Cancer Res* 2012; 196:215–26.
21. Bertleff MJ, Lange JF. Laparoscopic correction of perforated peptic ulcer: first choice? A review of the literature. *Surg Endosc* 2010; 24:1231–9.
22. Harbison SP, Dempsey DT. Peptic ulcer disease. *Curr Probl Surg* 2005; 42:346–454.
23. Palmer K, Nairn M. Management of acute gastrointestinal blood loss: summary of SIGN guidelines. *BMJ* 2008; 337:a1832.

PART 2.4

Hepatobiliary and pancreatic

CHAPTER 2.4.1

Hepatobiliary and pancreatic disorders

Robert P. Jones, Declan Dunne, and Graeme J. Poston

The gallbladder

Gallstones

Cholelithiasis, or gallstones, are found in 10% of people and are classified by content. Around 80% of gallstones are predominantly cholesterol, with the remaining 20% made of primary bile salts. The majority (> 80%) of people with gallstones are asymptomatic, and gallstones are often identified incidentally during imaging for other conditions.[1] Ultrasound remains the investigation of choice for cholelithiasis, with sensitivity in excess of 98%.

Complications of gallstones

Biliary colic

Biliary colic is the commonest complication of gallstones, and is caused by the gallbladder constricting against a stone impacted in Hartmann's pouch or the cystic duct. Patients with biliary colic typically report acute right upper quadrant abdominal pain during the attack. Symptoms often last for several hours, and colic is therefore a misnomer. The pain may be associated with nausea and vomiting.

In uncomplicated biliary colic the blood inflammatory markers and liver function tests are normal. An ultrasound scan is recommended to confirm the diagnosis of gallstones, and exclude bile duct dilation associated with common bile duct stones. Treatment is aimed at relieving symptoms, with most patients offered laparoscopic cholecystectomy to prevent further episodes of pain.

Acute cholecystitis

Acute cholecystitis, or acute inflammation of the gallbladder, presents with right upper quadrant pain similar to that seen in biliary colic, although usually of increased severity. Recurrent impaction of a gallstone into Hartmann's pouch or the cystic duct leads to chemical inflammation, which may then progress to bacterial infection from gastrointestinal organisms.

Patients often present with right upper quadrant tenderness and guarding. Murphy's sign (inspiratory arrest during subcostal palpation) is considered pathognomonic of acute cholecystitis. There may be associated signs of systemic sepsis such as pyrexia and tachycardia. An elevated white cell count and C-reactive protein are frequently found with acute cholecystitis. Very rarely, mild elevations in serum bilirubin and the transaminases may be indicative of severe inflammation resulting in extraluminal biliary obstruction by the enlarged gallbladder and inflammatory mass (Mirizzi syndrome).

Initial management consists of symptom control and broad-spectrum antibiotics to prevent septic complications. In the majority of cases this strategy will manage and control the acute attack. Complications of acute cholecystitis include gangrenous cholecystitis with perforation, biliary obstruction, gallstone ileus, and non-resolving sepsis. These complications may necessitate urgent surgical or endoscopic intervention.

As for biliary colic, definitive management involves laparoscopic cholecystectomy. The timing of cholecystectomy for acute cholecystitis is the subject of much debate, with many groups advocating immediate cholecystectomy at the time of initial presentation.[2] Conservative management of the acute episode with a delayed elective cholecystectomy is an alternative and justifiable management strategy.

Choledocholithiasis

Common bile duct stones (choledocholithiasis) are present in 10% of patients with gallstones. Common bile duct stones are often asymptomatic and only become apparent when they cause a degree of obstruction to the biliary tract. Choledocholithiasis can present with asymptomatic elevation of blood liver function tests (predominantly raised bilirubin and alkaline phosphatase), colic-like symptoms, obstructive jaundice, cholangitis, or acute pancreatitis. Routine abdominal ultrasound is poor at visualizing common bile duct stones (< 10%), but may identify dilatation of the intrahepatic and extrahepatic biliary tree if obstructed by the stone. Other imaging modalities are therefore used to identify the presence or absence of common bile duct stones, including magnetic resonance cholangiopancreatography (MRCP) and endoscopic ultrasound (EUS).

Even when asymptomatic, removal of all common bile duct stones is indicated due to the risk of serious complications. The primary method for retrieval is endoscopic retrograde cholangiopancreatography (ERCP). In 80% of cases, ERCP with balloon or basket trawl will be effective at retrieving all stones. Occasionally, more advanced methods of removal such as lithotripsy or formal surgical exploration may be required. In patients with concomitant gallbladder and common bile duct stones, experienced laparoscopic surgeons can offer laparoscopic cholecystectomy combined with laparoscopic bile duct exploration.[3]

Cholangitis

Infected obstructive jaundice (cholangitis) occurs when there is an obstruction to normal biliary drainage, and is usually a complication of common bile duct stones. Patients typically present with jaundice, right upper quadrant pain, and rigors (Charcot's triad). Treatment is with antibiotics and urgent decompression of the biliary tree (usually by ERCP).

The autoimmune condition sclerosing cholangitis can also give rise to a similar presentation, with multiple inflammatory fibrous strictures throughout the biliary tree. The natural progression of this disease results in secondary biliary cirrhosis; 10% of patients will also develop coincidental cholangiocarcinoma. The diagnosis is confirmed by a characteristic 'beads on a string' appearance on cholangiography.

Gallbladder cancer

Gallbladder cancer is relatively rare, with an incidence of 3/100 000 in the United Kingdom. Risk factors include the presence of a large (> 1 cm) adenomatous polyp, female gender, advancing age, cigarette smoking, and severe chronic cholecystitis. Around 85% of cases occur in the presence of gallstones.[4] Presentation is non-specific, with patients often reporting vague symptoms suggestive of chronic cholecystitis. Unfortunately, gallbladder cancer is normally asymptomatic until the advanced stages of the disease.

In patients with early (Tis, T1A, T1B, or T2) stage disease (often detected incidentally at laparoscopic cholecystectomy), surgical resection offers the only possibility of cure. If suspected at the time of surgery, the procedure should be abandoned and the patient referred to a specialist unit to ensure the best possible outcome.[5] Where the cancer has invaded only the lamina propria or muscular layer (Tis or T1A) then simple cholecystectomy may be curative. In patients with more advanced disease (T1B or T2) resection of the surrounding hepatic tissue and formal lymphadenectomy has been advocated.[6] Where patients have cancer diagnosed on histopathological examination after laparoscopic cholecystectomy, port site excision may be considered because of the high incidence of port site seeding.[7] For irresectable disease, palliative chemotherapy with gemcitabine and cisplatin remains the gold standard.[8] The overall 5-year survival for patients with gallbladder cancer is poor, at just 5%. However, those with early disease amenable to resection have a 5-year survival in excess of 60%.[5]

The liver

Benign liver lesions

Cysts

Simple benign cysts are common, generally solitary, and occur more frequently in women. Most are incidental findings, and have a characteristic blue hue when seen at laparoscopy. Indications for surgical intervention include symptoms, rupture, haemorrhage, infection, or indeterminate diagnosis. Surgical resection typically involves laparoscopic deroofing, with oversewing of the cyst wall.[9]

Polycystic liver disease is less common. It is an autosomal dominant condition, more frequently seen in women, and around half of patients will also have polycystic kidney disease, and less frequently, polycystic pancreas. Indications for surgical intervention are broadly similar to simple cysts, although the large number of lesions means that deroofing a single cyst is unlikely to relieve symptoms, and rarely, liver transplantation might be considered.

Haemangiomas

Haemangiomas are the commonest benign tumours of the liver, caused by a proliferation of vascular endothelial cells. They are more common in females and are generally asymptomatic, but may occasionally cause pain related to mass effect. Rupture is very rare. Diagnosis is usually incidental, and surgical resection only recommended if patients are symptomatic or the diagnosis remains uncertain on imaging.

Adenomas

Adenomas are benign liver tumours seen almost exclusively in women aged between 25 and 50 years. These well-defined and vascular lesions are classically associated with the use of the oral contraceptive pill, and are generally solitary. The majority are found incidentally on imaging, although up to a third may present with pain because of rupture. Adenomas are recognized as having malignant potential, with up to 10% developing into hepatocellular carcinoma. The risk of rupture and malignancy means that surgical excision is generally recommended if continuing to enlarge and in particular if greater than 5 cm in diameter, although some lesions may regress after discontinuation of the oral contraceptive pill.

Follicular nodular hyperplasia

Commonly confused radiologically with adenomas, follicular nodular hyperplasia (FNH) characteristically displays a central stellate scar on imaging. Generally affecting young women, FNH has no potential for rupture or malignant transformation, and so management is conservative unless patients are symptomatic, or the diagnosis remains uncertain.

Malignant liver lesions

Hepatocellular carcinoma

Hepatocellular carcinoma (HCC) is the second commonest cause of cancer-related death worldwide and accounts for over 80% of all primary liver malignancies. The overwhelming majority of HCCs arise in patients with chronic liver disease, with 5% of cirrhotic patients developing HCC.[10] There is marked geographical variation in incidence, with much higher rates in Africa and southeast Asia.[10] This geographical distribution reflects the underlying prevalence of hepatitis B and C infection. In the United Kingdom, the incidence of HCC is increasing as the incidence of viral and alcoholic hepatitis rises.[11]

Increasingly, patients with HCC are identified at an early stage as high-risk groups are entered into screening programmes.[12] These patients often have little in the way of symptoms. Patients presenting with symptomatic HCC typically have advanced disease and the associated symptoms are those of advanced malignancy. Occasionally, patients present with abdominal pain and haemodynamic instability after spontaneous rupture of an HCC.

Imaging is complicated by background liver disease, which may demonstrate a heterogeneous appearance with nodular regeneration, and so in the setting of chronic liver disease any nodule of 1 cm or greater detected on imaging should be considered an HCC.[12]

Treatment depends on both the stage of disease and the underlying aetiology. In the absence of cirrhosis, solitary tumours limited to a single liver lobe may be treated by resection.[13] However, resection in the presence of cirrhosis is considered exceedingly high risk as surgery can result in liver decompensation. Localized treatments such as thermal ablation[14] or transarterial chemoembolization[15] may be used, but are associated with high rates of recurrence. Transplant is considered where tumour load is limited (one tumour of a maximum diameter of 5 cm, or up to three tumours with a cumulative maximum of the sum of their diameters not exceeding 5 cm), and has the advantage of addressing not only tumour but also the underlying parenchymal disease.[16] However, its use is limited by the availability of donor organs. Palliative chemotherapy with sorafenib has been shown to have a survival advantage of around 3 months, and is currently the mainstay of treatment for advanced disease but only in patients whose cirrhosis is graded Child–Pugh A.[17]

Cholangiocarcinoma

Cholangiocarcinomas arise from intra- and extrahepatic biliary epithelial cells and are the commonest malignancy arising from the biliary tract. The incidence is increasing, and most commonly occurs in men over 50 years of age. Cholangiocarcinomas are classified according to their location in the biliary tree. Tumours are described as intrahepatic, extrahepatic, or perihilar (so-called Klatskin tumours, which form at the confluence of the left and right hepatic ducts). A number of risk factors for the development of cholangiocarcinoma have been identified, including primary sclerosing cholangitis with or without chronic ulcerative colitis, chronic hepatitis C, liver cirrhosis, and parasitic biliary infections.[18]

Like many primary liver cancers, cholangiocarcinomas are relatively asymptomatic and typically present late. However, patients with Klatskin or distal extrahepatic cholangiocarcinomas may present with obstructive jaundice at an earlier stage.

The investigation and staging of this disease is aimed at defining surgical resectability, as this offers the only chance of cure.[19] CT is the primary diagnostic investigation for cholangiocarcinoma and can define resectability in the majority of cases by assessing hepatic inflow and outflow structures. ERCP and percutaneous transhepatic cholangiopancreatography (PTC) are also useful in defining the biliary duct involvement of peri-hilar tumours. Staging laparoscopy is routinely carried out before proceeding to laparotomy because of the high rate of unidentified peritoneal metastases, although its role is increasingly being questioned as the diagnostic yield of imaging improves.[20]

Because of late presentation, only 20% of cholangiocarcinomas are resectable with curative intent.[19] Surgery aims to resect the entire malignancy with an adequate negative margin (frequently threatened by extensive lympho-vascular invasion) whilst maintaining sufficient viable healthy liver tissue. Hilar carcinomas may necessitate complex surgery, with resection combined with reconstruction of the biliary tree and hepatic arterial and venous supply.[21] However, such an aggressive approach is worthwhile with 5-year survival between 40% and 60%, compared to less than 5% for those treated with systemic chemotherapy.[22]

Secondary liver metastases

Because it uniquely drains the portal venous system, the liver is the main site of metastasis for many gastrointestinal cancers and liver metastases remain the most common type of liver cancer. Tumours that frequently metastasize to the liver include colorectal, lung, breast, melanoma (cutaneous and ocular), neuroendocrine tumours and renal cell carcinomas. Imaging techniques such as computed tomography (CT) scanning are often used to identify hepatic metastases.

Liver resection for metastases other than colorectal cancer has shown limited benefit. However, for patients with resectable colorectal liver metastases, surgical resection is now associated with a 50% 5-year survival.[23] By contrast, patients with unresectable metastases have a 5-year survival of less than 5%. Liver resection is safe, with operative mortality consistently under 1%, and guidance from the UK National Institute for Health and Care Excellence now states that a liver surgeon must review all patients with liver-limited metastatic colorectal cancer.

Resectability with curative intent is defined as the ability to successfully remove all residual disease from the liver with clear surgical margins whilst leaving adequate (about 30% future liver remnant) disease-free liver. Current UK guidance gives no absolute contraindications to surgery, but suggested that liver resection should not be carried out in the presence of:

◆ non-treatable primary tumour

◆ widespread pulmonary disease

◆ locoregional recurrence

◆ uncontrollable peritoneal disease

◆ extensive nodal disease, such as retroperitoneal or mediastinal lymph nodes

◆ bone or central nervous system metastases.

Chemotherapy for advanced colorectal cancer has also changed dramatically over the last 15 years. Previously, patients with unresectable metastatic colorectal cancer were treated solely with the aim of prolonging life. There is now growing recognition that some patients with liver limited disease who may not be resectable at presentation become resectable after chemotherapy, as the size of their liver lesions shrink. This approach is often referred to as 'induction' or 'conversion' chemotherapy. Resectability rates after chemotherapy for initially irresectable disease vary widely, with modern regimens achieving conversion rates approaching 60%.[24] Attempting to bring unresectable disease to resection is worthwhile, with overall 5-year survival comparable between patients resectable at presentation and those converted to resectability after systemic chemotherapy.[25]

The pancreas

Acute pancreatitis

There are many causes of acute pancreatitis. The exact mechanism for each of these causative mechanisms remains unclear, but is thought to involve the auto-activation of pancreatic enzymes leading to pancreatic inflammation and autodigestion. Pancreatitis can present at any age. Pain is usually of rapid onset, severe, constant, and often radiates from the epigastrium to the back. Repeated retching is common. Rarely, patients may develop bluish discolouration of the loins (Grey Turner's sign) caused by extravasation of blood stained pancreatic fluid into the retroperitoneum.

Causes of acute pancreatitis

The most common causes of acute pancreatitis are gallstones (~45%) and alcohol (~35%).[26] Because of the high incidence of gallstone pancreatitis, all patients admitted with pancreatitis should receive an abdominal ultrasound scan to diagnose or exclude the presence of gallstones. Other causes of acute pancreatitis are outlined in Box 2.4.1.1.

Box 2.4.1.1 Causes of acute pancreatitis

- Alcohol
- Gallstones
- Iatrogenic:
  - ERCP
  - Operative intervention in the region of the pancreas
- Neoplastic
- Viral infection
  - Mumps
  - Cytomegalovirus
  - Coxsackie B
- Trauma
- Hyperlipidaemia
- Metabolic disorders:
  - Hypercalcaemia
  - Hyperparathyroidism
  - Cushing's syndrome
- Hypothermia
- Drugs:
  - Corticosteroids
  - Azathioprine
  - Sulphonamides
  - Tetracyclines
  - Diuretics
- Pregnancy
- Idiopathic.

Assessment of acute pancreatitis

The diagnosis of acute pancreatitis is made by elevation of serum pancreatic amylase, in conjunction with the clinical history and examination. Elevated serum pancreatic enzymes tend to peak early in the episode of pancreatitis, so should always be interpreted in light of the onset of acute abdominal pain. If there is any doubt about the diagnosis, CT scanning may be used to establish the diagnosis and to exclude other diagnostic differentials such as a bowel perforation.

Once the diagnosis of acute pancreatitis has been made there is a need to establish the severity and cause of the disease. Mortality in severe pancreatitis is high, and such cases should be managed in an intensive care environment where complications can be more easily recognized and managed. Scoring systems to assess severity include the APACHE score, Glasgow score, and Ranson score.[27] The degree of amylase elevation is not predictive of severity. Early identification of severe cases allows aggressive management, ideally in a critical care environment.

Management of acute pancreatitis

Treatment is generally supportive and non-operative, and is outlined in Table 2.4.1.1.

Table 2.4.1.1 Management of acute pancreatitis

Treatment	Rationale
Analgesia	Relief of pain
Fluid replacement	Large volumes of fluid are sequestered during an episode of acute pancreatitis, and require replacement. Urinary catheterization aids assessment of fluid balance
Nutrition	Early feeding is appropriate if tolerated. For severe cases, total parenteral nutrition may be appropriate
Endoscopic sphincterotomy	For severe gallstone pancreatitis, ERCP may be indicated to allow urgent decompression. An early interval cholecystectomy is indicated

Complications of acute pancreatitis

CT scanning should be performed in non-resolving acute cases to identify complications. These include abscess formation with parenchymal necrosis and pyrexia, peri-pancreatic collections and pseudocyst formation, gastrointestinal bleeding, multi-organ dysfunction syndrome, and pancreatic insufficiency. Patients developing complications from acute pancreatitis, including multi-organ failure, should be managed in conjunction with a specialist pancreatic centre.[28]

Surgery is rarely indicated in the management of the acute attack, and should be avoided where possible. Percutaneous drainage of collections or abscesses may be useful, and often requires multiple drains. Failure to resolve despite percutaneous drainage may be an indication for surgical debridement (necrosectomy).[29]

Patients presenting with mild pancreatitis rarely suffer complications from the disease, and mortality is low, compared with severe pancreatitis (mortality of 20–30%).

Chronic pancreatitis

Chronic pancreatitis is characterized by the gradual destruction of pancreatic tissue by repeated attacks of pancreatitis. Alcohol abuse is the most common cause (70%).[30] Patients typically present with recurrent abdominal pain. Other presentations include steatorrhoea caused by pancreatic insufficiency, type 1 diabetes mellitus, and obstructive jaundice. For patients with obstructive jaundice, differentiating between chronic pancreatitis and head of pancreas carcinoma may be difficult (around 2% of patients with chronic pancreatitis will develop a pancreatic malignancy).[31] Serum amylase during attacks of pain may be elevated, but in long-standing disease amylase levels may be normal because of a lack of normal functioning pancreatic tissue. CT might demonstrate enlargement and irregular consistency of the gland, as well as calcification and ductal changes including dilatation and intraductal calculi.

Management should be in specialized units, and pain control is often the most difficult aspects of caring for these patients. If attacks are very frequent, surgery may be indicated for pain relief. Surgery is also considered where it is not possible to differentiate between an inflammatory mass and malignancy.

Pancreatic cancer

Pancreatic cancer occurs in approximately 1/10 000 people, and is more common in men. Ninety per cent of pancreatic tumours are ductal in origin, with the majority (>60%) arising in the head of the

Table 2.4.1.2 Exocrine pancreatic neoplasms

Tumour	Features	Usual site	Diagnosis	% malignant	Treatment
Insulinoma	Hypoglycaemia	Throughout pancreas	Fasting glucose and insulin levels	10%	Resection
Gastrinoma	Multiple peptic ulcers	Head of pancreas	Secretin stimulation test	50%	Resection, proton pump inhibitor
VIPoma	Watery diarrhoea, hypokalaemia, achlorhydria	Body/tail of pancreas	Elevated pancreatic polypeptide/ vasoactive intestinal polypeptide	>50%	Resection, octreotide
Glucagonoma	Diabetes	Body/tail pancreas	Fasting glucagon	>80%	Resection
Somatostatinoma	Diabetes	Periampullary head of pancreas	Fasting somatostatin	>90%	Resection
Non-functional	Mass, pain, jaundice, weight loss	Throughout pancreas	CT/MRI	50–90%	Resection/chemotherapy

pancreas.[32] Pancreatic adenocarcinomas typically metastasize to lymph nodes, liver, and peritoneum. The majority of patients present non-specifically, with weight loss and abdominal pain. Other symptoms might include jaundice, abdominal pain, nausea, anorexia, hepatomegaly, or vomiting due to gastric outlet obstruction. Head of pancreas lesions classically present earlier as they give rise to obstructive jaundice, whereas tail lesions remain asymptomatic for longer.

Laboratory tests may show a raised bilirubin and alkaline phosphatase. Non-specific tumour markers such as CA 19-9 and carcinoembryonic antigen might also be raised. Assessment of pancreatic lesions relies on contrast-enhanced CT, MRCP, ERCP, and EUS.[33]

The only potentially curative treatment of pancreatic cancer is surgery, but is appropriate in only a minority of cases. Technical contraindications to resection include liver and peritoneal metastases, as well as tumour invasion of the superior mesenteric artery. Resectability is definitively determined at laparotomy, but can be predicted preoperatively by assessing vascular involvement on CT and magnetic resonance imaging (MRI) as well as levels of CA-19-9.[34] Laparotomy allows formal assessment, although laparoscopy is often used in combination with laparoscopic ultrasound to assess vascular invasion and nodal involvement.[35]

The type of pancreatic resection performed depends on tumour location. Tumours of the head of the pancreas require a Whipple resection (pancreaticoduodenectomy), whilst tumours of the tail or body are treated by distal pancreatectomy. Adjuvant treatment with fluorouracil (5-FU) or gemcitabine is associated with improved overall survival.[36]

Postoperative complications of pancreaticoduodenectomy include delayed gastric emptying, pancreatic fistula (10–20%), infection, bile leak, and pancreatitis. Postoperative prognosis is affected by lymph node involvement, vascular invasion, as well as positive resection margins.

For patients with irresectable disease, treatment with gemcitabine and 5-FU has been shown to prolong survival.[37] However, palliative surgical intervention may be required to relieve gastric outlet obstruction or jaundice.

Endocrine pancreatic neoplasms

These tumours are rare, occurring at fewer than five cases per million, and can be broadly classified as functional (secreting hormones, giving rise to classical symptoms) or non-functional (presenting with pain, weight loss, or jaundice) (Table 2.4.1.2). Functional hormones are produced from amine precursor uptake and decarboxylation (APUD) cells, with some functional tumours associated with multiple endocrine neoplasia 1 syndrome.

Trauma

The spleen

Trauma remains the primary indication for splenectomy. Much rarer indications include hereditary spherocytosis, idiopathic thrombocytopenic purpura, thrombotic thrombocytopenic purpura, and splenic abscess (often caused by haematogenous spread of bacterial infection after intravenous drug abuse).

Patients with splenic trauma typically present following a blunt abdominal trauma with signs of hypovolaemia and peritonism from progressive blood loss. Splenic injuries are graded according to severity (Table 2.4.1.3), with some surgeons advocating conservative management for grade I–III injuries.[38] However, splenectomy is indicated for all grade IV/V injuries and where there is evidence of active bleeding on CT. In any cases where the patient is unstable or the diagnosis is unclear, immediate laparotomy is mandatory.

Patients with a contained subcapsular splenic haematoma should be monitored closely. They are at risk of delayed rupture, where a weakened splenic wall spontaneously ruptures several days after the initial trauma.

Liver

Liver injury in the United Kingdom is predominantly due to blunt abdominal trauma, but increasingly elsewhere in the world due to penetrating injury. Liver trauma is likewise graded although nearly all (the vast majority presenting with grades I–IV) can be managed conservatively if the patient remains haemodynamically stable. Surgery is only indicated in cases of ongoing haemodynamic instability despite adequate resuscitation and failure of interventional radiology interventions, or in grade V (hepatic vein disruption) or grade VI (hepatocaval disruption and usually rapidly fatal).

The other common cause of hepatobiliary injury is iatrogenic bile duct injury during cholecystectomy. This occurs when the surgeon gets lost, either as a result of failure to appreciate the degree of pericholecystitis resulting in the loss of Calot's triangle due to fibrosis, or fails to appreciate one of the many common variants of

Table 2.4.1.3 Grading system for splenic trauma

Grade	Description of injury
I	Subcapsular haematoma < 10% surface area, < 1 cm capsular tear
II	< 50% surface area, < 5 cm tear
III	Large > 50% surface area, > 5 cm tear, expanding haematoma
IV	Laceration involving hilar vessels
V	Hilar avulsion or shattered spleen

Reproduced from Ernest E. Moore *et al.*, Organ Injury Scaling: Spleen and Liver (1994 Revision), The *Journal of Trauma and Acute Care Surgery*, Volume 38, Issue 3, Copyright © 1994, with permission from Lippincott Williams & Wilkins.

biliary anatomy that are present in over 50% of people, so mistaking common hepatic duct or right hepatic duct for cystic duct. Steps to avoid such an injury include using intraoperative cholangiography (although 50% of such injuries occur before the cholangiogram when employed), or dissecting to the 'critical view of safety', that is, not clipping or dividing any tubular structure until the surgeon has dissected the gallbladder off the gallbladder fossa so far that it is inconceivable that the hepatic duct(s) crosses the operative field. If it is not possible to define the biliary anatomy, then either perform a subtotal cholecystectomy, leaving a cuff of Hartmann's pouch to protect the hepatic duct or a cholecystostomy and gallstone removal. In either case, the patient needs to be informed of their risk of further gallstone development. If there is any concern either intra- or postoperatively that a bile duct injury might have occurred then referral to a specialist hepatobiliary unit is mandatory.

Pancreas

Pancreatic trauma is uncommon and usually associated with blunt abdominal trauma directly to the epigastrium (e.g. handle-bar injuries in cyclists). The commonest finding is pancreatic transection, usually at the junction of neck and body of pancreas. As with liver trauma, most can be managed conservatively, and the expected complications are similar to those seen with severe acute pancreatitis. Surgery (usually distal pancreatectomy, but occasionally pancreatojejunostomy Roux-en-Y) may be necessary for a persistent pancreatic fistula but should only be considered in a pancreatic surgery centre.

References

1. Reshetnyak VI. Concept of the pathogenesis and treatment of cholelithiasis. *World J Hepatol* 2012; 4(2):18–34.
2. Young AL, Cockbain AJ, White AW, *et al.* Index admission laparoscopic cholecystectomy for patients with acute biliary symptoms: results from a specialist centre. *HPB (Oxford)* 2010; 12(4):270–6.
3. Sgourakis G, Lanitis S, Karaliotas Ch, *et al.* [Laparoscopic versus endoscopic primary management of choledocholithiasis. A retrospective case-control study]. *Chirurg* 2012; 83(10):897–903.
4. Pilgrim CH, Groeschl RT, Christians KK, *et al.* Modern perspectives on factors predisposing to the development of gallbladder cancer. *HPB (Oxford)* 2013; 15(11):839–44.
5. Cavallaro A, Piccolo G, Panebianco V, *et al.* Incidental gallbladder cancer during laparoscopic cholecystectomy: managing an unexpected finding. *World J Gastroenterol* 2012; 18(30):4019–27.
6. Shirai Y, Sakata J, Wakai T, *et al.* 'Extended' radical cholecystectomy for gallbladder cancer: long-term outcomes, indications and limitations. *World J Gastroenterol* 2012; 18(34):4736–43.
7. Maker AV, Butte JM, Oxenberg J, *et al.* Is port site resection necessary in the surgical management of gallbladder cancer? *Ann Surg Oncol* 2012; 19(2):409–17.
8. Valle J, Wasan H, Palmer DH, *et al.* Cisplatin plus gemcitabine versus gemcitabine for biliary tract cancer. *N Engl J Med* 2010; 362(14):1273–81.
9. Jabłońska B. Biliary cysts: etiology, diagnosis and management. *World J Gastroenterol* 2012; 18(35):4801–10.
10. Forner A, Llovet JM, Bruix J. Hepatocellular carcinoma. *Lancet* 2012; 379(9822):1245–55.
11. Sherman M. Hepatocellular carcinoma: new and emerging risks. *Dig Liver Dis* 2010; 42 Suppl 3:S215–22.
12. Trinchet JC. Surveillance for hepatocellular carcinoma in cirrhotic patients: from official recommendations to the real life. *J Hepatol* 2011; 54(6):1310–11.
13. Huang J, Yan L, Cheng Z, *et al.* A randomized trial comparing radiofrequency ablation and surgical resection for HCC conforming to the Milan criteria. *Ann Surg* 2010; 252(6):903–12.
14. Yu NC, Lu DS, Raman SS, *et al.* Hepatocellular carcinoma: microwave ablation with multiple straight and loop antenna clusters—pilot comparison with pathologic findings. *Radiology* 2006; 239(1):269–75.
15. Lammer J, Malagari K, Vogl T, *et al.* Prospective randomized study of doxorubicin-eluting-bead embolization in the treatment of hepatocellular carcinoma: results of the PRECISION V study. *Cardiovasc Intervent Radiol* 2010; 33(1):41–52.
16. Mazzaferro V, Regalia E, Doci R, *et al.* Liver transplantation for the treatment of small hepatocellular carcinomas in patients with cirrhosis. *N Engl J Med* 1996; 334(11):693–9.
17. Llovet JM, Ricci S, Mazzaferro V, *et al.* Sorafenib in advanced hepatocellular carcinoma. *N Engl J Med* 2008; 359(4):378–90.
18. Razumilava N, Gores GJ. Classification, diagnosis, and management of cholangiocarcinoma. *Clin Gastroenterol Hepatol* 2013; 11(1):13–21.e1.
19. Deoliveira ML, Kambakamba P, Clavien PA. Advances in liver surgery for cholangiocarcinoma. *Curr Opin Gastroenterol* 2013; 29(3):293–8.
20. Ruys AT, Busch OR, Gouma DJ, *et al.* Staging laparoscopy for hilar cholangiocarcinoma: is it still worthwhile? *Ann Surg Oncol* 2011; 18(9):2647–53.
21. Lim JH, Choi GH, Choi SH, *et al.* Liver resection for Bismuth type I and type II hilar cholangiocarcinoma. *World J Surg* 2013; 37(4):829–37.
22. Nagino M, Ebata T, Yokoyama Y, *et al.* Evolution of surgical treatment for perihilar cholangiocarcinoma: a single-center 34-year review of 574 consecutive resections. *Ann Surg* 2013; 258(1):129–40.
23. Taylor A, Primrose J, Langeberg W, *et al.* Survival after liver resection in metastatic colorectal cancer: review and meta-analysis of prognostic factors. *Clin Epidemiol* 2012; 4:283–301.
24. Folprecht G, Grothey A, Alberts S, *et al.* Neoadjuvant treatment of unresectable colorectal liver metastases: correlation between tumour response and resection rates. *Ann Oncol* 2005; 16(8):1311–19.
25. Adam R, Avisar E, Ariche A, *et al.* Five-year survival following hepatic resection after neoadjuvant therapy for nonresectable colorectal. *Ann Surg Oncol* 2001; 8(4):347–53.
26. Spanier BW, Dijkgraaf MG, Bruno MJ. Epidemiology, aetiology and outcome of acute and chronic pancreatitis: an update. *Best Pract Res Clin Gastroenterol* 2008; 22(1):45–63.
27. Brisinda G, Vanella S, Crocco A, *et al.* Severe acute pancreatitis: advances and insights in assessment of severity and management. *Eur J Gastroenterol Hepatol* 2011; 23(7):541–51.
28. Cruz-Santamaría DM, Taxonera C, Giner M. Update on pathogenesis and clinical management of acute pancreatitis. *World J Gastrointest Pathophysiol* 2012; 3(3):60–70.
29. Raraty MG, Halloran CM, Dodd S, *et al.* Minimal access retroperitoneal pancreatic necrosectomy: improvement in morbidity and mortality with a less invasive approach. *Ann Surg* 2010; 251(5):787–93.
30. DiMagno MJ, DiMagno EP. Chronic pancreatitis. *Curr Opin Gastroenterol* 2012; 28(5):523–31.

31. Klöppel G, Adsay NV. Chronic pancreatitis and the differential diagnosis versus pancreatic cancer. *Arch Pathol Lab Med* 2009; 133(3):382–7.
32. Raimondi S, Maisonneuve P, Lowenfels AB. Epidemiology of pancreatic cancer: an overview. *Nat Rev Gastroenterol Hepatol* 2009; 6(12):699–708.
33. Kaneko OF, Lee DM, Wong J, *et al.* Performance of multidetector computed tomographic angiography in determining surgical resectability of pancreatic head adenocarcinoma. *J Comput Assist Tomogr* 2010; 34(5):732–8.
34. Halloran CM, Ghaneh P, Connor S, *et al.* Carbohydrate antigen 19.9 accurately selects patients for laparoscopic assessment to determine resectability of pancreatic malignancy. *Br J Surg* 2008; 95(4):453–9.
35. Doran HE, Bosonnet L, Connor S, *et al.* Laparoscopy and laparoscopic ultrasound in the evaluation of pancreatic and periampullary tumours. *Dig Surg* 2004; 21(4):305–13.
36. Neoptolemos JP, Dunn JA, Stocken DD, *et al.* Adjuvant chemoradiotherapy and chemotherapy in resectable pancreatic cancer: a randomised controlled trial. *Lancet* 2001; 358(9293):1576–85.
37. Sultana A, Smith CT, Cunningham D, *et al.* Meta-analyses of chemotherapy for locally advanced and metastatic pancreatic cancer. *J Clin Oncol* 2007; 25(18):2607–15.
38. Franklin GA, Casós SR. Current advances in the surgical approach to abdominal trauma. *Injury* 2006; 37(12):1143–56.

PART 2.5

Colorectal

CHAPTER 2.5.1

Colorectal

Adam Kimble and Kenneth B. Hosie

Introduction

The lower gastrointestinal (GI) tract commences at the ligament of Treitz, at the duodenojejunal flexure, and finishes at the anus. Colorectal surgery as a specialty deals with malignant and benign diseases of the lower GI tract including the small bowel, appendix, colon, rectum, and anus. However, acute disease of the lower GI tract contributes substantially to the work of the emergency general surgeon. Indeed, the operative mortality for emergency colonic resection is two to four times that of elective resection, and so it is important for the non-colorectal specialist to be aware of the principles of assessment, resuscitation, and management of lower GI pathology to ensure optimum patient care.

Colorectal cancer

Colorectal cancer (CRC) is the third most common cancer in the United Kingdom, accounting for 13% of all new cancer cases. In 2009, there were 41 142 new cases, of which 64% were colonic.[1] Most rectal cancers occur in men (60%), whilst colonic cancers are approximately evenly divided (53% male). The overall male:female ratio is 12:10. The 5-year survival rate in 2005–2009 was approximately 55%, having risen from 22% in 1971–1975[1]. In 2010, there were 16 013 deaths from CRC in the United Kingdom. More than 90% of CRCs are adenocarcinomas.

Aetiology

The majority of CRC arises from pre-existing adenomatous polyps, the so-called adenoma-carcinoma sequence.[2] The stimuli to carcinogenesis remain unclear. There is an interaction between an individual's genotype and the environment to which they are exposed. Genetic factors demonstrate a spectrum of risk with high-risk individuals belonging to a family with a known inherited disorder, for example, familial adenomatous polyposis (FAP—characterized by hundreds of colorectal adenomatous polyps at a young age, multiple extraintestinal manifestations, and an almost 100% risk of CRC), or Lynch syndrome (hereditary non-polyposis colorectal cancer (HNPCC)—characterized by early-onset CRC which are often multiple, right-sided, poorly differentiated, and associated with extracolonic cancers such as endometrial, stomach, and ovarian). Genetic factors also play a role in sporadic CRC, as do environmental factors such as diet, exercise, obesity, and smoking. Long-standing inflammatory bowel disease also increases the risk of CRC.

Presentation

The presentation of CRC is determined by the anatomical site of the tumour: 60% of CRC are left sided or rectal and present with a change in bowel habit (increased frequency and/or looser stools), or rectal bleeding (in the absence of anal symptoms), whereas more proximal tumours present with iron-deficiency anaemia, or as an emergency with intestinal obstruction. Guidelines have been developed to identify patients presenting to primary care as either high or low risk of CRC, warranting either urgent referral and investigation in secondary care, or expectant management.[3]

Population screening

CRC is a suitable candidate for population screening. Screening is able to detect and treat adenomas before malignant transformation takes place, and also detects CRC at an early stage when survival rates after treatment are highest. Screening is dealt with in Chapter 2.15.1.

Once-only flexible sigmoidoscopy has been shown to reduce CRC incidence by 33% and mortality by 43% in those attending screening.[5] A national screening programme of flexible sigmoidoscopy for 55-year-olds has now begun.

Investigation and preoperative staging

Outside of a screening programme, bowel symptoms suggestive of malignancy are best investigated by direct visualization of the bowel mucosa either with colonoscopy (risk of perforation and a 10% incompletion rate), computed tomography (CT) colonography (less invasive, but does not allow biopsy of any lesions identified), or double-contrast enema (largely superseded by CT). Histology confirms the diagnosis.

Once a diagnosis of CRC is made, an important step is to stage the disease with preoperative CT to determine the local extent of the disease, and the presence of metastases. Patients with rectal cancer should have magnetic resonance imaging (MRI) of the pelvis to stage the tumour and assess the risk of local recurrence by determining the anticipated resection margins.[6] Endoanal ultrasound should be performed when local excision is considered or MRI is contraindicated.

Management

All patients diagnosed with CRC should be managed within a colorectal multidisciplinary team (MDT).[5,6]

Management of early cancer

Occasionally CRC is diagnosed at an early stage, particularly following the histopathological examination of an endoscopically resected polyp, which demonstrates an unanticipated invasive cancer. Small (<3 cm) tumours that do not invade past the submucosa are suitable for local excision by transanal endoscopic microsurgery or endoscopic submucosal resection. Following local excision, a proportion of patients will need to proceed to more radical surgery.[5]

Surgical management of advanced cancer

The mainstay of treatment of CRC is radical excision of the primary tumour along with the appropriate vascular pedicle and its lymphatic drainage. Surgery can be open or laparoscopic, and for caecal, ascending colonic, hepatic flexure, and proximal transverse colonic cancers a right hemicolectomy is performed. Distal transverse colonic and splenic flexure tumours are treated with an extended right hemicolectomy with an ileosigmoid anastomosis. Descending, sigmoid, and rectal cancers are treated with left hemicolectomy, sigmoid colectomy, and anterior resection with total mesorectal excision (TME) respectively. Low rectal cancers are treated with an ultra-low anterior resection with covering ileostomy, or abdominoperineal excision of rectum. The use of temporary ileostomies, or a Hartmann's procedure with TME, is advocated if there is any concern regarding an anastomosis (e.g. surgery on an obstructed colon). It is better to err on the side of caution than to risk faecal peritonitis following an anastomotic leak, and these stomas can be reversed at a later date. Covering stomas do not reduce the rate of leak, but mitigate the sequelae.

Locally advanced tumours may require en bloc resection of adjacent structures. Truly inoperable local disease may require ileocolic bypass formation (right-sided disease) or defunctioning stomas (distal colon).

Twenty per cent of operations for CRC are emergency procedures, and the operative mortality is 20%, compared with 5% for scheduled operations.[8] The commonest emergency presentation is obstruction. Diagnosis should be confirmed by CT to identify the site of obstruction and exclude pseudo-obstruction (see 'Acute colonic pseudo-obstruction'). Patients should be resuscitated appropriately and where possible any emergency surgery carried out in daylight hours by an experienced colorectal surgeon. Where there is local expertise, insertion of an expanding metal stent is an option, either as palliation or as a bridge to surgery—converting an emergency operation to a scheduled one with the attendant reduction in morbidity and mortality.

Around 25% of patients with CRC present with distant metastases, most commonly in the liver and lung. All such patients should be discussed at the appropriate MDTs to decide upon resectability. With careful patient selection, and following systemic treatment, hepatectomy for CRC metastases is associated with a 5-year survival of around 33%.[7]

Non-surgical treatment of colorectal cancer

Chemotherapy and radiotherapy have well-defined roles in CRC. They can be given as neoadjuvant, adjuvant, or palliative treatment.

The aim of neoadjuvant treatment in rectal cancer is twofold:

- Long-course chemoradiotherapy reduces tumour size, can downstage tumours, and improves the rate of curative resection.[9,10]
- Short-course preoperative radiotherapy reduces local recurrence rates.[11] Neoadjuvant chemotherapy is also used in the treatment of liver metastases to reduce size and improve surgical resection rates.

Improved disease-free survival rates are seen following adjuvant chemotherapy in node-positive disease.[12,13] There is also a small survival benefit in node-negative cancers. It is important to balance any potential benefits of treatment with the risk of toxicity.

Postoperative adjuvant chemoradiotherapy is advised in rectal cancers that did not receive neoadjuvant treatment and have positive circumferential resection margins or node positive disease.

For appropriately selected patients with unresectable metastatic disease, palliative chemotherapy increases survival.[5] Palliative radiotherapy is useful for symptomatic relief of advanced local disease or metastases.

Pathological staging

Pathological staging is important as a prognostic indicator and for planning further treatment. The TNM (tumour, node, and metastasis) system and Dukes' stage are two widely recognized classification systems, and a summary is given in Box 2.5.1.1. Age-adjusted 5-year survival rates are 93.2% for Dukes' A, 77% for stage B, 47.7% for Stage C, and 6.6% for stage D.[1]

Box 2.5.1.1 The TNM and Dukes' stage classification systems

TNM classification

T 0, no evidence of primary tumour

  1, invasion of submucosa

  2, invasion of muscularis propria

  3, invasion of mesorectal fat or adventitia but no serosal breach

  4a, direct invasion into adjacent structure

  4b, breaches serosa into peritoneal cavity

N 0, no lymph node metastasis

  1, metastasis in one to three pericolic or perirectal lymph nodes

  2, metastasis in four or more pericolic or perirectal lymph nodes

  3, metastasis in any lymph node along a named vascular trunk

M 0, no distant metastases

  1, distant metastases present.

Reproduced with permission from Edge, SB *et al.*, (Eds.), *AJCC (American Joint Committee on Cancer) Cancer Staging Manual*, Seventh Edition, Springer, New York, USA, Copyright © 2010.

Dukes' classification

A, invasive carcinoma not breaching the muscularis propria

B, invasive carcinoma breaching the muscularis propria, but not involving regional lymph nodes

C1, invasive carcinoma involving regional lymph nodes (apical node negative)

C2, invasive carcinoma involving regional lymph nodes (apical node positive)

(D), presence of distant metastases (not included in Dukes' original staging system, which was confined to the resection specimen).

From Dukes CE, The classification of cancer of the rectum, *Journal of Pathological Bacteriology*, Volume 35, pp. 35–323, Copyright © 1932 The Pathological Society of Great Britain and Ireland, with permission from John Wiley and Sons; and M. Whittaker, J. and Colicher C., The prognosis after surgical treatment for carcinoma of the rectum, *British Journal of Surgery*, Volume 63, Issue 5, pp. 384–388 Copyright © 1976 British Journal of Surgery Society Ltd., with permission from John Wiley and Sons.

Follow-up

The rationale for following up patients is to identify those in whom there is local recurrence, metastatic disease, and for early detection of metachronous cancers. This is achieved radiologically (CT), biochemically (serum carcinoembryonic antigen), and colonoscopically.[3]

Anal cancer

Anal cancer is rare and accounts for approximately 4% of large bowel cancers. Over 80% of anal cancers arise from the squamous epithelium of the anal canal and anal margin; adenocarcinoma and malignant melanoma are other rarer forms. Risk factors include genital warts and infection with human papilloma virus (HPV types 16, 18, 31, and 33).[14] There is an increase in the incidence of anal cancer in immunosuppressed populations (transplant recipients and HIV patients). In common with cervical or vulval cancer, it is thought that anal cancer may occur due to progression of dysplastic changes of anal intraepithelial neoplasia.[15]

Anal cancer typically presents with pain and bleeding of an ulcerated or mass lesion of the anus. Following staging, treatment is principally with combination chemoradiotherapy of fluorouracil (5-FU), mitomycin C, and high-dose external beam radiotherapy.[16,17] Surgery is reserved for small lesions at the anal margin or for salvage therapy after failure of primary chemoradiation. Spread is via the inguinal lymph nodes, which should be examined in all patients with anal lesions.

All patients diagnosed with anal cancer should be discussed by an anal cancer MDT.

Intestinal obstruction

Intestinal obstruction is any hindrance to the passage of intestinal contents, and is a common surgical emergency. It can be classified into two types:

+ *Dynamic obstruction*, in which peristalsis acts against a mechanical obstruction (this can be intraluminal, intramural, or extramural).

+ *Adynamic obstruction*, in which there is absent or disordered peristalsis (paralytic ileus, pseudo-obstruction).

For practical purposes, it is also useful to classify according to the site of the obstruction into small or large bowel obstruction.

Dynamic bowel obstruction

There are numerous causes of dynamic small bowel obstruction, but intra-abdominal adhesions secondary to previous surgery is the commonest aetiology in the developed world. In contrast, in the developing world the most common cause is hernia. Malignancy is the leading cause of dynamic large bowel obstruction worldwide (Table 2.5.1.1).

Small bowel obstruction
Adhesions

Intra-abdominal adhesions commonly form following abdominal surgery. Numerous causes have been identified, but in general, any peritoneal irritation leads to an inflammatory reaction resulting in fibrin production and subsequent adhesion formation. Open appendicectomy, colonic, and gynaecological surgery are known to result in an increased risk of adhesional small bowel obstruction (1–25%).[18] In the absence of previous abdominal surgery, congenital bands, such as an obliterated vitellointestinal duct, or omental adhesions to sites of previous intra-abdominal infection or inflammation can cause obstruction.

Hernia

Careful examination of the hernial orifices of any patient presenting in obstruction is mandatory. This includes any potential sites of incisional herniation, but the possibility of an internal hernia must also be considered. Potential sites of internal herniation include the foramen of Winslow, the paraduodenal fossae, congenital or acquired diaphragmatic defects, various postoperative mesenteric defects, and rarely the obturator foramina.

Large bowel obstruction
Malignancy

Malignancy accounts for between 50% and 60% of all cases of dynamic large bowel obstruction (LBO); however, only 8–29% of CRC present as an emergency with intestinal obstruction.[19] Disseminated intra-abdominal malignancy (e.g. from ovarian cancer) can also present as large or small bowel obstruction.

Diverticular disease

Diverticulosis is a common benign condition of the colon. It is more common in the Western world and is thought to be related to the relative lack of dietary fibre in these societies. This leads to increased intraluminal pressure and the subsequent herniation of the colonic mucosa through points of weakness in the muscle wall, that is, the site of penetration of the vasa recta. Incidence increases with advancing age (present in approximately two-thirds of 80-year-olds), the vast majority of whom are asymptomatic. Left-sided disease, particularly in the sigmoid colon, is the most common.

The main complication of diverticulosis is inflammation, thought to be caused by inspissated stool becoming stuck in the neck of the diverticulum. Diverticulitis can be graded according to the Hinchey classification:[20]

Table 2.5.1.1 The causes of dynamic bowel obstruction

	Small bowel	Large bowel
In the lumen	Gallstone ileus	Faeces
	Food bolus	Diaphragm disease
	Foreign body	(NSAID induced)
	Intussusception	
	Bezoars	
	Parasites	
In the wall	Crohn's disease	Carcinoma
	Tuberculosis	Diverticular disease
	Tumour (primary small bowel, caecal carcinoma)	Crohn's disease
Outside the wall	Adhesions (congenital and acquired)	Volvulus
	Hernia	Hernia
	Volvulus	(Adhesions)

Source: data from *The Lancet*, Volume 353, Issue 9163, Ellis H *et al.*, Adhesion-related hospital re-admissions after abdominal and pelvic surgery: a retrospective study, pp. 1476–9, Copyright © 1999 Elsevier Ltd. All rights reserved.

◆ *Stage I*—localized abscess

◆ *Stage II*—pelvic abscess (or other distant abscess)

◆ *Stage III*—purulent peritonitis

◆ *Stage IV*—faecal peritonitis.

Reprinted from *Advances in Surgery*®, Volume 12, Hinchey EJ et al., *Treatment of perforated diverticular disease of the colon*, pp. 85–109, Copyright © 1978 with permission from Elsevier, http://www.sciencedirect.com/science/journal/00653411/41

Repeated bouts of inflammation can lead to stricture formation and subsequent obstruction. Other complications include fistula formation, colonic bleeding, and perforation.

Volvulus

Volvulus is the axial rotation of the colon about its mesentery. It is most common in the sigmoid colon (76%), but also occurs in the caecum (22%) and transverse colon (2%).[21] Sigmoid volvulus commonly occurs in the frail elderly population, or those with chronic neurological conditions who are often institutionalized and have severe constipation.

Pathophysiology

Regardless of the aetiology, in dynamic obstruction, initially there is increased peristalsis as the bowel attempts to overcome the obstruction, leading to severe colicky abdominal pain. Subsequently, the bowel begins to dilate and there is a reduction in peristalsis and ultimately paralysis and flaccidity. The obstructed bowel fills with GI secretions and swallowed air, which results in increased intraluminal pressure and bowel wall oedema and further accumulation of electrolyte and protein-rich fluid within the bowel wall and lumen. Reduced oral intake, vomiting, and impaired gut absorption further exacerbate the fluid and electrolyte losses. In addition, impaired mucosal integrity can lead to bacterial translocation and subsequent bacteraemia and/or systemic inflammatory response.

Impairment of venous drainage leads to increased capillary pressure and progressive compromise of arterial flow. Left untreated, this leads to ischaemia, necrosis, and ultimately perforation. Closed-loop obstruction occurs when there is both proximal and distal obstruction such as in colonic obstruction in the presence of a competent ileocaecal valve, or volvulus.

Presentation

The four cardinal signs of dynamic intestinal obstruction are *pain, vomiting, abdominal distension*, and *absolute constipation*. These vary in their predominance according to the level of obstruction, the underlying pathology, and the presence of intestinal ischaemia. Distension and constipation are early features of more distal obstruction, whereas early vomiting is more common in proximal obstruction. Pain is usually the first symptom encountered and is usually severe and colicky in nature and is either central (small bowel) or lower abdominal (large bowel). The development of severe constant pain with localized tenderness is indicative of ischaemia. Peritonitis signifies infarction and/or perforation.

Late manifestations of all forms of intestinal obstruction include dehydration, oliguria, hypovolaemic shock, systemic inflammatory response syndrome, and peritonism.

Investigation

Investigations in suspected intestinal obstruction are aimed at assessing the general state of the patient, confirming the diagnosis and aetiology of the obstruction, and identifying those patients who should undergo early surgery or those in whom a non-operative approach is appropriate. Blood tests to identify anaemia, renal impairment, an inflammatory response, acidosis, pancreatitis, and a group and save are appropriate. Plain abdominal films identify approximately 60% of cases of intestinal obstruction, but do not distinguish the level or aetiology. Contrast radiology is useful in selected patients, In small bowel obstruction, water-soluble contrast studies can help identify those patients who are likely to need surgery or those in whom non-operative management is likely to be successful.[22] Rectal contrast studies in LBO can distinguish between mechanical obstruction and pseudo-obstruction. CT with oral and/or rectal contrast is arguably the most useful imaging modality as it provides information on the level of the obstruction, the possible aetiology, and can also stage malignant disease.

Management

The principles of the management of dynamic intestinal obstruction are GI decompression (facilitated by the placement of a large-bore nasogastric tube), replacement of fluid and electrolytes (which may be considerable), and relief of obstruction. The timing of surgical intervention depends on the clinical picture. Prolonged conservative management for up to 72 hours is reasonable in adhesional obstruction in the absence of pain or tenderness, and in up to 75% of cases, spontaneous resolution occurs. Indications for surgery include local or generalized peritonitis, an irreducible hernia, visceral perforation, the development of sepsis, a failure to improve with conservative measures, or the presence of an obvious obstructing lesion on imaging.

Principles of surgery are to identify the site and nature of the obstruction with an assessment of gut viability. Any adhesions are divided, any tumour is resected, bypassed, or decompressed proximally, any intraluminal foreign body or gallstone removed, an intussusception is reduced, and any volvulus decompressed and reduced. Following relief of the obstruction, the viability of the remaining gut is carefully assessed and any non-viable bowel resected.

Adynamic bowel obstruction

Paralytic ileus

Paralytic ileus affects the whole bowel, with failure of normal peristaltic activity. This stasis leads to accumulation of fluid and gas within the bowel with marked abdominal distension. Pain is not usually a feature. Ileus is classically seen postoperatively and is usually self-limiting, but other causes are intra-abdominal sepsis, metabolic disturbances such as hypokalaemia and uraemia, and some drugs (e.g. opiates).

Management is directed towards the cause, and particular attention is paid to the correction of any electrolyte abnormalities (hypokalaemia, hyponatraemia, and hypomagnesaemia), resolution of sepsis, and GI decompression with a nasogastric tube. Prolonged ileus warrants further investigation to rule out a mechanical cause.

Acute colonic pseudo-obstruction

Acute colonic pseudo-obstruction is also known as Ogilvie's syndrome and presents as acute LBO, although mechanical obstruction is absent. Ogilvie first described the syndrome in two patients with extensive retroperitoneal malignancy affecting the autonomic supply of the colon.[23] A typical patient is hospitalized for other reasons such as recent surgery, trauma, metabolic disorders, and cardiorespiratory disorders. The diagnosis rests on the exclusion of a mechanical cause of obstruction. Treatment involves correcting any underlying cause and avoiding any drugs that adversely affect gut motility such as opiates or anticholinergics. Nasogastric decompression is routinely used. Most cases resolve spontaneously but occasionally the colon requires colonoscopic decompression to avoid ischaemic perforation of the caecum. Intravenous neostigmine can be used to medically decompress the colon,[24] but risks bradycardia and caution should be taken in patients with cardiovascular disease. With continued colonic and caecal distension despite optimal non-operative measures surgery may be required to avoid perforation. This can be a simple caecostomy (percutaneous or trephine), or a full laparotomy and hemicolectomy.

Rectal bleeding

Lower GI haemorrhage is defined as any bleeding arising from the bowel distal to the ligament of Treitz. Bleeding from the colon and rectum accounts for 20% of all cases of acute GI haemorrhage, and is a common and distressing complaint. Most patients are elderly, often with significant co-morbidities. The site and cause of haemorrhage can be difficult to determine. Fortunately the bleeding settles spontaneously in the majority of patients. Severity of haemorrhage can be classified as occult, mild, moderate, or massive according to the amount of the circulating volume that is lost and loosely corresponds to the classes of haemorrhagic shock seen in trauma.[25]

Diverticular disease remains the commonest cause of lower GI haemorrhage in adults, accounting for approximately 50% of all cases. Bleeding can be life-threatening, but the vast majority stop spontaneously. Angiodysplasias are degenerative vascular malformations of the GI tract found predominantly in the right colon, and are the second most common cause of lower GI bleeds. Bleeding tends to be slow and recurrent. Other important causes of lower GI haemorrhage are colonic cancers, inflammatory bowel disease (usually presenting as bloody diarrhoea), ischaemic colitis, benign anorectal conditions such as haemorrhoids, fissures, fistulas, and anorectal varices. A massive upper GI haemorrhage may also present as fresh rectal bleeding.

Initial management is aimed at prompt resuscitation of the patient, with intravenous fluids and blood products given as necessary and any clotting abnormalities corrected. A history of previous GI bleeds, peptic ulcer disease, inflammatory bowel disease, non-steroidal anti-inflammatory drug (NSAID) or warfarin usage, liver disease, or aortic surgery should be elicited. Careful examination, including the anorectum, is important, and in massive rectal bleeding an upper GI source should be excluded with an upper GI endoscopy. Further investigation and management depends on the severity of the bleeding, and the local availability of expertise, and is aimed at locating the source of haemorrhage. Eighty per cent of bleeds will cease spontaneously and investigation can proceed electively, usually in the form of colonoscopy. If bleeding is ongoing then angiography is performed; CT angiography is a non-invasive preliminary investigation that can localize the bleeding and direct selective therapeutic angiography (embolization or vasopressin infusion) or surgery as necessary. If the bleeding is slow (i.e. 0.1 mL/min), it may not be evident on angiography and labelled red cell scanning may be useful to locate the site of bleeding. Embolization carries the risks of re-bleeding, bowel ischaemia, and renal failure secondary to intravenous contrast infusion. Colonoscopy, although very challenging, can also be performed in

the acute phase, where it can be both diagnostic and therapeutic (i.e. clip application, diathermy, adrenaline injection, or heater probes). Surgery is indicated if bleeding continues despite medical, endoscopic, and angiographic intervention. If the site of haemorrhage has been identified then segmental resection is the operation of choice. If not localized preoperatively, identification of the site of bleeding should be attempted intraoperatively with the use of surgeon-guided upper and lower GI endoscopy. If the cause remains unidentified, blind segmental resection should be avoided because of the high risk of re-bleeding and its associated morbidity and mortality; subtotal colectomy is the operation of choice.

Alterations in bowel habit

There is huge variation in individual bowel habit and much confusion over the words 'constipation' and 'diarrhoea'. To some patients, constipation means that their bowels are opening less frequently, and to others that their stools are harder than usual. Similarly, diarrhoea can mean either frequent defaecation, or loose stools. When assessing patients it is important to elicit what the patient actually means by these terms and relate them to their normal bowel habit and any associated symptoms such as abdominal pain, bloating, rectal bleeding, or weight loss. Diagnostic criteria for these terms (albeit for functional disorders) are given by the Rome III criteria as follows: [26]

Constipation—two or more of the following:

◆ Straining ≥ 25% of occasions

◆ Lumpy or hard stools ≥ 25% of occasions

◆ Sensation of incomplete evacuation ≥ 25% of occasions

◆ Sensation of anorectal obstruction/blockage > 25% of occasions

◆ Manual manoeuvres to facilitate evacuation ≥ 25% (e.g. digital evacuation, support of the pelvic floor)

◆ Fewer than three defaecations per week.

Diarrhoea:

◆ Loose (mushy) or watery stools without pain occurring ≥ 75% of stools.

Reprinted from Gastroenterology, Volume 130, Issue 5, Longstreth GF et al., *Functional bowel disorders*, pp. 1480–91, Copyright © 2006 The AGA Institute, with permission from Elsevier, http://www.sciencedirect.com/science/journal/00165085

The chronicity of any change in bowel habit is important as it gives vital clues to the aetiology. The 2015 guideline from the National Institute for Health and Care Excellence for the referral of suspected cancer[3] suggests urgent referral of all patients 60 years and older, with a change in bowel habit to looser stools and/or increased stool frequency persisting 6 weeks or more or iron deficiency anaemia, all patients 50 years and older who report unexplained rectal bleeding with associated symptoms, and 40 years and older with unexplained weight loss and abdominal pain.

Colorectal cancer rarely presents with constipation, but a persistent new change to constipation warrants exclusion of sinister pathology. A full list of the causes of constipation and diarrhoea is beyond the scope of this chapter, but the commonest and important causes are infective gastroenteritis, inflammatory bowel disease, colorectal cancer, diverticular disease, radiation enteritis, irritable bowel syndrome, coeliac disease, medications (opiates, antibiotics, laxatives, and atropine), metabolic derangements, pancreatic insufficiency, benign anorectal conditions, anxiety, and diet.

Functional constipation can be considered to be either due to slow transit within the gut or abnormal evacuation, or a combination of the two. Dietary advice and laxative use are the mainstays of treatment, but further investigation with transit studies, anorectal physiology, and defaecating proctography is often indicated in severe symptomatic constipation.

Obstructive defaecation may result from failure of the puborectalis muscle to relax (anismus, or pelvic floor dyssynergia), presence of an anterior rectocele and/or rectorectal intussusception. Biofeedback training is useful in anismus, whilst surgery can be helpful in rectocele and intussusception (see 'Rectal prolapse'), where the aim is to restore 'normal' anatomy and physiology to the pelvis. It has become increasingly recognized that the approach to such problems requires input from a specialized pelvic floor MDT.

Common perianal and rectal conditions

Anorectal sepsis

Anorectal sepsis is a common presentation on the acute surgical take. The cryptoglandular theory proposed by Parks[27] suggests that abscesses result from the obstruction of the anal glands and ducts. Subsequent pus formation travels along the path of least resistance. This can be in one of three planes—vertical, horizontal, or circumferential—and collects in the potential anorectal spaces—perianal, ischiorectal, intersphincteric, and supralevator. Circumferential spread results in the formation of a horseshoe abscess. Other causes of anorectal sepsis include inflammatory bowel disease (especially Crohn's disease), trauma (including surgery), foreign bodies, malignancy, radiation, and primary infection of the skin and soft tissues.

Presenting features are usually pain and a palpable tender lump with or without malaise and fever. Intersphincteric abscesses may present with pain alone and only become evident upon examination under anaesthetic. Treatment of acute anorectal sepsis is incision and drainage. In experienced hands, a careful search for potential fistulous tracks can be made and treated appropriately (see 'Fistula-in-ano'). Delay in diagnosis and treatment, or inadequate drainage of anorectal abscesses risks life-threatening necrotizing infection.

Fistula-in-ano

Fistula-in-ano and anorectal abscesses share a common aetiology. Abscess formation represents the acute phase, with subsequent epithelialization of the track leading to the establishment of a fistula. However, not all anorectal abscesses go on to form fistulas.

Sir Alan Parks devised the most widely used classification based on a study of 400 fistulas treated at St Mark's Hospital, London.[28] This describes four main groups in relation to the internal and external anal sphincters:

+ Intersphincteric
+ Trans-sphincteric
+ Suprasphincteric
+ Extrasphincteric.[28]

Patients with a fistula will often give a history of an abscess that was drained surgically or spontaneously with continued bloody or purulent discharge.

The assessment of a fistula-in-ano requires the identification of the internal and external openings, the course of the primary track, the presence of any secondary extensions, and the presence of other diseases complicating the fistula.

Goodsall's rule states that an external opening seen posterior to the transverse anal line will open into the anal canal in the midline posteriorly, and an anterior external opening is usually associated with a radial track. An exception to the rule is the anterior external opening lying greater than 3 cm from the anus which may represent an extension of a posterior horseshoe fistula.

The principles of treatment are to drain sepsis, eliminate the fistula, prevent recurrence, and preserve sphincter function. Recurrence occurs in up to 25% of fistulas, and in many cases is due to undrained sepsis at primary surgery. MRI is useful in reducing this recurrence by accurately demonstrating the anatomy of the fistula track in relation to the anal sphincter complex.

Laying open of the fistula (fistulotomy), is the most effective treatment, but requires the division of at least some of the internal sphincter and therefore risks incontinence, so patients should be counselled accordingly. There are multiple sphincter-preserving procedures for high or complex fistulas including tissue glues, collagen plugs, and mucosal advancement flaps, but all are associated with high rates of recurrence. A seton is a loop drain usually of silastic or silk through the fistula track which can be tight or loose. This option provides good long-term control of sepsis and symptoms with preservation of continence and an acceptable long-term cure rate.

Haemorrhoids

Haemorrhoids arise from the anal cushions which are normal vascular structures within the anal canal that provide the fine control of continence of liquids and gases. They characteristically lie in the 3, 7, and 11 o'clock positions (with the patient in the lithotomy position). Haemorrhoids, or piles, are said to occur when these anal cushions bleed, prolapse, or both. Haemorrhoids can be classified as follows:

+ First degree: bleeding alone
+ Second degree: prolapse with spontaneous reduction
+ Third degree: prolapse requiring manual reduction
+ Fourth degree: irreducible prolapse.

Bleeding from haemorrhoids is classically painless, bright red, and seen on the toilet paper when wiping or can drip into the toilet pan. A flexible sigmoidoscopy to rule out other more proximal causes should be considered.

Reassurance, dietary advice (increased fibre and fluid intake), treatment of any underlying constipation, and modification of defaecatory habits (e.g. avoiding straining and prolonged defaecation) will resolve most haemorrhoidal symptoms. Outpatient treatment with rubber band ligation, or injection sclerotherapy, is the treatment of choice for second-degree haemorrhoids and is also a useful primary treatment for third-degree haemorrhoids. Surgery should be reserved for third- or fourth-degree haemorrhoids, or recurrent haemorrhoids.[29] Traditionally, surgery has involved excisional haemorrhoidectomy. There are variations to the technique (e.g. open or closed), but risks of postoperative pain, bleeding, sepsis, and incontinence remain similar. Newer techniques of stapled haemorrhoidectomy and haemorrhoidal artery ligation are alternatives to conventional surgery with reported good resolution of symptoms,[30,31] although long-term efficacy is yet to be fully elucidated.

Anal fissure

An anal fissure is a longitudinal ulcer in the squamous epithelium of the anus distal to the dentate line, and in 90% of cases lies in the posterior midline. It is characterized by pain on defaecation and anal bleeding. The aetiology of the typical chronic anal fissure remains unclear, but the most consistent finding is that of hypertonia of the internal anal sphincter (IAS), which when combined with the relatively poor blood supply to the posterior midline of the anoderm, suggests an ischaemic cause. Historically, fissures were thought to be due to the passage of a hard stool causing a tear in the anal mucosa which caused pain and the reflex IAS spasm. Treatment is directed at lessening IAS spasm, which improves blood supply, with subsequent relief of symptoms and healing of the fissure. A stepwise approach to treatment has been shown to be effective in healing fissures, with topical nitrates or calcium channel blockers, followed by botulinum toxin injections favoured before surgery.[32] Lateral internal sphincterotomy remains the most effective treatment for fissures, but carries with it a risk of faecal incontinence in up to 30% of patients, and is reserved for the 5–26% of patients whose symptoms persist after non-surgical options have failed.[32] Fissurectomy, when used in combination with botulinum toxin, heals over 90% of chemically resistant fissures while avoiding the risk of a sphincterotomy. An important subtype of anal fissures has normal resting IAS pressures, and there is some evidence that occult rectal prolapse could be implicated in the aetiology. Multiple fissures or those in unusual positions (i.e. not the midline) should prompt the consideration of alternative diagnoses such as inflammatory bowel disease, tuberculosis, syphilis, or HIV.

Rectal prolapse

Rectal prolapse can be either mucosal, where only the rectal mucosal layer prolapses through the anus, or full thickness, with all linings of the rectal wall protruding. It is common in elderly multiparous women (with the attendant pelvic floor dysfunction), but occasionally occurs in young children following a diarrhoeal illness. Mucosal prolapse is initially treated with increasing dietary fibre and bulking laxatives, but it can also be treated in the outpatient setting with suction banding or sclerotherapy. Occasionally, endoluminal stapling techniques analogous to stapled haemorrhoidectomy can be employed. Full-thickness prolapse is almost exclusively treated surgically. This can be achieved either by the perineal or abdominal approach. Perineal surgery may involve mucosal resection and plication of the prolapsed rectal muscle (Delorme's procedure), or rectosigmoidectomy (Altmeier's procedure). Abdominal surgery can be open or laparoscopic, and the rectopexy can be achieved with either non-absorbable sutures or mesh, and can include resection of the sigmoid colon. Abdominal approaches have lower recurrence rates but the perineal approach is preferred in the frail elderly patient as it avoids the morbidity of an abdominal procedure.

Solitary rectal ulcer syndrome can occur in association with rectal prolapse. The anterior rectal ulcer is thought to form as a result of rectorectal intussusception or anterior mucosal prolapse causing symptoms of obstructive defaecation. Trauma secondary to anal digitation may also contribute. Treatment is with dietary modification, bulking agents, and biofeedback. Surgical intervention in the form of stapled mucosal resection, stapled transanal rectal resection, or an abdominal rectopexy is occasionally indicated.

Proctalgia fugax

Proctalgia fugax literally means 'fleeting rectal and/or anal pain', and is a condition characterized by severe cramping pain in the anorectal region. Individuals suffer attacks at irregular intervals up to five or six times in a year, but sometimes more often. Women are affected twice as often as men and symptoms usually start between 40 and 50 years of age. The frequency, intensity, and duration of attacks generally diminish with increasing age. The attacks of pain occur spontaneously, more commonly at night, and usually last between 30 seconds and 20 minutes.[26] The pain can be associated with the urge to defecate (without success), or with an erection in males. There is no clear aetiology, although it has been suggested that it is due to spasm of the levator ani. Diagnosis is made with a typical history in the absence of any physical findings. Management remains difficult, with no consistently effective treatment. Attacks are so sudden and short-lasting that oral medications are generally ineffective. Anecdotal success has been reported with biofeedback, tricyclic antidepressants, botulinum toxin, sacral nerve stimulation, and pudendal nerve block. Other manoeuvres such as taking a warm enema or bath may also help mitigate an attack.

Pruritus ani

Itching in the perianal region is a common problem. Virtually any perianal condition can result in pruritus, but often a primary cause is not identified. Commonly it is associated with a degree of faecal leakage either due to local pathology such as a fistula, fissure, or haemorrhoid, or due to a stool consistency or frequency, which makes perianal hygiene difficult. Irritants within the diet such as caffeine, alcohol, spices, and citrus fruits can be contributory factors as can tight fitting, non-absorbent undergarments that cause excessive sweating. In general, treatment is aimed at removing or correcting any identifiable cause in combination with basic hygiene measures to keep the perianal area clean and dry, and to prevent further irritation to the perianal skin.

In children, threadworm infestation should be excluded.

References

1. Cancer Research UK. *Bowel Cancer Statistics.* 2013. [Online] http://info.cancerresearchuk.org/cancerstats/types/bowel/
2. Leslie A, Carey FA, Pratt NR, *et al.* The colorectal adenoma-carcinoma sequence. *Br J Surg* 2002; 89:845–60.
3. National Institute for Health and Care Excellence. *Suspected Cancer: Recognition and Referral* [NG12]. 2015. [Online] https://www.nice.org.uk/guidance/ng12
4. NHS Cancer Screening Programmes. *The NHS Bowel Cancer Screening Programme.* [Online] http://www.cancerscreening.nhs.uk/bowel/
5. Association of Coloproctology of Great Britain and Ireland. *Guidelines for the Management of Colorectal Cancer* (3rd ed). London: Association of Coloproctology of Great Britain and Ireland; 2007.
6. National Institute for Health and Clinical Excellence. *Colorectal Cancer: The Diagnosis and Management of Colorectal Cancer.* Clinical Guideline 131. London: NICE; 2011. https://www.nice.org.uk/guidance/cg131

7. Garden OJ, Rees M, Poston GJ, *et al.* Guidelines for resection of colorectal liver metastases. *Gut* 2006; 55(Suppl III):iii1–8.

8. Mella J, Biffin A, Radcliffe AG, *et al.* Population-based audit of colorectal cancer management in two UK health regions. Colorectal Cancer Working Group, Royal College of Surgeons of England Clinical Epidemiology and Audit Unit. *Br J Surg* 1997; 84(12):1731–6.

9. Bosset JF, Collette L, Calais G, *et al.* Chemotherapy with preoperative radiotherapy in rectal cancer. *N Engl J Med* 2006; 355(11):1114–23.

10. Gerard JP, Conroy T, Bonnetain F, *et al.* Preoperative radiotherapy with or without concurrent fluorouracil and leucovorin in T3-4 rectal cancers: results of FFCD 9203. *J Clin Oncol* 2006; 24(28):4620–5.

11. Swedish Rectal Cancer Trial. Improved survival with preoperative radiotherapy in resectable rectal cancer. *N Engl J Med* 1997; 336(14):980–7.

12. QUASAR Collaborative Group. Comparison of fluorouracil with additional levamisole, higher-dose folinic acid, or both, as adjuvant chemotherapy for colorectal cancer: a randomised trial. *Lancet* 2000; 355(9215):1588–96.

13. Wolmark N, Wieand HS, Keubler JP. A phase III trial comparing FULV to FULV + oxaliplatin in stage II or III carcinoma of the colon: results of the NSABP protocol C-07. *J Clin Oncol* 2005; 23(Suppl):16s, Abstract 3500.

14. Palmer JG, Scholefield JH, Shepherd N, *et al.* Anal cancer and human papillomaviruses. *Dis Colon Rectum* 1989; 32:1016–22.

15. Scholefield J, Hickson W, Smith J, *et al.* Anal intraepithelial neoplasia: part of a multifocal disease process. *Lancet* 1992; 340:1271–3.

16. Nigro N, Vaitkevicius V, Considine B. Combined therapy for cancer of the anal canal. A preliminary report. *Dis Colon Rectum* 1974; 17(3):354–6.

17. UKCCR Anal Cancer Trial Working Party. Epidermoid anal cancer: results from the UKCCCR randomised trial of radiotherapy alone versus radiotherapy, 5-fluorouracil, and mitomycin. *Lancet* 1996; 348:1049–54.

18. Ellis H, Thompson JN, Parker MC, *et al.* Adhesion-related hospital readmissions after abdominal and pelvic surgery: a retrospective study. *Lancet* 1999; 353:1476–9.

19. Serpell JW, McDermott FT, Katrivessis H, *et al.* Obstructing carcinomas of the colon. *Br J Surg* 1989; 76:965–9.

20. Hinchey EJ, Schaal PG, Richards GK. Treatment of perforated diverticular disease of the colon. *Adv Surg* 1978; 12:85–109.

21. Ballantyne GH. Review of sigmoid volvulus: clinical pattern and pathogenesis. *Dis Colon Rectum* 1982; 36:508.

22. Chen S-C, Lin F-Y, Lee P-H, *et al.* Water soluble contrast study predicts the need for early surgery in adhesive small bowel obstruction. *Br J Surg* 1999; 86:1692–8.

23. Ogilvie H. Large intestine colic due to sympathetic deprivation: a new clinical syndrome. *Br Med J* 1948; 2:671–3.

24. Ponec RJ, Saunders MD, Kimmey MB. Neostigmine for the treatment of acute colonic pseudo-obstruction. *N Engl J Med* 1999; 341:137–41.

25. American College of Surgeons Committee on Trauma. *Shock: Advanced Trauma Life Support for Doctors* (8th ed). Chicago, IL: American College of Surgeons; 2008.

26. Longstreth GF, Thompson WG, Chey WD, *et al.* Functional bowel disorders, *Gastroenterology* 2006; 130:1480–91.

27. Parks AG. Pathogenesis and treatment of fistula-in-ano. *Br Med J* 1961; 1:463–9.

28. Parks AG, Gordon PH, Hardcastle JD. A classification of fistula-in-ano. *Br J Surg* 1976; 63:1–12.

29. Shanmugum V, Thaha MA, Rabindranath KS, *et al.* Rubber band ligation versus excisional haemorrhoidectomy for haemorrhoids. *Cochrane Database Syst Rev* 2005; 3:CD005034.

30. Mehigan BJ, Monson JR, Hartley JE. Stapling procedure for haemorrhoids versus Milligan-Morgan haemorrhoidectomy: randomised controlled trial. *Lancet* 2000; 355:782–5.

31. Dal Monte PP, Tagariello C, Sarago M, *et al.* Transanal haemorrhoidal dearterialization: nonexcisional surgery for the treatment of haemorrhoidal disease. *Tech Coloproctol* 2007; 11:333–9.

32. Sinha R, Kaiser AM. Efficacy of management algorithm for reducing need for sphincterotomy in chronic anal fissures. *Colorectal Dis* 2012; 14(6):760–4.

PART 2.6

Breast surgery

Sub-section editor: Malcolm W. R. Reed

CHAPTER 2.6.1

Clinical assessment and management of benign breast diseases

Amit Goyal and Malcolm W. R. Reed

Breast anatomy and development

Development

The breasts develop as an invagination of chest wall ectoderm. At puberty, alveoli sprout from the ducts and fatty infiltration takes place. With pregnancy there is significant development of the alveoli which secrete the fatty droplets of milk. After the menopause, the gland tissue atrophies and the breasts are predominantly comprised of fat.

Developmental abnormalities are not uncommon. The nipple may fail to evert and it is important to establish if this is a recent event or has been present since birth. Supernumerary nipples or even breasts may occur along the 'milk line', which extends from the axilla to the groin.

Location/anatomical boundaries

The female breast lies between the second and sixth ribs and between the sternal edge medially and midaxillary line laterally. Two-thirds of it rests on the pectoralis major, one-third on the serratus anterior, while its lower medial edge just overlaps the upper part of the rectus sheath. For descriptive purposes it is divided into four quadrants; the upper outer quadrant extends laterally into the axilla as the axillary tail.

Structure

The breast comprises 15–20 lobules of glandular tissue embedded in fat separated by fibrous septa running from the subcutaneous tissues to the fascia of the chest wall (the ligaments of Cooper). Malignant infiltration and fibrous contraction of these ligaments may result in dimpling of skin over a carcinoma. Each lobule consists of 10–100 alveoli, the basic secretory unit, and drains by its lactiferous duct on to the nipple. This area is lubricated by the areolar glands of Montgomery; these are large, modified sebaceous glands which may form sebaceous cysts which may, in turn, become infected.

Superficial pectoral fascia envelops the breast and is continuous with the superficial abdominal fascia of Camper. The undersurface of the breast lies on the deep pectoral fascia.

The male breast is rudimentary, comprising small ducts without alveoli and supported by fibrous tissue and fat; however, it is prone to most diseases that affect the female breast.

Blood supply

The axillary artery supplies blood via the superior thoracic artery, pectoral branches of the thoracoacromial artery, the lateral thoracic artery, and the subscapular artery. The internal mammary artery supplies perforating branches to the anteromedial part of the breast. The second to fourth anterior intercostal arteries supply perforating branches more laterally in the anterior thorax. The venous drainage is to the corresponding veins.

Innervation

Sensory innervation is primarily by the lateral and anterior cutaneous branches of the second to sixth intercostal nerves. The nipple is supplied from the anterior branch of the lateral cutaneous branch of T4 which forms an extensive plexus within the nipple.

Lymphatic drainage

The primary route of lymphatic drainage of the breast is through approximately 20 ipsilateral axillary lymph nodes. The sentinel lymph node is the first node receiving direct lymphatic drainage from a primary breast cancer and a tumour-free sentinel lymph node implies the absence of lymph node metastases in the remaining axillary nodes.

Axillary lymph nodes can be divided into levels based on location relative to the pectoralis minor muscle. Those lying below the pectoralis minor are the level 1 nodes, those behind the muscle are level 2, while the nodes between the medial border of pectoralis minor and the lower border of the clavicle are level 3.

A small amount of lymph drains to the internal mammary nodes in the intercostal spaces in the parasternal region. Sentinel node mapping has demonstrated that tumours in any quadrant may drain to the internal mammary nodes; however, the upper outer quadrant has a significantly lower rate of drainage.

Assessment of breast symptoms

Triple assessment

Triple assessment (clinical assessment, mammography and/or ultrasound imaging, and core biopsy/fine needle aspiration cytology) is mandatory in the preoperative diagnosis of breast cancer. It is best practice to carry out these assessments at the appointment. If

Table 2.6.1.1 Breast history

Presenting complaint	Lump—site, size, onset, duration, relationship to menstrual cycle, associated pain (cancer usually painless), nipple or skin changes
	Pain—cyclical or non-cyclical, bilateral, unilateral, or in part of one breast, duration, radiation
	Nipple discharge—frequency, duration, colour, spontaneous or expressed, single or multiduct, unilateral or bilateral
	Nipple or skin changes—unilateral or bilateral, duration, history of eczema
Family history	Breast or ovarian cancer
Menstrual and reproductive history	Age at menarche and menopause
	Parity
	Breastfeeding
Personal and drug history	Smoking
	Oral contraceptive
	Hormone replacement therapy
Past medical history	Trauma to breast, previous breast conditions and biopsies, pathology results and treatment received, previous mammograms

there is discordance between any of the tests, repeat biopsy or rarely open surgical biopsy is indicated.

History

Patients most commonly present with a breast lump, pain, nipple discharge, and nipple or skin changes. Table 2.6.1.1 summarizes the details that need to be gathered when taking a breast history.

Examination

Inspect the breasts with the patient in the upright position, initially with the arms and pectoral muscles relaxed, then with the pectoral muscles contracted, and finally, with the arms raised. Table 2.6.1.2 summarizes the key components of breast examination.

The patient's breast is examined in a semi-recumbent (45°) position with the ipsilateral arm raised above and behind the head. A diagram in the chart noting the examination findings is helpful. The features on clinical examination may be graded as P1, normal;

Table 2.6.1.2 Breast examination

Inspection	Symmetry, deformity, skin changes such as dimpling, erythema or oedema and scars, peau d'orange, nipple retraction, discoloration, inversion, ulceration, and eczematous changes
Palpation	Breasts
	Lump—site, size, surface, shape, texture, tenderness, fixation to skin or chest wall, and relationship to the nipple
	Nipple discharge—palpate around the areola and note where pressure elicits discharge, single or multiduct, appearance, and whether associated with a lump
	Lymphadenopathy—axillary, supraclavicular
	Hepatomegaly
Percussion	Spinal tenderness

P2, benign; P3, probably benign; P4, probably malignant; and P5, malignant.

Investigations

Imaging

The level of suspicion for malignancy on imaging is scored as 1, normal; 2, benign; 3, indeterminate/probably benign; 4, suspicious of malignancy; and 5, highly suspicious of malignancy. Prefixes to be used: mammography—M; ultrasound—U; and magnetic resonance imaging—MRI.

Mammography

Digital imaging has improved the sensitivity and specificity of mammography.

Screening A screening mammogram is performed in the asymptomatic patient and consists of two standard views, mediolateral oblique and craniocaudal. In the United Kingdom, women aged between 47 and 73 are invited for screening mammography every 3 years whereas the frequency of invitation is 2 years in most other national screening programmes.

Women with a substantially increased risk of breast cancer because of their family history or genetic mutation (*BRCA1* and/or *BRCA2* gene mutations) may be offered annual mammography or MRI scans of both breasts based on their age and estimated risk (Figure 2.6.1.1).

Symptomatic Bilateral mammogram is performed in the symptomatic patient (mediolateral oblique and craniocaudal views). The false-negative rate for mammography is 10–15% and therefore a normal mammogram in the presence of suspicious clinical abnormality does not exclude malignancy. Further workup with an ultrasound and core biopsy should be performed. Invasive lobular cancer in particular can be difficult to detect by mammography as it spreads by diffuse infiltration of malignant cells causing little disruption of the underlying anatomic structures.

Mammography is not as effective in younger women (< 40 years) because the density of the breast tissue makes it more difficult to detect problems and there is no additional diagnostic benefit. Mammography is not generally performed in these patients unless there are suspicious findings on clinical examination, ultrasonography, or pathology.

Ultrasonography

Ultrasound is the imaging technique of choice in women under 40 years with focal breast problems. Ultrasound is valuable in distinguishing between cystic and solid masses; benign lesions tend to have well-demarcated edges, while an ill-defined border is the hallmark of malignancy. In addition, ultrasound can delineate between a simple and a complex cyst (a cyst with internal echoes, septations, or solid component).

Magnetic resonance imaging

MRI is utilized if there is discrepancy in the extent of malignant disease between clinical examination and imaging, if breast density precludes accurate mammographic assessment, and to assess the tumour size if breast-conserving surgery is being considered for invasive lobular cancer (Figure 2.6.1.2).

Pathology

Core biopsy is preferred to fine-needle aspiration cytology (FNAC) because it provides architectural information, distinguishes *in situ*

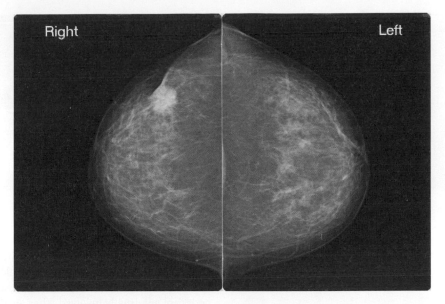

Fig. 2.6.1.1 Mammogram (craniocaudal view) showing spiculated right breast cancer with skin tethering.

from invasive disease, and gives a provisional indication of tumour grade. Biopsy should be performed under image guidance, preferably ultrasound, to ensure accurate sampling. Ultrasound guidance permits real-time demonstration of the needle traversing the lesion.

Fine-needle aspiration cytology

FNAC has been superseded by core biopsy in most centres. FNAC may be useful for sampling areas of nodularity where the imaging features are non-specific but there remains a degree of clinical concern (P3).

The level of suspicion for malignancy on cytology is scored as C1, inadequate for diagnosis; C2, benign; C3, atypia probably benign; C4, suspicious of malignancy; and C5, malignant.

Core biopsy

The availability of automated core biopsy guns and the very high sensitivity and specificity have resulted in more widespread use of image-guided core biopsy (Figure 2.6.1.3). The level of suspicion

for malignancy on core biopsy is scored as B1, unsatisfactory or normal breast tissue; B2, benign; B3, benign but of uncertain malignant potential; B4, suspicious of malignancy; and B5, malignant.

Stereotactic core biopsy

Stereotactic core biopsy is used to biopsy non-palpable, mammographically suspicious calcifications or lesions under radiographic control.

Vacuum-assisted biopsy

Vacuum-assisted core biopsy provides more tissue to the pathologist, and can remove small benign lesions such as fibroadenoma in the outpatient clinic. This device also has the ability to place a marking clip through the probe to allow for future identification of the biopsy site.

Open surgical biopsy

Open biopsy is rarely required, but non-diagnostic and insufficient biopsies from suspicious or indeterminate lesions should undergo open surgical biopsy. For impalpable lesions, needle localization biopsy is performed by placing a needle and hook-wire into the patient's breast adjacent to the lesion under mammographic guidance.

Pathology results should be reviewed at a multidisciplinary meeting to confirm concordance between clinical, imaging, and pathological findings.

Common benign breast symptoms and diseases

Thickening, nodularity, or lumpiness

Clinical features

Patients may present to the clinic with a thickening, nodularity, or lumpiness that may also be painful or tender and may fluctuate with the menstrual cycle. This is referred to as benign breast change, fibrocystic disease, or fibroadenosis. Clinical examination may demonstrate thickening, focal or generalized nodularity, and

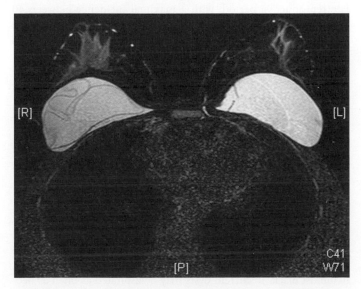

Fig. 2.6.1.2 MRI breast shows an intracapsular rupture of right silicone gel implant.

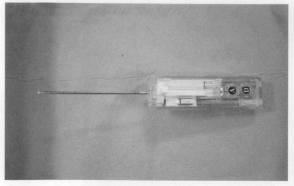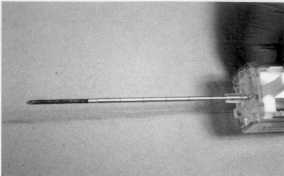

Fig. 2.6.1.3 Disposable core biopsy needle.

lumpiness. Re-examining the patient 1–2 weeks after the menses may demonstrate resolution of signs.

Investigations

Mammogram if aged 40 years or older, ultrasound scan of the focal abnormality, FNAC, or core biopsy if the abnormality is asymmetric and does not change with menstrual cycle as invasive lobular cancer may present as a thickening in the breast.

Management

Reassurance is all that is required if the triple test is negative. Treatment of associated breast pain is outlined in later sections. No further follow-up is required.

Palpable lumps

Solid fibroadenoma

Clinical features

Fibroadenoma is the most common discrete lump in women younger than 30 years although it occasionally occurs in older women. They present as smooth, round or lobulated, firm masses and may be multiple. The typical fibroadenoma has a well-defined capsule, giving the tumour great mobility (breast mouse). There is no increased risk of breast cancer in patients and most fibroadenomas remain static over several years following diagnosis, a few regress, and a small number grow.

Investigations

Ultrasound is the first line of investigation of fibroadenomas present in younger women where fibroadenomas appear as oval or round soft tissue densities with smooth or lobulated margins. Core biopsy is diagnostic but may be avoided in very young women (<25 years) with typical features.

Management

Excision is only required if associated with suspicious histology, the lump enlarges, or if the patient wants the lump to be removed. Lumps up to 25 mm can be removed using vacuum-assisted breast biopsy as an alternative to surgical excision.

Phyllodes tumour

Clinical features

Phyllodes tumours range from benign to malignant and often clinically mimic a fibroadenoma. Most present between 35 and 55 years and are usually unilateral, single, well-circumscribed, mobile, firm, bosselated, and benign. There may be a history of increase in size,

tumours may occupy the whole breast, and overlying skin may show large, dilated veins and pressure ulceration. The tumours are not fixed and remain mobile on the chest wall. The axillary lymph nodes are not usually involved. They are derived from stromal cells and because of their malignant potential are managed by surgical excision. They rarely develop into soft tissue sarcoma and may metastasize via the bloodstream.

Investigations

Ultrasound scan, mammogram if aged 40 years or older, and core biopsy. Imaging features are generally very similar to those of a fibroadenoma. Histological assessment is essential to exclude malignancy.

Management

These lesions must be excised completely with a surrounding rim of normal breast tissue to achieve an adequate margin. Large tumours may need mastectomy with or without immediate reconstruction to achieve adequate clearance. Failure to do so may result in local recurrence and the potential for malignant transformation.

Cysts

Clinical features

Cysts may be symptomatic or detected on mammographic screening (Figure 2.6.1.4). Cysts occur predominantly in the middle and late reproductive period, with a maximal incidence between 40 and 50 years. Cysts usually disappear after menopause, unless the patient is taking hormone replacement therapy. Cysts appear as smooth, well-defined, mobile lesions which are often multiple and bilateral. Cysts can appear suddenly, grow to any size, and may be associated with pain and tenderness. Cysts do not increase the risk of developing breast carcinoma.

Investigations

Ultrasound scan and mammogram if aged 40 years or older. Ultrasound is extremely reliable in distinguishing solid from cystic masses. On mammography, cysts appear as well-defined soft tissue densities. If a cyst appears to have a solid intracystic lesion, core biopsy should be performed.

Management

Symptomatic cysts should be aspirated to dryness under ultrasound guidance to ensure complete emptying for immediate relief. The cyst aspirate may be clear to turbid, and from green, light brown, to almost black. Recurrent cysts may be aspirated as often as necessary. There is no place for surgical excision. Cysts with a bloody

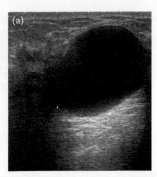

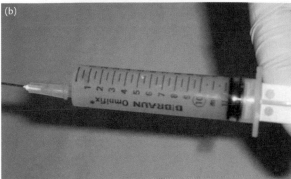

Fig. 2.6.1.4 (a) Ultrasound of a cyst. (b) Cyst fluid.

aspirate or any residual lump should be investigated by core biopsy to rule out intracystic papillary tumours. Cytological examination of cyst fluid is not otherwise required.

Breast pain

Clinical features

Most women experience some form of breast pain or discomfort during their lifetime. It is most common in women aged 30–50 years. Breast pain may be bilateral, unilateral, or in part of one breast. Pain may be cyclical (worse before a period) or non-cyclical (unrelated to the menstrual cycle), originating from the breast or the chest wall. The aetiology of cyclical mastalgia has not been established. Cyclical pain is often bilateral, usually most severe in the upper outer quadrants of the breast, and may be referred to the medial aspect of the upper arm. Non-cyclical pain may be caused by true breast pain or chest wall pain, located over the costal cartilages.

Tietze syndrome (costochondritis) is characterized by tender and swollen costal cartilages, and pain is felt in the overlying medial half of the breast. It has a chronic time course and increased pain occurs on pressure over the affected cartilage.

The best way to assess whether pain is cyclical is to ask the patient to complete a breast pain chart. A pain chart quantifies the patient's symptoms and has the added advantage of assessing effectiveness of therapy. Pain is rarely the presenting symptom of breast cancer and breast pain does not increase the risk of subsequent breast cancer.

Clinical examination is usually normal apart from breast or chest wall tenderness. Focal or generalized nodularity may be present. The chest wall should be examined by lifting the breast with one hand while palpating the underlying muscles and ribs with the other hand.

Investigations

In women aged over 40, mammography is performed. Women with asymmetric areas of focal nodularity, lump, or persistent localized pain will undergo ultrasound and if necessary FNAC or core biopsy.

Management

Reassurance that cancer is not responsible for the symptoms is the only treatment necessary in most women. Some women can improve their pain with simple measures such as wearing a well-fitting bra to support the breasts. Vitamin E, vitamin B_6, caffeine reduction, and progestogens (oral or topical) have not been shown to be of value in mastalgia. Evening primrose oil does not improve breast pain and can be considered to be an expensive placebo treatment. Women who start oral contraceptive or hormone replacement therapy may report breast pain, which usually settles with continued therapy. Topical or oral non-steroidal anti-inflammatory drugs (NSAIDs) are effective in relieving breast pain and should be considered as a first-line treatment. Women who do not respond to treatment are started on danazol 200 mg daily although this is associated with adverse androgenic side effects, including weight gain, deepening of the voice, menorrhagia, and muscle cramps. Surgery has no place in the management of breast pain.

Musculoskeletal pain often responds to oral or topical NSAIDs. Patients with persistent localized chest wall symptoms can be effectively treated by injection of a combination of local anaesthetic and steroid into the tender site. Injection of local anaesthetic confirms the correct identification of the painful area by producing complete disappearance of the pain.

Breast infection

Lactational breast abscess
Clinical features

The most common causative organism is *Staphylococcus aureus* from the infant's mouth via a sore and cracked nipple. The patient's breast is hard, swollen, erythematous, and painful. Fluctuation is a late sign or absent. There may be associated fever and chills.

Investigations

Ultrasound for diagnosis, excluding inflammatory cancer, and to guide aspiration. Patients will be too uncomfortable to endure the breast compression required to perform a mammogram.

Management

Women can continue breastfeeding or the infected breast should be emptied of milk using a breast pump. Treatment is with an appropriate antibiotic (flucloxacillin or co-amoxiclav—confirmed by culture and sensitivity) and repeated aspiration with ultrasound, every 2–3 days until no more pus is aspirated. Incision and drainage is performed if the overlying skin is necrotic, ideally as an outpatient procedure under local anaesthesia.

Periductal mastitis and fistula
Clinical features

Periductal mastitis presents with periareolar cellulitis or subareolar abscess. There may be associated nipple retraction and discharge, most commonly seen in young women, with a strong association with smoking. Patients often have a chronic relapsing course with multiple infections. A periductal fistula can form after spontaneous discharge of a periareolar abscess or develop after incision and drainage.

Investigations

Ultrasound to exclude inflammatory cancer, diagnose, and aspirate underlying pus collection.

Management

Management is similar to lactational breast abscess (Figure 2.6.1.5) except that the antibiotic should cover both aerobes and anaerobes (co-amoxiclav or flucloxacillin and metronidazole). Patients should be advised to stop smoking. For women who experience recurrence, treatment is total duct excision. Periductal fistula is treated by excision of the fistula and diseased duct or ducts once acute infection resolves. Recurrence is common after surgery.

Nipple discharge

Clinical features

Patients may present with spontaneous or expressed, unilateral or bilateral, single or multiduct clear, milky, blood stained, green, brown, or black discharge. There may be associated breast lump or nipple retraction. A clear, serous discharge may be physiological in a parous woman. The most common causes of bloody nipple discharge are intraduct papilloma, duct ectasia, and ductal carcinoma *in situ*/carcinoma. A green discharge is usually due to duct ectasia.

Investigations

Mammogram if older than 40 years and ultrasound of any palpable lump. Cytological examination of the nipple discharge is not useful in diagnosis. Medical workup of galactorrhoea (e.g. serum prolactin levels) is done when the discharge is milky, persistent, and bilateral.

Management

In the absence of a breast lump, management depends on the presence of blood in the discharge. For persistent bloody discharge, the affected duct/s should be excised to exclude malignancy (microdochectomy). When the duct of origin of nipple discharge is uncertain or when there is bleeding from multiple ducts, total duct excision (Hadfield's procedure) is advisable. For non-blood stained discharge, reassurance may be sufficient but if the discharge is proving intolerable, microdochectomy or total duct excision is performed.

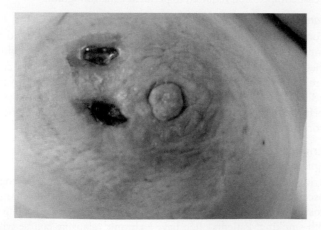

Fig. 2.6.1.5 Periareolar abscess which has burst spontaneously.

Nipple retraction

Clinical features

Long-standing nipple retraction is very common and of no significance. The commonest cause of new-onset nipple retraction in older women is duct ectasia; however, underlying breast cancer may present with nipple retraction.

Investigation

Mammogram if older than 40 years and ultrasound scan (and biopsy if appropriate) to exclude malignancy.

Management

Once cancer is excluded, treatment is usually unnecessary.

Gynaecomastia

Clinical features

Gynaecomastia is the benign enlargement of male breast ductal tissue. There is soft, elastic, or firm, disk-like growth under the nipple areola, which may be bilateral and tender. Physiological gynaecomastia occurs in neonates, at puberty, with obesity, and ageing. Non-physiological gynaecomastia develops with disorders or drugs associated with low testosterone levels (e.g. Klinefelter's syndrome and hyperprolactinemia), testosterone conversion to oestrogen (e.g. thyrotoxicosis and liver disease), high oestrogen levels (e.g. Sertoli cell or Leydig cell tumour and human chorionic gonadotropin (hCG)-producing tumour), and high sex hormone-binding globulin levels resulting in low free testosterone (e.g. hyperthyroidism). Body builders who use anabolic steroids frequently develop gynaecomastia. Gynaecomastia has been associated with a large number of drugs (e.g. digoxin and atorvastatin).

Investigations

If an adolescent or adult presents with acute onset of painful gynaecomastia without an obvious cause, serum hCG, testosterone, luteinizing hormone, and oestradiol levels should be measured to rule out other causes, although no abnormalities are detected in the majority of patients.

Management

Physiological gynaecomastia requires no treatment unless accompanied by pain or significant embarrassment. Withdrawing an offending drug or treating an underlying disorder may be sufficient for regression of the breast enlargement during the proliferative phase. Tamoxifen, 10 mg per day, may be prescribed (off-licence indication) during the rapid, proliferative phase, manifested clinically as breast pain and tenderness. If the gynaecomastia has not regressed by 1 year, or in patients who present with long-standing gynaecomastia who are troubled by their appearance, liposuction and/or subcutaneous mastectomy are the best options.

Further reading

Department of Health. *Best Practice Diagnostic Guidelines for Patients Presenting with Breast Symptoms*. London: Department of Health; 2010. http://www.associationofbreastsurgery.org.uk/media/4585/best_practice_diagnostic_guidelines_for_patients_presenting_with_breast_symptoms.pdf

Mansel RE, Webster DJT, Sweetland HM (eds). *Benign Disorders and Diseases of the Breast*. London: Elsevier; 2009.

Breast cancer treatment

Amit Goyal and Malcolm W. R. Reed

Introduction and epidemiology

Breast cancer is the most common cancer in women worldwide and in the United Kingdom, with about 50 000 new cases diagnosed and 11 500 deaths recorded each year. In men, breast cancer is rare, with about 400 cases diagnosed and 70 deaths in the United Kingdom each year. It is the second most common cause of cancer death among women in the United Kingdom, after lung cancer.

The lifetime risk of developing breast cancer is one in eight for women in the United Kingdom. The incidence is strongly related to age, being very rare in women under 30 years, with increasing incidence over the age of 50 not reaching a peak until age over 80 years. The peaks and troughs of incidence for women aged 50 and over may partly be explained by the impact of screening for breast cancer.

Incidence rates are high in Western societies, moderate in Asia, and low in most African countries but here breast cancer incidence rates are also increasing due to increasing life expectancy, urbanization, and adoption of Western lifestyles. The survival rates vary greatly, ranging from 80% or over in the United States, Sweden, and Japan to around 60% in middle-income countries, and below 40% in low-income countries.

Risk factors

A number of factors are associated with an increased risk of breast cancer. The majority of women (around 90%) with established breast cancer risk factors (except the high-risk genetic mutations) will never develop breast cancer.

Age

The strongest risk factor after gender for breast cancer is increasing age which is likely to be a surrogate for accumulated DNA damage with loss of tumour suppressor gene function.

Environment and lifestyle

Women in affluent and Western populations and in subpopulations of higher socioeconomic status within countries are at increased risk of breast cancer partly due to having fewer children and a limited duration of breastfeeding. Breast cancer incidence for migrants and their offspring approaches the rates of their adopted homeland rather than their country of origin, emphasizing the importance of environment in addition to hereditary factors.

Family history

Women with a family history of breast cancer are more likely to develop breast cancer, depending on the number and degree of relatedness of the family members affected. Women with a mother, sister, or daughter with breast cancer are, on average, at twice the risk of those with no affected first-degree relative. The risk increases when the relative is diagnosed below the age of 50. However, most women who have first-degree relatives with a history of breast cancer will never develop breast cancer.

Only 5–10% of all breast cancers are related to inherited mutation, the majority are in the autosomal dominant *BRCA1* and *BRCA2* genes (more common in women of Ashkenazi Jewish descent), less commonly in *p53*, *PTEN*, or *ATM* genes. The lifetime breast cancer risk for BRCA1 or -2 mutation carriers is 60–85%, lifetime ovarian cancer risk is 20–40% for BRCA1 mutation carriers and 10–20% for BRCA2 mutation carriers. Male BRCA2 mutation carriers have 100-fold increased risk of breast cancer.

Previous breast cancer or benign proliferative disease

Women diagnosed with invasive breast cancer are at two to six times the population risk of developing cancer in the contralateral breast. Ductal carcinoma *in situ* (DCIS), lobular carcinoma *in situ* (LCIS), atypical ductal hyperplasia, and increased mammographic breast density are associated with an increased risk of invasive breast cancer.

Hormonal risk factors

A prolonged or increased exposure to oestrogen is associated with an increased risk for developing breast cancer, whereas reducing exposure is protective. There is an increased likelihood for developing breast cancer with early age at menarche, nulliparity, and late onset of menopause whilst pregnancy and prolonged breastfeeding are protective.

Age at menarche and menopause

Women who had their first menstrual period at age 12 or later have a slightly lower risk of breast cancer than women who had their first menstrual period earlier. Late menopause increases the risk of breast cancer. Post-menopausal women have a lower risk of breast cancer than premenopausal women of the same age and childbearing pattern. Risk increases by almost 3% per year of delay in menopause (natural or induced by surgery), so that women aged 55 or older at menopause have about twice the risk of breast cancer than those aged 45 or under.

Pregnancy history and breastfeeding

Parous women with a younger age at first pregnancy (before 25 years) are at lower risk than women who are older at first pregnancy (after 29 years). Each term pregnancy after the first results in a small additional reduction in breast cancer risk.

Women who breastfeed are at reduced risk compared with those who do not breastfeed. Risk is reduced by 4% for every 12 months of breastfeeding. The longer a woman breastfeeds, the greater the protection.

Oral contraceptive and hormone replacement therapy use

The use of oral contraceptives increases the risk of breast cancer in current and recent users, but there is no significant excess risk 10 or more years after stopping use.

In current users of hormone replacement therapy (HRT), the risk of breast cancer increases with total duration of use. Five years of HRT use is associated with a 10% increase in risk and every additional 5 years of use doubles the increase in risk. When HRT is discontinued, this risk returns to that of a never-user within 5 years.

Diet, obesity, physical activity, and alcohol intake

The role of dietary fat in breast cancer remains unclear. Associations between dietary total or saturated fat and breast cancer have been inconsistent in prospective studies.

The major source of oestrogen in postmenopausal women is from the conversion of androstenedione to oestrone by the aromatase enzyme primarily in adipose tissue; thus, obesity is associated with a long-term increase in oestrogen exposure and higher breast cancer risk.

Physical activity has been proposed as a means of reducing breast cancer risk because of its potential effects on hormone profiles and weight gain. There is a lower breast cancer risk among more active women.

Breast cancer risk increases with both the amount and duration of alcohol consumption, possibly due to increase in serum levels of oestradiol.

Ionizing radiation

Ionizing radiation increases the risk of breast cancer particularly during breast development. Young women who received mantle radiation for Hodgkin's lymphoma have a markedly increased risk for developing breast cancer.

Pathology

Breast cancer is subdivided into two major categories, *in situ* disease, mainly in the form of DCIS, and invasive cancer.

Classification

Non-invasive:

A. DCIS

B. LCIS (lobular neoplasia)

Invasive (infiltrating):

A. Invasive ductal carcinoma ('NOS—not otherwise specified') 70–80%

B. Invasive lobular carcinoma 10–20%

C. Other types e.g. tubular, medullary 5–10%.

Ductal carcinoma *in situ*

Non-invasive carcinoma is confined to the mammary ducts or lobules and is classified as either DCIS or LCIS, respectively. Both are confined by a basement membrane and therefore incapable of metastasis. The incidence of DCIS is around 20% of malignant lesions diagnosed by screening mammography, primarily because of the detection of calcified necrotic debris or secretory material. DCIS rarely presents as a palpable or radiologically detectable mass. DCIS is a precursor to invasive ductal carcinoma and when carcinoma develops, it is usually in the same breast and of ductal histology.

Lobular carcinoma *in situ*

LCIS is typically an incidental finding in a breast biopsy specimen, does not form masses, and is not usually associated with calcifications. It may be multifocal or bilateral. It is not a true pre-invasive lesion but an indicator for increased breast cancer risk. Approximately one-third of women with LCIS will eventually develop invasive carcinoma. The invasive carcinoma may be ductal or lobular. Unlike DCIS, subsequent invasive carcinomas may arise in either breast.

Invasive ductal carcinoma

About 80% of all breast cancers fall into this group. Most of these tumours excite a pronounced fibroblastic stromal reaction to the invading tumour cells producing a palpable mass. The tumours range from well differentiated (grade 1), in which there is glandular formation, to poorly differentiated, containing solid sheets of pleomorphic neoplastic cells (grade 3). The *HER2* gene is a member of the epidermal growth factor receptor family, and its overexpression is associated with a poor prognosis. About two-thirds of invasive ductal carcinoma express oestrogen (ERs) or progesterone receptors (PRs) and about one-third overexpress HER2 protein.

Invasive lobular carcinoma

Often associated with adjacent LCIS, lobular carcinoma cells invade individually into the stroma and are often aligned in strands or chains ('Indian file pattern'). Lobular carcinomas are also more frequently multicentric and bilateral (10–20%). Almost all invasive lobular carcinomas express oestrogen receptors, but HER2 protein overexpression is very rare.

Molecular subtypes

More recently, breast cancers have been classified based on gene expression profiling into up to ten molecular subtypes. Four of these—luminal A (ER/PR positive, HER2 negative, low grade), luminal B (ER/PR positive, HER2 positive, and/or high grade), triple negative/basal-like (ER, PR, and HER2 negative), HER2 type (ER/PR negative, HER2 positive)—are associated with different outcomes and treatment protocols, used increasingly in clinical practice.

Clinical presentation

Symptomatic

Breast cancer is often discovered by the woman or her doctor as a discrete, solitary, painless, and mobile lump. The upper outer quadrant is the most common site. Palpability is influenced by size of tumour, density of surrounding breast tissue and distance from skin surface. Advanced cancers may cause dimpling of the skin, ulceration, retraction of the nipple, or fixation to the chest wall. Breast pain alone is not usually a sign of breast cancer.

Inflammatory carcinoma is characterized by an enlarged, swollen, erythematous breast, usually without a palpable mass. The skin is thickened and oedematous (peau d'orange). Tumour emboli within dermal lymphatics result in the typical skin appearance. Many of these tumours have distant metastases at presentation, and a poor prognosis.

Screening

With mammographic screening, breast cancers are frequently detected before they become palpable. The mammogram may show a mass, architectural distortion, or suspicious calcification. The average invasive carcinoma found by screening is around 1 cm in size and less than 20% of these have nodal metastases.

Investigations

Diagnosis is made by triple assessment (see Chapter 2.6.1). Preoperative ultrasound evaluation of the axilla should be performed for all patients being investigated for early invasive breast cancer and, if morphologically abnormal lymph nodes are identified, ultrasound-guided fine-needle aspiration (FNA) or core biopsy should be performed.

The use of magnetic resonance imaging of the breast is increasingly recommended particularly in lobular invasive cancer patients to exclude multifocal or bilateral disease.

Staging

Current staging of breast cancer is based on the TNM (tumour, node, metastasis) staging system but in clinical practice, alternative prognostic tools (e.g. Adjuvant! Online, PREDICT, or Nottingham Prognostic Index) are used to plan treatment and estimate prognosis.

Distant metastasis occurs through lymphatic and haematogenous routes typically to the skeleton, liver, lungs, and brain. All patients should have baseline full blood count and liver function tests. Early-stage breast cancer patients (stages I, II, and IIIA) have a low incidence of distant metastases and in the absence of abnormal blood results or specific signs or symptoms do not need further tests to identify metastatic disease before surgery. Bone and liver scans should be considered only in patients with a high risk of metastases.

Multidisciplinary assessment

Breast cancer diagnosis, staging, and treatment should comply with evidence-based guidelines and be discussed in a multidisciplinary team including specialist surgeons, pathologists, radiologists, oncologists, and specialist nurses, before discussing with the patient. Treatment should take into account patients' needs and preferences with the support of clinical nurse specialists.

Management

Ductal carcinoma *in situ*

The treatment is complete surgical excision—breast-conserving surgery (BCS) or mastectomy. Axillary staging is not necessary for small areas (<5 cm) of DCIS but sentinel node biopsy (SNB) is performed for patients with larger areas undergoing mastectomy due to the low incidence of unsuspected invasive disease with lymph node metastases.

Following BCS, radiotherapy is recommended in patients found to have high-grade DCIS. For pure DCIS, there is no added benefit from endocrine treatment although it may reduce the risk of future breast cancer in patients with ER-positive DCIS.

Invasive breast cancer

The treatment comprises removal of the tumour—BCS or mastectomy and axillary lymph node staging/clearance, followed by appropriate adjuvant therapy (radiotherapy, chemotherapy, endocrine).

Surgery

Breast-conserving surgery (wide local excision, lumpectomy)

BCS comprises removal of the tumour and a margin of surrounding healthy normal tissue, aiming for a 1 mm margin. If the lump is not palpable (e.g. screen detected cancer), a guidewire is inserted under ultrasound or mammographic guidance preoperatively to mark the area to be removed (Figure 2.6.2.1). BCS is followed by radiotherapy to the breast in patients with invasive breast cancer and high-grade DCIS to decrease local recurrence. BCS may be offered to patients with a favourable tumour:breast size ratio. For

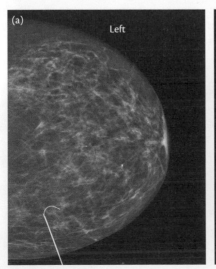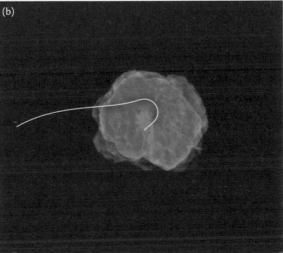

Fig. 2.6.2.1 (a) Left breast screen-detected impalpable invasive cancer marked with a wire; and (b) Specimen X-ray following wide local excision.

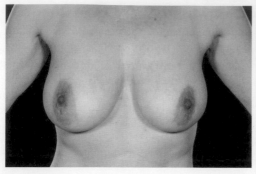
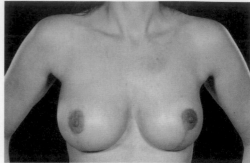

Fig. 2.6.2.2 Pre- and postoperative views of a patient undergoing right vertical scar therapeutic mammoplasty and left breast reduction. Right breast scars are barely visible after radiotherapy.

patients with large tumours who desire BCS, neoadjuvant (preoperative) chemotherapy or hormonal therapy may be offered to reduce the size of the tumour.

Oncoplastic techniques such as breast reduction can be modified to perform wide local excision for much larger tumours than those traditionally treated with BCS (therapeutic mammoplasty). This is a good option for patients who have large breasts and wish them to be smaller (Figure 2.6.2.2). A contralateral breast reduction is usually required for symmetry.

Radiotherapy is administered to the breast typically 5 days a week for 3 weeks, often with a boost to the tumour bed.

BCS is contraindicated in women with multiple primary tumours in separate quadrants, prior radiation therapy to the breast (radiotherapy cannot be given twice to a body area), large tumour in a small breast in which resection would result in significant cosmetic deformity, persistently positive margins after multiple attempts at complete resection, and connective tissue diseases (e.g. scleroderma) that are sensitive to radiation therapy.

The most frequent complications of BCS are infection, bleeding, and seroma. There is a potential risk of breast contour deformity and asymmetry.

Mastectomy

Mastectomy removes all of the breast tissue and skin, including the nipple and areola (simple mastectomy). For women undergoing immediate reconstruction, a skin-sparing mastectomy with or without sparing the nipple is performed to improve the reconstruction outcome.

More radical mastectomy operations (e.g. including underlying pectoral muscles) may rarely be performed for locally advanced disease or palliative surgical treatment.

The most frequent side effects are seroma, infection, bleeding, and pain or numbness of the skin of the chest wall or inner arm. Smokers are at increased risk of mastectomy skin flap necrosis.

Choosing between breast-conserving surgery and mastectomy

Many women with DCIS and early-stage invasive cancers can choose between BCS and mastectomy. Whilst mastectomy rates vary between centres and nations, the majority of women with early-stage disease opt for BCS rather than mastectomy. BCS preserves the breast but radiation treatment is needed after surgery for patients with high-grade DCIS and invasive cancer. However some women with invasive cancer who undergo mastectomy will

also need radiation and up to one in five women undergoing BCS need a reoperation (re-excision of margins or mastectomy) because of incomplete excision of cancer or inadequate clearance margins. BCS is associated with a higher local recurrence rate but there is no difference in overall survival.

Axillary surgery

Most women with early-stage invasive breast cancer are node negative. However, it is important to stage the axilla at the time of breast surgery as axillary lymph node involvement is the most important prognostic factor and has an impact on adjuvant therapy decisions. SNB has replaced the more morbid axillary lymph node dissection (ALND) and four-node sampling for axillary nodal staging. SNB is associated with less arm morbidity (lymphoedema, pain, numbness, shoulder function impairment) and better quality of life. ALND is reserved for patients with proven axillary lymph node involvement.

Sentinel node biopsy

SNB is performed using a combination of blue dye (e.g. patent blue V) and radioisotope colloid, through a 2–3 cm axillary incision. The tracer(s) is injected in intradermal, subdermal, subareolar, or peritumoural position. All blue-stained nodes and nodes with radioactive counts of 10% or greater of the hottest node are defined as sentinel nodes (Figure 2.6.2.3). The surgeon uses a hand-held gamma camera intraoperatively to identify 'hot' sentinel nodes (nodes with radioactivity). The goal is to remove a median of one to two sentinel nodes per patient.

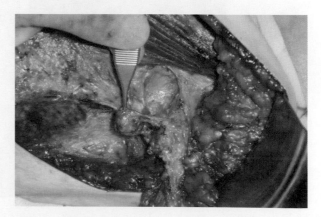

Fig. 2.6.2.3 Sentinel node.

The patient whose sentinel node is tumour free does not require further axillary-specific treatment. A quarter of patients are found to have sentinel node metastases. These patients return for a second operation, ALND, or receive axillary radiotherapy as there is a risk that higher order nodes may be involved with metastatic disease.

Axillary lymph node dissection

ALND is removal of lymph nodes up to the level of axillary vein in patients found to have cancer spread in the axillary nodes after preoperative, ultrasound-guided FNA/core biopsy of suspicious node(s) or after SNB. An adequate dissection should remove at least ten lymph nodes.

During ALND, there is a potential risk of damage to the long thoracic, medial pectoral, intercostobrachial nerves, axillary vein, and thoracodorsal pedicle. Postoperatively, the most frequent complications are wound infection and seroma. Following ALND, one in five patients develop upper limb lymphoedema, and one in five have impairment of shoulder movement. Sensory changes and pain may occur in up to one in three patients.

Breast reconstruction

Despite an increasing trend towards BCS, some women will require or choose a mastectomy. Breast reconstruction may be performed at the time of mastectomy or as a delayed procedure after completion of adjuvant treatments. It should be offered to all suitable patients undergoing mastectomy, unless there are significant contraindications. Women who are diabetic, hypertensive, heavy smokers, and morbidly obese are at high risk of wound complications.

Oncological principles should always take precedence and not be compromised. Breast reconstruction does not increase the likelihood of cancer recurrence or make it harder to check for recurrence.

Immediate breast reconstruction

Immediate breast reconstruction does not adversely affect breast cancer outcome.

The breast can be reconstructed at the time of cancer surgery in appropriately selected women with good cosmetic results. It allows preservation of breast skin (skin sparing mastectomy) and inframammary fold to give a better cosmetic outcome. There is the psychological and aesthetic advantage to immediate reconstruction although it is essential that patients are fully informed and have realistic expectations of the outcome. The drawback of immediate reconstruction is that it requires a longer surgery and recovery than having mastectomy alone, complications may delay adjuvant treatment, and

if radiotherapy is needed following surgery, the reconstruction may be adversely affected, particularly after implant-based procedures.

Delayed breast reconstruction

Delayed reconstruction may be preferable in patients who are not ready to make a decision at the time of cancer diagnosis and would like to focus on cancer treatment. Patients with multiple co-morbidities may benefit from a staged procedure to minimize the risks of surgery. The risk of surgical complications is less with delayed reconstruction and it avoids any potential delay of adjuvant treatment. However, delayed breast reconstruction requires a separate operation with replacement of a larger amount of breast skin.

Techniques

Breast reconstruction can be performed using either breast implants or tissue taken from elsewhere in a woman's body (autologous). Each breast reconstruction method has advantages and disadvantages. The choice of method depends largely on individual preference and cancer treatment plan, but other factors can influence the type of reconstructive surgery a woman chooses. All appropriate reconstruction options should be offered and discussed with patients.

Reconstruction using only an implant

A tissue expander (adjustable prosthesis) is inserted under the pectoralis major superiorly and subcutaneously in the inferior pole. The volume is adjusted by inflating the tissue expander with saline in the outpatient clinic to stretch the chest wall tissues and skin, and later a permanent implant is inserted. Alternatively, in selected patients one-stage immediate reconstruction may be performed in conjunction with skin-sparing mastectomy using a silicone implant and acellular dermal matrix (ADM)/synthetic mesh or autologous dermal sling (Figure 2.6.2.4) to support the implant inferiorly as a hammock.

Latissimus dorsi flap reconstruction

The latissimus dorsi (LD) flap (Figure 2.6.2.5) based on the thoracodorsal artery can be used to transfer well-vascularized muscle, fat, and skin island to the anterior chest wall to reconstruct the breast. It can provide tissue replacement of breast volume without the need for an implant in patients with small breast volume (autologous LD reconstruction). Women with moderate to large breasts generally need a tissue expander or implant to further supplement the volume of the breast and may need a matching procedure to obtain symmetry.

The loss of LD muscle function does not result in significant upper extremity weakness as teres major and subscapularis muscles compensate its actions. Complications include bleeding, infection, and seroma formation. Partial flap necrosis occurs in less than 5%

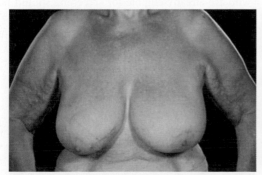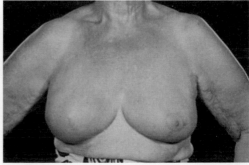

Fig. 2.6.2.4 Pre- and postoperative views of a patient undergoing one-stage right breast dermal sling and implant reconstruction along with left breast reduction.

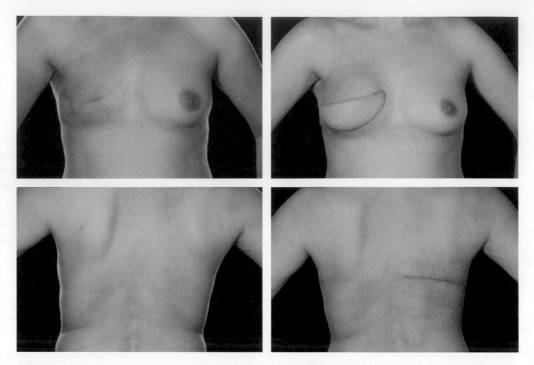

Fig. 2.6.2.5 Pre- and postoperative views of a patient undergoing right delayed latissimus dorsi flap and implant reconstruction.

of patients whilst total flap loss is rare (0.25%). Chronic pain is rare but can cause significant functional disturbance.

Reconstruction using lower abdominal flaps

A sizeable, natural looking and feeling breast reconstruction can be created using skin and fat, with or without muscle from the lower abdomen. This procedure tightens the lower abdominal wall and the umbilicus is re-sited. There are several types of lower abdominal flaps depending on which blood vessels are used, whether blood vessels remain connected (pedicled flap) or are detached and reattached at the recipient site by microvascular anastomosis (free flap), and whether muscle is transferred:

- Pedicled or free transverse rectus abdominis flap (TRAM): skin, fat, and rectus abdominis muscle are tunnelled under the skin to the mastectomy defect based on superior epigastric artery (pedicled TRAM flap). In free TRAM flap, the blood supply is the deep inferior epigastric artery and its venae comitantes which are divided at their origin. These vessels are anastomosed microsurgically to the thoracodorsal or internal mammary vessels.

- Free deep inferior epigastric artery perforator (DIEP) flap (Figure 2.6.2.6): this is similar to the free TRAM flap, but the blood supply is based on one or two perforator arteries of the deep inferior epigastric artery. This procedure requires dissection of perforators within the rectus abdominis muscle but does not require harvest of the muscle, resulting in less abdominal wall morbidity (e.g. abdominal wall bulging or hernia).

Other flaps

Alternative options for autologous tissue transfer are free superior and inferior gluteal artery perforator flaps and free transverse upper gracilis flap from inner thigh. These are less commonly used but are an option in patients not suitable for other autologous techniques or who want a scar in a less obvious body part.

Patients who undergo reconstruction often need additional outpatient or day-case procedures for nipple reconstruction, tattooing, and contour adjustments.

Follow-up imaging

Most locoregional recurrences occur in the first 2–3 years after surgery. Annual mammography is offered to all patients with early breast cancer, including DCIS, until invitation to the Breast Screening Programme. Patients diagnosed with early breast cancer who are already eligible for screening should have annual mammography for 5 years.

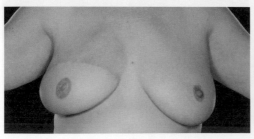
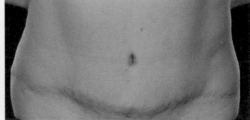

Fig. 2.6.2.6 Patient who underwent delayed DIEP flap right breast reconstruction.

Adjuvant treatment

For non-surgical and adjuvant treatment of breast cancer see Chapter 2.6.3.

Prognosis and survival

The 5-year relative survival rate for breast cancer is around 75% in the United Kingdom. Prognosis is dependent on age at diagnosis, stage, tumour grade, histological type, ER and HER2 status. Specialized types of breast carcinomas (tubular, medullary, mucinous) have a somewhat better prognosis than ductal carcinomas. The presence of hormone receptors confers a better prognosis. Overexpression of HER2 protein is associated with a poorer prognosis.

Paget's disease of the nipple

Paget's disease is an uncommon presentation of breast cancer. It occurs most commonly in postmenopausal women. The characteristic histopathological feature is the presence of Paget cells which are large cells with pale, clear cytoplasm and enlarged nucleoli located within the epidermis and along the basal layer. Most cases are accompanied by an underlying malignancy, either invasive ductal carcinoma or DCIS. The initial presentation of Paget's disease is an eczematous-like lesion limited to the nipple or extended to the areola, refractory to usual topical treatments. The nipple may be ulcerated, retracted, or destroyed (Figure 2.6.2.7). Palpable masses are present in some patients because of underlying invasive cancer. Early changes including scaling and redness may be mistaken for eczema or contact dermatitis but Paget's disease is very rarely bilateral.

The diagnosis can be made from a wedge biopsy or punch biopsy of the nipple under local anaesthetic. Mammography and ultrasound should be performed to identify an underlying carcinoma. Paget's disease can be treated with mastectomy or more frequently BCS with excision of the nipple–areolar complex, followed by radiation therapy with prognosis determined by the underlying malignancy.

Breast cancer during pregnancy

The majority of breast lesions identified during pregnancy are benign. Pregnancy-associated cancers tend be ER negative and carry a similar prognosis to other breast cancers when matched for stage and age. Physiological breast changes associated with pregnancy, including engorgement, hypertrophy, nodularity, and nipple discharge obscure detection by the patient and physician and delay in diagnosis is common, leading to more advanced stage at diagnosis.

Triple assessment should be done for a clinically suspicious or persisting breast mass during pregnancy. Ultrasonography should be the first diagnostic test in a pregnant woman, since it is non-ionizing and has high sensitivity and specificity. Mammography has a high false-negative rate during pregnancy. Adequate shielding can reduce fetal radiation exposure.

Treatment

Counselling is crucial because of the complexity of the issue and to allow patient the opportunity to make an informed decision on the fate of her pregnancy.

Treatment should be discussed in a multidisciplinary meeting and strategies are determined by tumour biology, tumour stage, gestational stage, and the patient's and her family's wishes whilst adhering to the standard for non-pregnant patients wherever possible allowing for the risk to the fetus in the first trimester associated with chemotherapy.

Surgery can be done safely during any stage of pregnancy. Radiotherapy after BCS is not usually a concern since most women receive chemotherapy with delay of radiotherapy until after delivery. SNB can be performed safely using radioisotope but blue dye should be avoided during pregnancy as it is associated with a risk of an anaphylactic reaction.

Adjuvant systemic therapies particularly tamoxifen and trastuzumab should be deferred until after delivery.

Breast cancer in the elderly

Breast cancer is common in the elderly with 30% occurring in women over 70 years in high-income countries. The cancers are biologically less aggressive with the majority being ER-positive invasive ductal carcinomas.

The majority of women present with a palpable lump as routine invitation to breast screening is not undertaken in elderly patients. The stage at presentation is therefore frequently more advanced in the elderly women, offsetting the benefit of less aggressive tumour biology.

Diagnosis is by triple assessment, ultrasound scan, mammogram, and core biopsy as for younger patients.

There is a limited evidence base for the management of older women with breast cancer but in principle the treatment options

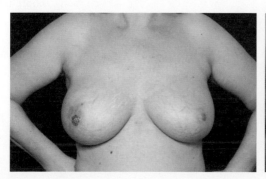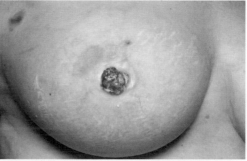

Fig. 2.6.2.7 Paget's disease, right nipple.

should be as for younger women but take full account of physiological age, life expectancy, co-morbidities, potential benefit:risk balance, treatment tolerance, and patient preference. There is evidence that adjuvant chemotherapy is effective in patients up to approximately 75 years of age but little or no evidence of benefit for older patients where toxicity may be a more significant risk. For the most frail elderly patients, optimal treatment lies between reduced surgery (e.g. BCS under local anaesthetic) or primary endocrine therapy alone for those with ER-positive cancer.

Breast cancer in men

Breast cancer in men accounts for less than 1% of male cancers and less than 1% of all breast cancers. Male breast cancer can occur at any age but mean age is 65 years. BRCA2 mutations are associated with approximately 4–6% of these cancers. Men typically have more advanced breast cancer at diagnosis than women.

Patients generally present with a non-tender eccentric hard mass with irregular margins. This contrasts with unilateral gynaecomastia, which is usually firm, central, and tender. Malignant lesions are often associated with nipple retraction. Ultrasound scan, mammogram, and core biopsy are used for diagnosis as in female patients.

Mastectomy is the surgical procedure of choice. SNB should be performed to stage the axilla in clinically/ultrasound node-negative patients. Men with FNA-, core biopsy-, or SNB-proven lymph node metastases should undergo axillary node dissection.

Most malignancies are infiltrating ductal carcinoma and are positive for ER. Adjuvant hormonal, radiotherapy, and chemotherapy treatment parallels that used in women. Although aromatase inhibitors are commonly prescribed instead of tamoxifen, experience is limited. When men and women are matched for tumour stage and histology, no sex difference is found in tumour-specific survival. Overall survival is shorter in men, possibly because they tend to be older and have more co-morbid conditions. The management of metastatic and recurrent disease is similar to that in women.

Further reading

Association of Breast Surgery at BASO 2009. Surgical guidelines for the management of breast cancer. *Eur J Surg Oncol* 2009; 35 Suppl 1:1–22. http://www.associationofbreastsurgery.org.uk/media/4565/surgical_guidelines_for_the_management_of_breast_cancer.pdf

Association of Breast Surgery, British Association of Plastic, Reconstructive and Aesthetic Surgeons. *Oncoplastic Breast Reconstruction: Guidelines for Best Practice.* 2012. [Online] http://www.associationofbreastsurgery.org.uk/media/23851/final_oncoplastic_guidelines_for_use.pdf

National Institute for Health and Care Excellence. *Early and Locally Advanced Breast Cancer: Diagnosis and Treatment.* Clinical Guideline 80. London: NICE; 2009 (Reviewed 2012). http://www.nice.org.uk/guidance/CG80

National Institute for Health and Care Excellence. *Familial Breast Cancer: Classification and Care of People at Risk of Familial Breast Cancer and Management of Breast Cancer and Related Risks in People with a Family History of Breast Cancer.* Clinical Guideline 164. London: NICE; 2013. http://www.nice.org.uk/guidance/CG164

CHAPTER 2.6.3

Non-surgical treatment of breast cancer

Mymoona Alzouebi and Matthew Q. F. Hatton

Treatment modalities

Radiotherapy

Radiotherapy is the use of high-energy ionizing radiation such as X-rays, electrons, and protons to kill tumour cells with DNA being the principal target for the biological effects. Radiation causes direct damage by inducing breaks in the DNA helical structure and indirect damage by the production of unstable, highly reactive, and short-lived free radicals that in turn damage the normal DNA. Radiation-induced damage can either be lethal and irreversible, which leads to cell death, or sublethal, in which case the cellular damage can be partially or completely repaired. The probability of a lethal cell injury is dependent on the amount of radiation energy deposited in the tissues and the 'type' of radiation used (i.e. X-ray, electrons, or other particles).

The early development of radiation treatment showed one large radiation dose had profound effects on tumours, but equally profound effects on normal tissues, limiting clinical usefulness. This limitation led to the development of fractionated treatments, utilizing the radiobiological principles of repair, redistribution, resistance, repopulation, and re-oxygenation to enhance the radiation effects on rapidly dividing tumour cells in comparison to more slowly dividing normal tissues. These factors have led to the classical radiation schedule, delivering 1 fraction per day (1.8–2 Gy per fraction), 5 days per week, over 5–6 weeks with the outcome of treatment depending on the total dose delivered.

Total dose is the main determinant of the effects of radiotherapy but increasing the radiation dose is a challenge for the radiotherapist due to the tolerance of several vital normal tissues—lung, heart, and brachial plexus—that must be taken into account. Most early side effects are predictable (tiredness, skin erythema, and local discomfort) but it is the irreversible late treatment effects causing significant morbidity (e.g. cardiac mortality and radiation neuropathy) which give most concern. Total dose is the main determinant of the risk of late effects, but these risks are made greater by increasing treatment volume and fraction size.

Improvements in radiotherapy schedules centre on reduction of the risk of late effects and aim to improve the local control rates leading to a reduction in distant metastasis and improved survival. Non-conventional fractionation schedules, initially developed on an empirical basis, look to take advantage of different radiobiological properties of tumour and normal tissues and, combined with new technologies reducing the volume of normal tissue being treated, to maintain (or increase) the biological tumour dose.

Chemotherapy

The systemic treatment of cancer is a critical component of management and reduces the risk of local recurrence and systemic metastasis. Chemotherapy is treatment using specific cytotoxic agents targeted at dividing cancer cells and distinguished from the forms of systemic treatment that have specific cellular targets (e.g. hormone therapy).

Cytotoxic drugs produce their effect by direct DNA damage, prevention of DNA synthesis and replication, or inhibition of cell division through damage to the mitotic spindle. As cytotoxic drugs have specific actions, the effectiveness of treatment can be increased by combining drugs to synergize killing effects by acting on different phases of the cell cycle. Like radiotherapy, chemotherapy is 'fractionated' to maximize tumour kill as normal tissue is expected to repair and recover before the tumour. Therefore, chemotherapy regimens are often administered at 3-weekly intervals using a combination of drugs that have been selected to give the optimal dose of each individual drug without overlapping toxicity. The use of therapeutic doses of cytotoxic drugs will involve the development of side effects which can be immediate (e.g. nausea, vomiting, and allergic reactions), acute (e.g. neutropenia, diarrhoea, and stomatitis) or late as a result of prolonged use of drugs (e.g. nephro-, cardio-, and neurotoxicity).

Targeted systemic treatments

Molecular-targeted cancer therapies are drugs that stop the growth and spread of cancer by interfering with specific molecular targets. As Figure 2.6.3.1 demonstrates, the pathways which promote cancer cell growth are complex and by identifying the specific molecular changes in these pathways targeted cancer therapies may prove more effective and less harmful to normal cells than cytotoxic chemotherapy. Hormonal treatment has a long history of use in breast cancer and recent developments have increased the range of targets for which we now have drugs that can interfere with cell growth signalling, tumour blood vessel development, promote apoptosis, stimulate the immune system, or target the delivery of toxic drugs to cancer cells. Figure 2.6.3.1 shows some of the pathways implicated in breast cancer and its management.

Hormone therapy

George Beatson pioneered 'systemic' treatment when he reported regression of breast tumours after oophorectomy. This first hormonal manipulation deprived cancer cells of an oestrogenic proliferative

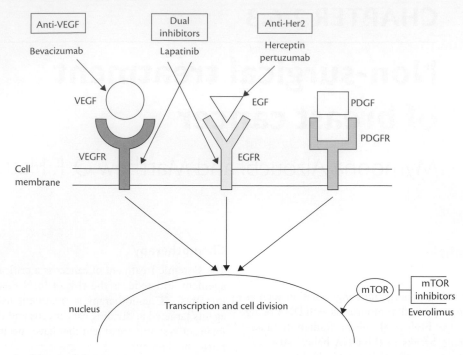

Fig. 2.6.3.1 Pathways and molecular targets in breast cancer.

stimulus by lowering plasma oestrogen levels. Oestrogen is a steroid hormone that in premenopausal women is made primarily in the ovaries. The smaller amounts made by other tissues, including the adrenals and adipose tissue, become the primary sources in postmenopausal women. Oestrogen crosses the plasma membrane of cells and enters the nucleus to bind with the oestrogen receptor (ER) proteins. This ER complex then binds to specific sequences of DNA and regulates the expression of numerous genes involved in cell growth. By lowering of oestrogen levels or by blocking their action at a receptor level, hormone-dependant tumour cell proliferation is reduced and apoptotic (programmed cell death) pathways increased.

Approximately two-thirds of women with breast cancer have oestrogen-positive tumours and it is this presence or absence of the ER that predicts responsiveness of a tumour to hormone treatment. Current treatment options still include ovarian ablation which can be achieved by oophrectomy, radiation treatment, or the use of analogues of luteinizing hormone-releasing hormone such as goserelin. More commonly used alternatives are the selective oestrogen receptor modulators (SERMs) such as tamoxifen, which compete with oestrogen and selectively bind to the cytoplasmic component of the oestrogen receptor. Further options are the pure antioestrogens (e.g. fulvestrant) which downregulate ER without the oestrogen agonist effects that can be seen with SERMs and aromatase inhibitors in postmenopausal women where oestrogen production is by the peripheral conversion of androgens mediated by aromatase enzymes.

Other molecularly targeted therapies

Manipulations of other driver pathways that have been identified in breast cancer have found applications in diagnosis and staging (e.g. immunohistochemistry and radio-immunodetection) as well as treatment. The HER2/neu (erbB2) receptor pathway and over-expression of this epidermal growth factor receptor is seen in

around 20% of breast cancers and associated with a more aggressive form of the disease.[1] Drugs targeting the HER2 pathway include trastuzumab, a humanized monoclonal antibody. Trastuzumab targets the extracellular domain of HER2, inhibiting signal transduction, and is the established treatment in this form of the disease. Other pathways for which there are targeted treatments in current use include vascular endothelial growth factor inhibitors such as bevacizumab and the activation of the mechanistic target of rapamycin (mTOR) intracellular signalling pathway as a mechanism of resistance to endocrine therapy with evidence for the use of mTOR inhibitors (e.g. everolimus) in combination with aromatase inhibitors in that situation.[2]

Treatment of breast cancer

A number of terms are used to describe the intent of non-surgical cancer therapy. Neoadjuvant (primary) treatment given in the preoperative period to 'downstage' the primary tumour, local lymph involvement, and treat any distant microscopic disease. Adjuvant therapy refers to treatment given after the macroscopic disease has been resected to remove any residual microscopic tumour cells. Palliative treatment is used to prolong and maintain quality of life in patients with incurable disease that has spread to distant organs or whose co-morbidities prevent potentially curative treatment being given.

Adjuvant treatment

The presence of undetected micrometastases at the time of diagnosis means all breast cancer patients are at risk of relapse following surgery. Prognostic information can predict the risk of recurrence for an individual patient and the most commonly used scores in the United Kingdom are the Nottingham Prognostic Index (NPI) and Adjuvant! Online.[3] NPI is based on tumour size, grade, and number of positive lymph nodes and Table 2.6.3.1 illustrates the variation

Table 2.6.3.1 The North Trent Cancer Network adjuvant treatment guideline recommendations (2012)

	ER strongly +ve	ER weakly +ve	ER −ve
Premenopausal			
Excellent risk (NPI < 2.4) 5% patients	3% 10-yr BCM Tamoxifen	Tamoxifen	6% 10-yr BCM No adjuvant treatment
Very good risk (NPI 2.4–3.39) 15% patients	9% 10-yr MCM Tamoxifen +/− OS	Tamoxifen +/− OS	14% 10-yr BCM HER2 +ve FEC × 4, then Herceptin
Good risk (NPI 3.4–4.39) 30% patients	15% 10-yr BCM Tamoxifen +/− OS HER2 +ve FEC × 4, then Herceptin	Tamoxifen +/− OS FEC × 6 with trastuzumab in HER 2 + ve	30% 10-yr BCM FEC × 6 with trastuzumab in HER 2 + ve
Intermediate risk (NPI 4.4–5.39) 30% patients	33% 10-yr BCM Tamoxifen +/− OS HER2 −ve. FEC × 6 HER2 +ve. Taxane-based chemo × 6 + trastuzumab	Tamoxifen +/− OS HER2 −ve. FEC × 6 HER2 +ve. Taxane-based chemo × 6 + trastuzumab	40% 10-yr BCM HER2 −ve. FEC × 6 HER2 +ve. Taxane-based chemo × 6 + trastuzumab
Poor risk # (NPI ≥ 5.4) 20% patients	50% 10-yr BCM Tamoxifen +/− OS HER2 −ve FEC or Taxane × 6 HER2 +ve. Taxane-based chemo × 6 + trastuzumab	Tamoxifen +/− OS HER2 −ve FEC or Taxane × 6 Taxane based chemo × 6 + trastuzumab	60% 10-yr BCM HER2 −ve. TAC × 6 HER2 +ve. TAC × 6 + Herceptin trastuzumab
Postmenopausal			
Excellent risk (NPI < 2.4) 5% patients	3% 10-yr BCM Tamoxifen	Tamoxifen	6% 10-yr BCM No adjuvant treatment
Very good risk (NPI 2.4–3.39) 20% patients	6% 10-yr BCM Tamoxifen / AI switch	Tamoxifen / AI switch	10% 10-yr BCM HER2 + ve FEC × 4, then Herceptin
Good risk (NPI 3.4–4.39) 30% patients	15% 10-yr BCM AI HER2 +ve FEC × 4, then trastuzumab	AI FEC × 6 with trastuzumab in HER 2 + ve	30% 10-yr BCM FEC × 6 with trastuzumab in HER 2 + ve
Intermediate risk (NPI 4.4–5.39) 35% patients	30% 10-yr BCM AI HER2 −ve. FEC × 6 HER2 +ve. FEC × 6 + trastuzumab	AI HER2 −ve. FEC × 6 HER2 +ve. FEC × 6 + trastuzumab	40% 10-yr BCM HER2 −ve. FEC × 6 HER2 +ve. Taxane-based chemo × 6 + trastuzumab
Poor risk # (NPI ≥ 5.4) 10% patients	55% 10-yr BCM AI HER2 −ve. FEC × 6 HER2 +ve. Taxane-based chemo × 6 + trastuzumab	AI HER2 −ve. FEC × 6 HER2 +ve. Taxane-based chemo × 6 + trastuzumab	60% 10-yr BCM HER2 −ve FEC or Taxane × 6 HER2 +ve. FEC or Taxane × 6 + trastuzumab

10 yr BCM, 10-year breast cancer mortality rate; AI, aromatase inhibitor; NPI, Nottingham Prognostic Index; OS, ovarian suppression.

Anthracycline-based chemotherapy: FEC (5FU, epirubicin, cyclophosphamide), TAC (docetaxel, epirubicin, cyclophosphamide).

Source: data from *Referral and Management Guidelines for Breast Cancers within North Trent*, North Trent Breast Cancer Group, NHS, UK, Copyright © 2012, available from http://www.yhscn.nhs.uk/media/PDFs/cancer/Breast%20docs/NEW%20NTBreast%20NSSG%20Guidelines%20revision%20Aug%2012%20REC%20FINAL%20FINAL.pdf

of 10-year breast cancer mortality across subgroups and demonstrates the complexity of adjuvant treatment options and decisions. The recommended treatment for each patient is guided by their risk of relapse and other factors including hormone receptor and HER2 status are important considerations in treatment selection. The increasing use of genetic tumour profiles (e.g. oncotype DX) will continue to refine these prognostic systems and may be able to tease out groups of patients for whom current guidelines risk over-treatment as they are already at low risk of recurrence following surgery.[4]

Adjuvant hormone therapy

In the early 1970s, tamoxifen and other antioestrogen adjuvant therapy was shown to reduce overall mortality from breast cancer in women with ER-positive disease. The Early Breast Cancer Trialists' Collaborative Group (EBCTCG) showed that 5 years of tamoxifen therapy reduced annual recurrence rates by almost half and breast cancer mortality by one-third.[5] These trials established a standard of 5 years of adjuvant tamoxifen therapy by showing this was superior to 2 years of treatment. The recently reported ATLAS study (Adjuvant Tamoxifen, Longer Against Shorter) now suggests there may be benefit in prolonging treatment further (8–10 years) in selected patients with 29% lower breast cancer mortality compared with women who stopped tamoxifen after 5 years.[6]

Tamoxifen is the mainstay of adjuvant treatment in ER-positive premenopausal women and in male breast cancer. There is some evidence to suggest that combined hormonal treatments in premenopausal women by the addition of ovarian suppression may be beneficial but this approach awaits the outcome of trials like the SOFT study (ovarian suppression + tamoxifen or exemestane) before it can be considered a standard approach.[7]

In postmenopausal women, large-scale studies comparing tamoxifen with aromatase inhibitors found significant improvements in disease-free survival and reduced toxicity from thromboembolic disease and endometrial cancer. Typically an aromatase inhibitor prolongs disease-free survival and reduces distant metastases by 14% but improvement in overall survival is yet to be documented.[8] Aromatase inhibitors show similar improvements when patients are 'switched' from tamoxifen halfway through the 5-year treatment[9] and when adjuvant treatment is extended by using an aromatase inhibitor for a further 3 years after the 5-year adjuvant tamoxifen treatment finishes.[10]

The role of adjuvant hormonal therapy following resection of ductal carcinoma *in situ* (DCIS) is less clear as tamoxifen offers a very small reduction in the risk of invasive breast cancers but no overall survival benefit.[11] Studies like the IBIS-II study which compares anastrozole and tamoxifen in postmenopausal women with ER-positive DCIS will define the role of aromatase inhibitors in this form of the disease.

It should be remembered that side effect profiles can influence the decision about adjuvant hormonal treatment. Menopausal symptoms are common to all and while tamoxifen protects against postmenopausal bone loss and lowers cholesterol it is associated with an increased risk of endometrial cancer and thromboembolic events. The latter are less of a concern with aromatase inhibitors but there are effects on bone that require monitoring and often treatment to prevent osteoporosis.

Adjuvant chemotherapy

The EBCTCG/Oxford overview summarize the improvements in disease-free and overall survival seen with adjuvant chemotherapy in breast cancer.[12] The absolute gains from chemotherapy are in proportion to the risk of recurrence and benefits are greatest in women with poor prognosis disease as indicated by young age (< 35 years), large tumour size, node positivity, high grade, hormone receptor negativity, and HER2 expression. The absolute benefit can be difficult to quantify and the use of prognostic scoring systems like the NPI and Adjuvant! Online[3] can be particularly helpful for individual patients with the latter system delivering results in simple graphical formats that helps guide the decision-making process for many women.

The general principles demonstrated in the Oxford overview are that single-agent adjuvant chemotherapy is inferior to combination chemotherapy treatment and treatment over 3–6 months

(four to eight cycles) offers the optimal balance between benefits and side effects. The benefit of adjuvant chemotherapy was first demonstrated with the CMF regimen (cyclophosphamide, methotrexate and 5-fluorourcil) in node-positive patients. Subsequently, trials demonstrated that the addition of an anthracycline gave further reduction in breast cancer recurrence and mortality.[12] Anthracycline-containing regimens are the current cornerstones of adjuvant chemotherapy though more recent trials have demonstrated the addition of a taxane to be a further improvement[13] and the UK National Institute for Health and Care Excellence (NICE) recommends the use of docetaxel in high-risk patients like those with lymph node-positive disease.[14]

Adjuvant trastuzumab

The biggest change in adjuvant treatment over the past 10 years has been the introduction of trastuzumab for patients with HER2-positive tumours. Studies showed it reduced the risk of relapse by 50% with associated survival benefits.[15] Trastuzumab is generally well tolerated but does have cardiac toxicities and cardiac monitoring is required during treatment and the drug should be used with caution in patients with known left ventricular systolic dysfunction. The current focus for trials is the duration of adjuvant trastuzumab and the role of newer drugs targeting the HER2 receptor pathway.

Adjuvant radiotherapy

Postoperative radiotherapy can be administered once the operative wound has healed and chemotherapy is complete, taking into account the type of surgery, pathology, breast size, and the presence of a prosthesis, and conventionally delivers 2 Gy fractions to doses of 50–60 Gy in 25–30 fractions over 5–6 weeks. It has been recognized to reduce locoregional recurrence for over 40 years with a constant relative risk reduction of approximately 50% for patients with invasive carcinoma or DCIS. However, the early radiotherapy techniques gave significant doses to the heart and the improvements in breast cancer mortality were exactly balanced by increases in cardiac mortality. Modifications in the radiotherapy fields and improvements in technology have reduced these toxicities and the EBCTCG meta-analysis of breast-conserving surgery followed by radiotherapy now shows a reduction in local recurrence, breast cancer deaths, and overall mortality at 15 years.[16,17]

The technological advances illustrated in Figures 2.6.3.2 and 2.6.3.3 contribute to the development of non-conventional

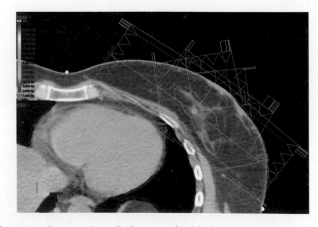

Fig. 2.6.3.2 Postoperative radiotherapy to the right breast using IMRT, showing a five-field plan.

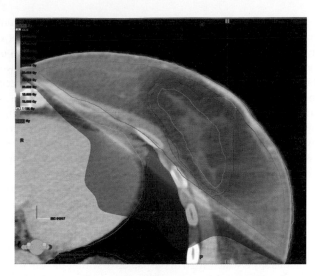

Fig. 2.6.3.3 Same patient as Figure 2.6.3.2 illustrating dose distribution using a colourwash.

fractionation schedules. Results from the START trial have shown hypofractionation using fewer, larger fractions to be as safe and effective as the standard schedule.[18] This has led to 40 Gy delivered in 15 fractions over 3 weeks becoming standard practice in the United Kingdom with more accelerated schedules that use a 5-fraction schedule to deliver treatment over 1 week being investigated in the FAST and FAST Forward trials, with the former (30 Gy in five once-weekly fractions) comparable to 50 Gy in 25 fractions in terms of adverse events.[19] An alternative approach being explored is intraoperative radiotherapy which has been investigated in the TARGIT study which assesses whether the use of partial breast irradiation using intraoperative techniques is equivalent to whole-breast irradiation in women undergoing conservation surgery without any adverse histopathological features.

Indications for radiotherapy
Conservation surgery
All patients with invasive carcinoma should be considered for radiotherapy to the breast once clear circumferential resection margins have been confirmed pathologically. There are relative contraindications including poor performance status, significant respiratory or cardiovascular impairment, and local anatomical factors such as poor shoulder movements or large pendulous breasts which may make the practical administration of radiotherapy difficult.

Radiotherapy boost to the tumour bed
In patients with invasive breast cancer who have undergone breast conserving surgery and whole-breast radiotherapy, the EORTC study showed 5-year local recurrence rates of 4.3% with boost radiotherapy versus 7.3% in no boost (reduction of 40%). Greatest benefit was seen in younger women (under the age of 40) though breast cosmesis may be adversely affected.[20] Standard practice is to give the boost sequentially in a 5- or 8-fraction course of radiotherapy. However, new radiotherapy technologies (intensity modulated radiotherapy (IMRT)) reduce the volume of normal tissue being treated and allow novel fractionations to increase the biological tumour dose. An example where this is being tested are IMPORT trials which aim to match the radiation dose to the differing risks of recurrence across the breast and in effect deliver the boost dose

concomitantly to the tumour bed during the standard 3-week treatment regimen.

Post mastectomy
Radiotherapy to the chest wall after mastectomy for invasive disease has been shown to improve local control with improvements in overall survival in selected patients.[21] These patients have been identified as having T3/T4 primary tumours, four or more positive lymph nodes, or positive resection margins. There are other factors recognized to increase the chance of local recurrence including vascular invasion, grade III tumour, and one to three nodes positive, and the ongoing SUPREMO trial (Selective Use of Post-operative Radiotherapy after Mastectomy) will determine the benefits of radiotherapy in these patients.[22]

Axilla
This should be managed surgically and radiotherapy to the axilla after axillary node clearance is not recommended due to the significant morbidity associated with lymphoedema of the arm. It can be considered if the patient with invasive breast cancer refuses/is unfit for axillary surgery or known residual microscopic disease after surgery has been performed.

Supraclavicular fossa
Radiotherapy has been shown to reduce the risk of nodal recurrence in the supraclavicular fossa and improve survival in patients with heavy (four or more) positive axillary nodes.

Ductal carcinoma *in situ*
DCIS comprises 15–20% of all screen-detected breast cancers and despite the lack of randomized trial evidence it is widely recognized that mastectomy is over-treatment for many and breast conservation is increasingly offered. Evidence from prospective randomized trials[23,24] and the EBCTCG[25] indicates that radiotherapy after breast-conserving surgery for DCIS approximately halved the local recurrence rate with an absolute 10-year risk reduction of 15%, half due to a reduction in the recurrent DCIS and half invasive breast cancer. With conservation surgery and radiotherapy becoming the standard of care in DCIS, the challenge is now to identify a subgroup with small tumours and good surgical margins at low risk for recurrence for whom adjuvant radiotherapy could be omitted. Retrospective studies by the National Surgical Adjuvant Breast Project indicate nuclear grade, necrosis, size, and margin width are important in predicting recurrence.[26] Historical recurrence data have led to various predictive tools to aid patient selection for adjuvant treatment, the Van Nuys Prognostic Index being the most widely recognized, but these tools have not been prospectively validated. The results of the large prospective trials have so far failed to identify the subgroups in whom radiotherapy is not needed and the specific studies[27,28] that have tried to address this question have struggled to accrue and are unlikely to provide any definitive answers.

Neoadjuvant treatment
Primary chemotherapy or hormone therapy is now commonly offered in locally advanced, inflammatory, or large operable breast cancer and allows the *in vivo* assessment of response to treatment and the opportunity to change therapy early if no response is seen. Studies comparing this approach to adjuvant treatment have shown equivalent survival[29–31] which has allayed the perceived disadvantages of delaying definitive local surgery. The clear advantage

to neoadjuvant systemic treatment is downstaging the primary tumour which for some women allows breast-conserving surgery where mastectomy was otherwise required.

Pathological complete response rates have proved a good marker of prognosis in this situation and that is seen in around 10% for anthracycline-based chemotherapy, 20% when a taxane is added, and in HER2-positive patients the addition of trastuzumab which can significantly increase pathological complete response rates to approaching 50%.[32] Clearly patients have to be monitored closely during treatment with clinical assessment following each cycle and ultrasound assessment after two cycles with ultrasound-guided insertion of marker clips for tumour bed localization. Post-treatment magnetic resonance imaging is recommended in those patients being considered for breast-conserving surgery.

Primary endocrine therapy

When compared to chemotherapy, endocrine approaches are associated with a slower response to treatment and lower complete response rate but for patients who are ER positive and unfit for chemotherapy, an aromatase inhibitor can downstage inoperable disease. Patients presenting with ER-positive operable disease but who are elderly and unfit for surgical treatment should be considered for primary hormonal therapy. Studies have shown complete and partial response rates of 12% and 35% respectively with clinical benefit gained in 98% of patients on first-line therapy.[33] Response to first-, second-, and third-line hormonal therapies often last 24 months, 12 months, and approximately 9 months on average.

Metastatic breast cancer

About 15–20% of patients with breast cancer have metastatic disease at the time of diagnosis and with advances in treatment of early invasive breast cancer women are surviving longer. They are then at increasing risk of developing metastases even 10–20 years after surgery. Metastatic disease remains an incurable disease and treatment is given with palliative intent aiming to control symptoms and improve quality of life and prolong time to the progression of disease and death. The likelihood of metastasis is strongly linked to the presence and quantity of positive axillary lymph nodes, and the grade and size of the tumour.[34] The role of preoperative screening remains debatable though most units will consider CT scanning in the presence of histologically confirmed nodal involvement at diagnosis. When distant metastases are found, prognostic factors including age, site of metastasis, and hormonal status are valuable for predicting survival. While the overall median survival from the time of diagnosis of metastatic disease has risen to around 24–30 months, certain groups like those with ER-positive disease and bone-only metastasis will do significantly better.

Hormonal treatment is the preferred first modality in patients with ER-positive disease because of the better side effect profile in comparison to chemotherapy. In premenopausal women, tamoxifen or ovarian suppression/ablation are used first line whereas an aromatase inhibitor would be used in the postmenopausal patient. Patients in whom the disease initially responds to endocrine therapy can be offered further lines of hormonal treatment with the expectation of a 25% response rate in the second line and 10–15% third line.

Chemotherapy would be preferred in ER-negative disease, rapidly progressive or ER-positive disease that is rapidly progressing, particularly when visceral metastases are present and it has a role for patients who are failing to respond to hormones. Combination chemotherapy can offer higher response rates but at the cost of extra toxicity in a palliative setting. The 2009 NICE guidelines on advanced breast cancer recommend anthracyclines first, followed by taxanes on progression, with single-agent vinorelbine or capecitabine in the third-line setting.[35]

HER2-directed treatment should be added in HER2-positive patients with trastuzumab the standard treatment considered. However, this is a large-molecular-weight protein that does not cross the blood–brain barrier and has a high rate of cerebral relapse. When relapse does occur, trials are reporting a number of drugs are active and target different parts of the HER2 pathway. Examples that have activity confirmed in phase III trials include pertuzumab (monoclonal antibody inhibiting receptor dimerization),[36] mertansine DM1 (cytotoxic attachment delivered using the trastuzumab antibody,[37] and lapatinib, a tyrosine kinase inhibitor.[38]

Radiotherapy is widely used in the palliative setting and can reduce symptoms at a range of metastatic disease sites. It is most widely used as a treatment for bone metastasis when one fraction can improve pain in 70–80%; other commonly used scenarios include the treatment of brain and spinal cord metastasis where it is used to maintain function and reduce corticosteroid requirements. More fractionated treatment (5–10 fractions) can be used to treat uncontrolled local disease and improve pain, bleeding, and other symptoms.

Over the past 10 years, the use of specific bone-directed treatments has become standard in patients with bone metastases and reduces skeletal-related events of fractures, cord compression, and prevention of malignant hypercalcaemia. Bisphosphonates such as zoledronic acid are the current standard but recent developments in metastatic bone research have identified the receptor activator of nuclear factor kappa-B ligand (RANKL) as a primary mediator of osteoclast activity. Denosumab, a fully human monoclonal antibody that reduces osteoclast-mediated bone destruction by inhibiting RANKL, has been shown to be superior to zoledronate and has recently been approved by NICE for the prevention of skeletal-related events.[39] In addition, there is also some intriguing data suggesting that the addition of these treatments may have a role in the adjuvant setting offering a further treatment option that can reduce the risk of recurrence following surgery.[40]

References

1. Kallioniemi OP, Holli K, Visakorpi T, *et al.* Association of c-erbB-2 protein over-expression with high rate of cell proliferation, increased risk of visceral metastasis and poor long-term survival in breast cancer. *Int J Cancer* 1991; 49:650–5.
2. Baselga J, Campone M, Piccart M, *et al.* Everolimus in postmenopausal hormone-receptor-positive advanced breast cancer. *N Engl J Med* 2012; 366:520–9.
3. Adjuvant! Online. *Decision Making Tools for Health Care Professionals.* [Online] http://www.adjuvantonline.com
4. Ishibe N, Schully S, Freedman A, *et al.* Use of oncotype DX in women with node-positive breast cancer. *PLoS Curr* 2011; 3:RRN1249.
5. Early Breast Cancer Trialists' Collaborative Group. Tamoxifen for early breast cancer: an overview of the randomised trials. *Lancet* 1998; 351(9114):1451–67.
6. Davies C, Pan H, Godwin J, *et al.* Adjuvant Tamoxifen: Longer Against Shorter (ATLAS) Collaborative Group. Long-term effects of continuing adjuvant tamoxifen to 10 years versus stopping at 5 years after diagnosis of oestrogen receptor-positive breast cancer: ATLAS, a randomised trial. *Lancet* 2013; 381; 9869:805–16.

7. International Breast Cancer Study Group. *Suppression of Ovarian Function Trial (SOFT). A Phase III Trial Evaluating the Role of Ovarian Function Suppression and the Role of Exemestane as Adjuvant Therapies for Premenopausal Women with Endocrine Responsive Breast Cancer.* [Online] http://www.ibcsg.org/Public/Health_Professionals/Closed_Trials/IBCSG_24-02/Pages/IBCSG24-02BIG2-02(SOFT).aspx

8. Howell A, Cuzick J, Baum M, *et al.* ATAC Trialists. Results of the ATAC (Arimidex, Tamoxifen, Alone or in Combination) trial after completion of 5 years' adjuvant treatment for breast cancer. *Lancet* 2005; 365(9453):60–2.

9. Coombes RC, Hall E, Gibson LJ, *et al.* A randomized trial of exemestane after two to three years of tamoxifen therapy in postmenopausal women with primary breast cancer. *N Engl J Med* 2004; 350:1081–92.

10. Goss PE. Letrozole in the extended adjuvant setting: MA.17. *Breast Cancer Res Treat* 2007; 105(1):45–53.

11. Allred DC, Anderson SJ, Paik S, *et al.* Adjuvant tamoxifen reduces subsequent breast cancer in women with estrogen receptor-positive ductal carcinoma in situ: a study based on NSABP protocol B-24. *J Clin Oncol* 2012; 30(12):1268–73.

12. Palmieri C, Jones A, Early Breast Cancer Trialists' Collaborative Group. The 2011 EBCTCG polychemotherapy overview. *Lancet* 2012; 379 (9814):390–2.

13. Martin M, Pienkowski T, Mackey J, *et al.* Breast Cancer International Research Group 001 Investigators. Adjuvant docetaxel for node-positive breast cancer. *N Engl J Med* 2005; 352:2302–13.

14. National Institute for Health and Care Excellence. *Early and Locally Advanced Breast Cancer: Diagnosis and Treatment.* London: NICE; 2009. http://www.nice.org.uk/CG80

15. Piccart-Gebhart M, Proctor M, Leyland-Jones B, *et al.* Trastuzumab after adjuvant chemotherapy in HER2-positive breast cancer. *N Engl J Med* 2005; 353:1659–72.

16. Early Breast Cancer Trialists' Collaborative Group (EBCTCG), Darby S, McGale P, *et al.* Effect of radiotherapy after breast-conserving surgery on 10-year recurrence and 15-year breast cancer death: meta-analysis of individual patient data for 10,801 women in 17 randomised trials. *Lancet* 2011; 378(9804):1707–16.

17. Clarke M, Collins R, Darby S, *et al.* Effects of radiotherapy and of differences in the extent of surgery for early breast cancer on local recurrence and 15-year survival: an overview of the randomised trials. *Lancet* 2005; 366:2087–106.

18. Bentzen SM, Agrawal RK, Aird EG, *et al.* The UK Standardisation of Breast Radiotherapy (START) Trial B of radiotherapy hypofractionation for treatment of early breast cancer: a randomised trial. *Lancet* 2008; 371(9618):1098–107.

19. FAST Trialists group, Agrawal RK, Alhasso A, *et al.* First results of the randomised UK FAST Trial of radiotherapy hypofractionation for treatment of early breast cancer. *Radiother Oncol* 2011; 100(1):93–100.

20. Bartelink H, Horiot JC, Poortmans PM, *et al.* Impact of a higher radiation dose on local control and survival in breast-conserving therapy of early breast cancer: 10-year results of the randomized boost versus no boost EORTC 22881-10882 trial. *J Clin Oncol* 2007; 25(22):3259–65.

21. Danish Breast Cancer Cooperative Group, Nielsen HM, Overgaard M, *et al.* Study of failure pattern among high-risk breast cancer patients with or without postmastectomy radiotherapy in addition to adjuvant systemic therapy: long-term results from the Danish Breast Cancer Cooperative Group DBCG 82 b and c randomized studies. *J Clin Oncol* 2006; 24(15):2268–75.

22. SUPREMO. *Selective Use of Post-operative Radiotherapy After Mastectomy.* [Online] http://www.supremo-trial.com

23. Fisher B, Dignam J, Wolmark N, *et al.* Lumpectomy and radiation therapy for the treatment of intraductal breast cancer: findings from National Surgical Adjuvant Breast and Bowel Project B-17. *J Clin Oncol* 1998; 16(2):441–52.

24. Julien JP, Bijker N, Fentiman IS, *et al.* Radiotherapy in breast-conserving treatment for ductal carcinoma in situ: first results of the EORTC randomised phase III trial 10853. EORTC Breast Cancer Cooperative Group and EORTC Radiotherapy Group. *Lancet* 2000; 355(9203):528–33.

25. Early Breast Cancer Trialists' Collaborative Group (EBCTCG), Correa C, McGale P, *et al.* Overview of the randomized trials of radiotherapy in ductal carcinoma in situ of the breast. *J Natl Cancer Inst Monogr* 2010; 2010(41):162–77.

26. Fisher E, Dignam J, Tan-Chiu E, *et al.* Pathologic findings from the National Surgical Adjuvant Breast Project (NSABP) eight-year update of Protocol B-17. *Cancer* 1999; 86:429–38.

27. Motwani SB, Goyal S, Moran MS, *et al.* Ductal carcinoma in situ treated with breast-conserving surgery and radiotherapy: a comparison with ECOG study 5194. *Cancer* 2011; 117(6):1156–62.

28. Millar J, Rodger A. Adjuvant radiotherapy for DCIS. *Lancet* 2000; 355(9220):2072.

29. Fisher B, Bryant J, Wolmark N. Effect of preoperative chemotherapy on the outcome of women with operable breast cancer. *J Clin Oncol* 1998; 16:2672–85.

30. Mauri D, Pavlidis N, Ioannidis J. Neoadjuvant versus adjuvant systemic treatment in breast cancer; a meta-analysis. *J Natl Cancer Inst* 2005; 97(3):188–94.

31. Mieog JS, Van der Hage JA, Van de Velde CJ. Neoadjuvant chemotherapy for operable breast cancer. *Br J Surg* 2007; 94:1189–200.

32. Rastogi P, Anderson SJ, Bear HD, *et al.* Preoperative chemotherapy: updates of national surgical adjuvant breast and bowel project protocols B-18 and B-27. *J Clin Oncol* 2008; 26(5):778–85.

33. Al-Khyatt W. Primary endocrine therapy for early operable primary breast cancer in elderly women: a large series from a single institution. *J Clin Oncol* 2009; 27:15s, abstr 630.

34. Largillier R, Ferrero JM, Doyen J, *et al.* Prognostic factors in 1,038 women with metastatic breast cancer. *Ann Oncol* 2008; 19(12):2012–19.

35. National Institute for Health and Care Excellence. *Advanced Breast Cancer (Update): Diagnosis and Treatment.* Clinical Guideline 81. London: NICE; 2009. http://www.nice.org.uk/CG81

36. Baselga J, Cortes J, Kim S, *et al.* CLEOPATRA Study Group. Pertuzumab plus trastuzumab plus docetaxel for metastatic breast cancer. *N Engl J Med* 2012; 366:109–19.

37. Verma S, Miles D, Gianni L, *et al.* EMILIA Study Group. Trastuzumab emtansine for HER2-positive advanced breast cancer. *N Engl J Med* 2012; 367:1783–91.

38. Geyer C, Forster J, Lindquist D, *et al.* Lapatinib plus capecitabine for HER2-positive advanced breast cancer. *N Engl J Med* 2006; 355:2733–43.

39. National Institute for Health and Care Excellence. *Denosumab for the Prevention of Skeletal-Related Events in Adults with Bone Metastases from Solid Tumours.* NICE Technology Appraisal Guidance TA265. London: NICE; 2012. http://www.nice.org.uk/guidance/ta265

40. Gnant M, Mlineritsch B, Schippinger W, *et al.* ABCSG-12 Trial Investigators. Endocrine therapy plus zoledronic acid in premenopausal breast cancer. *N Engl J Med* 2009; 360:679–91.

PART 2.7

Vascular surgery

Sub-section editor: Michael G. Wyatt

CHAPTER 2.7.1

Chronic arterial insufficiency

Christopher M. Butler

Introduction

Chronic arterial insufficiency (CAI) is a term used to describe a spectrum of symptoms usually affecting the lower limbs. The terms peripheral arterial disease and peripheral vascular disease also appear in the literature and are essentially describing the same conditions. The vast majority of cases are caused by atherosclerosis. It is a common condition with 15–20% of 70-year-olds affected. It usually presents as intermittent claudication (IC): typically a pain in the calf muscles of the lower limb, which comes on with walking and is relieved by rest. IC is an important marker for increased risk of vascular disease, which may be asymptomatic, in the coronary and cerebrovascular circulation. Many cases can be treated adequately in primary care with risk factor modification and simple treatment. These aim to prevent disease progression, which can lead to critical limb ischaemia (CLI) with pain at rest, ulceration, and gangrene. In recent years, the rapid expansion of vascular surgery and interventional radiology have led to the development of a wide range of possible interventions. In an attempt to establish sensible guidelines for treatment, consensus documents have been produced representing the best available advice and evidence. In the United Kingdom, the National Institute for Health and Care Excellence (NICE) has produced guidelines (2012) for the diagnosis and management of PAD.

Chronic arterial insufficiency

Incidence

Objective testing in population studies has estimated that the total incidence of CAI is between 3% and 10%, rising to 15–20% in people over the age of 70. Most patients will present with IC, a muscular leg pain which will come on reproducibly with exercise and is relieved by rest. Not all patients with CAI will present with IC symptoms, as they have other medical conditions, which limit their ability to walk or they have a very sedentary lifestyle. Best estimates of the prevalence of symptomatic IC in the general population suggest it is present in 3% of the population at the age of 40, rising to 6% at age 60. In the younger ages, males predominate, but beyond the age of 60 there is an equal gender distribution.

Risk factors for chronic arterial insufficiency

A number of important risk factors, some of which may be modifiable by appropriate treatment, have been established by large population studies. These include, race (more common in non-Hispanic black people), gender (male > female), age (increase in incidence with age), smoking, diabetes mellitus, hypertension, dyslipidaemia,

hyperviscosity/hypercoagulability of blood, chronic renal insufficiency, and hyperhomocysteinaemia.

Pathophysiology

The majority of lower limb CAI is due to atherosclerosis. This is a condition in which the wall of an artery thickens and hardens as the result of a deposition of fatty materials producing atheromatous ('lump of gruel' from Greek) plaques. Details of the pathology of atherosclerosis can be found in Chapter 1.4.1.

In the peripheral circulation, atherosclerotic plaques are often found at points of bifurcation in the arterial circulation; typically this involves carotid, aortic, iliac, and femoral arteries resulting in areas of turbulence and loss of laminar blood flow.

The expansion of atheromatous plaques can be very chronic and will only produce a reduction in downstream blood flow when 50% of the arterial lumen is occluded. In most situations a figure of 75% stenosis within a vessel is associated with clinically significant symptoms.

Atherosclerotic plaques may be stable or unstable. The unstable plaques are likely to be clinically significant, as the fibrous cap, which separates the lesion from the arterial wall, is weak and prone to rupture. This exposes thrombogenic material, such as collagen, to the circulation and thrombus develops. This will usually lead to an occlusion of the affected artery.

In the lower limbs, atheromatous plaques generally develop slowly, allowing time for the development of an adequate collateral circulation, which can mitigate against the effects of the thrombosis on the distal tissues. The thrombosis may, however, cause deterioration in symptoms such as walking distance and may precipitate the development of CLI. Rarer causes of occlusive arterial disease are given in Box 2.7.1.1.

Natural history of chronic arterial insufficiency

Available evidence suggests that of all the patients who present with IC, only about a quarter will develop significant deterioration in symptoms. This stabilization of symptoms is due to a number of factors including the development of an adequate collateral circulation, metabolic adaptations of ischaemic muscle, and gait alterations by the patient. The remaining 25% of patients presenting with IC will experience measurable deterioration in their walking distance. This tends to be worst in the first year after diagnosis (7–9%) compared with 2–3% per year later. It is important to note that, with the exception of diabetics, major amputation is a rare outcome of patients with CAI presenting with IC.

Patients presenting with IC have a high risk of other cardiovascular problems, with 20% having had a non-fatal myocardial

Box 2.7.1.1 Rarer causes of occlusive arterial disease

- Arteritis
- Congenital or acquired aortic coarctation
- Endofibrosis of the external iliac artery (seen in cyclists)
- Fibromuscular dysplasia
- Peripheral emboli
- Thrombosed popliteal aneurysm
- Popliteal artery adventitial cysts
- Popliteal entrapment syndrome
- Primary tumours of arteries
- Remote trauma or radiation injuries
- Takayasu's disease
- Thromboangiitis obliterans.

infarction (MI) or stroke (CVA) within 5 years and 10–15% dying, of which 75% will be from MI or CVA.

Critical limb ischaemia

The most serious manifestation of CAI is the development of CLI. This comprises a number of symptoms including pain in the foot at rest, vascular ulcers, and poor healing of minor trauma to the limbs, and may progress to gangrene. The process may be a chronic progression from IC to ischaemic pain in the foot at rest or patients may present with fairly sudden onset of symptoms without a previous history of IC.

The onset of CLI is a serious problem and, in the developed world, patients will normally be investigated and undergo interventional treatment to try and prevent limb loss. Because up to 90% of patients will have some form of active treatment, the natural history of the condition is not known. The 1-year outcomes of patients presenting with CLI are poor with only 45% being alive with two limbs, 30% alive after having a major amputation, and 25% will have died (the large majority from MI or CVA).

The diagnosis of chronic arterial insufficiency

This requires the taking of a thorough history, a clinical examination, and a number of appropriate diagnostic tests.

History

The presenting complaint will often be of IC. This is a cramping, aching discomfort in the calf muscles coming on reproducibly with walking and relieved by rest within 10 minutes. Usually the pain will develop earlier if walking faster or going uphill. Less commonly the claudication pain can affect the thigh and buttock muscles or the arch of the foot. The symptoms will indicate the level of the disease in the arterial circulation. It is important to determine the characteristics of the pain, its reproducibility, the effects of exercise, the effects of rest, and the effects of position. This will help distinguish IC from other conditions which affect the lower limb and can cause exercise-related problems.

Patient should be asked to estimate their pain-free walking distance and the amount of rest required for symptoms to disappear. The

effect of the symptoms on the patient's lifestyle is important. A 100-yard claudication distance in an 80-year-old may be of little practical significance, but would have major implications for a 50-year-old manual worker. Patients should be asked about any skin changes, ulcers, and if they develop pain in their feet at night. Typically, if they have rest pain, they will have to hang their feet out of bed at night and may find relief by putting their feet on a cold surface.

Care should be taken to establish a clear past medical history and this along with the systems review should be directed at establishing what co-morbidities the patient has. It is particularly important to ask about cardiac symptoms, strokes or transient ischaemic attacks, diabetes, hypertension, lipid problems, arthritis, and inflammatory conditions like rheumatoid arthritis.

A full drug history is important, as some agents (e.g. beta blockers) can have an effect on symptoms. Family history may be relevant and social history should document smoking and drinking history as well as home circumstances, which may be affected by the disease (e.g. impotence).

Physical examination

This should assess the whole circulatory system and include measurement of blood pressure in both arms, an assessment of cardiac murmurs and heart rhythms, and an abdominal examination to check for aortic aneurysm.

There should be a thorough inspection of the arms, hands, and the front and back of both of the lower limbs looking for colour differences, ulcers or other trophic changes, decreased hair growth, muscle atrophy, nail hypertrophy, and capillary refilling (Figures 2.7.1.1 and 2.7.1.2).

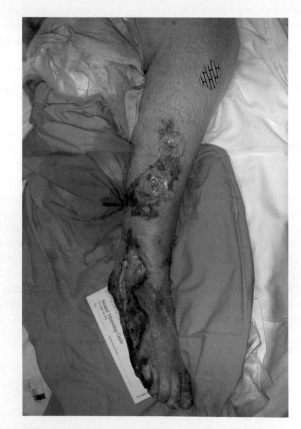

Fig. 2.7.1.1 Critical limb ischaemia, gangrene with extensive tissue loss.

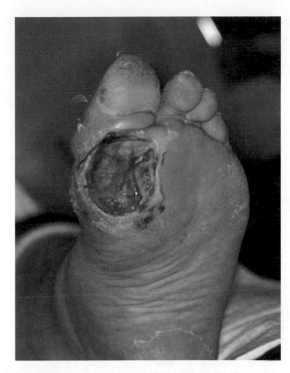

Fig. 2.7.1.2 Typical neuropathic foot ulcer in a diabetic patient.

Palpation should be used to assess temperature differences along limbs and between opposite hands and feet. The radial, ulnar, brachial, carotid, femoral, dorsalis pedis, and posterior tibial pulses should be graded as absent, diminished, or normal. A particularly prominent pulse in the femoral or popliteal arteries should raise the possibility of an aneurysm.

Pulses will normally be absent in the arterial segment above the muscle group that the patients have claudication symptoms in. For example, if the patient has claudication in the calf the femoral pulse will be normal and it will not be possible to feel normal popliteal or foot pulses. In patients with thigh and buttock claudication, the femoral pulse will also be absent.

Auscultation is used to listen for arterial bruits over the aorta, carotid, and femoral arteries. The presence of a bruit may indicate turbulence and be a sign of significant vascular disease. The absence of a bruit, however, does not exclude vascular disease.

The widespread availability and ease of use of the simple hand-held Doppler ultrasonic velocimeter has enabled the clinician to use this device as part of their routine clinical examination. This device is particularly useful in enabling clinicians with a little training to perform a measurement of the ankle–brachial pressure index (ABPI). An experienced clinician can also use the audible signals to assess the blood flow in peripheral vessels with a high degree of reliability.

The ABPI can provide an objective indicator of the severity of the CAI and should be a standard part of the assessment of the vascular patient. Care should be taken to ensure the measurement is taken in a reproducible way. Typically the patient should be at rest on an examination couch with a normal room ambient temperature. An appropriately sized sphygmomanometer cuff is placed just above the ankle to occlude the circulation. The Doppler probe is used to indicate at what pressure flow is re-established in the artery as the cuff is deflated. The measurement should be repeated for both dorsalis pedis and posterior tibial vessels in both feet. These

pressures are then normalized to the highest of the two arm pressure measurements.

In normal circumstances the ABPI is very reliable; however, care should be exercised in using it for the assessment of patients who may have significant vascular calcification such as diabetics or those with chronic renal disease. In these circumstances the cuff may not occlude the vessels and this will lead to a very high ankle pressure and a falsely elevated ABPI. The ABPI figure of less than 0.9 at rest is taken as the cut-off point for the diagnosis of CAI. It has proved a very useful diagnostic and prognostic tool for the vascular clinician and provides useful objective data when assessing the effects of treatment on patients.

Special investigations

In all cases blood should be sent for full blood count, renal function, liver function, cholesterol, lipids, and C-reactive protein. If arteritis is suspected, an erythrocyte sedimentation rate and antibody screening may be useful. Urine may be tested for sugar as a screen for diabetes mellitus. An electrocardiogram should be performed to look for signs of cardiac ischaemia and abnormal heart rhythms. A chest X-ray to look for cardiopulmonary abnormalities is also useful.

In patients suspected on clinical examination of having aneurysmal disease, ultrasound imaging of the area will confirm or exclude the diagnosis. Patients found to have a carotid bruit(s) should be referred for colour duplex imaging of their carotid arteries.

Patients suspected of having an iliac stenosis, which does not cause reduced femoral pulses at rest, should have an exercise test. This can demonstrate a significant fall in the ABPI and enable confirmation of the diagnosis. Patients suspected of having CAI in whom the ABPI is falsely elevated should have colour duplex imaging of their peripheral arteries to confirm the diagnosis.

Management of chronic arterial insufficiency

The majority of patients with IC will not require any interventional treatment and can be satisfactorily managed with simple risk factor modifications. These should include stopping smoking (with full support including cessation classes and pharmacological assistance), optimal diabetic control, regular exercise (± supervised exercise programmes), weight reduction, lipid control, and antiplatelet medication (clopidogrel/aspirin). A number of pharmacological agents, including cilostazol, naftidrofuryl, and carnitine, have been found to be of some benefit in the treatment of claudication. However, at present only naftidrofuryl is approved by NICE for use in England and Wales.

Patients with CLI and those with severe lifestyle-limiting claudication will require additional investigations with a view to determining an appropriate intervention to improve symptom control and reduce the risk of limb loss. All of these patients should be investigated under the supervision of a multidisciplinary specialist vascular team (MDT), which should include vascular surgeons, interventional radiologists, specialist nurses, and physiotherapists. Ideally patients with diabetes should be supervised by a clinic, which is jointly run by vascular surgeons, diabetic physicians, podiatrists, and physiotherapists.

In recent years, considerable advances have been made in the development of non-invasive techniques for high-quality imaging of the arterial system. These tests should only be performed in patients in whom a revascularization procedure is being considered.

Colour duplex imaging produces excellent results when performed by an experienced operative, particularly in the limb peripheries. However, this test is often inadequate in imaging the aorta/iliac vessels if disease is suspected at these sites.

Contrast-enhanced magnetic resonance (MRA) and computed tomography angiography (CTA), both give excellent imaging of the whole of the arterial tree. MRA is preferred, if tolerated, due to the radiation risk associated with CTA. These images will be studied at the multidisciplinary meeting and, dependent on the patient's symptoms and pattern of disease, treatment will be planned, guided by the severity of the symptoms.

Because interventional treatments are at risk of worsening the symptoms, only patients with severe IC should be considered for interventional treatment. They should all have had a full risk factor assessment and modification and have attended a supervised exercise programme (or equivalent).

Radiological intervention in severe IC involves angioplasty and stenting. More recently, drug-eluting balloons and stents have been used, but evidence for improvement of results is awaited. Bypass surgery can be considered in patients with severe lifestyle-limiting IC if angioplasty has failed or is unsuitable and imaging has confirmed that bypass surgery is feasible.

All patients with CLI should be considered for intervention and given adequate pain relief. They may require referral to a specialist pain management service if their pain is not being adequately controlled and revascularization is inappropriate or impossible, or ongoing high opiate doses are being required and if the pain persists after revascularization or amputation.

There are many interventional options now available for the treatment of patients with CLI. These include balloon angioplasty, which may be combined with primary bare-metal stent placement (± drug elution), endarterectomy, bypass surgery, and primary amputation. Bypasses may be anatomical (aortoiliac or femoropopliteal) or extra-anatomical (axillofemoral or femorofemoral crossovers).

The MDT will decide on the most appropriate form of intervention, depending on the fitness of the patient and suitability of the disease for a particular operation. Usually bypass surgery above the inguinal ligament can be satisfactorily performed using pre-formed grafts made of Dacron®. In the femoropopliteal segment, the best material is autologous vein using either long or short saphenous or arm veins. In cases where adequate vein is not available, prosthetic grafts (PTFE/Dacron®) may be used in combination with a vein cuff at the distal anastomosis.

Some patients will have unreconstructable disease and this coupled with extensive tissue loss may require primary amputation. This should only be performed in cases that the MDT has considered all options for revascularization. Amputation may also be required in combination with revascularization, usually at a more local level, in cases with tissue loss. Every effort should be made to amputate below the knee, as this will give the patient the best chance of successful rehabilitation with a prosthetic limb.

Further reading

Adam DJ, Beard JD, Cleveland T, *et al.* Bypass versus angioplasty in severe ischaemia of the leg (BASIL): multicentre, randomised controlled trial. *Lancet* 2005; 366(9501):1925–34.

American Diabetes Association. Peripheral arterial disease in people with diabetes. *Diabetes Care* 2003; 26(12):3333–41.

Boccalon H, Lehert P, Mosnier M. Effect of naftidrofuryl on physiological walking distance in patients with intermittent claudication. *Ann Cardiol Angeoil (Paris)* 2001; 50(3):175–82.

Bradbury AW, Cleveland TJ. Vascular and endovascular surgery. In Garden OJ, Bradbury AW, Forsythe JLR, Parks RW (eds) *Principles and Practice of Surgery* (6th ed). Edinburgh: Churchill Livingstone Elsevier; 2012:368–86.

Criqui M, Langer R, Fronck A, *et al.* Mortality over a period of 10 years in patients with peripheral arterial disease. *N Engl J Med* 1992; 326:381–6.

Criqui MH, Fronck A, Barrett-Connor E, *et al.* The prevalence of peripheral arterial disease in a defined population. *Circulation* 1985; 71(3):510–51.

Criqui MH, Vargas V, Denenberg JO, *et al.* Ethnicity and peripheral arterial disease: the San Diego population study. *Circulation* 2005; 112(17):2703–7.

Dormandy JA, Murray GD. The fate of the claudicant – a prospective study of 1969 claudicants. *Eur J Vasc Surg* 1991; 5(2):131–3.

Fowkes FG, Housley E, Cawood EH, *et al.* Edinburgh artery study: prevalence of asymptomatic and symptomatic peripheral arterial disease in the general population. *Int J Epidemiol* 1991; 20(2):384–92.

Hirsch AT, Haskal ZJ, Hertzer NR, *et al.* ACC/AHA 2005 guidelines for the management of patients with peripheral arterial disease. *J Am Coll Cardiol* 2006; 47:1239–312.

Murie JA. Arterial disorders. In Williams NS, Bulstrode CJK, O'Connell PR (eds) *Bailey and Love's Short Practice of Surgery* (25th ed). London: Hodder Arnold; 2008:899–924.

Murray CJ, Lauer JA, Hutubessy RC, *et al.* Effectiveness and costs of interventions to lower systolic blood pressure and cholesterol: a global and regional analysis on reduction of cardiovascular-disease risk. *Lancet* 2003; 361(9359):717–25.

National Institute for Health and Care Excellence. *Lower Limb Peripheral Arterial Disease: Diagnosis and Management.* Clinical Guideline 147. London: NICE; 2012. https://www.nice.org.uk/guidance/cg147

Norgren L, Hiatt WR, Dormandy JA, *et al.* Inter-society consensus for the management of peripheral arterial disease (TASC II). *J Vasc Surg* 2007; 45 Suppl:S5–67.

Stewart K, Hiatt W, Regensteiner J, *et al.* Exercise training for claudication. *N Engl J Med* 2002; 347(24):1941–51.

Taylor PR, Murie JA, Thompson MM, *et al.* The arteries. In Burnand KG, Young AE, Lucas J, *et al.* (eds) *The New Aird's Companion in Surgical Studies* (3rd ed). Oxford: Elsevier Churchill Livingstone; 2005:193–269.

Weitz JI, Byrne J, Clagett P, *et al.* Diagnosis and treatment of chronic arterial insufficiency of the lower extremities: a critical review. *Circulation* 1996; 94:3026–49.

Widmer L, Biland L. Risk profile and occlusive peripheral arterial disease. In *Proceedings of 13th International Congress of Angiology,* Athens; 1985:28.

CHAPTER 2.7.2

Acute limb ischaemia

Timothy A. Beckitt and Frank C. T. Smith

Introduction

There is no accepted international definition of acute limb ischaemia (ALI). The key feature is a sudden onset of limb-threatening ischaemia. The incidence of ALI may be as high as 15 cases/100 000/year; however, there is evidence that the incidence may be declining as a result of risk factor management.[1] Historically the outcome of ALI is poor, with a significant risk of limb amputation, and mortality that has been reported as high as 22%.[2]

Pathophysiology

ALI is the result of occlusion of a native artery or bypass graft. The most common causes are *in situ* thrombosis and embolism.

Causes of thrombotic occlusion

- Atherosclerosis
- Popliteal aneurysm
- Trauma (including iatrogenic injury)
- Intrinsic thrombotic condition
- Paraneoplastic
- Cystic adventitial disease
- Popliteal entrapment.

Thrombosis *in situ* at the site of an underlying atherosclerotic lesion is the principal cause of ALI. Other thrombotic causes include occlusion of a pre-existing bypass graft or endovascular stent, and occlusion of an underlying popliteal aneurysm. ALI can also be a feature of upper and lower limb trauma either due to thrombosis or arterial disruption. In particular, the brachial artery is at risk of injury in association with supracondylar fractures of the humerus, and the popliteal artery, in association with proximal tibial 'bumper' fractures. The femoral artery may be injured in femoral shaft fractures (Figure 2.7.2.1). Iatrogenic arterial occlusion caused by thrombosis or intimal dissection may be a consequence of radiological or cardiological endovascular interventions.

Thrombosis can also be the result of external compression. In the young patient, popliteal artery occlusion may be a result of entrapment, in which the popliteal artery lies in an abnormal anatomical position, passing around the medial head of the gastrocnemius muscle as opposed to between the two heads. Acute thrombotic occlusion has also been described as a result of cystic adventitial disease of the popliteal artery, a rare condition that characteristically presents with intermittent claudication in men in their fourth or fifth decade. Spontaneous arterial thrombosis may also occur in the absence of a vessel wall abnormality as a result of a thrombophilia such as antiphospholipid syndrome, or activated protein C and S deficiencies. Occult neoplasia may be responsible for prothrombotic states, warranting investigation for underlying malignancy. Underlying malignancy may be identified in 11.5%[3] of cases and the outcome of ALI in this group of patients is poor.[4]

Causes of arterial embolus

- Atrial fibrillation
- Cardiac mural thrombus
- Valvular vegetations
- Proximal aneurysmal disease
- Proximal atherosclerotic plaque
- Atrial myxoma.

ALI may also be the result of arterial embolism. Atrial fibrillation has replaced rheumatic mitral valve disease as the most common cause of arterial embolism. Atrial fibrillation affects between 1% and 2% of the population and carries an annual risk of ALI of 0.4%. Other cardiac sources of embolus include mural thrombosis following myocardial infarction, and valvular vegetations. The left atrium is the most common site of the rare cardiac myxoma. These benign tumours are seen in 0.03% of postmortem examinations and can predispose to embolization of both thrombus and tumour. Non-cardiac emboli may arise from proximal aneurysms or atherosclerotic plaques. Emboli from non-cardiac sources are often small and such lesions may be responsible for the phenomenon of cholesterol emboli. Small particles may pass to the distal circulation causing painful digital infarction known as the 'blue toe syndrome'.

Clinical features

Clinical assessment should include consideration of the severity, site, and the cause of ALI.

Clinical features of ALI

Key clinical features are described by the six Ps:

- Pain
- Paraesthesia
- Paralysis
- Pallor
- Perishing with cold
- Pulselessness.

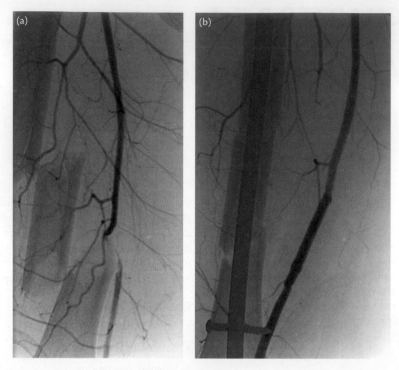

Fig. 2.7.2.1 (a) Femoral shaft fracture in a motorcyclist, with disruption of the superficial femoral artery requiring (b) reversed vein interposition graft.

Many of these features overlap with those of chronic critical ischaemia and it is essential when assessing the acutely ischaemic limb to determine viability. The presence of sensory loss and muscle weakness is the key discriminator in distinguishing the viable from the immediately threatened limb. The classification of the Society of Vascular Surgery/International Society of Cardiovascular Surgery[5] has been widely accepted. It divides ALI into three categories. A simplified version of this classification is presented in Table 2.7.2.1. Increasing severity of ischaemia results in both progression of the severity of symptoms, from altered sensation (paraesthesia) to anaesthesia, and in their distribution.

Alongside pallor, inspection of the limb may reveal venous guttering on elevation and skin mottling. With progression to irreversible ischaemia, this skin mottling may progress to fixed skin staining, which fails to blanch to digital pressure. The presence of muscle tenderness suggests a threatened limb and tense compartments are indicative of severe and potentially irreversible ischaemia.

The likely cause of ALI can often be derived from the clinical history. A prior history of intermittent claudication is highly suggestive of thrombosis *in situ*. History taking should identify risk factors for emboli such as recent myocardial infarction, a history of palpitations, arrhythmias, or valvular heart disease. Examination of pulses may help, not only to determine the site of the occlusion, but also the likely pathology. Emboli typically lodge at an arterial bifurcation where there is a change in vessel diameter such as the common femoral, below-knee popliteal, or brachial arteries. The absence of pulses in the contralateral limb is also a useful indicator of underlying peripheral arterial disease that may suggest the underlying pathology is *in situ* thrombosis as opposed to embolus. Caution should be urged in obtaining reassurance from detection of pedal hand-held Doppler signals, as while the absence of arterial signals is an indicator of limb-threatening ischaemia, venous signals can still be audible in an acutely threatened limb, as seen in Table 2.7.2.1.

Upper limb

Acute ischaemia of the upper limb is most commonly the result of embolism of intracardiac thrombus, with *in situ* thrombosis being

Table 2.7.2.1 Rutherford classification

Category		Sensory loss	Muscle weakness	Doppler signals	
				Arterial	**Venous**
I. Viable		None	None	Audible	Audible
II. Threatened	a. Acutely	Altered—limited to foot	None	None	Audible
	b. Immediately	Extensive paraesthesia	Mild to moderate	None	Audible
III. Irreversible		Anaesthetic	Paralysis	None	None

Adapted from *Journal of Vascular Surgery*, Volume 26, Issue 3, Rutherford RB *et al.*, Recommended standards for reports dealing with lower extremity ischemia: Revised version, pp. 517–538, Copyright © 1997 Society for Vascular Surgery and International Society for Cardiovascular Surgery, North American Chapter, with permission from Elsevier, http://www.sciencedirect.com/science/journal/07415214

relatively rare. Embolism or thrombosis can, however, also arise in subclavian aneurysmal disease or from atherosclerotic plaque in the proximal circulation. Subclavian aneurysms are rare and may result secondarily as a post-stenotic dilatation beyond a region of extrinsic compression in thoracic outlet syndrome, or as a primary atherosclerotic process. As in the leg, smaller emboli from a proximal stenosis can present with painful digital infarction or blue finger syndrome. In contrast to lower limb ischaemia, however, it is common for upper limb ischaemia to present with paraesthesia and coolness, but without features of limb-threatening ischaemia. There is a paucity of data regarding long-term outcome of these patients when managed non-operatively[6] and many cases are managed by local anaesthetic thromboembolectomy.

Management

The high mortality rate of ALI is partly a result of these patients' co-morbidities—ischaemic heart disease, heart failure, and tachyarrhythmias—that contribute to the aetiology. Multidisciplinary treatment may be required. Alongside resuscitation with oxygen and intravenous fluid, a bolus and subsequent infusion of intravenous heparin should be administered to reduce thrombus propagation. There is some evidence that heparin may improve outcome.[7] Antiplatelet agents are known to be effective in acute coronary syndrome[8] and are advisable in peripheral arterial disease for secondary prevention. Nevertheless, in ALI, there are concerns that in the acute setting, antiplatelet agents could increase risk of bleeding for patients receiving thrombolysis, and there is no convincing evidence to support administration of an antiplatelet agent alongside heparin.[9] Rapid assessment of the limb is required, as those patients with immediately limb-threatening ischaemia will require rapid surgical intervention (Figure 2.7.2.2). It is important to recognize irreversible limb ischaemia as these patients are at risk of myoglobinuria and acute kidney injury (key predictors of mortality[10]), and may require urgent amputation.

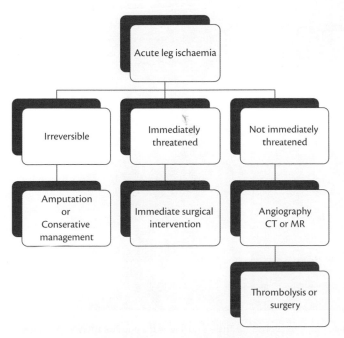

Fig. 2.7.2.2 A scheme for the immediate management of acute leg ischaemia.

Immediately threatening limb ischaemia with sensory and motor deficits requires urgent intervention. In the case of the acutely ischaemic limb with no prior history of claudication, it is often appropriate to proceed to surgical embolectomy with on-table angiography without delay for prior imaging. When the limb is not immediately threatened, it may be more appropriate to undertake imaging, as catheter embolectomy is often fruitless in the presence of *in situ* thrombosis with underlying atherosclerotic disease. In these patients, thrombolysis with subsequent percutaneous endovascular intervention or bypass surgery is often indicated. Refinements in computed tomography angiography have made this a rapid and effective technique in order to plan subsequent intervention, but caution is required as hyperosmolar iodinated contrast agents are potentially nephrotoxic. Magnetic resonance angiography is an alternative, but is time-consuming and there are concerns of an association with nephrogenic fibrosing dermopathy in patients with renal impairment.[11]

Surgical embolectomy

Surgical embolectomy is the primary treatment of ALI secondary to pure embolus. The Fogarty balloon embolectomy catheter[12] was introduced in 1963. The artery is approached surgically and controlled proximally and distally with elastic slings, avoiding clamping to prevent fragmentation of thrombus. In the case of the common femoral and brachial arteries, this can be achieved under local anaesthetic, but the assistance of an anaesthetist is advised for monitoring the patient, analgesia and, if necessary, sedation. The arteriotomy is made over the arterial bifurcation to permit access to distal branches. In the case of a pure embolus, a transverse arteriotomy is made as primary closure can then subsequently be achieved without narrowing the vessel lumen. When approaching a small below-knee popliteal artery, it may be necessary to use a longitudinal incision, closing the vessel subsequently with a vein patch. The embolectomy balloon is passed into the proximal and distal vessels until no further thrombus is retrieved. Success is heralded by the return of inflow and back-bleeding. However, completion angiography is usually required as there may be residual thrombus in 30% of cases; completion angiography has been shown to reduce amputation rates.[13] If distal embolectomy is unsuccessful, then consideration should be given to on-table administration of tissue plasminogen activator (t-PA) through an umbilical catheter for thrombolysis, leaving the agent *in situ* for 30 minutes.[14]

Thrombolysis

Catheter-directed thrombolysis (CDT) is an alternative to surgery when ALI is not immediately limb threatening. t-PA stimulates the conversion of plasminogen into the active protease plasmin and is more effective in intra-arterial thrombus resolution than streptokinase, resulting in a higher 30-day limb salvage rate.[15] In contrast to systemic thrombolysis used in acute stroke and in myocardial infarction, CDT requires a lower dose as it is delivered selectively to the occluded vessel via a catheter. The main predictor of success in CDT is the ability to cross the lesion with a guidewire in order to be able to place an infusion catheter within the thrombus. The main limitation of thrombolysis is the long infusion time required and resulting delayed limb reperfusion. Patients require management in a high dependency setting because of the risk of haemorrhage whilst catheter and introducer sheath remain in the vessel. Prolonged low-dose t-PA regimens of 0.5–1.0 mg/h for 18 hours have now been largely replaced with accelerated infusions of up to 3.5 mg/h following initial bolus treatment, with no reduction in efficacy.[16] The most serious complication of thrombolysis is intracranial haemorrhage and in the UK national audit, a 75% limb salvage rate was reported at the cost of a 2.3% risk of stroke.[17] The following contraindications to thrombolysis exist:

Absolute contraindications:

- Ischaemic or haemorrhagic stroke within 2 months
- Recent gastrointestinal bleeding
- Neurosurgery or intracranial trauma within 3 months.

Relative contraindications:

- Major surgery or trauma within 10 days
- Cardiopulmonary resuscitation within 10 days
- Uncontrolled hypertension
- Intracranial tumour, atrioventricular malformation or aneurysm
- Recent ophthalmic surgery.

Minor contraindications:

- Hepatic failure
- Pregnancy
- Diabetic haemorrhagic retinopathy.

Following successful thrombolysis, completion angiography is indicated and any underlying stenosis requires treatment with angioplasty and/or stenting. A Cochrane review of five randomized trials of catheter-guided thrombolysis[18] found no difference in limb salvage or mortality rates between thrombolysis and surgery at 30 days, 6 months, or 1 year. There was, however, an increased risk of major haemorrhage, of 8.8% versus 3.3% in surgical patients.

Percutaneous thrombectomy devices

The main limitation of CDT is the requirement for prolonged infusion and the resulting delay in reperfusion. A number of mechanical thrombolysis aids have been designed. Aspiration catheters can be placed into the thrombus and then repeatedly withdrawn under vacuum, but whilst case series have reported successful aspiration in up to 86%,[19] there are concerns about damage to the vessel intima resulting from repeated catheter passage. Newer technologies combine pharmacological and mechanical thrombectomy. The Angiojet™ system (Possis Medical) uses hydrodynamic thrombus fragmentation with high-pressure heparinized saline, alongside simultaneous aspiration. Success rates of 93% have been reported[20] when used within 14 days of onset; however, it should be noted that 50% of patients require subsequent CDT and these technologies still require full clinical evaluation.

Popliteal aneurysms

Popliteal aneurysms are the most common peripheral arterial aneurysms but in contrast to abdominal aortic aneurysms, rupture is rare. Instead they are at risk of thromboembolism and acute occlusion. The occluded popliteal aneurysm presenting as ALI is a particular challenge, as there is often pre-existing embolization of the calf vessels and as a result the risk of limb loss is high (14%).

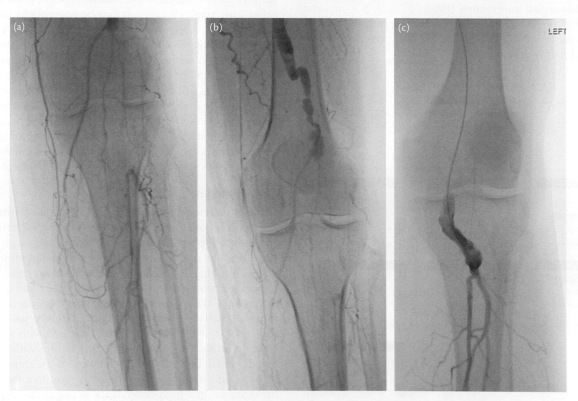

Fig. 2.7.2.3 Antegrade femoral angiogram showing occluded popliteal aneurysm treated with thrombolysis. (a) There is no flow in the popliteal artery, with filling seen in the posterior tibial artery from collaterals only. (b) Following initial thrombolysis, some restoration of flow in the above-knee popliteal artery is seen. (c) Restoration of flow in the below-knee popliteal, posterior tibial, and peroneal arteries is evident.

Historically these have been treated with emergency thrombectomy of the calf vessels and femoropopliteal or femorodistal exclusion bypass grafting, with intraoperative thrombolysis if necessary. There may also be a role for preoperative intra-arterial thrombolysis followed by surgical or endovascular aneurysm exclusion (Figure 2.7.2.3). As with other causes of ALI, patients with immediately limb-threatening ischaemia (Rutherford IIb) require prompt surgery and cannot wait for thrombolysis. There are no randomized control trials comparing these two approaches; however, systematic review of the literature[21] suggests that where possible a policy of preoperative thrombolysis may improve long-term graft patency.

Complications of revascularization

Compartment syndrome

Whether revascularization is surgical or radiological, successful reperfusion is associated with muscle compartment swelling. Acute compartment syndrome can occur as muscle oedema causes a rise in myofascial compartment pressures, initially impeding venous return, and subsequently, capillary blood flow.

Clinical features

◆ Pain out of proportion to clinical signs

◆ Tense myofascial compartment

◆ Pain on passive movement

◆ Paraesthesia.

It is particularly important to note that peripheral pulses and Doppler signals are maintained even in severe compartment syndrome. If the compartment pressure exceeds 30 mmHg for more than 6 hours, the limb may not be salvageable. Clinicians should have a high index of suspicion and, if there is any concern, prompt fasciotomy should be undertaken taking care to decompress of all four lower limb fascial compartments (Figure 2.7.2.4). Prophylactic fasciotomy should be considered following revascularization after prolonged and severe ischaemia.

Reperfusion injury

The other potential complication of revascularization is reperfusion injury. At its worst, reperfusion of a large volume of ischaemic muscle may result in a systemic inflammatory response syndrome with resulting pulmonary oedema and multiple organ failure, highlighting the importance of not attempting to revascularize an irreversibly ischaemic limb (Table 2.7.2.1). The resulting acute kidney injury can be exacerbated by myoglobinuria, and alongside amputation if revascularization has failed, these patients may require renal protection in the form of fluid resuscitation. The practice of alkalinizing the urine with sodium bicarbonate and maintaining a diuresis with mannitol does not have a sound evidence base[22] and patients may require early haemodialysis for renal protection.

Further management

There is a significant risk of re-thrombosis following successful revascularization of ALI. Not only is there a short-term risk of propagation of residual thrombus, but there is also a risk of further embolization from the same source. Clear guidelines exist for anticoagulation of patients with atrial fibrillation but in

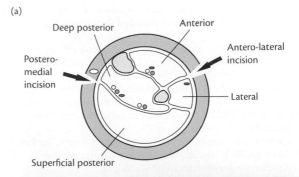

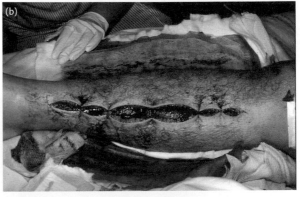

Fig. 2.7.2.4 (a) The four lower limb fascial compartments and sites for fasciotomy incisions. (b) Fasciotomies undertaken for the patient in Figure 2.7.2.1.

addition there is some evidence that anticoagulation may confer long term benefit even in the absence of a clear cardiac embolic source.[23] Independent of the decision for oral anticoagulation in view of the high mortality in this group, all patients should be offered best medical management of their risk factors, particularly in the form of antiplatelet, antihypertensive, and lipid-lowering medication.

Further reading

Working Party on Thrombolysis in the Management of Limb Ischemia. Thrombolysis in the management of lower limb peripheral arterial occlusion; a consensus document. *J Vasc Interv Radiol* 2003; 14(9):S337–49.

References

1. Heart Protection Study Collaborative Group. MRC/BHF Heart Protection Study of cholesterol lowering with simvastatin in 20,536 high-risk individuals: a randomised placebo-controlled trial. *Lancet* 2002; 360:7–12.
2. Campbell WB, Ridler BM, Szymanska TH. Current management of acute leg ischaemia: results of an audit by the Vascular Surgical Society of Great Britain and Ireland. *Br J Surg* 1998; 85(11):1498–503.
3. El Sakka K, Gambhir RP, Halawa M, *et al.* Association of malignant disease with critical leg ischaemia. *Br J Surg* 2005; 92(12):1498–501.
4. Javid M, Magee TR, Galland RB. Arterial thrombosis associated with malignant disease. *Eur J Vasc Endovasc Surg* 2008; 35(1):84–7.
5. Rutherford RB, Baker JD, Ernst C. Recommended standards for reports dealing with lower extremity ischemia: revised version. *J Vasc Surg* 1997; 26(3):517–38.
6. Turner EJ, Loh A, Howard A. Systematic review of the operative and non-operative management of acute upper limb ischemia. *J Vasc Nurs* 2012; 30(3):71–6.

7. Blaisdell FW, Steele M, Allen RE. Management of acute lower extremity arterial ischemia due to embolism and thrombosis. *Surgery* 1978; 84(6):822–34.

8. Berger JS, Bhatt DL, Cannon CP, *et al.* The relative efficacy and safety of clopidogrel in women and men a sex-specific collaborative meta-analysis. *J Am Coll Cardiol* 2009; 54(21):1935–45.

9. Sobel M, Verhaeghe R. Antithrombotic therapy for peripheral artery occlusive disease: American College of Chest Physicians Evidence-Based Clinical Practice Guidelines (8th Edition). *Chest* 2008; 133(6):815S–43S.

10. Lewington A, Kanagasundaram S. *Acute Kidney Injury.* The Renal Association; 2011. [Online] http://www.renal.org/guidelines/modules/acute-kidney-injury#sthash.iA5OA78N.dpbs

11. Grobner T. Gadolinium—a specific trigger for the development of nephrogenic fibrosing dermopathy and nephrogenic systemic fibrosis? *Nephrol Dial Transplant* 2006; 21(4):1104–8.

12. Fogarty TJ, Cranley JJ, Krause RJ, *et al.* A method for extraction of arterial emboli and thrombi. *Surg Gynecol Obstet* 1963; 116:241–4.

13. Bosma HW, Jorning PJ. Intra-operative arteriography in arterial embolectomy. *Eur J Vasc Surg* 1990; 4(5):469–72.

14. Beard JD, Nyamekye I, Earnshaw JJ. Intraoperative streptokinase: a useful adjunct to balloon-catheter embolectomy. *Br J Surg* 1993; 80(1):21–4.

15. Berridge DC, Gregson RH, Hopkinson BR, *et al.* Randomized trial of intra-arterial recombinant tissue plasminogen activator, intravenous recombinant tissue plasminogen activator and intra-arterial streptokinase in peripheral arterial thrombolysis. *Br J Surg* 1991; 78(8):988–95.

16. Plate G, Jansson I, Forssell C. Thrombolysis for acute lower limb ischaemia—a prospective, randomised, multicentre study comparing two strategies. *Eur J Vasc Endovasc Surg* 2006; 31(6):651–60.

17. Earnshaw JJ, Whitman B, Foy C. National Audit of Thrombolysis for Acute Leg Ischemia (NATALI): clinical factors associated with early outcome. *J Vasc Surg* 2004; 39(5):1018–25.

18. Berridge DC, Kessel D, Robertson I. Surgery versus thrombolysis for acute limb ischaemia: initial management. *Cochrane Database Syst Rev* 2002; 3:CD002784.

19. Wagner HJ, Starck EE, Reuter P. Long-term results of percutaneous aspiration embolectomy. *Cardiovasc Intervent Radiol* 1994; 17(5):241–6.

20. Ansel GM, George BS, Botti CF, *et al.* Rheolytic thrombectomy in the management of limb ischemia: 30-day results from a multicenter registry. *J Endovasc Ther* 2002; 9(4):395–402.

21. Kropman RH, Schrijver AM, Kelder JC, *et al.* Clinical outcome of acute leg ischaemia due to thrombosed popliteal artery aneurysm: systematic review of 895 cases. *Eur J Vasc Endovasc Surg* 2010; 39(4):452–7.

22. Brown CV, Rhee P, Chan L, *et al.* Preventing renal failure in patients with rhabdomyolysis: do bicarbonate and mannitol make a difference? *J Trauma* 2004; 56(6):1191–6.

23. Campbell WB, Ridler BM, Szymanska TH. Two-year follow-up after acute thromboembolic limb ischaemia: the importance of anticoagulation. *Eur J Vasc Endovasc Surg* 2000; 19(2):169–73.

Venous and lymphatic disease

Katy A. L. Darvall and Andrew W. Bradbury

Varicose veins

Epidemiology

Varicose veins (VV) are common, affecting up to 40% of the population.[1] VV are part of a spectrum of disorders usually called chronic venous insufficiency (CVI), although this term is often used to denote the presence of 'complicated' VV including skin changes and chronic venous ulceration (CVU).

Aetiology and pathophysiology

The aetiology of VV is unclear. The most widely held view is that a defect in the vein wall (which may be in part genetic), in addition to increased venous pressure (e.g. with obesity, prolonged standing, or pregnancy), leads to progressive dilatation of the vein and secondary disruption of the venous valves resulting in valvular incompetence. Valvular incompetence can occur in the deep veins but is usually secondary to direct damage from deep vein thrombosis (DVT).

Normally, when ambulating, the calf muscles pump venous blood out of the leg and reverse flow with gravity is prevented by valve closure. When the valves are damaged the pressure in the calf veins is increased, so-called ambulatory venous hypertension. In some cases the ambulatory venous hypertension is caused by deep venous obstruction (outflow obstruction) secondary to DVT or, more rarely, extrinsic compression.

Clinical presentation

The relationship between VV and various lower limb symptoms is complex. Some people with extensive VV can be asymptomatic while, in others, quite minor VV are troublesome. The lower limb symptoms typically related to venous disease include pain or ache, heaviness, itching, a feeling of swelling, heaviness, tingling, and restless legs. Venous symptoms are typically worse at the end of the day and after prolonged standing.[1]

The patient should be examined standing up, and viewed from in front and behind. Inspection may reveal telangiectasia or spider veins (superficial in the dermis, < 1 mm), reticular veins (deep in the dermis, < 4 mm), and true VV (> 4 mm and palpable). The distribution (and likely source) may be obvious at this point, that is, posterior calf VV from small saphenous vein (SSV) incompetence, medial thigh and calf VV from great saphenous vein (GSV) incompetence, or anterior/posterior thigh VV. The lower leg should then be inspected for the skin changes of CVI. Varicose (venous) eczema is red and intensely itchy. Lipodermatosclerosis is indurated, hardened, and inflamed. Haemosiderin deposition appears as brown discoloration, usually in the gaiter area (Figure 2.7.3.1).

Palpation will confirm the 'woody' feeling of lipodermatosclerosis and will aid detection of VV which may not be visible in the larger leg.

Investigations

Tourniquet tests are obsolete. Hand-held Doppler is also an inaccurate and incomplete examination technique, which has been superseded by duplex ultrasound. Portable duplex machines used in clinic permit a 'one-stop' diagnostic service. Recent guidance from the UK National Institute for Health and Care Excellence (NICE) states that all patients with VV should have a venous duplex to aid diagnosis and treatment options.[2]

Duplex ultrasound provides a 'map' of both the deep and superficial veins. Deep veins are assessed for patency (including evidence of a previous DVT) and competency. Superficial veins, and their junctions with the deep system (saphenofemoral junction, saphenopopliteal junction, and perforators), are also assessed for patency and competency. Duplex ultrasound also helps to determine the most appropriate treatment for an individual patient and is an integral part of endovascular interventions.

Other investigations such as plethysmography are only used as research tools, and invasive tests such as venography are rarely indicated.

Management

Conservative

The mainstay of conservative management for VV has been compression hosiery and lifestyle modification, including weight loss and avoiding prolonged standing. Compression hosiery, however, is only now recommended by NICE when interventional treatment is unsuitable.[2]

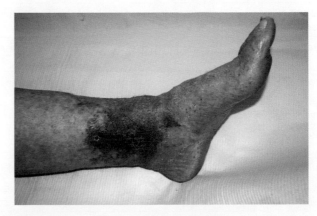

Fig. 2.7.3.1 Haemosiderin deposition, lipodermatosclerosis, eczema, and ulceration.

Surgery

Traditionally the mainstay of treatment for VV has been superficial venous surgery (SVS), but more recently there have been many developments in endovenous techniques which seek to improve the side effect profile of traditional surgery, shorten recovery times, and also to give greater durability.

SVS that aims to remove visible VV and correct axial superficial and perforator (deep to superficial) incompetence has been considered the 'gold standard' for many decades, although recent NICE guidance states that SVS should now only be performed in patients who are not suitable for either endothermal ablation or ultrasound-guided foam sclerotherapy (UGFS).[2]

In patients with GSV incompetence, the saphenofemoral junction is ligated and the GSV is stripped out from the groin to the knee. In patients with SSV incompetence, the saphenopopliteal junction is ligated, but not usually stripped to avoid damage to the sural nerve. Any remaining varices are removed through several tiny stab incisions (avulsions or phlebectomies).

Endovenous ablation

The most frequently used, and studied, endovenous techniques are endovenous laser ablation, radiofrequency ablation, and UGFS; all of which can be performed on an outpatient basis using local anaesthesia. Endovenous laser ablation and radiofrequency ablation both utilize specialist fibres and catheters placed within the vein to be treated. Endothelial damage (leading to fibrosis) occurs as a result of heat generation at the tip of the fibre or catheter which is gradually withdrawn to treat the entire length of vein.

UGFS involves injection of a liquid sclerosant, usually mixed with air, into the incompetent veins. The sclerosant acts immediately to cause endothelial damage that evolves to fibrosis.

Leg ulceration

Epidemiology

Up to 3–11% of patients with VV will develop the sequelae of severe venous insufficiency including ulceration. The lifetime risk of developing CVU is usually quoted at 1% in Northern Europe, with an estimated point prevalence of 0.1% (10% of those affected will have an open ulcer at any one time).[3]

The overall prognosis of CVU is poor, with delayed healing and recurrent ulceration being common. Venous ulceration has a profound effect on quality of life and social functioning, and the effect on healthcare spending is vast. It is estimated that up to 2% of the total annual healthcare budget in Western countries is spent on the treatment of chronic venous disease—around £600 million per annum in the United Kingdom. In addition, 22% of district nurses' time is spent treating leg ulcers.[3,4]

There are many risk factors considered to be associated with the development of CVI, including family history, increasing age, obesity, parity, prolonged standing, physical inactivity, and previous leg injury.[5,6]

Aetiology and pathophysiology

The term CVI encompasses the skin changes that occur as a result of ambulatory venous hypertension and poor venous drainage. These are hyperpigmentation (haemosiderin deposition), lipodermatosclerosis (subcutaneous tissue fibrosis), atrophe blanche (areas of devascularized skin), and eventually CVU.[6]

There are a number of proposed pathophysiological mechanisms. The most popular of these are the fibrin cuff hypothesis and the white-cell trapping theory, which result in localized chronic inflammation, tissue oedema, microcirculatory thrombosis, and hypoxia.

Clinical assessment

The majority of leg ulcers (>70%) are venous and a further 15–20% are of mixed arterial and venous aetiology. Clinical assessment is essential in determining the likely aetiology of the ulcer, thus guiding further investigations (Table 2.7.3.1, Figure 2.7.3.2). All patients should have their pulses assessed and an ankle–brachial pressure index measured.

Investigations

Investigations for venous ulcer are as for VV, with duplex ultrasound being the most useful modality.

Table 2.7.3.1 Differential diagnosis of leg ulceration

Clinical features	Arterial ulcer	Venous ulcer
Age and gender	Usually men > 60 years	Often women
Risk factors and past medical history	Smoking, diabetes, dyslipidaemia, and hypertension; often a history of cardiovascular disease	Previous DVT (confirmed or occult), thrombophilia, VV
Symptoms	Severe pain is present (unless there is diabetic neuropathy) and may be relieved by dependency	Pain only in about 30%, but usually not severe and may be relieved with elevation
Site	Usually on pressure areas (malleoli, heel, metatarsal heads, 5th metatarsal base)	Medial (70%), lateral (20%), or both malleoli and gaiter area
Edge	Regular, 'punched-out', indolent	Irregular, with neo-epithelium (whiter than mature skin)
Base	Sloughy or necrotic with no granulation tissue; may involve tendon, bone and joint	Pink with granulation tissue; but may be covered in yellow-green slough
Surrounding skin	Features of severe limb ischaemia, e.g. thin, dry skin, pallor, reduced temperature	Lipodermatosclerosis, varicose eczema, haemosiderin deposition
Veins	Empty, 'guttering' on elevation	Full, usually varicose
Swelling	Usually absent	Often present

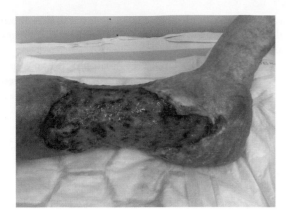

Fig. 2.7.3.2 Chronic venous ulceration.

Management

The management of patients with CVU requires a holistic approach: managing the ulcer in the context of the whole leg, the leg in the context of the whole patient, and the patient in the context of their social and cultural circumstances. Measures such as leg elevation to reduce oedema, weight loss, and exercise programmes should be encouraged.

The mainstay of treatment for venous ulceration is elasticated, multilayer, graduated compression bandaging, and it is very effective at healing the majority of venous ulcers[7] (Figure 2.7.3.3). After healing of the ulcer with bandaging, the patient should be placed in graduated compression hosiery to reduce the risk of recurrence. There is also evidence that when venous ulceration occurs in association with superficial venous reflux, SVS can reduce the risk of recurrence.[8]

It is generally accepted that the type of dressing used has little effect on healing. Larval therapy and negative-pressure dressing systems improve debridement but do not shorten the time taken to healing (or increase the number of ulcers that ultimately heal).[9,10]

Swollen leg

Differential diagnosis of the swollen leg

There are many different conditions that can cause chronic leg swelling (Box 2.7.3.1), but the two most common are CVI and lymphoedema. Unilateral leg swelling is more likely to be due to a local cause than a systemic condition.

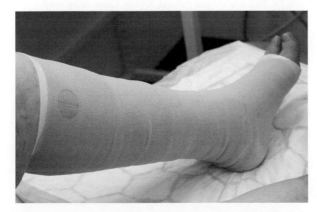

Fig. 2.7.3.3 Compression bandaging.

Lymphoedema

Epidemiology

Lymphoedema is a debilitating condition, has no cure, affects up to 1–2% of the population,[11] and is characterized by the accumulation of protein-rich fluid in the skin and subcutaneous tissues due to a defect in the lymphatic system.

Aetiology and pathophysiology

Lymphoedema can be primary or secondary and should be differentiated from other causes of limb swelling. In primary lymphoedema the cause is unknown (or at least uncertain) and it can be classified based on the age of onset. Women are more commonly affected and it usually occurs in the lower limbs.

Lymphoedema congenita is present at birth and can be autosomally inherited (Milroy's disease). It is more likely to be bilateral and to involve the whole leg. Lymphoedema praecox presents up to the age of 35 years, usually during adolescence. Most patients have unilateral limb involvement and it usually extends only to the knee. Lymphoedema tarda presents after the age of 35 years and is often associated with obesity. All subgroups of primary lymphoedema are likely to represent a spectrum of disease due to defective lymphatic drainage (aplasia, hypoplasia, hyperplasia, or fibrosis).

Secondary lymphoedema is the commonest form and occurs when the lymphatic vessels become occluded by an acquired pathology. The lymphatic channels distal to the obstruction become dilated and the lymphatic valves secondarily incompetent. The commonest cause worldwide is filariasis caused by infestation with the parasite *Wuchereria bancrofti*. The commonest cause in the Western world is neoplasia and its treatment, resulting in damage or removal of lymph nodes, for example, post-mastectomy lymphoedema of the upper limb.

The lymphatic system removes excess water and protein from the interstitial space and returns it to the intravascular space. Failure of this mechanism results in stagnation of protein-rich fluid in the interstitial space, and the resultant oncotic pressure causes accumulation of more water, leading to dilatation of the lymphatic vessels and lymphatic valvular incompetence.[12]

Box 2.7.3.1 Differential diagnosis of chronic leg swelling

- Venous disease:
  - Primary superficial and/or deep venous incompetence
  - Previous DVT (post-thrombotic syndrome)
  - Arteriovenous malformations
  - Venous outflow obstruction (intrinsic or extrinsic)
- Lymphoedema
- General disease:
  - Congestive cardiac failure
  - Pretibial myxoedema
  - Hypoproteinaemia (e.g. nephrotic syndrome)
  - Hepatic failure
  - Lipoedema
  - Dependency/disuse.

Clinical assessment

The initial presentation is with peripheral oedema. A detailed history and examination of the patient may help to differentiate primary from secondary lymphoedema, and exclude other causes of limb swelling. Initially the oedema is pitting and shows diurnal variation, but over time it becomes non-pitting due to fibrosis of the subcutaneous tissues. Unlike other forms of oedema, lymphoedema characteristically involves the foot. As the oedema progresses, skin complications develop including bacterial and fungal infection.

Investigations

Duplex ultrasound can be used to exclude concomitant venous disease but lymphoedema can usually be diagnosed on the basis of history and examination alone. Investigation is usually only indicated if there is uncertainty about the diagnosis, surgery is being considered, or there are concerns about underlying malignancy.

Lymphangioscintigraphy (isotope lymphangiography) is the most commonly performed investigation. The test involves injecting a radiolabelled colloid into a webspace and taking gamma-camera pictures at intervals to determine lymphatic transit. If it is negative, lymphoedema is effectively ruled out. Lymphangioscintigraphy defines anatomy, evaluates dynamics, and determines severity.

The main role of computed tomography is to diagnose malignancy, either primary or secondary, as a cause of lymphoedema. Recurrent disease should be sought in patients with a previous history of pelvic or abdominal malignancy. Magnetic resonance imaging can give clear images of the lymph channels and nodal architecture. It can distinguish between lymphatic and venous swelling but gives less information than lymphoscintigraphy.

Management

The treatment aims of lymphoedema management are to reduce limb swelling, reduce infection risk, and improve function. Conservative measures are more likely to be successful when used early in the disease process. Maintenance is an important part of the long-term management. Surgery is rarely indicated and is palliative, not curative.[11]

There is no cure for lymphoedema and this should be explained to the patient. General measures include skin care to reduce infection risk, limb elevation and avoidance of tight clothing, exercise, weight reduction, and simple massage. Manual lymphatic drainage is performed by specially trained therapists and uses massage to stimulate the flow of lymph from an abnormal area to an adjacent normal area.

Graduated compression is used both in the initial treatment phase (usually achieved with multilayer bandaging) and during the maintenance phase (usually compression stockings). Intermittent pneumatic compression works best before subcutaneous fibrosis

occurs. The affected limb is placed in a sleeve that is alternately inflated and deflated, to create a pressure gradient thereby moving fluid out of the limb.

Surgery is only indicated in a very small proportion of patients in whom conservative measures have failed, and there is severe disability or gross deformity, and can be by debulking or bypass.

Further reading

Burnand KG. The physiology and hemodynamics of chronic venous insufficiency of the lower limb. In Gloviczki P, Yao JS (eds) *Handbook of Venous Disorders* (2nd ed). New York: Arnold; 2011, 49–57.

Eklof B, Rutherford RB, Bergan JJ, *et al.* American Venous Forum International Ad Hoc Committee for the Revision of the CEAP Classification. Revision of the CEAP classification for chronic venous disorders: consensus statement. *J Vasc Surg* 2004; 40:1248–52.

Nicolaides AN. Investigation of chronic venous insufficiency: a consensus statement. *Circulation* 2000; 102:e126–63.

References

1. Evans CJ, Allan PL, Lee AJ, *et al.* Prevalence of venous reflux in the general population on duplex scanning: the Edinburgh vein study. *J Vasc Surg* 1998; 28:766–76.
2. National Institute for Health and Care Excellence. *Varicose Veins in the Legs: The Diagnosis and Management of Varicose Veins.* Clinical Guidance 168. London: National Institute for Health and Care Excellence; 2013.
3. Rabe E, Pannier F. Societal costs of chronic venous disease in CEAP C4, C5, C6 disease. *Phlebology* 2010; 25 Suppl 1:64–7.
4. Ruckley CV. Socioeconomic impact of chronic venous insufficiency and leg ulcers. *Angiology* 1997; 48:67–9.
5. Fowkes FG, Evans CJ, Lee AJ. Prevalence and risk factors for chronic venous insufficiency. *Angiology* 2001; 52:S5–15.
6. Bradbury AW. Epidemiology and aetiology of C4-6 disease. *Phlebology* 2010; 25 Suppl 1:2–8.
7. O'Meara S, Cullum NA, Nelson EA. Compression for venous leg ulcers. *Cochrane Database Syst Rev* 2009; 1:CD000265.
8. Barwell JR, Davies CE, *et al.* Comparison of surgery and compression with compression alone in chronic venous ulceration (ESCHAR study): randomized controlled trial. *Lancet* 2004; 363:1854–9.
9. Palfreyman SJ, Nelson EA, Lochiel R, *et al.* Dressing for healing venous leg ulcers. *Cochrane Database Syst Rev* 2006; 3:CD001103.
10. Darvall KAL, Bradbury AW. The management of venous ulceration. In Earnshaw JJ, Murie JA (eds) *The Evidence for Vascular Surgery* (2nd ed). Shrewsbury: TFM Publishing; 2007:207–15.
11. International Society of Lymphology. The diagnosis and treatment of peripheral lymphedema: consensus document of the International Society of Lymphology. *Lymphology* 2003; 36:84–91.
12. Lees TA, Bhutia SG, Balakrishnan A, *et al.* Chronic leg swelling. In Beard JD, Gaines PA (eds) *A Companion to Specialist Surgical Practice: Vascular and Endovascular Surgery* (4th ed). Edinburgh: Saunders; 2009:323–40.

Aneurysms

Robert Davies and Robert Sayers

Introduction

An arterial aneurysm is defined as a 50% or greater increase in the diameter of a vessel whereas an increase of less than 50% is ectasia. The infrarenal abdominal aorta is the commonest site for an arterial aneurysm and abdominal aortic aneurysms (AAAs) account for almost 12 000 hospital admissions per year in England. Popliteal artery aneurysm (PAA) is the most common peripheral artery aneurysm.

Arterial aneurysms rarely occur in isolation and their aetiology is multifactorial, including a genetic preponderance. The majority of arterial aneurysms are asymptomatic at the time of presentation, but the 5-year complication rate of aneurysms that are more than twice the size of the normal vessel diameter is high.

Complications associated with aneurysms relate to their size, including mass effect on surrounding structures and rupture, and thromboembolization. Aneurysm rupture is a life-threatening event and 6000 deaths per year in England and Wales result from ruptured AAA. Therefore, the general principle for treating all asymptomatic arterial aneurysms is quantifying the risk of an aneurysm developing complications and weighing this up against the risk associated with elective repair.

Abdominal aortic aneurysm

Incidence

The incidence of AAA, defined as an enlargement of at least 3 cm, increases with age and affects approximately 4% of the elderly general population ($\geq$ 65 years) within the United Kingdom. The age-specific prevalence is six times greater in men than women with an estimated prevalence of 5–8% for men aged 65–80 years old.[1–3]

Pathophysiology

AAA represents a chronic inflammatory pathology and is usually characterized by the presence of a biologically active mural thrombus directly proportional to the maximum AAA diameter.[4] Ten per cent of AAAs are classed as 'inflammatory' referring to the presence of a dense retroperitoneal inflammatory reaction with a thick 'rind' of fibro-inflammatory tissue overlying the native vessel.

Patients with an AAA demonstrate a high incidence of cardiovascular disease and associated risk factors including male gender, cigarette smoking, hypercholesterolaemia, and hypertension. Diabetes mellitus appears to be protective for AAA. There appears to be a genetic preponderance for the development of AAA with 20% of patients having a positive family history; a variant in the *LRP1* gene has recently been implicated as a potential causal gene.

Symptoms and signs

The majority of AAAs affect the infrarenal aorta and 75% are asymptomatic at the time of presentation having been identified incidentally during routine health checks or investigations for other pathologies.

Alternatively, the patient with a symptomatic non-ruptured AAA may present with (a) symptoms/signs resulting from the growth/mass effect of the AAA itself, for example, lumbar-sacral or loin pain, constitutional illness including malaise and fatigue, and a pulsatile abdominal mass, or (b) acute or chronic limb ischaemia resulting from distal embolization. Inflammatory aneurysms associated with retroperitoneal fibrosis may cause ureteric or duodenal obstruction. The patient with a ruptured AAA presents with the classic triad of lumbar/loin pain, haemodynamic instability/collapse, and a pulsatile abdominal mass. Rarely AAAs present with primary aortoenteric or aortocaval fistulae.

Management

When to repair

The natural history of AAA is that of gradual accelerating, asymptomatic expansion until rupture occurs. The best-known predictor of rupture rate is the maximum AAA diameter; the annual risk of rupture for an aneurysm with a diameter greater than 7 cm may be as high as 25% (Table 2.7.4.1).[5]

Approximately 2500 men aged 60 years or older die as a result of a ruptured AAA (rAAA) in England and Wales per year; 2.5% of all deaths in males aged 60 years or older. Of these deaths, approximately half occur prior to hospital treatment.[5,6] For patients who survive to reach hospital alive, despite advances in perioperative management, in-hospital mortality rates following emergency open surgery for rAAA remain devastatingly high. Open surgical repair of rAAA is associated with an in-hospital mortality rate of 40%.[7] Therefore in the United Kingdom elective repair of an infrarenal AAA, in a suitably fit patient, is recommended when the aneurysm measures 5.5 cm or more, or greater than 4.5 cm with a growth rate greater than 0.5 cm/6 months.[5]

Preoperative investigation

Investigation of the patient with an AAA is aimed at (a) assessing the AAA, and (b) assessing the physiological fitness of the patient.

Assessing the AAA

Duplex Doppler ultrasonography (DDU) is an ideal imaging modality to confirm or screen for the presence of an AAA and can be performed within the emergency department. In skilled hands, aneurysm morphology and relationship to the renal arteries can be assessed although views may be limited as a result of

Table 2.7.4.1 AAA rupture rates based on maximum transverse diameter

Diameter	5-year risk of rupture
<5 cm	5%
5–6 cm	25%
6–7 cm	35%
>7 cm	75%

Source: data from *The Lancet*, Volume 352, Issue 9141, The UK Small Aneurysm Trial Participants, Mortality results for randomised controlled trial of early elective surgery or ultrasonographic surveillance for small abdominal aortic aneurysms, pp. 1649–55, Copyright © 1998 Elsevier Ltd, http://www.sciencedirect.com/science/journal/01406736

obesity or overlying bowel gas. A computed tomographic aortogram (CTA) that includes the arterial tree from the aortic arch to the femoral arteries should be performed in all patients found to have a large AAA (≥5.5 cm). Precise AAA anatomical configuration is vital when assessing the suitability of an AAA for endovascular aneurysm repair (EVAR). For patients found not to be anatomically suitable for EVAR, CTA provides valuable information for planning an open surgical repair including the presence of anatomical variants such as a retro-aortic left renal vein or horseshoe kidney. AAAs are frequently associated with aneurysmal disease affecting the peripheral arteries with 10% and 5% of patients found to have concomitant popliteal and femoral artery aneurysms respectively.

Assessing the patient

Both open surgical repair and EVAR cause considerable physiological insult to patients' cardiorespiratory and renal systems; 20–25% of patients undergoing elective open AAA repair or EVAR suffer perioperative myocardial injury as determined by raised cardiac troponin levels. Thus, it is vitally important to assess a patient's physiological fitness and ability to survive a major operation, and weigh this up against the risk of not intervening, that is, risk of rupture. Recently, cardiopulmonary exercise testing has been trialled as a risk stratification tool. Anaerobic exercise threshold and maximum oxygen uptake (VO_2) are measured preoperatively as a measure of cardiopulmonary function. Although initial reports are encouraging, further robust and standardized studies are required before its widespread adoption can be fully supported.

Identifying, investigating, and physiologically optimizing at-risk patients should be undertaken in the multidisciplinary team setting involving surgeons, radiologists, anaesthetists, and, when indicated, cardiologists, respiratory physicians, and nephrologists.

Open surgical repair

Open surgical repair is traditionally performed transperitoneally through a midline or transverse incision under general anaesthesia. The posterior peritoneum is incised with the duodenum and small bowel retracted to the right and the transverse colon superiorly. The left renal vein is identified and the underlying aortic neck is dissected sufficiently to allow the safe application of a clamp. Dependent on the extent of the AAA, the common iliac arteries or iliac bifurcations are dissected and controlled. The iliac arteries are then clamped, followed by the aorta. The aneurysm sac is opened longitudinally and any back-bleeding from the lumbar or inferior mesenteric arteries oversewn. Inlay graft reconstruction using a straight or bifurcated prosthetic graft is then performed. It is important to note that cross-clamping of the aorta places considerable strain on the myocardium by dramatically increasing systemic vascular resistance and arterial pressure. Furthermore, upon re-establishing flow into the lower limbs, significant hypotension may occur resulting in further myocardial or nephric injury.

Elective, open infrarenal AAA repair is associated with a perioperative mortality rate of 3–10%, with the majority secondary to micro- and macrovascular thrombosis causing myocardial injury, thromboembolism, and multiple organ failure.[8–12] Meticulous preoperative planning, intraoperative technique, and postoperative care are vital to achieve good outcomes. The use of preoperative beta blockers, intraoperative cell salvage, and heparin, and early postoperative extubation has been reported to improve results.

Endovascular aneurysm repair

EVAR provides a less invasive and safer alternative treatment to open surgical repair in the fit and anatomically suitable patient. The EVAR-1, EVAR-2, and DREAM trials reported EVAR was associated with a 3% absolute risk reduction in perioperative mortality when compared to open surgical repair. However, exponents have argued that these initial operative mortality benefits are offset by the long-term economic cost due to late graft-related complications.

Endoleak is a complication unique to EVAR and results in perfusion of the aneurysm sac and subsequent risk of rupture (Table 2.7.4.2). The EVAR-1 trial reported 22% of EVARs were complicated by endoleak and 35% require a secondary procedure to maintain complete aneurysm exclusion within 3 years of the procedure. However, the endoleak rate is influenced by a variety of factors including preprocedural planning, type of stent graft deployed, aortic morphology, and technical expertise.[13] For these reasons, and the risk of other stent-related complications including stent migration, regular outpatient follow-up with CTA or DDU combined with abdominal radiographs is necessary to identify aneurysm exclusion failure. Thus, the short-term perioperative mortality/morbidity benefits of EVAR may be outweighed by its long-term morbidity in terms of re-intervention as well as the associated economic burden.

The UK National Health Service AAA screening programme has recently been implemented in an attempt to reduce the risk of death from AAAs in men aged 65 years and over by 50%. Men in their 65th year are invited to attend screening, which consists of a DDU of the abdominal aorta. It is calculated that 192 men need to be scanned to prevent one rupture AAA death over a 10-year period. However, for every 1660 men scanned, one extra postoperative

Table 2.7.4.2 Classification of endoleak

Type I	Failure of stent graft to seal against the aortic wall proximally (type Ia) or against the iliac arteries distally (type Ib)
Type II	Retrograde blood flow through one (type IIa) or more (type IIb) normal branches of the excluded aortic segment, e.g. inferior mesenteric artery or lumbar arteries
Type III	Structural failure of the stent graft secondary to fabric disruption (type IIIa), separation of modular components (type IIIb), suture holes in fabric (type IIIc)
Type IV	Caused by graft porosity typically identified at the time of stent graft deployment

death will occur. Therefore, for every 10 000 men scanned, 65 AAA ruptures will be prevented saving 52 lives over a 10-year period.

Femoral artery aneurysms

Incidence

Femoral artery aneurysms (FAAs) are the second most common peripheral artery aneurysm to popliteal artery aneurysms. They are ten times more common in males and predominantly occur in patients aged over 65 years of age with risk factors for cardiovascular disease.[14] FAAs rarely occur in isolation (<10%) and are frequently associated with a contralateral aneurysm or/and aneurysmal disease affecting the aorta or other peripheral arteries.

Pathophysiology

Although not well understood, it is theorized that the initiating element for the majority of FAAs is atherosclerotic constriction at the level of the inguinal ligament causing a poststenotic dilatation of the common femoral artery (CFA). The resulting turbulent flow and pressure fluctuations within the CFA results in arterial wall vibration, clinically evident as a bruit or thrill. The arterial wall, pre-weakened by atherosclerosis, and subjected to long-term vibratory forces, progressively weakens and undergoes aneurysmal degeneration.[15,16]

Symptoms and signs

The majority of patients with FAAs present with localized symptomatology or lower limb ischaemia, although a third are asymptomatic and identified incidentally. FAAs are classically felt as smooth, fusiform, pulsatile swellings in the groin that may or may not be tender. Compression of adjacent neurovascular structures may result in lower limb chronic venous hypertensive changes, but dysaesthesia/paraesthesia from resultant femoral nerve compression is rare.

As with all aneurysms, thrombosis, distal embolization, and rupture may occur. In the case of FAAs, thromboembolization occurs more commonly than rupture reflecting the protective nature of the constraining femoral sheath. In cases of acute thrombosis, patients may present with a 'threatened' leg that requires emergency treatment, which is often made more complex due to previous 'silent' embolic occlusion of the crural vessels.

Investigation

Only 20% of FAAs are reliably identified on clinical examination.[17] Thus a high index of suspicion is required and all patients with AAAs or peripheral artery aneurysms should undergo imaging assessment of their lower limb vasculature as routine.

DDU is an adequate screening tool in both the emergency and elective setting. Upon identification, the authors recommend further assessment of the lower limb arterial tree utilizing CTA and/or magnetic resonance angiography (MRA) to allow accurate planning of future interventions. In the acutely ischaemic limb, lengthy preoperative investigations may be detrimental to the success of limb salvage surgery; in these circumstances a combination of DDU and on-table angiography are key.

Management

All symptomatic aneurysms, or aneurysms complicated with thromboembolism or rupture, should be offered primary surgical repair. There is considerable debate relating to the treatment of asymptomatic FAAs, as their natural history is unknown. In practice, modern vascular surgeons will consider a FAA measuring greater than 2.5 cm or enlarging on serial imaging for elective repair.

The majority of FAAs are isolated to the CFA (type I). These are best repaired with a straight inlaid, interposition graft with the redundant sac plicated over the graft. Autologous vein should be utilized where there is a suspicion of infection otherwise a prosthetic conduit may be used. Aneurysms that extend into the superficial femoral artery or profunda femoris artery (type II) require individually tailored solutions depending on the anatomy. Similarly, for those patients in whom multilevel aneurysmal disease occurs, the most clinically pressing disease should be addressed at the initial operation whilst simultaneously planning for any necessary future vascular reconstructions.

Femoral artery pseudoaneurysms

Pathophysiology

The wall of a pseudoaneurysm consists of thin fibrous tissue as opposed to all three tunica (intima, media, and adventitia) layers, as is the case with a true aneurysm. This fibrous pseudocapsule develops as a result of an arterial wall or anastomotic defect that allows extravasation of blood at systemic pressure into the perivascular soft tissues.

Iatrogenic, post-catheterization pseudoaneurysm formation is the commonest cause of femoral artery pseudoaneurysms (FAPs) with a reported incidence of 1–6%.[18,19] Risk factors include coagulopathies, including antiplatelet and warfarin therapy, hypertension, and factors that reduce the effectiveness of post-procedural vessel compression or closure devices including obesity, heavily calcified arteries, cannulation of the superficial femoral or profunda femoris arteries, and a sheath size greater than 7 Fr.[20]

Infection, particularly in the drug abuser population, and femoral para-anastomotic failure may also lead to pseudoaneurysm formation. Anastomotic pseudoaneurysms complicate 8% of aortobifemoral bypasses and 2.5% of all femoral anastomoses at a median follow up of 8 years.[21,22]

Symptoms and signs

FAP may present as a pulsatile groin mass that may or may not be painful. The weakened pseudocapsule when subjected to systemic blood pressure may gradually expand causing localized compression and/or erosion of adjacent structures, distal embolization, or rupture. Mycotic aneurysms present as a painful, erythematous groin mass often with a concurrent purulent/sanguineous discharge and represent a surgical emergency due to the high risk of bleeding.

Investigation

Investigation is primarily aimed at (1) confirming the clinical diagnosis, (2) assessing the size of the pseudoaneurysm, and (3) assessing the size and location of the arterial/anastomotic defect. DDU is the initial investigation of choice and can be used to plan treatment in isolation when an uncomplicated post-catheterization pseudoaneurysm occurs. In cases in which complex reconstructive surgery may be required, for example, anastomotic pseudoaneurysm, CT angiography should be utilized as an adjunct to DDU.

Treatment

The majority of small post-catheterization pseudoaneurysms undergo spontaneous thrombosis. Pseudoaneurysm size and anticoagulation status are the two most important predictors of spontaneous thrombosis; approximately 90% of pseudoaneurysms measuring 3 cm or less thrombose within 1 month without intervention.[23] Thus an initial conservative management strategy for small pseudoaneurysms (≤3 cm) with serial DDU remains advocated by some authors.

The use of minimally invasive techniques for treating FAP, particularly iatrogenic, post-catheterization pseudoaneurysms, has gained widespread acceptance. Ultrasound-guided compression in isolation has reported success rates of 63–100%.[20] Concomitant systemic anticoagulation and/or pseudoaneurysm size greater than 3 cm are independent predictors of failure, and complications including pseudoaneurysm rupture, femoral vein thrombosis, and acute limb ischaemia have been reported in up to 4% of cases.[20]

The use of ultrasound-guided percutaneous thrombin injection into the pseudoaneurysm sac is now widespread with reported success rates of greater than 90%. Unlike ultrasound-guided compression, the patient's anticoagulation status does not adversely affect outcome.[24] Complications including distal embolization are reported in 4% or less of cases and may be further reduced with the adjunct use of an intra-arterial balloon protection devices in pseudoaneurysms with wide necks.

Minimally invasive percutaneous treatments have confined the indications for open surgical repair to those pseudoaneurysms that are rapidly expanding, mycotic, causing neurovascular compression, skin necrosis, or have undergone failed percutaneous treatment—*complex* pseudoaneurysms. Non-infected pseudoaneurysms are repaired primarily with interrupted non-absorbable sutures or with an autologous vein patch-angioplasty depending on the size of the arterial defect. However, the surgical treatment of mycotic pseudoaneurysms is more complex with surgical goals being (a) the excision of infected tissues, and (b) preservation of the distal circulation. The use of extra-anatomical autologous vein grafts is often required, whilst in some cases of gross suppurative infection and systemic decompensation, primary ligation of the femoral vessels as a 'bail-out' procedure may become necessary with a 30% risk of subsequent amputation.

Popliteal artery aneurysms

Incidence

PAAs are the most common peripheral artery aneurysm being diagnosed predominantly in males during their seventh decade of life. The presence of a PAA often reflects a systemic aneurysmal preponderance; 50% are bilateral and 40% are associated with an AAA. Conversely, 10% of patients with an AAA have a concomitant popliteal artery aneurysm.

Pathophysiology

The majority of PAAs result from atherosclerotic disease affecting the tunica media. Non-atherosclerotic causes of aneurysmal degeneration are infrequent and include the vasculitides and connective tissue disorders. Mechanical causes including poststenotic dilatation secondary to popliteal entrapment syndrome or repetitive trauma, as in the case of horse riding boots, may also result in aneurysmal change.

Symptoms and signs

Two-thirds are symptomatic at the time of diagnosis, with 90% of patients presenting with features of limb ischaemia; symptoms secondary to neurovascular compression or aneurysm rupture are rare.

Clinical examination may reveal an obvious pulsatile mass arising from the popliteal fossa. However, more often than not it is the clinical symptomatology in conjunction with the absence of the normal concavity of the popliteal fossa on examination that alerts the clinician to the possibility of a PAA. Differential diagnoses should include Baker cyst, lymphadenopathy, and pseudoaneurysm.

Acute thrombosis and/or distal embolization causing critical limb ischaemia are the most common complications of PAAs. Occasionally, a more insidious onset of claudication and critical limb ischaemia may occur due to repeated 'showering' of emboli into the distal arterial tree. Asymptomatic 'silent' thrombosis and/or embolization may be identified through reduced ankle–brachial pressure indices or loss of pedal pulses during a routine medical check-up.

Large aneurysms may compress surrounding neurovascular structures causing lower limb swelling and paraesthesia. However, due to the relative mobility of the popliteal artery, tethered at the adductor hiatus proximally and the soleal muscular arch distally, rupture is rare. When aneurysm rupture does occur, limb salvage rates are poor with more than two-thirds of patients undergoing subsequent amputation (Figure 2.7.4.1).

Investigation

Radiological investigations are aimed at (a) confirming the clinical diagnosis, (b) assessing the extent of the aneurysm, and (c) assessing the inflow and run-off vessels for concomitant stenotic/occlusive or aneurysmal disease. DDU performed by a skilled sonographer can provide excellent and expedient information regarding inflow, outflow, diameter, sac thrombus, and venous thrombosis compression. The authors recommend the use of CTA or MRA to further assess the proximal and distal arterial trees in line. Specifically, detailed assessment of the run-off vessels is required as they directly relate to the urgency and success of future surgical and endovascular reconstruction.

Management

There are no randomized controlled trials to establish clear indications for intervention for PAAs. It is widely accepted that all symptomatic PAAs require intervention to prevent limb loss; however, indications for intervention in an asymptomatic popliteal aneurysm remain controversial. It is reported that the majority of asymptomatic popliteal artery aneurysms eventually develop thromboembolic complications with associated amputation rates of 67%.[25,26] Furthermore, graft patency and limb salvage rates are much better when performed in the asymptomatic limb with results superior to that for occlusive disease. Thus, the authors would recommend all fit patients with a PAA measuring 2 cm or more in maximum diameter with an available suitable autologous conduit be considered for intervention.

Surgical reconstruction

The two main approaches to the popliteal aneurysm are the medial and posterior approach.

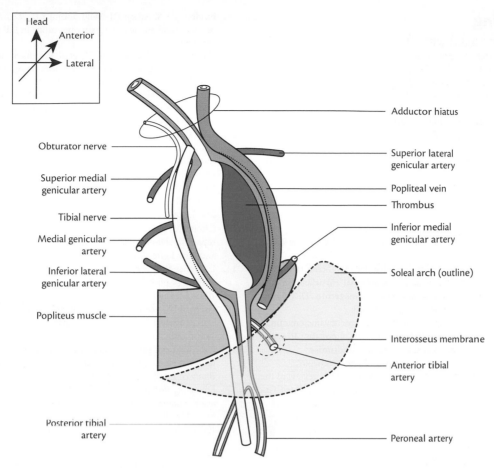

Fig. 2.7.4.1 Diagrammatic representation of a right popliteal artery viewed from behind.

The *posterior approach* involves an 'S'-shaped incision in the popliteal fossa with dissection of the aneurysm from other popliteal structures followed by inlay, interposition grafting. The advantages of the posterior approach are (a) the ability to freely ligate feeding geniculate branches thereby preventing future endoleak and sac expansion that may occur following simple ligation and bypass, and (b) the sac may be excised which is especially important in cases of neurovascular compression. The disadvantage of this approach, however, is the difficulty in exposing the crural vessels and the superficial femoral artery should the extent of reconstruction be more complex that preoperatively anticipated. Harvesting the long saphenous vein for use as a conduit is more difficult in the prone position; a preoperatively marked basilic vein may be utilized as an alternative in these cases.

The *medial approach* employs the same exposure technique as one would use for a femoral below-knee popliteal bypass and is thus considered more familiar if not easier by some surgeons. The popliteal artery is ligated above and below the aneurysm with a non-absorbable suture and a femoral below-knee popliteal bypass reconstruction is performed. This approach should be employed for aneurysms that are not isolated to the popliteal artery or in cases where femoral-distal arterial reconstruction is anticipated. Although technically challenging, it is possible to ligate the geniculate vessels utilizing this approach and thus the perceived drawback to this approach of potential sac expansion due to an 'endoleak' is negated if endoaneurysmorrhaphy is performed.

Both techniques can be combined with intra-arterial thrombolysis or crural vessel thromboembolectomy in the acutely ischaemic limb. In a chronically ischaemic leg, thrombolysis and/or embolectomy are unlikely to resolve a mature (>21 days) thromboembolic occlusion in the run-off vessels and therefore a crural or pedal bypass may be required.

Endovascular reconstruction

A preoperatively planned covered stent (endograft) is deployed through a transfemoral approach with 'landing zones' being healthy artery proximal and distal to the aneurysm. Endograft reconstruction is less traumatic than open reconstruction, resulting in smaller wounds, a reduced hospital stay, and therefore reduced cost in the short term. Furthermore, initial reports of early stent kinking/fracture/thrombosis as a result of repeated knee extension and flexion have diminished with stent technology improvements. However, there remains a paucity of evidence, particularly long-term follow-up data, to support the use of endograft and the authors reserve their use to the 'unfit' symptomatic patient.

Further reading

Antonello M, Frigatti P, Battocchio P, *et al.* Open repair versus endovascular treatment for symptomatic popliteal artery aneurysm: results of a prospective randomized study. *J Vasc Surg* 2005; 42(2):185–93.

Davies RS, Wall M, Rai S, *et al.* Long-term results of surgical repair of popliteal artery aneurysm. *Eur J Vasc Endovasc Surg* 2007; 34(6):714–18.

EVAR trial participants. Endovascular aneurysm repair and outcome in patients unfit for open repair of abdominal aortic aneurysm (EVAR trial 2): randomised controlled trial. *Lancet* 2005; 365(9478):2187–92.

EVAR trial participants. Endovascular aneurysm repair versus open repair in patients with abdominal aortic aneurysm (EVAR trial 1): randomised controlled trial. *Lancet* 2005; 365(9478):2179–86.

Galland RB, Magee TR. Management of popliteal aneurysm. *Br J Surg* 2002; 89(11):1382–5.

Lederle FA, Wilson SE, Johnson GR, *et al.* Immediate repair compared with surveillance of small abdominal aortic aneurysms. *N Engl J Med* 2002; 346(19):1437–44.

Prinssen M, Verhoeven EL, Buth J, *et al.* A randomized trial comparing conventional and endovascular repair of abdominal aortic aneurysms. Dutch Randomized Endovascular Aneurysm Managemtn (DREAM) Trial Group. *N Engl J Med* 2004; 351(16):1607–18.

Thompson SG, Ashton HA, Gao L, *et al.* Multicentre Aneurysm Screening Study Group. Screening men for abdominal aortic aneurysm: 10 year mortality and cost effectiveness results from the randomised Multicentre Aneurysm Screening Study. *BMJ* 2009; 338:b2307.

Young EL, Karthikesalingam A, Huddart S, *et al.* A systematic review of the role of cardiopulmonary exercise testing in vascular surgery. *Eur J Vasc Endovasc Surg* 2012; 44(1):64–71.

References

1. Scott RA, Ashton HA, Kay DN. Abdominal aortic aneurysm in 4237 screened patients: prevalence, development and management over 6 years. *Br J Surg* 1991; 78(9):1122–5.
2. Collin J, Araujo L, Walton J, *et al.* Oxford screening programme for abdominal aortic aneurysm in men aged 65 to 74 years. *Lancet* 1988; 2(8611):613–15.
3. O'Kelly TJ, Heather BP. General practice-based population screening for abdominal aortic aneurysms: a pilot study. *Br J Surg* 1989; 76(5):479–80.
4. Hans SS, Jareunpoon O, Balasubramaniam M, *et al.* Size and location of thrombus in intact and ruptured abdominal aortic aneurysms. *J Vasc Surg* 2005; 41(4):584–8.
5. The UK Small Aneurysm Trial Participants. Mortality results for randomised controlled trial of early elective surgery or ultrasonographic surveillance for small abdominal aortic aneurysms. *Lancet* 1998; 352(9141):1649–55.
6. Wilmink TBM, Quick CRG, Hubbard CS, *et al.* The influence of screening on the incidence of ruptured abdominal aortic aneurysms, *J Vasc Surg* 1999; 30:203–8.
7. Davies RS, Dawlatly S, Clarkson JR, *et al.* Outcome in patients requiring renal replacement therapy after open surgical repair for ruptured abdominal aortic aneurysm. *Vasc Endovascular Surg* 2010; 44(3):170–3.
8. Bradbury AW, Adam DJ, Makhdoomi KR, *et al.* A 21-year experience of abdominal aortic aneurysm operations in Edinburgh. *Br J Surg* 1998; 85(5):645–7.
9. Dardik A, Lin JW, Gordon TA, *et al.* Results of elective abdominal aortic aneurysm repair in the 1990s: a population-based analysis of 2335 cases. *J Vasc Surg* 1999; 30(6):985–95.
10. Kazmers A, Jacobs L, Perkins A, *et al.* Abdominal aortic aneurysm repair in Veterans Affairs medical centers. *J Vasc Surg* 1996; 23(2):191–200.
11. Sayers RD, Thompson MM, Nasim A, *et al.* Surgical management of 671 abdominal aortic aneurysms: a 13 year review from a single centre. *Eur J Vasc Endovasc Surg* 1997; 13(3):322–7.
12. Dueck AD, Kucey DS, Johnston KW, *et al.* Long-term survival and temporal trends in patient and surgeon factors after elective and ruptured abdominal aortic aneurysm surgery. *J Vasc Surg* 2004; 39(6):1261–7.
13. Ghouri M, Krajcer Z. Endoluminal abdominal aortic aneurysm repair: the latest advances in prevention of distal endograft migration and type 1 endoleak. *Tex Heart Inst J* 2010; 37(1):19–24.
14. Lawrence PF, Lorenzo-Rivero S, Lyon JL. The incidence of iliac, femoral, and popliteal artery aneurysms in hospitalized patients. *J Vasc Surg* 1995; 22(4):409–15.
15. Graham LM, Zelenock GB, Whitehouse WMJr, *et al.* Clinical significance of arteriosclerotic femoral artery aneurysms. *Arch Surg* 1980; 115(4):502–7.
16. Gow BS, Legg ML, Yu W, *et al.* Does vibration cause poststenotic dilatation in vivo and influence atherogenesis in cholesterol-fed rabbits? *J Biomech Eng* 1992; 114:20–5.
17. Diwan A, Sarkar R, Stanley JC, *et al.* Incidence of femoral and popliteal artery aneurysms in patients with abdominal aortic aneurysms. *J Vasc Surg* 2000; 31(5):863–9.
18. Katzenschlager R, Ugurluoglu A, Ahmadi A, *et al.* Incidence of pseudoaneurysm after diagnostic and therapeutic angiography. *Radiology* 1995; 195(2):463–6.
19. Lumsden AB, Miller JM, Kosinski AS, *et al.* A prospective evaluation of surgically treated groin complications following percutaneous cardiac procedures. *Am Surg* 1994; 60(2):132–7.
20. Morgan R, Belli AM. Current treatment methods for post-catheterization pseudoaneurysms. *J Vasc Interv Radiol* 2003; 14(6):697–710.
21. Marković DM, Davidović LB, Kostić DM, *et al.* False anastomotic aneurysms. *Vascular* 2007; 15(3):141–8.
22. Biancari F, Ylönen K, Anttila V, *et al.* Durability of open repair of infrarenal abdominal aortic aneurysm: a 15-year follow-up study. *J Vasc Surg* 2002; 35:87–93.
23. Toursarkissian B, Allen BT, Petrinec D, *et al.* Spontaneous closure of selected iatrogenic pseudoaneurysms and arteriovenous fistulae. *J Vasc Surg* 1997; 25(5):803–8.
24. Corriere MA, Guzman RJ. True and false aneurysms of the femoral artery. *Semin Vasc Surg* 2005; 18(4):216–23.
25. Dawson I, van Bockel JH, Brand R, *et al.* Popliteal artery aneurysms. Long-term follow-up of aneurysmal disease and results of surgical treatment. *J Vasc Surg* 1991; 13:398–407.
26. Shortell CK, DeWeese JA, Ouriel K, *et al.* Popliteal artery aneurysms: a 25-year experience. *J Vasc Surg* 1991; 14(6):771–6.

Transient ischaemic attack and stroke

A. Ross Naylor

What is a stroke/transient ischaemic attack?

A stroke is a focal (occasionally global) loss of cerebral function that persists for more than 24 hours and which is ultimately found to have a vascular aetiology. A transient ischaemic attack (TIA) has a similar definition but lasts less than 24 hours. The term 'neurologically asymptomatic' refers to patients who do not report any prior focal neurological symptoms. However, this is not an exact definition as patients can suffer a short-lived TIA whilst asleep (of which they may not be aware) and up to 25% of 'neurologically asymptomatic' patients will have evidence of 'silent' infarction on computed tomography (CT) or magnetic resonance imaging (MRI).

Risk factors for stroke/transient ischaemic attack

Modifiable risk factors include hypertension, atrial fibrillation, raised cholesterol, smoking, excess alcohol consumption, diabetes, physical inactivity, obesity, prior stroke/TIA, and peripheral vascular disease. Non-modifiable risk factors include increasing age, male gender, and race. Only 15% of stroke patients will report a prior TIA or minor stroke.

Aetiology of stroke/transient ischaemic attack

If you consider the next 100 strokes destined to happen in a Western community, 80 will be ischaemic, whilst 20 will be haemorrhagic (intracranial, subarachnoid). Of the 80 ischaemic strokes, about 60 will affect the carotid territory and about 20 will affect the posterior circulation (vertebrobasilar). Of the 60 carotid territory ischaemic strokes, 30 will follow thrombosis of the internal carotid artery and/or embolism of atherothrombotic material from a carotid stenosis into the middle or anterior cerebral arteries.

Of the remaining 30 carotid territory ischaemic strokes, 15 will be due to small vessel disease, 9 will follow cardiac embolism, 3 will be secondary to haematological conditions (polycythaemia, myeloma, or thrombocytosis), and 3 will be due to non-atherosclerotic pathologies (fibromuscular dysplasia, arteritis, or aneurysm).

Clinical presentation of stroke/transient ischaemic attack

Table 2.7.5.1 summarizes the 'classical' symptoms associated with carotid and vertebrobasilar territory TIAs or stroke. It also details those (non-hemispheric) symptoms that are sometimes wrongly considered to be clinical manifestations of TIA or stroke (unless they coexist with one or more of the classical symptoms). Most carotid territory events are embolic (only 2% of strokes are haemodynamic). However, a haemodynamic aetiology should be considered in any patient who reports symptoms that occur after a meal or on getting out of a hot bath.

Two clinical entities require further clarification. 'Crescendo' TIAs means that the patient is reporting one or more frequent focal events, but the key clinical issue is that there is full neurological recovery in-between each event. This contrasts with 'stroke in evolution' or 'stuttering stroke' where there are frequent neurological events with incomplete recovery between each one.

Investigation of stroke/transient ischaemic attack

The protocol for investigating patients with a suspected TIA or minor stroke is completely different to a decade ago. The key issue now is the provision of daily 'rapid access' TIA clinics where patients are investigated and treatment initiated as soon as possible

Table 2.7.5.1 Clinical presentation of stroke and TIA

Carotid territory symptoms	Vertebrobasilar territory symptoms	Non-hemispheric symptoms that cannot be attributed to TIA/minor stroke
Hemisensory/motor signs	Hemi- or bilateral motor/sensory signs	Isolated syncope (blackout or drop attack)
Monocular visual loss	Bilateral visual loss	Presyncope (faintness)
Dysphasia, visuospatial neglect	Dysarthria	Isolated dizziness
	Problems with gait and stance	Isolated diplopia
	Homonymous hemianopia	Isolated vertigo
	Diplopia, vertigo, nystagmus (not in isolation)	

Table 2.7.5.2 The ABCD^2 scoring system for triaging referrals to rapid access TIA clinics

Parameter			Score
A	Age	>60 years	1
B	Blood pressure	Systolic > 140 or diastolic > 90 mmHg	1
C	Clinical features	Unilateral weakness	2
		Speech disturbance (no weakness)	1
		Retinal symptoms	0
D	Duration	>60 minutes	2
		10–59 minutes	1
		<10 minutes	0
D	Diabetes	Diabetes present	1
Maximum score			7

Source: data from *The Lancet*, Volume 369, Issue 9558, Johnston SC *et al.*, Validation and refinement of scores to predict very early stroke risk after transient ischaemic attack pp. 283–292, Copyright © 2007 Elsevier Ltd. All rights reserved.

after the index event. This is because the risk of recurrent stroke is very high in the first few days after onset of symptoms.[1]

Most patients will be referred to a 'rapid access' TIA clinic via their family doctor or the emergency department. Most centres now use the ABCD^2 scoring system[2] to triage referrals (Table 2.7.5.2). A low ABCD^2 score (0–3) is associated with a 1% risk of recurrent stroke at 7 days and these patients do not need to be seen urgently. However, a moderate score (4–5) or a high score (6–7) is associated with 6% and 12% stroke rates at 7 days respectively. Consequently, patients with an ABCD^2 score of 4 or more are triaged to be seen the same day or the following morning.

In the TIA clinic, most patients will undergo a chest X-ray (to exclude cardiomegaly and lung tumour), an electrocardiogram (to check for arrhythmias, left ventricular hypertrophy, and evidence of pre-existing ischaemic heart disease), and baseline bloods. About 5% of all strokes are secondary to a haematological problem and a full blood count will exclude polycythaemia or thrombocytosis. Younger patients (< 50 years) are more likely to have a vasculitis, which may be associated with a raised plasma viscosity. It is also important to identify modifiable risk factors such as undiagnosed or poorly controlled diabetes.

The role of the rapid access TIA clinic is to identify the most likely underlying aetiology (e.g. carotid stenosis, cardiac embolism, or small vessel disease) and then treat accordingly. Functional imaging can now be performed in everyone because of advances in access and availability of MRI and CT. This may reveal areas of embolic (cortical) infarction or lacunar infarction. The latter is defined as small areas of brain injury in the deeper brain structures that are typical of small vessel occlusion (e.g. the lenticulostriate end-arteries). Functional imaging will also identify the rare TIA patient whose event was secondary to a small haemorrhage.

It is important to identify patients with a significant carotid stenosis, as they will benefit from an expedited surgical intervention. Intra-arterial angiography is never used routinely (1–2% risk of

procedural stroke) and everyone should undergo some form of non-invasive carotid imaging (magnetic resonance angiography (MRA), CT angiography (CTA), or Duplex ultrasound scanning (DUS).

DUS is usually the first-line investigation in most rapid access TIA clinics and many surgical units are happy to operate on the basis of ultrasound alone. Some prefer corroborative imaging with CTA or MRA and that is acceptable provided it does not lead to delays in offering a carotid intervention. If, however, carotid artery stenting (CAS) is being considered, more extensive imaging with CTA or MRA is necessary in order to plan any procedure (e.g. severity of aortic arch disease, excessive vessel calcification, or excessive carotid tortuosity).

Anyone preferring to use DUS (alone) prior to carotid endarterectomy (CEA) should be aware that corroborative CTA or MRA imaging is necessary in any patient where DUS suggests possible tandem inflow or outflow disease.

Randomized trials of carotid interventions

Symptomatic carotid disease

The Carotid Endarterectomy Trialists Collaboration (CETC) combined all the data from 6000+ patients randomized within the NASCET, ECST, and VA Trials,[3] which compared CEA with best medical therapy (BMT). Its main findings are summarized in Table 2.7.5.3. Surgery conferred significant benefit in patients with moderate (50–69%) or severe (70–99%) stenoses, but conferred no benefit in symptomatic patients with 0–49% stenoses or in those with near occlusion (small channel extending towards skull base).

Subgroup analyses from the CETC also identified clinical and imaging features that predicted a higher risk of stroke if treated medically. Clinical factors included male gender, increasing age, hemispheric symptoms, recent symptoms, and increasing co-morbidity. Imaging predictors included contralateral occlusion, increasing stenosis severity, and an irregular plaque surface.

Carotid artery stenting has now emerged as an alternative to CEA. A number of randomized trials have compared CEA with CAS in symptomatic patients and most have consistently shown that the procedural risk (30-day death/stroke) is nearly two times higher following CAS.[4] This is partially offset by a higher risk of perioperative myocardial infarction (MI) after CEA, but there is also consistent evidence that CAS is significantly more risky when

Table 2.7.5.3 Carotid Endarterectomy Trialists collaboration: 5-year risk of any stroke (including 30-day stroke/death) from the VA, ECST, and NASCET trials

Stenosis	5-year stroke after CEA	5-year stroke on BMT	Absolute risk reduction	Relative risk reduction
0–30%	18.4%	15.7%	−2.7	No benefit
30–49%	22.8%	25.5%	+2.7%	10%
50–69%	20.0%	27.8%	+7.8%	28%
70–99%	17.1%	32.7%	+15.6%	48%
Sub-occlusion	22.4%	22.3%	−0.1%	No benefit

BMT, best medical therapy; CEA, carotid endarterectomy.

Source: data from *The Lancet*, Volume 363, Issue 9413, Rothwell PM *et al.*, Endarterectomy for symptomatic carotid stenosis in relation to clinical subgroups and timing of surgery, pp. 915–24, Copyright © 2004 Elsevier Ltd. All rights reserved.

treating patients in the hyperacute period after onset of symptoms (threefold excess risk of stroke[5]).

Asymptomatic carotid disease

This remains an enduringly controversial subject. Two large trials (ACAS[6] and ACST[7]) randomized 4500 patients to CEA or BMT and observed that surgery conferred a 50% relative risk reduction in late stroke from approximately 12% down to 6% at 5 years. The benefit was maximal in males and those aged under 75 years. ACAS and ACST recruited patients almost two decades ago and the current controversy is fuelled by a growing awareness that the risk of stroke in patients with significant carotid disease (on BMT alone) has fallen from about 2–3% per year to 1% (possibly less).[8] If true, this would render many of the ACAS and ACST trial findings obsolete.

A number of randomized trials are currently comparing CEA with CAS in asymptomatic patients, but only two intend to include a medical limb. This is unfortunate as it is essential that we are able to identify the 'high-risk for stroke' cohort in whom to target CEA or CAS.

Management of stroke/transient ischaemic attack

'Best medical management'

In the 1980s (i.e. when the randomized trials were recruiting), the concept of BMT essentially meant 'stop smoking and take aspirin'. The whole concept of what constitutes BMT has now radically changed. The key components to BMT in patients presenting with a stroke/TIA include (a) long-term control of hypertension, (b) high-dose statin therapy, and (c) dual antiplatelet therapy. The European Stroke Initiative Guidelines[9] recommend aspirin plus dipyridamole, the National Institute for Health and Care Excellence (NICE) recommends aspirin and modified release dipyridamole for TIA and clopidogrel for ischaemic stroke. In addition, lifestyle modification is also recommended (stop smoking, reduce alcohol intake, take exercise, and dietary changes).

One key finding has been the importance of starting medical therapy as soon as possible after onset of symptoms.[11] Most rapid access TIA clinics now recommend that the family doctor or emergency department staff give the patient 300 mg aspirin and 40 mg simvastatin when they are first seen. At the TIA clinic, a CT/MRI scan will exclude haemorrhage and the patient is then administered a further 300 mg aspirin, 75 mg clopidogrel, and 40 mg simvastatin. If the blood pressure is elevated, the family doctor is advised to treat this.

Role of carotid surgery and carotid stenting

The key issue is to offer CEA (or CAS) as soon as possible after onset of symptoms.[12] This is because (in patients with 50–99% stenoses) the 7-day risk of recurrent stroke is 10%. For most UK centres, this will mean the patient undergoing CEA, as the procedural stroke risk (compared with CAS) is significantly lower. However, NICE has advised that where high-volume CAS centres can perform CAS with procedural risks comparable to CEA in the hyperacute period (i.e. <14 days), stenting can be considered to be alternative treatment strategy.[13]

Certain recently symptomatic patients may be considered 'high risk for CEA' and may be better treated with CAS. These might include previous neck irradiation, very high carotid disease, severe medical co-morbidity, and a contralateral recurrent laryngeal palsy (bilateral palsies can be fatal).

Management of asymptomatic carotid disease

'Best medical management'

As stated earlier, improvements in the modern concept of BMT have been associated with reductions in the annual rate of stroke in patients with asymptomatic carotid stenoses over the last decade.[8] Accordingly, irrespective of whether you believe that CEA or CAS confers significant benefit in the modern era, it is essential that asymptomatic patients receive guidance on optimal BMT as soon as possible. This would include the same lifestyle modifications (as for symptomatic patients), careful blood pressure control, and high-dose statin therapy. There are conflicting guidelines regarding antiplatelet therapy. Some recommend aspirin (alone), while others advise aspirin and dipyridamole. The main reason for the lack of consensus is the simple fact that no randomized trials have been undertaken.

Role of carotid surgery and carotid stenting

Given the controversy, it would probably be better to avoid performing CAS in asymptomatic patients until the ongoing randomized trials report. This is currently NICE guidance.[14] The decision to offer CEA will depend upon a number of factors, not least one's interpretation of the current role of CEA. Clinical and/or imaging features (based on previous research) that might support a pro-interventional approach include age under 75 years, male sex, progressive stenosis, a history of contralateral TIA, renal impairment, silent infarction on CT scan, and spontaneous embolization on transcranial Doppler ultrasound.[8]

Complications of carotid interventions

Table 2.7.5.4 summarizes the major procedural risks associated with CEA and CAS in symptomatic patients, as observed in CREST[15] and a meta-analysis of three European randomized trials.[5] CAS was associated with a doubling of the risk of stroke/death;

Table 2.7.5.4 Procedural complications after carotid endarterectomy (CEA) and carotid artery stenting (CAS)

Complication	Source	CEA	CAS
Death/stroke	CSTC	5.8%	8.9%
	CREST	3.2%	6.0%
Death/stroke/myocardial infarction	CREST	5.4%	6.7%
Cranial nerve injury	CSTC	6.0%	
	CREST	4.3%	
Severe haematoma	CSTC	1.9%	0.7%

CSTC is the Carotid Stenting Trialists Collaboration who combined data from three European randomized trials (EVA-3S, SPACE, and ICSS).

CREST was the North American randomized trial.

Source: data from Brott TG et al., Stenting versus endarterectomy for treatment of carotid-artery stenosis, *New England Journal of Medicine*, Volume 363, Number 1, pp. 11–23, Copyright © 2010 Massachusetts Medical Society. All rights reserved.

CEA was associated with a doubling of the risk of perioperative MI; there was no-difference in the composite endpoint of death/stroke/MI; significant bleeding was rarely encountered; and CEA was associated with a 4–6% risk of cranial nerve injury. One important finding from the International Carotid Stenting Study (ICSS) was that CAS was associated with a fivefold excess risk of new post-operative ischaemic lesions on diffusion-weighted MRI, compared with CEA.[16] Studies are currently evaluating whether these lesions confer harm to the patient (e.g. dementia).

Long-term outcomes after carotid interventions

It was previously thought that CAS would be associated with a significantly higher rate of restenosis and that this would be associated with a higher risk of late ipsilateral stroke. There have been conflicting data on restenosis rates, but the consistent message from each of the large randomized trials is that following successful CAS, late stroke rates are identical to those following CEA[4] (i.e. CAS is durable). This is a very important finding and indicates that the main determinant for determining what intervention should be recommended to the patient remains the procedural risk.

CREST observed that CEA was associated with an increased risk of perioperative MI (clinical and biomarker) and that this was associated with reduced long-term survival.[17] This has become a very controversial subject, but further subgroup analyses have shown that there is no difference in long-term survival in patients who suffer a perioperative MI as opposed to a perioperative stroke (i.e. the risk of perioperative MI should not assume greater importance in patient selection). In reality, more patients will suffer death or disabling stroke through delayed interventions as opposed to reduced life expectancy following a perioperative MI.

Conclusion

Despite the controversy surrounding the management of asymptomatic carotid disease, the key message for stroke prevention is the rapid investigation and treatment of patients suffering a TIA or minor stroke. Delay may make the surgeon or interventionist look good, but it confers little benefit to the patient.[12]

Further reading

Furie KL, Kasner SE, Adams RJ, et al. Guidelines for the prevention of stroke in patients with stroke or transient ischaemic attack: a guideline for healthcare professionals from the American Heart Association/American Stroke Association. *Stroke* 2011; 42:227–76.

References

1. Giles MF, Rothwell PM. Risk of stroke after transient ischaemic attack: a systematic review and meta-analysis. *Lancet Neurol* 2007; 6:1063–72.
2. Johnston SC, Rothwell PM, Nguyen-Huynh N, *et al*. Validation and refinement of scores to predict very early stroke risk after transient ischaemic attack. *Lancet* 2007; 369:283–92.
3. Rothwell PM, Eliasziw M, Gutnikov SA, *et al*. Endarterectomy for symptomatic carotid stenosis in relation to clinical subgroups and timing of surgery. *Lancet* 2004; 363:915–24.
4. Economoupoulos KP, Sergentanis TN, Tsivgoulis G, *et al*. Carotid artery stenting versus carotid endarterectomy: comprehensive meta-analysis of short and long-term outcomes. *Stroke* 2011; 42:687–92.
5. Carotid Stenting Trialists Collaboration. Short term outcome after stenting versus carotid endarterectomy for symptomatic carotid stenosis: pre-planned meta-analysis of individual patient data. *Lancet* 2010; 376:1062–73
6. Executive Committee for the Asymptomatic Carotid Atherosclerosis Study. Endarterectomy for asymptomatic carotid artery stenosis. *JAMA* 1995; 273:1421–61.
7. Halliday A, Mansfield A, Marro J, *et al*. Prevention of disabling and fatal strokes by successful carotid endarterectomy in patients without recent neurological symptoms: randomized trial. *Lancet* 2004; 363:1491–502.
8. Naylor AR. Time to rethink management strategies in asymptomatic carotid disease. *Nat Rev Cardiol* 2011; 9(2):116–24.
9. The European Stroke Initiative Executive Committee and the EUSI Writing Committee. European Stroke Initiative recommendations for stroke management—Update 2003. *Cerebrovasc Dis* 2003; 16:311–37.
10. National Institute for Health and Clinical Excellence. *Clopidogrel and Modified-Release Dipyridamole for the Prevention of Occlusive Vascular Events*. NICE Technology Appraisal Guidance 210. London: NICE; 2010. https://www.nice.org.uk/guidance/ta210
11. Rothwell PM, Giles MF, Chandratheva A, *et al*. Effect of urgent treatment of transient ischaemic attack and minor stroke on early recurrent stroke (EXPRESS Study): a prospective population based sequential comparison. *Lancet* 2007; 370:1–11.
12. Naylor AR. Delay may reduce the procedural risk, but at what price to the patient? *Eur J Vasc Endovasc Surg* 2008; 35:383–91.
13. National Institute for Health and Clinical Excellence. *Carotid Artery Stent Placement for Symptomatic Extracranial Carotid Stenosis*. NICE Interventional Procedure Guidance 389. London: NICE; 2011. http://www.nice.org.uk/guidance/ipg389
14. National Institute for Health and Clinical Excellence. *Carotid Artery Stent Placement for Asymptomatic Extracranial Carotid Stenosis*. NICE Interventional Procedure Guidance 388. London: NICE; 2011. http://www.nice.org.uk/guidance/ipg388
15. Brott TG, Hobson RW, Howard G, *et al*. Stenting versus endarterectomy for treatment of carotid-artery stenosis. *N Engl J Med* 2010; 363:11–23.
16. Bonati LH, Jongen LM, Haller S, *et al*. New ischaemic brain lesions on MRI after stenting or endarterectomy for symptomatic carotid stenosis: Substudy of the ICSS. *Lancet Neurol* 2010; 9:353–62.
17. Blackshear JL, Cutlip DE, Roubin GS, Hill MD, *et al*. Myocardial infarction after carotid stenting and endarterectomy: results from the Carotid Revascularization Endarterectomy versus Stenting Trial. *Circulation* 2011; 123:2571–8.

PART 2.8

Cardiac and pulmonary surgery

CHAPTER 2.8.1

Cardiac surgery

J. R. Leslie Hamilton

Introduction

In the United Kingdom, our specialty is cardiothoracic surgery and in the past surgeons did both cardiac and thoracic surgery, often on the same operating list. With increasing subspecialization, the practice of consultant surgeons is separating into cardiac and thoracic surgery; training is still undertaken jointly but during the later phase of their training, trainees are concentrating on one or the other.

This chapter relates to cardiac surgery and encompasses surgery on the heart and ascending aorta. It does not include surgery on the descending aorta (part of vascular surgery) or discussion of congenital heart defects (this is a topic in its own right and is beyond the scope of this textbook), even though the first operations in the 1950s in cardiac surgery were undertaken on patients with congenital heart defects (see 'Historical background').

Historical background

In the mid 1940s, a paediatrician, Helen Taussig, was faced with a child with tetralogy of Fallot (one of the commonest cyanotic congenital heart defects in which there is reduced blood flow to the lungs). She persuaded a surgeon (Alfred Blalock) to create a shunt by anastomosing the left subclavian artery to the left pulmonary artery. Their report of three cases of Blalock–Taussig shunts was a landmark in our specialty and heralded the beginning of the modern era of cardiac surgery.

In the early 1950s, a number of surgeons undertook closure of atrial septal defects using a technique known as hypothermia and in-flow occlusion; the patient would be anaesthetized, placed in a bath of iced water, and cooled to about 30°C. Then, using a short period where the superior and inferior vena cava were clamped, the surgeon would open the atrium and close an atrial septal defect.

The most important advance occurred in 1953 when John Gibbon used a heart–lung machine (cardiopulmonary bypass) to maintain the circulation while he closed successfully an atrial septal defect. This represented about 30 years of dedicated research by him. The 1950s and 1960s saw a huge explosion of interest in open heart surgery using cardiopulmonary bypass to allow access to the inside of the heart to repair congenital defects.

In 1961, Albert Starr successfully replaced a mitral valve using an artificial prosthesis (Starr–Edwards valve, a ball bearing in a cage). Another leap forward was in 1967, when Rene Favaloro constructed a coronary artery bypass graft (CABG) using a segment of long saphenous vein. However, the main focus at this time was on valve surgery because of the residual effects of rheumatic fever and

in 1971, Alain Carpentier used a pig's aortic valve mounted on a frame (the tissues strengthened by treatment with glutaraldehyde) as a bioprosthesis.

Surgical access

The chest may be opened in a number of ways:

Median sternotomy

The typical route where the sternum is divided down the middle using an oscillating saw. It is very important to stay in the midline of the sternum as deviating to one side will leave little bone to allow closure at the end of the operation with the sternal wires.

Mini-sternotomy

An increasing number of surgeons are using a limited upper sternotomy to perform an aortic valve replacement.

Thoracotomy

A left thoracotomy may be used for operations on the descending aorta or in an emergency to get at the pericardium—it is important not to go too low as the diaphragm comes up quite high. A right thoracotomy can be used for access to the mitral valve (the left atrium is at the back of the heart). Cardiopulmonary bypass is established using cannulation of the femoral artery and vein.

Clam shell

A submammary incision is created on either side in the fourth or fifth intercostal space and joined across the midpoint of the sternum. Typically used for bilateral lung transplantation in patients with intrathoracic adhesions.

Port access/minimally invasive surgery

Increasingly used in modern practice for access to the mitral valve. Ports are placed for thoracoscopic instruments on the right side of the chest and cardiopulmonary bypass is achieved using the femoral artery and vein access.

Cardiopulmonary bypass

A technique in which a machine does the work of the heart and lungs. Essentially the oxygenated blood is removed from the right atrium, drained back to the bypass machine, passed through an artificial lung (to allow gas exchange to take place), then a heater-cooler, and then pumped back into the arterial circulation, usually via a cannula in the ascending aorta.

Venous drainage

If the heart does not have to be opened (e.g. in CABG surgery), the venous blood is drained by a single cannula placed in the right atrium—traditionally a two-stage cannula with the tip in the inferior vena cava and the upper drainage holes in the right atrium itself. If the proposed operation requires access to the inside of the heart, separate cannulae are placed directly into the superior and inferior vena cavae and a tape is placed around the vena cava and pulled tight onto the cannula, so taking all the venous return directly back to the machine.

Arterial return

This is typically through a cannula in the ascending aorta just before the origin of the innominate artery. Alternative sites are the femoral, the right axillary or even the carotid arteries.

Hypothermia

The bypass circuit delivers non-pulsatile flow in contrast to the natural pulsatile flow delivered by the heart. To allow for this and also allow for a margin of safety in case of problems with the circuit, many surgeons will cool the patient using the heat exchanger in the bypass circuit—typically to 34°C, 32°C, or even 28°C.

Myocardial protection

To operate successfully, the surgeon needs a still, bloodless operating field. To achieve this the surgeon places a clamp on the ascending aorta proximal to the aortic cannulation site and gives an injection of cardioplegia (a cold solution of either crystalloid or blood containing potassium) into the aortic root, which puts the heart into asystole. The combination of lack of myocardial activity and hypothermia gives 'myocardial protection'; some would say, more properly regarded as damage limitation. For CABG procedures, an alternative is to induce ventricular fibrillation (to give a relatively still operating field). The short period of ischaemia needed to construct the coronary anastomosis (8–15 minutes) is well tolerated.

Special circumstances

Re-do surgery

Because the heart may be stuck to the back of the sternum by adhesions, the surgeon may wish to place the patient on cardiopulmonary bypass before opening the chest. The venous drainage cannula can be placed in the femoral vein (usually by direct exposure of the vessel and the Seldinger technique) with arterial return through a cannula into the femoral artery via the same cut-down site.

Deep hypothermia and circulatory arrest

In certain circumstances the surgeon may wish to stop the circulation. For example, the surgeon may need to expose the aortic arch and use an open anastomosis technique to place a graft. If the patient's temperature is sufficiently low then no circulation is necessary (similar to the situation when a patient is found in snow or cold water). The patient would be cooled on bypass to 18°C and at this temperature the circulation may be stopped for up to 30 minutes. In this situation, some surgeons prefer to use cerebral perfusion via a cannula in the carotid artery.

'Off-pump' surgery (CABG)

It is recognized that cardiopulmonary bypass induces a 'total body inflammatory response' which in some patients can cause significant problems. A lot of work has been done in recent years to develop ways to allow the surgeon to operate on the surface of the beating heart (the coronary arteries run on the epicardial surface). By careful positioning of the heart and using stabilizers it is possible to isolate the portion of the coronary artery to allow construction of a graft; small shunts are placed in the lumen of the open artery to expose it and limit bleeding. It was generally expected that avoiding bypass would bring significant benefits but randomized studies have not been convincing. There is evidence that fewer grafts are performed in 'off-pump' cases. At present in the United Kingdom, 15–20% of CABG cases are done 'off pump' with some enthusiasts doing almost 100% and others using it in selected cases.

Preoperative assessment

Fitness for surgery

This is aimed at addressing the fitness of the patient for surgery/anaesthesia by identifying co-morbidities. Typical co-morbidities in patients with cardiac disease are:

- chronic obstructive pulmonary disease/emphysema
- diabetes
- renal disease
- carotid disease—past history of stroke/transient ischaemic attack (carotid Doppler studies are performed)
- peripheral vascular disease—limb ischaemia and bowel ischaemia are rare but significant postoperative complications
- obesity—increases the risk of respiratory complications and sternal wound dehiscence.

In patients undergoing CABG, assessment also includes the conduit for grafting: long saphenous vein, short saphenous vein, or radial artery.

Risk stratification

Monitoring an individual surgeon's/team's performance by looking at patient outcomes after surgery (in every surgical specialty) is an important part of modern practice. As professionals we owe it to our patients. To do this in a fair manner, some form of risk stratification is needed. The most widely used one is 'EuroSCORE' (http://www.euroscore.org) although the Americans have developed the 'STS score'. The EuroSCORE is calculated by allocating points for both patient- and operation-related factors and a predicted mortality can be calculated. Thus performance can be plotted as expected versus observed mortality.

Postoperative care

Cardiac surgery is a major insult to the body's physiological homeostasis. This is especially so with the increasing age profile of patients who have associated co-morbidities. Traditionally the patients are nursed in an intensive care unit with a 1:1 ratio of nurse to patient. Rather than reverse the anaesthesia at the end of the procedure as in other surgical specialties, the anaesthetic is allowed to wear off gradually (typically 3–4 hours) and so the patient is ventilated during this time.

Following cardiac surgery we want to know how well the heart is working and that it is pumping the appropriate amount of blood around the body. Cardiac output can be measured (see 'Cardiac output') but this is invasive and usually we monitor the progress of the patient with other surrogate measures of cardiac output; no one parameter is specific but when put together like a jigsaw, a picture is obtained. The following parameters are monitored:

Monitoring

Heart rate/electrocardiogram

Cardiac output is heart rate × stroke volume (the volume of blood pumped out with each beat) and so control of heart rate is important. Chronotropic drugs can be used to increase or decrease heart rate. Additionally a patient will have temporary pacing wires placed on the right ventricle +/− right atrium to allow control of heart rate including any episodes of complete heart block. Atrial fibrillation occurs in up to 30% of patients in the early postoperative period.

Blood pressure

Usually via an arterial line in the radial artery (or femoral artery). It must be remembered that blood pressure is cardiac output × peripheral resistance and therefore a normal blood pressure does not necessarily indicate a normal cardiac output.

Peripheral resistance (systemic vascular resistance)

In a stable patient, this is assessed clinically by feeling the peripheral temperature in the hands and feet and looking at capillary return. In an ill patient, it can be calculated using a Swan–Ganz catheter (see 'Cardiac output').

Right atrial pressure/central venous pressure

Stroke volume depends on pre-load and the pre-load of the right ventricle is easily measured using a central venous catheter via the internal jugular vein in the superior vena cava/right atrium.

Left atrial pressure

If there are specific concerns about the left ventricular function then a direct left atrial line may be placed to the right superior pulmonary vein to give a direct left atrial pressure. However, there is a risk of bleeding when this is removed.

Urinary output

The kidneys are very sensitive to blood pressure and cardiac output and so a normal urinary output (minimum of 1 mL/kg/h) is reassuring.

Cardiac output

A long flotation catheter (Swan–Ganz) is placed via a sheath in the right internal jugular vein. It is passed into the right atrium and then via the tricuspid valve into the right ventricle. A balloon at the tip is inflated and the flow usually directs this through the pulmonary valve and out into the pulmonary artery. With the balloon inflated and occluding the distal pulmonary artery, a pressure monitor at the tip will give an indication of left atrial pressure (pulmonary artery wedge pressure), with the balloon wedged in the pulmonary artery. The cardiac output can be measured using a thermodilution technique. A bolus of ice-cold saline is injected through a port in the catheter in the right atrium and the computer calculates the cardiac output by assessing the time taken for the cold bolus to reach the tip of the catheter in the distal pulmonary artery. From these calculations the peripheral resistance can be calculated (systemic vascular resistance).

Intra-aortic balloon pump

In patients with impaired left ventricular function, the circulation can be assisted by a balloon catheter placed in the femoral artery and positioned in the descending thoracic aorta just beyond the left subclavian artery. The balloon inflation is triggered by the electrocardiogram to inflate in diastole. Blood is forced backwards into the coronary arteries in diastole improving coronary perfusion and distally into the peripheral circulation thus reducing systemic vascular resistance and so the work of the heart.

Tamponade

In the early postoperative period, bleeding can cause compression of the heart thus reducing the cardiac output; typical signs are a falling blood pressure, reducing urinary output, and a rising central venous pressure. This may occur gradually in which case there is time to take the patient back to theatre. Alternatively it may occur acutely with a sudden bleed requiring opening of the chest in the intensive care unit.

Coronary artery disease

Coronary artery anatomy

Anatomically there are two coronary arteries:

- *The right coronary artery*: arises from the anterior/right coronary sinus and passes in the groove between the right atrium and right ventricle onto the inferior surface of the heart where it gives its *posterior descending branch* (and sometimes a significant branch to the back of the left ventricle).

- *The left coronary artery*: arises from the left posterior sinus of the aorta and the first portion (the *left main stem*) passes behind the pulmonary artery. It then bifurcates. The *left anterior descending coronary artery (LAD)* emerges on the left border of the main pulmonary artery and passes in the anterior groove between right ventricle and left ventricle. It gives *diagonal branches* to the anterior wall of the left ventricle. The *circumflex coronary artery (Cx)* passes posterior in the groove between left atrium and left ventricle and gives *obtuse marginal branches* to the lateral wall of the left ventricle.

Investigations

Coronary angiography

The traditional investigation for patients with coronary disease. A catheter is passed via the radial or femoral artery and is positioned at the origin of each artery and contrast medium injected. Lesions are assessed visually (remembering that three-dimensional lesions are being assessed in two dimensions). Anything more than 70% narrowing is taken to be significant. Coronary lesions can be assessed more accurately using intravascular ultrasound or fractional flow reserve (FFR: a small transducer wire is passed into the coronary artery and into the lesion and the pressure drop assessed on pullback). Computed tomography (CT) coronary angiography with multislice fast scanners is now possible and is being used as a screening tool—a 'calcium score' is calculated.

Left ventricular function

Impaired left ventricular function is an important risk factor for surgery. It is typically assessed using ejection fraction on echocardiography—more than 50% is regarded as normal. However, it can also be assessed using a left ventricular angiogram, isotope myocardial perfusion scanning, or magnetic resonance imaging.

Revascularization

Indications

Flow-limiting lesions in the coronary arteries typically cause angina though there is no relationship between the degree of disease and the severity of symptoms. Improving blood flow to the myocardium relieves angina but in some cases also improves prognosis. In 2010, the European Association for Cardiothoracic Surgery (EACTS) and the European Society of Cardiology (ESC) produced joint guidelines on all aspects of myocardial revascularization (see 'Further reading').

Syntax trial

One of the major drivers for these guidelines was the landmark Syntax trial, a real-life, randomized study in patients with three-vessel disease (including left main stem lesions). Patients were considered by cardiologists and a surgeon and, if felt suitable for both methods of revascularization, were randomized. Those patients felt to be unsuitable for one or the other were placed in a Registry. As time goes on, the survival curves are increasingly separating in favour of surgery. See 'Further reading' for more details.

Procedures

Coronary artery bypass grafts

Throughout the 1970s and 1980s this operation achieved widespread acceptance and was the most commonly performed surgical procedure throughout the world. In essence, conduits are used to bypass obstructive lesions in the coronary arteries (identified by coronary angiography).

Conduit for grafting

The original graft was a portion of reversed *long saphenous vein* and this has been the mainstay of treatment over the years. The vein is harvested through a long incision directly over the vein (starting at the medial aspect of the ankle), but many patients have problems with wound healing and discomfort. A technique has been developed which uses an endoscopic system but there is some concern about damage to the vein using this technique.

Vein grafts are prone to occlusion and it is estimated that approximately 50% of grafts will be occluded by 10 years postoperatively. The major change in approach came in the 1970s following work at the Cleveland Clinic, Cleveland, Ohio, USA using the *left internal mammary artery* (LIMA), a branch of the left subclavian artery, to graft the left anterior descending artery. Studies showed that it gave longer patency and increased patient survival. This prompted interest in other arterial grafts and surgeons have used the right internal mammary artery or the *radial artery*. It should be noted that the mammary arteries are elastic in character whereas the radial arteries are muscular arteries and are prone to spasm.

Percutaneous coronary intervention

Over the last two decades cardiologists have performed an increasing number of coronary angioplasties (percutaneous coronary intervention: PCI). The cardiologists, as the ones who undertake the investigations, are the gatekeepers. There has been concern about the appropriateness of the rapidly increasing numbers of PCIs.

Valve surgery

The Joint Task Force on the Management of Valvular Heart Disease of the ESC and EACTS produced guidelines in 2012 which provide a comprehensive review of valve disease (see 'Further reading').

Aortic valve replacement

Aortic stenosis

Aortic stenosis is seen with increasing prevalence with increasing age. Many patients have congenitally bicuspid aortic valves and so tend to present earlier. The indications for surgery are symptoms (shortness of breath, syncope, angina) in the presence of echocardiographically estimated severe aortic stenosis (peak velocity > 4 m/s; mean gradient > 40 mmHg; area < 1 cm^2).

Transcatheter aortic valve implantation (TAVI)

Cardiologists have developed a technique of crimping a tissue valve onto a balloon catheter which can be passed via the femoral artery or via the left ventricular apex and positioned inside the native aortic valve. Despite heavy calcification (most surgeons predicted this would never work), the valve can then be expanded (some are self-expanding, some are balloon expanded) and are held in position by the radial force.

Aortic regurgitation

The indication for surgery is symptoms (shortness of breath on exertion) and the onset of impairment of left ventricular function or a dilating left ventricle (see guidelines in Further reading').

Mitral valve surgery

As rheumatic fever has disappeared, it is rare to find patients with rheumatic mitral valve stenosis. The vast majority of patients presenting with mitral valve disease in current practice have regurgitation due to degeneration of their own mitral valve. There is good evidence to show that left ventricular function is better preserved if the patient's own mitral valve can be repaired rather than a rigid prosthesis placed in the annulus. There is a range of techniques used in mitral valve repair and this has become a subspecialist area—one measure of the quality of care in a unit is the mitral valve repair rate. Intraoperative repair is guided and assessed by transoesophageal echocardiography.

Port access

As noted earlier, some surgeons are increasingly developing a minimal access technique for carrying out mitral valve repair.

Percutaneous catheter-based repair

One repair technique which most surgeons predicted would never work is the Alfieri 'edge-to-edge' technique. He simply stitched the middle of each cusp together creating a dual orifice valve which cured the regurgitation. Cardiologists have now developed a percutaneous technique to mimic this, the MitraClip®.

Prosthetic valves

Although a small number of surgeons use human valves (homografts), prosthetic valves essentially fall into two groups: bioprostheses and mechanical prostheses.

Bioprostheses

The original valve was a pig's aortic valve mounted on a stent. In current practice there are also valves constructed out of bovine pericardium fashioned around a stent/frame (Figure 2.8.1.1). Tissue valves have the big advantage that they do not require formal anticoagulation (a small dose of aspirin is sufficient) but have the disadvantage that they do wear out in time. As each valve is a unique biological construct, the long-term function of each valve cannot be

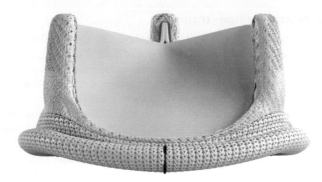

Fig. 2.8.1.1 Carpentier–Edwards PERIMOUNT Magna Ease® aortic heart valve.
Image Copyright © Edwards Lifesciences. Reproduced with permission.

predicted. The current generation of valves appear to last an average of 15 years in patients over 70 years of age. Re-replacement in the future should be possible by transcatheter aortic valve implantation (see earlier section).

Mechanical prostheses

The original Starr–Edwards valve was a ball bearing in a cage but the current generation are bi-leaflet valves constructed of a very hard carbon material (Figure 2.8.1.2). The main advantage is that they do not wear out and so it is rare for the patient to require further surgery (on rare occasions tissue may grow into and obstruct the orifice). The main disadvantage is that they require formal anticoagulation—at present with warfarin with all its attentive problems; it may be possible in future to use the new generation of antithrombin anticoagulants, which do not require monitoring. In addition, these valves make a soft clicking sound during function, which can be off-putting to some patients.

Aortic surgery

Ascending aorta

Patients with long-term hypertension or more commonly patients with connective tissue disorder can develop aneurysms of the ascending aorta. If the aortic valve annulus is dilated, this will induce aortic regurgitation. The indication for surgery is an ascending aortic diameter of greater than 5.5 cm in patients with hypertension and 5 cm in patients with connective tissue (Marfan's/Erhlos–Danlos syndrome). In some patients, it is only the ascending aorta,

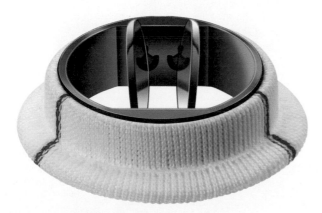

Fig. 2.8.1.2 Sorin Carbomedics Top Hat® aortic valve.
Image Copyright © Sorin Group. Reproduced with permission.

which has to be replaced, but some (with aortic regurgitation) require replacement of the aortic root using a composite prosthesis with a valve *in situ*, which requires re-implantation of the coronary arteries.

Descending aorta

Aneurysms of the descending aorta are typically due to degenerative disease and are more the area of expertise of the vascular surgeon.

Heart failure

As our population ages, more and more patients are presenting with heart failure unresponsive to medical therapy. The options are as follows.

Surgery

Some operations have been developed to excise part of the dilated left ventricle thus restoring normal geometry (the Dor procedure/Batista) but these have not achieved widespread popularity.

Heart transplantation

This is the mainstay of surgical treatment for end-stage heart failure. However, the number of donors is limited and indeed has decreased markedly in recent years (due to the change in management of severe head injuries and increasingly safe motor vehicles). In adults, the 50% survival in patients following heart transplantation is approximately 12–14 years. Patients require lifelong antirejection therapy, which has side effects of hypertension, renal failure, and malignancy.

Left ventricular assist devices

Originally introduced as a 'bridge to transplantation'. Technology has developed to such an extent that they are becoming a destination therapy. A number of models are available based on continuous flow by an axial pump placed in the apex of the left ventricle with a graft to the ascending aorta. The main complications are thromboembolism and infection (related to the percutaneous driveline). As technology improves, the thromboembolic rate will get less and ultimately a transcutaneous power source will eliminate the need for a percutaneous driveline/electrical source.

Total artificial heart

Most patients have left ventricular failure but a small number will require replacement of both. Until recently these had an element of science fiction but a number of models are being trialled at present.

Pericardium

The pericardium is a tough sac totally enclosing the heart. It is important in two situations in cardiac surgery:

◆ *Tamponade*: if fluid collects it will compress the heart (especially the right side) thus limiting venous return and so cardiac output. This can be chronic (usually relieved by a thoracic surgeon using a thoracoscopic technique) or acute due to bleeding after cardiac surgery.

◆ *Constrictive pericarditis*: an inflammatory process (in the past caused by tuberculosis) in which the pericardium infiltrates into the heart, compressing it and restricting pulmonary and systemic venous return. It is difficult to diagnose and the surgery (removal of as much of the pericardium as possible) is challenging.

Emergencies

Most emergencies in cardiac surgery relate to acute postoperative problems with bleeding (requiring emergency re-opening in the intensive care unit) or ischaemia (requiring urgent coronary angiography). However there are a number of specific circumstances.

Post-infarction ventricular septal defect

A situation where a myocardial infarction affects the interventricular septum and a ventricular septal defect typically occurs a week to 10 days following the acute infarct. Now that ST-segment elevation myocardial infarctions are treated using primary angioplasty, this is a rarely seen complication. Surgery involves an incision through the infarcted area of muscle in the left ventricle and a patch on the ventricular septal defect. As the muscle is very oedematous and friable, mortality is high.

Acute mitral regurgitation

(Due to rupture of the mitral valve chordae.) Severe mitral regurgitation leads to pulmonary oedema and requires emergency mitral valve replacement.

Endocarditis

Infection on a heart valve is a rare, but serious event. It can affect either the native valve (usually left sided) or a prosthetic valve. Approximately 50% of patients who develop endocarditis will require surgery; the indications are heart failure, failure to control infection, and neurological events (emboli).

Aortic dissection

Related to hypertension or connective tissue disorders, although ideally patients with connective tissue disorders will be monitored and have surgery prophylactically. It is a true emergency with a high mortality in the first few hours. Dissection typically begins in the ascending aorta (type A dissection) and extends a variable distance through the arch and descending aorta and often into the femoral arteries. The aim of surgery is to replace the torn segment in the ascending aorta and surgery carries a significant mortality (up to 30%) and a risk of neurological injury. Type B dissections affect the descending aorta and in general are treated medically.

Aortic transection (trauma)

In trauma resulting in rapid deceleration, the aorta is flexed forwards at a point just beyond the origin of the left subclavian artery. This may result in a circumferential tear leaving only the adventitia holding the aorta together; many rupture completely, but some survive to reach hospital. Diagnosis is by thinking of the mode of injury (so considering the diagnosis) and then by CT scan. Treatment in the past was by open surgery (with or without cardiopulmonary bypass). Most of these patients have multiple injuries (especially head) and so are best managed by an interventional radiologist with an intravascular stent.

Pulmonary embolism

The initial treatment for a major pulmonary embolism causing haemodynamic instability is thrombolytic therapy. Failure of or contraindications to thrombolytic therapy are indications for surgery. Many patients have underlying medical problems (e.g. malignancy), which promote formation of venous thrombosis.

Emergencies from the catheter laboratory

In the past we saw problems with perforation or dissection of coronary arteries or tamponade due to perforation of the ventricular wall. However, these complications are now rare as cardiologists can usually seal perforations using a transcatheter technique.

Further reading

Chikwe J, Cooke D, Weiss A. *Cardiothoracic Surgery* (2nd ed). Oxford: Oxford University Press; 2013.
Kaiser LR, Kron IL, Spray TL (eds). *Mastery of Cardiothoracic Surgery* (3rd ed). Philadelphia, PA: Lippincott Williams and Wilkins; 2013.

Guidelines on myocardial revascularization

Mohr FW, Morice MC, Kappetein AP, *et al*. Coronary artery bypass graft surgery versus percutaneous coronary intervention in patients with three-vessel disease and left main coronary disease: 5-year follow-up of the randomised, clinical SYNTAX trial. *Lancet* 2013; 381:629–38.
The Joint Task Force on the Management of Valvular Heart Disease of the European Society of Cardiology (ESC) and the European Association for Cardiothoracic Surgery, Guidelines on the Management of Valvular Heart Disease (2012). *Eur J Cardiothorac Surg* 2012; 42:S1–44. http://ejcts.oxfordjournals.org/content/early/2012/08/21/ejcts.ezs455.extract
The Task Force on Myocardial Revascularization of the European Society of Cardiology (ESC) and the European Association for Cardio-Thoracic Surgery (EACTS). *Eur J Cardiothorac Surg* 2010; 38:S1–52.

Pulmonary surgery

Sasha Stamenkovic

History

Hippocrates is recorded as performing the first chest drainage for pleural infection. Since then, chest surgery largely was confined to operations for parapneumonic infections and war injuries. In the twentieth century, thoracic surgery continued to evolve as the treatment of tuberculosis (TB), and with parallel advances in anaesthesia in between the world wars, was in the domain of general surgeons who were starting to develop a specialist interest in the chest. With the advent of antituberculous drugs, thoracic surgeons used the inventions of double-lumen intubation and positive-pressure ventilation to manage patients with lung cancer. The first pneumonectomy for bronchogenic lung cancer was performed in 1933 and since then the surgical goal has been complete clearance of cancer with as much lung preservation as possible. The result is a decrease in pneumonectomies over the last 20 years and the increase of smaller lung resections.

Thoracic surgeons manage patients with many conditions other than lung cancer, and the spectrum of operations is from tracheal resection for post-tracheostomy stenosis to chest wall reconstruction for cosmetic reasons. There is a move, as with many other specialties, to embrace minimally invasive techniques for more and more thoracic operations and this is even more meaningful for chest surgery, as these techniques aim to reduce potentially the worst pain a surgeon can cause.

Reasons for resection

Diagnostic operations

Histology is taken to inform the relevant team and to ensure the patient follows the correct therapeutic pathway. Often this is done after less invasive biopsies and non-diagnostic results.

Treatment operations

Treatment may be undertaken for a number of reasons:

- Curative intent: to remove cancer or infection
- Debulking: with adjuvant chemotherapy and/or radiotherapy
- Damage limitation in the case of trauma
- Palliative: for treatment of pain, temperature, and breathlessness
- Transplantation.

Chest imaging is necessary for planning. Operations in the chest are performed either with an open or video-assisted thoracoscopic surgery (VATS) technique. More and more operations are being done by VATS.

Types of resection

- Wedge resection: this is removal of the smallest amount of lung including tumour with good clearance
- Segmentectomy: anatomical dissection of an anatomical segment of a lobe, separating bronchus, artery, and vein
- Lobectomy: anatomical resection of a whole lobe
- Sleeve lobectomy: anatomical resection of whole lobe including a portion of the major airway to the lobar bronchus, with anastomosis of the two ends
- Pneumonectomy: resection of whole lung.

Imaging

Chest X-ray, computed tomography (CT) chest, CT head, positron emission tomography (PET)-CT, ventilation/perfusion (V/Q), and magnetic resonance imaging (MRI) scans can all be useful.

Chest X-ray

Chest X-ray is the simplest imaging technique, allowing the distinction of air versus bone and soft tissue shadows.

- *Posterior-anterior film* (PA): film immediately in front of the patient, camera behind. These are taken in the X-ray department and used for ambulant patients. The scapulae should be out of the way (raised arms). The lung edges and vascular shadows can be interpreted.
- *Anterior-posterior film* (AP): film behind and camera in front. These are used for bed-bound patients. There is magnification of the mediastinum, making it difficult to interpret aortic size and cardiomegaly.
- The horizontal fissure is visible on PA or AP films.
- Areas are labelled in zones: upper, mid, and lower. The reason for this is that it is often difficult to identify which lobe a lesion is in—the apex of lower lobe is actually quite high and the middle lobe/lingula can touch the diaphragm.
- *Lateral chest X-ray*: the oblique and horizontal fissures, the relative heights of the hemi-diaphragms, and the actual lobes can be seen. It is, therefore, possible to determine which lobe a lesion sits in. This modality has been largely superseded by other more modern imaging techniques.

CT chest scan

CT chest scans give a lot more information than chest X-rays.

Axial views are commonest, with 'slices' made through the body. Other options include CT chest/abdomen, high-resolution CT, and CT pulmonary angiogram (CTPA) Mediastinal windows show contrast in vascular structures against grey areas of non-contrast (e.g. lymph nodes (LNs)). Lung windows show which lobe the abnormality is in and show disease (e.g. bullous emphysema or fibrosis).

CT head

This is performed to stage cancer.

Some metastases may be asymptomatic. Symptomatic patients with negative CT head should have an MRI head scan.

Positron emission tomography (PET and PET-CT fusion scanning)

These are performed if radical cancer treatment (surgery or radical radiotherapy) is planned. The superimposition of CT onto the PET scan gives functional information.

In PET scans, glucose isomer is taken up by metabolizing tissue, resulting in hot spots.

The amount of 'heat' is graded and given in a systemic uptake value (SUV). The higher the SUV, the more likely the lesion is to be cancerous, but exceptions exist (e.g. slowly growing tumours, abscesses, and granulomata). In LNs, a higher SUV is likely to be malignant, with the same exceptions.

Ventilation/perfusion scan

This used to be the gold standard to diagnose pulmonary embolism, but now CTPA is used instead. V/Q scans are performed to aid understanding of the lung function. Most scans are Q scans—how much blood (perfusion) to which part of the lungs—which helps the surgeon to determine if the patient will manage with one lung deflated. These scans also help to determine if lung resection possible.

Nuclear magnetic resonance imaging

This is used to examine soft tissues, often at the peripheries of the chest, for example, a mass close to vertebrae (MRI to show relation with spinal cord) or a lesion at apex of chest (MRI to show brachial plexus involvement).

Preoperative work-up

This should include the following:

◆ Stage—imaging gives clinical stage of lung cancers (cTNM):
  • T defines tumour size and fixity; N shows type of lymph node involvement; M, metastasis.
◆ Fitness—assessed by lung function testing:
  • Forced expiratory volume in 1 second:
    • Gives idea of postoperative ability to cough
    • Used to predict postoperative breathlessness
  • Total lung carbon monoxide transfer—more accurate to assess risk of resection
  • 6-minute walk test—assesses level of deconditioning and desaturation
  • Arterial blood gases on air, pO_2/pCO_2
  • Cardiopulmonary exercise test—test VO_2 max and anaerobic threshold

◆ Resectability: is the mass attached to vital structures—T4 does not mean irresectable
◆ Preassessment clinic (PAC): to allow anaesthetist review of patient.

Enhanced recovery

Enhanced recovery relies on the following components:

◆ PAC is done before admission, permitting assessment of risk, further investigations, optimization of chronic illnesses (diabetes), cessation of drugs (antiplatelets/anticoagulants), planning for difficult airway, epidural, etc.
◆ Physiotherapy exercise information is given
◆ A planned day of surgery admission (DOSA) is arranged
◆ Carbohydrate loading is organized
◆ Nil-by-mouth/intravenous fluid management is organized.

Anaesthetic room preparation

Preparation includes the following steps:

◆ Premedication is not routine, especially if DOSA
◆ Operating department professional accepts patient and prepares equipment
◆ World Health Organization surgical safety checklist
◆ Preoxygenation, rigid bronchoscopy is often performed.
◆ Intubation—double-lumen tube or single tube with bronchial blocker. The desired effect is to deflate the operated side and ventilate the non-operated side
◆ Arterial/central venous lines, bispectral index (cerebral monitoring), urinary catheter
◆ Positioning—commonly lateral position, rubber wedges are used to prevent pressure area damage. A break in in the table maximizes rib separation, and therefore minimizes pain from operation
◆ Intercostal block, paravertebral or epidural catheter
◆ Application of diathermy plate and body warming.

Theatre preparation

This should include the following:

◆ Lighting, suction, and diathermy connection
◆ Imaging on display
◆ Exposure—depends on whether emergency or elective. Emergency operations may be for salvage, in which case optimal positioning may not be possible. To minimize difficulty with the operation and complications to the patient, positioning the patient correctly is vital. For thoracic surgery, this needs a degree of imagination as there are several axes of view into the chest (chest X-ray, CT, bronchoscopic, transcervical, anterior/posterior VATS, robotic).

Surgical anatomy

A review of current imaging will show the height of the diaphragm, enabling the correct incision to be made into the chest.

Choosing the correct rib space and making the incision in the correct obliquity will allow an easier operation. Upper lobectomies require a 'hockey-stick' incision to permit access to the upper hilum. Lower lobectomies can be achieved through a more horizontal incision.

Anterior rib spaces are wider than posterior ones and therefore in a VATS operation, the anterior space is used as the utility port to remove lobes.

Apical tumours may be approached by an incision that runs more posteriorly and cranially.

VATS operations also require careful planning, as all operating will have to be performed through ports, and no rib spreading will be possible to gain more exposure.

The oblique and horizontal fissures are key anatomical landmarks to find to make identification of different lobes of the lung possible.

The anatomy of the lung hila follows a pattern. The anatomy of the pulmonary veins is mostly constant, whereas that of the pulmonary artery branches is variable. The inferior vein and the vagus nerve are at the posterior hilum and the superior veins and phrenic nerve are at the anterior hilum, on both sides. On the right, cranial to the inferior vein, is the intermediate bronchus, then continuing in a clockwise direction is the right main bronchus with the azygous vein arching around it, then the truncus branch of the pulmonary artery overlapped by the upper lobe vein at the anterior hilum, and the middle lobe vein most inferiorly. On the left, cranial to the inferior vein, is the left main bronchus, then continuing in a anti-clockwise direction is the left pulmonary artery with the aorta arching around it, and at the anterior hilum is the upper lobe vein and at the lingular vein.

There is a condensation of pleura attaching lung to diaphragm, known as the inferior pulmonary ligament, which when stripped cranially reveals a LN (number 9) and then the inferior vein, and so is often the starting point of any pulmonary surgery. Stripping this after an upper lobectomy also allows the lower lobe to ascend in the chest during re-inflation. The heads of the ribs are visible posteriorly and the sympathetic trunk can be seen descending on each of these. The internal thoracic artery is seen anteriorly on the chest wall just lateral to the edge of the sternum. Apically the pulsation of the subclavian artery is visible which helps to delineate the outline of the first rib.

Open versus video-assisted thoracoscopic surgery

Open operations allow a hands-on and hands-in approach. Tactile feedback permits knowledge of how thin/thick tissues are, finger-and-thumb circumnavigation around structures, easy retraction of lobes, and arguably quicker dissection as a result.

However, open operations necessarily mean significant rib spreading, which can result in worse and longer-standing neuropraxic injury, due to compression of the intercostal nerve. They can only afford the view under the incision, and shadows can be cast even with the use of a head-light. It takes longer to open and close an incision from an open operation.

VATS operations can give a 360°, magnified, high definition well-illuminated view of the chest internally. There is no rib spreading, so this minimizes the possibility of neuropraxic injury. It is quick to open and close port incisions. An operation started as VATS (video-assisted thoracoscopic assessment) allows the finding of surprise features that have not been seen on prior imaging, preventing unnecessary and potentially damaging exploratory thoracotomies (open-close), for example, pleural metastases or tumour too close to the hilum for permitted resection. VATS allow planning of subsequent thoracotomy in cases of chest wall resection.

VATS operations reduce the amount of tactile feedback in that only a finger can be placed into the chest. Small nodules and those more centrally in a lobe are therefore more difficult to find by VATS. No finger-and-thumb circumnavigation is possible.

VATS instruments are longer as they are used through the fulcrum of the ports, so there is more movement of the distal end relative to the proximal end—this means more judicious smaller movements are required by the operator's hand. The points of the instruments are needed to be more thought about if not always on-screen, as the potential for collateral damage to other structures is always present. Similarly all metallic conducting surfaces of instruments with diathermy attached have to be kept in full view to prevent inadvertent touching of surrounding tissues.

The precise and delicate nature of VATS operations acts as a challenge to some surgeons and a reward to others, and this probably explains why the majority of thoracic surgeons worldwide perform open operations. This will probably change in the near future due to more home-TV gaming, better technology, and the possible increase in the use of robotic surgery.

Operating kit and strategy

To gain entry into the chest, rib resection is sometimes necessary. After this, a retractor cranks open the ribs to allow a large thoracotomy. Duval forceps hold onto the lung, a 'fish-slice' lung retractor holds back lung, and a swab-on-a-stick holds back other structures. 'Peanut' dissection is done with the use of pledgets (mini-swabs) if tissue planes are thin whereas the use of diathermy and scissors is necessary for fibrous tissues. To go around structures before taping, tying, or stapling, a right-angle Leahy, O'Shaughnessy, or Sem forceps is used. If the plan is anatomical resection of the lung, it is usual to start with hilar dissection and it is advisable to dissect the more proximal tissues first to allow 'proximal control' before turning attention to fissural dissection. There is no difference in strategy for VATS operations.

A whole industry of stapling devices is available to the thoracic surgeon. In open operations, linear staplers with staples either side and a sliding knife are used to divide fissures. Artery and vein branches, if large enough, can be divided with right-angle staplers. These come with staples on one side and require the other side to be tied off before using a knife to divide. The alternative is to double ligate and cut in-between. VATS operations are carried out using laparoscopic devices. The VATS stapling is done with staples either side with a sliding knife between. Stapler articulation is designed to make placement easier. Energy sources such as ultrasound and heat can also be used in both open and VATS operations.

Transplantation

Most lung transplant operations involve removal of a whole lung and anastomosis of a donor lung in its place. However, lobar lung transplantation allows an adult lobe to replace a small adult/child lung.

Single- or double-lung transplantation can be performed on or off cardiopulmonary bypass, depending on the patient's saturations and blood pressure, and also the degree of difficulty.

Worldwide, the majority of lung transplantations are for emphysema, but in the United Kingdom, there is a large population of patients with cystic fibrosis and pulmonary fibrosis. Rarely, this is also performed for primary pulmonary hypertension.

Reasons for difficulty and helpful hints

The commonest reason for a difficult operation is poor preparation. Careful review of the individual patient's investigations and imaging is imperative. The imaging will often show signs of adhesions, or a raised hemidiaphragm, and so it is helpful in the planning of the correct rib space.

Prior medical/surgical and occupational history might predict a lung being stuck. Pleurisy/empyema or previous rib fractures may cause adhesions of the lung to the chest wall including diaphragm. A previous operation means the possible use of another rib space to enter the chest. Miners and stonemasons have exposure to mineral dusts that can lead to adhesions and very fibrotic tissue planes around LNs. Asbestos exposure can lead to asbestos plaques, which may also cause significant adhesions.

In particularly adherent lungs, a posteriorly placed nasogastric tube can help delineate the plane between lung and oesophagus, thus limiting the chance of viscus perforation. Similarly, a fibreoptic bronchoscope can be used to shine down a bronchus to allow easier dissection around it.

Non-surgical issues that affect a successful operation

Tube position is critical to allow a fully deflated lung, but patients' airways differ in width and length and sometimes a double-lumen tube just does not fit as it should. A lot of effort goes into placing and checking the position of the tube in the anaesthetic room, but it may still not be perfect, and the turning of the patient and manipulation of the lung may potentially change the tube position.

Tube herniation can occur. There are two cuffs to a double-lumen tube. One is in the tracheal tube, the other in the distal bronchial tube. The bronchial cuff can herniate to occlude the end of that lumen, resulting in poor ventilation of the contralateral lung, and desaturation as a result.

Pulmonary hypertension can result in right ventricle strain during one-lung-ventilation. This shows in electrocardiogram changes and also a drop in blood pressure. Some anaesthetists use pulmonary vasodilators such as nitric oxide to facilitate a safe operation. Pulmonary hypertension also can cause more bleeding of suture/staple lines.

A factor out of the anaesthetist's control is shunting, that is, good perfusion of a lung that is deflated, resulting in significant desaturation. This often happens in fit patients with good lung function tests, and there is no predictability. It means that one-lung ventilation is not possible and the operation has to be performed with the lung inflated most of the time. The anaesthetist will check the tube position and ensure there is no herniation of the tube cuff reducing ventilation of the contralateral lung, as this also causes significant desaturation.

Systematic lymph node dissection

In cancer cases, systematic nodal dissection (SND) is imperative. Up to the operation, the clinical stage is decided by imaging and biopsies. At operation, the surgeon has the ability to check this stage by looking for metastases in the chest that were not evident before. Once this is ruled out and a successful lung resection has been performed, attention is given to the LNs. A knowledge of drainage patterns is needed to understand why SND is so important.

There is a standard LN map accepted by all lung cancer doctors. Cancer drains from a lobe of a lung into intralobar then interlobar LNs. After this they may drain into hilar LNs and then on into mediastinal LNs. Dissecting all LNs will give an accurate staging and, therefore, the patient will have the correct adjuvant treatments and the correct prognosis.

All LNs are therefore collected and labelled separately. At VATS operations, it is easier to see LNs as they are magnified, and SND is standard practice. In operations where the diagnosis is not known, it is wise to include SND. Similarly, even in patients where anatomical lung resection is not possible due to fitness or other issues, SND is important to do—these patients may not get adjuvant treatments but the prognosis would be clearer.

When LNs are matted or stuck onto structures, it might imply that there is extranodal spread. This might mean a more proximal dissection is required if the patient is sufficiently fit. Calcified LNs implies long-standing presence and often the cause is old TB.

Haemostasis

There is no substitute for careful dissection, as this will minimize the amount of haemostatic manoeuvres required.

If the patient is particularly hypertensive during opening, there will need to be time spent to carefully stop bleeding from subcutaneous and muscle layers. It may be possible for the anaesthetist to lower the blood pressure temporarily. Prolene™ 3/0 is often kept on standby for the scrub nurse to give to the surgeon. This is in case staples have failed or a suture tie has fallen off.

Unipolar diathermy is used to incise tissues and to stop bleeding from a pedicle of tissue. It can be applied to appropriate VATS dissectors also. Solid haemostatic agents with a cellulose polymer are used to pack spaces where there is a low-pressure focal ooze, and syringed or sprayed haemostatic sealants can be used for more diffuse areas.

If a lobectomy is performed, a certain amount of tamponade can be achieved by the lung re-inflating at the end of the procedure. If a pneumonectomy has been performed, it is imperative to ensure that there is no bleeding at all as there is no tamponade effect of the lung. If a rib resection has been performed, then bone-wax can be used to seal the ends and if a rib fracture has occurred during retraction of the thoracotomy, careful closure is required.

Irrigation

This follows a logical process. All irrigation should be with warm solutions to avoid any bradyarrhythmias. If the operation is for cancer, surgeons prefer to use water to act as an osmotic killer of any residual cancer cells. In mesothelioma surgery, some surgeons go one step further, using hyperthermic solutions or chemotherapy irrigations. If the operation is for infection, surgeons will use saline or dilute concentrations of povidone-iodine or tauroline.

After any resection, it is appropriate to test suture/staple lines with positive pressure up to 30 cm water, particularly if there is a bronchial stump, as this allows any repair to be performed immediately, and prevents the unnecessary complication of other-lung contamination.

Drains

After lung resection, other than pneumonectomy, the purpose of draining the hemithorax is to allow lung re-expansion, as well as monitoring pleural fluid/blood loss, and air leak.

There is much written about two versus one drain post resection.

After pneumonectomy, the drain is there to monitor blood loss. It is clamped for the majority of the hour, and unclamped for the last 5 minutes to see how much blood drains. It also acts as a portal for injecting air into the pneumonectomy space if there is gross mediastinal shift.

Surgical analgesia

A paravertebral catheter (PVC) does not involve the epidural space and, therefore, has no hypotensive effects. It may better be termed an extrapleural catheter, as it perfuses this space with regional local anaesthetic to bathe the intercostal nerves. If placed correctly and working well, this offers good analgesia to patients' thoracic and drain wounds. If an extrapleural dissection has been necessary to remove lung or tumour from the chest wall, there is less chance of a PVC working well and alternatives have to be considered (e.g. epidural).

Phrenic nerve block involves a small volume injection of periphrenic tissue and may reduce the amount of referred pain from drains. Intercostal nerve blocks involve an injection of 5 mL of local anaesthetic into the intercostal bundle in the groove of the rib, as much as two rib spaces above and two below the incision, taking care to aspirate to avoid intravascular injection.

Closure

The most important part of closure is to communicate with the scrub nurse to ensure that all instruments, needles, and swabs are accounted for. The break in the table is taken down to facilitate rib approximation. All layers are individually sutured with specific-sized needles to ensure strength of closure. Extra local anaesthetic is sometimes placed into the wounds and drain sites at the end.

Complications

Complications include the following:

- Air leak: the commonest complication (up to 25%)
- Infection: chest greater than urinary greater than wound risk
- Atrial arrhythmias: more common if pericardium dissected
- Acute coronary syndrome: due to latent coronary artery disease
- Stroke
- Venous thromboembolism: vital to check prophylaxis is being given
- Bronchopleural fistula: different to air leak, as that is parenchymal lung leak
- Lobar torsion: commonest is middle lobe after upper lobectomy.

Further reading

British Thoracic Society, Society for Cardiothoracic Surgery in Great Britain and Ireland Lung Cancer Guideline Group. Guidelines on the radical management of lung cancer. *Thorax* 2010; 65 Suppl III:iii1–iii27.

De Wever W, Ceyssens S, Mortelmans L, *et al.* Additional value of PET-CT in the staging of lung cancer: comparison with CT alone, PET alone and visual correlation of PET and CT. *Eur Radiol* 2007; 17:23–32.

Goldstraw P, Ball D, Jett JR, *et al.* Non-small cell lung cancer: *Lancet* 2011; 378:1727–40.

Kim AW, Johnson KM, Detterbeck FC. The lung cancer stage page: there when you need it—staginglungcancer.org. *Chest* 2012; 141:581–6.

Varela G, Jiménez MF, Novoa N, *et al.* Estimating hospital costs attributable to prolonged air leak in pulmonary lobectomy. *Eur J Cardiothorac Surg* 2005; 27:329–33.

PART 2.9

Genitourinary surgery

Sub-section editor: Ian Eardley

CHAPTER 2.9.1

Stones and infections

Benjamin Hughes and Neil Burgess

Stones

Epidemiology

The lifetime risk of developing a urinary tract stone is 10–20% with a peak incidence occurring between the ages of 30 and 50 years. The recurrence rate is approximately 50% over 10 years and the incidence of stone disease is increasing. According to Hospital Episode Statistics the number of UK hospital episodes due to upper urinary tract stones has increased by 63% to 83, 050 per year over the past 10 years.[1] A recent study of more than 5000 patients undergoing non-contrast computerized tomography (CT) found incidental asymptomatic renal stones in approximately 8% of patients.[2]

Stone types and mechanisms of formation

Approximately 80% of stones are composed of calcium oxalate and/ or calcium phosphate; approximately 10% are composed of uric acid; approximately 10% are composed of struvite (magnesium, ammonium, phosphate); and approximately 1% are composed of cystine. Calcium oxalate and cystine stones tend to be hard, pure urate stones tend to be brittle and radio-lucent, whereas struvite stones are soft. Calcium oxalate stones form when the urine becomes supersaturated with calcium and oxalate and natural inhibitors of stone formation such as citrate and magnesium become ineffective. Uric acid is a by-product of purine metabolism; it is insoluble in acidic urine and soluble in alkaline urine.[3]

Struvite stones are formed when certain Gram-negative bacteria in urine split urea into ammonium ions, which raise urine pH and combine with phosphate and magnesium. The usual causative organisms include *Proteus mirabilis*, *Pseudomonas aeruginosa*, and *Klebsiella* species. Cystinuria is an inherited disorder of amino acid transport in the intestine and renal tubule causing high levels of insoluble cystine in the urine of affected patients.

Risk factors

There are several risk factors associated with stone development:

Sex

Males are more likely to be affected, with a male to female preponderance of 2.5 : 1.

Diet

Low fluid intake and high salt and animal protein intake all predispose to stone formation, whereas contrary to popular perception, a restricted dietary calcium intake is not protective.

Environmental conditions

There is a higher incidence of stone disease during the summer months and in those who work in hot conditions.

Medical disease

Hyperparathyroidism and distal renal tubular acidosis cause hypercalciuria and thus calcium stone formation. Hyperoxaluria (primary or enteric) causes oxalate stones, whereas type 2 diabetes mellitus, obesity, and gout predispose to uric acid stones. Chronically infected urine, especially in patients with indwelling catheters or impaired bladder emptying, predisposes to struvite stone formation.

Metabolic investigation

All of the above factors should be considered during the workup of a stone patient. Basic metabolic investigations should include stone analysis (when possible), serum electrolytes including calcium and urate, and mid-stream urine for pH and culture. Recurrent stone formers and those at high risk of stone disease should also have a 24-hour urine collection with analysis for volume, potassium, sodium, calcium, oxalate, phosphate, citrate, uric acid, and cystine.

Renal/ureteric colic

Renal or ureteric colic describes the pain associated with a urinary tract stone causing partial or complete obstruction. It is excruciatingly painful and accounts for approximately 50% of all emergency urological referrals. A stone passing down the ureter causes prostaglandin-mediated smooth muscle spasm, obstruction to urine flow, and urinary tract dilatation. The pain is intermittent and is classically described as 'loin to groin' but can radiate to the genitalia. It is associated with nausea and often vomiting due to the common innervation pathway of the renal pelvis, stomach, and intestines. A patient with renal colic often describes being unable to get comfortable due to pain, whereas in comparison a patient with peritonitis tries to lie still as movement exacerbates peritoneal irritation. At least 90% will have haematuria (visible or non-visible) and the presence of lower urinary tract symptoms such as strangury, urgency, and frequency may indicate a stone in the intramural ureter causing bladder irritation.

Analgesia

The severity of the pain often precludes initial thorough history taking and examination so immediate management should focus on analgesia. Non-steroidal anti-inflammatory drugs have been shown to have better analgesic efficacy than opioids, although combined use is often necessary.[4,5] They induce less vomiting and are best given as a suppository. They reduce ureteric smooth muscle spasm and renal blood flow and reduce glomerular filtration by causing afferent arteriolar vasoconstriction, which reduces the pressure in the pelvi-calyceal system. The use of antispasmodics such as hyoscine butylbromide (Buscopan®, Boehringer Ingelheim) has not been shown to add any analgesic benefit[6] and forced diuresis with intravenous fluids is unnecessary.[7]

Investigations and imaging

Once analgesia has been achieved the patient's history can be more easily obtained and an examination performed. The main differential diagnoses are pyelonephritis, acute appendicitis, cholecystitis, diverticulitis, ectopic pregnancy, and a leaking abdominal aortic aneurysm. A basic metabolic stone screen as described above should be sent, the patient's urine should be dipstick tested to rule out infection and ascertain pregnancy status, and the patient's temperature should be checked. The diagnosis of a urinary tract stone should be determined with a non-contrast CT scan that has a sensitivity and specificity approaching 100%[4,8] for all stone types. Ultrasound remains the investigation of choice in children. Intravenous urograms are almost obsolete. Non-contrast CT avoids the use of intravenous contrast agents and has the advantage of being able to determine the exact stone burden in patients with multiple stones, the presence of upper tract dilatation, and can detect other relevant non-urological pathologies. If a stone is to be managed conservatively then checking if the stone is visible on the scout film of the CT should enable plain kidney, ureter, and bladder (KUB) X-ray to be used for monitoring stone passage without exposing the patient to further CT scans.

Ureteric stone management

The size and location of the stone in the ureter determines the likelihood of it passing spontaneously. A stone less than 4 mm has a greater than 90% chance of passing, whereas a 5 mm to 10 mm stone has an approximately 50% chance of passing. A stone presenting in the lower ureter has a far greater chance of passing than one presenting in the upper ureter.[4,9]

Patients undergoing a trial of conservative management are ideally seen in a urology outpatient clinic within 2 weeks. Unless there is good evidence that the patient has passed their stone (the absence of pain should not be taken as proof of stone passage) they should have further imaging. If a plain KUB X-ray is not conclusive then a stone at the vesico-ureteric junction can sometimes be seen using ultrasound with a full bladder. A limited intravenous urogram can also be useful but often a repeat CT is necessary. Failed conservative therapy warrants intervention, which will be discussed in the section on treatment options for stone disease.

There are certain situations when conservative management of a ureteric stone is not appropriate: These include patients with a solitary kidney or bilateral ureteric stones, patients with refractory pain or evidence of acute kidney injury, and patients with concurrent urinary tract infection (UTI) raising the possibility of a pyonephrosis. Airline pilots and some other professionals are not allowed to work until they are stone free. All of these patients should be discussed with the urology team and are likely to be admitted to hospital for interventions such as primary ureteroscopy or insertion of a ureteric stent or nephrostomy tube.

Pyonephrosis

An obstructed infected kidney is a urological emergency. Patients in whom this is suspected should be promptly referred to the urology team, should be started on broad-spectrum intravenous antibiotics according to local microbiology guidelines, and should be given intravenous fluid resuscitation. Patients with urosepsis refractory to fluid resuscitation should be managed in a critical care facility in conjunction with intensive care physicians. The mainstay of treatment is to relieve the obstruction either by inserting a retrograde ureteric stent in the operating theatre under general anaesthetic or by inserting a nephrostomy tube in the interventional radiology suite under local anaesthetic. The method used to drain an infected obstructed kidney is the source of great debate amongst urologists and radiologists and is dependent on local facilities and expertise. There is limited evidence that one treatment is better than the other and each has its advantages and disadvantages.[10,11]

Treatment options for stone disease

Treatment options for stone disease depend on patient factors (e.g. co-morbidities, obesity, infection, coagulopathies, and pregnancy status) and stone factors (e.g. size, position, obstruction, and, if known, stone composition). Treatment also depends on local facilities and expertise. The three main treatment modalities are extracorporeal shockwave lithotripsy, ureteroscopy (semi-rigid and/or flexible) and laser fragmentation, and percutaneous nephrolithotomy. Each has its advantages and disadvantages, indications and contraindications but this discussion is beyond the scope of this text.

Staghorn calculi

These are defined as stones occupying the renal pelvis and one or more calyceal systems. They are usually struvite stones formed as a result of chronic UTI. Left untreated, patients with staghorn stones have a significantly higher morbidity and mortality than those managed surgically.[12] Treatment is with percutaneous nephrolithotomy, which can be challenging and should be performed in a unit with appropriate surgical and interventional radiology expertise so as to achieve maximum stone clearance with minimal morbidity.

Infection

Epidemiology

UTIs affect females more than males except at the extremes of age where the incidence is similar. The lifetime risk of a UTI for a female is approximately 30% and so UTIs represent a significant proportion of emergency and outpatient urological referrals.

Definitions

A *UTI* can be defined as an urothelial inflammatory response to bacteria. *Bacteriuria* is defined as the presence of bacteria in the urine and can be symptomatic or asymptomatic. Traditionally, the diagnosis of a UTI implies the presence of $>10^5$ colony-forming units (CFU) per millilitre of mid-stream urine (MSU), but a significant proportion of patients will have a symptomatic UTI with 10^2 CFU/mL.[13] *Asymptomatic bacteriuria* normally only requires treatment in pregnant women and those patients about to undergo urinary tract instrumentation. *Pyuria* describes the presence of white blood cells in the urine and implies an inflammatory response usually, but not always, to bacteriuria. *Sterile pyuria* describes the presence of white blood cells but not bacteriuria and can be associated with urinary tract stones, carcinoma *in situ*, tuberculosis, interstitial cystitis, or a partially treated UTI.[13]

A *complicated UTI* occurs in the presence of a structurally or functionally abnormal urinary tract or in the presence of disease that affects the host's response to infection. A *recurrent UTI* is defined as two infections in 6 months or three within 1 year and can be due to *re-infection* with a different bacteria or *persistence* of the same organism.[14]

Microbiology

The most common organism responsible for a UTI is *Escherichia coli*, a Gram-negative bacillus, which accounts for approximately 85% of community-acquired UTIs and approximately 50% of hospital-acquired UTIs.[13] Other Gram-negative microorganisms implicated in UTIs are *Klebsiella, Proteus mirabilis*, and *Pseudomonas aeruginosa*. Common Gram-positive causative bacteria are *Enterococcus faecalis* and *Staphylococcus saprophyticus*.

The most common route of UTI is bacterial ascent from the perineum up the urethra, and for this reason women (with comparatively short urethras) and those with indwelling urinary catheters are at increased risk. Bacterial virulence mechanisms include: adhesion to the urothelium via specialized fimbriae on the bacterial surface called pili; production of cytotoxic cytokines; and production of β-lactamases that hydrolyse the β-lactam bond of certain antibiotics rendering them ineffective. Host defence mechanisms include the antegrade flow of urine; low urinary pH; a bladder surface mucin layer consisting of a protective glycosaminoglycans layer; and in women the breakdown of glycogen by lactobacilli in well-oestrogenized vaginal epithelial cells causes a protective acidic environment.[15] The relative paucity of oestrogen in perimenopausal women increases susceptibility to UTIs and is the rationale behind topical oestrogen therapy in treating recurrent UTIs in these patients.

Presentation and diagnosis

A lower tract UTI (cystitis) usually causes storage lower urinary tract symptoms such as frequency, urgency, and dysuria. Cystitis can cause haematuria and may be associated with systemic symptoms such as fever, rigors, and malaise. An upper tract UTI (pyelonephritis) is a clinical diagnosis made in the presence of flank pain, flank tenderness, and fever. It is usually preceded by symptoms of a lower tract UTI and often associated with nausea and vomiting, general malaise, and raised serum inflammatory markers.

Dipstick testing of a fresh sample of MSU looking for leucocytes and nitrites is mandatory. Many Gram-negative bacteria convert nitrates to nitrites in urine. The specificity of the nitrite dipstick test for detecting bacteriuria is approximately 90% whereas the sensitivity is 35–85%.[13] Thus a positive nitrite test strongly suggests the presence of UTI; however, a negative test does not rule out a UTI. False negatives can occur if the UTI is caused by non-nitrate converting bacteria or if the bacterial count in the MSU is low, which can be caused by frequency of micturition.

Management

Any antibiotic therapy for UTIs should be prescribed in accordance with sensitivities and local microbiology guidelines in order to maximize efficacy and reduce resistance. Cystitis can be managed as an outpatient with a short course of appropriate antibiotics. A patient with suspected pyelonephritis is usually managed in hospital with a short course of intravenous antibiotics followed, upon discharge, by 1 to 2 weeks of oral antibiotics. They should have an ultrasound scan of their urinary tract to exclude obstruction, a *perinephric abscess*, or a potentially contributory renal tract anomaly such as a duplex kidney. The presence of UTI with obstruction

(*pyonephrosis*) is a urological emergency and is described in the Pyonephrosis section. Pyelonephritis that does not settle after 3 to 4 days of appropriate treatment warrants repeat imaging to rule out the development of an abscess or pyonephrosis.

Specific urological infections

Emphysematous pyelonephritis

This is a rare and severe form of upper tract UTI with a 40–50% mortality rate. It usually occurs in diabetic patients, often in the presence of an obstructing urinary tract stone. It is caused by gas-forming organisms such as *E. coli* and *Klebsiella*, and the presence of this air in and around the kidney is often visible on CT or plain X-ray. Patients with this condition are usually managed in a critical care facility and emergency nephrectomy may be required if the sepsis does not respond to conservative measures.

Xanthogranulomatous pyelonephritis

This is a chronic form of upper tract infection that causes renal parenchymal destruction and subsequent loss of function. It usually affects 40 to 60 year olds with a 4 : 1 female-to-male preponderance. Seventy-five per cent of cases are associated with urinary tract stones, and causative organisms include *E. coli* and *Proteus mirabilis*. The kidney becomes enlarged and contains areas of pus, haemorrhagic necrosis, and yellowish nodules,[13] changes that can mimic the radiological appearance of a renal cell carcinoma.

Orchitis

This is defined as inflammation of the testis and often occurs with inflammation of the epididymis. Orchitis can develop in 20–30% of postpubertal patients with mumps virus infection. The diagnosis is supported by a recent history of parotitis and evidence of IgM antibodies in the serum.[14] A small proportion of cases are bilateral and if this results in testicular atrophy it can cause sub-fertility.

Epididymitis

This inflammatory condition of the epididymis is almost always the result of bacterial infection. It causes pain and swelling of the epididymis and often the spermatic cord. It is usually unilateral and relatively acute in onset. The majority of cases of epididymitis in sexually active males aged younger than 35 years are due to sexually transmitted organisms such as *Chlamydia trachomatis*, whereas in older patients it is usually due to urinary pathogens and may be associated with voiding difficulties. A preceding history of urethritis or dysuria may help make the diagnosis but it is imperative to exclude testicular torsion as a differential diagnosis. In cases where there is doubt, surgical exploration to exclude testicular torsion is mandatory.

The microbial aetiology of epididymitis may be determined by obtaining a sample of MSU prior to treatment with antibiotics. Most laboratories offer nucleic acid amplification testing of urine to detect sexually transmitted pathogens; however, if this is not available a urethral swab should be obtained. The choice of antibiotics should be based on the likely pathogen. In cases of *Chlamydia trachomatis* epididymitis, the sexual partner should also be treated.

Fournier's gangrene

This is a rapidly progressive synergistic polymicrobial necrotizing fasciitis affecting the genitals and perineum. It causes small vessel occlusion, ischaemia, and gangrene of the skin and subcutaneous tissues and has a mortality of 20–40%. The most common primary infection is usually genitourinary but can also be colorectal in origin. It is more common in immunocompromised patients such as diabetic and alcoholic patients. The diagnosis should be considered in any septic patient with a perineal or genital infection causing skin discolouration and/or crepitus. It is a surgical emergency that requires prompt recognition and a multidisciplinary approach to treatment. Broad-spectrum antibiotics to cover Gram-negative and Gram-positive, aerobic and anaerobic organisms should be started expeditiously together with intravenous fluid resuscitation. The amount of subcutaneous tissue damage is often more extensive than the superficial appearance would suggest, and prompt radical surgical debridement back to healthy tissue is required. The testicles are often spared due to their intra-abdominal blood supply. Surgery should be performed in conjunction with urologists, and the colorectal and plastic surgery teams as patients may require a suprapubic catheter, colostomy faecal diversion, and skin grafting. These factors should be considered when obtaining consent for surgery.

References

1. Turney BW, Reynard JM, Noble JG, et al. Trends in stone disease. *BJU Int* 2012;109(7):1082–7.
2. Boyce CJ, Pickhardt PJ, Lawrence EM, *et al.* Prevalence of urolithiasis in asymptomatic adults: objective determination using low dose noncontrast computerized tomography. *J Urol* 2010;183(3):1017–21.
3. Reynard J, Brewster S, Biers S. Stone disease. In: *Oxford Handbook of Urology*. Oxford: Oxford University Press; 2006: 349–400.
4. European Association of Urology Guidelines 2012. *Urolithiasis*. http://www.uroweb.org/gls/pdf/20_Urolithiasis_LR%20March%2013%20 2012.pdf (accessed March 2013).
5. Holdgate A, Pollock T. Nonsteroidal anti-inflammatory drugs (NSAIDs) versus opioids for acute renal colic. *Cochrane Database Syst Rev* 2005;18;(2):CD004137.
6. Holdgate A, Oh CM. Is there a role for antimuscarinics in renal colic? A randomized controlled trial. *J Urol* 2005;174(2):572–5.
7. Springhart WP, Marguet CG, Sur RL, *et al.* Forced versus minimal intravenous hydration in the management of acute renal colic: a randomized trial. *J Endourol*;20(10):713–6.
8. Niemann T, Kollmann T, Bongartz G. Diagnostic performance of low-dose CT for the detection of urolithiasis: A meta-analysis. *Am J Roentgenol* 2008;191(2):396–401.
9. Miller OF, Kane CJ. Time to stone passage for observed ureteral calculi: a guide for patient education. *J Urol* 1999;162(3 Pt 1):688–90.
10. Pearle MS, Pierce HL, Miller GL, *et al.* Optimal method of urgent decompression of the collecting system for obstruction and infection due to ureteral calculi. *J Urol* 1998;160(4):1260–4.
11. Mokhmalji H, Braun PM, Portillo FJ, *et al.* Percutaneous nephrostomy versus ureteral stents for diversion of hydronephrosis caused by stones: A prospective, randomized clinical trial. *J Urol* 2001;165(4):1088–92.
12. Teichman JM, Long RD, Hulbert JC. Long-term renal fate and prognosis after staghorn calculus management. *J Urol* 1995;153(5):1403–7.
13. Reynard J, Brewster S, Biers S. Infections and inflammatory conditions. In *Oxford Handbook of Urology*. Oxford: Oxford University Press; 2006: 135–65.
14. European Association of Urology Guidelines 2011. *Urological infections*. http://www.uroweb.org/gls/pdf/17_Urological%20infections_ LR%20II.pdf (accessed March 2013).
15. George NJR. Urinary tract infection. In Mundy A, Fitzpatrick JM, Neal DE, George NJR (eds) *Scientific Basis of Urology*, 2nd edition. London: Informa Healthcare; 2004: 165–203.

Genitourinary malignancies

Aidan Noon and James Catto

Introduction

Genitourinary cancers include some of the most common and most expensive human malignancies to treat. The outcomes from these cancers vary from excellent (low-risk prostate cancer) to poor (metastatic bladder and renal cancer). Most of these cancers increase in incidence with ageing, and overall more men are affected by these cancers than women. This reflects the fact that prostate cancer is male specific, and that urothelial and renal cancers are linked to occupational exposure or cigarette smoking. Systematic screening programmes (for prostate cancer) and opportunistic testing for haematuria (urinalysis) or abdominal pain (widespread use of ultrasound scans) have increased the detection of most genitourinary cancers and induced a migration to lower-stage disease. Current challenges facing clinicians include the overtreatment of indolent disease (Figure 2.9.2.1) and improving the treatment of advanced incurable cancers.

Kidney cancer

Incidence

In the UK, kidney cancer is the seventh and ninth most common malignancy in men and women, respectively. It has a peak incidence in the sixth and seventh decade (Figure 2.9.2.1) and is more common in men than women (2:1 ratio).[1] Recognized risk factors include obesity and smoking. Approximately 4% of cancers are hereditary.[2]

Pathology

Kidney tumours include renal cell carcinoma (RCC) originating from the parenchyma (80% of all tumours), urothelial carcinoma (arising from the renal pelvis: 18%), and rare tumours (such as lymphoma [1–2%] or sarcoma [<1%]). There are histological variants of RCC, of which clear cell (ccRCC 75%), papillary (12%), and chromophobe (4%) are the most common. Patients with Von Hippel–Lindau (VHL) syndrome inherit a mutant VHL gene. Loss of this tumour suppressor predisposes patients to ccRCC (often bilateral). Approximately 60% of ccRCCs harbour loss of VHL expression and this leads to overexpression of angiogenic transcription factors (large ccRCC are often highly vascular).[3,4]

Renal tumours grow locally through the capsule and renal fat, and have the propensity to invade the renal vein, inferior vena cava, and even reach the right atrium with tumour thrombus. The lungs are the most common site for metastatic spread, followed by lymph nodes, the liver, and skeleton. RCC is staged according to the TNM classification and graded by the Fuhrman system (I–IV). Survival decreases for patients as stage or grade increases.

Clinical presentation

Currently most tumours are detected incidentally through imaging for unrelated abdominal symptoms or the investigation of haematuria. Patients with advanced disease present with a classic triad of loin pain, haematuria, and a mass. For smaller lesions less than 3 cm, there can be diagnostic uncertainty (20–30% of lesions are benign). Renal biopsy can help clarify the diagnosis. RCC is associated with a number of paraneoplastic syndromes: hypercalcaemia, anaemia, hyponatraemia, elevated erythrocyte sedimentation rate, polycythaemia, and Stauffer's syndrome (abnormal liver function tests, hepatic necrosis, thrombocytopenia, fever, weight loss).

Management

Localized disease

Tumours confined to the kidney (pT2) may be managed by surveillance,[5] partial nephrectomy (termed nephron sparing surgery) if anatomically possible, ablation (using energy to destroy the tissue) if small and exophytic, or by radical nephrectomy (typically for larger tumours). The desire for long term nephron-preservation has made partial nephrectomy the treatment of choice in suitable patients.[6]

Locally advanced and metastatic disease

Locally advanced tumours, particularly with tumour thrombus involving the vena cava, are mostly removed by open or robotic radical nephrectomy. RCC is resistant to chemotherapy. Patients with metastatic disease are treated with targeted molecular therapy (sorafenib, sunitinib and temsirolimus) or immunotherapy (PD-1 inhibitors).[7–9]

Bladder cancer

Incidence

Bladder cancer (BC) is the fourth most common malignancy in men and seventh most common malignancy in females. Risk factors include smoking (accounts for 50% of BC), occupational carcinogen exposure (10%), cyclophosphamide, pioglitazone, and pelvic irradiation. Squamous carcinoma may arise following chronic inflammation (e.g. long-term indwelling catheters, bladder stones, and schistosomiasis). BC is more common in males than females.[10]

Pathology

Histologically most BC are urothelial cell carcinoma (UCC; 90%), followed by squamous cell carcinoma (5%), adenocarcinoma (2%), and rare pathologies (sarcoma, lymphoma, etc.). BC is staged using

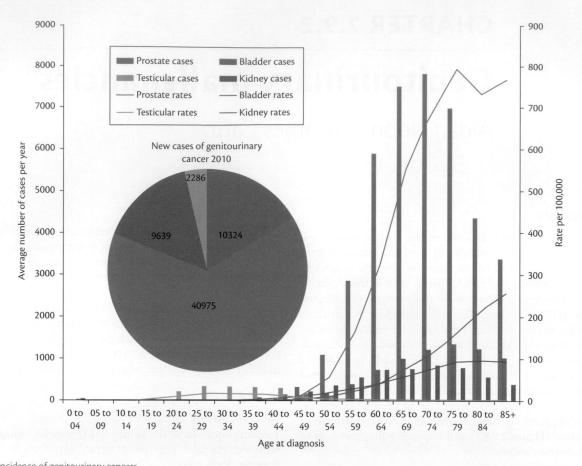

Fig. 2.9.2.1 Incidence of genitourinary cancers.

Source: data from Cancer Research UK, *Latest cancer statistics publications*, Copyright © Cancer Research UK 2013, available from http://www.cancerresearchuk.org/cancer-info/cancerstats/incidence/

the TNM classification. Around 80% of tumours are non-muscle invasive at diagnosis (NMI = CIS, pTa and pT1). Tumours are graded according the World Health Organization (WHO) 1977 (G1, G2, and G3) and the WHO 2004 (low or high grade) systems. BC commonly metastases to pelvic lymph nodes and the lungs.[3]

Clinical presentation

Painless visible and non-visible haematuria are the most common presentations. Other presenting symptoms include irritative urinary symptoms and recurrent or difficult to treat UTIs.

Management

Investigation of haematuria includes a flexible cystoscopy and evaluation of the upper tracts (such as computed tomography urogram). Patients with tumours then proceed to transurethral resection of tumour (TURT). Subsequent management depends on the tumour stage, grade, multiplicity and the state of the flat urothelium.

Non-muscle-invasive disease

NMI tumours are treated by TURT and a single dose of intravesical mitomycin C (to reduce future recurrences).[11] Tumour excision should include underlying muscle (and sampling of the flat urothelium in high-grade cases). For high-grade NMI disease (any grade 3), patients may undergo re-resection within 6 to 10 weeks to ensure the tumour has been fully excised.[12]

Muscle-invasive disease

Treatment options for muscle-invasive disease include radical cystectomy and radical radiotherapy. Cure rates with cystectomy are improved with neo-adjuvant chemotherapy.[13] Pelvic lymphadenectomy is performed at the time of cystectomy to fully stage the disease and in an attempt to remove micrometastatic disease. Excised nodes include the obturator and the external and internal iliac chains. Radical cystectomy in the male involves removing the prostate (cystoprostatectomy) and in females involves removing the uterus, cervix, and anterior vagina (anterior pelvic exenteration). Following cystectomy, urinary reconstruction may be through formation of an ileal conduit (most common), construction of an orthotopic neo-bladder (around 25%),[14] catheterizable continent urinary pouch, or formation of a ureterosigmoidostomy (both rare). Less fit patients or those seeking bladder preservation may be treated with radical external beam radiotherapy.

Systemic treatments

Patients with symptomatic metastatic disease may be treated with palliative cisplatin-based chemotherapy, although UCC is relatively drug resistant.

Upper tract disease

Urothelium lines the collecting system of the kidney and ureters, and these areas are also susceptible to upper tract UCC in at-risk individuals. Patients commonly present with haematuria (occasionally clot colic) or incidentally on cross-sectional imaging. Treatment is normally by radical nephroureterectomy (laparoscopic or open). Patients with mid to lower ureteric lesions and single renal units may be amenable to segmental ureteric excision and reimplantation/reconstruction. These patients require surveillance as they are at high risk of recurrence within the bladder or the contralateral upper tract.[15]

Prostate cancer

Incidence

Prostate cancer is the most common male malignancy and the second leading malignant cause of death in men in the UK. The incidence of the disease is increasing reflecting opportunistic screening using prostate-specific antigen testing (PSA) and the ageing population (<0.1% of cases occur in men < 50 years of age). Post-mortem studies reveal many men have small well-differentiated prostate cancers (termed latent or insignificant; found in half of 50 year olds and the majority of 70 year olds) and so the key clinical challenge is to discriminate between indolent and aggressive tumours. Approximately 10% of cancers have an inherited genetic component.[16,17]

Pathology

Most prostate cancers are adenocarcinoma and are staged according to TNM: T1 disease is non-palpable (diagnosed from TURP or needle biopsy); T2 is palpable disease confined to the prostate; T3 is extracapsular extension beyond the prostate; and T4 is invasion into adjacent organs. Gleason grading evaluates the architectural disruption of the cancer and assigns two scores between 1 (best differentiated) to 5 (worst) for the two most common disease patterns (e.g. 3 + 4 = 7). Prostate cancer metastasizes to pelvic lymph nodes and the axial skeleton. Visceral metastases are uncommon and usual herald a poor prognosis.[18]

Clinical presentation

Localized disease

Most localized tumours are detected through PSA testing. Otherwise, localized cancers rarely cause lower urinary tract symptoms (mostly due to benign prostatic enlargement) but can be found in the tissue removed during TURP, or during investigation of haematuria, or other symptoms. PSA is a serine protease important for liquefying the ejaculate. PSA is produced by prostate tissue and in cancer there is architectural disruption of the glands that allows PSA to reach the circulation. Screening using PSA testing has been shown in randomized controlled trials to decrease prostate cancer mortality, but at the expense of over detection and over treatment.[19] As such, screening has not yet been introduced in the UK. Glandular architectural disruption (leading to an elevated serum PSA) is also found with infection, instrumentation of the lower urine tract, and ejaculation. Thus, PSA has a low specificity (25% of men with elevated PSA have cancer) and low sensitivity (25% of cancers have a PSA < 4.0 ng/μL) for the disease.

In patients thought likely to benefit from treatment, histological confirmation is provided by needle biopsy of the prostate using a transrectal or transperineal approach guided by a rectal ultrasound probe. Not all patients are diagnosed by their first set of biopsies. If clinical suspicion remains, patients may be subjected to multiple biopsy procedures with the chance of detecting clinically important disease falling after each biopsy. Diffusion-weighted MRI and template biopsy protocols can be used amongst other techniques to try to detect lesions that might be missed using a standard prostatic biopsy protocol. It is important to note that prostatic biopsy carries a risk of severe sepsis (<1%) and for this reason the decision to pursue a histologically diagnosis of prostate cancer must be balanced against this risk.[18]

Locally advanced and metastatic disease

Patients with more advanced disease may present in a number of ways depending on the effect of the tumour. An enlarging prostatic cancer can cause hydronephrosis and obstructive nephropathy resulting in overt renal failure. Patients with skeletal metastases may present with bone pain, acute spinal cord compression, symptoms of bone marrow failure, or hypercalcaemia.

Management

The management of prostate cancer depends on the patient (performance status, age, symptoms) and the tumour (extent judged by PSA, clinical stage, and Gleason grade).

Treatments with curative intent

In low-risk cases, patients should consider a period of active surveillance (close observation using protocols with serial PSA measurement, interval re-biopsy, and MRIs) rather than risking the side effects of radical treatment. Triggers for radical intervention are a rapidly rising PSA or a 10 ng/uL threshold, or an increase in grade/stage. Patients with locally confined (≤pT2) and locally advanced (pT3) tumours are suitable for radical treatment. These include radical prostatectomy (the gold standard treatment) that may be performed via an open, laparoscopic, or robotically assisted technique, and radical radiotherapy in the form of external beam or brachytherapy (for certain tumours). Side effects of surgery include stress urinary incontinence (1–5% at 1 year) and erectile dysfunction (common). Both can be reduced by nerve-sparing procedures in suitable tumours. Focal ablative techniques exist in the form of cryotherapy, high intensity focused ultrasound, or photodynamic treatments.[20]

Systemic and palliative treatments

Patients with incurable disease (metastatic or not suitable for curative treatments) may be managed expectantly (watchful waiting). In this setting palliative treatments are initiated when a patient becomes symptomatic. Systemic treatments normally start with androgen deprivation by surgical castration or hormone manipulation. Testosterone release may be stopped by supraphysiological non-cyclical administration of luteinizing hormone-releasing hormone (LHRH) agonists (note: these cause an initial testosterone surge) or an LHRH antagonist. Patients presenting with spinal cord compression due to a hormone naïve prostate cancer should have urgent castration (emergency orchidectomy) and if performed early enough, this offers a rapid and dramatic improvement to the patients' symptoms.[21] Patients that develop symptoms during hormone treatment or display a biochemical relapse (successively rising PSAs) may be offered second-line hormone manipulation (anti-androgens). Other options include taxane chemotherapy, abiterone. Radiotherapy or Zoledronic acid can be used for bone pain.[20]

Testicular carcinoma

Incidence

Testicular cancer is responsible for 1% of male tumours in the UK. The lifetime male risk is 1:500 for a normally descended testicle.

The major risk factors for this disease are testicular maldescent, first-degree relative with the disease, subfertility, Kleinfelter's syndrome, and Kallman's disease.[22]

Pathology

Ninety-five per cent of tumours derive from germ cells and the remainder are non-germ cell tumours (3% Leydig cell and 1% Sertoli cell). Germ cell tumours are divided into seminomatous (70%: classic, spermatocytic, or anaplastic) and non-seminomatous germ cell tumours (NSGCTs: 30%). NSGCTs are subdivided according the WHO classification (mature teratoma, immature teratoma, embryonal carcinoma, choriocarcinoma, yolk-sac tumour, or mixed). Elevated serum testicular tumour markers (alpha-fetoprotein produced by yolk-sac elements, beta subunit of human chorionic gonadotrophin produced by syncytiotrophoblasts, and lactate dehydrogenase) are seen in 50% of tumours. Testicular tumours metastasize first to the para-aortic lymph node chain.[22]

Clinical presentation

Testicular carcinoma most commonly presents as a hard mass arising within the body of testicle. Patients with advanced disease may manifest abdominal swelling (enlarged lymph nodes), breathlessness (lung metastases), or weight loss.[23]

Management

Testicular carcinoma is diagnosed clinically and confirmed ultrasonically. Patients with obvious signs of metastatic disease should be referred to oncologists for consideration of immediate chemotherapy. Radical inguinal orchidectomy is the gold standard treatment.[23,24]

Post-orchidectomy management

Patients undergo cross-sectional imaging with a computed tomogram scan. The stage of their disease, including tumour marker status, is combined with histological information to risk stratify the patients. Motivated patients with low-risk disease are suitable for regular clinic surveillance. Patients at high risk of recurrence may be offered radiotherapy (not NSGCTs, which are radio-insensitive), chemotherapy, or prophylactic lymph node dissection. Patients with metastatic disease may be offered radiotherapy or chemotherapy with surgical lymph node excision being reserved for residual disease.[23,24]

Penile cancer

Penile carcinoma is a rare condition with an incidence of 1/100 000 population (approximately 350 men/year in the UK). Risk factors include human papilloma virus 16, 18, 31, and 33. Patients present with a lesion or thickening of the glans or prepuce. There are a number of recognized premalignant lesions, for example erythroplasia of Queryat, Bowen's disease, and leukoplakia.[25] Penile carcinoma progresses in a step-wise manner with metastases to the inguinal and then pelvic lymph nodes. Patients may present (30–60%) with enlarged inguinal lymph nodes and assessment of these will reveal malignancy in approximately 50% of cases. The majority of tumours are squamous cell cancers (95%) and there are a number of recognized subtypes. Three growth patterns are commonly observed: superficial spreading, nodular, and verrucous (exophytic). Initial management requires biopsy of the penile lesion and assessment of the lymph nodes.

Treatment of the lesion depends on the grade and stage of the tumour. Carcinoma *in situ* can be treated by topical ointments (imiquimod or 5-fluorouracil cream), laser ablation, cryotherapy, phytotherapy, or surgical resurfacing. Ta/T1 lesions can be treated by glandular resurfacing, wide local excision, or glansectomy. For T2 lesions affecting the corpus spongiosum, glansectomy is the treatment of the choice and partial penectomy is employed for lesions affecting the corpus cavernosum. T3 lesions are treated by radical penectomy, and T4 lesions can be treated with neo-adjuvant chemotherapy with salvage surgery if sufficient down staging is achieved.

Management of the lymph nodes depends on their size (i.e. palpable or not palpable). Impalpable nodes can be sampled using sentinel lymph node biopsy (injecting a blue dye/radiolabelled nanocolloid around the tumour to locate the first lymph node draining the lesion). Patients with positive lymph nodes undergo lymph node dissection.[26]

References

1. Cancer_Research_UK. 2014 [cited 2014 1.2.14]; Available from: http://www.cancerresearchuk.org/cancer-info/cancerstats/incidence/
2. Motzer RJ, Bander NH, Nanus DM. Renal-Cell Carcinoma. *N Engl J Med* 1996; 335: 865–75.
3. Lopez-Beltran A, Scarpelli M, Montironi R, et al. 2004 WHO classification of the renal tumors of the adults. *Eur Urol* 2006; 49: 798–805.
4. Vira MA, Novakovic KR, Pinto PA, et al. Genetic basis of kidney cancer: a model for developing molecular-targeted therapies. *BJU Int* 2007; 99: 1223–9.
5. Jewett MA, Mattar K, Basiuk J, et al. Active surveillance of small renal masses: progression patterns of early stage kidney cancer. *Eur Urol* 2011; 60: 39–44.
6. Russo P. Partial nephrectomy for renal cancer: Part I. *BJU Int* 2010; 105: 1206–20.
7. Motzer RJ, Hutson TE, Tomczak P, et al. Overall survival and updated results for sunitinib compared with interferon alfa in patients with metastatic renal cell carcinoma. *J Clin Oncol* 2009; 27: 3584–90.
8. Motzer RJ, Hutson TE, Tomczak P, et al. Sunitinib versus interferon alfa in metastatic renal-cell carcinoma. *N Engl J Med* 2007; 356: 115–24.
9. Motzer RJ, Bukowski RM. Targeted therapy for metastatic renal cell carcinoma. *J Clin Oncol* 2006; 24: 5601–8.
10. Burger M, Catto JW, Dalbagni G, et al. Epidemiology and risk factors of urothelial bladder cancer. *Eur Urol* 2013; 63: 234–41.
11. Sylvester RJ, Oosterlinck W, van der Meijden AP. A single immediate postoperative instillation of chemotherapy decreases the risk of recurrence in patients with stage Ta T1 bladder cancer: a meta-analysis of published results of randomized clinical trials. *J Urol* 2004; 171: 2186–90, quiz 435.
12. Herr HW. The value of a second transurethral resection in evaluating patients with bladder tumors. *J Urol* 1999; 162: 74–6.
13. Advanced Bladder Cancer Meta-analysis C. Neoadjuvant chemotherapy in invasive bladder cancer: a systematic review and meta-analysis. *Lancet* 2003; 361: 1927–34.
14. Studer UE, Varol C, Danuser H. Orthotopic ileal neobladder. *BJU Int* 2004; 93: 183–93.
15. Roupret M, Zigeuner R, Palou J, et al. European guidelines for the diagnosis and management of upper urinary tract urothelial cell carcinomas: 2011 update. *Eur Urol* 2011; 59: 584–94.
16. Gronberg H. Prostate cancer epidemiology. *Lancet* 2003;361:859–64.
17. Hsing AW, Chokkalingam AP. Prostate cancer epidemiology. *Front Biosci* 2006;11:1388–413.

18. Heidenreich A, Bastian PJ, Bellmunt J, *et al*. EAU guidelines on prostate cancer. part 1: screening, diagnosis, and local treatment with curative intent-update 2013. *Eur Urol* 2014; 65: 124–37.

19. Schroder FH, Hugosson J, Roobol MJ, *et al*. Screening and prostate-cancer mortality in a randomized European study. *N Engl J Med* 2009; 360: 1320–8.

20. Heidenreich A, Bastian PJ, Bellmunt J, *et al*. EAU guidelines on prostate cancer. Part II: Treatment of advanced, relapsing, and castration-resistant prostate cancer. *Eur Urol* 2014; 65: 467–79.

21. Sharifi N, Gulley JL, Dahut WL. Androgen deprivation therapy for prostate cancer. *JAMA* 2005; 294: 238–44.

22. Winter C, Albers P. Testicular germ cell tumors: pathogenesis, diagnosis and treatment. *Nature Rev Endocrinol* 2011; 7: 43–53.

23. Krege S, Beyer J, Souchon R, *et al*. European consensus conference on diagnosis and treatment of germ cell cancer: a report of the second meeting of the European Germ Cell Cancer Consensus group (EGCCCG): part I. *Eur Urol* 2008; 53: 478–96.

24. Krege S, Beyer J, Souchon R, *et al*. European consensus conference on diagnosis and treatment of germ cell cancer: a report of the second meeting of the European Germ Cell Cancer Consensus Group (EGCCCG): part II. *Eur Urol* 2008; 53: 497–513.

25. Arya M, Kalsi J, Kelly J, *et al*. Malignant and premalignant lesions of the penis. *BMJ* 2013; 346: f1149.

26. Pizzocaro G, Algaba F, Horenblas S, *et al*. EAU penile cancer guidelines 2009. *Eur Urol* 2010; 57: 1002–12.

CHAPTER 2.9.3

Benign prostatic hyperplasia and obstructive uropathy

Mary Garthwaite

Pathogenesis

Regulation of prostatic growth

Testosterone and its metabolite dihydrotestosterone (DHT) play an important role in the regulation of prostatic growth (Figure 2.9.3.1). Testosterone diffuses into prostatic stromal and epithelial cells. Within epithelial cells it binds directly to androgen receptors and initiates the transcription of growth factors required for prostate cell division and proliferation. In stromal cells only a small proportion of testosterone binds directly to the androgen receptors, whereas the remainder binds to 5-alpha–reductase, an enzyme located on the stromal cell nuclear membrane, and is converted to DHT. DHT has a far greater affinity for the androgen receptor and is therefore more potent than testosterone. DHT also has the ability to diffuse out of the stromal cells and into adjacent epithelial cells where it can also bind to the androgen receptors and initiate growth factor production.

Development of benign prostatic hyperplasia

Benign prostatic hyperplasia (BPH) is characterized by hyperplasia of both stromal and epithelial cells within the periurethral area (or transition zone) of the prostate. This increase in cell number results in the formation of nodules of tissue, which can constrict the prostatic urethra and lead to bladder outflow obstruction (BOO) and the development of lower urinary tract symptoms (LUTS).

It is not clear whether this increase in cell number reflects epithelial and stromal cell proliferation, impairment of programmed cell death, or a combination of both. However, the development of new epithelial glands seen in BPH mirrors that seen during the embryological development of the prostate and has led to the concept of 'reawakening'.[1]

Symptoms of benign prostatic hyperplasia

Lower urinary tract symptoms

The relationship between BPH and LUTS is complex as not all men with histological BPH will develop LUTS significant enough to lead them to seek medical intervention, even with the presence of BOO secondary to prostatic enlargement (Figure 2.9.3.2). LUTS can also occur in the absence of BPH due to a variety of other causes, including detrusor overactivity, urethral stricture, and adenocarcinoma of the prostate (Box 2.9.3.1).

Table 2.9.3.1 summarizes the classification of LUTS into storage-associated and voiding-associated symptoms. It is postulated that increased prostatic resistance underlies voiding symptoms, whereas storage symptoms result from secondary

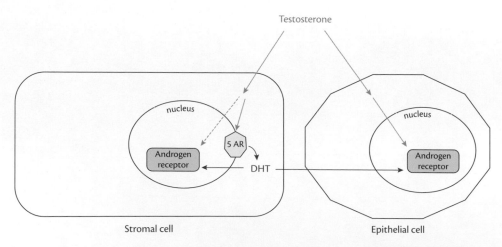

Fig. 2.9.3.1 Regulation of prostatic cell growth and proliferation via interactions with androgen receptors in both epithelial and stromal cells. DHT is produced in the stromal cells where it has an autocrine action on androgen receptors, but also diffuses into nearby epithelial cells where it exerts a paracrine effect.
5AR, 5-alpha-reductase; DHT, dihydrotestosterone.

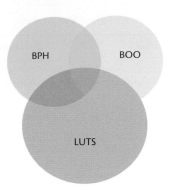

Fig. 2.9.3.2 The relationship between BPH, LUTS and BOO. The cause of LUTS is multifactorial, however, they remain the usual trigger for men to seek medical attention and may led to a diagnosis of BPH, with or without evidence of BOO. BPH, benign prostatic hyperplasia; BOO, bladder outflow obstruction; LUTS, lower urinary tract symptoms.

Box 2.9.3.1 Causes of lower urinary tract symptoms

Benign prostatic hyperplasia BPH
Detrusor overactivity (idiopathic or neuropathic)
Detrusor hypocontractility
Urethral stricture
Prostatic adenocarcinoma
Transitional cell carcinoma of the bladder
Nocturnal polyuria
Recurrent urinary tract infections

---

hypertrophy of the detrusor muscle and development of detrusor overactivity.

Symptom scores

Several symptom scores have been developed to rate the severity of LUTS.[2] In the UK the validated International Prostate Symptom Score is the most widely used and is based on the answers to seven questions concerning urinary symptoms and one question concerning quality of life. Questions regarding urinary symptoms cover both storage and voiding symptoms (Table 2.9.3.2) and allow the patient to choose one out of six answers indicating increasing severity. The answers are assigned points from 0 to 5. The total score can therefore range from 0 to 35. The severity of symptoms can be classified according to the total score with ≤7 classed as mild, 8–19 moderate, and a score of ≥20 as severe. The form also includes a single question regarding quality of life rated from 0 to 6, where 0

Table 2.9.3.1 Classification of lower urinary tract symptoms

Storage symptoms	Voiding symptoms
Frequency	Hesitancy
Urgency	Weak stream
Nocturia	Intermittency
Incontinence	Straining
	Incomplete emptying

Table 2.9.3.2 International Prostate Symptom Score urinary symptom range

Question	Symptom
1	Incomplete emptying
2	Frequency
3	Intermittency
4	Urgency
5	Weak stream
6	Straining
7	Nocturia

Source: data from *Journal of Urology*, Volume 148, Issue 5, Barry MJ *et al.*, The American Urological Association symptom index for benign prostatic hyperplasia: The Measurement Committee of the American Urological Association, pp. 1549–57, Copyright © 1992.

indicates that the patient's symptoms cause them no bother at all and 6 indicates that they are intolerable.

Assessment of benign prostatic hyperplasia

Examination

When examining the patient with presumed BPH it is important to look for signs of other potential causes of LUTS and of the possible complications of BPH. Table 2.9.3.3 summarizes the important findings that can be made on clinical examination. Although digital rectal examination allows for estimation of prostate volume, which is known to be a risk factor for BPH progression, it is unfortunately associated with considerable measurement error and can underestimate the actual volume by up to 55%.[3,4]

Clinical investigations

Initial investigations are aimed at excluding other possible causes of LUTS, assessing the severity of the disease, and identifying the presence of complications. Studies have shown that serum prostate-specific antigen (PSA) level correlates well with prostate volume and is a useful predictor of BPH progression and the development of acute urinary retention.[5] However, the use of PSA testing in BPH remains controversial and should only be performed after

Table 2.9.3.3 The importance of findings on clinical examination

Clinical finding	Importance
Palpable bladder	If palpable after voiding suggests significant BOO and retention of urine
Phimosis	Possible cause of LUTS
Meatal stenosis	Possible cause of LUTS
Hard irregular prostate	Possibility of adenocarcinoma of the prostate
Signs of anaemia	Possibly due to chronic obstructive nephropathy secondary to BOO and chronic retention of urine
Signs of neurological disease	Potential cause of LUTS

BOO, bladder outflow obstruction; LUTS, lower urinary tract symptoms.

Table 2.9.3.4 Indications for recommended baseline tests

Test	Indication	Comments
Urine dipstick analysis	Identification of infection, haematuria or sterile pyuria	Send MSU to confirm presence of infection and quantify sterile pyuria
Flow rate analysis	Pattern of flow can suggest presence of BOO, detrusor hypocontractility or urethral stricture	Voided volumes ≤150 mL make interpretation difficult
Post-void residual volume measurement	To assess bladder emptying	Volumes greater than 200ml warrant further investigation to rule out hydronephrosis and renal impairment
Frequency-volume chart	To identify other causes of LUTS including excessive daily fluid intake and nocturnal polyuria	Completed over a minimum of three consecutive days. Provides a guide for conservative management of LUTS
Serum electrolytes	Identification of renal impairment	Even if normal at presentation baseline results are important in surveillance of disease progression

MSU, mid-stream urine; BOO, bladder outflow obstruction; LUTS, lower urinary tract symptoms.

appropriate counselling regarding the implications of an abnormally raised PSA, including the possible diagnosis and management of prostatic adenocarcinoma.

Baseline tests

Table 2.9.3.4 summarizes the recommended baseline tests in the investigation of men with LUTS and possible BPH.

Optional tests

Further investigations, which are not recommended as routine, may be required depending on the result of initial assessment and investigation (Table 2.9.3.5).

Progression of benign prostatic hyperplasia and associated complications

Definition of progression and associated risk factors

BPH progression is defined as worsening of symptoms, deterioration of urinary flow rate, increase in prostate volume as well as outcomes such as acute urinary retention (AUR), and the need for surgery either for AUR or symptoms.[6] Several factors have been linked with the risk of BPH progression including age and prostate volume, reduced urinary flow, increased symptom score, and increased bother. These factors can be used to stratify the risk of BPH progression and identify patients who would most benefit from treatment.[7]

Complications

Table 2.9.3.6 lists the complications associated with BPH.

Table 2.9.3.5 Indications for further investigations

Test	Indication	Comments
PSA	As a proxy for prostate volume or in the assessment of possible prostatic adenocarcinoma	Patients must be fully informed regarding the implications of an abnormally raised PSA and the possible diagnosis and treatment of prostatic adenocarcinoma
Transrectal ultrasound	Accurate assessment of prostate volume	Transabdominal estimation of prostate volume is not as accurate
Renal tract ultrasound	To identify or exclude hydronephrosis	Also used to investigate cause of recurrent urinary tract infections or sterile pyuria
Cystoscopy	Investigation of haematuria, sterile pyuria and recurrent infections	Also recommended when symptoms are persistent/painful despite other tests being normal
Urodynamic studies	To confirm BOO and exclude detrusor hypocontractility when other investigations are equivocal. In complex cases (e.g. history of prostate surgery or neurological disease)	

PSA, prostate-specific antigen; BOO, bladder outflow obstruction.

Table 2.9.3.6 Complications of BPH

Complication	Comments
Acute urinary retention (AUR)	Painful
Chronic urinary retention (CUR)	Painless
Acute-on-chronic urinary retention	A sudden inability to void on a background of CUR
Overflow incontinence	Usually occurs at night and denotes the presence of CUR
Urinary tract infection (UTI)	Often a consequence of incomplete bladder emptying
Bladder stones	A consequence of incomplete bladder emptying +/- recurrent UTI
Hydronephrosis	High pressures within the bladder lead to obstruction of the flow of urine from the kidneys producing a standing column of urine
Renal failure	Renal damage occurs when the high bladder pressures are transmitted to the upper tracts
Haematuria	The overgrowth of benign prostatic tissue is highly vascular with friable superficial blood vessels

Treatment options

Surveillance

Surveillance combined with conservative measures is an acceptable option for men with mild to moderate LUTS and a low degree of bother. Such patients can be easily managed in the primary care setting. Conservative measures may include optimization of fluid intake, avoidance of caffeine and alcohol, smoking cessation, weight loss, and double voiding. Some patients opt to self-treat with plant extracts (phytotherapies) that are commercially available without prescription. Such therapies have a long tradition in European countries such as France and Germany; however, their precise mechanisms of action *in vivo* remain unclear and the clinical efficacy of these agents remains largely unproven.[8]

Medical therapy

Over the last 15 years there has been a steady decline in the rates of BPH-related surgery, which is largely due to the concurrent advance in medical therapy.

Alpha-blockers

Prostatic and bladder neck smooth muscle contain a predominance of alpha-1_A-adrenoreceptors, which induce contraction when stimulated. Inhibition of alpha-mediated stimulation can be achieved with an alpha-antagonist (alpha-blocker) and is postulated to promote relaxation of prostatic and bladder neck smooth muscle and thereby alleviate BOO. Alpha-blockers have a very rapid onset of action of within hours to days, but their full effect can take a number of weeks to develop. Typical improvements in symptom scores of 30–40% after 3 months' treatment have been demonstrated.[9,10] They appear to be effective regardless of symptom severity, prostate size, and age, making them a useful first-line treatment.

The two most commonly prescribed alpha-blockers in the UK are tamsulosin and alfuzosin. Another alpha-blocker more usually prescribed for the control of hypertension is doxazosin.

5-Alpha-reductase inhibitors

There are two 5-alpha-reductase inhibitors available for the treatment of BPH: finasteride and dutasteride. 5-Alpha-reductase exists in two isoforms and type 2 has predominant expression and activity within the prostate. Finasteride is a selective inhibitor of 5-alpha-reductase type 2 whereas dutasteride inhibits both types 1 and 2. By inhibiting the conversion of testosterone to its more potent metabolite dihydrotestosterone they prevent cell proliferation and may induce apoptosis. Consequently a reduction in prostate size of about 15–25% and circulating PSA levels of about 50% is seen after 6 to 12 months of treatment. The effect on circulating PSA is predictable and therefore does not jeopardize the role of PSA testing in the investigation and management of prostate adenocarcinoma.

Combination therapy

The rationale for combination therapy is based on the complementary effects of alpha-blockers and 5-alpha-reductase inhibitors. While alpha-blockers offer rapid symptomatic relief without targeting the underlying disease process, 5-alpha-reductase inhibitors provide good mid- to long-term symptom relief as well as a reduction in the risk of BPH progression.

Combination therapy has been shown to be superior to monotherapy in two large randomized studies (MTOPS and CombAT) with regards to both symptom relief and prevention of overall clinical progression.[11,12] It is therefore offered as first-line medical treatment to men at high risk of disease progression (large prostate volume, significant LUTS, and reduced flow rate).

Surgical options

Indications for surgery

The most frequent indication for surgical management is the presence of bothersome LUTS refractory to medical management. The following complications of BPH are also considered strong indications for surgery:

- refractory urinary retention
- recurrent urinary tract infection
- recurrent haematuria refractory to medical treatment with 5-alpha-reductase inhibitors
- renal impairment secondary to obstructive uropathy
- bladder stones.

Transurethral resection of the prostate (TURP)

TURP was first performed in 1932 and has continued to provide durable long-term improvement in LUTS. Despite recent modifications to the equipment used, the basic principle of TURP has remained unchanged. The aim of TURP is to remove the obstructing overgrowth of tissue causing BOO and to reduce LUTS.

One of the most important and recent modifications has been the introduction of bipolar technology. Utilization of a specialized resectoscope loop, which incorporates both the active and return electrodes, allows both tissue cutting in a conductive saline medium (rather than glycine) and coagulation. Table 2.9.3.7 reviews the complications of TURP.

Laser enucleation, resection, and vaporization

It is impossible to directly compare clinical results and outcome data for the different laser modalities and equipment used in the treatment of BPH, as the effects caused by laser energy vary according to the wavelength, applied energy, fibre architecture, and tissue properties.

Table 2.9.3.7 Complications of TURP

Complication	Risk	Comments
Retrograde ejaculation	75%	Permanent
Erectile dysfunction	10%	May be related to compounding factors such as age
Urinary retention	5%	–
Haemorrhage requiring transfusion	≤5%	–
Urethral stricture	4%	–
Urinary incontinence	4%	May be temporary or permanent
UTI	4%	–
TUR syndrome	≤1%	Associated with large prostates, excessive bleeding and prolonged operating time
Death	≤0.1%	–

Holmium lasers

Holmium lasers are widely used for a variety of endourological applications in soft tissues and for the treatment of stones. The 2140 nm wavelength of the Ho:YAG (holmium:yttrium-aluminum-garnet) laser is strongly absorbed by water, which limits the area of tissue coagulation to 3–4 mm, allowing for precision cutting and adequate haemostasis. Holmium laser resection of the prostate (HoLRP) is usually performed when the prostate is smaller than 60 mL, while holmium laser enucleation (HoLEP) is used for larger glands.

Green light lasers

Vaporization of prostatic tissue is achieved by a sudden increase in temperature of the tissue, from 50°C to 100°C following the application of laser energy. This rapid increase in tissue temperature results in intracellular vacuoles and an increase in intracellular pressure, which ultimately causes the cell to burst or 'vaporize'. Green light lasers emit a wavelength of 532 nm, which lies within the effective range for tissue vaporization (500–580 nm).

Minimally invasive techniques

Various devices have been developed that allow direct application of either low-level radiofrequency energy or microwave radiation to the periurethral area of the prostate in order to treat BOO secondary to BPH.

Transurethral microwave thermotherapy (TUMT) works by heating prostatic tissue to >45°C to cause coagulation necrosis. The treatment is delivered via a specially designed catheter, which is passed urethrally, and can be performed under local anaesthetic or sedation.[13] Cystoscopy is required pre-treatment to exclude the presence of a large middle lobe or a short prostatic urethra, both of which would render TUMT an inappropriate treatment modality.

Transurethral needle ablation (TUNA™) of the prostate delivers low-level radiofrequency energy to the prostate via needles inserted transurethrally causing coagulation necrosis.[13] Needles are placed under direct vision using a modified cystoscope.

Both techniques have been shown to have low morbidity, but they have higher rates of irritative voiding symptoms and urinary retention after the procedure, compared with standard TURP. Their long-term durability remains unclear and re-treatment rates are high.

Open prostatectomy

Open prostatectomy is the oldest surgical treatment modality for BPH causing BOO. It is the most invasive technique, but also the most effective as the obstructive prostatic adenomas are completely enucleated using the index finger, either through the anterior prostatic capsule (Millin procedure) or from inside the bladder (Freyer procedure). With the advent of laser enucleation techniques, open prostatectomy has become a rarely performed procedure, but in the absence of such facilities it remains an option for large volume prostates (≥80 mL).

Catheterization

Long-term catheterization may be the only option for patients with severe symptoms, chronic urinary retention (CUR) or recurrent AUR who have failed medical management or who are unfit for surgery. Intermittent self-catheterization is preferable to an indwelling catheter, but is dependent on good cognition and manual dexterity.

Management of acute urinary retention

AUR is characterized by a sudden onset of an inability to void and is associated with intense pain. Urethral catheterization is the initial treatment and the amount of urine drained from the bladder should be recorded. Following catheterization, initial investigations include serum electrolytes and a catheter specimen of urine for culture together with a digital rectal examination assessment of the prostate. If the serum creatinine is elevated then an ultrasound of the renal tract should be performed to exclude hydronephrosis, which may be present in cases of acute-on-chronic urinary retention.

Any precipitating cause for AUR, such as a urinary tract infection or constipation, should be treated prior to a trial without catheter. If the patient does not appear to have any precipitating cause other than BPH and is treatment naive, consideration can be given to commencement of medical therapy prior to a delayed trial without catheter. Patients who fail a trial without catheter or who progress to AUR despite maximal medical therapy have the option of either surgery or long-term catheterization (indwelling or intermittent self-catheterization).

Management of chronic urinary retention associated with renal impairment

This condition is often referred to as high-pressure CUR, which relates to the aetiology of the renal impairment. It is a painless condition and patients are usually completely unaware of a problem until they present unable to void and are therefore little prepared for the long-term impact on their voiding function. Urgent catheterization is indicated to relieve the obstruction and to allow recovery of residual renal function, but particular attention must be given to three immediate clinical sequelae: sepsis, decompression haematuria, and post-obstructive diuresis.

Patients with CUR often have infected urine and passage of a catheter may trigger sepsis. Antibiotic cover and close observation post-catheterization are advised.

Decompression haematuria can develop within minutes of catheterization, but usually settles within 24 to 48 hours. In most cases no extra investigation or treatment is required.

Post-obstructive diuresis can be significant and prolonged, with the passage of between 6 and 12 litres of urine per 24 hours lasting for several days. It is thought to reflect maintenance of glomerular filtration despite inadequate recovery of tubular reabsorption. Careful monitoring of fluid balance and serum electrolytes is essential and intravenous fluid supplementation may be necessary.

It is unsafe to perform a trial without catheter until definitive treatment has been undertaken. Prolonged over-distension of the bladder can lead to detrusor hypocontractility or acontractility necessitating long-term catheterization. Surgery is only an effective option if there is evidence of recovery of detrusor function and urodynamic studies may be necessary to confirm this.

Further reading

American Urological Association Education and Research, Inc. Guideline on the management of benign prostatic hyperplasia (BPH). Linthicum (MD): American Urological Association Education and Research, Inc.;2010:34 http://guideline.gov/content.aspx?id=25635.

Speakman MJ, Kirby RS, Joyce A, *et al*. Guideline for the primary care management of male lower urinary tract symptoms. *BJU Int* 2004; 93: 985–90.

References

1. Oesterling JE. Benign prostatic hyperplasia: a review of its histogenesis and natural history. *Prostate Suppl* 1996; 6: 67–73.

2. Barry MJ. Evaluation of symptoms and quality of life in men with benign prostatic hyperplasia. *Urology* 2001; 58(6A); 25–32.

3. Roehrborn CG. Accurate determination of prostate size via digital rectal examination and transrectal ultrasound. *Urology* 1998; 51(Suppl.1): 19–22.

4. Roehrborn CG, Girman CJ, Rhodes T, *et al*. Correlation between prostate size estimated by digital rectal examination and measured by transrectal ultrasound. *Urology* 1997; 49: 548–57.

5. Roehrborn CG, Malice M, Cook TJ, *et al*. Clinical predictors of spontaneous acute urinary retention in men with LUTS and clinical BPH: A comprehensive analysis of the pooled placebo groups of several large clinical trials. *Urology* 2001; 58: 210–6.

6. Emberton M, Andriole GL, de la Rosette J, *et al*. Benign prostatic hyperplasia: a progressive disease of aging men. *Urology* 2003; 61: 267–73.

7. Emberton M, Fitzpatrick JM, Rees J. Risk stratification for benign prostatic hyperplasia (BPH) treatment. *BJU Int*. 2011; 107: 876–80.

8. Oelke M, Bachmann A, Descazeaud A, *et al*. Guidelines on the management of male lower urinary tract symptoms (LUTS), including benign prostatic obstruction (BPO). European Association of Urology Uroweb 2012 http://www.uroweb.org/gls/pdf/12_Male_LUTS_LR%20May%209th%202012.pdf (accessed on 1st March 2013).

9. Djavan B, Chapple C, Milani S, *et al*. State of the art on the efficacy and tolerability of alpha1-adrenoceptor antagonists in patients with lower urinary tract symptoms suggestive of benign prostatic hyper- plasia. *Urology* 2004; 64: 1081–8.

10 Nickel JC, Sander S, Moon TD. A meta-analysis of the vascular-related safety profile and efficacy of a-adrenergic blockers for symptoms related to benign prostatic hyperplasia. *Int J Clin Pract* 2008; 62(10): 1547–59.

11. McConnell JD, Roehrborn CG, Bautista O, *et al*; Medical Therapy of Prostatic Symptoms (MTOPS) Research Group. The long-term effect of doxazosin, finasteride, and combination therapy on the clinical progression of benign prostatic hyperplasia. *N Engl J Med* 2003; 349(25): 387–98.

12. Roehrborn CG, Siami P, Barkin J, *et al*; CombAT Study Group. The effects of combination therapy with dutasteride and tamsulosin on clinical outcomes in men with symptomatic benign prostatic hyperplasia: 4-year results from the CombAT study. *Eur Urol* 2010; 57(1): 123–31.

13. Blute ML, Larson T. Minimally invasive therapies for benign prostatic hyperplasia. *Urology* 2001; 58(6A): 33–40.

CHAPTER 2.9.4

Benign scrotal and penile conditions

Ian Eardley

Disorders of the foreskin

Phimosis

The most common disorder of the foreskin is phimosis. This is a condition where the foreskin is tight and will not retract fully. At birth the foreskin is adherent to the glans penis. These adhesions gradually loosen such that the foreskin becomes progressively retractile. The foreskin is at least partially retractile in the majority of boys by the age of five. The term 'physiological phimosis' refers to a foreskin that is supple, non-scarred but is not yet fully retractile. Such a foreskin does not require treatment. In contrast, a pathological phimosis refers to a foreskin that is scarred and non-retractile. The usual cause in children is balanitis xerotica obliterans (BXO), which is a condition of unknown aetiology associated with scarring of the foreskin and occasionally with scarring of the glans penis and urethral meatus (Figure 2.9.4.1).

Paraphimosis refers to a condition where a tight foreskin has been retracted behind the glans penis. This results in obstruction to the venous outflow from the glans with oedematous swelling such that the foreskin becomes 'stuck' behind the glans. Treatment involves manual compression of the glans penis and restoration of the foreskin to the normal position. Adjunctive measures that are occasionally helpful are cold compresses of the penis, local anaesthetic blocks, and hyperosmotic applications to the glans. In severe cases a dorsal slit or circumcision is necessary.

Balanoposthitis is an infection of the glans penis and prepuce. It can arise secondary to phimosis, but can also occur in association with a normally retractile foreskin. It usually resolves with simple cleansing measures but on occasions antibiotic treatment is required.

Phimosis in adults

In adult men the most common causes of phimosis are scarring of the prepuce secondary to recurrent infections and BXO. Men usually present with a foreskin that is painful on intercourse or in severe cases with ballooning of the foreskin at the time of micturition. Complications of a tight foreskin include balanoposthitis, paraphimosis, and, under rare circumstances, carcinoma of the penis.

Circumcision

Indications for circumcision in a child include a pathological foreskin secondary to BXO, phimosis associated with repeated episodes of balanoposthitis, and repeated paraphimosis. There is some evidence that circumcision may be helpful in preventing urinary tract infections in young boys with vesicoureteric reflux or posterior urethral valves although this is contentious.

Cultural circumcision is widely practiced in Islamic and Jewish cultures. Surgery is usually performed in the community by practitioners who are skilled in its practice. There are occasions, however, when significant damage to the penis can be caused by poorly performed cultural circumcision and this occasionally presents acutely to the medical team.

In adults, indications for circumcision include phimosis that causes problems at the time of micturition or during intercourse,

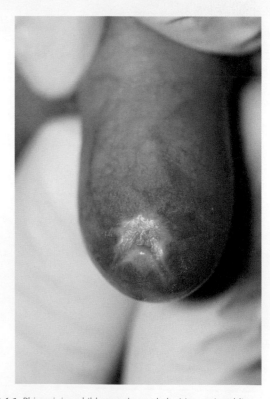

Fig. 2.9.4.1 Phimosis in a child secondary to balanitis xerotica obliterans.
Reproduced from Hamdy F and Eardley I (eds.), *The Oxford Textbook of Urological Surgery*, Oxford University Press, Oxford, UK, Copyright © Oxford University Press [forthcoming], by permission of Oxford University Press.

phimosis associated with episodes of paraphimosis, BXO, and in those men where there is a palpable, hard lesion under the foreskin that might be malignant and where a biopsy is needed.

Circumcision can be performed under local or general anaesthesia. It is important to remember that a circumcision is a cosmetic procedure and a careful surgical technique is essential. The most common error in a circumcision is to take too much skin. In children there are a variety of other approaches including the plastibell technique.

Frenulum breve

In frenulum breve the frenulum is short and tight. This may be secondary to BXO but more commonly simply reflects a frenulum that has been torn, usually during sexual intercourse. When it heals it does so with a scar that makes it tighter and more likely to tear. The patient typically presents with pain on erection and recurrent tearing of the frenulum. The appropriate treatment is frenuloplasty under local or general anaesthesia. Frenuloplasty utilizes the Heineke Mikulicz principle whereby the frenulum is incised transversely and repaired longitudinally.

Hypospadias

Hypospadias is a condition where the urethral meatus is more proximally placed than usual, lying anywhere between the glanular and the perineal urethra (Figure 2.9.4.2). There is associated hooded foreskin and a degree of chordee (a ventral deformity of the penis

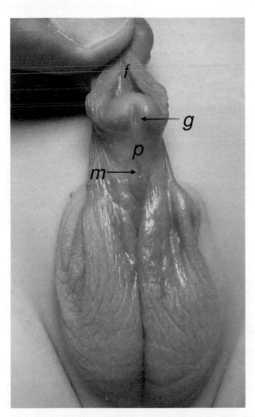

Fig. 2.9.4.2 Hypospadias: a ventral urethral meatus located on the penile shaft (m). Urethral plate distal to the meatus (p) and dorsal hooded foreskin (f). Shallow glans groove and distal glanular pit (g).

Reproduced from Hamdy F and Eardley I (Eds.), *Oxford Textbook of Urological Surgery*, Oxford University Press, Oxford, UK, Copyright © Oxford University Press [forthcoming], by permission of Oxford University Press.

on erection). The most common site of the meatus is at or around the coronal sulcus. There are a variety of surgical techniques to treat hypospadias that are beyond the scope of this book but which are ideally undertaken before the age of 2 years.

Disorders of the penis

Erectile dysfunction

The inability to attain or maintain an erection is called erectile dysfunction (ED). It is a common condition that is associated with increasing age, and it has a variety of causes including vascular, neurological, psychological, psychiatric, and endocrine disease. The most common cause is atherosclerosis, and ED is therefore associated with diabetes, hypertension, dyslipidaemia, smoking, obesity, and lack of exercise.

Clinical management focuses upon identification and treatment of these risk factors, if present, and first-line treatment involves the use of phosphodiesterase type 5 inhibitors such as sildenafil. If these drugs fail, then alternative treatments include intracavernosal injection therapy, vacuum devices, and penile implant surgery.

Penile deformity

The most common cause of penile deformity is Peyronie's disease, which is a condition of unknown aetiology characterized by a combination of penile deformity, palpable plaques of fibrotic tissue within the penis, ED, and pain upon erection. The condition has two phases. In the first phase (the 'active' phase), there is progressive deformity of the penis as the fibrotic plaques enlarge and mature. This phase is associated with pain on erection. After about 12 to 18 months the condition enters a 'chronic' phase where the fibrotic plaques cease to progress, the deformity becomes stable, and the pain disappears. The ED is caused by a variety of factors including impaired arterial inflow, abnormal venous leakage around the fibrotic plaques, and the psychological consequences of the penile deformity.

The patient presents with a penile bend. He will often give a history of trauma although there is no clear evidence that trauma causes this condition. The deformity is most usually a dorsal deformity and may be severe (Figure 2.9.4.3). The diagnosis is usually apparent upon physical examination when the palpable plaques can be easily identified within the body of the penis.

During the acute phase of the condition there is no evidence that any intervention can treat or improve the condition. It is important to encourage the patient to maintain sexual activity if the deformity allows him to do so. When the condition has stabilized the central issue is whether the deformity interferes with sexual activity. If it does then some form of corrective surgery is appropriate. The usual technique is the Nesbit procedure where a wedge of tunica albuginea on the convex side of the penis is excised. The plication of the remaining edges of the tunica albuginea pulls the deformity straight. There is a consequent loss of length, perhaps up to 2 cm, and in a small proportion of men the quality of erections postoperatively is diminished.

Occasionally, young men present with a penile deformity that is not due to Peyronie's disease. This is an unusual condition called congenital curvature of the penis. The deformity is usually a ventral deformity and there are no palpable plaques. The treatment is as for Peyronie's disease, namely some form of penile plication procedure.

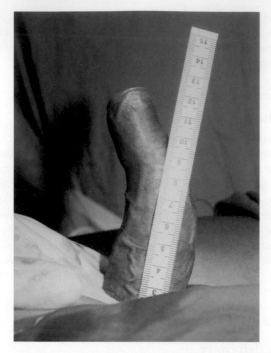

Fig. 2.9.4.3 Peyronie's disease: a perioperative photograph of an artificial erection in a man with Peyronie's disease, demonstrating a severe dorsal deformity.

Priapism

A persistent erection lasting longer than 4 hours is known as a priapism. The most common type is an 'ischaemic' priapism where there is sludging of blood within the venous system of the penis. This results in relative ischaemia of the penile tissues. The most common causes are drugs, including psychotropic agents used to treat schizophrenia or severe depression. Intracavernosal injection of alprostadil, which is a treatment for ED, is also a cause. Hypercoagulability of the blood can lead to priapism with causes including sickle cell disease, acute leukaemia, and myeloma.

Patients present with a painful erection and the diagnosis is confirmed either by aspiration of penile blood (confirming the hypoxia, hypercapnia, and acidosis) or by Doppler scanning the penis that confirms the lack of penile blood flow. Treatment is an emergency and should be instituted within 4 to 6 hours of presentation. If resolution of the priapism is delayed there will be permanent damage to the penis with endothelial damage and loss of smooth muscle tissue. Beyond 24 hours treatment is usually unsuccessful and the man is typically rendered permanently impotent.

Initial measures include aspiration of blood from the penis and irrigation with heparinized saline. If this fails, intracavernosal injection of sympathomimetic agents such as phenylephrine is appropriate. Such approaches are usually successful but if they fail, surgical shunting is necessary.

A less common type of prolonged erection is 'high-flow' priapism. This occurs following an injury to the penis or perineum where there is damage to the penile artery resulting in a fistula between the artery and the sinusoidal tissues of the corpus cavernosum. This results in excessive blood flow through the penis. Typically the erection is painless and is fluctuant in severity. Diagnosis can be made by aspiration of penile blood with normal oxygen saturations seen, while Doppler scanning will typically demonstrate the

fistula. Treatment of the 'high-flow' priapism is not an emergency and should be undertaken in specialist units where there is facility for selective penile arteriography and embolization.

Disorders of the urethra

Meatal stenosis

Meatal stenosis is uncommon and is usually secondary to BXO. It results in diminution and spraying of the urinary stream and may result in urinary tract obstruction and infection. It is important to assess the whole of the urethra to exclude the presence of more proximal urethral strictures. If the condition is due to BXO then topical steroid treatment is appropriate. Surgical treatment is necessary in resistant cases and in cases not due to BXO. There are a number of surgical procedures described but all increase the tendency of the urine to spray.

Urethral stricture

The most common disorder of the urethra is a urethral stricture. This is an area of narrowing and scarring within the urethra resulting in a diminished urinary flow. Causes include sexually transmitted diseases. Gonorrhoea was an important cause of urethral stricture a hundred years ago, although it is less common nowadays. Perineal trauma is also a cause although the majority of strictures are idiopathic in origin. BXO is a rare cause of stricture affecting typically the penile urethra.

The patient typically complains of a poor urinary stream with post micturition dribbling and often with recurrent episodes of urinary tract infection. The condition is usually diagnosed on the basis of a poor urinary flow rate and can be confirmed either with a urethrogram or at the time of cystoscopy.

The usual first-line treatment is optical urethrotomy or urethral dilatation. These approaches are designed to open up the urethra at the area of narrowing. They cure the problem in around 50% of cases but for the remaining patients the stricture will recur and require more definitive treatment. Recurrence is more likely when the stricture is long (greater than 2 cm) and when it is located within the penile urethra.

The treatment of recurrent urethral strictures is usually urethroplasty. For short strictures of the bulbar urethra it is possible to excise the stricture with an end-to-end anastomotic urethroplasty. For more extensive strictures of the bulbar urethra and for strictures in other parts of the urethra some form of skin flap or graft is required to reconstruct the urethra. Currently buccal mucosa is the most commonly used graft under these circumstances. When the patient declines urethroplasty, repeated urethrotomy with or without long-term intermittent self-dilatation is an option.

Disorders of the testicles

Undescended testicles

The testis develops within the genital ridge between the sixth to eighth weeks of gestation. Its descent under androgenic control in the third trimester is mediated by contraction of the gubernaculum that guides the testis into the scrotum. The testis should be within the scrotum by term. It is accompanied by a pouch-like extrusion of the peritoneal cavity called the processus vaginalis that normally closes but remains open in around 5% of boys at the time of birth. This creates the potential for a communicating hydrocele or inguinal hernia. Most will close during the first year of life.

The germ cells of the testicle mature from around 6 months of age but only if the testis is within the scrotum, which is 2 to 3 degrees centigrade cooler than an intra-abdominal location. Failure to descend therefore is associated with delayed or incomplete maturation of the germ cells.

The incidence of undescended testicle is around 1.5% in term infants. In preterm infants the incidence is considerably higher depending upon the degree of prematurity. They are classified by their location: intra-abdominal, intracanalicular, inguinal, or intrascrotal. Ascending testicles are testicles that have descended fully at birth but subsequently undergo secondary ascent during childhood into an inguinal position. A retractile testicle is a *normally* descended testicle that 'retracts' into the neck of the scrotum following contraction of the cremasteric muscle. Most commonly seen in boys between the ages of 3 and 7 years it does not need treatment.

Examination is best undertaken in a warm environment and should include careful inspection of the scrotum to assess the position of the testicles prior to palpation. When the testicle is impalpable, ultrasound, computed tomography, and laparoscopy are useful in identifying the testicle. Of these, laparoscopy has the advantage of also allowing initial surgical treatment of an intra-abdominal testicle.

Orchidopexy, the surgical procedure that mobilizes the testicle and fixes it within the scrotum is most commonly performed around 12 months of age. It is performed under general anaesthetic as a day case and is a straightforward procedure for inguinal, high scrotal, and intracanalicular testes. Intra-abdominal testes require more complex procedures that may require a staged approach.

Orchidopexy at an early age appears to maximize fertility. This is particularly true in bilateral cases. Testes that have been retained in the groin or abdomen into adult life carry an increased risk of malignancy and it seems likely that *early* orchidopexy can reduce the risk of testicular cancer, while it also reduces the risk of torsion and protects the testicle from trauma. If the testicle is atrophic then an orchidectomy is performed.

Testicular torsion

Testicular torsion occurs when the testicle twists on the spermatic cord such that there is obstruction initially to the venous outflow and secondarily to the arterial inflow. This causes ischaemia and testicular infarction.

The most common form of testicular torsion is intra-vaginal torsion where the testicle twists within the tunica vaginalis through 180°, 360°, 540°, or 720°. The greater the twist, the more rapid and severe the ischaemia. Animal evidence shows that there is significant ischaemic damage within 6 hours.

Extra-vaginal testicular torsion is seen only in neonates. Here the testis and its covering twist in their entirety. The usual presentation is of a neonatal scrotal swelling, and almost invariably the testicle is dead at the time of diagnosis.

Intra-vaginal torsion most commonly occurs in children in adolescence but is occasionally seen in adults. It can be precipitated by exercise and the patient presents with acute testicular pain. On examination the testicle is extremely tender, is often 'high-riding', and is associated with erythema of the scrotal skin.

The differential diagnosis is a torted hydatid of Morgagni, epididymo-orchitis, and idiopathic scrotal oedema. A torted hydatid of Morgagni is usually seen in young boys and is often distinguishable by seeing a blue-black torted hydatid through the scrotal skin. Epididymo-orchitis is extremely uncommon in children and

adolescence although it is a viable differential diagnosis in adults. Idiopathic scrotal oedema is a rare condition seen only in children.

Although ultrasound and Doppler scanning can sometimes be helpful in making a diagnosis, because of the incidence of false negative and false positive results, if in *any* doubt at all, the diagnosis should be confirmed by scrotal exploration. This is a surgical emergency and surgery needs to be performed within 6 hours of the onset of the pain if the testicle is to be reliably saved.

At operation the testicle is exposed and untwisted. If there is a return of blood flow then the testicle is fixed in position. Because of the risk of contralateral torsion it is standard practice to fix both testicles. If, following untwisting of the testicle, there is no recovery in blood flow then an orchidectomy is performed, although the contralateral testicle is still fixed. Three-point fixation using non-absorbable suture material is routine in order to prevent recurrence of the twist.

Following surgery for testicular torsion there may be delayed atrophy of the testicle. This is particularly true when surgery has been undertaken after 6 hours even if the testicle appears to be viable at operation.

Scrotal swellings

A common clinical problem is a patient who presents with a scrotal swelling. The clinical assessment of such patients is important and it is important to examine the patient both when they are lying and when that are standing. Both testicles should be examined, usually starting with the unaffected testicle. It is important to be gentle with the patient because testicular examination can be uncomfortable and tender. During the course of the examination the clinician should ask themselves a number of questions:

◆ Firstly, is it possible to get above the scrotal swelling? If not, that raises the possibility of an inguinal hernia or a varicocoele.

◆ Secondly, the examiner should ascertain whether the testicle is separate from the swelling. If the swelling appears to enclose the testicle then the differential diagnosis is a hydrocele or possibly a haematocele.

◆ Thirdly, if the testicle itself is palpable then the exact location of the swelling should be identified. If the swelling is clearly epididymal then epididymal cyst or epididymitis become possible diagnoses. If the lump is testicular this raises the possibility of a tumour.

◆ Finally, the clinician should attempt transillumination. If the swelling transilluminates brightly this makes hydrocele or epididymal cyst a possibility, depending on the location of the swelling.

A useful adjunct in all cases of testicular swelling is the use of ultrasound, which will often clarify the diagnosis even when clinical examination has been inconclusive.

Hydrocoele

A hydrocoele is a collection of fluid within the tunica vaginalis surrounding the testicle. There are two main types: those that communicate with the peritoneal cavity and those that do not. The former are known as patent processus vaginalis (PPV) and are most typically seen in children. The latter is non-communicating and is usually a primary hydrocoele associated with no specific testicular pathology, although it can be secondary to trauma, tumour, or infection.

In children, most PPVs close within the first year of life but if they are present thereafter then they are best treated by surgery. Surgery is performed by ligation of the PPV and evacuation of the fluid from around the testicle.

In adults indications for treatment include discomfort and cosmetic concerns. Ultrasound is particularly useful to confirm the presence of a normal testicle. Aspiration is usually ineffective because the fluid rapidly reappears. There are a number of surgical procedures described for the treatment of hydroceles. The most commonly performed are the 'Jaboulay' procedure where the hydrocoele sac is everted behind the testicle or the 'Lord's' procedure where the sac is opened and plicated around the testicle to produce a collar of tunica vaginalis. Complications include haematoma and wound infection with an incidence of recurrence of around 5%.

Epididymal cyst

An epididymal cyst is a cystic swelling of the epididymis. The exact aetiology is unknown and the cyst is usually full of clear fluid. They are often multiple and may be of variable size from small pea-like swellings up to cysts that are several centimetres in diameter. The diagnosis is usually straightforward on clinical grounds but can be confirmed on ultrasound scan. When the fluid is milky, it is called a spermatocoele.

Indications for treatment include discomfort and concerns about cosmesis. Small cysts that cause no discomfort do not require treatment. Aspiration of the fluid is usually pointless because the fluid rapidly re-accumulates. Treatment of a single cyst is surgical excision, but if there were multiple or recurrent cysts then a partial epididymectomy is appropriate. The patient should be warned that the surgery will affect the fertility of that testicle. Complications include haematoma and recurrence.

Varicocoele

A varicocoele is a collection of varicose veins around the testicle. Most commonly seen on the left side there are various grades ranging from grade 1 where the varicocoele is palpable during a Valsalva manoeuvre, grade 2, which is palpable at rest but not visible, and grade 3, which is visible and palpable at rest (Figure 2.9.4.4).

Varicocoeles are found in 15–20% of healthy men and are harmless in the vast majority of patients. Occasionally they can cause aching of the testicle, particularly when the patient has been standing for a long time. When present in adolescence they can cause testicular atrophy and there is a long-standing controversy regarding their role in male infertility. Diagnosis can be confirmed by testicular ultrasound. One particular point to note is that the acute onset of a varicocoele in a middle-aged man can be associated with obstruction either of the left renal vein or occasionally of the inferior vena cava by tumour thrombus from a renal tumour.

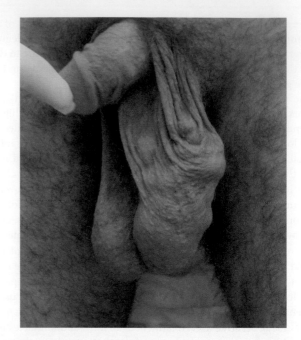

Fig. 2.9.4.4 A varicocoele that is visible within the left hemiscrotum.
Reproduced from Hamdy F and Eardley I (Eds.), *Oxford Textbook of Urological Surgery*, Oxford University Press, Oxford, UK, Copyright © Oxford University Press [forthcoming], by permission of Oxford University Press.

Accordingly, when presenting at this age it is prudent to organize an ultrasound scan of the kidneys.

Most varicocoeles do not require treatment. Indications for treatment include testicular atrophy in an adolescent, aching discomfort for which no other cause can be found, and occasionally in cases of infertility. Treatment is either by radiological embolization of the vein or by laparoscopic or open ligation of the vein.

Further reading

Blandy JP, Kaisary A. *Lecture Notes in Urology*. Oxford: Blackwell Publishing, 2009.

Cox AM, Patel H, Gelister J. Testicular torsion. *Br J Hosp Med* 2012;73(3):C34–6.

Hatzimouratidis K, Eardley I, Giuliano F *et al*. EAU guidelines on penile curvature. *Eur Urol* 2012;62(3):543–52.

Pinto K. Circumcision controversies. *Pediatr Clin N Am* 2012; 59(4):977–86.

Masson P, Brannigan RE. The varicocele. *Urol Clin N Am* 2014;41(1):129–44.

Mundy AR, Andrich DE. Urethral strictures. *BJU Int* 2011;107(1):6–26.

Salonia A, Eardley I, Giuliano F, *et al*. European Association of Urology guidelines on priapism. *Eur Urol* 2014;65(2):480–9.

Thomas DFM, Duffy PG, Rickwood AMK. *Essentials of Paediatric Urology*. London: Informa Publishing, 2008.

PART 2.10

Orthopaedic surgery

CHAPTER 2.10.1

Common fractures and complications

Hemant Sharma and Kevin Sherman

Introduction

This chapter presents the principles of the management of the patient with a fracture with some illustrative examples of common fractures. This chapter is not intended to be an exhaustive text on the management of fractures.

The management of the patient with a fracture involves not only selecting the most appropriate treatment for the bony injury, but also the management of the adjacent soft tissues, which will in many cases have a major influence on the eventual outcome, affecting both the healing of the bony injury itself and any eventual disability.

General principles

Complications of fractures

It is useful to consider potential complications first.

Damage to adjacent structures such as blood vessels, nerves, articular surfaces, ligaments, tendons, and in the case of children, the growth plate, may have a profound influence on the eventual outcome.

Bones will naturally attempt to heal when broken. Treatment involves facilitating this natural healing process and the avoidance (or management) of complications. Fracture healing is a biological process that depends upon an adequate blood supply. A fractured bone that has been stripped of soft tissue will be much slower to heal, or may not heal at all. Infection will also impede healing.

The aim of treatment of a fracture in a limb is to end up with a well-aligned, pain free, functioning limb in the shortest feasible time, with minimal disruption to the patient's lifestyle during the healing process.

Complications can be considered as 'early' or 'late'. Early complications include:

- vascular damage
- compartment syndrome
- nerve injury
- skin loss
- infection of soft tissues and/or bone (acute).

Late complications include:

- delayed union (union not achieved in the expected time but still potential for healing)

- non-union (evidence that the fracture will not heal without intervention)
- malunion (fracture heals but in unacceptable alignment)
- post-traumatic osteoarthritis
- complex regional pain syndrome
- chronic osteomyelitis
- muscle contracture
- joint contracture.

Assessment of the patient with a fracture

The initial assessment of a patient with a possible fracture involves the detection and diagnosis of the bony injury, and the evaluation of the adjacent anatomical structures.

In keeping with Advanced Trauma Life Support[1] principles, priority must be given to life- or limb-threatening injuries, which will usually be those with major associated vascular injury, spinal cord injury, or severe muscle crushing.

Diagnosis of a fracture

The classical signs of a fracture are: swelling, deformity, localized bony tenderness, abnormal movement, and crepitus. Abnormal movement and crepitus should not be sought actively.

Localized bony tenderness indicates the need for radiological investigations, usually radiographs in a minimum of two planes. Computed tomography or magnetic resonance imaging scans may also be necessary.

Classifications of fractures

Fractures can be classified as:

- open/closed
- transverse/spiral/oblique
- non-comminuted or comminuted
- extra-articular or intra-articular.

There are many classifications of fractures at individual anatomical sites. Some are useful for treatment decisions or for establishing a prognosis, and others are mainly for research.

Examples of useful therapeutic classifications are the Gustilo[2,3] classification of open fractures (Table 2.10.1.1) and the Salter-Harris classification of growth plate injuries[4] (Box 2.10.1.1).

Table 2.10.1.1 Gustilo Anderson classification of open fractures

	Wound	Contamination	Soft tissue	Bone	Vascular injury
Grade 1	1 cm	None	Minimal	Simple	
Grade 2	>1 cm	minimal	moderate	Simple—minimal comminution	
Grade 3 A	>10 cm	high	Severe with crushing	Comminuted/segmental—soft tissue cover possible	
Grade 3 B	>10 cm	High	Severe with crushing	Comminuted—soft tissue cover not possible	
Grade 3 C	>10 cm	High	Severe with crushing	Comminuted	Yes

Adapted with permission Gustilo, RB and Anderson JT, Prevention of infection in the treatment of one thousand and twenty-five open fractures of long bones, *The Journal of Bone and Joint Surgery*, Volume 58, Issue 4, pp. 453–458, Copyright © 1963. All Rights Reserved, The Journal of Bone and Joint Surgery, Inc. STRIATUS Orthopaedic Communications 1976; and Gustilo RB et al, Problems in the management of type III (severe) open fractures: A new classification of type III open fracture, *Journal of Trauma*, Volume 24, Issue, pp. 742–746, Copyright © 1984, with permission from Lippincott, Williams & Wilkins.

Assessment of the soft tissues

It is essential to make a systematic assessment of the adjacent soft tissue structures:

+ vascular
+ nerves
+ skin
+ ligaments
+ tendons.

Vascular injuries

Bleeding from major vessels may be life or limb threatening and must be dealt with immediately. Management of these injuries is dealt with in the section on major trauma.

Box 2.10.1.1 Salter-Harris classification of growth plate injuries

Type I: fracture passes across the growth plate leaving the proliferative zone, where the cells divide, intact. Except in the case of epiphyses that lie within the joint (e.g. the femoral head) these fractures heal well.

Type II: fracture passes partly along the growth plate and then involves part of the metaphysis. The proliferative zone remains intact. These behave in a similar fashion to type I fractures. The metaphyseal fragment can be useful radiographically in demonstrating the position of the epiphysis in injuries occurring before the epiphyseal ossification centre has formed.

Type III: fracture passes partly along the growth plate and then angles across the epiphysis. These fractures disrupt the proliferative layer of the growth plate and the articular surface. They require accurate reduction to prevent growth disturbance and/or osteoarthritis. These fractures tend to occur in partially closed growth plates.

Type IV: fracture crosses the growth plate, involving both the metaphysis and the epiphysis. The complications and treatment are as for type III.

Type V: crushing of the growth plate. The diagnosis is suspected on the basis of the history.

Reproduced with permission from Salter R, Harris W, Injuries involving the epiphyseal plate, *The Journal of Bone and Joint Surgery*, Volume 45, Issue 3, pp. 587–622, Copyright © 1963. All Rights Reserved The Journal of Bone and Joint Surgery, Inc. STRIATUS Orthopaedic Communications.

Arteries may be damaged by direct external trauma or by compression from displaced fractures, for example in displaced supracondylar fractures of the elbow.

In addition to looking for signs of external or internal bleeding and loss of pulses distal to the injury, the circulation to muscle compartments must be evaluated. If the differential between the arteriolar pressure and the venule pressure falls below the pressure within a fascial compartment there will be no capillary circulation to the contents of the compartment despite intact distal pulses. The symptoms and clinical signs of compartment syndrome include:

+ severe pain
+ palpable tightness of the muscle compartment
+ increased pain on stretching the ischaemic muscles within the compartment
+ loss of sensation in areas supplied by cutaneous nerves passing through the compartment.

Compartment syndrome may also occur after prolonged compression of an artery that is then released, such as following a displaced supracondylar fracture of the elbow.

Nerve injuries

Nerve injury may be present from the time of injury or may develop subsequently, either due to the secondary effects of the injury or from iatrogenic causes.

Nerves may be damaged by:

+ direct external injury (open or closed)
+ stretching resulting from displaced or angulated fractures or dislocations
+ pressure or laceration from displaced bone ends
+ traction or compression during attempts to reduce fractures or during definitive fracture treatment
+ pressure from external sources such as operating table components
+ ischaemia in compartment syndrome.

Nerve injury may range from bruising with temporary loss of function to complete division of the nerve. Seddon's[5] classification (1942) is useful:

+ Neuropraxia: conduction block and myelin injury, axons intact. There is no permanent damage to nerve fibre and full recovery is expected.

Box 2.10.1.2 Sunderland's classification of nerve injuries

First degree: equivalent to Seddon's neuropraxia

Second degree: axons disrupted

Third degree: axons and endoneurium damaged

Fourth degree: axons, endoneurium, and perineurium damaged

Fifth degree: complete division of the nerve trunk (equivalent to neurotmesis

Reproduced from Sunderland S., A Classification of Peripheral Nerve Injuries Producing Loss of Function, *Brain*, Volume 74, Issue 4, pp. 491–516, Copyright © 1951 Oxford University Press, by permission of Oxford University Press.

◆ Axonotmesis: nerve fibre damage with complete Wallerian degeneration, but the connective tissue structure is intact. Slow recovery takes place.

◆ Neurotmesis: disruption of nerve structures leading to cessation of nerve conduction. Recovery of function does not occur.

Axons are covered by endoneurium, fascicles by perineurium, and peripheral nerves by epineurium. Sunderland[6] classified nerve injuries into five degrees based on this anatomy (Box 2.10.1.2).

Nerves are vulnerable to injury where they either lie in a superficial position, particularly where they are close to bone, or where they are tethered to bone.

Some common sites for nerve injuries are listed in Table 2.10.1.2. This list is not exhaustive.

Any neurological impairment must be documented before intervention.

Skin

The term 'open' is preferable to 'compound' for fractures or dislocations in which the overlying skin is breached.

Open fractures are classified by the degree of contamination and soft tissue damage. Open wounds should be photographed and covered prior to expeditious early cleaning and debridement; they should not be repeatedly be exposed for inspection. Antibiotics should be commenced where a wound overlies a fracture or joint.

In closed injuries, skin viability must be preserved. Skin under pressure from displaced fractures may become ischaemic, leading to subsequent necrosis and infection. Where there is obvious deformity with skin under pressure it is appropriate to gently realign the limb to ease skin pressure and also tension on nerves and vessels prior to radiological investigations.

Ligaments and tendons

An attempt should be made to assess the integrity of the ligaments around a joint, but in some cases the diagnosis of ligament injury can only be made by evaluation under anaesthesia, or after fracture stabilization.

Radiological investigations such as magnetic resonance imaging scanning or ultrasound may be useful.

Tendons may be damaged by incision or by avulsion of their insertions or origins, often with some attached bone.

Fracture patterns

The radiographic fracture pattern is a useful indicator of the mechanism of injury and the probable stability of any reduction. In most

Table 2.10.1.2 Common sites for nerve injuries

Site	Nerve	Clinical signs
Dislocation of shoulder	Axillary nerve	Numbness in 'regimental badge' area
Humeral neck injury	Axillary nerve	Numbness in 'regimental badge' area
Humeral shaft fracture	Radial nerve	Wrist and finger drop, numbness in dorsum of first web space
Radial neck fracture	Posterior interosseous nerve	Finger drop, intact brachioradialis function
Elbow fractures/dislocations	Ulnar nerve	Numbness ulnar border of hand, weakness of little finger abduction
Carpal fractures or dislocations, distal radius fractures	Median nerve	Numbness in volar aspect of radial three and a half digits of hand
Hip dislocations	Sciatic nerve	Weakness of dorsiflexion and plantarflexion of foot and ankle, numbness in leg distal to knee
Fibular neck fractures	Common Peroneal nerve	Drop foot, numbness over dorsum of foot
Anterior compartment syndrome in leg	Deep peroneal nerve	Drop foot, numbness in first web space of foot

cases fractures are reduced by disimpacting the fracture and then reversing the original mechanism.

◆ Transverse fractures usually indicate a simple bending force – if angulated they can be reduced and held by three-point fixation.

◆ Spiral fractures indicate a twisting force – they are often stable when reduced and held by two twisting forces (a turning couple).

◆ Oblique fractures usually indicate a combination of compression and angulation and are usually unstable when reduced.

Pathological fractures

Pathological fractures occur in weakened bone. When a fracture occurs following relatively minor trauma the differential diagnosis may include:

◆ genetic disorders: for example, osteogenesis imperfect (Box 2.10.1.3)

◆ metabolic bone disease: including osteomalacia, osteoporosis and many rarer metabolic disorders (Figure 2.10.1.1)

◆ benign localized lesions of bone: tumours or cysts

◆ malignant disease: primary or secondary.

Fragility fractures are discussed in Box 2.10.1.3[7,8]

Initial treatment of fractures

The initial treatment of a patient involves: suitable analgesia and immobilization to prevent further damage and for pain relief, and appropriate treatment of any wound.

Definitive treatment options for a bony injury[9]

Bone will heal if the bone ends are viable and if there is appropriate control of movement at the fracture site. Rigid fixation will lead to 'primary bone healing' (bone remodelling) that is slow and only

Box 2.10.1.3   Fragility fractures

In the UK osteoporosis is the most common cause of fragility fractures and due to demographic factors the incidence is predicted to rise, with considerable social and economic impact.

Common sites for fragility fractures include the distal radius, the spine, and the femoral neck.

Osteoporosis is diagnosed if the bone mineral density of the patient is <2.5 SD below that of a sex- and race-matched control group of young adults (T-score) on a DEXA (dual intensity X-ray absorptiometry).

Treatment of patients with fragility fractures may differ from that for other fractures because of the concomitant medical conditions frequently found in the typical age group, the difficulty of obtaining good internal fixation in weak bone, and the need to investigate and treat the underlying condition to prevent further fractures.

Locking plates and screws are popular for the treatment of many fragility fractures (e.g. proximal humeral and distal radial fractures) as they are less prone to pull-out of the screws but they are more expensive than conventional metalwork.

occurs if there is no significant gap between the bone ends. The most rapid healing is that occurring by 'secondary bone healing', which involves the formation of callus, but excessive movement will damage the ingrowing blood vessels. The ideal strain at the fracture site for secondary bone healing to occur is between 2% and 10%.

Treatment may be non-operative or operative. The choice of treatment methods includes:

* no specific treatment
* traction
* support (e.g. broad arm sling)
* external casting
* internal fixation
  * wires
  * screws

* plates
  * intramedullary nails
* external fixation.

Traction

Traction may utilize external weights, the weight of a body part, or counter pressure against some other part of the body. The collar and cuff sling, for example, uses the weight of the arm to produce traction.

Simple support and/or splinting

Simple support or splinting is used for stable fractures to give pain relief. Examples include splinting of a greenstick fracture of the distal radius or a broad arm sling for an impacted humeral neck fracture.

Formal casting

Casting can be used to maintain correction of a deformity at a fracture site.

Casting avoids the need for an invasive operation but there is a risk of pressure sores or compartment syndrome. In most cases the joints above and below the fracture must be immobilized (usually necessary to control rotation) and there is therefore a risk of joint stiffness.

Internal fixation[10]

Internal fixation may be performed using wires, screws, plates, and screws or with intramedullary nails.

The advantages of internal fixation are:

* The amount of movement ('strain') at the fracture site can be controlled for optimal healing.
* Accurate reduction of the fracture can be achieved, which is important, for example, in intra-articular fractures.
* The adjacent joints can be mobilized early, with reduced risk of joint stiffness, contractures or muscle wasting, and with earlier return of function.

The disadvantage of internal fixation are:

* Infection risk.
* Potential to cause further damage to the soft tissues including nerves, etc.
* May need to have surgical metalwork removed with risk of re-fracture or other operative complications.

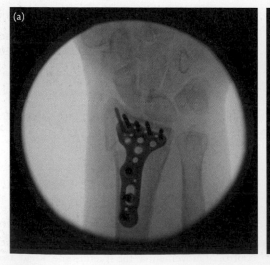
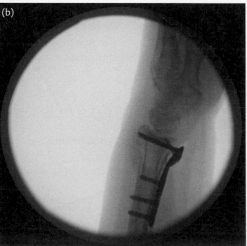

Fig. 2.10.1.1 Locking plate used to fixed unstable distal radius fracture in osteoporotic bone.

Plates may be used in many different ways; as buttresses, as neutralization plates to protect a compression screw, to bridge a comminuted fracture, and so on.

Intramedullary nails are load-sharing devices with less risk of re-fracture after removal.

External fixation

External fixation can be used for emergency stabilization of a fracture to allow repairs to other structures, such as arteries, or it may be the definitive treatment.

External fixation devices[11] can be constructed in a number of configurations. The fixation to bone may be with large diameter pins, as used in uniaxial constructs, or with fine wires under tension that pass through the bone and are fixed to a frame (e.g. Ilizarov frames).

External fixation wires or pins must be inserted along 'safe corridors' to avoid damage to nerves, blood vessels, or joints.

There is a risk of infection at the pins sites and good pin track care is essential.

Fine-wire fixation frames are used for complex deformity correction, lengthening of bone, or to 'transport' bone as part of a corrective procedure.

Examples

Fractures of the distal radius

Distal radius fractures are common, with peak prevalence at about 10 years' of age and in the over 60s (where osteoporosis is a factor).

Restoration of length and alignment of the distal radius is important for normal function. In the adult the radial styloid lies, on average, 11 mm distal to the tip of the ulnar styloid. The slope of the articular surface of the distal radius should be approximately 22° in the frontal plane, with volar angulation of approximately 12°.

The common 'Colles' fracture has the following deformity:

* radial angulation and translation
* dorsal angulation and translation
* shortening.

The term Smith's fracture is applied to a fracture with volar angulation. The term Barton's fracture (volar or dorsal) is used to refer to fractures that involve part of the distal radial articular surface.

It is important to establish whether the fracture is intra- or extra-articular, whether it is stable or unstable and whether there are features predicting a poor outcome.

Complications

* Stiffness of wrist or fingers due to prolonged immobilization or casts that extend beyond the metacarpophalangeal joints.
* Persisting pain often due to malunion, especially radial shortening leading to pain near the distal ulna.
* Complex regional pain syndrome, type I (secondary to nerve damage) or type II (no nerve damage).
* Osteoarthritis due to joint incongruity affecting either the distal radius articular surface or the distal radio-ulnar joint.
* Median nerve compression.
* Ulnar nerve injury.

* Compression of the radial nerve from casts.
* Late rupture of extensor pollicis longus at Lister's tubercle (more common in undisplaced fractures).

Median nerve injury may be immediate or delayed, due to swelling in the carpal tunnel. Sensory loss, other than minor, should be treated by release of all constricting casts and bandages, and elevation of the limb. If the symptoms do not improve early surgical decompression is indicated.

Factors to consider in planning treatment

These fractures cover a wide spectrum and no single approach will suffice for every fracture. The 'personality' of the fracture and patient factors will determine the optimum treatment.

Fracture 'personality' includes comminution, stability, articular depression, and osteoporosis. Patient factors include age, functional demands, and occupation. Functional demands are more important than chronological age.

Treatment
Non-operative

Stable undisplaced fractures, and some displaced fractures, can be treated non-operatively with carefully applied casts, following reduction if necessary. Casts for 'Colles' fractures should not have excessive volar angulation as this can cause median nerve compression. To avoid finger stiffness casts must not extend beyond the distal palmar crease.

Loss of reduction is not uncommon, often as the swelling subsides and the cast becomes loose, or when the cast molding is inadequate.

Operative treatment

Operative treatment can be with Kirschner wires or plates. External fixation is only occasionally used.

Kirchner wire fixation usually involves inserting two or three wires. In the Kapanji[12] technique the first wire is passed through the fracture site on the dorsal and radial side and used to lever the distal fragment into position, and then by obtaining purchase against the opposite cortex used to buttress the fracture.

Internal fixation

Fixed-angle volar locking plates have recently become very popular for unstable fractures (Fig 2.10.1.1). Plates have following advantages:

* stabilize multifragmentary/unstable fracture
* option of holding radial styloid fragment
* prevent late collapse
* usually no plaster required
* early mobilization.

Disadvantages include soft tissue problems, median nerve damage (main trunk and palmar branch), and iatrogenic damage to the distal radial articular surface.

Femoral neck fractures

Fractures of the neck of femur are common; the incidence in the UK being 70 000 to 75 000 with the majority being 'fragility fractures' associated with osteoporosis. Many patients have multiple co-morbidities and the outcome of treatment will, to a large extent, depend on their general physical and mental condition and their medical management. They are therefore best managed jointly between trauma surgeons and elderly care physicians. The 30-day mortality is 10% and 12-months mortality 33%, with mortality after 1 year being the same as age matched controls.

The National Institute for Health and Care Excellence[13] has produced guidelines for managing these fractures; which include surgical treatment as soon as general health has been optimized.

Fractures of the neck of femur can be loosely divided into intracapsular and extracapsular fractures.

Intracapsular fractures

The femoral head receives its blood supply form three main sources: the intra-osseous supply; the artery to the ligamentum teres; and the retinacular vessels that arise from the trochanteric anastomosis, formed from the ascending branches of the lateral and medial circumflex arteries plus branches from the superior and inferior gluteal arteries. The ligamentum teres supply is often poor in the elderly and the interosseous source is damaged by subcapital fractures. The blood supply then relies on the intracapsular retinacular vessels, particularly the lateral ones, which can be damaged especially if the fracture is displaced. As a result, these fractures are prone to two main complications: avascular necrosis and non-union. Avascular necrosis may not become apparent for more than 2 years following fracture.

The Garden classification is the one most commonly used for these fractures (Box 2.10.1.4).

Garden types I and II generally have a good prognosis and can potentially be treated non-operatively but require careful monitoring as some will displace late; for this reason operative fixation is often performed with two or three parallel cancellous screws, or a dynamic hip screw with or without a de-rotation screw. The rationale for operative fixation is that a relatively small operation is performed for an undisplaced fracture rather than a possible larger one later if the fracture displaces.

Garden types III and IV are treated operatively unless the patient is too unfit for surgery. In young patients, internal fixation can be attempted but there is a high risk of avascular necrosis. In the elderly treatment is usually with either a hemiarthroplasty (cemented or uncemented) or sometimes with total hip replacement for physically active patients. Bipolar hemiarthroplasties are modular and can be converted to total hip replacements if acetabular wear later occurs.

Extracapsular fractures

In extracapsular fractures the risk of avascular necrosis is very small and non-union is uncommon (<2%). The treatment rationale is based on the risk of malunion, potentially leading to severe shortening and rotation.

Extracapsular fractures can be described as two, three or four part, where the femoral head and neck is one part, the femoral shaft another part, and the greater and lesser trochanters are the third and fourth parts.

Evans described type I and type II fractures. In type I fractures the fracture line runs upwards and outwards from the lesser to the greater trochanter. In type II fractures the fracture line passes distally and laterally from the lesser trochanter. Type II fractures are unstable. Type I fractures are unstable if they are four part or if they are three part with posteromedial comminution.

Box 2.10.1.4 Garden classification of intracapsular fractures

Type I: Incomplete fracture with lateral compression (inferior trabeculae still intact)

Type II: complete but undisplaced

Type III: complete with some displacement but some soft tissue attachment (trabeculae of femoral head and acetabulum do not line up)

Type IV: completely displaced (trabeculae of femoral head and acetabulum line up because femoral head assumes normal position in acetabulum)

Reproduced with permission and Copyright © of the British Editorial Society of Bone and Joint Surgery. Garden R. S., Low-angle fixation in fractures of the femoral neck, *Journal of Bone and Joint Surgery*, Volume 43-B, pp. 647–663, Copyright © 1961.

Stable fractures are usually treated with a sliding ('dynamic') hip screw device ('DHS'), which allows controlled collapse at the fracture site, ensuring good bony contact and compression. In unstable fractures a high valgus angle is often used and the posteromedial buttress must be reconstructed.

An intramedullary device (e.g. cephalocondylar nail) is an alternative.

Ankle fractures

Ankle stability depends on the bony contours and three sets of ligaments: the deltoid ligament; the lateral ligament complex; and the syndesmotic ligaments (anterior and posterior tibiofibular ligaments and interosseous ligament).

The skin is at risk of necrosis in highly displaced fractures and/or dislocations, and pressure on the skin from underlying bone must be relieved by gentle reduction of severe angulation/displacement towards neutral alignment.

Stability of the ankle mortice must be assessed in all injuries.

The outcome of ankle fractures is highly influenced by the accuracy of reduction of any displacement. The aim of treatment is to maintain a congruent joint and fibular length. Failure to maintain congruence and alignment may lead to stiffness, pain, and early onset osteoarthritis (often within 2 years).

Radiological assessment of the ankle should include lateral and a 'mortice view' (AP with the ankle 20° internally rotated). The medial joint space should be equal to the superior joint space and 4 mm or less; widening of the medial joint space indicates instability of the

---

Box 2.10.1.5 Danis-Weber classification of ankle fractures

Type A: fibular fracture below level of syndesmosis

Type B: fibular fracture at level of syndesmosis

Type C: fibular fracture above the level of the syndesmosis

Source: data from Danis R., Les fractures malleolaires, in Danis R. (Ed), *Théorie et pratique de l'osteosynthese*, Masson, Paris, Copyright © 1949; and Weber B. G., *Die verletzungen des oberen sprunggelenkes*, Second Edition, Verlag Hans Huber, Berne, Switzerland, Copyright © 1972.

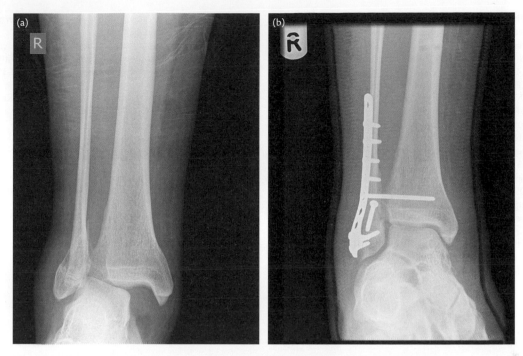

Fig. 2.10.1.2 (a) Unstable Weber B fracture before fixation. (b) Unstable Weber B fracture after fixation including diastasis screw.

talus within the mortice of the ankle joint. Instability results from a combination of:

- fracture of the medial malleolus or rupture of the deltoid ligament
- fracture of the fibula at any level
- disruption of the syndesmosis.

It is important to identify those cases where the fibula is fractured proximally (e.g. at the fibular neck). Lateral shift of the talus in combination with a high fibular fracture indicates extensive damage to the interosseous ligament.

Classification

The Danis-Weber classification of ankle fractures is useful (Box 2.10.1.5).

Type A fractures are stable, type C are unstable, and the stability of type B fractures depends on whether there is damage to the syndesmosis.

Type A fractures and stable type B fractures can be treated non-operatively, usually with a below-knee walking cast for 6 weeks, although good results[14] have been reported for stable type B fractures treated with a support bandage and early weight bearing.

Treatment

Unstable fractures are usually treated operatively, although non-operative treatment is potentially possible[15] with careful attention to casting and follow-up.

Surgical techniques usually involve fixation with plates and screws. For fibular fractures the length and rotational alignment is restored and the fracture fixed with a 'lag' (compression) screw and a neutralization plate, which protects the lag screw fixation. The integrity of the syndesmosis must be checked by external rotation stress views with or without a direct pull on the lateral malleolus with a hook. If unstable the syndesmosis is stabilized with one or more screws or other commercial fixing devices (Fig 2.10.1.2).

Medial malleolar fractures are fixed with screws, ensuring that the articular surface is congruent. Posterior malleolar fractures only require internal fixation if they involve more than one third of the articular surface.

Further reading

Baumgaertner MR, Curtin SL, Lindskog DL, *et al.* The value of tip-apex distance in predicting failure of fixation of peritrochanteric fractures of the hip. *J Bone Joint Surg Am* 1995; 77(7): 1058–64.

Browner B, Jupiter J, Levine A, et al. (eds). *Skeletal Trauma* 5th edition. Philadelphia: Saunders Elsevier, 2015.

Flynn JM, Skaggs DL, Waters PM (eds) *Rockwood and Wilkins' Fractures in Children* 8th edition New York: Lippincott Williams & Wilkins, 2009.

McQueen M. Court-Brown CM. Compartment monitoring in tibial fractures; the pressure threshold for decompression M. *J Bone Joint Surg Br* 1996; 78: 99–104.

Murray IR, Amin AK, White TO, *et al.* Proximal humeral fractures: Current concepts in classification, treatment and outcomes. *J Bone Joint Surg Br* 2011; 93: 1–11.

National Institute of Health and Care Excellence. Hip fractures. London: NICE http://www.nice.org.uk/nicemedia/live/13489/54921/54921.pdf (accessed November 2013).

Novack V, Jotkowitz A, Etzion O, *et al.* Does delay in surgery after hip fracture lead to worse outcomes? A multicenter survey. *Int J Qual Health Care* 2007; 19(3): 170–6.

Robb JE. The pink, pulseless hand after supracondylar fracture of the humerus in children. *J Bone Joint Surg Br* 2009; 91: 1410–12.

References

1. *Advanced Trauma Life Support (ATLS) Course Manual* 9th edition. Chicago: American College of Surgeons, 2012.
2. Gustilo R, Anderson J. Prevention of infection in the treatment of one thousand and twenty-five open fractures of long bones. *J Bone Joint Surg Am* 1976; 58A: 453–8.

3. Gustilo RB, Mendoza RM, Williams DM. Problems in the management of type III (severe) open fractures. A new classification of type III open fractures. *J Trauma* 1984; 24: 742–6.

4. Salter R, Harris W. Injuries involving the epiphyseal Plate: *J Bone Joint Surg Am* 1963; 45(3): 587–622.

5. Seddon HJ. A classification of nerve injuries. *BMJ* 1942; 2(4260): 237–9.

6. Sunderland S: *Nerve and Nerve Injuries* 2nd edition. London: Churchill Livingston, 1978.

7. National Institute of Health and Clinical Excellence (NICE) Guidelines. Fragility fractures. London: NICE http://publications.nice.org.uk/osteoporosis-assessing-the-risk-of-fragility-fracture-cg146 (accessed November 2013).

8. National Osteoporosis Foundation. Clinician's Guide to Prevention and Treatment of Osteopororsis. Washington DC: National Osteoporosis Foundation. http://nof.org/files/nof/public/content/file/344/upload/159.pdf (accessed November 2013).

9. Solomon L, Warwick D, Nayagam S. *Apley's System of Orthopaedics and Fractures* 9th edition. London: Hodder Arnold 2010.

10. Orthopaedic Trauma Association. Basic principles and techniques of internal fixation of fractures. Rosemont, IL: Orthopaedic Trauma Association. http://ota.org/media/29257/G10_Internal_Fix_Principles.ppt (accessed November 2013).

11. Orthopaedic Trauma Association. Principles of external fixation. Rosemont, IL: Othorpaedic Trauma Association. http://ota.org/media/29260/G11-Ex-Fix-Principles-JTG-rev-2-4-10.ppt (accessed November 2013).

12. Trumble T, Wagner W, Hanel D, *et al.* Intrafocal (Kapandji) pinning of distal radius fracture with and without external fixation. *J Hand Surg* 1998; 23A: 381–94.

13. NICE. Guidelines for fracture neck of femur. London: NICE. http://www.nice.org.uk/nicemedia/live/13489/54921/54921.pdf (accessed November 2013).

14. Port A, McVie J, Naylor G, *et al.* Comparison of two conservative methods of treating an isolated fracture of lateral malleolus. *J Bone Joint Surg Br* 1996; 78: 568–72.

15. Makwana N, Bhowal B, Harper W, *et al.* Conservative versus operative treatment for displaced ankle fractures in patients over 55 years of age: A prospective randomized study. *J Bone Joint Surg Br* 2001; 83: 525–9.

CHAPTER 2.10.2

Degenerative and inflammatory joint disease

Pierre Nasr and Vikas Khanduja

Introduction

Arthritis encompasses a variety of both non-inflammatory and inflammatory conditions that affect synovial joints. In order to understand both inflammatory and degenerative arthritides as a disease process, the normal structure and function of articular cartilage must be understood.

Structure and function of articular cartilage

Articular cartilage is a type of hyaline (glass like) cartilage, which is the most common variety of cartilage. Hyaline cartilage is also found in costal cartilage, the fetal skeleton, and epiphyseal plates. It is composed of chondrocytes that make up 5% of the wet weight of articular cartilage and produce collagen within an extracellular matrix.[1] Cartilage is avascular, aneural, alymphatic, and is relatively non-immunogenic. It contains predominantly type II collagen with lesser amounts of types IX and XI, which constitute 10–20% of the wet weight of articular cartilage. It functions to provide resistance to compressive and shear forces across a joint, the collagen fibres being arranged in layers (Figure 2.10.2.1). Mutations in type II collagen cause chondrodysplasias, which are a group of disorders characterized by dwarfism and a spectrum of joint deformities.[2]

Synovial fluid nourishes cartilage and decreases the coefficient of friction and, therefore, the wear of the joint.[3] Synovial fluid is a dialysate of blood plasma synthesized by synoviocytes in the synovium of joints. Normal joints have little friction with movement and do not wear out under physiological load, overuse, or trauma.

Chondrocytes have the longest cell cycle in the body, similar to central nervous system and muscle cells.[4] Cartilage health and function depend on the compression and relaxation associated with weight bearing and locomotion. Compression causes fluid to egress from the cartilage into the joint space and ultimately into the capillaries and venules.[5] Relaxation allows the cartilage to re-expand, increase its hydration, and absorb necessary electrolytes and nutrients.

The largest constituent of extracellular matrix is water, which comprises 75% of the wet weight of articular cartilage, held together by proteoglycans that comprise 10–15% of the wet weight. It contains substances such as hyaluronic acid, collagenases, glycoproteins, proteinases, and lubricin that allow it to have lubricant properties.[6] Hyaluronic acid is a glycosaminoglycan composed of a complex sugar that acts as a barrier permitting metabolites to pass through via diffusion[7] (Figure 2.10.2.2).

It can behave like a viscous material under low-velocity movements but changes to behave like an elastic material under high-velocity movements. It is, therefore, termed a viscoelastic material. Synovial fluid also provides a nourishment function for the chondrocytes.[8]

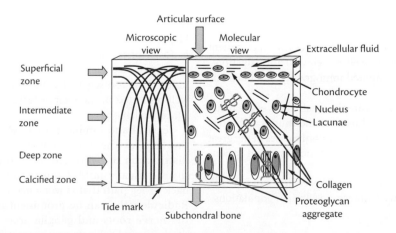

Fig. 2.10.2.1 Schematic representation of the microscopic and molecular structure of articular cartilage.
Reprinted from Mark Miller, Stephen Thompson, and Jennifer Hart, *Review of Orthopaedics*, Sixth Edition, Saunders, Philadelphia, USA, Copyright © 2012 by Saunders, an imprint of Elsevier Inc., with permission from Elsevier.

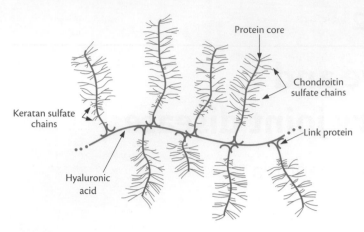

Fig. 2.10.2.2 Structure of a proteoglycan aggregate.
Reprinted from Mark Miller, Stephen Thompson, and Jennifer Hart, *Review of Orthopaedics*, *Sixth Edition*, Saunders, Philadelphia, USA, Copyright © 2012 by Saunders, an imprint of Elsevier Inc., with permission from Elsevier.

Osteoarthritis

Definition

Osteoarthritis (OA) is a common, chronic arthropathy characterized by disruption and potential loss of articular cartilage and exposure of subchondral bone associated with bone hypertrophy (osteophyte formation), subchondral cyst formation, and subchondral sclerosis. These changes are often evident on plain radiographic imaging as narrowing of the joint space. There is no worldwide-accepted definition, however, the National Institute for Health and Care Excellence has described it as a disorder of synovial joints characterized by focal areas of damage to the articular cartilage, remodelling of underlying bone, and the formation of osteophytes and mild synovitis.[9]

Incidence

OA is the most common joint disorder, which often becomes symptomatic around the fourth and fifth decades and is nearly universal, although not always symptomatic, by the age of 80. Only half of patients with pathologic changes of OA have symptoms. Below age 40, most OA occurs in men and results from traumatic injuries. Women predominate from age 40 to 70, after which men and women are equally affected.[10]

Diagnosis

The diagnosis is based on a large array of sources, such as patient history, physical examination, as well as relevant investigations, including plain radiographs, computed tomography, and magnetic resonance imaging.

The most common joints affected are the small joints of the hand, especially the metacarpophalangeal joint of the thumb and interphalangeal joints of the hand. OA also commonly arises in the great toe metatarsophalangeal joint, facet joints of the spine, and various compartments of the hip and knee.[11]

There are various ethnic differences in the prevalence of OA with low rates seen in black Africans, Chinese, and Indian populations.

Classification

The classification system for OA is based on whether it is primary or secondary. Primary OA is commonly referred to as idiopathic

OA as the aetiology is unknown in most cases, although OA in the hip is now thought that it may be secondary to subtle anatomical abnormalities caused by slipped upper femoral epiphyses and acetabular labral tears. The natural history is not fully understood but OA is likely to represent the end point of a variety of processes at both a macroscopic and microscopic level.

Pathophysiology of osteoarthritis

OA is often simply referred to as 'wear-and-tear' arthritis. However, the disease process is much more complicated with changes occurring at a cellular level that causes joints to fail in their attempts to repair damaged cartilage.

OA, as well as other degenerative and inflammatory diseases of joints, needs to be understood in terms of its biochemical, histological, and mechanical changes that deviate from normal structure and function.

OA begins with tissue damage from mechanical injury such as from a torn meniscus. This causes inflammatory mediators from the synovium to attack cartilage and derange cartilage metabolism. The tissue damage stimulates chondrocytes to attempt repair by increasing the production of proteoglycans and collagen. However, efforts at repair also stimulate the enzymes that degrade cartilage as well as inflammatory cytokines that are normally present in small amounts. Inflammatory mediators trigger an inflammatory cascade that further stimulates the chondrocytes and synovial lining cells, eventually breaking down articular cartilage.[12] Chondrocytes undergo programmed cell death (apoptosis). Once cartilage is destroyed, exposed bone becomes eburnated and sclerotic.

Subchondral bone then stiffens and undergoes infarction as well as developing subchondral cysts. Attempts at bony repair cause subchondral sclerosis and osteophytes at the periphery of joints. The osteophytes develop in an attempt to stabilize the joint. The synovium becomes inflamed and thickened and produces synovial fluid with less viscosity and greater volume. Periarticular tendons and ligaments become stressed, resulting in tendonosis and can cause joint contractures and deformity. As the joint becomes less mobile, surrounding muscles atrophy and ligaments fail in their ability to support the skeleton.

OA of the spine can cause marked thickening and proliferation of the posterior longitudinal ligaments, which are posterior to the vertebral body but anterior to the spinal cord. The result can be transverse bony bridges that encroach on the anterior spinal cord. Hypertrophy and hyperplasia of the ligamentum flavum, which is posterior to the spinal canal, can compress the posterior canal, causing lumbar spinal stenosis. In contrast, the anterior and posterior nerve roots, ganglia, and common spinal nerve are relatively well protected in the intervertebral foramina where there is more space available.

Cervical and lumbar spinal OA may lead to myelopathy (at the level of the spinal cord) or radiculopathy (dermatomal distribution of pain). However, the clinical signs of myelopathy are usually mild. Lumbar spinal stenosis may cause lower back or leg pain that is worsened by walking or back extension. Radiculopathy can be prominent but is less common because the nerve roots and ganglia are well protected. Insufficiency of the vertebral arteries, infarction of the spinal cord, and dysphagia due to oesophageal impingement by osteophytes occasionally occur.

Rheumatoid arthritis

Definition

Rheumatoid arthritis (RA) is a chronic, inflammatory disease mediated by an autoimmune process that affects synovial joints. RA is a symmetric polyarthritis that erodes and deforms joints.

Incidence

RA affects around 2% of the adult female population and 0.5% of the adult male population in the United Kingdom. Its prevalence (indicated by consultation rate) is 40–80 in every 10 000 of the population with women being more affected than men.[13]

Diagnosis

It classically presents with joint inflammation, early morning stiffness, and a typical pattern of disease that affects the wrists and small joints of the hands and feet. There is associated warmth and erythema of these joints.

Joint damage in RA causes earlier joint disease than in OA with characteristic bony erosions, joint destruction, and subsequent characteristic clinical deformities. Rheumatoid nodules are found around the extensor aspects of the elbows and forearm and are present in around 25% of patients with RA.[14]

There are also systemic features such as general lethargy, low-grade fever, weight loss, and tenosynovitis. Over a variable period of months and years, functional impairment ensues causing difficulty with fine dexterous tasks at work or within activities of daily living.

The diagnosis is based on a typical history, physical examination, and relevant special investigations. The American College of Rheumatologists has used the particular criteria published in 2010 to diagnose RA (see Table 2.10.2.1). Greater than or equal to 6 points confidently diagnoses RA.[15]

It is important to be able to distinguish RA from other inflammatory arthropathies.

Systemic manifestations of RA occur in up to 5% of patient and can cause symptoms that can be confused with sepsis or malignancy.[16] Immunoglobulin M rheumatoid factor occurs in around 80% of patients with RA but can be found in 5% of the normal population. Immunoglobulin G and A are also found and correlate with a more severe and destructive form of RA.[17]

Due to improved understanding of the disease process, new treatments and therapeutic strategies are constantly being initiated. Recent studies have shown that early, aggressive intervention with disease modifying anti-rheumatic drugs (DMARDs) in the first 2 years can limit joint involvement and improve radiological appearances.

Pathophysiology of rheumatoid arthritis

The role of cytokines in the disease process in RA must be understood. They are produced by activated immune cells that can both enhance and inhibit the immune response. Pro-inflammatory cytokines include interleukin-2, interferon gamma, and tumour necrosis factor alpha. These cytokines stimulate synovial cells to proliferate and synthesize collagenase, which breaks down collagen within articular cartilage. Collagenase also causes resorption of bone and inhibition of proteoglycan synthesis. Matrix metalloproteinases are also involved in perpetuation of the inflammatory

Table 2.10.2.1 American College of Rheumatologists diagnostic criteria for rheumatoid arthritis (2010)

◆ **Joint distribution (0–5)**	
◆ 1 large joint	0
◆ 2–10 large joints	1
◆ 1–3 small joints (large joints not counted)	2
◆ 4–10 small joints (large joints not counted)	3
◆ >10 joints (at least one small joint)	5
◆ **Serology (0–3)**	
◆ Negative RF AND negative ACPA	0
◆ Low positive RF OR low positive ACPA	2
◆ High positive RF OR high positive ACPA	3
◆ **Symptom duration (0–1)**	
◆ <6 weeks	0
◆ ≥6 weeks	1
◆ **Acute phase reactants (0–1)**	
◆ Normal CRP AND normal ESR	0
◆ Abnormal CRP OR abnormal ESR	1

A score ≥6 confidently diagnoses RA. ACPA, anticyclic citrullinated peptide antibodies; CRP, C-reactive protein; ESR, erythrocyte Sedimentation Rate; RF, rheumatoid factor.

Reproduced with permission from Daniel Aletaha et al., Rheumatoid arthritis classification criteria: An American College of Rheumatology/European League Against Rheumatism collaborative initiative, *Arthritis and Rheumatism*, Volume 62, Number 9, pp. 2569–2581, Copyright © 2010 by the American College of Rheumatology.

cascade. Newer treatments target specific cytokines in order to down regulate the effects of specific cytokines to suppress the immune dysfunction present in the disease process.

Seronegative spondyloarthritis

These are a heterogeneous group of inflammatory diseases that present with joint pain, especially in the spine and peripheral joints. They can be associated with cardiac, ocular, and mucocutaneous system manifestations. The group includes Ankylosing spondylitis (AS), Psoriatic arthritis, reactive arthritis, and enteropathic arthritis associated with inflammatory bowel diseases.

AS is a chronic inflammatory disease of the axial skeleton that characteristically affects young adult males and usually presents with back pain and progressive stiffness. Radiographs show squaring of the vertebrae and ankylosis (fusion) of the spine. There is commonly an increase in the erythrocyte sedimentation rate and C-reactive protein. There are associations with the HLA-B27 allele in 95% of patients (the general populations prevalence of this gene is 5–10%). The goals of therapy are to provide symptom relief and prevent irreversible joint destruction but as the disease is poorly understood, treatment has not been as successful as the treatment of RA.[18] Psoriatic arthritis is another chronic inflammatory disease that affects 30% of patients with psoriasis. Peripheral joints are mainly affected and to a lesser extent, the spine. Patients are often treated with non-steroidal anti-inflammatory drugs (NSAIDs) and DMARDs, and there is emerging evidence that anti-tumour necrosis factor-α agents may improve the immune-mediated component to this disease.[19]

Symptoms and signs of degenerative and inflammatory joint disease

Symptoms of degenerative and inflammatory joint disease have certain characteristics that are common to all and others than are characteristic of specific conditions due to their unique disease processes.

Common symptoms include gradually developing pain, which is the earliest symptom, often described as a dull and deep ache. The pain is aggravated or triggered by activity and relieved by rest but can become so obtrusive as to cause night pain that wakes the patient from sleep.

Symptoms and signs from OA in general may also derive from subchondral bone, ligamentous structures, synovium, periarticular bursae, capsules, muscles, tendons, intervertebral discs, and periosteum, all of which are pain sensitive. Venous pressure may increase within the subchondral bone marrow and cause pain (sometimes called bone angina).

Osteoarthritis is associated with stiffness lasting less than 30 minutes on awakening and after inactivity. Younger patients often complain that the pain and stiffness affects their ability to perform sports, and as the disease process worsens the pain prevents patients from walking distances that they were previously able to achieve with ease. Hobbies and activities of daily living are ultimately affected as joint destruction proceeds. It is important to glean an accurate history of the pain in order to differentiate it from other sources, such as neurogenic pain originating from the spine, referred pain from joints more proximally, vascular insufficiency causing claudication, and pain emanating from different systems of the body. The site of the pain can give clues, such as groin pain from arthritis of the hip, which must be distinguished from a spinal source and even hernias.

As arthritis progresses, motion of the joint is restricted , which can impact on a patient's ability to rise from a chair, kneel, squat, perform fine dexterous tasks with their hands, or to adequately attend to perineal hygiene.

A detailed social history is extremely important in every orthopaedic patient. Questions asked must include a patient's occupation, their hand dominance (for patients presenting with symptoms in the upper limb), whether a patient lives in a house and how they cope with stairs, whether they use mobility aids, who does their shopping, and whether the patient still drives a car. A patient's social network is also important to appreciate, as this has an impact on their ability to adapt to a decrease in mobility and also how they may cope after an operation.

Physical signs occurring in patients with RA include soft tissue swellings, tender joints (especially affecting the proximal interphalangeal joints of the hands, as compared to Heberden's and Bouchard's nodes seen in OA), stiffness (morning stiffness can persist for an hour or more), erythema, and increased warmth. Flexor tenosynovitis of the long finger flexors may be present and there is also an association with carpal tunnel syndrome. Characteristic deformities such as Swan neck and Boutonnière commonly develop together with radial deviation at the wrist and ulnar deviation at the metacarpophalangeal joints.

RA also affects the foot and can cause metatarsalgia, deformities of the forefoot, and collapse of the midfoot transverse arch and valgus malalignment of the hindfoot. RA is associated with extraarticular manifestations that can affect a large number of organ systems including the cardiovascular, respiratory, neurological, haematological, and immune systems that predispose to pericarditis, pulmonary fibrosis, sensory peripheral neuropathy, normochromic normocytic anaemia, and increase risk of infection respectively.

Physical examination should be tailored to the specific joint and the author refers the reader to other more detailed texts that deal specifically with clinical examination.

Investigations

The diagnosis of OA is confirmed on radiographic examination taken in two planes. Typical features include joint space narrowing, subchondral sclerosis, subchondral cysts, and periarticular osteophytes.[20] Radiographic features of OA may be coincidental and the severity of symptoms sometimes does not correlate with the severity of the radiograph. The diagnosis of RA must take into account both the history and serological markers as well as radiological features common with OA.

Magnetic resonance imaging is becoming important in being able to visualize articular cartilage and adjacent soft tissues as well as intra-articular pathology such as meniscal injury and ligamentous abnormalities. Arthroscopic evaluation, under a general anaesthetic, normally via two small portals can visualize the joint surfaces directly but the procedure is normally reserved for cartilage and soft tissue debridement. Joint aspiration is reserved for cases where septic arthritis or crystal arthropathy such as gout or pseudogout is suspected.

Treatment

Treatment involves a stepwise approach to alleviate symptoms. This starts with conservative measures such as a weight loss reduction programme with the input of a dietician, modification of activities and even changes to the type of employment a patient is involved in, for example, cessation of manual labour. This then progresses to physiotherapy that loads the joint to improve diffusion of synovial fluid and improve the metabolism of articular cartilage. Specific exercises to improve particular muscle groups can have a beneficial effect, for example, the strengthening of the quadriceps in patients with OA of the knee. Patient education is important in order to empower them to manage their own treatment strategies.

Oral visco-supplementation in the form of nutritional supplements such as glucosamine and chondroitin sulphate may in some instances lead to improvement in symptoms.[21] Both are glycosaminoglycans that have been shown to reverse the inhibition of proteoglycan synthesis by interleukin-1. Intra-articular visco-supplementation is aimed at increasing hyaluronan and improves the visco elastic properties of articular cartilage.

Drug treatments to reduce pain can take the form of topical creams, oral analgesics, and patch therapy. Oral paracetamol is the first line, followed by NSAIDs, codeine-based preparations, and finally opioids. NSAIDs can cause unacceptable side effects such as gastrointestinal upset and renal toxicity, especially if used on a long-term basis.

Surgical treatment is again approached in a stepwise manner to improve pain and mobility. Exposed subchondral bone can, if subjected to a microfracturing technique during arthroscopy, enable undifferentiated mesenchymal stem cells to 'repair' cartilage defects by replacing exposed bone with fibrocartilage. It is a very crude repair technique that produces fibrocartilage, which has less resistance to shear stresses but may improve symptoms for a few years.

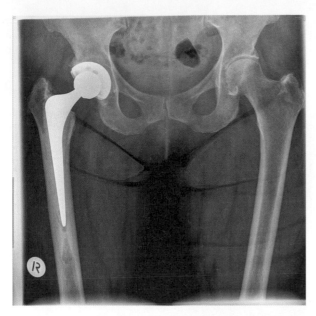

Fig. 2.10.2.3 Plain AP radiograph of the pelvis showing a Hybrid Total Hip Replacement (uncemented acetabular component and a cemented femoral stem).

Full-thickness osteochondral autografts can be harvested from the least weight-bearing periphery of the articular surface and transplanted into the defective area. Cadaveric osteochondral allograft has some viable chondrocytes that can synthesize collagen with structural integrity being provided by the osseous part of the graft.

Mesenchymal stem cells can be extracted from bone marrow in culture plates. These cells are then placed in a three-dimensional matrix of collagen gel and allowed to differentiate into chondrocytes that are then transplanted into the cartilage defect to form hyaline cartilage. Autologous chondrocyte implantation harvests a small amount of cartilage from the articular surface; the cells are isolated and proliferate in tissue culture to be reimplanted at a subsequent operation.[22]

Joint realignment procedures such as an osteotomy can also be carried out to offload the affected side of the joint and improve pain and also correct deformity simultaneously.

Ultimately, surgery can be performed for these diseases to address the joint destruction. Joint arthroplasty involves worn surfaces being excised and replaced by metal or plastic (Figure 2.10.2.3). Joint replacements, unfortunately have a finite lifespan that is increasing the burden of revision procedures once the replaced bearing surfaces wear or are subject to septic or aseptic loosening.

In some instances, soft tissue procedures must also be undertaken to attempt to correct deformities and ensure that muscle and tendon function across a joint is maximized, for example, performing tendon transfers in patients suffering from RA of the hands.

Complications

Patients need to be fully informed of the possible complications related to all their orthopaedic procedures. All surgeons must be aware of medical, anaesthetic, and surgical complications. Surgical complications can be grouped into immediate, early, and late complications (Box 2.10.2.1).

Box 2.10.2.1 Complications related to orthopaedic procedures

Immediate:

- Bleeding, infection, nerve injury

Early:

- Infection, deep vein thrombosis, pulmonary embolism, dislocation of prosthesis, rupture of repaired tendons/ligaments, metalwork failure, Non-union/malunion of osteotomy

Late:

- Infection, wear of bearing surfaces and subsequent aseptic loosening of the prosthesis

---

Conclusion

Degenerative and inflammatory joint diseases encompass a large variety of chronic destructive conditions that affect articular cartilage. Once the basic structure and function of articular cartilage is understood, the clinician will better be able to understand the current and future therapeutic strategies to deal with these common and debilitating diseases.

Further reading

Kasser JR (ed.) *Orthopaedic Knowledge Update 5*, 163–75. Rosemeont, IL, American Academy of Orthopaedic Surgeons, 1996.

Mankin HJ. Current concepts review: The response of articular cartilage to mechanical injury. *J Bone Joint Surg Am* 1982; 64: 460–6.

Pivec R, Johnson AJ, Mears SC, *et al*. Hip arthroplasty. *Lancet*. 2012 Nov 17; 380(9855): 1768–77.

Van Manen MD, Nace J, Mont MA. Management of primary knee osteoarthritis and indications for total knee arthroplasty for general practitioners. *J Am Osteopath Assoc* 2012; 112(11): 709–15.

References

1. Pearle AD, Warren RF, Rodeo SA. Basic science of articular cartilage and osteoarthritis. *Clin Sports Med* 2005; 24(1): 1–12.
2. Kannu P, Bateman J, Savarirayan R. Clinical phenotypes associated with type II collagen mutations. *J Paediatric Child Health* 2012; 48(2): E38–43.
3. Schmidt TA, Sah RL. Effect of synovial fluid on boundary lubrication of articular cartilage. *Osteoarthr Cartilage* 2007; 15(1):35–47.
4. Wilsman NJ, Farnum CE, Green EM, *et al*. Cell cycle analysis of proliferative zone chondrocytes in growth plates elongating at different rates. *J Orthop Res* 1996; 14(4): 562–72.
5. O'Hara BP, Urban JP, Maroudas A. Influence of cyclic loading on the nutrition of articular cartilage. *Ann Rheum Dis* 1990; 49(7): 536–9.
6. Sophia Fox AJ, Bedi A, Rodeo SA. The basic science of articular cartilage: structure, composition, and function. *Sports Health* 2009; 1(6): 461–8.
7. Fraser JR, Laurent TC, Laurent UB. Hyaluronan: its nature, distribution, functions and turnover. *J Intern Med* 1997; 242(1): 27–33.
8. Ulrich-Vinther M, Maloney MD, Schwarz EM, *et al*. Articular cartilage biology. *Acad Orthop Surg* 2003; 11(6): 421–30.
9. National Institute for Health and Clinical Excellence. Osteoarthritis. The care and management of osteoarthritis in adults. NICE clinical guideline 59. February 2008
10. Woolf A, Pfleger B. Burden of major musculoskeletal conditions. *Bull World Health Organ* 2003; 81(9): 646–56.

11. National Collaborating Centre for Chronic Conditions. *Osteoarthritis: National Clinical guideline for care and management in adults.* London: Royal College of Physicians, 2008.

12. Goldring MB. The role of cytokines as inflammatory mediators in osteoarthritis: lessons from animal models. *Connect Tissue Res* 1999; 40(1): 1–11.

13. Symmons D, Turner G, Webb R, *et al.* The prevalence of rheumatoid arthritis in the United Kingdom: new estimates for a new century. *Rheumatology* 2002; 41(7): 793–800.

14. Ziff M. The rheumatoid nodule. *Arthritis Rheum* 1990; 33:761–7.

15. Aletaha D, Neogi T, Silman AJ, *et al.* 2010 Rheumatoid arthritis classification criteria: an American College of Rheumatology/European League Against Rheumatism collaborative initiative. *Arthritis Rheum* 2014; 62(9): 2569–81.

16. Turesson C, O'Fallon WM, Crowson CS, *et al.* Extra-articular disease manifestations in rheumatoid arthritis: incidence trends and risk factors over 46 years. *Ann Rheum Dis* 2003; 62(8): 722–7.

17. Halvorsen EH, Pollmann S, Gilboe IM, *et al.* Serum IgG antibodies to peptidylarginine deiminase 4 in rheumatoid arthritis and associations with disease severity. *Ann Rheum Dis* 2008; 67(3): 414–7.

18. Tam L-S, Gu J, Yu D. Pathogenesis of ankylosing spondylitis. *Nat Rev Rheumatol* 2010; 6: 399–405.

19. Gladman DD, Antoni C, Mease P, *et al.* Psoriatic arthritis: epidemiology, clinical features, course and outcome. *Ann Rheum Dis* 2005; 64(Suppl II):ii14–ii17.

20. Kellgren JH, Lawrence JS. Radiological assessment of osteo-arthrosis. *Ann Rheum Dis* 1957; 16(4): 494–502.

21. Kahan A, Uebelhart D, De Vathaire F, *et al.* Long-term effects of chondroitins 4 and 6 sulfate on knee osteoarthritis: the study on osteoarthritis progression prevention, a two-year, randomized, double-blind, placebo-controlled trial. *Arthritis Rheum* 2009; 60(2): 524–33.

22. Crawford DC, DeBerardino TM, Williams RJ3rd. NeoCart, an autologous cartilage tissue implant, compared with microfracture for treatment of distal femoral cartilage lesions: an FDA phase-II prospective, randomized clinical trial after two years. *J Bone Joint Surg Am* 2012; 94(11): 979–89.

Joint and bone infections

Jehangir Mahaluxmivala and Daoud Makki

Septic arthritis

Background

Septic arthritis is an infectious process within the joint. In native joints, it often occurs following haematogenous spread but can also result from penetrating injuries or surgery. The incidence is around 5 cases per 100,000 person-years with the knee being the most common.[1]

Prosthetic joint infections occur in 1 per 100 cases[2] and present in three forms:[3]

1. Acute: occur within 4 weeks following surgery.

2. Acute haematogenous: acute onset of pain and swelling in a previously asymptomatic joint replacement.

3. Chronic: present beyond 4 weeks following surgery.

Pathophysiology

When a host's defence mechanisms are disrupted either systemically (immunocompromised patients) or locally (osteoarthritis or rheumatoid arthritis), synovial fluid will fail to resist bacterial invasion.

Bacterial colonization of synovial fluid and membrane triggers an inflammatory reaction. Destruction of the articular cartilage can then ensue from high concentrations of cytokines, collagen-degrading enzymes (metalloproteinase), and pressure from the effusion. Prompt intervention is therefore paramount to salvage of the articular cartilage.

Aetiology

Although all types of microorganisms might be involved, bacterial infection with coagulase-negative *Staphylococcus aureus* remains the most common and serious form in adults and children older than 2 years. This affinity of staph aureus to articular cartilage is linked to collagen binding factor (CNA gene product).[4]

Mycobacterial infections are encountered in patients from endemic areas, intravenous drug users, and following prolonged use of antibiotics.

Common bacteria, with risk factors, are shown in Table 2.10.3.1.

Presentation

Painful joint effusions should be considered septic until proven otherwise. Children might solely present with a reluctance to mobilize the affected limb or to weight bear.

Clinical examination should follow a look, feel, and move sequence. Effusion might be obvious in some joints (e.g. knee, ankle, and wrist), but not in others (e.g. hip). In hip septic arthritis,

effusion will cause flexion and external rotation of the leg in order to maximize joint volume.

Affected joints exhibit local warmth with a reduced range of motion. It is important to examine adjacent joints for simultaneous involvement. For instance, pain in the knee could be referred from the hip and vice versa.

Pre-patellar bursitis should not be mistaken for septic arthritis of the knee. Attempted aspiration of the knee joint could lead to inoculation with bacteria and cause septic arthritis.

Investigation

In children, clinical prediction for hip septic arthritis has been based on four variables:[5] inability to weight bear, pyrexia, erythrocyte sedimentation rate (ESR) > 40 mm/hr and white cell count (WCC) > 12000. There is 99% chance of septic arthritis when all of these criteria are present and 93% if three are present. The chance decreases to 40% if two criteria are present and to 3% when only one criterion is met.

Investigation should include plain radiographs, blood cultures, WCC, C-reactive protein (CRP), and ESR. In general WCC has a better sensitivity than ESR, but both have low specificity compared to joint aspirate WCC. The sensitivity of an ESR of >15 mm/hour is 66% and that of a CRP of >80 mg/L is 90%.[6] Both combined have better sensitivity. CRP normalizes quicker than ESR and is therefore useful to monitor response to treatment.

Joint aspiration, using an aseptic technique, constitutes the mainstay of diagnosis. Aspirate should be processed for urgent Gram

Table 2.10.3.1 Microorganisms in septic arthritis and the associated risk factors

Organism	Age	Risk factors
Staphylococcus aureus	Adults and children older than 2 years	Rheumatoid arthritis, Immunosuppressive drugs, Prosthetic joints
Streptococcus B	Infants (<3months)	Malignancy, DM
Other streptococci	Elderly	
Neisseria gonorrhoeae	Young adults	Sexual activities
Gram negative rods		
Pseudomonas	Adult	Immunosuppression,
H. influenza	Infants (6–24months)	IVDU, DM
Aeromonas	Adult	Leukaemia
Salmonella	Any age	Sickle cell disease

DM, diabetes mellitus; IVDU, intravenous drug user.

staining and cell count. Culture will guide future antibiotic therapy and the search for crystals will help reveal other diagnoses (Gout, pseudogout).

In prosthetic joints, urgent aspiration should be considered when sepsis is present and must be carried out in theatre. In the absence of sepsis, an arthroplasty surgeon can undertake aspiration and further management.

Management

Figure 2.10.3.1 shows the algorithm for the initial management of patients with suspected septic arthritis. The timing of washout depends on the index of suspicion and the results of joint aspirate. Empirical antibiotics are required when systemic sepsis is present. Following parenteral administration, high serum concentration is achieved rapidly whereas synovial penetration remains slow and poor.

Native joint septic arthritis is managed by arthroscopic or open washout followed by a course of antibiotics intravenously for 2 to 4 weeks then orally for 4 to 8 weeks.[7] This varies according to local hospital policies and type of microorganism.

The management of prosthetic joint infections depends on the mode of presentation. In acute and haematogenous forms, joint washout with retention of the prosthesis might be considered. In chronic infections, the presence of a biofilm on the implant protects bacteria against antibiotics and renders eradication difficult without removal of the prosthesis. Two-stage procedures are therefore considered; the first stage involves removal of prosthesis and cement, debridement, and then the insertion of a temporary spacer to maintain soft tissue balance. This is followed by a course of antibiotics for at least 6 weeks.

The second stage is a re-implantation procedure, the timing of which is based on the clinical response combined with a progressively decreasing CRP. A repeat joint aspiration might precede the second stage.

Some surgeons advocate one-stage revision under certain specific circumstances, such as when a single infecting organism has been identified and where the organism has known antibiotic sensitivity.

Long-term suppressive antibiotic therapy can be considered in patients who are medically unfit for revision procedures.

Osteomyelitis

Acute osteomyelitis

Background

Osteomyelitis is an infective process that affects bone or bone marrow with an incidence of 10-100/100,000 population per year.[8] Microorganisms can enter bone through the bloodstream or by direct inoculation from surrounding tissues. In adults, haematogenous osteomyelitis is common within the spine (vertebrae and discs). Long bone osteomyelitis is often posttraumatic in adults (tibia) and haematogenous in children.[9]

Pathophysiology

During bacteraemia, seeding within the bone occurs particularly when local integrity is disrupted by trauma or recent surgery. Direct contamination can occur in open fractures, deep wounds (human or animal bites) and diabetic foot ulcers. Bone oedema can cause breakdown of trabeculae leading to necrosis.

Aetiology

S. aureus is the most common microorganism. Infections with Gram negative bacteria can follow urinary sepsis or surgery. *Pseudomonas* infections are encountered in intravenous drug users and anaerobes in diabetic feet or following bites (human or animal).

Clinical presentation

Diagnosing osteomyelitis can be challenging due to the paucity of symptoms and signs. Patients might present with malaise, fatigue, and fever. Focal signs, if present, include localized pain, erythema, and swelling. A detailed history concerning other co-morbidities and recent injury or surgery will help point to the diagnosis.

Investigations

Blood cultures are positive in only 50% of cases.[9] WCC, CRP, and ESR are of value, but do not distinguish osteomyelitis from other

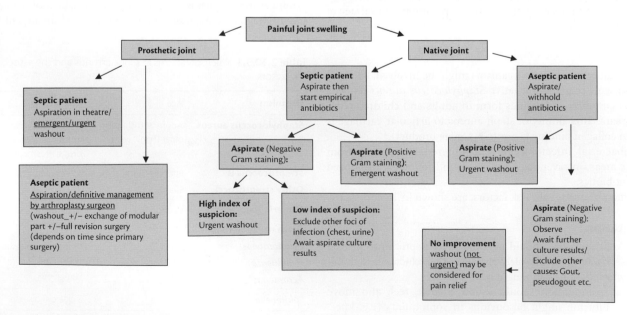

Fig. 2.10.3.1 Algorithm for the management of patients with suspected joint septic arthritis.

diagnoses.[10] CRP helps monitor the response to treatment once the diagnosis is confirmed.

Plain radiographs remain essential in excluding tumours or previous fractures. Changes of acute osteomyelitis may take 3 weeks to become apparent.

Other imaging studies include:

◆ Ultrasound scan: In children detects periosteal thickening or subperiosteal collection and can guide aspiration or biopsy.

◆ Computed tomography scan (CT) scan: detects early changes but involves substantial radiation and lacks soft tissue contrast.

◆ Magnetic resonance imaging: Detects bony changes as early as 3 days. [10] It delineates the extent of infection and guides surgical debridement if required. However, it may not be tolerated by young patients and produces artefactual images in the presence of prostheses or other metal.

◆ Three-phase technetium radionuclide bone scan can detect early changes showing enhanced uptake of the radioisotope on the three phases due to increased local blood flow. There is no interference from prostheses or metalwork. However, it has a low specificity and does not differentiate osteomyelitis from other inflammatory conditions or malignancies.

Bone biopsy with histological examination is considered the gold standard for the diagnosis of osteomyelitis. Microbiology cultures performed on bony aspirates from radiologically suspected osteomyelitis are positive only in 30% of cases[11] and thus care must be taken when interpreting negative results. Biopsy or aspiration could be obtained by open approach or percutaneously under CT or ultrasound guidance.

Management

If clinical sepsis is present, empirical antibiotics should be started, once blood samples have been taken for cultures. Empirical antibiotics should be guided by each individual case and according to local hospital guidelines as this might warrant the combination of broad-spectrum agents (see Table 2.10.3.2).

The definitive antibiotic spectrum can be narrowed once the identity of pathogen and susceptibility data becomes available. Intravenous antibiotics are often required for at least 6 weeks,[9] and

this might be extended or followed by oral antibiotics. Treatment in the community has been facilitated by the use of peripherally inserted central catheters.

Surgical debridement or decompression might be considered in addition to antibiotics. Tissue sampling is then required to identify the responsible microorganism.

Chronic osteomyelitis

Even when treated optimally, acute osteomyelitis can progress to chronicity in about 10% of cases. Chronic osteomyelitis is characterized by recurrent symptoms, varying in severity, and which are often quiescent along with normal inflammatory markers. Radiological changes might become apparent and include:

◆ Sequestrum: a localized area of devitalized bone, which is being replaced by purulent material and granulation tissue.

◆ Involucrum: new bone formation that surrounds the sequestrum.

◆ Cloacae: perforations within the involucrum where drainage occurs from a sequestrum.

◆ Sinuses: tracts reaching the skin and that discharge the debris of sequestrum.

◆ Brodie's abscess: is a bone abscess that is a sharply delineated focus of infection.

Treatment options include surgical debridement, resection of the diseased bony segment followed by bone transport or acute shortening with re-lengthening. Adequate skin and soft tissue cover warrants plastic surgical input with local or free flaps. Recurrent relapses within a limb along with significant functional compromise might warrant amputation; such an option is regarded as the last resort and requires a multidisciplinary team input.

Complications of osteomyelitis

Residual symptoms include swelling, stiffness, and localized bony destruction leading to pathological fractures. Malignant transformation of skin at the site of draining sinus can lead to squamous cell carcinoma.

Table 2.10.3.2 Commonly used antibiotics in osteomyelitis

Microorganism	Drug name	Comments
Methicillin-*susceptible* Staphylococcus aureus, coagulase-negative staphylococci (CNS), β-haemolytic streptococci	Penicillin G (benzylpenicillin)	Drugs of choice/first line treatment
	Penicillin(β-lactamase inhibitors): Ampicillin, flucloxacillin	
	Ceftriaxone	Advantage of once daily dose
	Fusidic acid	Combined with Rifampicin to prevent resistance, good bone penetration
	Clindamycin, trimethoprim	Oral bioavailability (can be used to switch from parenteral to oral treatment)
	Rifampin	
Methicillin-resistant *Staphylococcus aureus* (MRSA)	Vancomycin, teicoplanin	Can be used for methicillin-susceptible S. aureus in penicillin-allergic patients
Gram negative (*E. coli, P. aeuroginosa*)	Gentamycin, ciprofloxacin	Increased resistance

Further reading

Prosthetic joint infections

Haddad FS, Bridgens A. Infection following hip replacement: solution options. *Orthopedics* 2008; 31(9): 907–8.

Segawa H, Tsukayama DT, Kyle RF, *et al.* Infection after total knee arthroplasty. A retrospective study of the treatment of eighty-one infections. *J Bone Joint Surg Am.* 1999; 81(10): 1434–45.

Acute osteomyelitis

Pineda C, Espinosa R, Pena A. Radiographic imaging in osteomyelitis: the role of plain radiography, computed tomography, ultrasonography, magnetic resonance imaging, and scintigraphy. *Semin Plast Surg* 2009; 23(2): 80–9.

Chronic osteomyelitis

Louie KW. Ilizarov method. *West J Med* 1991; 155(2): 170.

References

1. Goldenberg DL. Septic arthritis [review]. *Lancet* 1998, 351: 197–202.
2. Blom AW, Taylor AH, Pattison G, *et al.* Infection after total hip arthroplasty. The avon experience. *J Bone Joint Surg Br* 2003; 85: 956–9.
3. Haddad FS, Bridgens A. Infection following hip replacement: solution options. *Orthopedics* 2008; 31(9): 907–8.
4. Xu Y, Rivas JM, Brown EL, *et al.* Virulence potential of the staphylococcal adhesin CNA in experimental arthritis is determined by its affinity for collagen. *J Infect Dis* 2004; 189(12): 2323–33.
5. Kocher MS, Zurakowski D, Kasser JR. Differentiating between septic arthritis and transient synovitis of the hip in children: an evidence-based clinical prediction algorithm. *J Bone Joint Surg Am* 1999; 81(12): 1662–70.
6. Ernst AA, Weiss SJ, Tracy LA, *et al.* Usefulness of CRP and ESR in predicting septic joints. *South Med J* 2010; 103(6): 522–6.
7. Mathews CJ, Coakley G. Septic arthritis: current diagnostic and therapeutic algorithm. *Curr Opin Rheumatol* 2008; 20(4): 457–62.
8. Berend, AR, McNally M. Osteomyelitis In Warrel DA, Cox TM, Firth JD (eds) *Oxford Textbook of Medicine*, 5th edition, volume 3. Oxford University Press, 2010, 3788-95
9. Paluska SA. Osteomyelitis. *Clin Fam Pract* 2004; 6: 127–56.
10. Kocher M S, Lee B, Dolan M, *et al.* Pediatric orthopedic infections; early detection and treatment. *Pediatr Ann* 2006; 35: 112–22.
11. Sehn JK, Gilula LA. Percutaneous needle biopsy in diagnosis and identification of causative organisms in cases of suspected vertebral osteomyelitis. *Eur J Radiol* 2012; 81(5): 940–6.

Back pain and sciatica

David Sharp

Introduction

Back pain

Back pain is common in the general population, affecting up to 80% of people at some time in their lives. Most cases are minor and self-limiting, managed in primary care with analgesics and physical therapy, requiring no investigation.

Back pain may be broadly defined as mechanical and non-mechanical pain.

- Mechanical back pain is usually related to structural changes in the spine (most commonly degenerative), induced or exacerbated by physical activities, and relieved with rest.

- Non-mechanical back pain (such as pain due to inflammatory conditions, infection, or tumour) typically is unrelated to activities, may be present at rest, and disturb sleep.

Pain in the back is, therefore, the presentation of a wide variety of pathologies.

The role of the surgeon in the management of back pain is diagnosis and treatment when there is (i) severe and/or prolonged pain, interfering with activities of daily living or work, with or without associated neurological symptoms and signs, or (ii) indication of more serious pathology.

It is then essential to define the cause in order to plan specific treatment.

Sciatica

Sciatica is pain in the distribution of the sciatic nerve, which may or may not be associated with back pain.

The most common cause is nerve compression in the spine, either due to a disc protrusion or stenosis.

There are, however, a wide range of causes that must be considered when a spinal cause is not found.

The role of the surgeon is to investigate the cause and then plan treatment.

The management of both back pain and sciatica require a wide range of treatment modalities, ideally as part of a multidisciplinary team, and the important role of surgery is only required in a minority of patients.

Back pain

Causes

The causes of back pain are spinal and non-spinal.

Spinal causes

Spinal causes of back pain may be best considered using the classical list of the aetiology of disease.

Trauma

This may be soft tissue or bony. *Soft tissue injuries* involving the iliolumbar and sacroiliac ligaments will cause low back pain, which may also be of myofascial origin. *Bony injuries* may following acute trauma or present spontaneously or following apparently minor injuries as a result of pathological fractures due to osteoporosis, tumour or infection.

Degeneration

All degenerative conditions of the spine (spondylosis) may cause back pain, most commonly as pain originating in degenerative discs or facet joint osteoarthritis.

Inflammatory back pain

Back pain may be caused by inflammation affecting the spinal joints (sacroiliac and facet joints). The most common cause is ankylosing spondylitis, but it may also be associated with psoriatic arthritis, ulcerative colitis, and Crohn's disease.

Spinal inflammatory conditions have a characteristic presentation, with back pain associated with prolonged early morning stiffness, improved by exercise, occurring in a young age group (20–30 years), men more frequently affected, and a family history (with a genetic association with HLAB27).

Infection

Infection of the spine is usually blood-borne from a primary source (e.g. chest and genitourinary infections), but may also be iatrogenic, following intradiscal spinal injections (spinal biopsy or discography), surgery, or epidural catheter.

Infection may cause infective discitis, vertebral osteomyelitis, or epidural abscess.

Infective discitis The most common infection of the spine is infective discitis.

The most common causative organisms are staphylococci, coliforms, and streptococci. Indolent infections may be caused by organisms with low-grade pathogenicity, typically coagulase negative staphylococci, and *Streptococcus viridans*.

Vertebral osteomyelitis The incidence of vertebral osteomyelitis is 1:100–250,000, highest in seventh decade. Risk factors include:

- debilitation, obesity, and malnutrition

- smoking

- immunodeficiency and steroids

- diabetes

- septicaemia

- drug addicts and alcoholics
- human immunodeficiency virus infection
- renal failure
- urethral/bladder surgery
- malignancy
- radiotherapy

Therefore spinal infection should be considered in patients with these conditions, but also they should be considered when spinal infection has been diagnosed.

Unusual spinal infections such as *Salmonella*, tuberculosis (TB), fungal, and parasitic infections may develop in immunocompromised patients. *Salmonella* infections may also occur in sickle cell disease.

TB is the most common cause of vertebral body osteomyelitis in many parts of the world; the incidence is increasing in the UK. There is a history of visceral TB in 50% of patients, and the extrapulmonary site of TB is the spine in 50% of cases (50% occurring in the thoracic spine, 25% cervical, and 25% lumbar).

It starts in the metaphyseal bone, causing vertebral body destruction. The disc is spared until advanced disease. It spreads under the anterior longitudinal ligament to adjacent segments. Skip lesions occur in 15%, and abscesses in 50% of cases.

The *Mycobacterium* is present in TB abscesses in low concentration, which may make confirmatory diagnosis from aspiration difficult.

A characteristic feature of TB of the spine is that it spares the disc.

Epidural abscess Epidural abscesses may occur without associated spinal infection, or may be secondary to infective discitis or vertebral body osteomyelitis.

They are serious infections because of an increased risk of infective thrombosis in the spinal canal and thus serious neurological complications, and therefore require urgent and thorough management.

Tumours

The majority of spinal tumours are metastatic, being 40 times more common than primary tumours, occurring in 20% of those with bony metastases.

The vertebral body is 20 times more often involved than the posterior elements, which has important implications for spinal stability and its management (if the posterior elements are surgically excised to decompress the spine, supplementary stabilization is essential).

The majority of spinal metastases occur in the thoracic spine (70%), cervical in 20%, and lumbar spine in 10%. It is important to note that 86% are multiple level.

The majority (84%) involve the bone and are extradural, while the minority are purely osseous or extradural, and just 1% are intradural.

Spinal metastases are the presenting feature in 8% of cancers, and present with either back pain and/or neurological involvement (either radicular or spinal cord). The pain is caused by the release of chemical mediators, mechanical pain of instability (causing back pain in 10% of patients with cancer), or nerve root compression.

Five primary tumours account for 80% of spinal metastases: thyroid, breast, lung, kidney, and prostate.

Bone pain affects 70% of myeloma patients, usually involving the spine and ribs.

Other causes

Spondylolisthesis (forward slip of one vertebra on another) may present with low back pain. It is classified into five types.

1. dysplastic (congenital)

2. isthmic (lesion in the pars)

3. degenerative

4. post-traumatic

5. pathologic (generalized or local bone disease).[1]

There are three grades: grade I, a slip of less than 25%; grade II, a slip of 25–50%; and grade III, a slip of greater than 50%.

Non-spinal causes

Extra-spinal pathology in the posterior chest, abdomen, and pelvis causing back pain must always be considered (to include aortic aneurysm, renal disease, and tumours such as pancreatic cancer).

Natural history

Epidemiological studies show that up to 30% of people report daily back pain, 40% report pain in the last month, and 80% report back pain at some time in their life. However, most acute episodes settle rapidly, with considerable improvement over the first 4 weeks, but of these only 30% will be pain free and 20-25% will still have substantial activity limitations.

A study of patterns of prevalence of back pain in a 12-month period demonstrates three groups: group 1, 62% are free of back pain; group 2, there is intermittent or less disabling low back pain in 32%; and group 3, 6% have had long-standing or seriously disabling low back pain. It can therefore be seen that only a minority of cases lead on to chronic disabling pain.[2,3]

Assessment

Because of the wide variety of causes, the clinical assessment of the patient presenting with back pain necessitates a complete medical history and examination. The history will yield much information. Pain may be acute (spontaneous or following injury) or chronic. It may be constant unaffected by activity (an indication of potentially serious pathology), or mechanical (e.g. sharp catching pain related to instability or facet joint). Pain exacerbated by walking (claudicant back pain) may be related to stenosis, with or without claudicant lower limb pain.

Where there is associated lower limb dysfunction and pain, pathology at more than one level must be considered (e.g. concurrent cervical myelopathy).

Examination must include the spine, the general musculoskeletal system, foot pulses, abdomen, and neurological system.

Red and yellow flags

The critical initial clinical decision to be made in a case of back pain is whether there is serious pathology. Therefore, a system of red flags for physical risk factors, and yellow flags for psychosocial risk factors, have been developed.[4,5]

The *red flags*, requiring urgent investigation, are:

- age 16< or >50 with new onset pain

- features of cauda equina syndrome

- significant trauma
- weight loss
- history of cancer
- recent significant infection, fever
- intravenous drug use
- steroid use
- thoracic pain
- pain worse when lying down
- severe unremitting night time pain.

Yellow flags: in cases of back pain, there may biopsychosocial factors influencing the perception of pain. Yellow flags highlight the risk of chronicity, which may be prevented by early treatment. These are:

- *Attitude*: does the patient feel that help will enable return to normal activities?
- *Beliefs*: does the patient feel they have a serious cause ('catastrophization')?
- *Compensation*.
- *Diagnosis*: inappropriate communication leading to misunderstanding.
- *Emotions*: depression and anxiety.
- *Family*: over bearing or under supportive families.

Investigation

The baseline set of investigation is full blood count, electrolytes, bone chemistry, inflammatory markers (erythrocyte sedimentation rate, C-reactive protein), and magnetic resonance imaging (MRI) scan.

The inflammatory markers lack specificity. Erythrocyte sedimentation rate lags in recovery; C-reactive protein is the best indicator for progression of disease of inflammatory or infective origin.

MRI scan is the investigation of choice for excluding or confirming the diagnosis.

When red flags are present, urgent investigation is essential.

The further investigation will be guided by the clinical findings and the results of the baseline investigations, and may include infection screens (e.g. urine and blood culture, echocardiogram in intravenous drug abusers), myeloma screen, isotope scanning, and biopsy.

Management

The management of back pain potentially requires a wide range of treatment modalities, from simple analgesia to surgery. Treatment is dependent on the cause, involving a multidisciplinary team approach including physiotherapists, pain specialists, rheumatologists, spinal surgeons, and physiotherapists with a view to the application of pain management techniques, transcutaneous electrical nerve stimulation, drugs for neuropathic pain (amitriptyline, gabapentin, and pregabalin), and nerve root, epidural and facet joint injections.

Surgery is required in a minority of cases where all else has failed.[6]

There is no such thing as 'surgery for low back pain', only surgery aimed at specific diagnoses that culminate in low back pain, to include discogenic pain, instability secondary to degenerative change, trauma,

infection, and tumours. Other conditions causing low back are usually, but not exclusively, associated with sciatic or claudicant leg pain, when the primary aim is usually to relieve the leg pain.

The long-running controversy concerning surgery for low back pain centres on the treatment of discogenic pain, several studies over the past decade mainly demonstrating at best minor increased success compared to physical therapy.[7,8] Considerable problems continue, the most fundamental being the difficulty of confirming the diagnosis.

Sciatica

Anatomy of the sciatic nerve

The sciatic nerve is a mixed nerve which is supplied by the L4 to S3 spinal nerve roots. The sciatic nerve emerges into the buttock lying on the ischium. It supplies the hamstring compartment and then separates into the tibial and common peroneal nerves to supply the flexor, extensor, and peroneal compartments of the lower leg, and dorsum and sole of the foot.

The motor and dermatomal supply to the lower limb is critical to making a clinical diagnosis in spinal radicular conditions. The concept of 'spinal centres for joint movements'[9] provides an easy aide memoire for motor supply:

Hip	L2L3	Flex
	L4L5	Extend
Knee	L3L4	Extend
	L5S1	Flex
Ankle	L4L5	Dorsiflex
	S1S2	Plantarflex

Causes of sciatica

Sciatica is caused by spinal and extra-spinal causes.

The most common *spinal causes* are disc protrusion or stenosis at the L3/4, L4/5, or L5/S1 levels. Stenosis may be lateral recess and/or foraminal. The most common causes of this are facet joint hypertrophy and spondylolisthesis. It may also be caused by trauma, infection and tumour.

Non-spinal causes are compressive or other conditions of the nerve outside the spine. These include lateral disc protrusions, sciatic nerve tumours (neurofibroma), trauma (a direct blow, or an injection placed too low and medial in the buttock) or buttock haematoma (notably associated with anti-coagulants), pelvic pathology (to include tumour and endometriosis), and finally conditions affecting the nerve, to include sciatic neuritis.

Presentation

Sciatica is typically unilateral, presenting with pain with or without paraesthesia, numbness, or motor deficit in the distribution of the sciatic nerve to the lower leg and foot. It may also include low back and buttock pain. Differentiation from referred pain from the spine or hip is required (the latter being typically into the thigh without lower leg involvement).

Examination

The examination is as discussed in the section for back pain.

Neurological examination is for radicular tension signs with a straight leg raise (Lasègue's sign) and sciatic nerve stretch test by dorsiflexion of the foot (these reproducing sciatic pain), and motor, sensory and reflex examination of the lower limbs.

Lasègue's sign is performed with the patient lying supine, and is positive when sciatica is reproduced with the straight leg at 30–70°. However, while its sensitivity is 91%, it should be remembered that specificity is only 26%.[10]

Lower limb symptoms and dysfunction may be caused by pathology at any level of the spine, especially in the more elderly patient. Therefore examination includes testing for upper motor neurone signs (increased tone, brisk reflexes, clonus, and extensor plantar response) and long tract signs (Rhomberg's Test, and loss of proprioception, vibration, coordination).

Investigation

The fundamental examination is lumbar spine MRI, which will demonstrate a disc protrusion or stenosis. It will also exclude other pathology such as trauma, infection, and tumour. Full blood count and inflammatory markers are routine.

Further investigation is according to the clinical findings.

Management

In a new case of sciatica, if red flags are excluded and if the pain can be adequately controlled and there are no progressive neurological signs, then conservative treatment for approximately 6 weeks is standard practice in the UK. This is because the majority of cases of disc protrusions causing sciatica resolve within 6-8 weeks. Bed rest is not advised, there being no difference of outcome compared with active treatment.

The next stage is nerve root injections as a day case procedure.

Finally, surgery with a posterior decompression is indicated when all these measures fail and the pain and degree of disability are sufficiently severe. Surgical treatment of sciatica due to a disc protrusion effects early relief, but the results even of this commonly performed procedure remain controversial.[11]

Cauda equina syndrome

Cauda equina syndrome (CES) is the only cause of sciatica due to a disc protrusion which requires urgent management, such are the devastating consequences of delayed diagnosis and treatment.

The cauda equina ('horse tail') is formed by the nerve roots passing from the conus down to the lumbar and sacral neural foraminae. These include the autonomic supply to the bladder, rectum, and sexual function, and sensation to the saddle area (S3 + S4).

CES is compression of the cauda equina causing impaired autonomic function in the pelvis. Permanent dysfunction will result if not decompressed urgently.

The symptoms of CES are back pain, bilateral leg pain, bladder dysfunction, and perianal and saddle area sensory changes. Bladder symptoms include loss of bladder sensation, abnormal sensation on

passing urine, retention (more common in men), or incontinence (more common in women).

With any combination of these symptoms, urgent assessment the same day with full neurological examination and rectal examination for perianal sensation and anal tone, MRI, and surgery if cauda equina compression is confirmed, are mandatory.

There is some controversy over the timing of decompressive surgery for CES; some surgeons advocate surgery within 24 hours whereas there is some literature evidence to suggest that 48 hours is the critical time.[12] It is important to look for any perineal sparing or residual bladder function as incomplete CES (CES-I) has better prospects for recovery than complete CES with retention (CES-R) and therefore should be treated surgically with great priority.

Further reading

Gardner A, Gardner E, Morley. Cauda equina sydrome: a review of the current clinical and medico-legal position. *Eur Spine J* 2011; 20(5): 690–7.

References

1. Newman PH, Stone KH. The etiology of spondylolisthesis. *J Bone Joint Surg* 1963;.45B: 39–59.
2. Papageorgiou AC, Croft PR, Ferry S, *et al*. Estimating the prevalence of low back pain in the general population. Evidence form the South Manchester back pain survey. *Spine* 1995; 20: 1889–94.
3. Papageorgiou AC, Croft PR, Thomas E, *et al*. Influence of previous pain experience on the episode incidence of low back pain: results from the South Manchester Back Pain Study. *Pain* 1996; 66: 181–5.
4. *Clinical Practice Guideline: Acute Low Back Problems in Adults: Assessment and Treatment (AHCPR)*. National Health Committee, Wellington: New Zealand, 1996.
5. *Guide to Assessing Psychosocial Yellow Flags in Acute Low Back Pain*. National Health Committee, Wellington: New Zealand, 1996.
6. National Institute for Health and Care Excellence (NICE). *Low Back Pain. Early Management of Persistent Non-Specific Low Back Pain*. NICE Clinical Guideline 88. London: NICE, 2008.
7. Fairbank J, Frost H, Wilson-MacDonald J, *et al*. Randomised controlled trial to compare surgical stabilisation of the lumbar spine with an intensive rehabilitation programme for patients with chronic low back pain: the MRC spine stabilisation trial. *BMJ* 2005; 330: 1233.
8. Fritzell P, Hägg O, Wessberg P, *et al*. Chronic low back pain and fusion: a comparison of three surgical techniques: a prospective multi-center randomized study from the Swedish Lumbar Spine Study Group. *Spine* 2002; 27: 1131–41.
9. Last RJ. *Anatomy: Regional and Applied*. Edinburgh: Churchill Livingstone, 1999.
10. Speed C. Low back pain. *BMJ* 2004; 328: 1119–21.
11. Gibson JN, Waddell G. Surgical interventions for lumbar disc prolapse: updated Cochrane Review. *Spine* 2007; 32(16): 1735–47.
12. Ahn U, Ahn NU, Buchowski JM, *et al*. Cauda equina syndrome secondary to lumbar disc herniation: A meta-analysis of surgical outcomes. *Spine* 2000: 25(12): 1515–22.

Malignant and metastatic bone disease

Helen Cattermole

Introduction

Malignant bone disease is a common presentation to the orthopaedic surgeon. It can be thought of in three ways: metastatic bone disease, caused by tumour cells spreading to bone from another primary site in the body (common); malignant disease where the primary tumour is in the blood or bone marrow (common); or primary bone cancer, arising in the bone tissue itself (rare).

Metastatic bone disease

Bone is the third most common site for metastatic spread, after lung and liver. The most common cancers giving rise to metastatic bone disease are shown in Table 2.10.5.1.

Other cancers such as colon, bladder, and gynaecological cancers also spread to bone, but it is less common for this to happen.

Other common malignancies giving rise to skeletal complications (although not strictly metastatic, since the disease is a blood cell cancer arising in the bone marrow) are myeloma and lymphoma.

Clinical presentation of metastatic bone disease

Bone pain: Often an unremitting dull ache, which may be exacerbated by movement or weight bearing.

Pathological fracture: A fracture in abnormal bone occurring after minimal trauma

Spinal cord compression (URGENT): There are symptoms of saddle anaesthesia, bilateral motor deficit, and urinary or bowel disturbance. The patient requires URGENT investigation (magnetic resonance imaging [MRI]) and referral for surgery or radiotherapy.

Hypercalcaemia: Symptoms of confusion, dehydration, polyuria and constipation

Incidental finding on X-ray or scan: This may present in a patient with a previously known cancer (with or without known bone metastases) or in a patient where the diagnosis of cancer was previously unknown (Figure 2.10.5.1).

Assessment and management of patient with suspected bone metastases

History

Take a full patient history including current symptoms, history of cancer, and treatments to date. If there is no history of cancer then a careful systems enquiry will be required. Assess for symptoms of cord compression or hypercalcaemia.

Examination

A full physical examination is necessary including, in women, examination of breasts and axillae; rectal examination is important in both sexes. Examine for a primary tumour and other manifestations of malignancy.

Differential diagnosis

This includes benign and degenerative bone and joint disease, metabolic bone disease and infection.

Investigations

The following investigations should be carried out:

Bloods: Full blood count, biochemical profile (particularly serum calcium), Prostate Specific Antigen (in men) and serum electrophoresis.

Urinalysis: Test for blood and protein, and send for cytology.

Imaging: Plain radiographs (two planes) are always required. Isotope bone scan can detect whether the lesion is single or multiple. Computerized tomography scan of chest/abdomen/pelvis

Table 2.10.5.1 Cancers giving rise to metastatic bone disease

Site of primary tumour	Percentage of patients with bone metastases found at autopsy	Comments
Breast	60%	Long survival with disease so skeletal complications are common
		May be lytic, sclerotic or mixed lesions
Prostate	60%	Long survival with disease so skeletal complications are common
		Usually sclerotic lesions
Thyroid	40%	
Lung	35%	
Kidney (renal cell)	35%	Isolated metastases have good survival if treated by *en bloc* resection

Source: data from Eccles SA, General Mechanisms of Metastasis, pp. 3–25, in C. Jasmin *et al.* (Eds.), *Textbook of Bone Metastases*, John Wiley and Sons, Chichester, UK, Copyright © 2005.

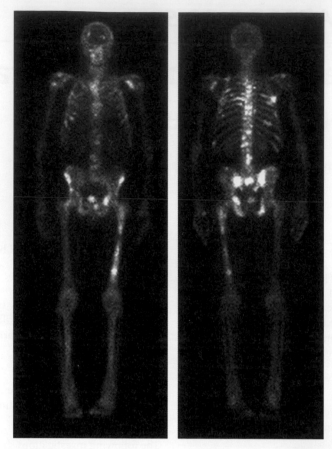

Fig. 2.10.5.1 Multiple bony metastases from prostate cancer.

can detect a previously unknown primary. MRI of affected area is useful if surgery is contemplated. Skeletal survey is needed if myeloma is suspected.

Bone marrow biopsy: May be required if myeloma or other haematological malignancy is suspected.

Biopsy: *Only* if investigations show an accessible lesion with multiple metastases. Solitary bone lesions require discussion with a tertiary referral centre BEFORE biopsy.

Clinical decision making

Important clinical decisions must be made after investigation and BEFORE surgery. The most important judgment is to decide whether this is a *solitary or multiple lesion*. Solitary lesions should be approached with caution (engage brain before surgery!) since they may (rarely) be primary lesions arising in the bone, and/or have a good prognosis if treated in a specialist centre. *Identification of a primary site* can give valuable information about the likely prognosis, and therefore the extent of surgery that should be considered. Some tumours (e.g. renal cancer and its skeletal metastases) can bleed excessively and may therefore benefit from preoperative embolization. The *presence or absence of visceral metastases* helps with determining the prognosis which may alter surgical management.

Team work and planning

This will depend upon the clinical situation but may include any or all of the following:

Specialist referral for diagnosis e.g. respiratory medicine for bronchoscopy, breast surgery for needle biopsy.

Oncology/haematology referral: The patient may already be known to an oncologist or haematologist. They may be on chemotherapy which needs stopping in the perioperative period. The treating team may wish to alter treatment in the light of the metastatic disease. A guide to prognosis can often be obtained from discussion with the oncologist. If the patient is not already known to a particular team, there is often an acute oncology service to advise.

Radiology discussion: For timely investigation and interpretation of imaging. Occasionally biopsy under imaging is required (not for suspected primary bone tumours).

Vascular interventional radiology: If angiography and embolization are needed before surgery.

Musculoskeletal interventional radiology: For consideration of vertebroplasty/kyphoplasty if multiple vertebrae are involved.

Palliative care: For symptom control, psychological support and ongoing care.

Multidisciplinary team (MDT) referral and discussion: Cancer MDT discussions usually involve surgeons from appropriate specialties, oncologists with appropriate specialty interests, radiologists, pathologists, and specialist nurses and ensure that treatment decisions and follow-up plans are multidisciplinary, recorded, and communicated. There may be a site-specific MDT such as a lung cancer MDT, urology MDT, etc., where care of patients with this disease is coordinated. An 'unknown primary MDT' (where a primary source has not been found) is often set up in cancer centres, and in some hospitals there is a specific bone metastasis MDT.

Tertiary referral: If a primary bone tumour is suspected, or an isolated metastasis is found that requires biopsy, the patient should be referred to a specialist tertiary centre. Referral should be made BEFORE any invasive investigation since a poorly thought-out biopsy can compromise the outcome.

Clinical trials/audits: if appropriate, the patient can be discussed with a trials coordinator (often this takes place alongside MDT meetings).

Communication skills

In what may be difficult and emotionally charged circumstances, communication skills are very important. The most common areas where difficulties arise are breaking bad news and communication with colleagues.

Consent

There are some specific issues that arise with metastatic bone disease, which should be discussed in addition to the usual operative risks. The risk of *infection* is high due to immunosuppression, marrow involvement with disease, and chemotherapy. Disseminated malignancy predisposes patients to *venous thromboembolism*. Diseased marrow may be displaced during bony surgery (particularly nailing) and cause *tumour embolus*, which can give rise to hypoxia, perioperative arrhythmias, and death on the table. *Metalwork failure* is more of a problem than in normal fracture surgery due to the fracture not healing. Finally, *pathological fracture* during or after surgery is a potential issue due to the abnormal bone.

Perioperative care

Patients with metastatic bone disease, by definition, are high risk due to their disseminated malignancy. Skilled surgical, anaesthetic, nursing, and ward medical care will be needed. Particular care should be taken to address, monitor, and treat *hypercalcaemia* and monitor fluid balance. Patients are at high risk of *venous thromboembolism* and may be on therapeutic anticoagulation. Consider inferior vena cava filtration in the perioperative period. *Pain control* can be an issue; patients may be accustomed to opiate analgesia and require higher than usual postoperative doses. Careful monitoring of potential *neurological deficit* is essential.

Principles of management of metastatic bone disease

Fracture risk assessment

If a patient presents with a bone lesion secondary to metastatic cancer, it is important to assess the fracture risk if it has not already fractured. Patients can be spared the trauma, inconvenience, and uncertain clinical course of a pathological fracture if these can be accurately predicted and appropriate measures taken to prevent fracture. These measures include protection of the site by walking aids and other appliances, treatment by bisphosphonates, desnosumab or other drugs, external beam radiotherapy, and surgery.

Mirels' scoring system is commonly used to assess the facture risk (see Table 2.10.5.2).

Table 2.10.5.2 Prediction of fracture risk: Mirels' scoring system

Site of lesion	Score
Upper limb	1
Lower limb	2
Peritrochanteric	3
Size of lesion	
<1/3 diameter	1
1/3–2/3 diameter	2
>2/3 diameter	3
Type of lesion	
Blastic	1
Mixed	2
Lytic	3
Pain	
Mild	1
Moderate	2
Functional	3

Prophylactic surgery should be considered in lesions scoring more than 8 out of 12 as this indicates a high risk of pathological fracture.

Reproduced from Mirels H., Metastatic Disease in long bones: A proposed Scoring System for diagnosing impending pathologic fracture, *Clinical Orthopaedics and Related Research*, Volume 249, pp. 256–264, Copyright © 1989 Lippincott-Raven Publishers, with permission from Lippincott Williams and Wilkins.

Prophylactic surgery

Patients with impending pathological fracture (see Table 2.10.5.2) should ideally be assessed by an MDT team to determine a suitable course of action. In many cases, surgery can be offered to try and prevent pathological fracture. This has the advantage of planning surgery when a patient is well, and can often reduce the length of stay and postoperative recovery compared to a similar operation done for fracture.

Principles of management of pathological fractures

Assume that pathological fractures *will not heal*. Operative treatment usually offers better quality of life, as controlling the fracture in a cast or brace may be difficult and uncomfortable for the lifespan of the patient. Because the fracture will not heal, fixation should be designed to be *load bearing*, not load sharing, and sufficient stability should be provided by the fixation to *allow immediate weight bearing*. Bone defects should be augmented where possible (e.g. with bone cement), and fixation should last the lifetime of the patient.

All lesions in the affected bone should, where possible, be stabilized. Spinal lesions usually require decompression and stabilization. Proximal fractures usually need prosthetic replacement (e.g. proximal femoral replacement rather than internal fixation), particularly if the prognosis is good. Complete workup of the patient is more important than rushed surgery.

Primary bone tumours

Malignant primary bone tumours are serious, but very rare (<0.2% of all cancers), and will not therefore be discussed in detail. Key points to remember are: *benign lesions* are far more common than malignant ones, *infection* can mimic bone tumours and vice versa, and *early diagnosis* and *specialist treatment* are essential.

The characteristic features of primary bone tumours are shown in Table 2.10.5.3. There are, however, certain principles of management that apply to all types of primary bone tumours.

Oncological principles

Early referral to tertiary centre: Because these tumours are rare, expertise is concentrated in only a few sites. Suspected primary bone tumours should be discussed BEFORE any intervention (including biopsy) is undertaken; advice is always freely and quickly given about investigation and management.

Avoidance of contamination of field/compartment: Patient survival and limb salvage can both be compromised by inappropriate biopsy and surgery. Prevention is far better than cure, and experienced teams make fewer mistakes than occasional tumour surgeons. Refer early and do not meddle!

Wide excision including any biopsy track: It is essential that biopsy tracks are excised along with the tumour, and therefore it is in the patient's best interests that the surgeon doing the biopsy is the one who also performs the cancer surgery.

Avoidance of pitfalls: Although primary bone tumours are rare, surgeons need to be aware of the possibility of these conditions when planning surgery. An isolated bone lesion without any evidence of a primary lesion elsewhere, or other secondary lesions, should be treated with extreme caution. It is not uncommon for primary lesions to be unrecognized; for example, a primary chondrosarcoma of the femur with a pathological fracture, if inadequately investigated, can easily be mistaken for a metastasis and nailed. The tumour is then spread along the medullary canal, with devastating consequences. Another frequent mistake is performing an arthroscopy on a symptomatic knee without first obtaining an X-ray; the diagnosis subsequently turns out to be a giant cell tumour just below the articular surface.

Table 2.10.5.3 Features of primary bone tumours

Tumour type	Age	Incidence	Bones commonly affected	Site within bone	Radiological features	Treatment
Osteosarcoma	5–20 Adult	56% of children's bone cancers 28% of adult bone cancers	Femur Tibia	Metaphysis	Codman's triangle Sunray spicules Periosteal reaction New bone formation	Multimodal ◆ Neo-adjuvant chemotherapy ◆ Limb salvage surgery ◆ Endoprosthetic replacement ◆ Postoperative chemotherapy
Ewing's sarcoma	10–20 Adult	34% of children's bone cancers 8% of adult bone cancers	Pelvis Femur Tibia	Diaphysis	Onion skin periosteal reaction Lytic, central lesion Endosteal scalloping Needs CT and MRI	Multimodal ◆ Preoperative chemotherapy and/or radiotherapy ◆ Wide surgical excision ◆ Postoperative chemotherapy
Chondrosarcoma	Adult Average age at diagnosis is 51	>40% of adult bone cancers 6% of children's bone cancers Fewer than 5% of chondrosarcomas develop in children <20 years	Pelvis Femur Humerus Scapula Ribs	Surface tumour or intramedullary	Fusiform, lucent defect Endosteal scalloping Bone destruction Periosteal reaction Stippled cartilage calcification Soft tissue extension	Wide surgical excision
Chordoma	Adult Peak age 40–70	10% of adult bone cancers Fewer than 5% of chordomas develop in children <20 years	Sacrum Coccyx Base of skull	Notochord remnant	Solitary, midline Bone destruction Soft tissue extension/mass Needs CT and MRI	Surgical excision if possible (difficult locations)
Malignant Fibrous Histiocytoma	Adult	4% of adult bone cancers May arise secondary to another process such as surgery, radiotherapy	Distal femur Proximal tibia Proximal femur Proximal humerus	Metaphysis Diaphysis	Permeative Destructive High signal on bone scan	Pre-op chemotherapy Limb-sparing surgery

CT, computerized tomography; MRI, magnetic resonance imaging.

Neo-adjuvant Chemo therapy: Many primary bone tumours are treated with neo-adjuvant chemotherapy prior to surgery. This shrinks the tumour and makes surgical excision more straightforward. The response to chemotherapy may provide a predictor of prognosis.

Life-saving versus limb-sparing surgery: Where possible, limb-saving surgery should be carried out. The tumour, with its surrounding soft tissues, is excised with wide margins. It is often necessary to replace large parts of the bone with a custom-made prosthesis. Occasionally the only way to obtain disease-free margins is to excise the whole limb (i.e. amputation).

Further reading

British Orthopaedic Association. *Metastatic Bone Disease: A Guide to Good Practice*. http://www.boa.ac.uk/publications/documents/metastatic_bone_disease.pdf (accessed 21/02/13).

Capanna R, Campanacci DA. Indications for the surgical treatment of long bone metastases. In Jasmin C, Coleman RE, Coia LR, *et al.* (eds) *Textbook of Bone Metastases* Chichester: John Wiley & Sons, 2005, pp 135–45.

Dennis K, Vassiliou V, Balboni T, Chow E. Management of bone metastases: recent advances and current status. *J Radiat Oncol* 2012; 1: 201–10.

Eccles SA (2005). General mechanisms of metastasis. In Jasmin C, Coleman RE, Coia LR et al. (eds) *Textbook of Bone Metastases*. Chichester: John Wiley & Sons Ltd, 2005, pp. 3–25.

Halpin RJ, Bendok BR, Liu JC. Minimally invasive treatments for spinal metastases: vertebroplasty, kyphoplasty, and radiofrequency ablation. *J Support Oncol* 2004; 2(4): 339–51; discussion 352–5.

Harvey N, Ahlmann ER, Allison DC, *et al.* Endoprostheses last longer than intramedullary devices in proximal femur metastases Clin Orthop Rel Res 2012; 470: 684–91.

Jasmin C, Coleman RE, Coia LR, *et al.* (eds) *Textbook of Bone Metastases* Chichester: John Wiley & Sons, 2005.

Karnofsky DA, Burchenal JH. The clinical evaluation of chemotherapeutic agents. In McLeod E (ed), *Evaluation of Chemotheraputic Agents*. New York: Columbia University Press, 1949.

Metastatic Bone Disease web page, American Academy of Orthopaedic Surgeons http://orthoinfo.aaos.org/topic.cfm?topic=a00093 (accessed 11/09/2013).

Mirels H. Metastatic disease in long bones. A proposed scoring system for diagnosing impending pathologic fracture. *Clin Orthop Rel Res* 1989; 249: 256–64.

Molloy AP, O'Toole GC. Orthopaedic perspective on bone metastasis. *World J Orthop* 2013; 4(3): 114–9.

Neilson OS, Munro AJ, Tannock IF. Bone metastases: pathophysiology and management policy. *J Clin Oncol* 1991; 9(3): 509–24.

NICE Clinical Guideline: Metastatic spinal cord compression: Diagnosis and management of adults at risk of and with metastatic spinal cord compression. CG75 (2008). National Institute for Health and Care Excellence. http://publications.nice.org.uk/metastatic-spinal-cord-compression-cg75 (accessed 11/09/13).

NICE Clinical Knowledge Summary: Hypercalcaemia (2010). National Institue for Health and Care Excellence. http://cks.nice.org.uk/hypercalcaemia#!topicsummary (accessed 12/09/2013).

NICE Technology appraisal guidance: Denosumab for the prevention of skeletal-related events in adults with bone metastases from solid tumours. TA265 (2012). National Institute for Health and Care Excellence. http://publications.nice.org.uk/denosumab for-the-prevention-of-skeletal-related-events-in-adults-with-bone-metastases-from-solid-ta265 (accessed 11/09/13).

Ratasvuori M, Wedin R, Keller J, *et al.* Insight opinion to surgically treated metastatic bone disease: Scandinavian Sarcoma Group Skeletal Metastasis Registry report of 1195 operated skeletal metastasis. *Surg Oncol* 2013; 22: 132–8.

Rosenthal DI (1997). Radiologic diagnosis of bone metastases. *Cancer* 1997; 80: 1595–607.

Schwab JH, Springfield DS, Raskin KA, *et al.* (2012). What's new in primary bone tumors. *J Bone Joint Surg Am* 2012; 94(20): 1913–9.

Tokuhashi Y, Matsuzaki H, Toriyama S, *et al.* Scoring system for the pre-operative evaluation of metastatic spine tumor prognosis. *Spine* 1990; 15: 1110–3.

PART 2.11

Skin and soft tissue masses

Benign and malignant skin lesions

Mandeep Kang and David Ward

Benign skin lesions

Benign skin lesions can be classified according to their physical characteristics such as their colour, shape, and contour.

Macular lesions

Macules are non-palpable lesions that represent a change in the colour of the skin. They are not raised or atrophic.

Campbell de Morgan spot
Clinical features

Campbell de Morgan spots or 'cherry angiomas' are common benign skin macules that are usually 1 to 3 mm in diameter. They are typically bright cherry red in colour and are non-blanching (Figure 2.11.1.1a). Their aetiology is unknown but they are lesions of advancing age and approximately 75% of the population over 75 years old acquire them.[1]

Pathological features

Campbell de Morgan spots are formed by abnormal proliferating, dilated capillaries, and post-capillary venules.

Actinic keratosis
Clinical features

Actinic keratosis or 'solar keratosis' is an area of chronically sun-damaged skin that appears as a scaly patch. Some are skin coloured, and others are pink or red (Figure 2.11.1.1b). They more commonly affect older patients.[2]

Pathological features

There are focal areas of abnormal keratinocyte proliferation and differentiation with epithelial dysplasia. Actinic keratoses carry a low risk of progression to invasive squamous cell carcinoma – less than one in 1000 per annum.[3]

Papular lesions

Papules are well circumscribed lesions, with solid elevation of the skin.

Dermatofibroma
Clinical features

Dermatofibromas or 'benign fibrous histiocytomas' are hard solitary slow-growing papules occurring four times more commonly in women.[4] They are often elevated and vary in colour from brown to tan.

Pathological features

They are composed of an overgrowth of abnormal collagen laid down by fibroblasts in the dermal layer of the skin.

Seborrhoeic keratosis
Clinical features

Seborrhoeic keratoses are slow-growing skin lesions that occur most commonly on the back or chest. They are often multiple and can vary in colour from tan to brown or black. The lesions thicken over time and have a rough wart-like texture with a grainy, uneven surface that crumbles easily. They can vary in size from 1 to 30 mm in diameter.

Pathological features

They occur because of an abnormal proliferation of epidermal cells and can show increased melanin pigmentation of the lesional keratinocytes.

Keratoacanthoma
Clinical features

Keratoacanthomas rapidly grow over a few weeks to months, followed by a slow spontaneous resolution that can take up to one year. They are usually solitary and begin as a firm, round, skin-coloured or reddish papule that rapidly progresses to a dome-shaped nodule with a smooth shiny surface, often with a crusty central core. They can mimic squamous cell carcinomas in appearance and distinguishing the two can be difficult clinically.

Pathological features

A keratoacanthoma is a growth that originates in the pilosebaceous glands at the neck of a hair follicle.

Pyogenic granuloma
Clinical features

A pyogenic granuloma appears as a small, raised, red vascular papule (Figure 2.11.1.1c). It typically bleeds very easily on contact due to the proliferation of blood vessels at the site.

Pathological features

The exact cause is unknown but it is often found at the site of a recent injury. It is characterized by abnormal angiogenic vascular proliferation, so can be classed as a lobular haemangioma.

Cutaneous horn
Clinical features

Cutaneous horns present as hard, conical projections above the surface of the skin.

Pathological features

Cutaneous horns are formed by a proliferation of keratin. This hyperkeratosis develops over the surface of a hyperproliferative

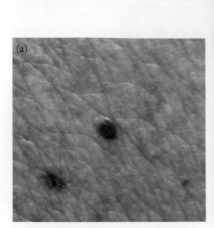
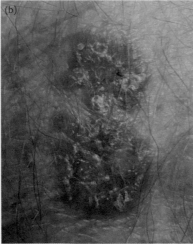
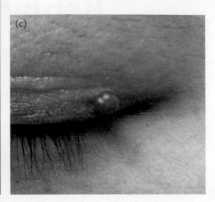

Fig. 2.11.1.1 Examples of common benign skin lesions. (a) Campbell de Morgan spot on the anterior chest wall. (b) Actinic keratosis on the dorsum of the wrist. (c) Pyogenic granuloma on the upper eyelid.

lesion. Most often this is a verruca or seborrhoeic keratosis. A squamous cell carcinoma can develop undetected at the base of a cutaneous horn in up to 20% of lesions.[5]

Macular-papular lesions

These are lesions that can exist as flat or raised areas on or within the skin. The most common are melanocytic naevi that are benign lesions that typically appear in early childhood, reach maximal size and number in early adulthood, and then tend to disappear with advancing age. Congenital melanocytic naevi are present at birth and can be very large (giant or bathing trunk naevus).

There are three types of common acquired melanocytic naevi: junctional, compound, and intradermal. These are composed of melanocytic clusters and are classified according to the histological location of these clusters.

Junctional naevus

Junctional naevi exist as flat macular lesions that are uniformly pigmented, with colours varying from tan to brown to black. They can occur anywhere on the body but tend to lie more commonly in sun-exposed areas. They are regularly shaped and can vary in size from 1 to 10 mm in diameter.

Histology shows clusters of melanocytes that develop within the epidermis, forming nests that lie at the dermo-epidermal junction at the bases of rete ridges.

Compound naevus

Compound naevi present as raised, smooth papules or small nodules that are less than 10 mm in diameter. They can exhibit a varying amount of pigment. These naevi often have regular, well demarcated edges, and can contain terminal hairs.

Histology shows nests of melanocytes within both the epidermis and dermis.

Intradermal naevus

Intradermal naevi present as well demarcated papules, less than 10 mm in diameter with a soft, rubbery texture. They are deficient in pigment and therefore are skin coloured or tan. They are typically not seen until the third decade and may become peduculated.

Histology shows nests of melanocytes in the dermis.

Treatment of benign skin lesions

In most patients benign lesions do not require any treatment unless the patient is concerned about the lesion's cosmetic appearance or there are suspicions of an alternative diagnosis, such as the development of a squamous cell carcinoma in the base of a sebaceous horn or a keratoacanthoma being a squamous cell carcinoma. They carry a relatively low risk of transformation into malignant lesions but if a lesion changes in size, shape or colour it should be examined with a view to excision biopsy for histological diagnosis.

Alongside complete surgical excision various other treatments are available: topical creams such as 5-fluorouracil, laser ablation, curettage and cautery, shave excision, and cryotherapy.

Premalignant skin lesions

Bowen's disease

Bowen's disease, also known as 'intraepidermal squamous cell carcinoma', is a premalignant growth that is confined to the epidermis and does not invade the basal layer into the dermis. It is a histological diagnosis. It typically presents as an asymptomatic, slow growing, and sharply demarcated, scaly, and erythematous plaque in older patients. Approximately 3% of Bowen's disease transform to malignant squamous cell carcinoma.[6] Unless there has been transformation, treatment includes topical creams such as 5-fluorouracil, cryotherapy, and curettage and cautery. For well-defined small lesions where excision and direct closure can be achieved, or when transformation is suspected, surgical excision can be considered. Bowen's disease is radiosensitive and radiotherapy can be used as primary treatment for large or multiple lesions. If the lesion has been adequately treated then no formal follow-up is required.[6]

Lentigo maligna

Lentigo maligna (LM) (Hutchinson's melanotic freckle) is a premalignant melanoma *in situ* where the cells are confined to the tissue of origin, the epidermis. Conversion to invasive melanoma (lentigo maligna melanoma, LMM) occurs when the cells of malignant melanoma invade into the dermis or deeper. This occurs in 3% to 10% of cases. LM usually presents with a large diameter greater than 6 mm and has an irregular shape and border. The pigmentation can be variable and the lesion usually has a smooth surface. The diagnosis is histological. LM has an unusually high risk of recurrence of up to 20%. To achieve best-cure rates LM should undergo surgical excision unless contraindicated. Less effective treatments include radiotherapy, cryotherapy, and imiquimod cream. If the LM has been completely excised then no outpatient follow-up is required.

Malignant skin lesions

Basal cell carcinoma

Basal cell carcinomas (BCCs) or 'rodent ulcers' are the most common skin malignancies in Caucasians. They are slow-growing non-melanocytic epidermal skin tumours that rarely metastasize but can cause significant destruction and disfigurement by local invasion of surrounding tissues. Subtypes include nodular, superficial, morphoeic/infiltrative, pigmented, and baso-squamous.

Aetiology

The exact cause of BCCs is unknown but there are environmental and genetic factors that are believed to predispose patients to BCC such as increasing age, male sex, and skin types I and II. Chronic ultraviolet (UV) light exposure (i.e. sunlight) increases the risk of BCC development. Immunosuppressed patients and patients who suffer from albinism, xeroderma pigmentosum, or epidermodysplastic verruciformis also show an increased lifetime risk for BCC formation, as do patients with Gorlin's syndrome (basal cell naevus syndrome).

Clinical presentation

The anatomical distribution of BCCs varies. Seventy per cent occur on the head with the most common location being the nose,[7] and 25% occur on the trunk. BCCs can vary greatly in appearance: they may appear as cystic nodules with telangiectasia or as scaly plaques. Most BCCs are painless lesions that can bleed, itch, and fail to heal completely (Figure 2.11.1.2).

Diagnosis

Usually this is clinical by examining the appearance of the lesion, which varies according to the subtype. Confirmation of diagnosis is achieved by incision or excision biopsy and histological analysis.

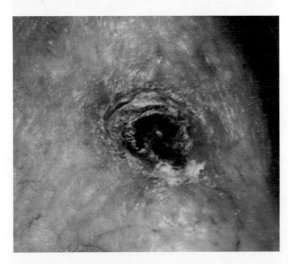

Fig. 2.11.1.2 Basal cell carcinoma on the nose.

Pathological features

BCCs are thought to arise from the pleuripotential cells in the basal layer of the epidermis or follicular structures. Tumours usually arise from the epidermis and occasionally arise from the outer root sheath of a hair follicle.

Surgical treatment

Most BCCs are treated by surgical excision. Adequate peripheral and deep margins of normal tissue are required for complete excision. A 5 mm margin gives about 95% complete excision but morphoeic/infiltrative lesions need a wider margin or excision by Moh's micrographic surgery.[8] The defect may require a graft or flap.

Minimally invasive and non-surgical treatment

Curettage can be employed to 'scrape' away the BCC and the skin surface is then cauterized. Cryotherapy with liquid nitrogen may be used to freeze superficial BCCs. Topical treatment with imiquimod or photodynamic therapy may be used for certain types of superficial BCCs. Radiotherapy may also be used as primary treatment in patients with significant co-morbidities or on anticoagulants, or as an adjunct to surgical excision when margins of excision are close or incomplete.

Prognosis

For BCCs with complete surgical excision the prognosis is extremely good. However, all patients are at some risk of local recurrence, especially if the original lesion was infiltrative or morphoeic. The risk of development of another primary BCC at a different site is relatively low at 2% over 2 years.[9]

Follow up

National guidelines recommend that no long-term follow-up is required for patients who have had their first and only primary BCC treated with complete excision.[10] For patients that have had incomplete excisions or have multiple BCCs, further treatment may be required or outpatient surveillance maybe indicated for 1 to 3 years.

Squamous cell carcinoma

Squamous cell carcinoma (SCC) is the second most common skin cancer after BCC. It is non-melanocytic, locally invasive, and has the potential to metastasize, usually to regional lymph nodes. Subtypes include papillary, verrucous, large cell keratinizing, large cell non-keratinizing, small cell keratinizing, spindle cell, adenoid, intraepidermal, and lymphoepithelial.

Associated conditions

Squamous cell carcinoma may develop from Bowen's disease, a sunlight-induced skin disease and a premalignant lesion for SCC, or in chronic non-healing ulcers or wounds (Marjolin's ulcer).

Aetiology

SCCs are more common in men than women and rarely appear before the age of 50 years. Chronic exposure to UV light and sunlight are significant aetiological factors, especially in fair-skinned patients. Skin injuries and wounds, chronic infections, and skin inflammation can give rise to these carcinomas. There is also a significantly higher incidence in immunosupressed patients and a correlation with the human papilloma virus.

Clinical presentation

SCCs can vary in their appearance but usually present as indurated keratinizing nodular or crusted tumours that may ulcerate or bleed. Most are found on sun-exposed sites and can vary in size from a few millimetres to several centimetres in diameter (Figure 2.11.1.3). There may be regional lymph node enlargement.

Diagnosis

The diagnosis is usually clinical but incision biopsy for histological diagnosis may be required before deciding on the mode of treatment. Imaging is not routinely indicated unless regional lymphadenopathy is present or there are associated symptoms (e.g. neurological symptoms indicating invasion) – in these cases a staging computed tomography scan is warranted. Staging is along the TNM classification.

Pathological features

The histological hallmark of SCC is the presence of keratin. The histology report should include the subtype, degree of differentiation, tumour depth, and level of dermal invasion (Clark's level). Poor prognostic features include poor differentiation, perineural invasion, and lymphovascular invasion.

Surgical treatment

Most cutaneous SCCs are treated by surgical excision, ensuring adequate peripheral and deep surgical margins with a margin of 4 to 6 mm.[11] Metastatic disease involving regional lymph nodes requires staging and, if operable, regional lymph node dissection, followed sometimes by non-surgical adjunctive therapy (i.e. radiotherapy or chemotherapy).

Minimally invasive and non-surgical treatment

Curettage of the lesion with accompanying cautery can aid removal of lesions, particularly in patients with extensive co-morbidities. Cryotherapy gives good short term cure rates but is not suitable for locally recurring or highly invasive tumours. Radiotherapy can be used as an adjunct to surgical excision or as primary treatment.

Prognosis

This is dependent on metastatic potential, which is influenced by various factors. SCCs arising at sun-exposed areas have the lowest metastatic potential compared to those arising in areas of radiation or injury, chronic ulcers/inflammation, or Bowen's disease. Tumours greater than 2 cm in diameter are twice more likely to recur locally and three times as likely to metastasize than smaller tumours.[12] Tumours greater than 4 mm in depth or extending beyond the subcutaneous tissue are more likely to recur and metastasize.[12] Poorly differentiated tumours have a poorer prognosis, with more than double the local recurrence rate and triple the metastatic rate of better differentiated SCC.

Follow-up

Seventy-five per cent of local recurrences and metastases are detected within 2 years and 95% within 5 years.[13] National guidelines recommend follow-up in outpatients for a minimum of 2 years.

Malignant melanoma

Cutaneous malignant melanomas (CMM) are carcinomas of the melanin producing melanocytes of the skin. They are classified as follows:

Superficial spreading melanoma represents 70% of all melanomas. Characteristic signs are an irregular border, differential pigmentation and progressive central depigmentation. They are also usually flat and may be greater than 1 cm in diameter (Figure 2.11.1.4).

Nodular melanoma represents 10% of all melanomas. This type is the most aggressive of all melanomas. It presents as a firm papule, nodule, or plaque and up to 50% are hypomelanotic or amelanotic and pink-red in colour.

Lentigo maligna melanoma represents 5% to 15% of all melanomas. They arise from a LM precursor lesion.

Acral lentiginous melanoma represents 5% of all melanomas and occurs on the palms, soles, or beneath the nails.

Aetiology

CMM is a malignancy with multifactorial aetiology, the major environmental factor being exposure to sources of UV radiation such as sunlight and sunbeds. An important host risk factor in fair-skinned people is the presence of both common acquired and dysplastic melanocytic naevi, which transform to CMM. Patients with a family history of CMM are also at an increased risk.

Clinical presentation

CMM lesions are more likely than benign lesions to be asymmetrical, to have irregular borders, a greater variation in colour, and to be

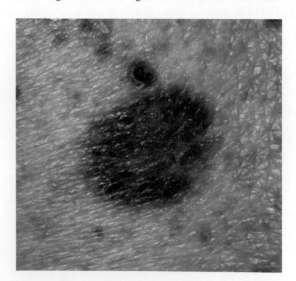

Fig. 2.11.1.4 Superficial spreading malignant melanoma on the lower back.

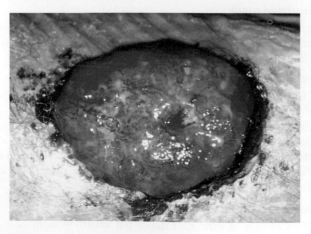

Fig. 2.11.1.3 Large fungating squamous cell carcinoma on the forearm.

larger with a diameter usually greater than 6 mm. Regional lymph node examination is required to assess for metastatic spread.

Diagnosis

Clinical examination of the suspected lesion may include dermoscopy if there is doubt about the diagnosis. Excisional biopsy to confirm the diagnosis is indicated before initiating treatment regimes. Imaging (i.e. computed tomography or magnetic resonance imaging) is not routinely indicated unless regional lymphadenopathy is present or there are associated symptoms indicating further invasion. Sentinel lymph node biopsy may be indicated to assess possible metastatic disease. Staging is along the TNM classification.

Pathological features

Although no single feature is pathognomonic for a melanoma, characteristic features exist. Upward growth of melanocytes is seen, with them no longer being confined to the basal layer (Pagetoid spread). It may grow by radial or vertical growth. 'Clark's level' defines the level of invasion in local tissues and 'Breslow thickness' is the total vertical height of the tumour.

Treatment

All treatment regimens should be discussed with a specialist skin cancer multidisciplinary team.

Lesions suspected to be CMM should be excised with a margin of normal surrounding skin and assessed for histological diagnosis and staging. Incision biopsy is usually contraindicated because of the risk of sampling a benign area of a lesion and difficulty with histological interpretation. Wider local excision will then be indicated, dependent on the Breslow thickness: lesions less than 1 mm thick require excision of the scar with a 1 cm margin, lesions 1 to 2 mm thick have a 1 to 2 cm margin, and lesions over 2.1 mm have a 2 to 3 cm margin.[14]

If there is lymph node involvement, then a regional lymph node dissection may be indicated after staging. Sentinel lymph node biopsy to help staging is often offered to patients with CMM between 1 mm and 4 mm thick, although it does not offer a survival advantage.

The role of adjuvant therapy is limited. Melanomas are not radiosensitive. The role of interferon is still controversial and clinical trials are on-going.

Prognosis and follow-up

Prognosis for patients with CMM is primarily determined by the thickness of the tumour and the presence and extent of metastatic disease. Patients with CMM less than 1 mm Breslow thickness have a 5-year disease free survival rate of over 90% or better, therefore follow-up for 1 year is suggested by guidelines.[15] All other stages of CMM have a relatively high risk of recurrence from between 40% and 90%, over 2 to 4 years, depending on the thickness of tumour and metastatic spread.[16] These patients require a follow-up for 5 years.

Other

Merkel cell carcinoma

Merkel cell carcinoma (MCC) is a rare and aggressive malignancy. It arises from abnormal growth of Merkel cells in the skin whose key function is as touch receptors. MCC arises most often on sun-exposed areas in patients over the age of 50 years. It usually appears as a firm, painless lesion and tumours can vary in size. Diagnosis is made following biopsy of a lesion – histological analysis with special stains is required. Multimodal treatment is required for MCC: surgical excision of the primary lesion and any involved regional lymph nodes, radiotherapy, and sometimes chemotherapy. Mortality from MCC occurs within the first 3 years of diagnosis.[17] Due to its rarity survival is difficult to predict but patients require close clinical follow-up.

Further reading

Luba M, Bangs S, Mohler A, et al. Common benign skin tumours. Am Acad Fam Phys 2003; 67(4): 729–38.

References

1. Kim JH, Park HY, Ahn SK. Cherry angiomas on the scalp. Case Rep Dermatol 2009; 1(1): 82–6.
2. de Berker D, McGregor J, Hughes B. Guidelines for the management of actinic keratoses. Br J Dermatol 2007; 156: 222–30.
3. Marks R, Rennie G, Selwood TS. Malignant transformation of solar keratoses to squamous cell carcinoma. Lancet 1988; i: 795–7.
4. Joseph C, Pierson DM. 'Dermatofibroma'. eMedicine. WebMD [online]. Available from: http://emedicine.medscape.com/article/1056742-overview. [Accessed 3rd March 2013].
5. Sandbank M. Basal cell carcinoma at the base of cutaneous horn (cornu cutaneum). Arch Dermatol 1971; 104(1): 97–8.
6. Cox N, Eedy D, Morton C. Guidelines for management of Bowen's disease: update 2006. Br J Dermatol 2007; 151: 11–21.
7. Erba P, Farhadi J, Wettstein R, et al. Morphoeic basal cell carcinoma of the face. Scand J Plast Reconstr Hand Surg 2007; 41(4): 184–8.
8. Fresini A, Rossiello L, Severino BU, et al. Giant basal cell carcinoma. Skinmed. 2007; 6(4): 204–5.
9. Bower C, Lear J, de Berker D. Basal cell carcinoma follow-up practices by dermatologists: a national survey. Br J Dermatol 2001; 145: 949–56.
10. Telfer N, Colver G, Morton C. Guidelines for the management of basal cell carcinoma. Br J Dermatol 2008; 159:35–48.
11. Motley R, Preston P, Lawrence C. Multi-professional guidelines for the management of the patient with primary cutaneous squamous cell carcinoma. Br J Dermatol 2009; 146: 18–25.
12. Clayman G, Lee J, Holsinger C, et al. Mortality risk from squamous cell carcinoma. J Clin Oncol 2005; 23: 759–65.
13. Rowe D, Carroll R, Day C. Prognostic factors for local recurrence, metastasis and survival rates in squamous cell carcinoma of the skin, ear and lip. J Am Acad Dermatol 1992; 26: 976–90.
14. Marsden J, Newton-Bishop J, Burrows L, et al. Revised UK guidelines for the management of cutaneous melanoma 2010. Br J Dermatol 2010; 163: 238–56.
15. Einwachter-Thompson J, MacKie R. An evidence base for reconsidering current follow-up guidelines for patients with cutaneous melanoma less than 0.5mm thick at diagnosis. Br J Dermatol 2008; 159: 337–41.
16. Newton-Bishop J, Bataille V, Gavin A, et al. The prevention, diagnosis, referral and management of melanoma of the skin: concise guidelines. Royal College of Physicians and British Association of Dermatologists Concise Guidelines to Good Practice Series. London: Royal College of Physicians, 2007, 7.
17. Lyhne D, Lock-Anderson J, Dahlstrom K, et al. Rising incidence of Merkel cell carcinoma. J Plast Surg Hand Surg 2011; 45: 274–80.

CHAPTER 2.11.2

Soft tissue masses

Mandeep Kang and David Ward

Introduction

Soft tissue masses (STMs) are benign or malignant growths that occur in the subcutaneous and connective tissues beneath the skin; adipose tissue, muscles, tendons, and vasculature. STMs are common, with a large majority being benign and outnumbering malignant STMs by a factor of 100. Malignant soft tissue tumours amount to less than 1% of all malignant tumours and there are more than 50 histological subtypes.[1] An STM is often asymptomatic during the early stages of development, but as it grows discomfort may occur when pressure is exerted upon surrounding tissues or nerves.

Aetiology

In most STMs there is no known definitive cause for their development. Sometimes the origin may be genetic. Hereditary conditions that can contribute to STM development include Garner syndrome, neurofibromatosis, and inherited retinoblastoma. A Kaposi sarcoma is an STM found in some immunocompromised patients and is associated with the human herpes virus 8. Additional causal factors may include exposure to chemicals (e.g. herbicides, vinyl chloride) or exposure to radiation. Soft tissue sarcomas arising in scar tissue have also been reported.

Diagnosis

Despite the diversity associated with soft tissue tumour development and prognosis, all diagnoses carry similar symptoms and treatment options. After taking a complete history and physical examination, imaging and a biopsy are usually required to aid diagnosis and to tailor treatment regimes.

Radiographs

Plain radiographs may identify calcified areas within the mass. This can initially help to identify the subtype of tumour.

Computed tomography (CT)

Assessment via CT allows for staging of the tumour locally and assessment of metastatic spread.

Magnetic resonance imaging (MRI)

MRI is the modality of choice for detecting, characterizing, and staging STMs. MRI provides the best tissue discrimination between normal and abnormal tissues. MRI biopsies can also be conducted to aid diagnosis by histological confirmation.

Positron emission tomography (PET)

This technique can be used selectively to distinguish benign tumours from high-grade sarcomas, to evaluate local recurrence, and to determine the biological activity of STMs.

Angiography

Angiography can identify feeding vessels to a mass for preoperative or intraoperative embolization.

Biopsy

A biopsy is necessary if histological confirmation of the diagnosis is needed before planning treatment, unless the STM is clearly benign, such as a sebaceous cyst or a lipoma. The management plan can then be tailored to the predicted pattern of local growth and risk of metastasis. Small tumours may be sampled using fine needle aspiration. A core biopsy or incisional biopsy, which involves excision of a larger portion of the mass, may also be conducted.

Types

The many types of STMs are summarized in Table 2.11.2.1. Gross classifications encompassing both benign and malignant subtypes are as follows:

- **Adipocytic tumours** arise from fat/adipose tissue and account for 30% of all STMs.
- **Fibrous tumours** arise from fibrous tissue. Malignant fibrous histiocytoma is the most common mesenchymal malignancy and accounts for approximately 24% of all soft tissue sarcomas.[2]
- **Muscle tumours**: there are two types of muscle tissue tumours. Smooth muscle tumours arise from the involuntary smooth muscle found in internal viscera. Skeletal muscle tumours arise from voluntary skeletal muscle.
- **Pericytic (perivascular) tumours** grow around blood vessels but do not arise from the vasculature.
- **Vascular tumours** arise from blood vessels.
- **Tumours of uncertain differentiation** are STMs that cannot be correlated histologically to any specific normal tissue.

Common benign

Of the benign soft tissue tumours 99% are superficial and 95% are less than 5 cm in diameter.[3]

Table 2.11.2.1 World Health Organization (WHO) classification of soft tissue tumours[1]

Tumour subtype	Benign	Intermediate	Malignant
Adipocytic	Lipoma Lipomatosis (of nerve) Lipoblastoma Angiolipoma Myolipoma Chondroid lipoma Extrarenal angiomyolipoma Extra-adrenal myelolipoma Spindle cell/pleomorphic lipoma Hibernoma	Aytpical lipomatous tumour/ well differentiated liposarcoma	Dedifferentiated liposarcoma Myxoid liposarcoma Round cell liposarcoma Pleomorphic liposarcoma Mixed liposarcoma Liposarcoma
Fibroblastic/myofibroblastic	Nodular fasciitis Proliferative fasciitis Proliferative myositis Myositis ossificans fibro- osseous pseudotumour of digits Ischaemic fasciitis Elastofibroma Fibrous hamartoma of infancy Myofibroma/myofibromatosis Fibromatosis colli Juvenile hyaline fibromatosis Inclusion body fibromatosis Fibroma of tendon sheath Desmoplastic fibroblastoma Mammary-type myofibroblastoma Calcifying aponeurotic fibroma Angiomyofibroblastoma Cellular angiofibroma Nuchal-type fibroma Gardner fibroma Calcifying fibrous tumour Giant cell angiofibroma	Superficial fibromatoses Desmoid-type fibromatoses Lipofibromatosis Solitary fibrous tumour Inflammatory myofibroblastic tumour Low-grade myofibroblastic sarcoma Myxoinflammatory fibroblastic sarcoma Infantuke fibrosarcoma	Adult fibrosarcoma Myxofibrosarcoma Low-grade fibromyxoid sarcoma hyalinizing spindle cell tumour Sclerosing epithelioid fibrosarcoma
Fibrohistiocytic tumours	Giant cell tumour of tendon sheath Diffuse-type giant cell tumour Deep benign fibrous histiocytoma	Plexiform fibrohistiocytic tumour Giant cell tumour of soft tissues	Pleomorphic 'MFH' Giant cell 'MFH' Inflammatory 'MFH'
Smooth muscle	Angioleiomyoma Deep leiomyoma Genital leiomyoma		Leiomyosarcoma
Pericytic (perivascular)	Glomus tumour Myopericytoma		Malignant glomus tumour
Skeletal muscle	Rhabdomyoma		Embryonal rhabdomyosarcoma Alveolar rhabdomyosarcoma Pleomorphic rhabdomyosarcoma
Vascular	Haemangiomas Epithelioid haemangioma Angiomatosis Lymphangioma	Kaposiform haemangioendothelioma Retiform haemangioendothelioma Papillary intralymphatic angio-endothelioma Composite haemangioendothelioma Kaposi sarcoma	Epithelioid haemangioendothelioma Angiosarcoma of soft tissue

(continued)

Table 2.11.2.1 (*Continued*)

Tumour subtype	Benign	Intermediate	Malignant
Chondro-osseous	Soft tissue chondroma		Mesenchymal chondrosarcoma
			Extraskeletal osteosarcoma
Uncertain differentiation	Intramuscular myxoma	Angiomatoid fibrous histiocytoma	Synovial sarcoma
	Juxta-articular myxoma	Ossifying fibromyxoid tumour	Epithelioid sarcoma
	Deep angiomyxoma	Mixed tumour/ myoepithelioma parachordoma	Alveolar soft part sarcoma
	Pleomorphic hyalinizing angiectatic tumour		Extraskeletal myxoid chondrosarcoma
	Ectopic hamartomatous thymoma		PNET/extraskeletal Ewing tumour
			Desmoplastic small round cell tumour
			Extrarenal rhabdoid tumour
			Malignant mesenchymoma
			Neoplasms with perivascular epithelioid cell diff
			Intimal sarcoma

Source: data from Fletcher *et al.* (eds), *Pathology and Genetics of Tumours of Soft Tissue and Bone*, International Agency for Research on Cancer (IARC), IARC Press, Lyon, France, Copyright © 2002.

Lipoma

Aetiology

Lipomas are the most common benign soft tissue tumour to present and are composed of adipose tissue retained within a capsule. Their cause is not completely understood: a tendency to develop may be inherited and minor injuries and trauma may also trigger growth.

Classification

Lipomas can arise within the subcutaneous tissue or within deep tissue and therefore can be classified initially according to their anatomical location: subcutaneous, intramuscular, and intermuscular. Deep-seated lipomas (i.e. intramuscular, intermuscular) are usually larger and less well-defined than subcutaneous lipomas. Subtypes of lipoma include simple subcutaneous lipoma, angiolipoma, spindle cell/pleomorphic lipoma, lipoblastoma, hibernoma, angiomyolipoma, and chondroid lipoma.

Clinical presentation

Lipomas are usually slow growing and present as painless STMs with normal skin overlying. The more subcutaneous in their orientation the more mobile the masses are. Approximately 5% of patients present with multiple lipomas (Dercum's disease).[4]

Treatment

Lipomas generally do not require treatment until they become symptomatic (i.e. if the lipoma becomes painful, infected, or interferes with function). They can then be excised surgically.

Sebaceous cyst

Aetiology

Sebaceous glands lie in close relation to hair follicles and produce a substance called sebum. Sebaceous cysts are thought to occur as a result of trauma or occlusion of this pilosebaceous unit.

Clinical presentation

A sebaceous cyst can occur anywhere on the body except from the palms of the hand and soles of the feet. The more common areas are the scalp, ears, back, and face. It presents as a mobile fluid-filled ball lying beneath, and sometimes tethered to, the skin. The cyst is usually filled with keratin and can have a punctum visible on the skin. These cysts can become infected and leave resultant scar tissue (Figure 2.11.2.1).

Treatment

Sebaceous cysts generally do not require any treatment unless they are symptomatic (i.e. painful, infected, or have a poor cosmesis). Symptomatic cysts can be incised and drained, but this does not remove the cyst capsule and the cyst may recur. Surgical excision where the cyst lining and its contents are removed reduces the risk of recurrence greatly, but is best not done if the cyst is acutely inflamed.

Common malignant: soft tissue sarcoma (STS)

Incidence

STS is an umbrella term used to describe any malignant neoplasm of connective tissue. STSs account for approximately 1% of all

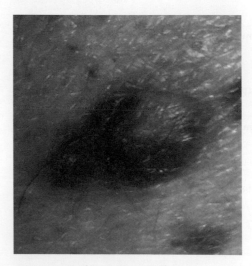

Fig. 2.11.2.1 Infected sebaceous cyst on the lower back.

malignant tumours. The majority affect the limbs or trunk but they can be found in other sites including the skin, uterus, stomach, and breast. Some, such as angiosarcomas, are very rare, less than 1% of STSs.[5] Synovial sarcomas and leiomyosarcomas each account for up to 10% of STSs, and malignant fibrous histiocytomas are the most common at about 24%. Approximately 2300 patients were diagnosed annually with STS in England between 1990 and 2007. There is no specific sex preponderance. More than 65% occur in people aged 50 and over.[5]

Aetiology

The exact cause is unknown but there are several risk factors that are thought to be related to the development of STSs. Some inherited conditions exhibit an increased risk for STS formation. These include neurofibromatosis, Li Fraumeni syndrome, and retinoblastoma. Radiotherapy treatment or exposure to radiation can cause STSs to develop at the site of treatment in 3% of patients that present with an STS. A radiation-induced STS usually has delayed development 5 to 10 years after the original treatment. Patients who have undergone lymph node dissection may develop chronic lymphoedema of a limb, which can progress rarely to a lymphangiosarcoma or Stewart-Treves syndrome. Immunosuppressed patients are at an increased risk when compared to patients with normal immunity. Kaposi's sarcoma is an angiosarcoma that has an association with acquired immunodeficiency syndrome and impaired immunity. Epstein Barr virus has been linked to leiomyosarcomas in children. Several chemicals are thought to increase the risks of some types of sarcoma (e.g. vinyl chloride, dioxins, and chlorophenols).

Classification

STSs are classified according to the tissue of origin. This is summarized under malignant STMs in Table 2.11.2.1.

Histological grading

Histological diagnosis should be made according to the latest World Health Organization (WHO) classification as shown in Table 2.11.2.1. Grading, based on histological parameters only, evaluates the degree of malignancy and indicates the probability of distant metastasis. Staging based both upon histology and clinical parameters provides better information on the extent of the tumour. One of the most widely used systems for grading is the FNCLCC (French Federation Nationale des Centres de Lutte Contre le Cancer) system, summarized in Table 2.11.2.2.

Clinical presentation

In their early stages, STSs are usually asymptomatic. Tumours can grow quite large, pushing aside normal tissue before causing symptoms. They tend to present late as a painless mass or with pain and neuropathic discomfort from pressure on nearby nerves and muscles. Rarely an STS can ulcerate overlying skin, causing surface wounds and risk of infection.

Diagnosis

The mass is assessed by imaging, with MRI being the mode of choice for accurate analysis of the mass and its anatomical relations.[6] The diagnosis is determined by fine needle aspiration or incisional biopsy of the mass, and the tumour's subtype and grade elicited by histological examination of the biopsy. Low-grade

Table 2.11.2.2 French Federation Nationale des Centres de Lutte Contre le Cancer (FNCLCC) grading system: definition of parameters

Tumour differentiation	
Score 1	Sarcomas closely resembling normal adult mesenchymal tissue
Score 2	Sarcomas for which histological typing is certain
Score 3	Embryonal and undifferentiated sarcomas
Mitotic count	
Score 1	0–9 mitoses per 10 HPF (high power field)
Score 2	10–19 mitoses per 10 HPF
Score 3	>20 mitoses per 10 HPF
Tumour necrosis	
Score 0	No necrosis
Score 1	<50% tumour necrosis
Score 2	>50% tumour necrosis
Histological grade	
Grade 1	Total score 2,3
Grade 2	Total score 4,5
Grade 3	Total score 6,7,8

HPF, high power field.

Reproduced with permission from Fletcher, C.D.M., Unni, K.K., Mertens, F., *World Health Organization Classification of Tumours: Pathology and Genetics of Tumours of Soft Tissue and Bone*, IARC Press, Lyon, France, Copyright © 2002.

sarcomas are less likely to metastasize than high grade sarcomas. A staging CT scan is indicated if metastatic disease is suspected or requires elimination.

Staging

This is done in concordance with the TNM staging system summarized in Table 2.11.2.3. It incorporates histological grade as well as tumour size and depth (T), regional lymph node involvement (N), and distant metastasis (M). The higher the stage of the STS the poorer the prognosis.

Treatment

A multidisciplinary approach involving pathologists, radiologists, surgeons, and oncologists is mandatory in all cases.[7] Treatment is dependent on the stage of the STS, which is based upon the size and grade of the tumour and whether there is any metastatic disease. The mainstay of treatment for STSs is surgical excision. The tumour is excised with a safe margin of normal tissue to increase the likelihood of complete excision of the neoplasm and to reduce the risk of recurrence. If the tumour is high grade, and palliation rather than cure is the aim of treatment, surgical debulking of the tumour may allow symptomatic control. Radiotherapy can be preoperative to shrink the tumour before excision, postoperative to increase the cure rate, or a primary treatment in patients where surgery is contraindicated or deemed not appropriate. Chemotherapy is used as an adjunct to treatment, usually in combination with surgery and radiotherapy. Metastatic deposits may require surgical excision if amenable and regional lymph node dissection may be warranted.[8]

Table 2.11.2.3 TNM classification for soft tissue sarcoma[1]

Primary tumour (T)	
TX	Primary tumour cannot be assessed
T0	No evidence of primary tumour
T1	Tumour < 5cm in greatest dimension
T1a	Superficial tumour (located exclusively above fascia without invasion)
T1b	Deep tumour
T2	Tumour > 5cm in greatest dimension
T2a	Superficial tumour
T2b	Deep tumour
Regional lymph nodes (N)	
NX	Regional lymph nodes cannot be assessed
N0	No regional lymph node metastasis
N1	Regional lymph node metastasis
Distant metastasis (M)	
M0	No distant metastasis
M1	Distant metastasis

Reproduced with permission from Fletcher, C.D.M., Unni, K.K., Mertens, F., *World Health Organization Classification of Tumours: Pathology and Genetics of Tumours of Soft Tissue and Bone*, IARC Press, Lyon, France, Copyright © 2002.

Prognosis

The prognosis differs according to the histological subtype of STSs. The most important prognostic factors for survival are the completeness of the surgical resection and the histological type and grade.[9] For the majority of patients treatment is palliative and not curative. The majority of metastases and local recurrences occur within 3 years.[10] There are no UK statistics for the outcomes by stage of sarcoma. Statistics from the USA suggest 5-year survival for stage 1 STS is 90%, stage 2 is 75%, and stage 3 is 54%.[11]

Follow-up

Due to the relative rarity of STS and the number of subtypes and their clinical presentations, there is no published data to indicate the optimal routine follow-up policy of surgically treated patients with localized disease. However, patients with an STS do need close follow-up after treatment. The surgically treated high-grade disease patient may be followed up 3-monthly for the first 3 years, then 6-monthly up until year 5, then once a year thereafter until year 10. Low-grade sarcoma patients may be followed for local relapse every 3 months, with radiographs or CT scans at more widely spaced intervals in the first 3 to 5 years, then yearly.[12]

References

1. Fletcher C, Unni K, Mertens F. *World Health Organization Classification of Tumours: Pathology and Genetics of Tumours of Soft Tissue and Bone*. Lyon: IARC Press; 2002.
2. Salisbury J. Malignant fibrous histiocytoma. *Postgrad Med J* 1989; 65: 872–4.
3. Bancroft L, Kransdorf M, Peterson J, *et al.* Benign fatty tumours: classification, clinical course, imaging appearance, and treatment. *Skeletal Radiol* 2006; 35(10): 719–33.
4. Hakim E, Kolander Y, Meller Y, *et al.* Gigantic lipomas. *J Plast Reconstruct Surg* 1994; 94(2): 369–71.
5. Fletcher C, Ryndolm A, Singer S, *et al.* World Health Organization Claassification of Tumours: Soft Tissue Tumours: Epidemiology, Clinical Features, Histopathological Typing and Grading. Lyon: IARC Press, 2006, pp. 10–18.
6. Bland K, McCoy D, Kinard R. Application of magnetic resonance imaging and computerized tomography as an adjunct to the surgical management of soft tissue sarcomas. *Ann Surg* 1987; 205(5): 473–81.
7. Wardelmann E, Chemnitz J, Wendtner C. Targeted therapy of soft tissue sarcomas. *J Oncol* 2012; 35(1): 21–7.
8. Fong Y, Coit D, Woodruff J. Lymph node metastasis from soft tissue sarcoma in adults. Analysis of data from a prospective database of 1772 sarcoma patients. *Ann Surg* 1993; 217(1): 72–7.
9. Jensen O, Hogh J, Ostgaard S. Histopathological grading of soft tissue tumours. Prognostic significance in a prospective study of 278 consecutive cases, *J Pathol* 1991; 163(1): 19–24.
10. Hashimoto H, Daimaru Y, Takeshita S. Prognostic significance of histologic parameters of soft tissue sarcoma. *Cancer* 1992; 70(12): 816–22.
11. Scoggins C, Pisters P. Diagnosis and management of soft tissue sarcoma. *Adv Surg* 2008; 42:219–28.
12. Demetri G, Antonia S, Robert B, *et al.* Soft tissue sarcoma. *J Natl Compr Cancer Netw* 2010; 8: 630–74.

PART 2.12

Head and neck surgery

Sub-section editor: Maurice Hawthorne

Benign and malignant lesions of the head and neck

Yujay Ramakrishnan and Maurice Hawthorne

Head and neck cancer

History

An accurate history is fundamental and must be based on a working knowledge of the likely pathology and possible risk factors.

Symptoms can be otological, rhinological, related to the pharynx or larynx, or systemic. Depending on the spread of tumour, there can also be neurological or orbital symptoms. Occasionally, there can be a single symptom signifying more sinister pathology. For example, otalgia in the setting of a normal otological examination could be referred from larynx or pharyngeal cancer. Unilateral hearing loss (due to glue ear) can be due to postnasal space pathology like nasopharyngeal carcinoma blocking the Eustachian tube.

Risk factors include smoking and alcohol. There are also specific risk factors for certain cancers:

- sinonasal carcinoma: hard wood industry and exposure to water soluble chrome salts

- oropharyngeal cancer: human papilloma virus (HPV)

- thyroid cancer: familial, ionizing radiation, Hashimoto thyroiditis

- skin cancer: ultraviolet radiation, type of skin, immunosuppression, familial.

Examination

A full ear, nose, and throat examination including the skin of the scalp needs to be undertaken. Neck examination should be performed systematically. The lymph node groups are divided into six levels, which can point to the origin of the primary tumour due to the predictable patterns of lymphatic spread (Figure 2.12.1.1). Fibreoptic endoscopy gives an excellent view of the nasal cavity, postnasal space, and larynx.

The identification of the difficult airway is essential, as patients with head and neck cancers can present with airway obstruction. Investigations should be deferred until the airway is secure. Medical management with steroids, antibiotics, nebulized adrenaline, and heliox (a mixture of helium and oxygen) can buy time, allowing a tracheostomy to take place under controlled conditions. The airway should be secured by an experienced anaesthetist, with the surgeon ready to perform an emergency tracheostomy. If intubation is likely to risk the airway, then a tracheostomy under local anaesthetic is the safest option.

Investigations

Any suspected head and neck cancer must be confirmed by biopsy. Imaging may be indicated depending on the site of the tumour, to assess the extent of the primary, neck nodes, and distant metastases as well as synchronous tumours. This can involve radiographs (e.g. chest X-ray, orthopantogram), ultrasound, computed tomography (CT), magnetic resonance imaging (MRI), and positron emission tomography–computed tomography (PET-CT) fusion scan. CT scans are useful to assess bony invasion whereas MRI gives excellent soft tissue detail.

Biopsies can range from a punch biopsy, fine needle aspirate (FNA) cytology, core biopsy, and incisional or excisional biopsy. The accuracy of the FNA depends on the quality of the sample and the cytologist. Progressively larger samples must be obtained if FNA cytology is inadequate. Incisional biopsies of a neck lump for a suspected squamous cell carcinoma should not be performed due to risk of spread to the skin; any future neck dissection will need to incorporate the scar of the incisional biopsy with concomitant loss of skin.

The extent of spread of the tumour can be assessed through a number of staging systems. In the UK, the TNM (Tumour, Nodal, Metastasis) staging provides the best prognostic indicator of treatment outcome. There are two components to the TNM staging, the clinical (pre-treatment) classification (cTNM) and pathological (post-surgical histopathological) classification (pTNM). The cTNM is vital to select the appropriate treatment, whereas the pTNM helps calculate prognosis. The validity of the TNM classification depends on the diagnostic methods employed and this is reflected in the certainty (C) factor (C1–5). Clinical staging is equivalent to C1, C2, and C3, pathological classification C4, whereas C5 is evidence from autopsy.

Treatment

The treatment of any head and neck cancer depends on certain broad principles and depends on a number of factors involving the tumour, patient, and local expert. It can be curative or palliative with the primary treatment options including:

- surgery: open or minimally invasive (e.g. endoscopic, transoral)

- radiotherapy or chemoradiotherapy

- biological agents.

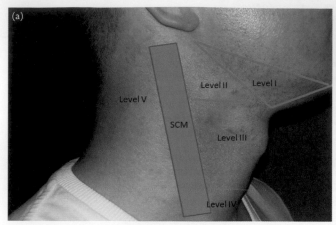
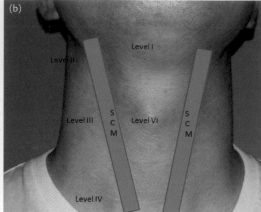

Fig. 2.12.1.1 Neck nodal levels. (a) Lateral view; (b) anteroposterior view. SCM, sternocleidomastoid.

In advanced tumours, multimodality treatment is employed to achieve improved loco-regional disease control and survival. Recurrent tumours have a guarded prognosis and salvage treatments include surgery, radiotherapy or chemotherapy.

Prognosis

The prognosis depends on tumour (grade, stage, biology of the tumour, local perineural or lymphovascular invasion, and extracapsular nodal spread) and patient (co-morbidity, performance status) factors as well as the effectiveness of treatment (completeness of surgical excision, shrinkage of tumour by radiotherapy, or chemotherapy).

Skin cancer

Skin cancers are named according to the type of skin cell from which they arise; basal cell carcinoma (BCC) from the basal layer of the epidermis, squamous cell carcinoma (SCC) from the middle layer of the epidermis and melanoma from the melanocytes (Figure 2.12.1.2). They can be categorized into melanoma and non-melanoma skin cancers.

Predisposing factors include:

+ chronic ultraviolet (sunshine) exposure

+ genetic: Gorlin's syndrome presents with multiple BCC, Li Fraumeni

+ skin type

+ immunosuppression: transplant patients, haematological malignancies

+ chronic inflammation in wounds—(SCC).

Basal cell carcinoma and squamous cell carcinoma

There are a number of BCC subtypes. Nodular BCC is the most common, while morphoeic BCC are found exclusively around the head and neck. Low-grade BCC (nodular, superficial, cystic, pigmented) are associated with less local tissue destruction compared to high risk BCC (morphoeic, micronodular, infiltrative, and basosquamous).

Typically nodular BCCs present with an indurated nodule ± ulceration. Morphoeic BCC have indistinct margins. Cutaneous

SCC usually presents with an indurated nodular keratinizing, crusted tumour that may ulcerate, or an ulcer without evidence of keratinization. They can occasionally present with a metastasis to the parotid gland and be mistaken for a primary parotid tumour.

Diagnosis is usually clinical, but can be confirmed with a punch biopsy. High risk BCCs include:

+ size > 2 cm

+ indistinct margins

+ morphoeic form

+ high-risk areas: central face, eyes, nose, lip, and ears

+ recurrent tumours

+ high-risk individuals: immunosuppression, genetic conditions.

Histological adverse features include certain histological subtypes (morphoeic, micronodular, infiltrative, basosquamous) as well as perineural and/or perivascular involvement. In addition, high-risk cSCC include > 2 cm size, depth > 4 mm thickness, Clark level V or beyond, as well located near the ear, non-hair-bearing lip, or scalp.

National Institute for Health and Care Excellence guidelines advise that the following patients are discussed at the skin multidisciplinary team meeting:

+ high-risk tumours: all cSCCs or high-risk BCCs with positive margins or recurrent disease

+ high-risk patients: immunocompromised and genetic predisposed patients

+ patients undergoing Mohs' surgery

+ those who may benefit from radiotherapy

+ those who may be eligible for entry into clinical trials.

The treatment of skin cancers is discussed in the chapter on benign and malignant skin conditions (Chapter 2.11.1).

Melanoma

Cutaneous melanoma is a malignant tumour of the cutaneous melanocytes. Despite rising incidence, the prognosis has improved mainly due to earlier diagnosis attributable to increased disease awareness amongst patients and healthcare professionals.

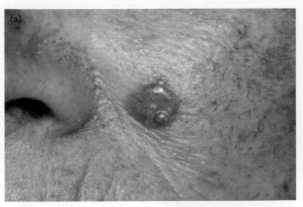

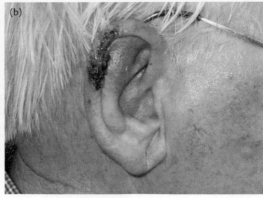

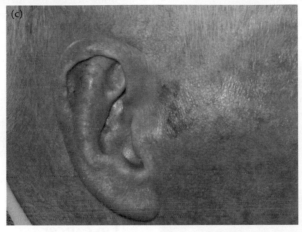

Fig. 2.12.1.2 (a) Basal cell carcinoma (pearly appearance and telangiectasia). (b) Squamous cell carcinoma (crusting and ulceration). (c) Melanoma (irregular border and pigmentation).
Images reproduced courtesy of Mr V Paleri and Mr S Anari.

The aetiology of cutaneous melanoma is complex, with ultraviolet radiation in susceptible individuals playing a key role. Other risk factors include family history (*CDKN2A* gene), giant pigmented hairy naevi, as well as atypical or dysplastic naevi.

There are several subtypes including:

◆ superficial spreading: most common

◆ nodular: can bleed or ulcerate

◆ lentigo maligna melanoma: pre-invasive phase termed lentigo maligna

◆ acral lentiginous melanoma: least common; on palms, soles, and under nails

◆ desmoplastic neurotropic melanoma: higher local recurrence thought to be secondary to perineural spread.

Clinical diagnosis can be challenging and should be assessed using the seven-point checklist (*major features*: change in size, irregular border, and pigmentation; *minor features*: inflamed, itch/altered sensation, lesion larger than others, oozing/crusting of lesion) or ABCDE (*a*symmetry, irregular *b*order, irregular *c*olour, *d*iameter >6 mm, *e*levation of lesion).

The treatment and prognosis is greatly influenced by the thickness of the tumour. Accurate tumour thickness can be assessed with an excision biopsy (2–5 mm margin) or punch biopsy at the thickest part of the lesion. Staging scans like CT of the head, chest, abdomen, and pelvis, MRI, and PET-CT may be performed prior to definitive surgery, depending on the stage of the lesion.

Wide local excision of the primary tumour is recommended. Excision margins vary depending on the Breslow thickness and can range from 5 mm (*in-situ* lesion) to 3 cm (>4 mm Breslow thickness). Clearly, there are certain anatomical and cosmetic constraints that may preclude this degree of clearance in the head and neck (e.g. near the eye or ear). Mohs' microsurgery is a surgical technique for the removal of certain cutaneous carcinomas that allows precise microscopic marginal control by using horizontal frozen sections. It may, therefore, have a role in cutaneous melanomas of the face. If primary closure is not possible, the reconstructive ladder options should be explored (skin grafts, local flaps, distant flaps). If the neck nodes are positive, a neck dissection is performed. There is no role for prophylactic neck dissection in node-negative patients. Sentinel node biopsy maybe considered in specialist centres for node-negative patients.

Oral cavity neoplasm

The oral cavity comprises the tongue, palate, floor of mouth, gingiva, and buccal region.

Lesion can be benign or malignant:

◆ benign

• papilloma

• salivary gland origin (e.g. pleomorphic adenoma)

• haemangioma

* premalignant
  * leukoplakia
  * erythroplakia
* malignant
  * SCC (majority; Figure 2.12.1.3)
  * salivary gland origin (mucoepidermoid, adenocarcinoma, adenoid cystic carcinoma).

The majority of malignant tumours of the oral cavity are SCCs. In order of frequency, the regions affected are anterior two-thirds of the tongue > floor of mouth > buccal mucosa > retromolar trigone > hard palate and gingivae.

Smoking and alcohol are the main risk factors, although betel nut chewing and HPV also play a small, significant role in certain lesions. Carcinoma of the oral cavity usually arises *de novo* or from a premalignant dysplastic lesion such as leukoplakia or erythroplakia. Early lesions can be rather subtle (flat and discoloured). Typically, a mass or a non-healing ulcer is the main presentation. Invasion of the surrounding structures can lead to loose teeth, trismus, referred otalgia, and neck lump.

Following biopsy and imaging of the lesion, there are two major treatment options:

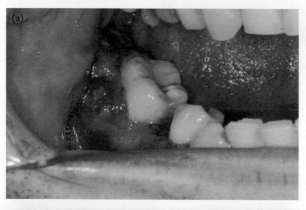
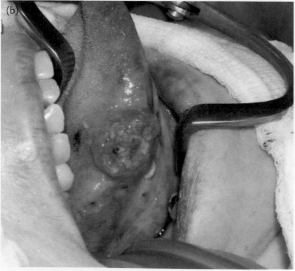

Fig. 2.12.1.3 (a) Gingival squamous cell carcinoma. (b) Tongue squamous cell carcinoma.

* surgery ± reconstruction ± neck dissection ± adjuvant radiotherapy
* radiotherapy or chemoradiotherapy.

Oral cavity tumours can be approached transorally. However, larger posterior tumours may need to be removed through a lingual release or mandibulotomy. Treatment options can be cold steel, laser, or coblation. A margin of 1 cm is ideal, vital structures permitting. 'Close margins' (pathological margin <5 mm) require further resection or adjuvant radiotherapy. Where there is bony involvement, periosteal stripping or partial mandibulectomy may be necessary. The defect may be reconstructed using the reconstructive ladder, ranging from local, pedicled flap to free flaps. Bony defects may be reconstructed with autologous bone grafts, but more commonly free flaps (fibula, radius, iliac crest, or scapula) are employed. Adjuvant radiotherapy may be indicated in large tumours with adverse histological features as well as advanced neck disease. The addition of chemotherapy (concurrent chemoradiation) is recommended in tumours with positive margins or extracapsular spread to improve local control rates.

Prognosis depends on a variety of factors; tumour thickness (>4 mm tongue SCC is associated with increased risk of lymph node metastasis), pattern of invasion (non-cohesive, perineural), positive margin, and extracapsular spread of nodes are all associated with a poorer prognosis. In addition, certain subtypes of SCC may have a better prognosis (e.g. verrucous SCC has a better prognosis compared to basaloid SCC).

Lip cancer

Lip cancer is the most common head and neck cancer. Over 90% lesions arise from the lower lip, with SCC being the most common lesion. Other cancers include BCC and salivary gland tumours. Ultraviolet radiation is the main risk factor, although smoking and viruses may play a contributory role in certain cases. The clinical behaviour is similar to skin cancer.

Early stage lip cancer can be treated equally well by surgery or radiation, though the cosmetic results with the latter may be inferior. For small lesions, wedge excisions and primary closure, or advancement flaps are employed. Larger lesions may be reconstructed by rotating adjacent tissue (e.g. opposite lip, advancement flaps) or free flaps. Apart from cosmesis, the functional outcome with regard to lip sensitivity and muscle function needs to be taken into account.

Oropharynx

The oropharynx is composed of the following subsites: base of tongue, tonsil, soft palate (includes uvula), and pharyngeal walls (posterior and lateral). Histologically, the majority of oropharyngeal cancers are SCC (OPSCC), although lymphoma can also occur.

Although smoking and alcohol are the main risk factors for OPSCC, this disease is appearing in younger non-smoking individuals, related to HPV acquired through oral sex or perinatal transmission.

Early cancers can be treated with surgery (trans-oral laser/robotic surgery) or chemoradiation. Trans-oral surgery is associated with faster recovery and improved speech and swallowing outcomes. Advanced stage cancer can be treated with primary chemoradiation or surgery plus adjuvant treatment. Intensity-modulated radiation therapy is associated with less xerostomia due to sparing of the parotid gland.

HPV status is an important prognostic factor; retrospective analysis has shown HPV-positive patients have improved survival rates compared to their HPV-negative counterparts when treated with radiotherapy or chemoradiotherapy. Prophylactic vaccination may lead to reduced incidence of this cancer. Two vaccines are currently available on the market: the bivalent Cervirax® vaccine (Merck) and quadrivalent Gardasil®.

Nasopharyngeal neoplasm

Most benign tumours originate from the minor salivary glands and tumours of epithelial origin are rare. Occasionally, juvenile angiofribroma can present as a vascular mass in the nasopharynx. Malignant lesions include nasopharyngeal carcinoma, lymphoma and salivary gland tumours.

Nasopharyngeal carcinoma (NPC) is frequent in patients of southern Chinese, north African and Alaskan origin, with a median age of presentation of 50 years. The incidence is far higher in the east ranging between 20 and 30/100 000 per year compared to 1/100 000 per year in the western countries. NPC is believed to be due to a combination of genetic and environmental factors (salted fish, Epstein Barr virus). NPC is classified according the World Health Organization classification into the following subtypes:

+ type 1: keratinizing SCC
+ type 2a: non-keratinizing SCC
+ type 2b: undifferentiated SCC.

The majority of patients present with a neck lump (neck metastasis). Other symptoms include nasal obstruction, epistaxis, hearing loss (glue ear), as well cranial nerve palsies due to skull base involvement.

Investigations include biopsy as well as staging CT and MRI. Radiotherapy is the mainstay of treatment. Concurrent chemoradiotherapy has been shown to significantly improve loco-regional control and survival in advanced stage disease. Patients are followed up clinically (endoscopically) and with CT, MRI, or PET-CT imaging. Patients with recurrence may undergo salvage nasopharyngectomy (± neck dissection) and receive further radiation and chemotherapy.

Sinonasal neoplasms

Sinonasal neoplasms can be benign or malignant:

+ benign:
  • epithelial: inverted papilloma (most common), warts
  • non-epithelial:
    a. salivary gland (pleomorphic adenoma)
    b. haemangioma (e.g. juvenile angiofibroma)
    c. pyogenic granuloma: friable polypoid lesion that bleeds
    d. schwannoma
    e. osteoma
    f. chordoma
    g. fibroma

+ malignant:
  • epithelial: SCC, melanoma, olfactory neuroblastoma, sinonasal undifferentiated
  • non-epithelial:
    a. salivary gland origin (adenocarcinoma, adenoid cystic carcinoma)
    b. rhabdomyosarcoma
    c. lymphoma
    d. vascular origin (haemangipericytoma)
    e. chondrosarcoma
    f. teratoma

The most common benign growth in the nasal cavity is the inverted papilloma. It is locally aggressive and CT may reveal erosion of the lateral nasal wall and extension into the maxillary sinus. These tumours are excised endoscopically, occasionally supplemented with Caldwell Luc approach for areas with limited access. Lifelong follow-up is essential due the risk of malignant transformation (5–10%).

Juvenile angiofibroma presents with unilateral nasal obstruction and epistaxis in adolescent males. It is a benign highly vascular and locally invasive tumour, usually arising at the sphenopalatine foramen. It can extend into the paranasal sinus, orbit, skull base, and intracranially. It is treated endoscopically (if small/accessible) or surgically (with preoperative embolization), with radiotherapy reserved for inoperable, residual, or recurrent tumours.

A patient with sinonasal carcinoma typically present with a unilateral nasal mass, nasal blockage or epistaxis. Risk factors related to occupation (wood dust exposure, heavy metals, leather tanning) should be elucidated. A full ear, nose, and throat examination including flexible nasoendoscopy and orbital and neurological examination is carried out along with a staging CT/MRI and biopsy. Surgery can be endoscopic or open, and adjuvant radiotherapy or chemotherapy may be considered. Diligent tumour surveillance by flexible nasoendoscopy and interval imaging is necessary in the post-treatment phase.

Larynx neoplasms

Benign laryngeal neoplasms include, laryngeal papilloma, salivary gland benign neoplasm, chondroma, haemangioma (e.g. subglottic), and schwannoma. The majority of malignant tumours are SCC (Figure 2.12.1.4), but chondrosarcoma and salivary gland malignancy can also occur. Alcohol and smoking are major risk factors for laryngeal cancer.

Treatment depends on multiple factors including the tumour, patient, and local expertise. Early stage laryngeal cancers (T1 and T2) can be managed with surgery or radiotherapy. T3 lesions tend to be managed non-surgically (radiation or concurrent chemoradiation therapy) and transoral laser in selected cases. Most T4 lesions are treated with concurrent chemoradiation therapy unless there is complete thyroid cartilage invasion, where a total laryngectomy is performed. Where indicated, concurrent chemoradiation should be applied due to improved loco-regional control and survival (approximately 10%). In patients unable to tolerate chemotherapy, cetuximab (a monoclonal antibody against epidermal

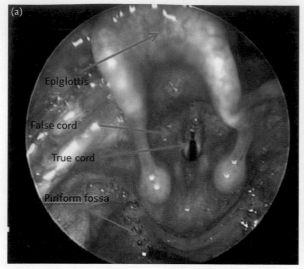

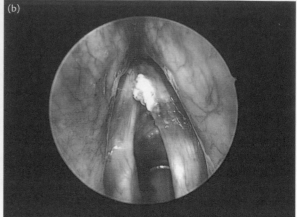

Fig. 2.12.1.4 (a) Endoscopic view of normal larynx. (b) Early laryngeal cancer.

growth factor receptor) appears to improve oncological outcomes compared to radiotherapy alone.

Salivary neoplasm

Salivary gland neoplasms are rare, accounting for approximately 3% of head and neck cancers. They are unique compared to other head neck cancers, due to the diverse range of histological and clinical behaviour. They can be either benign or malignant. Most lesions are benign, though the incidence of malignancy is inversely proportional to the size of the gland, being higher in in the submandibular and minor salivary glands compared to the parotid gland. Although salivary tumours are rare in children, a greater proportion (20–30%) are malignant (usually low grade mucoepidermoid carcinomas).

Parotid neoplasm

Benign lesions (80%) include pleomorphic adenoma, adenolymphoma (Warthin tumour), and haemangioma. Malignant tumours can be classified as mucoepidermoid carcinoma, adenocarcinoma, adenoid cystic carcinoma, acinic cell carcinoma, malignant mixed tumour, lymphoma, or metastatic.

Most parotid neoplasms present with a palpable lump or with accompanying symptoms suggestive of malignancy (Figure 2.12.1.5). Parotid lumps are investigated using ultrasound-guided FNA; core biopsy may be indicated if the FNA is non-diagnostic. Imaging (CT or MRI) is not generally performed for benign lesions unless it is a large tumour with deep lobe extension. Staging CT is warranted for all malignant tumours.

The treatment of parotid lymphomas is non-surgical. Other tumours are excised, the extent varying between a superficial and complete parotidectomy. Patients with confirmed neck metastasis will undergo a neck dissection and dissection of an N0 (node-negative) neck may be indicated in certain high-grade tumours. Radiotherapy may be used primary for palliation or adjuvantly post-surgery (high grade or large tumours >4 cm, adenoid cystic carcinoma, incomplete margins, extracapsular spread, recurrent disease).

Parapharyngeal neoplasms

Primary parapharyngeal neoplasms are rare (<0.5% of head neck cancers) and 80% are benign. The most common tumour is the pleomorphic adenoma followed by neurogenic tumours (schwannoma, paraganglioma, neurofibroma). Any of the cranial nerves and sympathetic chain in the parapharyngeal space are capable of giving rise to schwannoma.

They present with a neck lump near the angle of the mandible, intraoral lump due to displacement of the tonsil or cranial nerve palsies. The post-styloid lesion can compress the 9th, 10th, 11th, and 12th nerve causing hoarseness, dysphagia, dysarthria, and weakness of the shoulder or Horner's syndrome. Compression of the carotid vessels can also lead to cerebrovascular events. A very small proportion of paranagangliomas can secrete catecholamines, leading to episodic hypertension manifesting as headaches and palpitations. The key to investigation is to differentiate between vascular and non-vascular lesions using non-invasive magnetic

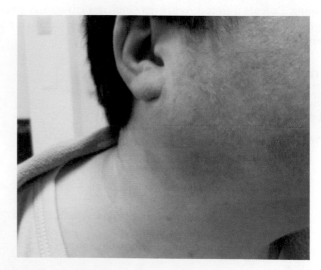

Fig. 2.12.1.5 Parotid lump.
Image reproduced courtesy of Jai Manickavasagam.

resonance angiography or invasive angiography, alongside MRI and CT. The mainstay of treatment is embolization, surgery, and radiotherapy.

Further reading

Ang KK, Harris J, Wheeler R, *et al.* Human papillomavirus and survival of patients with oropharyngeal cancer. *N Engl J Med* 2010; 363, 24–35.

Pignon JP, Bourhis J, Domenge C, *et al.* Chemotherapy added to locoregional treatment for head and neck squamous-cell carcinoma: three meta-analyses of updated individual data. MACH-NC Collaborative Group. Meta-Analysis of Chemotherapy on Head and Neck Cancer. *Lancet* 2000; 355, 949–55.

Posner MR, Wirth LJ. Cetuximab and radiotherapy for head and neck cancer. *N Engl J Med* 2006; 354, 634–6.

Roland NJ, McRae RDR, McCombe AW. *Key Topics in Otolaryngology.* London: Informa Healthcare, 2000.

The British Thyroid Association and the Royal College of Physicians. *Guidelines for the management of thyroid cancer* (2nd ed). London: Royal College of Physcians, 2007.

Upper airway obstruction

Himanshu Swami and Maurice Hawthorne

Introduction

Upper airway obstruction is defined as any abnormal condition of the mouth, nose, or larynx that interferes with breathing when the rest of the respiratory system is functioning normally. Upper airway obstruction can be acute or chronic. Acute airway obstruction is one of the most serious emergencies faced as delay of a few minutes in restoring the airway can lead to pulmonary oedema, cardiac arrest, or irreversible brain damage.[1] Chronic airway obstruction, on the other hand, can lead to obstructive sleep apnoea, hypertension, stress, and other mental disturbances. If no timely intervention is done it may progress to acute obstruction. There are various causes for upper airway obstruction and the line of management depends on the aetiology and condition of the patient at time of presentation.

Aetiopathogenesis

The aetiology of upper airway obstruction is different in the paediatric age group where most pathological processes that result in upper airway compromise are a consequence of infection, trauma, or aspiration (see Box 2.12.2.1). Trauma and neoplasms are the leading causes in adults. Narrowing of the upper respiratory tract has an exponential effect on airflow because linear airflow is a function of the fourth power of the radius (Poiseuille's equation).[2] The anatomy of the paediatric airway differs from adults as they are obligatory nasal breathers, the larynx is located higher (C4, as compared with C6 in adults), and the narrowest part is the subglottis (as compared with the vocal cords in adults). This leads to different anatomical sites being involved in children than adults.

Upper airway obstruction can be classified in different ways as follows.[3]

According to aetiology

1. Congenital:

   - micrognathia
   - macroglossia (large tongue)
   - laryngeal web

Box 2.12.2.1 Aetiopathogenesis

- Can be anatomical or functional
- Infective causes and foreign body common in children
- Trauma and neoplasms common in adults
- Narrowing of airway has exponential effect on airflow

   - vascular ring
   - vocal cord dysfunction
   - laryngomalacia.

2. Trauma:

   - laryngeal stenosis
   - tracheal stenosis
   - airway burn
   - acute laryngeal injury
   - facial trauma (mandibular or maxillary fractures)
   - haemorrhage.

3. Infections and inflammations:

   - suppurative parotitis
   - retropharyngeal abscess
   - tonsillar hypertrophy
   - Ludwig's angina
   - epiglottitis
   - laryngitis
   - laryngotracheobronchitis (croup)
   - diphtheria
   - sarcoidosis
   - Wegener's granulomatosis
   - relapsing polychondritis.

4. Iatrogenic causes:

   - tracheal stenosis post-tracheostomy
   - tracheal stenosis postintubation
   - mucous ball from transtracheal catheter.

5. Foreign bodies.

6. Vocal cord paralysis.

7. Tumours:

   - laryngeal tumours (benign or malignant)
   - laryngeal papillomatosis
   - tracheal stenosis (caused by intrinsic or extrinsic tumours).

8. Angioedema:

   - anaphylactic reactions

- C1 inhibitor deficiency
- angiotensin-converting enzyme inhibitors.

9. Neuromuscular:

- recurrent laryngeal nerve interruption (postoperative, inflammatory, tumour infiltration)
- obstructive sleep apnoea
- laryngospasm
- myasthenia gravis
- Guillain-Barre polyneuritis
- hypocalcaemia (causing vocal cord spasm)
- tetanus.

Anatomical site

1. Intrathoracic:

- fixed
- variable.

2. Extrathoracic:

- vixed
- variable

Acute or chronic

There are various other classifications that can be used to describe upper airway obstruction. There are different flow loop contours seen in patients with upper airway obstruction, which depend on the site of lesion (intrathoracic or extrathoracic) and whether the obstruction is fixed or variable. The intrathoracic airway dilates during inspiration as it is exposed to the outward force of negative intrapleural pressure. Positive intrapleural pressure during expiration causes compression and narrowing. The compliant extrathoracic airway, not exposed to intrapleural pressure, collapses during inspiration and increases in diameter during expiration Accordingly lesions can be classified into:

- fixed upper airway obstruction (intrathoracic or extrathoracic), e.g. postintubation strictures, goitres, and tracheal tumours
- variable extrathoracic obstruction, e.g. glottic strictures, tumours, and vocal cord paralysis
- variable intrathoracic obstruction, e.g. tracheal tumours and tracheomalacia.

Depending on the presentation, upper airway obstruction can also be classified into acute or chronic phase. Acute obstruction is an emergency but chronic obstruction can also progress to acute obstruction and respiratory failure.

Clinical features

Symptoms and signs vary depending on the aetiology. Children can present with different clinical features than adults and are more prone to develop acute respiratory failure and hence they should be monitored carefully.[4] History plays an important part in identifying the cause of obstruction. In acute cases a quick history of onset, preceding event and progression of symptoms should be taken with simultaneous management. A detailed history will lead to the diagnosis in most of the cases.

In chronic obstruction symptoms become more pronounced on exertion but an acute obstruction can precipitate symptoms quickly. Stridor is an abnormal, high-pitched sound produced by turbulent airflow through a partially obstructed airway at the level of the supraglottis, glottis, subglottis, and/or trachea. It implies reduction in airway to less than 5 mm in an adult. Stridor may be inspiratory, expiratory, or biphasic depending on its timing in the respiratory cycle. Inspiratory stridor suggests a laryngeal obstruction, whereas expiratory stridor implies tracheobronchial obstruction. Biphasic stridor suggests a subglottic or glottic anomaly. A triad of choking, cough, and wheezing is suggestive of foreign body inhalation in children. History of fever is suggestive of infective pathology. However, there are some common features of upper respiratory obstruction.

Common clinical symptoms

- Breathing difficulty on exertion or at rest
- Choking
- Wheezing
- Sweating
- Difficulty in speaking
- Panic
- Fever in infective aetiology

Common clinical signs

- Stridor—inspiratory, expiratory or biphasic
- Inspiratory retraction
- Cyanosis
- Altered consciousness
- Apathy
- Active abdominal contractions

Investigations

Acute airway obstruction is an emergency due to impending respiratory failure. In such cases establishing a safe and secure airway by intubation or surgical procedures such as tracheostomy or cricothyroidotomy is a priority and definitive management follows the primary condition (see Box 2.12.2.2). However, in patients who have mild respiratory obstruction there are certain diagnostic tools that are helpful in establishing the diagnosis and forming the line of management.

- **Bronchoscopy** is the procedure used to visualize the larynx, trachea, and main bronchi.
  - **Flexible bronchoscopy:** flexible scope has certain advantages. It can be done under local anaesthesia in outpatient settings.

Box 2.12.2.2 Investigations

- In acute conditions airway is established prior to investigations
- Bronchoscopy is the most valuable tool in diagnosis
- Virtual bronchoscopy

One can visualize up to the third generation of airway and it can be used for certain therapeutic procedures such as removal of small foreign bodies, delivering fibre optic laser, stents, etc. It is limited by the fact that simultaneous ventilation cannot be done. The condition of a patient with obstruction can deteriorate if the procedure is prolonged.

- **Rigid bronchoscopy** is mainly performed for therapeutic purpose. Due to ventilation channels the procedure can be performed for longer duration, moreover, it can provide access to the airway in emergency if negotiated carefully through the site of partial obstruction.

- **Computed tomography (CT) scan** is a useful tool to provide the site, size and extent of obstruction. It can also give information about the nature of the lesion such as vascularity and density. As the patient needs to be shifted to the facility for CT it is not advisable in acute cases prior to securing the airway.

- **Virtual bronchoscopy** involves using CT images of the chest to generate a three-dimensional model of the walls of the trachea and bronchi (airway passages). A protocol for virtual bronchoscopic assessment of a three-dimensional CT pulmonary image would have two main stages (i.e. pre-processing of image data and interactive image assessment). This is a relatively new technique and with improvement in software and technology it can provide valuable information in a non-invasive manner.

Treatment

If upper airway obstruction is suspected it should be taken as an emergency and an experienced otolaryngologist and anaesthetist should be involved immediately in the management. The approach to management depends on the age, site, severity, and chronic or acute nature of obstruction. Patients with slowly progressive or easily treatable causes of upper airway obstruction may be managed expectantly; signs of impending respiratory arrest dictate that the airway be secured immediately. In the paediatric age group condition may deteriorate rapidly as they fatigue early.[5] The presence of

a paediatrician is also important in ensuring that appropriate intervention takes place in such cases. Each patient requires an individual approach to management; universal recommendations are difficult.

We will discuss common aetiologies and their management in the paediatric and adult age groups.

Paediatric age group

Infective pathologies

Obstruction due to infection is common in infants and children. The subglottic area is the narrowest part of the paediatric airway and is particularly vulnerable to obstruction because the cricoid ring, being a complete ring, restricts the ability of this segment to expand. The loosely attached submucosa contains a high number of mucus glands and can rapidly decrease the airway calibre should inflammation and oedema occur. The clinical importance of acute upper airway obstruction derives from the fact that some cases can progress rapidly to cause severe hypoxia and even cardiorespiratory arrest.[6] The child's general appearance is the most reliable indicator of severity rather than vitals or scoring systems (see Table 2.12.2.1).

Foreign bodies

Foreign bodies in the tracheobronchial tree are usually encountered in the paediatric age group and more so in infants as they have a tendency to explore and put things in their mouths. In most children the aspiration is manifested by a triad of choking, coughing, and wheezing.[7] Site of lodgement of the foreign body can be the vocal cords and subglottis, which can cause acute respiratory distress. Aggressive management in form of direct laryngoscopy and removal of foreign body is required.

The Heimlich manoeuvre can be performed. The technique differs from adults.

- **Infants:** place the infant face down across your forearm (resting your forearm on your leg) and support the infant's head with your hand. Give four forceful blows to the back with the heel of your hand. You may have to repeat this several times until the obstructing object is coughed out.

Table 2.12.2.1 Infective causes in children

	Epiglotitis	Croup	Bacterial laryngotracheobronchitis
Anatomical site	Supraglottis	Larynx, trachea, bronchus	Larynx, trachea, bronchus
Organism	Bacterial *Haemophilus influenzae* type B (HIB) (most common)	Viral Parainfluenza virus type 1 (most common)	Bacterial *Staphylococcus aureus* (most common)
Clinical features	High fever, drooling, dysphagia, dysphonia and dyspnoea, 'tripod position', toxic	Fever ±-, inspiratory stridor, hoarseness, barky, seal-like cough	High fever, severe stridor, respiratory distress, able to lie supine and swallow
X-ray	Lateral neck: 'thumb sign' due to swollen epiglottis and AE folds	Anteroposterior neck: 'steeple sign' due to narrow subglottis	Non-specific Laryngoscopy: ulcerations and pseudomembrane formation in subglottis and trachea
Treatment	Intubation (short term) Intravenous antibiotics	Nebulized 1% L-epinephrine or 2.25% racemic epinephrine, oral steroids Rarely intubation	Intravenous antibiotics Intubation ±

- **Toddler:** use the heel of your hand to deliver five quick strikes to the child's back in an attempt to dislodge the obstruction. Aim for the middle of the back between the shoulder blades. Start the Heimlich manoeuvre by kneeling or standing behind the toddler. Make a fist with one hand to properly perform the Heimlich manoeuvre. Place your fist against the child's belly—slightly above the belly button—with the thumb-side closest to his stomach. Use your other hand to grip the fist near the child's belly. Thrust your fist quickly upward into the abdomen several times. Repeat back strikes and the Heimlich manoeuvre until the obstructed item is coughed out of the child's mouth. The child will start to cough and breathe heavily once the item is dislodged.

Fortunately, most foreign bodies pass the vocal cords and lodge in the *lower airways*. After a brief history of choking, which may go unnoticed, it may result in atelectasis, chronic pulmonary infections, abscess, bronchiectasis, or asthma. However, the presentation may be more subtle, resulting in prolonged and misguided therapy for asthma and pneumonia prior to correct diagnosis. Rigid or fibre optic brochoscopy is required for confirmation of diagnosis and treatment. Right main bronchus is a common site as it is wider and straighter than left main bronchus.

Adults

Most patients with upper airway obstruction require urgent establishment of a patent and secure airway. In emergencies a few steps are carried out for maintaining airway and breathing, this will include manually opening the patient's airway (head tilt-chin lift or jaw thrust) or possible insertion of oral (oropharyngeal airway) or nasal (nasopharyngeal airway) adjuncts, to keep the airway unblocked (patent). For breathing, this may include artificial respiration, often assisted by emergency oxygen or heliox.[8] The line of management will depend on the age group, history, physical examination, aetiology, and severity of obstruction. We will discuss some procedures which can be utilized in the management of upper airway obstruction:

Heimlich manoeuvre

The Heimlich manoeuvre is an emergency procedure for removing a foreign object lodged in the airway that is preventing a person from breathing. It can be performed under any setting. If the person is sitting or standing, stand behind him or her. Form a fist with one hand and place your fist, thumb-side in, just below the person's rib cage in the front. Grab your fist with your other hand. Keeping your arms off the person's rib cage, give four quick inward and upward thrusts. You may have to repeat this several times until the obstructing object is coughed out. If the person is lying down or unconscious, straddle him or her and place the heel of your hand just above the waistline. Place your other hand on top of this hand. Keeping your elbows straight, give four quick upward thrusts. You may have to repeat this procedure several times until the obstructing object is coughed out.

Airway manoeuvres

These are carried out in patients who are unconscious or require assistance in breathing. These procedures prevent the tongue from falling backwards.

- **Head tilt-chin lift:** The simplest way of ensuring an open airway in an unconscious patient is to use a head tilt-chin lift technique,

thereby lifting the tongue from the back of the throat. This can be done when cervical spine injury is not a concern.
- **Jaw thrust:** thumbs of both hands are used to push the posterior aspects of the mandible upwards which causes tongue to be pulled forwards. This procedure can be done in patients with cervical injury.
- **Oropharyngeal airway:** These are curved plastic devices that prevent the tongue falling backwards, which causes airway obstruction.

Intubation

This can be using the orotracheal or nasaotracheal route. The indications for intubation can be acute infections of the upper airway, such as epiglottis, parapharyngeal or retropharyngeal abscess, Ludwig's angina, etc. Intubation is also required when mucosal oedema of the upper airway, as in inhalational injuries and angioneurotic oedema, leads to obstruction. Another indication for intubation is a fall in consciousness level due to increasing respiratory failure.

Nebulization

This is an effective technique to reduce the oedema of inflamed mucosa in the upper airway. The various drugs used for this purpose include racemic a and corticosteroids.

Cricothyroidotomy

This is done as an emergency procedure. An opening is created in the cricothyroid membrane which is superficial and an airway is introduced into the trachea to maintain oxygen saturation. It is fast, requiring less than 30 seconds, and can be done under any clinical setting. Its utility is restricted by the fact that prolonged use of a cricothyroidotomy can lead to subglottic stenosis. In addition it may not be possible to get a wide enough bore airway for even short-term use.

Tracheostomy

This procedure requires expertise. Emergency tracheostomy is rarely performed nowadays for upper airway obstruction. It can be considered in cases of laryngeal trauma where intubation may aggravate the pre-existing mucosal injury.[9] In cases of tumours obstructing the airway above the cricoid, tracheostomy can be performed in an emergency under local anaesthesia if the patient is severely compromised and intubation is not possible due to the bulk of tumour. Alternatively, it is performed to provide anaesthesia to facilitate definitive surgery for the lesion. In laryngectomy permanent tracheostomy is part of the procedure itself, whereas in some cases pre-emptive tracheostomy is done in view of impending airway obstruction such as excision of lesions from base of tongue or partial laryngectomies.

Further reading

Pracy P. Upper airway obstruction. In: Gleeson M, Browning GG, Martin JM *et al.* (eds) *Scott-Brown's Otorhinolaryngology Head and Neck Surgery,* 7th edition. London: Hodder Arnold, 2008.

Pracy P. Tracheostomy In: Gleeson M, Browning GG, Martin JM *et al.* (eds) *Scott-Brown's Otorhinolaryngology Head and Neck Surgery,* 7th edition. London: Hodder Arnold, 2008.

Pitkin L. Laryngeal trauma and stenosis. In: Gleeson M, Browning GG, Martin JM *et al.* (eds) *Scott-Brown's Otorhinolaryngology Head and Neck Surgery,* 7th edition. London: Hodder Arnold, 2008.

Swift A. Acute infections of the larynx. In: Gleeson M, Browning GG,
Martin JM *et al.* (eds) *Scott-Brown's Otorhinolaryngology Head and
Neck Surgery*, 7th edition. London: Hodder Arnold, 2008.

References

1. Jaiganesh T, Wiese M, Hollingsworth J, *et al*. Acute angioedema: recognition and management in the emergency department. *Eur J Emerg
Med* 2013; 20(1): 10–7.
2. Kotecha B. The nose, snoring and obstructive sleep apnoea. *Rhinology*
2011; 49(3): 259–63.
3. Dobbie AM, White DR. Laryngomalacia. *Pediatr Clin North Am* 2013;
60(4): 893–902.
4. Patino M, Sadhasivam S, Mahmoud M. Obstructive sleep apnoea in children: perioperative considerations. *Br J Anaesth* 2013; 111(Suppl 1): i83–95.
5. Pfleger A, Eber E. Management of acute severe upper airway obstruction in children. *Paediatr Respir Rev* 2013; 14(2): 70–7.
6. Leboulanger N, Garabedian EN. Airway management in pediatric head
and neck infections. *Infect Disord Drug Targets* 2012; 12(4): 256–60.
7. Foltran F, Ballali S, Rodriguez H, *et al*. Inhaled foreign bodies in
children: a global perspective on their epidemiological, clinical, and
preventive aspects. *Pediatr Pulmonol* 2013; 48(4): 344–51.
8. Moraa I, Sturman N, McGuire T, *et al*. Heliox for croup in children.
Cochrane Database Syst Rev 2013; 12: CD006822.
9. Byard RW, Gilbert JD. Potentially lethal complications of tracheostomy: autopsy considerations. *Am J Forensic Med Pathol* 2011; 32(4): 352–4.

CHAPTER 2.12.3

Ear pain and hearing loss

Maurice Hawthorne

Ear pain

Pain from the external ear

Most causes of pain in the external ear are obvious, such as acute otitis externa, trauma from a cut or a scald, a squamous cell carcinoma, or the rarer inflammatory condition of relapsing polychondritis that classically spares the ear lobe.

In addition to redness and swelling, moving the external ear exacerbates the pain and as such is a useful way of distinguishing pain from the middle ear.

In the early stages of a herpetic infection there may be little to see until vesicles appear.

Malignant otitis externa, on the other hand, usually presents in the immunosuppressed or the elderly. Initially pain with pus in the external auditory canal is the cardinal feature, which after a number of weeks progresses to the development of cranial nerve palsies, VII, IX, X, XI, and eventually XII. Bone destruction is clear on computed tomography (CT) scanning and a biopsy is required to exclude cancer.

Pain from the middle ear

Acute pain in the ear is usually accompanied by redness of the drum, a conductive hearing loss, and fluid in the middle ear. In acute infections the pain ceases when the ear drum ruptures.

Chronic pain accompanied by signs of inflammation can be due to chronic suppurative otitis media, though this condition is not characterized by severe pain, more a grumbling ache. Rarer inflammatory conditions such as Wegener's granulomatosis can present with severe relentless pain. Malignancy of the middle ear is rare and usually associated with many years of discharge and infection.

Pain from the petrous temporal bone and adjacent structures

Pain arising from the petrous temporal bone is usually a consequence of disease spreading from elsewhere or a systemic illness such as a vasculitis.

Primary tumours of the bone itself are rare, and so tumours that present with pain are nearly always secondary tumours usually of breast, prostate, and lung cancer. The more common benign tumours associated with petrous bone (e.g. paragangliomas, neuromas, schwannomas, and meningiomas) do not cause pain.

Osteitis arising from malignant otitis externa or middle ear suppuration is becoming increasingly common in the UK as the population ages.

Referred pain from elsewhere

As the ear has a complex nerve supply secondary to its embryology, referred pain to the ear is common. Characteristically there is no hearing loss and the ear examination is normal. Common 'innocent' causes include post-tonsillectomy pain, dental extraction or dental disease origin, arthritis in the upper cervical spine, temporomandibular joint syndrome, and benign ulcers of the mucosa of the oral cavity.

It is really important, however, not to miss tumours of the upper aerodigestive tract. Common examples include carcinoma of the tongue, tonsil, oropharynx, hypopharynx, larynx, and floor of mouth.

Investigation of earache

After taking a thorough history, a full ear, nose, and throat examination should take place. If the ear is normal, a fibre optic examination of the upper aerodigestive tract is mandatory. The tongue should be bimanually palpated and neck lumps searched for. The mouth should be carefully examined, paying particular attention to the back and sides of the tongue and the retromolar trigone.

In cases that do not follow the pattern of the typical upper respiratory infection, additional tests should be carried out: an erythrocyte sedimentation rate, immunoglobulin electrophoresis, and autoantibody assays (including the antinuclearcytoplasmic antibody).

Any prolonged ear discharge in which a diagnosis has not been confirmed requires a CT scan. If an occult malignancy is suspected, a magnetic resonance imaging (MRI) scan and/or a positron emission tomography (PET) scan can be of value.

Finally, in cases of intractable pain in which no diagnosis has been found after blood tests and scanning, removing the tonsil on the side of the ear pain and blind biopsies of the tongue and oropharynx should be considered, especially in those at high risk for cancer such as smokers and alcohol abusers.

Conductive hearing loss

External ear conditions

In conductive hearing loss, sound is not efficiently gaining access to the inner ear. Common conditions of the external ear that can cause this are:

- wax
- exostoses
- foreign body
- otitis externa both acute and chronic
- rare disorders are: congenital absence or stenosis of the external auditory canal, and tumours.

Middle ear disorders

Acute viral middle ear infection is by far the most common cause of mild conductive hearing loss. The eardrum can rupture if a secondary bacterial infection occurs. The usual outcome is complete resolution of the infection. In a minority of patients, a permanent perforation of the drum can occur or the infection can become chronic involving the whole middle ear cleft and eventually the bone in which the ear is housed. This is known as chronic suppurative otitis media of the tubotympanic type and once established pain is not a marked feature.

Painless chronic discharge can be due to cholesteatoma, which is basically a 'cyst'-like structure containing dead skin within the middle ear cleft. They can occur just with a conductive hearing loss and no discharge but the majority become infected. With time the disease destroys middle ear structures such as the ossicles and eventually the inner ear. They can present with a facial palsy.

Otosclerosis is an inherited disorder that usually presents with a conductive deafness and an otherwise normal ear on clinical examination. It is progressive, usually affecting both ears, and eventually will affect the cochlea causing a sensory deafness.

Endocrine disorders rarely affect the ear; however, rickets and osteomalacia may occur, usually presenting in an Asian patient with a conductive loss and tinnitus.

Inflammations such as vasculitis, Wegener's granulomatosis, and sarcoidosis all occur but are rare. Surprisingly rheumatoid arthritis does not appear to affect the synovial joints of the ossicles to any extent.

Specific infections such as tuberculosis and syphilis occur but are rare, as are tumours.

Trauma, however, is common. It can be direct (e.g. blast injury) or a penetrating wound. Changes in pressure can cause barotrauma and radiotherapy to the ear can cause an otitis.

Sensorineural hearing loss

Infections

Sudden hearing loss due to herpetic infection is quite common. Bacterial meningitis is another major cause of total loss of hearing. Other infections are rare but important to spot as they may be treatable (e.g. penicillin for tertiary syphilis).

Inflammations

The same inflammations that affect the middle ear can affect the inner ear, such as sarcoidosis and Wegner's granulomatosis.

Endocrine

Pendred's syndrome or deafness associated with an underactive thyroid in childhood can cause a severe sensorineural deafness. Diabetes mellitus does not cause deafness directly but it may be part of inherited syndromes such as DIDMOAD syndrome where it is joined by diabetes insipidus. It can cause hearing loss through the mechanism of stroke.

Vascular causes

The primary vascular cause of sensory deafness is vasculitis. Thrombosis can cause sudden deafness and is typically seen in young women on the oral contraceptive pill.

Iatrogenic

Apart from surgery, the primary cause of deafness inadvertently initiated by doctors is through ototoxic drugs (usually aminoglycosides) but occasionally through diuretics and certain chemotherapy

agents used in oncology. A common group that are vulnerable to iatrogenic damage are premature babies.

Tumours

Most tumours that cause deafness are benign with vestibular schwannoma and meningioma being the most common. Both are very slow growing and usually present with a VIII nerve isolated partial palsy.

Trauma

This is the same as for the middle ear, with the exception of barotrauma where the bends can cause sudden sensory deafness but this is rare.

An additional and important cause is noise. It is now a requirement that employers protect their staff from the effects of noise. Hearing protection should be provided where a worker is exposed to a mean noise level of 85 dB for 8 hours per day, and the wearing of protection should be enforced where the level is above 90 dB. Alternatively, prevention of hearing loss can be achieved by reducing the hours of exposure. The time of exposure should be halved for each 3 dB of additional sound pressure exposure. For example, the exposure time is 8 hours at 85 dB, 4 hours at 88 dB, and 2 hours at 91 dB.

Congenital and hereditary deafness

There are huge numbers of both congenital and hereditary forms of deafness. They can be non-syndromal or the deafness can form part of a syndrome of other congenital abnormalities that run in families. The detail of these forms of deafness is beyond the scope of this book.

Investigating hearing loss

The corner stone of investigating hearing loss is the pure tone audiogram. Inner ear function can be tested in isolation using a bone conductor. As humans have two ears it is possible for the non-test ear to be the one that is hearing the test thresholds and not the ear that the audiologist thinks they are testing. To avoid this problem, masking noise has to be played to the ear that is not being tested. The bone conduction gives the sensorineural hearing loss. However, the pure tone audiogram cannot tell whether the deafness is due to a cochlea problem (sensory) or a nerve of hearing problem (neural).

Sensory deafness is characterized by a reduction in the dynamic range of hearing. In a normal person the threshold of hearing is between 0 and 10 dB and the threshold for pain is about 90 dB to 100 dB. The difference between threshold for hearing and threshold for discomfort is known as the dynamic range. In the normal ear it is typically about 90 dB. In a sensory deafness it can be much reduced. The patient may notice that a small change in the volume of the sound now produces a marked increase in loudness compared to when they had normal hearing. This is seen in deafness of old age (presbycusis). An example of which is a nurse asking an elderly person 'Do you want a cup of tea dear,' and the elderly person saying 'Pardon, you'll have to speak up.' The nurse raises her voice slightly and the patient then says 'You don't have to shout, I'm not deaf you know!'

In neural deafness there is abnormal facilitation of sound. A normal-hearing person should be able to hear a tone at 5 dB above threshold for a minute. Those who require the test sound to be between 5 dB and 15 dB above threshold to hear the tone for a minute are borderline, and those that require it to be greater than 20 dB above threshold to hear a sound for a minute probably have a neural deafness. There are a number of tests that are based on the two phenomenon of reduced dynamic range and abnormal facilitation that can be used to differentiate between neural and sensory deafness (e.g. tone decay and loudness discomfort levels). In practical terms though, when a patient presents with asymmetric hearing these days they get an MRI scan in most Western countries.

MRI scans are useful at picking up soft tissue disease (e.g. a vestibular schwannoma) that may be causing a hearing loss. CT scans are useful for detecting bone destruction (e.g. in osteitis) or bone disease (e.g. otosclerosis).

If vasculitis is suspected then an erythrocyte sedimentation rate is a useful screening test before going on to look at autoantibodies.

If a bone disease is suspected then calcium, phosphate, and alkaline phosphatase assays should be undertaken, as well as measuring vitamin D levels. An assessment of renal function may also be required.

Treating hearing loss

Treating hearing loss is not just the provision of a hearing aid. Before prescribing a hearing aid advice should be given.

It is important to provide advice in order to avoid further loss. This could be advice on hearing protection in those that are exposed to noise. Infections can be reduced in those with otitis externa and a perforation of the eardrum can be avoided by keeping water out of the ear. Hygiene advice may be appropriate for those patients that have to wear hearing protection.

Careers advice is often essential, particularly in those of school and working age. If someone is 20 years old and has a progressive condition such as otosclerosis then working in an industry with strict hearing criteria may not be sustainable in the long term. Examples would include the armed forces, working on rail track, or in the off shore oil industry.

Middle ear effusion, which is common in childhood, can be treated surgically. Current NHS guidelines require the child to have a hearing loss in both ears present for at least 3 months. If this guideline is met then ventilation tubes can be inserted into both ears. Tubes may be also inserted to prevent recurrent earache. An exception to this guideline is children with trisomy 21 in which a hearing aid is recommended.

The effects of chronic suppurative otitis media and trauma due to blast or penetrating trauma can also be treated surgically. Myringoplasty or grafting holes in the eardrum has a success rate between 70% and 95%, with those cases due to trauma having the better results. An ossiculoplasty can be offered where there is ossicular discontinuity. If not too badly damaged, the patient's own ossicles can be used or alternatively an artificial ossicle can be used. These are usually made from hydroxylapatite or titanium. Provided the stapes superstructure is still present, success rates of 70% are common; however, the success rate drops to less than 30% when the stapes superstructure is absent.

The stapes is fixed in otosclerosis, causing a conductive loss. This can be corrected by replacing the stapes with a prosthesis. There are many different designs on the market but the Fisch 0.4 mm Teflon/steel prosthesis gives good results with a low rate of incus necrosis as a late complication.

In patients that cannot wear a conventional hearing aid and with reasonable cochlear function a bone anchored hearing aid can be used. This clips onto a permanently positioned titanium 'bolt' that is screwed into the skull.

While a vestibular schwannoma can be removed surgically, most patients opt for stereotactic radiosurgery due to its high success rate and low morbidity. The treatment does not, however, prevent further hearing loss but it does allow the patient to retain some hearing in the affected ear at least for a while.

For those patients with no hearing in both ears, and who have failed a trial of conventional hearing aids, a cochlear implant may be an option. As a general rule they are not suitable for those born profoundly deaf, with no recollection of sound, and are over 5 years of age. Children born profoundly deaf do best when implanted under the age of 2.

One group that require urgent referral to a cochlear implant team are those deafened by meningitis. Meningitis cases often have pus in the cochlear duct. This can organize and ossify, making it impossible to get an implant inserted into the cochlea.

One downside to cochlear implants is that MRI scanning is restricted. Before ordering an MRI scan in a patient with a cochlear implant the case should be discussed with radiology and the implant team. In some implants the magnet within the implant can be removed prior to scanning thus improving accuracy of diagnosis by reducing the artefact produced by the implants.

Monopolar diathermy is usually contraindicated in the presence of a cochlear implant; however, if it has to be used advice can be obtained from your local implant team on where to place the diathermy pad to minimize risk of damage to the implant. Bipolar diathermy can be used safely below the clavicles, but if it has to be used in the head advice should be obtained from your implant service.

Many patients derive considerable benefit from learning lip reading skills.

The profoundly deaf child does not have to be brought up with aids or a cochlear implant; some families may choose for their child to learn sign language. In the UK the dominant sign language is British Sign Language (BSL). Most hospitals and local authorities have access to BSL interpreters for important meetings and hospital appointments.

Environmental aids can also be very helpful to the deaf and hard of hearing. Examples are lights that flash when the doorbell is pushed or the telephone rings. Other gadgets include vibrating alarm clocks and voice apps for use with smart phones and electronic note pads such as the iPad®. A useful website is www.sarabec.com, where details on a wide range of devices for the hard of hearing and the deaf can be found.

Further reading

Araújo Eda S, Zucki F, Corteletti LC, et al. Hearing loss and acquired immune deficiency syndrome: systematic review. *J Soc Bras Fonoaudiol* 2012; 24(2): 188–92.

Awad Z, Huins C, Pothier DD. Antivirals for idiopathic sudden sensorineural hearing loss. *Cochrane Database Syst Rev* 2012; 8: CD006987.

Blaiser K. Supporting communicative development of infants and toddlers with hearing loss. *Semin Speech Lang* 2012; 33(4): 273–9.

Browning, G. Conditions of the pinna and external auditory canal. In: Gleeson M, Browning GG, Martin JM et al. (eds) *Scott-Brown's Otorhinolaryngology Head and Neck Surgery,* 7th edition. London: Hodder Arnold, 2008.

Browning, G. Conditions of the middle ear. In: Gleeson M, Browning GG, Martin JM *et al.* (eds) *Scott-Brown's Otorhinolaryngology Head and Neck Surgery,* 7th edition. London: Hodder Arnold, 2008.

Browning, G. Conditions of the cochlea. In: Gleeson M, Browning GG, Martin JM *et al.* (eds) *Scott-Brown's Otorhinolaryngology Head and Neck Surgery,* 7th edition. London: Hodder Arnold, 2008.

Browning, G. Management of hearing impairment. In: Gleeson M, Browning GG, Martin JM *et al.* (eds) *Scott-Brown's Otorhinolaryngology Head and Neck Surgery,* 7th edition. London: Hodder Arnold, 2008.

Campo P, Morata TC, Hong O. Chemical exposure and hearing loss. *Dis Mon* 2013; 59(4): 119–38.

Chau JK, Cho JJ, Fritz DK. Evidence-based practice: management of adult sensorineural hearing loss. *Otolaryngol Clin North Am* 2012; 45(5): 941–58.

Chen RC, Khorsandi AS, Shatzkes DR, *et al.* The radiology of referred otalgia. *AJNR Am J Neuroradiol* 2009; 30(10): 1817–23.

Conover K. Earache. *Emerg Med Clin North Am* 2013; 31(2): 413–42.

Dale OT, Clarke AR, Drysdale AJ. Challenges encountered in the diagnosis of tuberculous otitis media: case report and literature review. *J Laryngol Otol* 2011; 125(7): 738–40.

Deltenre P, Van Maldergem L. Hearing loss and deafness in the pediatric population: causes, diagnosis, and rehabilitation. *Handb Clin Neurol* 2013; 113: 1527–38.

Eshetu T, Aygun N. Imaging of the temporal bone: a symptom-based approach. *Semin Roentgenol* 2013; 48(1): 52–64.

Goh AY, Hussain SS. Sudden hearing loss and pregnancy: a review. *J Laryngol Otol* 2012; 126(4): 337–9.

Green K. The role of active middle-ear implants in the rehabilitation of hearing loss. *Expert Rev Med Devices* 2011; 8(4): 441–7.

Hong O, Buss J, Thomas E. Type 2 diabetes and hearing loss. *Dis Mon* 2013; 59(4):139–46.

Kari E, Friedman RA. Hearing preservation: microsurgery. *Curr Opin Otolaryngol Head Neck Surg* 2012; 20(5): 358–66.

Kuppler K, Lewis M, Evans AK. A review of unilateral hearing loss and academic performance: is it time to reassess traditional dogmata? *Int J Pediatr Otorhinolaryngol* 2013; 77(5): 617–22.

Leong SC, Youssef A, Lesser TH. Squamous cell carcinoma of the temporal bone: outcomes of radical surgery and postoperative radiotherapy. *Laryngoscope* 2013; 123(10): 2442–8.

Lustig LR, Akil O. Cochlear gene therapy. *Curr Opin Neurol* 2012; 25(1): 57–60.

Majumdar S, Wu K, Bateman ND, *et al.* Diagnosis and management of otalgia in children. *Arch Dis Child Educ Pract Ed* 2009; 94(2): 33–6.

McCormack A, Fortnum H. Why do people fitted with hearing aids not wear them? *Int J Audiol* 2013; 52(5): 360–8.

Mijovic T, Zeitouni A, Colmegna I. Autoimmune sensorineural hearing loss: the otology-rheumatology interface. *Rheumatology* 2013; 52(5): 780–9.

Neilan RE, Roland PS. Otalgia. *Med Clin North Am* 2010; 94(5): 961–71.

Rajguru R. Military aircrew and noise-induced hearing loss: prevention and management. *Aviat Space Environ Med* 2013; 84(12): 1268–76.

Rey-Dios R, Cohen-Gadol AA. Current neurosurgical management of glossopharyngeal neuralgia and technical nuances for microvascular decompression surgery. *Neurosurg Focus* 2013; 34(3): E8.

Rosenfeld RM, Schwartz SR, Cannon CR, *et al.* Clinical practice guideline: acute otitis externa. *Otolaryngol Head Neck Surg* 2014; 150(1 Suppl): S1–24. Erratum in: *Otolaryngol Head Neck Surg* 2014 Mar; 150(3): 504.

Siddiq MA, Samra MJ. Otalgia. *BMJ* 2008; 336(7638): 276–7.

Spielmann PM, Yu R, Neeff M. Skull base osteomyelitis: current microbiology and management. *J Laryngol Otol* 2013; 127(Suppl 1):S8–12.

Stew BT, Fishpool SJ, Williams H. Sudden sensorineural hearing loss. *Br J Hosp Med (Lond)* 2012; 73(2): 86–9.

Tarshish Y, Leschinski A, Kenna M. Pediatric sudden sensorineural hearing loss: diagnosed causes and response to intervention. *Int J Pediatr Otorhinolaryngol* 2013; 77(4): 553–9.

Uy J, Forciea MA. In the clinic. Hearing loss. *Ann Intern Med* 2013; 158(7): ITC4-1; quiz ITC4-16.

van As JW, van den Berg H, van Dalen EC. Medical interventions for the prevention of platinum-induced hearing loss in children with cancer. *Cochrane Database Syst Rev* 2012; 5: CD009219.

Venekamp RP, Sanders S, Glasziou PP, *et al.* Antibiotics for acute otitis media in children. *Cochrane Database Syst Rev* 2013; 1: CD000219.

Verbeek JH, Kateman E, Morata TC, *et al.* Interventions to prevent occupational noise-induced hearing loss. *Cochrane Database Syst Rev* 2012; 10: CD006396.

Vergison A, Dagan R, Arguedas A, *et al.* Otitis media and its consequences: beyond the earache. *Lancet Infect Dis* 2010; 10(3): 195–203.

Visvanathan V, Kelly G. 12 minute consultation: an evidence-based management of referred otalgia. *Clin Otolaryngol* 2010; 35(5): 409–14.

Viswanatha B. Lateral sinus thrombosis in children: a review. *Ear Nose Throat J* 2011; 90(6): E28–33.

Walling AD, Dickson GM. Hearing loss in older adults. *Am Fam Physician* 2012; 85(12): 1150–6.

Wei BP, Stathopoulos D, O'Leary S. Steroids for idiopathic sudden sensorineural hearing loss. *Cochrane Database Syst Rev* 2013; 7: CD003998.

Yoon PJ. Hearing loss and cochlear implantation in children. *Adv Pediatr* 2011; 58(1): 277–96.

Zimmerman E, Lahav A. Ototoxicity in preterm infants: effects of genetics, aminoglycosides, and loud environmental noise. *J Perinatol* 2013; 33(1): 3–8.

Neurosurgery

CHAPTER 2.13.1

Acute neurosurgical emergencies

Mark Wilson and Ian Sabin

Introduction

The Glasgow Coma Score (GCS) (Table 2.13.1.1) is commonly used in all forms of acute cranial neurosurgical emergency to assess level of consciousness.

Cranial trauma

Traumatic Brain Injury (TBI) is the world's leading cause of morbidity and mortality in individuals under the age of 45. The UK incidence of head injury is estimated to be 400 per 100 000/year (approximately 1.4 million/year). Of these, approximately 10% are classified as moderate or severe.

Classification and grading of brain injury

Primary/secondary injury

Primary injury is the damage done at the moment of impact. Secondary injury refers to all the injuries that evolve as a result of the primary injury, for example, hypoxia from the loss of airway, poor perfusion from hypotension, or continuing blood clot expansion and seizures. The clinician's job is to minimize these secondary injuries. The aim of TBI treatment should be that if the primary injury has not killed you, you should not die.

Brain injury severity

GCS is the scale adopted worldwide for monitoring conscious level in brain-injured patients. The initial GCS has been used as a tool to classify brain injury severity (mild = GCS 13–15, moderate = GCS 9–12, and severe = GCS <8). Approximately 30% of patients admitted to hospital with a GCS of <13 will die. If GCS is less than 8 this increases to 50%. However, while GCS may correlate with outcome in studies of large numbers of people, on an individual level it can be misleading. A head injury patient who is simply post-ictal (GCS 3) may have a normal brain on scan and return to normality. An expanding extra-dural haematoma can present very well (GCS 15) and yet cause death.

Basic pathophysiology

Table 2.13.1.2 outlines mechanisms of injury, pathology, and treatment for different forms of brain injury.

Basic principles of intracranial pressure

The skull is a 'closed box' and, since its volume is constant, if a substance (e.g., blood, swelling, and/or tumour) is added, another component must be displaced for pressure to remain constant. The accumulation of a haematoma results in ventricular effacement and displacement of cerebrospinal fluid (CSF) down the vertebral canal. Further accumulation results in additional displacement and possibly some displacement of venous blood. When

Table 2.13.1.1 Glasgow Coma Score and a paediatric version of verbal response for the under 5s

Eye opening (E)	
Spontaneous	4
To voice	3
To pain	2
None	1
Verbal response (V)	
Orientated	5
Confused conversation	4
Inappropriate words	3
Incomprehensible sounds	2
None	1
Motor response (M)	
Obeys commands (normal movement in children)	6
Localises pain	5
Normal flexion (withdrawal)	4
Abnormal flexion (decortiate)	3
Extension (decerebrate)	2
None (flaccid)	1
Paediatric verbal response (V)	
Best response for age (as before injury)	5
Confused or spontaneous irritable cries	4
Cries to pain	3
Moans to pain	2
None	1

Reproduced with permission from the British Paediatric Neurology Association (BPNA), *Child's Glasgow Coma Scale*, http://www.bpna.org.uk/audit/GCS.PDF. Adapted by permission from BMJ Publishing Group Limited: REFO:JARTA Tatman *et al.*, Development of a modified paediatric coma scale in intensive care clinical practice, *Archives of Disease in Childhood*, Volume 77, Issue 6, pp. 519–521, Copyright © 1997 BMJ Publishing Group Ltd & Royal College of Paediatrics and Child Health; and adapted from *The Lancet*, Volume 304, No. 7872, G Teasdale and B Jennett, Assessment of Coma and Impaired Consciousness, pp. 81–84, Copyright © 1974, with permission from Elsevier, http://www.sciencedirect.com/science/article/pii/S0140673614622595.

this buffering capacity reaches its limit, the system decompensates (Figure 2.13.1.1) with a sudden and rapid rise in intracranial pressure (ICP). When pressure rises, brain shifts occur (Figure 2.13.1.2).

The main principals of TBI management are to keep ICP normal or low.

Basic principles of cerebral perfusion pressure

Under normal circumstances, cerebral blood flow is autoregulated, however in head injury this autoregulation can be lost. Cerebral

Table 2.13.1.2 Different forms of brain injury

Diagnosis	Classic mechanism of injury	Pathology	Treatment	CT/MRI image
Extradural	Blow with hammer/bat to temporal region	Skull fracture ruptures branch of middle meningeal artery	If >30 cm^3 or >5 mm MLS craniotomy[a] If less and GCS 15, consider observation and serial CT	
Acute Subdural	Sudden deceleration/ rotation/shearing e.g. motorcyclist vs. road	Ruptured vein connecting brain and sagittal sinus	If >10 mm thick or causing >5 mm MLS, should be removed by craniotomy whatever GCS[a]	
Chronic Subdural	Elderly/Alcoholic minor head injury. Often on aspirin	Ruptured vein connecting brain and sagittal sinus	If neurologically compromised, burr hole drainage	
Contusion	Deceleration/energy transfer. Can be coup/contre-coup	Common in anterior/middle fossa with rough inner skull table. Evolve over time	ICP monitor. If ICP refractory, may benefit from decompression	

(continued)

Table 2.13.1.2 (Continued)

Diagnosis	Classic mechanism of injury	Pathology	Treatment	CT/MRI image
Intracerebral Haematoma	Direct blow or coalescence of contusion	Often the coalescence of a contusion	If >20 cm³ or progressive deterioration, operative treatment indicated[a]	
Traumatic Subarachnoid Blood	Sudden declaration causing small vessel rupture	Rupture of small vessel → blood tracks through subarachnoid space	Observe for hydrocephalus and EVD if required.	
Diffuse Axonal Injury	Shearing/sudden deceleration e.g. fall from motorbike/ horse	Shearing of grey and white matter → direct neuronal disruption (axonal retraction balls)	ICP Monitor. Optimal medical care. Can result in spectrum from normal outcome to persistent vegetative state	
Depressed skull fracture	Direct blow e.g. with hammer	Fracture of underlying skull	Elevate if > thickness of skull	

(continued)

Table 2.13.1.2 (Continued)

Diagnosis	Classic mechanism of injury	Pathology	Treatment	CT/MRI image
Base of Skull Fracture	Significant head injury (e.g. fall from height)	Fracture usually through middle fossa	Usually conservatively managed. Check facial nerve and hearing	

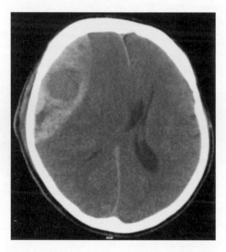

[a] Brief summary based on guidance from the Brain Trauma Foundation can be found online.[1]

CT, computed tomography; GCS, Glasgow Coma Scale; ICP, intracranial pressure; MLS, midline shift; MRI, magnetic resonance imaging.

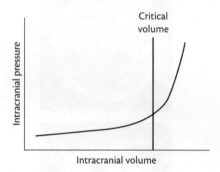

Fig. 2.13.1.1 The Monro-Kellie Doctrine: a graph of volume of additional mass and intracranial pressure.
Adapted from Volume Pressure Curve, *Advanced Trauma Life Support Student Course Manual, Ninth Edition*, American College of Surgeons, Chicago, USA, Copyright © 2012 American College of Surgeons.

perfusion pressure (CPP) is a calculated value—a balance of systemic blood pressure and intracranial pressure:

$$CPP = MAP - ICP$$

where MAP is mean arterial pressure.

The optimal CPP is unknown and probably varies for each of the pathologies listed in Table 2.13.1.2. The Lund concept aims to keep physiological variables normal. Previously there has been a vogue for increasing CPP to maintain perfusion to the penumbra of the injured area. However, maintaining CPP by lowering ICP as much as possible is probably the best technique.

Pre-hospital and emergency care

The optimal management of brain injury in the first hour is critical to minimizing secondary brain injury. Hypoxia and hypotension in this early phase are associated with a significant increase in morbidity and mortality.[2] Dispatching the correct resources, early

Fig. 2.13.1.2 Brain shifts resulting from accumulating intracranial mass. Lateral tentorial herniation causes the medial temporal lobe to compress the occulomotor nerve, the outer parasympathetic fibres of which therefore no longer cause pupil constriction, which results in unopposed sympathetic pupillary dilatation.
Reprinted from Kenneth W. Lindsay, Ian Bone, and Geraint Fuller, *Neurology and Neurosurgery Illustrated, Fifth Edition*, Churchill Livingston, Copyright © 2010 Elsevier Ltd., with permission from Elsevier.

establishment of head injury, and optimal management are vital. In advanced systems securing of the airway with endotracheal intubation often allows for more rapid transfer and computed tomography (CT) scanning as well as protecting the patient's lungs during transfer.[3] Once in the emergency department, continued resuscitation and early CT scan (within 30 minutes) should occur. If there is pupil dilatation, hypertonic saline or mannitol can be used. To date, no neuroprotective pharmacological intervention has been found to be of benefit; however, it is within the timeframe of minutes that such an intervention, if successful, would be required.

Intensive care management

Intensive care management comprises optimization of physiology to aid brain recovery. The following techniques can lower ICP:

- loosen cervical collar (optimal head position)
- head up 30 degrees
- full paralysis and sedation
- normal end tidal CO_2 ($EtCO_2$)
- optimal ventilation (minimal positive end expiratory pressure)
- osmotic diuretics (hypertonic saline/mannitol)
- cooling
- external ventricular drain (EVD) insertion
- craniectomy.

Other considerations

Seizure prevention should be instigated when there is a significant risk, for example with a depressed skull fracture breaching the dura, temporal/frontal haematoma, foreign body parenchymal irritation, and when a seizure has already occurred. There is no evidence of benefit of levetiracetam over phenytoin, hence the latter is usually the first choice. There is also no evidence of longer-term seizure risk reduction hence prophylaxis is usually only given for the first 10 days after injury.

Neurosurgical management

Intracranial pressure monitoring

The benefit of ICP monitoring over serial CT scanning has recently been brought into question.[4] However, ICP monitoring should alert clinicians to a developing intracranial pathology prior to the very late sign of pupil dilatation. There are a number of ICP monitor types, the gold standard being an EVD. The most common is an intraparenchymal monitor, which is usually placed on the non-dominant (usually right) coronal suture.

External ventricular drain placement

An EVD is a tube placed within the lateral ventricle to monitor ICP and allow drainage of CSF to lower ICP.

Burr holes

Burr hole placement is an emergency technique to relieve the pressure of an extra-axial haematoma. Using a perforator drill bit minimizes the risk of plunging that can occur with a traditional Hudson-Brace. While a burr hole may buy time in the management of an extradural haematoma, by itself it is unlikely to be adequate and progression to a formal craniotomy is almost always required. Figure 2.13.1.3 demonstrates the appropriate location of burr hole placement for immediate relief of an extradural haematoma.[5]

Craniotomy for mass lesions

To evacuate an extra-axial haematoma, an opening over the haematoma is required (craniotomy). An extradural haematoma should be washed off and any continued bleeding stopped. If subdural, the dura is incised and the haematoma removed.

If there is minimal parenchymal brain injury and the brain is sunken, it is safe to close the dura and replace the bone, holding it with screws/plates. If, however, if the brain swells, then it is safer

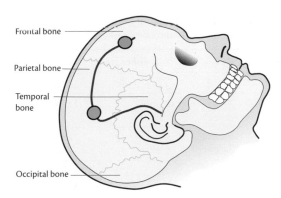

Fig. 2.13.1.3 Diagram of where to place burr holes for urgent relief of corresponding extradural haemorrhage. Three such holes can be joined together to create a trauma craniotomy.
Adapted with permission from Matthew D. Gardiner et al (Eds.), *Training in Surgery: The essential curriculum for the MRCS*, Figure 10.5, p. 263, Oxford University Press, Oxford, UKREFO:BK, Copyright © 2009, by permission of Oxford University Press.

to leave the bone out and close the dura and skin. The bone can be replaced once the swelling has receded.

Decompressive craniectomy for refractory intracranial pressure

The role of surgical decompression (e.g. bifrontal decompression) to relieve ICP is currently under investigation.[6] A recent study demonstrated that although it was an effective tool for reducing ICP, it did not improve outcome.[7]

Elevation of depressed skull fractures

Depressed skull fractures that are either compound or depressed greater than the thickness of the skull should be considered for operative treatment. Such wounds need to be cleaned. If there is no cosmetic concern or if the fracture is over the sagittal or transverse sinus (which would carry considerable operative risk) then conservative treatment should be considered.

Rehabilitation

Optimal TBI management requires early diagnosis and treatment. Early and high quality cognitive and physical rehabilitation is vital to obtain the best results.[8]

Vascular

Subarachnoid haemorrhage

Subarachnoid haemorrhage (SAH) accounts for 3% of all strokes affecting approximately 10.5/100 000 people/year. The weighted average case fatality is 51% with a 30-day mortality of 45%. Approximately one-third of survivors remain dependent.

Grading of subarachnoid haemorrhage

The World Federation of Neurological Surgeons grading system uses initial GCS as its grading system. Fisher established a grading system based on blood load on CT (Table 2.13.1.3).

Pathogenesis

Eighty-five per cent of SAHs are from saccular aneurysms. Other causes include perimesencephalic bleeds, trauma, arterial dissection, arteriovenous malformations, spinal vascular lesions, infective aneurysms, pituitary apoplexy, and cocaine use.

Table 2.13.1.3 World Federation of Neurological Surgeons (WFNS) grading system for subarachnoid haemorrhage

WFNS grade	GCS	Fisher grade	Blood on CT
I	15	0	Unruptured aneurysm
II	13–14 (no focal deficit)	1	No subarachnoid blood
III	13–14 (with focal deficit)	2	Diffuse or vertical layers <1 mm thick
IV	7–12	3	Localised clot and/or vertical layers >1 mm thick
V	3–6	4	Intracerebral or intraventricular clot

CT, computed tomography; GCS, Glasgow Coma Scale.

Adapted from Drake CG et al., Report of World Federation of Neurological Surgeons Committee on a Universal Subarachnoid Hemorrhage Grading Scale, *Journal of Neurosurgery*, Volume 68, Number 6, pp. 985–6, Copyright © 1998 American Association of Neurological Surgeons; and adapted from Fisher C et al., Relation of cerebral vasospasm to subarachnoid hemorrhage visualized by computerized tomographic scanning, *Neurosurgery*, Volume 6, Issue 1, pp. 1–9, Copyright © 1980 by the Congress of Neurological Surgeons, by permission of Lippincott, Williams, and Wilkinson.

Diagnosis

The clinical hallmark of SAH is a sudden onset severe headache. Approximately half have a period of unresponsiveness and 70% vomit. If the history suggests SAH, then a CT scan should be followed by a lumbar puncture (if CT negative).

- *CT Scan:* At best, a CT scan performed with <3 mm cuts within 12 hours of ictus has a 98% sensitivity. A CT angiogram will demonstrate 90–95% of aneurysms greater than 2 mm in diameter.

- *Lumbar puncture:* A lumbar puncture should be performed if CT is not possible or if it is negative with a convincing history. It is recommended not to perform this before 12 hours after ictus. Oxyhaemoglobin appears in CSF 4 to 10 hours after ictus and Bilirubin after 10 hours.

- *Digital subtraction angiography* is still considered the 'gold standard' in aneurysm investigations. This delineates the neck of aneurysm and assesses the local perforating vessels and collateral circulation.

Management

The immediate management of SAH is that of resuscitation if required followed by the investigations outlined above. The main risks to the patient are rebleeding, vasospasm, hydrocephalus and electrolyte disturbance and these should be treated appropriately.

Rebleeding

The risks of rebleeding are 12% at 1 week, rising to 20% at 2 weeks and 50% at 1 month. Because of this, 'securing' of the aneurysm is a priority, using either a coiling (radiology) or clipping (surgery) technique.[9,10]

Vasospasm

Vasospasm risk peaks between the first and second week after ictus. Although common on angiography, clinically relevant vasospasm only occurs in 20–30% of patients. Techniques to prevent it include

keeping the patient well filled and the use of nimodipine. If symptomatic, it can result in infarction hence 'Triple-H' treatment should be commenced:

- hypertension (in secured aneurysms, systolic BP of 200–220 mmHg, in unsecured, 140–160 mmHg)

- hypervolaemia with colloid

- haemodilution (target haematocrit of ~30–35%).

If still problematic then endovascular mechanical (balloon) or chemical (intra-arterial nicardipine/verapamil/nimodipine) can be given.

Hydrocephalus

Hydrocephalus affects ~25% of SAH patients and can be acute or delayed. If there is neurological deterioration, CSF diversion should be considered. Lumbar puncture can drain CSF if the fourth ventricle is patent. EVD allows monitoring of CSF drainage. If the patient continues to require CSF diversion, then a ventriculo-peritoneal shunt may be required.

Electrolyte disturbance

SAH patients commonly develop intravascular volume depletion. Hyponatreamia occurs in 30–45% and hypernatreamia in 20% of patients. Such disturbances can increase risks of vasospasm and cause neurological disturbance.

Intracerebral haemorrhage

Spontaneous intracerebral haemorrhage (ICH) affects 10–20/100 000 people per year and accounts for ~10–15% of all strokes. Common causes include: hypertension, vascular lesions (e.g. aneurysms, arteriovenous malformations, and cavernous malformations), coagulation disorders, haemorrhagic transformation of ischaemic stroke, brain tumours, vasculitidies, amyloid angiopathy, and substance abuse.

There is a very poor prognosis if the ICH volume is >60 mL (<90% survive 30 days), if GCS <9, or there is intraventricular blood.

Management

This depends on the underlying cause. Reversal of coagulopathy and blood pressure management are important parts of optimal medical management. Superficial haematomas >2 cm in size may be best managed surgically.[11]

The posterior fossa has less volume to accommodate ICH and can result in rapid brainstem compression or hydrocephalus. If there is obliteration of the fourth ventricle on CT, then early evacuation is recommended. If the fourth is partially patent, then observation and/or EVD insertion (to treat hydrocephalus) are reasonable.[12]

Infarction

Huge progress has been made in the early management of cerebral infarction with early thrombolysis. Neurosurgical involvement occurs either when this results in haemorrhagic change or when infarction leads to severe life threatening swelling. Both survival and modified Rankin scale functional outcome (a scale from 0 = no disability, through to 5 = severe disability, bed bound, nursing home, and 6 = dead) are improved with early (<48 hours) decompression.[13]

The surgical technique for acute decompression is similar to that described for the trauma craniotomy above. Since the main purpose of this technique is pressure relief, creating a large (>12 cm) craniotomy is essential.

Acute hydrocephalus

In this context, hydrocephalus refers to a failure of normal CSF circulation resulting in a rise of ICP.

Classification

Hydrocephalus is classified as:

• Obstructive (non-communicating) where CSF pathways are clearly obstructed. Causes vary with the location of obstruction; however, common causes in adults include colloid cysts, post-haemorrhagic (acutely post SAH) or post-infective (fibrosis), and obstruction due to tumours.

• Non-obstructive (communicating) where CSF reabsorption mechanisms (arachnoid granulations) are not functioning. Post-haemorrhagic (more prolonged after SAH) and post-ventriculitis (especially tuberculosis) are common causes. It can also sometimes follow trauma.

Rare and childhood causes of hydrocephalus are not discussed here.

Diagnosis

Diagnosis is usually made on CT scan where temporal horn dilatation is an early feature. If hydrocephalus has occurred over a period of weeks, papilloedema may be a demonstrable sign.

Treatment

The mainstay treatments involve CSF diversion although conservative treatment can be considered in minimally symptomatic patients where reversal is likely (e.g. post SAH).

• *Lumbar puncture* can be used as a temporizing measure in communicating hydrocephalus. It should not be used if the fourth ventricle is obstructed/obliterated as it risks creating a differential pressure between the supratentorial and spinal compartments, which could contribute to coning.

• *EVD insertion:* In the acute setting, rapid relief of hydrocephalus can be achieved through EVD insertion. While it is simple and allows continued drainage, prolonged EVD placement has considerable risk of ventriculitis hence 'internalization' as a shunt should be achieved as soon as possible.

• *Shunt insertion:* Shunting CSF from the ventricles to the peritoneum (VP) (or rarely to the pleura or right atrium) is the standard treatment. The proximal catheter is placed in the lateral ventricle (frontal or occipital horn). This is connected to a reservoir and a valve and sometimes an anti-siphon device. It is tunnelled and 'buried' within the peritoneum.

• *Endoscopic third ventriculostomy:* Suitable for treating obstructive hydrocephalus (aqueduct stenosis or tumours obstructing the third or fourth ventricles) and involves perforating the third ventricular floor.

Infection

The most common need for neurosurgical intervention in infection is to diagnose and reduce the volume of an abscess or empyema.

Other infective problems include mycotic aneurysms, sinus thrombosis, encephalitis, and ventriculitis. In Western medicine these rarely require a neurosurgeon; infection carries a much greater disease burden in South America and Africa. Cysticercosis is endemic in some areas with 50 million people being affected worldwide. Central nervous system infection occurs in 50–90% of these. Although the mainstay of treatment is albendazole, treatment for resulting hydrocephalus and/or cyst removal is sometimes required. There are 7-8 million new cases of tuberculosis worldwide each year. In the immunocompromised, toxoplasmosis and fungal infections commonly occur.

Bacterial abscess

The incidence of brain abscess is approximately 4 per million per year.

Pathogenesis

They arise either due to *direct spread* from the frontal sinus, dental infections, middle ear or mastoid air cells, or *haematogenous spread* from chest and urinary tract infections and bacterial endocarditis. Penetrating trauma can also result in abscess formation.

The stages of abscess formation include early (3 to 5 days) then late cerebritis (5 days to 2 weeks), and early (2 to 4 weeks) then late abscess (>4 weeks) formation when a collagenous wall and necrotic centre occurs.

Diagnosis

The classical triad of headache, fever, and focal neurology occurs in less than 50% of patients. The diagnosis is usually suspected from CT scan with enhancement occurring in the capsule. To distinguish it from other ring enhancing lesions, a diffusion-weighted MRI or magnetic resonance spectroscopy sequence can be performed.

Treatment

Although small areas of cerebritis can be treated with targeted antibiotic therapy, once the wall of an abscess has formed, surgical drainage is the usual treatment. If oedema and mass effect are causing immediate compromise, dexamethasone may be given to buy a few hours prior to surgery.

Subdural empyema

The most common causes are through direct spread following rhinogenic or otogenic infection. Occasionally it can occur following meningitis or direct trauma. The diagnosis is usually on CT scan, with enhancement if contrast is given. A common organism is *Streptococcus milleri*. Treatment is surgical (craniotomy/craniectomy) and prolonged antibiotics.

Acute spinal emergencies

Spinal cord trauma

The incidence of spinal cord injury is around 15–40 per million per year. Approximately half are quadriplegic and half paraplegic, with equal numbers being complete and incomplete. Road traffic accidents are the most common cause in most countries.

Basic pathophysiology

Mechanisms of spinal cord injury include direct pressure from fractures/dislocations, vascular compromise (e.g. from anterior

Table 2.13.1.4 Grade of spinal injury

Grade	Complete?	Definition
A	Complete	No sensory or motor function is preserved in the sacral segments S4–5
B	Sensory incomplete	Sensory but not motor function is preserved below the neurological level and includes the sacral segments S4–5 (light touch or pin prick at S4–5 or deep anal pressure) AND no motor function is preserved more than three levels below the motor level on either side of the body
C	Motor incomplete	Motor function is preserved at the most caudal sacral segments for voluntary anal contraction OR the patient meets the criteria for sensory incomplete status (sensory function preserved at the most caudal sacral segments [S4–5] by LT, PP or DAP), and has some sparing of motor function more than three levels below the ipsilateral motor level on either side of the body. (This includes key or non-key muscle functions to determine motor incomplete status.) For AIS grade C, less than half of key muscle functions below the single NLI have a muscle grade ≥3
D	Motor incomplete	Motor incomplete status as defined above, with at least half (half or more) of key muscle functions below the single NLI having a muscle grade ≥3
E	Normal	If sensation and motor function as tested with the ISNCSCI are graded as normal in all segments, and the patient had prior deficits, then the AIS grade is E. Someone without an initial SCI does not receive an AIS grade
	Using ND	To document the sensory, motor and NLI levels, the ASIA Impairment Scale grade, and/or the zone of partial preservation when they are unable to be determined based on the examination results

AIS C, ASIA Impairment Scale; DAP, Deep Anal Pressure; ISNCSCI, International Standards for Neurological Classification of Spinal Cord Injury; LT, Light Touch; ND, Not demonstrable (in their latest version this is NT Not Testable); NLI, Neurological Level of Injury; PP, Pin Prick; SCI, spinal cord injury.

Adapted with permission from *International Standards for Neurological Classification of Spinal Cord Injury (ISNCSCI)*, American Spinal Injury Association, Copyright © 2015 American Spinal Injury Association, available from http://www.asia-spinalinjury.org/elearning/ASIA_ISCOS_high.pdf

spinal artery injury), and actual axonal transection from penetrating injuries. The principles of management are the prevention of further injury (immobilization), maintenance of cord perfusion, decompression if incomplete, and immobilization/fixation of instability.

Spinal shock is the transient period of areflexia, flaccid paralysis, and sensory loss due to spinal cord 'shutdown' following injury. It usually lasts <24 hours, but may make it difficult to assess 'completeness'.

Neurogenic shock is the immediate loss of sympathetic tone that occurs after spinal cord injury resulting in hypotension and sometimes bradycardia.

Assessment

Injuries above C3 can result in loss of diaphragmatic innervation (C3,4,5) and hypoxia rapidly follows. Cervical and thoracic injuries can cause significant sympathetic disruption resulting in hypotension. If above T6, a compensatory tachycardia cannot be mounted hence hypotension with bradycardia should trigger thoughts of a spinal cord cause of shock. Priaprism is also common in complete injuries.

Assessment and treatment should occur concurrently. An American Spinal Injury Association (ASIA) chart should be completed at the earliest opportunity to document the level and completeness of the injury and to monitor for any progression (Table 2.13.1.4).

Immediate management

This involves immobilization (collar, blocks, tape) on a scoop stretcher, spinal board or trauma mattress, oxygen and the maintenance of cord perfusion by maintaining blood pressure (MAP ~ 85 mmHg) with intravenous crystalloid or inotropes (dopamine 2.5–20 mcg/kg/min or dobutamine 2.0–20 mcg/kg/min). If profound bradycardia exists, atropine should be considered.

Imaging

Although plain films can confirm spinal fractures in the majority of cases, CT and reconstruction of images to provide axial, sagittal, and coronal views has greater sensitivity and is more useful in understanding the injury and operative planning. MRI allows visualization of any cord impingement (e.g. from disc herniation), haematoma or ligamentous injury and should be obtained if the patient has neurological compromise, although this should not delay surgery.

Non-operative management

A cervical collar is required for cervical fractures that are relatively stable or in patients (e.g. the elderly) who will not tolerate surgery or a halo brace. For unstable cervical fractures where surgical treatment is not appropriate, halo application can be used. This comprises pins fixed to a frame that connects to a chest jacket. Traction for displaced fractures or facet joint dislocation can also be used. The Gardner-Wells tongs and a pulley technique uses graded additional weights with serial X-rays. Usually between 5–10 lb per vertebral level is used as the starting traction load, increasing to aim to reduce the fracture within 4 hours. If this measures two-thirds of the patient's body weight or new neurological symptoms develop, no further weight should be added.

There have been a number of studies that have prospectively investigated methylprednisolone in spinal injuries (NASCIS trials I, II, and III). Currently there is no evidence to support its use.

Operative management

The two main objectives of surgical management are decompression and fixation. There are many types of both anterior and posterior fixation that cannot be covered in this text and the timing of spinal decompression has been controversial. There is increasing evidence that early decompression (<24 hours) is both safe and associated with a significantly better neurological outcome at 6 months.

Cauda equina syndrome

Cauda equina syndrome usually occurs when a lumbar disc herniates resulting in significant thecal sac compression to cause bladder or bowel dysfunction. Urgent MRI and surgery are indicated.

Acute metastatic spinal cord compression

Acute metastatic spinal cord compression pathways now exist and urgent evaluation for surgery to preserve neurological function should occur.[14]

Further reading

Brain Trauma Foundation Guidelines Available online: https://www.brain-trauma.org/uploads/06/06/Guidelines_Management_2007w_book-marks_2.pdf (accessed 21 April 2016).

Fehlings MG, Vaccaro A, Wilson JR, *et al.* Early versus delayed decompression for traumatic cervical spinal cord injury: results of the Surgical Timing in Acute Spinal Cord Injury Study (STASCIS). *PloS One* 2012; 7(2): p.e32037.

Samandouras G. *The Neurosurgeon's Handbook.* Oxford: Oxford University Press, 2010.

Smith J, Greaves I, Porter K. *Oxford Desk Reference: Major Trauma.* Oxford: Oxford University Press, 2010.

References

1. Bullock MR, *et al.* Introduction. *Neurosurgery* 2006; 58(Suppl 2): 1–3.
2. Chesnut RMR, Marshall LF, Klauber MR, *et al.* The role of secondary brain injury in determining outcome from severe head injury. *J Trauma* 1993; 34(2): 216–22.
3. Bernard SA, Nguyen V, Cameron P, *et al.* Prehospital rapid sequence intubation improves functional outcome for patients with severe traumatic brain injury: a randomized controlled trial. *Ann Surg* 2010; 252(6): 959–65.
4. Chesnut RM, Temkin N, Carney N, *et al.* A trial of intracranial-pressure monitoring in traumatic brain injury. *N Engl J Med* 2012; 367(26): 2471–81.
5. Wilson MH, Wise D, Davies G, Lockey D. *et al* Emergency burr holes: 'How to do it'.*Scand J Trauma Resusc Emerg Med* 2012; 20: 24.
6. Hutchinson PJ, Kirkpatrick PJ, RESCUEicp Central Study Team. Craniectomy in diffuse traumatic brain injury. *New Engl J Med* 2011; 365: 375; author reply 376.
7. Cooper DJ, Rosenfeld JV, Murray L, *et al.*, 2011. Decompressive craniectomy in diffuse traumatic brain injury. *New Engl J Med* 2011; 364(16): 1493–502.
8. Thornhill SS, Teasdale GM, Murray GD, *et al.* Disability in young people and adults one year after head injury: prospective cohort study. *BMJ*, 2000; 320(7250): 1631–5.
9. Molyneux A, Kerr R, Stratton I, *et al.* International Subarachnoid Aneurysm Trial (ISAT) of neurosurgical clipping versus endovascular coiling in 2143 patients with ruptured intracranial aneurysms: a randomised trial. *Lancet* 2002; 360(9342): 1267–74.
10. Molyneux AJ, Kerr RS, Yu LM, *et al.* International subarachnoid aneurysm trial (ISAT) of neurosurgical clipping versus endovascular coiling in 2143 patients with ruptured intracranial aneurysms: a randomised comparison of effects on survival, dependency, seizures, rebleeding, subgroups, and aneurysm occlusion. *Lancet* 2005; 366(9488): 809–17.
11. Mendelow AD, Gregson BA, Fernandes HM, *et al.* Early surgery versus initial conservative treatment in patients with spontaneous supratentorial intracerebral haematomas in the International Surgical Trial in Intracerebral Haemorrhage (STICH): a randomised trial. *Lancet* 2005; 365(9457): 387–97.
12. Kirollos RW, Tyagi AK, Ross SA, *et al.* Management of spontaneous cerebellar hematomas: a prospective treatment protocol. *Neurosurgery* 2001; 49(6): 1378–86; discussion 1386–7.
13. Vahedi K, Hofmeijer J, Juettler E, *et al.* Early decompressive surgery in malignant infarction of the middle cerebral artery: a pooled analysis of three randomised controlled trials. *Lancet Neurol* 2007; 6(3): 215–22.
14. Patchell RA, Tibbs PA, Regine WF, *et al.* Direct decompressive surgical resection in the treatment of spinal cord compression caused by metastatic cancer: a randomised trial. *Lancet* 2005; 366(9486): 643–8.

CHAPTER 2.13.2

Neuro-oncology

Ian Sabin

Incidence

In 2010, 9156 new central nervous system tumours were registered in the UK (Office for National Statistics). This figure does not include metastases, which are much more common than primary tumours.

Their incidence has increased over the past three decades, which may be a genuine rise but may also be due to the increasing availability and quality of scanning and possibly also to changes in coding.

Of the tumours diagnosed in 2010, 54% were malignant and 46% benign. The definition of benign relates to histological appearances, but the behaviour of a 'benign' tumour may still lead to death. In the UK in 2011 there were 311 deaths from 'benign neoplasms of the meninges'.

For the Membership of the Royal College of Surgeons examination, a detailed knowledge of neuro-oncology is not required. The principles behind the mechanisms leading to presenting symptoms, basic patient examination, and appropriate investigations should, however, be understood.

Presentation

The presence of a growing mass within the cranium or spine may present in a limited number of ways:

- Generalized intracranial mass effect: headache, problems with memory/concentration, altered level of consciousness.

- Cerebral irritation: epileptic seizures.

- Hydrocephalus secondary to ventricular obstruction (non-communicating) or to diffuse carcinomatous meningitis (communicating): failure of memory/concentration, ataxia, visual obscurations, headache, incontinence and a depressed level of consciousness.

- Neurological deficit dependent on the location of the mass: hemiparesis, cranial nerve deficits, dysphasia, visual field deficits, personality change, quadriparesis, paraparesis, cauda equina syndrome.

Diagnosis

The history and examination will direct subsequent investigations, but these will normally include magnetic resonance imaging (MRI) and/or computed tomography (CT) scans. The appearances of lesions on scan may strongly suggest a diagnosis and in some cases (vestibular schwannoma/meningioma) are characteristic enough to allow treatment without a histological diagnosis, while others (lymphoma/low-grade glioma) may require a biopsy for confirmation.

Additional investigations may also be useful before planning any therapy, including functional MRI to delineate eloquent areas of cortex that may be at risk during treatment, tractography to determine the relationship of important fibre bundles to the mass, MR spectroscopy to determine the chemical composition, and positron emission tomography/CT in an attempt to differentiate areas of active tumour from radionecrosis in previously irradiated brain.

Management

There are essentially three options:

Observation

A watch-and-wait policy is often adopted for small, benign lesions with minimal or no referable symptoms.

Surgery

Surgical resection may be radical and complete, or subtotal depending on the biology of the tumour (encapsulated or diffusely infiltrating) and the location of nearby critical structures. Surgery remains a good treatment for relief of mass effect, confirmation of diagnosis, and, potentially, cure of suitably located benign tumours. The operating microscope significantly improved outcomes when introduced in the 1960s but the addition to the surgical armamentarium of ultrasonic aspirators, image guidance, high-speed drills, haemostatic agents, and, more recently, endoscopes have all helped to transform surgical techniques, aided by the impressive advances in neuro-imaging.

Radiotherapy/radiosurgery

Fractionated, conformal, external beam radiotherapy has been used for decades to treat malignant brain tumours. There have been technical advances in the planning software and linear accelerators delivering this mode of radiotherapy but the greatest change in practice in the treatment of benign tumours has been the emergence of 'stereotactic radiosurgery'. The term radiosurgery is used to imply surgical precision in the administration of radiation, giving a high dose to the target with a rapid fall off of dose to the surrounding structures. This accuracy requires high-resolution imaging to define the target and complex hardware to deliver multiple beams of radiation, which converge on that target. Radiosurgery is now internationally defined as treatment given in five fractions or less, with the gamma knife normally delivering single-fraction treatments and the CyberKnife often using three to five fractions.

Box 2.13.2.1 The World Health Organization 2007 classification of central nervous system tumours

The subclassification of CNS tumours above is complex, but the following subdivision is often used:

Brain
    Intrinsic (gliomas, metastatic deposits)
    Extrinsic (meningiomas, vestibular schwannomas)

Spine
    Intramedullary (ependymomas, gliomas)
    Extramedullary intradural (meningiomas, schwannomas)
    Extramedullary extradural (secondary deposits in the vertebral bodies)

Adapted with permission from David N Louis et al., The 2007 WHO Classification of Tumours of the Central Nervous System, *Acta Neuropathologica*, Volume 114, Issue 2, pp. 97–109, Copyright © Springer-Verlag 2007, reproduced under a Creative Commons license CC-BY.

Central nervous system tumours: intrinsic

Gliomas are the commonest primary intrinsic central nervous system (CNS) tumours, occurring in the brain, brainstem, and spinal cord. As the name implies, they arise from glial cells (usually astrocytes, oligodendrocytes or ependymal cells). Although grouped together as gliomas, there are significant differences in behaviour and response to treatment for the different subtypes shown in Box 2.13.2.1.

Astrocytomas

The World Health Organization (WHO) classification recognizes four grades (I–II low grade, III–IV high grade). Grade IV astrocytomas are also referred to as glioblastoma multiforme.

Although grade II lesions are considered low grade, they are not benign and will usually grow slowly over years before 'transforming' into grade III or IV with subsequent rapid growth.

True grade I tumours are uncommon and may be either diffusely infiltrating or discrete and encapsulated. These tumours are often histologically 'pilocytic' (formed of cells with long hair-like processes). A cystic/solid enhancing tumour in the cerebellum of a child is likely to be a juvenile pilocytic astrocytoma, which surgical resection alone may cure.

Grade II astrocytomas occur throughout the neuraxis and are diffusely infiltrating, slowly growing tumours.

In the spinal cord, they normally present by causing damage to the neural pathways leading to motor weakness, sensory disturbance, and proprioceptive loss in varying degrees. The level in the cord determines the pattern of weakness produced; quadriparesis or paraparesis.

In the brain, their presentation depends on location. Epilepsy is the most common initial symptom, but if they arise in an eloquent area, they may cause dysphasia, limb weakness, or hemianopia. In non-eloquent brain, particularly the frontal lobe, headache or other features of raised intracranial pressure such as disturbance of memory and concentration or changes in personality and behaviour may be the initial signs. A significant number are also now being discovered incidentally on scans for minor head injury or unrelated headache.

The management of grade II tumours remains controversial and has included biopsy followed by external beam radiotherapy, biopsy followed by simple observation, and more recently resection where possible, often during an 'awake craniotomy' in the hope of reducing the risk of iatrogenic deficits. Surgical debulking may have an effect in delaying malignant transformation, improving overall survival. This potential benefit has to be balanced against the surgical risk of neurological deficit and the knowledge that their diffuse nature makes complete resection unlikely.

Management of grade III (anaplastic) and grade IV (glioblastoma multiforme) tumours generally comprises surgical debulking where location allows, chemotherapy, and fractionated conformal external beam radiotherapy to a total dose of 55–60 Gy. Currently temozolomide is the chemotherapeutic agent of first choice for grade IV tumours. Methylguanine-DNA methyltransferase is an enzyme involved in DNA repair that may reduce the efficacy of temozolomide chemotherapy and consequently positivity for this in the histological specimen is considered an indicator of a poor response to the drug.

Oligodendrogliomas

Oligodendrogliomas are generally less aggressive than astrocytomas (median survival for low-grade oligodendroglioma 13 years versus 7.5 years for low-grade astrocytoma). They are more sensitive to systemic chemotherapy than astrocytomas of similar grade and have characteristic genetic markers, with most having deletions of the short arm of chromosome 1 (1p) and the long arm of chromosome 19 (19q). This co-deletion appears to predict sensitivity to chemotherapy.

Medulloblastoma

The most common malignant brain tumour of childhood, these normally present with signs and symptoms of raised intracranial pressure, including headache, nausea, vomiting, and altered level of consciousness. These symptoms are similar to meningitis and lumbar punctures have resulted in death from cerebellar tonsillar herniation. The finding of an enhancing midline cerebellar tumour on MRI scan is very suggestive and treatment generally comprises surgical resection, radiotherapy and chemotherapy. These tumours may disseminate throughout the subarachnoid space, with enhancing nodules visible over the brain surface, within the ventricles or in the spinal canal. Radiotherapy is usually given to the whole craniospinal axis to deal with this risk of dissemination. In children under the age of 3, however, radiotherapy is delayed in view of the very great risk of cognitive impairment when the growing brain is irradiated. Chemotherapy (often using four- or five-drug regimens) is given to infants under 3 years of age, but the result of treatment in terms of disease-free survival is not as good as in the older age groups, when radiotherapy is also given (60% versus 80%).

Metastases

It is estimated that between 10% and 30% of patients with disseminated malignancy will develop CNS secondary deposits, and this percentage may be increasing due in part to better imaging but possibly also to better systemic treatment of extracerebral disease. These lesions may be intracerebral or intraspinal, with intramedullary or subarachnoid spread around the spinal cord being commoner than previously thought.

In adults the most common primary tumours producing cerebral secondaries are breast, lung, melanoma, renal, and colon, occurring in:

◆ cerebrum (80%)

◆ cerebellum (15%)

◆ brainstem (5%).

This distribution is in keeping with the comparative size and blood flow of each of these regions and these deposits are characteristically at the junction of the grey and white matter.

Mass effect, intratumoural haemorrhage, or epilepsy are frequent presentations, but diffuse seeding throughout the cerebrospinal fluid spaces may lead to 'carcinomatous meningitis' causing hydrocephalus and multiple cranial nerve palsies.

MRI scans normally show multiple enhancing lesions, which may be solid or show 'ring' enhancement secondary to central necrosis or cyst formation.

Where the diagnosis is clear due to the presence of a known primary tumour, biopsy is not often indicated. Treatment may be surgery, with resection of suitable single lesions, or radiotherapy, either fractionated whole brain or stereotactic radiosurgery. Prognosis and decision making depends on:

◆ Karnofsky performance status/performance status (Box 2.13.2.2)

◆ type and extent of primary cancer

◆ volume load of CNS tumour

◆ age.

The best outcomes are seen in those patients with Karnofsky scores of >70, controlled or controllable systemic disease, and a small volume load of metastatic lesions. Without therapy the median survival is measured in months.

Treatment for multiple brain metastases in the UK has traditionally involved whole brain radiotherapy (WBRT), frequently given to a dose of 30 Gy in ten fractions. This has the advantage of being relatively cheap and relatively easy to administer. By irradiating the whole brain, there is a chance that microscopic deposits will be 'nipped in the bud'. The disadvantage, however, is the potential for damage to cognition, particularly where there is a reasonable expectation of long term survival, such as systemically controlled breast cancer.

More recently, stereotactic radiosurgery has been promoted as an alternative to WBRT and there is increasing evidence of efficacy in selected cases. The treatment is usually single fraction and day case, and some early data suggest less effect on cognition than with WBRT. The disadvantages are the possible development of new lesions outside the treatment field and the greater cost.

Central nervous system tumours: extrinsic

Meningioma

These account for approximately 30% of all primary brain and CNS tumours, with an estimated annual incidence of 2 per 100 000.

They are classified according to location (frontal convexity, cerebello-pontine angle, etc.) and histological grade (WHO I–III). Grade I tumours comprise more than 90% of the total, are histologically benign, normally very slowly growing, and if resected along with their dural origin have a low risk of recurrence. Grade II tumours account for approximately 5%, are more rapidly growing, and more prone to recurrence. Grade III lesions (around 3%) are

---

Box 2.13.2.2 Karnofsky performance status/performance status

The performance status and Karnofsky status are both now commonly used in referrals of patients with cancer.

Performance status

The World Health Organization (WHO) designed the scale that doctors use most often. It has categories from 0 to 4.

0: You are fully active and more or less as you were before your illness.

1: You cannot carry out heavy physical work, but can do anything else.

2: You are up and about more than half the day and can look after yourself, but are not well enough to work.

3: You are in bed or sitting in a chair for more than half the day and you need some help in looking after yourself.

4: You are in bed or a chair all the time and need a lot of looking after.

Adapted from Oken MM et al., Toxicity and response criteria of the Eastern Cooperative Oncology Group, *American Journal of Clinical Oncology*, Volume 5, Issue 6, pp. 649–55, Copyright © 1982 Lippincott-Raven Publishers, with permission from Wolters Kluwer Health, Inc. All rights reserved.

Karnofsky performance status

Similar to the WHO scale, but goes to up 100.

100: You don't have any evidence of disease and feel well.

90: You only have minor signs or symptoms but are able to carry on as normal.

80: You have some signs or symptoms and it takes a bit of effort to carry on as normal.

70: You are able to care for yourself but not able to carry on with all your normal activities or do active work.

60: You need help from time to time but can mostly care for yourself.

50: You need quite a lot of help to care for yourself.

40: You always need help to care for yourself.

30: You are disabled and may need to stay in hospital.

20: You are ill, in hospital and need a lot of treatment.

10: You are very ill and unlikely to recover.

Reproduced from Karnofsky DA and Burchenal JH, 'The Clinical Evaluation of Chemotherapeutic Agents in Cancer', p. 146, in MacLeod CM (Ed.), *Evaluation of Chemotherapeutic Agents*, Columbia University Press, New York, USA, Copyright © 1949, with permission from Columbia University Press.

frankly malignant, and usually rapidly fatal although some series show a 5-year survival of approximately 30%.

Many small tumours may be observed with serial scanning but where treatment is indicated, surgical resection including the dural origin is considered the gold standard. Sometimes their location precludes this due to the risk of damage to cerebral arteries or cranial nerves. In these cases, subtotal removal followed by radiotherapy (increasingly radiosurgery) gives excellent control, with radiosurgery leading to growth arrest in more than 90% of residual grade I tumours.

Vestibular schwannoma

With an annual incidence of approximately 2 per 100 000, vestibular schwannomas account for 80% of tumours within the cerebello-pontine angle. They arise, as their name suggests, from the vestibular nerves and generally present with hearing loss, tinnitus and disturbance of balance.

The current investigation of choice for unexplained, asymmetric sensorineural hearing loss is an MRI scan of the internal auditory meati. Most of these scans will be normal but a significant number will show classical schwannomas, growing both into the internal auditory meatus and the cerebello-pontine angle. These often demonstrate inhomogeneous enhancement, due to the presence of intratumoural cysts.

Schwannomas are normally slowly growing (1–2 mm per annum) with no need for urgent treatment. They may rarely present acutely, with haemorrhage or hydrocephalus, requiring rapid decompression or shunting, but most patients have time to make an informed decision about management.

With small tumours, a watch-and-wait policy is often adopted, with annual scanning to detect those that are uncommonly rapid in their growth. If treatment is recommended, it has to be emphasized that any hearing loss on the affected side will not be restored (and instead is likely to be sacrificed), that tinnitus is unlikely to be reduced, and that a good result is one which leaves them neurologically no worse.

Radiosurgery has become the treatment of choice over the past 15 years, except for tumours considered too large. Many surgeons will now debulk these tumours, attempting to preserve the facial nerve, and then treat the residual with radiosurgery. The control of growth with gamma knife treatment is approximately 95%, with few tumours escaping and requiring surgical resection. There is a small risk of malignant change, but this is estimated to be 1:5000 at most, and is much less than the risk of death from surgery.

Pituitary tumours

Intrasellar tumours include pituitary adenoma (the most common), meningioma, and craniopharyngioma. Their presentation may be with visual failure due to mass effect, or endocrine effects such as hypopituitarism, Cushing's disease, hyperprolactinaemia, or acromegaly. The typical visual field loss is a bitemporal hemianopia due to optic chiasm compression, usually with red fields being disproportionately impaired.

Patients may be managed conservatively if they harbour relatively small, non-functioning adenomas. Once the tumour reaches the optic chiasm, however, surgery is normally recommended unless the tumour is a prolactinoma as these respond very well to dopamine agonists such as cabergoline and shrink in response to medication alone. Other endocrine-active tumours are resected regardless of size, although there is currently a trend to pre-treat growth hormone secreting tumours with somatostatin analogues such as lanreotide or octreotide as these drugs will often shrink the tumour and may facilitate complete surgical resection.

Surgery now is almost exclusively trans-nasal, transphenoidal, and in many centres is entirely endoscopic as this gives an excellent view of the tumour cavity, the cavernous sinuses and the supra-sellar extension. Occasionally craniotomy is still recommended if the configuration of the tumour precludes adequate transphenoidal resection.

Spinal tumours

Benign tumours are usually slowly growing and will normally cause progressive limb weakness and sensory loss, which may be profound before diagnosis and treatment. Once decompressed in these circumstances, neurological recovery may be gratifying, often with excellent recovery of function. This is in marked contrast to metastatic disease, where severe deficits rarely recover despite decompression, possibly due to vascular compromise. Prompt diagnosis and, where indicated, treatment of spinal secondaries is required before there is significant neurological damage, in an attempt to preserve quality of life.

Spinal secondary deposits causing vertebral collapse are common and if treated surgically will often require decompression of the spinal cord followed by reconstruction and stabilization with adjuvant radiotherapy and chemotherapy.

Intradural tumours are generally managed in the UK by neurosurgeons and are usually resected using microsurgical techniques. The most common intradural tumours are meningiomas and schwannomas, with astrocytomas and ependymomas being found within the spinal cord and posing particular surgical challenges in the attempt to resect them without causing additional significant neural injury.

Further reading

Patten J. *Neurological Differential Diagnosis*. London, Springer, 1998.
Love S, Perry A, Ironside J, *et al.* (eds). *Greenfield's Neuropathology* (9th ed). London: Hodder Arnold 2015.

PART 2.14

Endocrine surgery

Endocrine surgery

Sheila Fraser and Mark Lansdown

Thyroid

Embryology

The thyroid is the first endocrine gland to develop, at day 24 of gestation. It develops from an endodermal thickening in the midline of the floor of the developing pharynx. This thickening grows downwards into the underlying mesenchyme as the thyroglossal duct. The duct is left elongated, extending from the foramen caecum at the base of the tongue, through the hyoid bone, to the final location of the thyroid, anterior to the trachea.

In the 7th week the thyroid completes its descent. As it descends it forms its mature shape of lateral lobes connected by a medial isthmus. The thyroglossal duct is obliterated early in fetal life, although the distal part may remain as the pyramidal lobe.

The parafollicular or C cells, which produce calcitonin, are of neural crest origin. These cells arise from the ultimobranchial bodies, from the fifth pharyngeal pouch, and fuse laterally within the thyroid lobes.

Anatomy

The anatomy of the thyroid gland is described in Chapter 1.1.5.

Developmental abnormalities

Thyroglossal cyst

Thyroglossal cysts are cystic remnants of the thyroglossal duct, and can occur at any point along the tract. They are commonly seen as a midline swelling closely related to the hyoid bone. The characteristic diagnostic sign is upwards movement of the swelling on protrusion of the tongue, as the thyroglossal duct is attached to the foramen caecum. These cysts are predisposed to infection so surgical excision is advised.

The classic operation is the Sistrunk procedure. This involves removal of the cyst and any associated tract, along with excision of the central portion of the hyoid bone. Failure to do this risks recurrence.

Lingual thyroid

Failure in descent of the thyroid may occur at any point along the thyroglossal duct. Most frequently, aberrant thyroid tissue is seen at the base of the tongue close to the foramen caecum as a lingual thyroid. A large mass of tissue in infants can cause respiratory or swallowing difficulties or even haemorrhage.

Ectopic thyroid

Ectopic thyroid tissue is rare and is defined as thyroid tissue located in a place other than its normal position. Ninety per cent of all ectopic thyroid tissue presents as a lingual thyroid. However, ectopic thyroid tissue can occur at any point along the thyroglossal duct and also outside this pathway of descent. It has rarely been reported in the thorax, trachea, and oesophagus.

Goitre

This is a non-specific term meaning 'visible or palpable enlargement of the thyroid gland', which can occur as diffuse or nodular enlargement. Goitres can expand anteriorly, as an obvious neck mass, or retrosternally. These might not be clinically obvious but can cause significant compressive symptoms. The thyroid may function normally (non-toxic goitre), be overactive (toxic goitre) or underactive (hypothyroid goitre). The thyroid is often physiologically enlarged and visible in thin women in both adolescence and pregnancy; very few will persist as a goitre.

There are multiple causes of goitre, but the most common worldwide is iodine deficiency. Iodine is an essential element in thyroxine production. If thyroxine levels are low, the pituitary releases thyroxine-stimulating hormone (TSH) to encourage follicular cells to increase iodine intake and so amplify thyroxine production. Goitre development begins as an adaptive process to low iodine levels, initially with diffuse enlargement, progressing to nodular change.

Other causes of goitre include Hashimoto's thyroiditis (now the most common cause in the UK), Grave's disease, thyroiditis, thyroid cancer, and other rare conditions.

A retrosternal goitre is defined as an enlarged thyroid with over 50% of the gland below the thoracic inlet. Retrosternal goitres are clinically important due to the compressive symptoms that can cause airway obstruction, dysphagia or obstruction of the major thoracic vessels (superior vena cava syndrome). Pemberton's sign demonstrates thoracic inlet obstruction caused by a large goitre: when asked to raise their hands as high as possible above their heads, patients develop facial flushing, a raised jugular venous pressure, distended superficial veins of the head and neck, and inspiratory stridor.

A chest X-ray may demonstrate a mediastinal mass or tracheal deviation. Computed tomography (CT) or magnetic resonance imaging (MRI) provide more detailed information regarding the size and extent of the goitre and tracheal narrowing. Unless known to be stable and asymptomatic large retrosternal goitres should be considered for surgery, to remove the risk of increasing airway obstruction, and for exact histopathological diagnosis if this is in doubt.

Solitary thyroid nodule

Thyroid nodules are very common, with up to 5% of the population having palpable nodules, and are more frequent in women. A thyroid nodule may be a true solitary nodule or a dominant nodule within a multinodular goitre. The differential diagnosis of a solitary nodule includes adenoma, cyst, or carcinoma. Although it was previously thought that multinodular goitres were less likely to be malignant, it is now recognized that a dominant nodule in a multinodular goitre has virtually the same risk of malignancy as a true solitary nodule.[1]

The main aim in investigating a thyroid nodule is to exclude malignancy, which occurs in approximately 5% of all nodules. The risk of malignancy is higher in men, children, and adults over 60 years of age. Other risk factors include a family history of thyroid cancer or other endocrine diseases and prior radiation exposure.

Voice change and hoarseness may suggest malignancy. Dysphagia, shortness of breath, and choking are more indicative of a multinodular goitre.

Examination should initially assess the general thyroid status of the patient, before focusing on the thyroid itself and the presence of any cervical lymphadenopathy, in both the central and lateral compartments.

Patients should be assessed biochemically for thyrotoxicosis, as this will usually need treatment before considering surgical options (Figure 2.14.1.1) and the section discussing the management of the thyrotoxic patient, p. 473).

The main investigation for any solitary nodule is FNAC (fine needle aspiration cytology) and is virtually mandatory, unless the patient is thyrotoxic. FNAC results are divided into five categories:

Thy 1: inadequate

Thy 2: benign

Thy 3: indeterminate

This category is now divided into:

Thy 3a: atypical features, but not enough to place in any other category

Thy 3f: follicular neoplasm suspected

Thy 4: suspicious of malignancy

Thy 5: diagnostic of malignancy

A Thy 1 result should be repeated, ideally under ultrasound guidance. If a nodule with a Thy 2 result is being considered for conservative management, a second FNAC is recommended to increase diagnostic accuracy and to ensure a malignancy is not overlooked.

If cystic lesions resolve after aspiration with negative cytology for malignant cells, no additional treatment may be necessary. However, cystic nodules can occasionally contain papillary carcinoma within the cyst wall and so recurrent cysts (aspirated twice or more), cystic nodules over 4 cm, and those with a bloodstained aspirate should be considered for diagnostic excision.

Most lesions with a FNAC result of Thy 3f or above are considered for surgery. In particular with follicular neoplasms cytopathology cannot differentiate between a follicular adenoma or carcinoma, and definitive histopathology is required. The latest thyroid cancer guidelines propose that not all benign appearing nodules need FNA but individual centres need to be aware of the diagnostic accuracy of their own scans if adopting this policy.

The most important supportive test in assessing a thyroid nodule is ultrasound. Its main role is to differentiate between a true solitary nodule and a multinodular goitre. Ultrasound can also assess the cystic nature of a lesion, demonstrate features suspicious of malignancy within a nodule, and detect cervical lymphadenopathy with great sensitivity.

Other imaging modalities are not routinely indicated in the investigation of a solitary nodule. In a thyrotoxic patient isotope scanning will distinguish between a solitary toxic adenoma

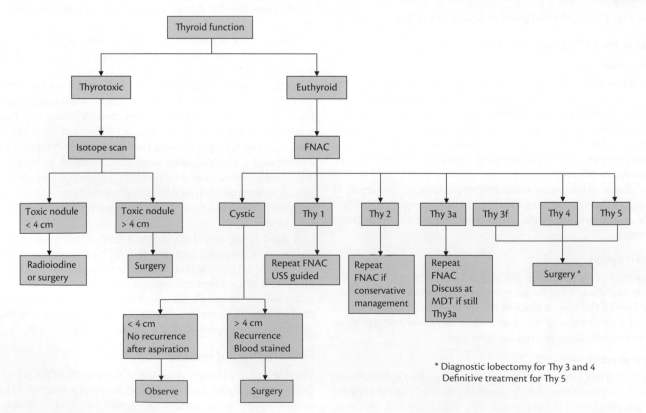

Fig. 2.14.1.1 Investigation of the solitary nodule.

and Graves' disease. CT and MRI have a role in evaluating the extent of a multinodular or retrosternal goitre and in patients with diagnosed thyroid malignancy, the incidence and extent of cervical lymphadenopathy and the presence of any pulmonary metastases.

Hyperthyroidism

In the UK around 1% of people are currently diagnosed with hyperthyroidism (also known as thyrotoxicosis) and the condition is six times more common in women. It occurs when excess thyroxine is produced by the thyroid gland, speeding up the body's metabolism resulting in increased heat production and oxygen consumption.

The three most common causes for hyperthyroidism are Graves' disease, a toxic multinodular goitre, and a toxic solitary nodule. Rarely hyperthyroidism can occur secondary to thyroiditis—inflammation of the thyroid gland causing excess hormone production—due to pregnancy, viral infection or drugs.

The signs and symptoms of hyperthyroidism result from the raised metabolic rate. Patients often complain of fatigue, heat intolerance, sweating, weight loss despite an increased appetite, diarrhoea, irritability, anxiety or emotional changes, and a tremor. Increased action of the sympathetic nervous system causes cardiac effects, which are often more troublesome in older patients, with tachycardia, palpitations, arrhythmias (especially atrial fibrillation), and cardiac failure.

The diagnosis is confirmed biochemically. Blood tests show elevated levels of thyroid hormones – T3 (tri-iodothyroxine) and T4 (thyroxine), and suppressed levels of TSH (thyroid-stimulating hormone).

Graves' disease

Nearly 80% of cases of hyperthyroidism are due to Graves' disease, an autoimmune disease. Thyroid-stimulating immunoglobulins bind to the TSH receptor and stimulate the thyroid gland to produce increased thyroid hormones. The gland usually becomes diffusely enlarged and hypervascular.

Graves' disease is confirmed by the presence of TSH-receptor autoantibodies in the blood, plus the biochemical abnormalities described above. Thyroid peroxidase autoantibodies are often demonstrated.

Patients with Graves' disease have complex immunological changes resulting in further signs and symptoms not seen with other causes of hyperthyroidism. Around one-third of patients suffer with eye problems, called 'Graves' ophthalmopathy'. This results in exophthalmos (bulging eyes), upper eyelid retraction, grittiness and soreness of the eyes and, rarely, double vision or sight loss. Pretibial myxoedema, proximal myopathy, and finger clubbing maybe present.

Toxic multinodular goitre (Plummer's disease)

This usually occurs on a background of a long-standing non-toxic multinodular goitre. One or more of the nodules within the goitre start to function autonomously, not responding to the background TSH levels.

Toxic solitary nodule

Like the nodules in a toxic multinodular goitre, in this case a solitary nodule becomes autonomous and is not subject to the normal autoregulation of the thyroid gland.

Treatment of hyperthyroidism

If the diagnosis of Graves' disease is without doubt, further investigations are not necessary. If there is clinical doubt an isotope scan can differentiate between a toxic solitary nodule and multinodular goitre.

There are three methods of treatment for Graves' disease: antithyroid drugs, radioactive iodine, and surgery. Antithyroid medications block the incorporation of iodine into tyrosine, and so prevent the synthesis of thyroid hormones. Commonly used medications are carbimazole and prophythiouracil. Although minor side effects are widespread, patients should be warned about the rare but serious risk of agranulocytosis.

Antithyroid drugs can be titrated slowly according to T3 and T4 levels over several weeks (titrated dose regime) or given at a higher rate in combination with levothyroxine replacement to maintain normal thyroxine levels (block and replace regime). Only around 30–40% of patients remain euthyroid after stopping antithyroid drugs and the majority require more definitive treatment.

Antithyroid medications are not usually considered a long-term solution in toxic multinodular goitres or solitary nodules. As the nodules function autonomously, hyperthyroidism will recur when the medication is discontinued. Such medication may be considered prior to definitive treatment or in elderly patients not fit for further treatment.

Beta-adrenergic blockers have a role in controlling the symptoms of hyperthyroidism, especially predominantly cardiac symptoms. Usually propranolol is used at a dose of 20–40 mg three times a day. Propranolol also reduces the peripheral conversion of T4 to T3, the active hormone.

Radioactive iodine (^{131}I) is used extensively to treat hyperthyroidism. The radioiodine is taken up selectively by the thyroid gland and destroys overactive tissue. It can take up to 6 months to destroy the tissue, and 50–80% of patients eventually develop hypothyroidism, requiring levothyroxine replacement. Radioiodine is a safe treatment with no evidence of an increased cancer risk, which many patients worry about. However, patients with Graves' disease should be warned that Graves' ophthalmopathy can worsen following radioiodine treatment.

Surgery is a definitive and effective treatment for patients with relapsed Graves' disease, significant eye disease, or large goitres. Patients need to be rendered euthyroid prior to surgery, otherwise there is a risk of a hyperthyroid crisis (thyrotoxic storm) during anaesthetic. A total thyroidectomy is performed with levothyroxine replacement postoperatively. Details of the surgical procedure and potential complications are described in the Thyroid surgery section.

In small multinodular goitres radioiodine can be effective, but for larger goitres a total thyroidectomy is recommended. Patients with a solitary toxic nodule less than 4 cm are often treated with radioiodine, whereas those with bigger nodules are referred for a thyroid lobectomy.

Thyroiditis

Thyroiditis is a general term referring to inflammation of the thyroid gland and can be due to range of different conditions.

Hashimoto's thyroiditis (autoimmune thyroiditis)

This is an autoimmune condition resulting in invasion and destruction of thyroid follicles by lymphocytes and plasma cells.

Antibodies against thyroid peroxidase and thyroglobulin are detected in the serum and used to confirm the diagnosis. There is often a past medical history or family history of associated auto-immune diseases. Postmenopausal women are most commonly affected.

Due to lymphocyte infiltration and fibrosis, the gland becomes diffusely enlarged and firm. Clinically patients are usually initially euthyroid but may be periodically hyperthyroid, as damage to thyroid follicles causes a temporary increased release of thyroid hormones. Gradual destruction of the gland eventually results in hypothyroidism.

Levothyroxine treatment is required for hypothyroidism and may shrink small goitres. Surgery is required for large goitres with compressive symptoms. There is an association between Hashimoto's thyroiditis and lymphoma. This should be excluded if rapid expansion of the gland or an asymmetrical nodular area should occur.

Granulomatous (de Quervain's thyroiditis)

This is the most common cause of a painful thyroid, often associated with fever, arthralgia, and malaise. It is thought to be of viral origin. Patients frequently report a sore throat or flu-like symptoms a couple of weeks before the start of the thyroid symptoms.

The acute phase of the illness presents with a painful thyroid, typically for 3 to 6 weeks. A small percentage of patients are briefly hyperthyroid as excess thyroid hormones are released when the gland is acutely inflamed and thyroid damage occurs. For the majority of patients the symptoms resolve after this stage. However, some patients will have a brief euthyroid stage before developing mild hypothyroidism, which can last for weeks to months before recovery.

Treatment is mainly symptomatic and non-steroidal anti-inflammatory drugs are extremely effective analgesia. In severe cases a short course of high-dose steroids (prednisolone) will settle symptoms within 72 hours. The hypothyroid stage is usually mild and transient and does not require treatment. In prolonged cases or symptomatic patients low-dose levothyroxine is started.

Riedel's thyroiditis

This is a rare condition, believed to be of autoimmune origin, where thyroid tissue is replaced by a dense fibrosis. The gland feels stony hard and the fibrosis can extend outside the thyroid capsule to involve adjacent structures, most seriously causing tracheal compression or oesophageal obstruction.

IgG4 levels are elevated in the plasma in nearly all cases, and Riedel's thyroiditis is now thought to be a manifestation of a systemic disease called IgG4-related disease. Other conditions may co-exist in patients, including sclerosing cholangitis and retroperitoneal, mediastinal, and retro-orbital fibrosis.

The condition is difficult to differentiate from thyroid cancer. FNAC is not usually helpful, showing fibrotic changes only that are also present in anaplastic cancer. An open biopsy is necessary for a definitive diagnosis: wedge resection of the isthmus is performed , which additionally decompresses the trachea and frees the airway.

Postpartum thyroiditis

This typically occurs around 2 to 6 months post pregnancy, due to immune changes during pregnancy. Women usually have an initial mild hyperthyroid stage, followed by hypothyroidism that can occur up to 12 months postpartum. Many women recover without treatment, but some will require temporary levothyroxine treatment and a few develop permanent hypothyroidism.

Amiodarone-associated thyroiditis

Amiodarone is a very effective anti-arrhythmic drug but has notable side effects, including thyroid dysfunction. Due to its high iodine content, amiodarone can be directly toxic to the thyroid and cause both hyperthyroidism and hypothyroidism, usually the latter. If possible in both hyperthyroid and hypothyroid patients amiodarone should be withdrawn and alternative medications considered.

Hypothyroidism

Hypothyroidism is a clinical state caused by a lack of thyroid hormones, resulting in a slowing of the body's metabolism. Congenital hypothyroidism (cretinism) is rare and the majority of cases are acquired in adult life. Iodine deficiency is the most frequent cause of hypothyroidism worldwide, but in the developed world Hashimoto's thyroiditis is more common. Occasionally secondary or tertiary hypothyroidism occurs, if either the pituitary gland or hypothalamus do not produce enough TSH or TRH (thyrotropin-releasing hormone). This is usually caused by a tumour, radiation, or surgery.

Signs and symptoms of hypothyroidism include fatigue, weight gain, constipation, cold intolerance, bradycardia, muscle cramps, infertility, and depression. Often hypothyroidism has an insidious onset and may not be diagnosed until symptoms are more overt.

Hypothyroidism is diagnosed biochemically, with raised levels of TSH and reduced levels of T3 and T4, although in secondary or tertiary hypothyroidism levels of all three will be low. The treatment for primary hypothyroidism is daily levothyroxine, with blood levels of TSH to check that patients are on the correct dosage.

Thyroid cancer

Although thyroid cancer makes up <1% of all malignancy, it is the most common endocrine cancer. Thyroid cancers are a heterogeneous group and are classified according to histopathological characteristics.

Differentiated thyroid cancer (DTC)

This category comprises the two most common types: papillary and follicular thyroid cancer. They have a better prognosis than other subtypes.

Papillary thyroid cancer (PTC)

This is the most common of the thyroid cancers, accounting for 70–80% of cases. It is usually seen in children and young adults below the age of 40 years. Risk factors include a history of ionizing or external beam radiation. PTC is seen more in iodine-rich areas.

Patients usually present with a nodule in the thyroid or enlarged lymph nodes in the neck, which may present as cystic swellings. Enlarged cervical lymph nodes are sometimes the only finding in patients with a 'microscopic' thyroid primary (defined as less than 1 cm) and were previously, mistakenly, termed 'lateral aberrant thyroid'.

PTC has early lymphatic spread to the paratracheal and cervical lymph nodes. Haematogenous invasion is late, with metastases usually to the lungs and bones. Tumours often extend directly into the soft tissues in the neck, especially the trachea and oesophagus, causing vocal cord palsy secondary to RLN (recurrent laryngeal nerve) invasion. Multifocality is common.

Follicular cancer

Between 10% and 20% of cases of thyroid cancer are follicular cancers. In contrast to papillary cancer, follicular cancer is more common in iodine-deficient areas. Patients are slightly older, with a mean age of 50 years.

Follicular cancer presents as a solitary, encapsulated nodule. It is not possible to distinguish on FNAC between a follicular adenoma and carcinoma. Vascular and or capsular invasion seen on histological examination of the whole nodule is required to diagnose carcinoma. A thyroid lobectomy is therefore required for definitive histological diagnosis of any Thy 3f lesion on FNAC.

Follicular cancer is divided into minimally and widely invasive cancer, with the latter being less common but more aggressive. Haematogenous spread to the lungs, liver, and bones is early, and may be present at diagnosis, whereas lymphatic spread is late.

Treatment of differentiated thyroid cancer

Patients with DTC can be divided into high- and low-risk groups in relation to predicted survival and recurrence. Several scoring systems have been developed to accurately identify into which group patients fall, including:

TNM—tumour, node metastases, distant metastases

AMES—age, metastases, extent, and size of tumour

AGES—age, grade, extent, and size of tumour

MACIS—metastases, age, completeness of surgical resection, extra-
thyroidal invasion, and size of tumour.

The majority of patients are classified as low-risk and have an excellent long-term prognosis. High-risk features include age (>40 or <10 years), male gender, tumour size (over 4 cm), histological grade, extra-thyroidal spread, and distant metastases.

PTC is often multifocal so a total thyroidectomy is recommended. The exceptions are low-risk patients with a tumour of <1 cm when a lobectomy and isthmusectomy is sufficient. If patients are categorized as high risk or have disease evident in the central compartment, a level VI node dissection should also be performed. A selective lateral neck dissection (levels II to V) is performed if there is evidence of disease in the lateral neck.[2]

If follicular carcinoma is diagnosed following lobectomy no further surgical treatment is required for low-risk female patients with a tumour <2 cm and minimal capsular or vascular invasion. There is debate regarding the extent of surgical treatment for low-risk patients with tumours from 2–4 cm and this is usually at the discretion of the multidisciplinary team. For high-risk patients with tumours >4 cm a total thyroidectomy is advised.

Radioiodine therapy is considered for most patients with DTC after total thyroidectomy. There is normally a small amount of residual tissue. The remnant thyroid tissue concentrates radioiodine, resulting in the destruction of residual thyroid cells.

Following a total thyroidectomy patients require life-long thyroxine-replacement treatment. Higher doses are prescribed to suppress TSH levels, to prevent the stimulation of any remaining thyroid cells by TSH.

Thyroglobulin (TG) measurement is used routinely as a tumour marker after total thyroidectomy. Elevated TG levels indicate disease progression or recurrence and should prompt further investigations.[1,3]

Medullary thyroid cancer

Medullary thyroid cancer (MTC) arises from the parafollicular C cells and is the third most common thyroid cancer, comprising 5–8% of cases. In approximately 80% of patients MTC is sporadic, but 20% have a genetic origin due to mutations in the RET proto-oncogene. Inherited syndromes include familial MTC and MEN2 (type II multiple endocrine neoplasia). Patients with sporadic MTC are usually aged 40 to 50 years, whereas those with inherited disease are younger. MTC in association with MEN2 is recognized to have the worst prognosis and is a more aggressive disease.

MTC usually presents with a thyroid mass. At diagnosis enlarged cervical lymph nodes are observed in 50% of patients. The cancer secretes calcitonin, which predominantly causes diarrhoea and sometimes flushing. It is an effective tumour marker and is used postoperatively to monitor recurrent disease. Carcinoembryonic antigen (CEA) is also produced by C cells, but is less sensitive as a tumour marker.

A thorough family history of thyroid cancer and other endocrine problems should always be taken when patients present with a thyroid nodule. The diagnosis of MTC is confirmed by FNAC and measurement of calcitonin levels. MEN2 must be excluded in patients presenting with MTC, as proceeding to surgery with an undiagnosed phaeochromocytoma can be fatal.

As the disease is multifocal a total thyroidectomy is recommended along with a central compartment lymph node dissection. For cancers over 2 cm an ipsilateral selective lateral neck dissection is performed. With inherited cancers more extensive surgery in the form of a bilateral lateral neck dissection is usually carried out. There is no role for radioiodine in MTC, but external beam irradiation is sometimes used in metastatic or recurrent disease.

Anaplastic cancer

This is aggressive but rare, comprising less than 5% of all thyroid cancers and occurring in older patients. It often arises on a background of pre-existing thyroid disease and frequently presents with rapid growth of a pre-existing goitre. Areas of follicular or papillary cancer are often demonstrated within an anaplastic cancer. It is therefore thought to develop from a previously unknown DTC.

The cancer grows rapidly and invades surrounding tissues, causing vocal cord palsy and compressive symptoms. Invasion of the cervical sympathetic nerves can cause Horner's syndrome (triad of miosis: constricted pupil, ptosis, and loss of sweating on one side of the face and neck). Pulmonary metastases are common and present in 50% of patients at diagnosis.

Curative surgery is not usually possible due to extensive local disease, but surgery may be required to relieve airway obstruction. Radiotherapy and chemotherapy have limited success and death is typically within 6 months of diagnosis.

Lymphoma

Primary lymphoma of the thyroid normally arises as a complication of Hashimoto's thyroiditis, although can rarely occur without a background of autoimmune disease. It is commonly non-Hodgkin's B-cell type. The majority present in elderly women, with a rapidly enlarging painless neck mass and associated cervical lymphadenopathy. It should be differentiated from anaplastic cancer as both are rapidly growing neck masses, but lymphoma is highly treatable. FNAC may provide an accurate diagnosis; if any doubt core biopsy should be performed.

Surgery is not necessary unless there is airway compromise, with chemotherapy and radiotherapy providing the mainstay of treatment. Although the prognosis is generally good for localized disease, it is influenced by the histological subtype.

Metastases to the thyroid

Thyroid metastases are rare. Many are not demonstrated until autopsy. Occasionally metastatic disease to the thyroid can present as a palpable nodule. Usually this is associated with disseminated disease and a poor prognosis. Surgical resection may be indicated if the thyroid is the only site of metastasis and the primary disease is under control. The most common primary cancers are kidney, breast, lung, and gastrointestinal.

Thyroid surgery

Thyroid surgery generally consists of a thyroid lobectomy or total thyroidectomy. Occasionally an isthmusectomy is performed, but a subtotal thyroidectomy is no longer recommended. Prior to thyroid surgery all patients should undergo a vocal cord check to exclude pre-existing asymptomatic recurrent laryngeal nerve palsy.

The patient is placed supine with slight extension of the neck. A transverse incision is made 2–3 cm above the sternal notch in a skin crease and the thin platysma muscle divided. Superior and inferior skin flaps are raised in front of the anterior jugular veins. The deep cervical fascia is separated vertically in the midline and the strap muscles dissected off the thyroid and retracted laterally.

The thyroid is retracted medially and the middle thyroid vein is ligated if evident. To fully mobilize the thyroid the superior pole vessels are divided, with care taken to avoid damage to the external branch of the superior laryngeal nerve. The inferior pole vessels are then ligated to free up the lower pole.

The RLN should be identified on both sides to avoid injury. On the left side the nerve has a relatively fixed position in the tracheo-oesophageal groove, but the course is more oblique on the right.

Finding the parathyroid glands is important. The inferior parathyroid is usually anterior and medial to the RLN near the lower thyroid pole. The superior parathyroid gland is typically within a 1 cm radius of the junction of the inferior thyroid artery and the RLN. However the position of the parathyroid glands can be highly variable.

Once the RLN and parathyroids have been identified, the thyroid lobe is dissected from the trachea. As in total thyroidectomy, thyroid lobectomy includes excision of the isthmus and pyramidal lobe but leaving the opposite lobe.

Meticulous haemostasis is vital.

Complications of thyroid surgery

Full informed consent is essential before any thyroid operation to ensure awareness of potential complications. Bleeding deep to the strap muscles can compress adjacent structures causing venous congestion and airway obstruction. Airway obstruction is probably due to subglottic and laryngeal oedema secondary to venous and lymphatic congestion, rather than direct tracheal compression by a haematoma. The first priority is to open the wound and evacuate the haematoma, before the patient is re-intubated and taken back to theatre to control the bleeding.

Damage to the RLN is rare, but serious. Temporary vocal cord paralysis occurs in about 5% of patients, due to neuropraxia from traction or bruising of the nerve intraoperatively. Recovery is expected within 3 months. Permanent injury or division of the nerve is uncommon, and normally happens when the nerve has not been identified within surgery. On postoperative laryngoscopy the vocal cord is revealed in the 'cadaveric' position, midway between the open and closed positions. Bilateral RLN is extremely rare but catastrophic as the patient develops stridor and a tracheostomy may be required.[4]

All patients undergoing a total thyroidectomy need life-long levothyroxine replacement treatment. Up to 20% of patients who have a thyroid lobectomy will develop hypothyroidism, necessitating levothyroxine supplementation.

Temporary bruising or removal of the parathyroid glands can cause postoperative hypoparathyroidism resulting in symptoms of hypocalcaemia, with tingling around the mouth and fingers and muscle tetany in severe cases. Classic signs of hypocalcaemia are Chvostek's and Trousseau's signs, which demonstrate neuromuscular excitability caused by hypocalcaemia. Chvostek's sign is described as twitching of the muscles of facial expression when tapping the facial nerve over the parotid gland. Trousseau's sign is more sensitive and specific: a blood pressure cuff is placed around the upper arm and inflated above systolic blood pressure for 3 minutes; the resulting ischaemia exacerbates hypocalcaemic neuromuscular excitability instigating carpopedal spasm (flexion of the wrist and metacarpophalangeal joints with hyperextension of the fingers and flexion of the thumb onto the palm).

Calcium levels must be checked following a total thyroidectomy. Any patient with symptoms of hypocalcaemia or an adjusted calcium level below 2.0 mmol/L should receive calcium supplementation. For severe hypocalcaemia vitamin D supplementation is also recommended. Patients seldom require intravenous calcium treatment, but it is needed in cases of falling calcium levels despite supplementation or tetany. For many patients calcium supplementation can be withdrawn as the parathyroid glands gradually recover function. If it is still required at 12 months postsurgery, permanent calcium treatment will be needed.[5]

Parathyroid

Embryology and anatomy

There are two pairs of parathyroid glands: a superior and inferior pair. The superior glands descend with the thyroid. They are usually found outside the thyroid's fibrous capsule at the upper pole of the thyroid, in a posterolateral position. Most commonly they are located just above the junction of the RLN and the inferior thyroid artery.

The inferior parathyroids descend caudally and anteriorly with the thymus and have a longer descent. They have a more variable location and can lie near the lower pole of the thyroid, within the thymus or in the upper mediastinum.

The pairs of parathyroid glands are typically symmetrically arranged on the two sides of the neck. Although most people have four glands, a small percentage will have supernumerary glands.

Parathyroid glands are small, tan-coloured, bean-shaped structures that can be difficult to differentiate from adjacent thyroid nodules or surrounding fat. Their blood supply is usually from the inferior thyroid artery, although some superior parathyroids receive their blood supply from the superior thyroid artery. Venous drainage is via the thyroid vein plexus.

Parathyroid hormone (PTH) and calcium regulation

The parathyroid glands produce PTH, a key regulator of serum calcium levels. The normal calcium range is 2.2–2.6 mmol/L. Small decreases in serum calcium levels activate calcium-sensing receptors on the parathyroid glands, instigating the synthesis and release of PTH to increase serum calcium levels.

PTH acts on the kidneys, bones, and gastrointestinal tract to increase serum calcium levels. In the kidney its action results in increased resorption of calcium with increased phosphate and bicarbonate excretion. The bones store 99% of calcium in the body; PTH triggers osteoblast and osteoclast activity, amplifying bone turnover and increasing the extracellular calcium pool.

PTH also stimulates the kidney to convert 25-hydoxyvitamin D to its active metabolite 1,25-dihydroxyvitamin D. Vitamin D is important in calcium regulation as it stimulates calcium and phosphate absorption by the gastrointestinal tract.

Calcitonin is the natural antagonist to PTH and is produced by the thyroid parafollicular C cells. It decreases osteoclast activity in the bones and reduces calcium resorption by the kidneys. However, in comparison to PTH, calcitonin only has a very minor role in regulating serum calcium levels in humans.

Primary hyperparathyroidism (PHPT)

Hyperparathyroidism is over-secretion of the PTH by the parathyroid glands, resulting in hypercalcaemia and hypophosphataemia. Despite high serum calcium levels there is a failure of negative feedback in reducing PTH secretion.[6]

PHPT is the most frequent cause of elevated PTH levels. In 87-90% of patients it is caused by a single adenoma, in 3% there is more than one adenoma, in 10% four-gland hyperplasia occurs and in <1% of cases it is due to parathyroid carcinoma.

Clinical features of PHPT

PHPT occurs more frequently in women and the incidence rises with age. Prior radiation exposure is a risk factor for parathyroid adenomas. Clinically the symptoms are those of hypercalcaemia and are extremely variable, ranging from asymptomatic to severe. Many patients are identified when asymptomatic on routine biochemical tests.

Symptoms of hypercalcaemia are classically known by the mnemonic 'bones, stones, abdominal groans, and psychiatric moans'. The most common presentation is with renal calculi and nephrocalcinosis, although excessive thirst and polyuria may be an early sign. PHPT is linked with osteoporosis and associated pathological fractures. The characteristic bone damage related to PHPT, osteitis fibrosa cystica (demineralization and sub-periosteal bone resorption typically in the fingers, with cysts in the long bones and jaws and a moth-eaten appearance of the skull), is now rarely seen.

Most patients report fatigue. Other symptoms include constipation, nausea and vomiting, muscle weakness, and psychotic symptoms. Hypercalcaemia is linked with increased acid secretion and peptic ulceration and pancreatitis.

Rarely, patients present with a hypercalcaemic crisis, usually with calcium levels over 3.5 mmol/L. The typical presentation is with confusion, nausea and vomiting, and abdominal pain. Vomiting can cause severe dehydration and renal failure, with worsening hypercalcaemia, which may result in fatal arrhythmias or coma if not urgently treated.

The aim of treatment is to aggressively rehydrate the patient and increase the renal excretion of calcium. PHPT and malignancy are the most common causes of hypercalcaemia and the correct diagnosis should be immediately sought. In addition to rehydration, the calcium levels can be reduced by a loop diuretic and bisphosphonate. Loop diuretics, such as furosemide, work by inhibiting calcium resorption in the loop of Henle, whereas bisphosphonates inhibit osteoclast activity.

Diagnosis

PHPT is confirmed biochemically by a raised serum calcium level and an inappropriate (non-suppressed or high) PTH level. A 24-hour urine collection is carried out to check for the presence of hypercalciuria. A low urinary calcium excretion indicates benign familial hypercalcaemic hypocalciuria, rather than PHPT (see Familial hypocalciuric hypercalcaemia section). Hypophosphataemia is often seen due to the increased renal excretion of phosphate.

Management

Surgery is the only curative treatment for PHPT. The gold-standard operation remains a bilateral neck exploration, with a cure rate of over 95%. All four glands are identified and examined, and enlarged glands removed.

Recently there has been a move towards minimally invasive surgery as PHPT is commonly caused by a single adenoma. This approach reduces potential complications since only one side of the neck is explored and gives a better cosmetic result.

For minimally invasive surgery the adenoma must be localized preoperatively by imaging studies. Initial imaging techniques are usually ultrasound and sestamibi scanning. CT, MRI, and selective venous sampling are typically reserved for patients needing re-exploration. Sestamibi scanning is the most sensitive method, but no technique is 100% sensitive and specific. For minimally invasive surgery at least two imaging studies are recommended with concordant results,[7] with consideration given to intraoperative PTH (IOPTH) measurement.

In patients with suspected multi-gland disease or equivocal imaging, bilateral neck exploration is advised. The initial approach to the neck is similar to thyroid surgery. The superior parathyroid glands are searched for on the posterior aspect of the upper pole of the thyroid by retracting the thyroid medially. The RLN should be identified to avoid damage and the inferior thyroid artery left intact. If a superior parathyroid gland is not found, it should be searched for along the path of potential migration. Abnormal superior parathyroid glands tend to migrate posteriorly and downwards and so should first be hunted for next to or behind the oesophagus.

The inferior parathyroid glands have a less consistent location. Initially the area from the inferior thyroid artery down to the lower pole of the thyroid should be explored. The inferior parathyroid gland in this region lies anterior to the RLN. If the inferior parathyroid is not visible, the thyro-thymic ligament and thymus should be examined. In contrast to the superior, the inferior parathyroid glands become more anterior the further they migrate in the neck.

Since a solitary adenoma is the most common cause of PHPT, removal of the affected gland will usually provide a cure. The normal weight of a parathyroid gland is 30–60 mg, anything over 75 mg is considered enlarged. If two or more glands are enlarged, both should be removed. In four-gland hyperplasia, a subtotal parathyroidectomy is usually performed, leaving a single vascularized gland remnant, with a weight approximately the same as a normal gland.

The aim of minimally invasive surgery is to target through a small incision a specific gland that has been detected on preoperative localization studies. A small, 2–3 cm incision is made over the medial border of sternocleidomastoid muscle, or in the suprasternal notch for suspected low inferior glands. Minimally invasive surgery can be performed using an intraoperative gamma probe, so the area of dissection corresponds with the level of radioactivity, and by endoscopic techniques.[8]

IOPTH monitoring is a useful adjunct, especially in minimally invasive surgery. It confirms removal of the correct parathyroid gland and excludes a double adenoma or hyperplasia. IOPTH monitoring works as PTH has a short half-life of only 3 to 5 minutes. An operation is considered successful if there is over 50% drop in IOPTH levels between baseline and the value 10 to 15 minutes after parathyroid removal.

Secondary hyperparathyroidism

This is virtually always seen in patients with chronic renal failure on long-term dialysis. PTH levels rise in response to reduced levels of activated vitamin D and hyperphosphataemia. As renal function reduces, the kidneys are unable to hydroxylate vitamin D to its active form, affecting calcium absorption from the gastrointestinal tract. The diminished kidney function means phosphate is not excreted sufficiently and so serum phosphate levels escalate. The increased serum phosphate binds to calcium, creating an insoluble calcium complex, decreasing serum calcium levels, and further stimulating PTH release.

Renal bone disease (renal osteodystrophy) can be problematic, with osteomalacia and osteitis fibrosa cystica. Extra-skeletal calcification occurs due to insoluble calcium complexes, mainly in the cardiovascular system, increasing cardiovascular morbidity and mortality. Calciphylaxis is a rare condition: calcification of small arteries of the skin takes place with resulting cutaneous ischaemia and necrosis. The mortality rate is high, with >50% of patients dying within 1 year of diagnosis, usually from septicaemia.

Patients are initially treated with activated vitamin D, followed by dietary phosphate restriction and phosphate-binding medications. Surgical treatment is indicated in refractory hyperparathyroidism, usually with PTH levels over 800 pg/mL. Cinacalcet, a calcimimetic agent, is currently only recommended by the National Institute of Health and Care Excellence for patients with very high PTH and calcium levels in whom surgery is contraindicated.

Surgical treatment aims to correct hyperparathyroidism, without inducing severe postoperative hypocalcaemia and avoiding persistent disease. The surgical approach is a subtotal or total parathyroidectomy. Supernumery parathyroid glands in the region of the thymus are not uncommon in chronic renal failure so the operation includes cervical thymectomy. Some renal units advocate total parathyroidectomy with autotransplantation of parathyroid tissue. All four glands are resected and small pieces of fresh parathyroid tissue placed into the brachioradialis muscle in the forearm. This site is recommended as hyperplasia of the transplanted parathyroid tissue can be more readily dealt with than if implanted in a neck muscle. Surgery on recurrent disease in the forearm can be achieved under local anaesthetic.

Tertiary hyperparathyroidism

This is continued excessive autonomous PTH secretion after renal transplantation in patients with long-standing secondary hyperparathyroidism. PTH and calcium levels usually fall within 1 year of transplantation. A failure to do so indicates autonomous PTH production. Surgery is necessary: either a subtotal parathyroidectomy or total parathyroidectomy with autotransplantation.

Parathyroid carcinoma

This is extremely rare, characterized by very high levels of PTH secretion and severe hypercalcaemia. Patients often have symptomatic hypercalcaemia and a palpable mass may be felt in the neck, virtually never present in benign disease.

Parathyroid carcinoma is linked with genetic syndromes, in particular type I multiple endocrine neoplasia, familial hyperparathyroidism, and familial hyperparathyroidism-jaw tumour syndrome.

The diagnosis is frequently made postoperatively, but may be suspected intraoperatively by the appearance of the parathyroid gland. It is typically a stony, hard mass with a dense fibrous capsule adhering to adjacent structures. The only definite diagnostic criteria for parathyroid carcinoma are local invasion and metastatic disease.

If the diagnosis of parathyroid carcinoma is established preoperatively, or strongly suspected intraoperatively, excision of the parathyroid plus an ipsilateral thyroid lobectomy, central neck dissection, and removal of any adherent tissue is advocated.

Patients are at risk immediately postoperatively of severe hypocalcaemia, as calcium and phosphate are deposited back into the bone after prolonged hyperparathyroidism ('hungry bone syndrome'). PTH levels are monitored for signs of recurrent or persistent disease. Further surgery may be required, as adjunct treatments have a limited role.

Parathyromatosis

It is important to remove parathyroid glands intact. Rare cases of recurrent hyperparathyroidism have been reported due to the spillage of parathyroid tissue intraoperatively. Spilled cells form hyperfunctional nodules. This is difficult to diagnose preoperatively and to treat surgically. Eventually the patient may die of uncontrollable hypercalcaemia.

Familial hypocalciuric hypercalcaemia (FHH)

FHH is an autosomal dominant condition characterized by asymptomatic mild to moderate hypercalcaemia. It is important to differentiate it from PHPT as FHH is not cured by surgery.[9]

The diagnosis is made by raised PTH and calcium levels with low calcium urinary excretion. A calcium/creatinine clearance ratio of less than 0.01 is highly suggestive of FHH.

Recurrent disease

Persistent disease postoperatively is often due to technical error. Too much tissue may have been left *in situ* during a subtotal parathyroidectomy or a double adenoma or ectopic parathyroid gland missed.

Occasionally a second adenoma can develop, usually in patients with a family history or prior neck irradiation. Recurrence in autotransplanted tissue has been reported and is more common after surgery for secondary or tertiary hyperparathyroidism.

Hypoparathyroidism

This is a common temporary complication of parathyroid surgery. Hyperfunction of the removed glands can result in suppression of the residual glands. Signs and symptoms are as described in the

'Complications of thyroid surgery' section. A significant number of patients suffer from hungry bone syndrome after prolonged hyperparathyroidism. Oral supplements are often required. In patients with severe symptomatic hypocalcaemia, intravenous replacement is occasionally necessary.

Adrenal glands

Embryology and anatomy

The adrenal glands are in close proximity to the upper pole of each kidney. In the adult each gland weighs about 5 g. Embryologically, the adrenal medulla develops from the neural crest. The medulla secretes adrenalin and noradrenalin, and is macroscopically distinct from the cortex. The three layers of the cortex develop from mesothelium and can be distinguished microscopically: the zona reticularis is nearest the medulla and secretes androgens; the zona fasciculata secretes glucocorticoids; the outermost layer, the zona glomerulosa, secretes mineralocorticoids.

Disorders of the adrenal glands

Referrals to endocrine surgery usually follow the discovery of an adrenal mass on cross-sectional imaging (the so-called 'incidentaloma') or diagnosis of hypersecretion of an adrenal hormone. Smaller numbers of patients are referred for consideration of adrenalectomy for isolated metastatic disease. Even in patients where the suspicion of metastatic disease is high, investigation of an unexpected adrenal mass aims to determine whether it is hyperfunctional, as well as whether or not it is malignant. Sometimes hypersecretion is subclinical but appropriate biochemical tests should determine if there is excess secretion of corticosteroids (a cause of Cushing's syndrome), aldosterone (Conn's syndrome), or catecholamines (phaeochromocytoma).

The risk of malignancy increases as these tumours enlarge, and continued enlargement itself may be a sign of malignancy. The rate of malignancy in adrenal tumours >6 cm in size is 15%. The finding of carcinoma in non-functional incidentalomas <4 cm is very rare. If a non-functional adrenal adenoma is 4 cm or greater, consideration should be given to adrenalectomy. If the adenoma is <4 cm re-evaluation with further imaging and biochemistry after 6 months then annually for 2 years is appropriate. Surgery is re-considered if the adenoma becomes hormonally active or if there is growth greater or equal to 1 cm.

The incidentaloma

For the approximate frequencies of the most common types of incidentaloma please see Table 2.14.1.1.

Haemorrhage into one or both adrenal glands has a variable appearance on CT depending on the time since the bleed. The history may be suggestive and the mass should reduce in size on serial CT scans. If a myolipoma or small benign cyst can be diagnosed with reasonable certainty resection is not required.

Adrenal myolipomas consist of fat and mature myeloid tissue in varying proportions. If there is a high fat content then diagnosis on CT or MRI is usually sufficient. It can be harder to distinguish from an adenoma if there is very little fat. Surgery is reserved for cases of doubt and those large enough to be symptomatic.

Simple adrenal cysts have a smooth, thin wall. On CT the contents are homogeneous and have the density of water. Ultrasound will confirm their cystic nature. Septation, variable wall thickness,

Table 2.14.1.1 Approximate frequencies of the most common types of incidentalomas[10]

Non-functioning adenoma	80%
Cushing's syndrome (subclinical)	5%
Phaeochromocytoma	5%
Hyperaldosteronism	1%
Adrenocortical carcinoma	<5%
Metastatic carcinoma	2.5%
Myolipomas, ganglioneuromas, and benign cysts, and haemorrhage make up the rest	

Reprinted from *Endocrine Practice*, Volume 15, #5; Author(s): Zeiger MA, Thompson GB, Duh QY, Hamrahian AH, Angelos P, Elaraj D; Title of Article: The American Association of Clinical Endocrinologists and American Association of Endocrine Surgeons Medical Guidelines for the Management of Adrenal Incidentalomas: Executive Summary of Recommendations; pages 1–20; Copyright ©2009, with permission from the American Association of Clinical Endocrinologists.

or a soft tissue component will raise suspicion of carcinoma. Larger symptomatic cysts may require surgery.

Adrenocortical carcinomas are rare, accounting for 0.02% of all cancers, but make up 1–5% of incidental adrenal lesions. Only about 50% of adrenocortical carcinomas are functional, most often secreting cortisol, but androgens are sometimes secreted causing virilization in female patients.[11]

Surgery offers the only potentially curative treatment for adrenocortical carcinoma. Incomplete resection is usually followed by rapid regrowth of the tumour. Some patients benefit from mitotane alone or in combination with other agents, but the results of chemotherapy are often disappointing.

Functional adenomas

Cushing's syndrome and Cushing's disease

The signs and symptoms of Cushing's syndrome are due to prolonged exposure to inappropriately high circulating cortisol levels. Cushing's disease is a term used only when excess cortisol is as a consequence of excess adrenocorticotrophic hormone (ACTH) production in the pituitary. Bilateral adrenalectomy is occasionally a treatment for Cushing's disease when pituitary interventions (surgery and or radiotherapy) have failed. In such patients continued enlargement of the pituitary and excess ACTH secretion (and melanocyte stimulating hormone from the same precursor peptide) can cause Nelson's syndrome with skin hyperpigmentation.

Ectopic ACTH secretion from tumours outside the pituitary can cause Cushing's syndrome. Exogenous steroids can produce the same symptoms and signs along with a 'Cushingoid' appearance.

In patients with established Cushing's syndrome due to an adrenal adenoma, surgery is usually the best form of treatment. In patients with subclinical Cushing's and an adenoma of <4 cm, surgery may be reserved for those with another indication such as abnormal glucose tolerance, osteoporosis, or hyperlipidaemia. After adrenalectomy for Cushing's, a period of steroid supplementation is often required and some patients need longer-term steroid replacement.

Conn's syndrome

The classic presentation of hyperaldosteronism is hypertension with unexplained hypokalaemia. Confirmation is made by measuring renin and aldosterone levels. Selective venous sampling will confirm which adrenal is responsible. Care should be taken to avoid surgery for a co-incidental non-functional adenoma in patients whose Conn's syndrome is due to bilateral nodular hyperplasia.

End organ damage from prolonged hypertension may not recover after adrenalectomy and many patients still require medication for ongoing hypertension, though management is easier.

Phaeochromocytoma

The prevalence of phaeochromocytoma is <1% and it is diagnosed in <1% of hypertensive patients. Most patients have symptoms such as palpitations and anxiety, but these can be absent and not all patients are hypertensive. There is a significant risk of sudden death in patients with undiagnosed and untreated phaeochromocytoma, especially during general anaesthesia or invasive procedures. All patients with an adrenal mass must be screened for phaeochromocytoma.

Diagnosis is usually confirmed by measuring 24-hour urinary fractionated metanephrines. If there is doubt, serum metanephrines can be measured in the resting patient. Adrenal phaeochromocytomas secrete predominantly noradrenalin with variable amounts of adrenalin or dopamine, and rarely ACTH. MIBG scans are normally performed after diagnosis to exclude metastatic or multiple phaeochromocytomas or paragangliomas, especially in patients with an inherited susceptibility.

About 90% of phaeochromocytomas are benign. Even in patients with metastases, surgery may play a role in symptom management.

Surgical approaches to the adrenal gland and preparation for theatre

There are a variety of approaches to the adrenal gland, both open and laparoscopic. Choice of approach should be determined by the characteristics of the patient and tumour, and referrals made to specialized teams of surgeons, endocrinologists, and anaesthetists.

Preoperative preparation of patients with functional tumours
Phaeochromocytoma

Patients should be rendered normotensive and normovolaemic. A useful regime has been published by the Society for Endocrinology.[12] An alpha-blocker is the initial treatment; beta-blockers are only required if the patient remains tachycardic.

Conn's syndrome

Treatment of hypertension should be optimized preoperatively and potassium deficiency corrected.

Cushing's syndrome

It is important to ensure optimize treatment of blood pressure and diabetes mellitus if present. Sometimes mitotane, which blocks cortisol synthesis, is necessary. Steroid replacement in the perioperative period allays concern about steroid deficiency due to suppression of the other adrenal.

Adrenal surgery
Open adrenalectomy

There are four approaches to open adrenalectomy: transabdominal, lateral, posterior, and thoraco-abdominal.

Transabdominal

This approach uses midline, subcostal, or bilateral subcostal incisions. It allows good access to both adrenal glands if necessary, plus extra-adrenal disease, adjacent organs, and synchronous pathology. The aorta and vena cava are accessible if needed for vascular control. It is a good option for adrenocortical carcinoma if resection of adjacent organs is required. The disadvantages include postoperative pain and higher morbidity. It is not the best approach for smaller benign tumours.

Lateral

An incision is made through the flank, as for a retroperitoneal nephrectomy. It gives better exposure than the posterior retroperitoneal approach but similar postoperative pain to the anterior approach. Bilateral surgery requires re-positioning.

Posterior

The posterior approach requires a smaller incision than the lateral approach, and is associated with less pain. Both adrenal glands are accessible through separate incisions but without re-positioning. It gives limited exposure so can be a disadvantage for larger tumours, especially when malignancy is suspected.

Thoraco-abdominal

This allows for maximum exposure but has greater morbidity. It is reserved for very large adrenal glands that cannot be safely approached by other routes and adrenal cortical carcinoma where resection of adjacent structures is required. It allows access to pulmonary metastases from phaeochromocytoma if they are on the same side. The more laterally the patient is positioned, the more difficult access is to the rest of the abdomen and the other adrenal gland.

Laparoscopic adrenalectomy

Laparoscopic adrenalectomy is appropriate for the majority of tumours. Opinion is divided on whether the approach is safe in adrenal cancer, with breaching of the tumour capsule and seeding quoted as particular risks. Other disadvantages include specific complications of laparoscopic surgery such as trochar injuries. Laparoscopic adrenalectomy can be transabdominal or retroperitoneoscopic.

Transabdominal

This is commonly performed with the patient in the lateral position. Re-positioning is required for access to the other adrenal.

Retroperitoneoscopic

If difficulty is encountered this approach can be converted to open for better access. It is best suited to small tumours and has the advantage that both adrenals can be accessed through separate approaches without re-positioning.

Pituitary

Anatomy and physiology of the anterior and posterior pituitary

The pituitary gland is not part of the brain but sits at the base, enclosed in a bony cavity, the sella turcica, covered superiorly by a fold of dura mater, the diaphragma sellae. The pituitary is connected to the hypothalamus by the pituitary stalk.

The pituitary is divided into two parts: the anterior pituitary (around 80%) (adenohypophysis) and posterior pituitary (neurohypophysis). The anterior pituitary arises from Rathke's pouch, an epithelial outgrowth from the pharynx. The posterior

Table 2.14.1.2 Hormones secreted by the anterior pituitary

Hormone released from the anterior pituitary	Neurohormone controlling release from hypothalamus
Thyroid-stimulating hormone	Thyrotropin-releasing hormone
Growth hormone	Growth hormone releasing hormone: stimulatory
	Somatostatin: inhibitory
Adrenocorticotrophic hormone	Corticotropin releasing hormone
β-Endorphin	Corticotropin releasing hormone
Luteinizing hormone	Gonadotropin releasing hormone
Follicle stimulating hormone	Gonadotropin releasing hormone
Prolactin	Prolactin-inhibiting factor

pituitary develops from neuroectoderm, as an extension of the hypothalamus.

The anterior pituitary synthesizes a range of hormones whose release is under the control of the neurohormones secreted from the hypothalamus; these reach the anterior pituitary by a portal venous system within the pituitary stalk (see Table 2.14.1.2).

The posterior pituitary does not synthesize hormones, but stores hormones produced in the supraoptic and paraventricular nuclei of the hypothalamus. The hormones are passed down axons in the pituitary stalk to terminal axons in the posterior pituitary, before being released into the blood. The posterior pituitary releases oxytocin and anti-diuretic hormone (vasopressin).

Anterior pituitary adenomas

The majority of pituitary adenomas are small (<10 mm) and termed microadenomas. Functional tumours often present while very small, due to the excess hormones. Adenomas >10 mm (i.e. macroadenomas) may present later if they are non-functional. Expanding adenomas can compress or herniate through the diaphragma sellae, compressing the optic nerve and causing visual defects.

Functional pituitary adenomas

There are three endocrine syndromes caused by functional pituitary adenomas that are surgically relevant: hyperprolactinaemia, Cushing's disease, and acromegaly.

Hyperprolactinaemia

Prolactin-secreting adenomas (prolactinomas) are the most common functional pituitary tumours, comprising 40% of all pituitary tumours.

Prolactinomas are more common in women and the majority present with galactorrhoea and amenorrhoea. In men the main features are gynaecomastia and impotence. The diagnosis is more obvious in women and is often made earlier.

Hyperprolactinaemia is diagnosed biochemically. Other causes of hyperprolactinaemia should always be considered, including pregnancy, medications, hypothyroidism (due to high TRH levels), chronic liver or kidney disease, and sarcoidosis.

MRI scanning is the most sensitive imaging method to assess the presence and size of a pituitary adenoma. Dopamine agonists, principally bromocriptine and cabergoline, are the medications of choice. They prevent the synthesis and secretion of prolactin and shrink the size of prolactinomas. Patients are considered for transsphenoidal surgery if they struggle with long-term medication, progress despite medical treatment, or prefer a surgical option.

Cushing's disease

Cushing's syndrome is covered in more detail in the adrenal section of this chapter. The key treatment for Cushing's disease is transsphenoidal surgery to remove the adenoma but leave functional pituitary tissue. Radiotherapy has a role, especially for relapsed disease after pituitary surgery.

Medications that inhibit steroid synthesis, including mitotane, ketoconazloe, metyrapone, and aminoglutethimide, are used for symptom control prior to surgery or after unsuccessful surgery. Bilateral adrenalectomy may also be considered.

Acromegaly

This is caused by excess growth hormone (GH) production by a pituitary adenoma, usually in middle-aged adults. It has an insidious onset and diagnosis is often delayed by several years. Characteristic features are soft tissue swelling, chiefly of the face, feet, and hands, with general thickening of the skin. Patients have a classically protruding lower jaw and pronounced brow with sweating. Hypertension, cardiovascular disease, and glucose intolerance or diabetes develop. Headaches and visual field defects can result from external compression by the adenoma.

The aim of treatment is to reduce GH levels and compressive effects. Usually a several treatments are required, with transsphenoidal surgery being the first choice. Patients should be warned that surgery may not be curative and further treatment may be necessary. Medical treatments consist of somatostatins (e.g. octreotide), dopamine agonists, and GH receptor antagonists. Radiation is used for refractory tumours but takes up to 10 years to work and can induce hypopituitarism.

Pituitary incidentalomas

Non-functional microadenomas, often found during CT or MRI scans for other conditions, are called incidentalomas. All patients should be checked for hormone hypersecretion or hypopituitarism. Visual field testing is recommended in incidentalomas close to the optic nerve or optic chiasm. Patients should be followed up clinically and radiologically to ensure there is no increase in size.

Familial endocrine syndromes

Multiple endocrine neoplasia (MEN) syndromes

MEN syndromes are inherited in an autosomal dominant fashion, with unpredictable penetrance and expression. They are characterized by benign or malignant tumours in multiple endocrine glands.[13]

Multiple endocrine neoplasia 1 (MEN1)

MEN1 should be considered in patients presenting with two endocrine tumours in the parathyroid, pancreas, and pituitary. Patients with a first-degree relative with MEN1 should have the diagnosis considered if a single endocrine tumour arises.

Patients with MEN1 have a heterozygous mutation of the MEN1 tumour suppressor gene. A further spontaneous mutation allows tumours to develop.

Tumours or hyperplasia typically occur in the parathyroid glands, pituitary gland, and islet cells of the pancreas. MEN1 is also associated with benign cutaneous tumours, including lipomas, angiofibromas, and collagenomas, carcinoid tumours of the lungs or gastrointestinal tract, and non-functional thyroid and adrenal tumours.

The most common clinical presentation is hypercalcaemia due to hyperparathyroidism. All four glands are usually hyperplastic, with asymmetric enlargement. Following a subtotal parathyroidectomy there is a high incidence of recurrence.

The majority of pituitary tumours are prolactinomas. These should be diagnosed and treated as discussed in the Pituitary section (p.36).

Generally, pancreatic tumours are non-functional and clinically silent. The most common functional tumours are gastrinomas and insulinomas. Approximately 20–30% of patients with a gastrinoma (Zollinger-Ellison Syndrome) have MEN1. Gastrinomas are gastrin-secreting tumours that are usually in the pancreas, but can be in the stomach or duodenum. Increased gastrin levels cause excess acid production, resulting in peptic ulceration and severe diarrhoea.

About 50–60% of gastrinomas are malignant and even small tumours can have lymph node metastases. Multicentric tumours are common and at diagnosis 50% patients have liver metastases. Diagnosis is made biochemically with a high fasting serum gastrin concentration (in the absence of other causes such as proton pump inhibitors). Treatment consists of acid suppression and surgery.

In contrast to gastrinomas, over 90% of insulinomas are within the pancreas and are usually solitary, benign tumours. They are typically very small (<2 cm) and can be difficult to localize. Excess insulin production causes symptoms of hypoglycaemia, often during the early morning. Up to 10% of patients with insulinomas have MEN1.

A biochemical diagnosis is made by a supervised 72-hour fast, with measurement of serum insulin, glucose, and C-peptide levels. Clinically symptoms usually appear within 24 hours when the blood glucose level drops below 2.5 mmol/L. The mainstay of treatment is surgery, although symptoms may be controlled medically with frequent feeds and diazoxide, which prevents insulin release. Surgical options include enucleation of the tumour or distal pancreatectomy if the lesion is in the tail of the pancreas. Laparoscopic surgery is offered in some centres.

Multiple endocrine neoplasia 2 (MEN2)

MEN2 is caused by a background heterozygous mutation in the RET proto-oncogene, before a second additional mutation. It is subdivided into MEN2A, MEN2B, and familial MTC (FMTC). MEN2B is the most aggressive form.

MEN2A is associated with MTC (over 90% patients), phaeochromocytomas (50–60%), and hyperparathyroidism (20–30%). MEN2B is associated with MTC, phaeochromocytomas, a marfinoid habitus, and mucosal and digestive neurofibromatosis. FMTC is a variant of MEN2. It is due to mutations in the RET proto-oncogene, but has no other detectable features of MEN2.

All three types of MEN2 have a high risk of developing MTC, although the age of onset varies. MTC generally occurs during early childhood in MEN2B, early adulthood in MEN2A, and middle age in FMTC. In families with a diagnosis of MEN2, genetic screening is offered for potentially affected children. A prophylactic total thyroidectomy in childhood can prevent MTC becoming clinically relevant.

Once MEN2 is diagnosed, patients are screened from childhood. In patients with MEN2A and MEN2B, catecholamines and catecholamine metabolites are checked annually, plus calcium and PTH levels in MEN2A patients.

Inherited conditions associated with phaeochromocytomas

Other autosomal dominant familial conditions associated with phaeochromocytomas include von Hippel-Lindau disease (VHL), neurofibromatosis type 1 (NF1), and familial paraganglioma syndromes.

von Hippel-Lindau disease (vHL)

This is a rare disease caused by mutations of the vHL tumour suppressor gene. It predisposes patients to multiple benign and malignant tumours. The most common tumours are haemangioblastomas, generally retinal, cerebellar, brainstem and spinal cord, in up to 75% of patients. Other frequent tumours found in 10–20% patients include renal cell carcinomas or cysts, pancreatic tumours or cysts, and phaeochromocytomas.

Phaeochromocytomas in vHL are typically less symptomatic than in MEN2 and predominantly secrete norepinephrine.

Neurofibromatosis type 1

NF1, also called von Recklinghausen disease, is due to a mutation of the NF1 tumour suppressor gene. About 50% of cases are inherited in an autosomal dominant pattern, the rest are spontaneous mutations.

There are strict criteria for the diagnosis of NF1.[14] Patients require two or more of the following symptoms:

- six or more *café au lait* spots
- axillary or inguinal freckling
- two or more neurofibromas or one plexiform neurofibroma
- optic glioma
- two or more Lisch nodules (iris hamartomas)
- an osseous lesion: kyphoscoliosis, sphenoid dysplasia, thinning of long bone cortex or pseudoarthritis
- first-degree relative with NF1.

Phaeochromocytomas are rare in NF1, seen in 1% patients. However 20–50% of NF1 patients with hypertension have a phaeochromocytoma, compared to 0.1% of the general population with hypertension.[15]

Familial paraganglioma syndromes

Phaeochromocytomas and paragangliomas are rare and caused by mutations in the succinate dehydrogenase (SDH) genes. There are three types: SDHB, SDHC, and SDHD. Tumours develop in paraganglioma tissue anywhere from the head and neck to the thorax, abdomen, and pelvis.

Not all paragangliomas secrete catecholamines. Only 5% in the head and neck are secretory, whereas virtually all abdominal paragangliomas are functional. SDHB mutations are often associated with intrathoracic or intra-abdominal tumours, with a higher chance of malignancy. SDHC mutations are most commonly linked with non-functioning head and neck tumours. SDHD mutations predispose to multifocal tumours, which can manifest anywhere.[16]

Non-medullary familial thyroid cancer

About 3–6% of non-medullary thyroid cancers are familial, principally PTC and FTC. Familial cancers are often more aggressive, bilateral, occur in younger patients, and can have mixed PTC and FTC features.

Non-medullary familial thyroid cancer is associated with other autosomal dominant tumour syndromes; including familial adenomatous polyposis (FAP), Cowden syndrome, Carney complex, and familial paraganglioma syndromes.

FAP is due to an *APC* gene mutation and is associated with PTC, generally in young women. Cowden syndrome is linked with a *PTEN* gene mutation, causing multiple hamartomas and an increased risk of breast, thyroid, and endometrial cancer. Carney complex is very rare and due to a *PRKAR1A* gene mutation. It predisposes individuals to cardiac and skin myxomas, endocrine tumours, and unusual skin pigmentation.

Further reading

Clark O, Duh Q-Y, Kebebew E. *Textbook of Endocrine Surgery* (2nd ed). London: Elsevier, 2005/
Hay ID, Wass JAH (eds). *Clinical Endocrine Oncology* (2nd ed). Oxford: Wiley, 2008.

References

1. Cooper DS, Doherty GM, Haugen BR, et al. Revised American Thyroid Association management guidelines for patients with thyroid nodules and differentiated thyroid cancer. *Thyroid* 2009; 19(11): 1167–214.
2. Holmes JD. Neck dissection: nomenclature, classification, and technique. *Oral Maxillofac Surg Clin North Am* 2008; 20(3): 459–75.
3. Perros P. Guidelines for the management of thyroid cancer. London: British Thyroid Association, Royal College of Physicians. Available from: www.british-thyroid-association.org.
4. Hayward NJ, Grodski S, Yeung M, et al. Recurrent laryngeal nerve injury in thyroid surgery: a review. *ANZ J Surg.* 2013; 83(1–2): 15–21.
5. Khan MI, Waguespack SG, Hu MI. Medical management of postsurgical hypoparathyroidism. *Endocr Pract* 2011; 6: 1–19.
6. Marcocci C, Cetani F. Clinical practice. Primary hyperparathyroidism. *N Engl J Med* 2011; 365(25): 2389–97.
7. Mihai R, Simon D, Hellman P. Imaging for primary hyperparathyroidism: An evidence-based analysis. *Langenbecks Arch Surg* 2009; 394(5): 765–84.
8. Mihai R, Barczynski M, Iacobone M, et al. Surgical strategy for sporadic primary hyperparathyroidism an evidence-based approach to surgical strategy, patient selection, surgical access, and reoperations. *Langenbecks Arch Surg* 2009; 394(5): 785–98.
9. Giusti F, Cavalli L, Cavalli T, et al. Hereditary hyperparathyroidism syndromes. *J Clin Densitom* 2013; 16(1): 69–74.
10. Zeiger MA, Thompson GB, Duh QY, et al. The American Association of Clinical Endocrinologists and American Association of Endocrine Surgeons medical guidelines for the management of adrenal incidentalomas. *Endocr Pract* 2009; 15(Suppl 1): 1–20.
11. Henley DJ, van Heerden JA, Grant CS, et al. Adrenal cortical carcinoma—a continuing challenge. *Surgery* 1983; 94(6): 926–31.
12. Society for Endocrinology. *Protocol using oral phenoxybenzamine to prepare patients with catecholaminesecreting phaeochromocytoma and paraganglioma for surgery.* http://www.endocrinology.org/policy/docs/10-10_Protocol_using_oral_phenoxybenzamine.pdf (accessed 06/05/2013).
13. Callender GG, Rich TA, Perrier ND. Multiple endocrine neoplasia syndromes. *Surg Clin North Am* 2008; 88(4): 863–95, viii.
14. National Institutes of Health Consensus Development Conference Statement: neurofibromatosis. Bethesda, MD, USA, July 13–15, 1987. *Neurofibromatosis* 1988; 1(3): 172–8.
15. Zografos GN, Vasiliadis GK, Zagouri F, et al. Pheochromocytoma associated with neurofibromatosis type 1: concepts and current trends. *World J Surg Oncol* 2010; 8: 14.
16. Young WF Jr, Abboud AL. Editorial: paraganglioma—all in the family. *J Clin Endocrinol Metab* 2006; 91(3): 790–2.

PART 2.15

Surgical oncology

CHAPTER 2.15.1

Cancer screening

Paul Sutton, Declan Dunne,
Anita Hargreaves, and Graeme J. Poston

Introduction

Cancer screening has increased over recent decades, and most countries with an established health service now offer screening for cervical, breast, and colorectal cancer.

The premise on which cancer screening is employed is that early detection is commensurate with better survival. This seemingly logical argument has led to widespread adoption of screening tests. It is important that the distinction between screening participants and patients is understood (i.e. participants in screening programmes are healthy individuals and subjecting them to investigation can be associated with both physical and psychological harm).

It is clear therefore that clinicians should have an understanding of cancer screening, including the history of its inception and the evidence upon which it is based, and be able to apply these to both populations as well as individual patients.

Principles of screening tests

A screening test is one that is applied to asymptomatic individuals that allows for early detection, therapeutic intervention, and decreased mortality from the disease which is being screened. Screening may be offered to a whole population, or targeted to those individuals deemed high risk on the basis of a set of criteria. In 1968 the World Health Organization published guidance on the development and adoption of screening tests:[1]

1. The condition should be an important health problem.

2. There should be a treatment for the condition.

3. Facilities for diagnosis and treatment should be available.

4. There should be a latent stage of the disease.

5. There should be a test or examination for the condition.

6. The test should be acceptable to the population.

7. The natural history of the disease should be adequately understood.

8. There should be an agreed policy on whom to treat.

9. The total cost of finding a case should be economically balanced in relation to medical expenditure as a whole.

10. Case-finding should be a continuous process, not just a 'once and for all' project.

Reproduced with permission from Jungner Wilson, Principles and practice of screening for disease, *Public Health Papers*, Number 34, Copyright © The World Health Organization 1978.

These principles were formative in the development of today's three key cancer screening programmes: cervical cancer, breast cancer, and, latterly, colorectal cancer.

Screening for cervical cancer

Cancer of the uterine cervix is the third most common cancer in women worldwide (11th most common in the United Kingdom), accounting for 9.8% of all new cancers.[2] The geographical distribution is uneven, with a greater incidence in developing countries. A marked reduction in incidence has been reported in developed countries following the introduction of widespread screening and early treatment. Two primary histological abnormalities account for the majority of cancers of the uterine cervix: squamous cell carcinoma (70%) and adenocarcinoma (30%). Squamous cell carcinoma arises from the transformation zone (squamo-columnar junction) and adenocarcinoma develops from the mucus producing cells of the endocervix.

Development of cervical cancer screening

Cervical cancer has precancerous changes defined as cervical intraepithelial neoplasia (CIN) grades 1–3 and carcinoma *in situ*. There is a 30% risk of subsequent invasion over a 5 to 10 year period. Cervical cancer is mainly secondary to chronic infection with strains of the human papilloma virus (HPV).

In 1941, Papanicolou and Trout introduced a simple and inexpensive method for diagnosing cervical cancer, the cytology smear. There was no evidence for this, yet experience yielded a high percentage of correct diagnoses. No randomized controlled trials (RCTs) have been performed; it was presumed that early detection of invasive disease would decrease cancer mortality and detection of pre-invasive lesions would decrease incidence.

The most convincing evidence to support widespread screening followed the introduction of screening programmes in Finland, Iceland, Sweden, and parts of Denmark and Norway in the 1970s. Declining trends in cervical cancer incidence and mortality were clearly observed.[3]

Following the formal establishment of the UK cervical cancer screening programme in 1988, there has been a significant decline in the incidence of the disease. In 1988 there were 4132 cases diagnosed in England (age standardized incidence rate of 16.2 per 100 000 population [CI 15.7–16.7]) and in 2008, 2369 cases were diagnosed (age standardized incidence rate of 8.3 per 100 000 population [CI 8.0–8.7]).[4]

While the results of the programme have largely been regarded as a success, there are a number of frequently encountered problems:

1. Inadequate sampling leading to an inability to confidently reach a diagnosis.

2. False negatives: inflammatory cells mask the presence of premalignant cells.

3. False positives: cytological changes induced by infection or hormones may be misinterpreted as premalignant or malignant.

4. Unnecessary treatment of premalignant lesions can lead to long-term complications—cervical stenosis, premature rupture of membranes and preterm delivery.

Controversies with cervical screening

Screening intervals

There are no RCTs to support the currently used screening interval. Evidence is based on modelling studies, which identified no significant difference in outcomes for screening at 2-year or 3-year intervals.[5] Women aged 30–65 years who are low risk and have had negative cytology can have an extended screening interval of 5 years.[6] Current UK screening is undertaken at 3-yearly intervals from 25 to 49 years and 5-yearly from 50 to 64 years.

Screening age

In 2003 the NHS raised the screening age to 25 years. This followed a study that demonstrated that screening older women led to a substantial reduction in cervical cancer, but screening women aged 20 to 24 had no impact on the rates of invasive cervical cancer at ages 25 to 29.[7] Following the change in screening age, the UK has seen a small rise in the incidence of cervical cancer within the younger age group. There has also been a significant rise in the incidence of sexually transmitted infection within the same time frame.

Liquid-based cytology

A recent RCT failed to demonstrate any difference in relative detection or absolute sensitivity or specificity for detection of CIN grades 2–3 between liquid-based cytology and conventional cytology. However, there was a lower proportion of unsatisfactory slides with liquid-based cytology.[8]

Human papilloma virus

HPV DNA was reported in most cervical cancer cells in the 1980s. Subsequent detection in virtually all samples of tumour tissue (99.7%) led to the conclusion that persistent HPV infection was a key risk factor in the development of cervical neoplasia. HPV testing as a primary screening tool has a higher sensitivity for CIN than cytology (96% versus 53% for CIN grade 3) but a lower specificity for younger women who have transient infection.[9]

The 'ARTISTIC UK' RCT evaluated cervical cytology versus cervical cytology and HPV testing over three screening rounds identifying prevalent and then incident and undetected disease. Routine primary HPV testing alone was found to be highly effective with a high negative predictive value.[10] This has led to six pilot centres within the UK trialing the use of HPV as a primary screening tool.

Screening for breast cancer

Worldwide the incidence of breast cancer is increasing. With over 1 million new diagnoses per year it is the most common cause of cancer-related death in women (15% of UK female cancer deaths).

Ninety-five per cent of breast cancers are sporadic and relate to environmental factors (early menarche, late menopause, prolonged use of the oral contraceptive pill/hormone replacement therapy, nulliparity, and obesity).

The prognosis of breast cancer is highly dependent upon primary tumour size, histological grade, and regional lymph node metastases. The current 5-year survival figures for breast cancer are: 98.6% for local disease, 83.8% for regional disease, and 23.3% for distant disease.[4] The presence of a preclinical detectable phase, which may also be pre-invasive, makes early detection through screening effective.

The ability of screening to advance diagnostic time is determined by the duration of the preclinical detectable phase and the sensitivity and specificity of the screening test. Reduction in mortality should be the primary end point of screening; however, decreased disease-specific incidence (following detection of pre-invasive disease) is an indicator of the efficacy of screening. We should not forget the secondary benefits of reduced surgical morbidity and a reduction in the need for adjuvant therapy. Assessing mortality rather than survival in screening studies helps to control bias. Screen-detected breast cancer advances the diagnosis by 2 to 3 years, thus survival will always be longer even if the disease course is unaffected by detection and treatment (lead time bias). Screening is more likely to detect pre-invasive or slowly progressing tumours as these will have a longer sojourn time. This is more pronounced in the prevalent (first) screening round.[11]

The evidence for breast cancer screening

Since 1963, a number of RCTs have been conducted on mammographic screening. The earliest RCT was the Health Insurance Plan and recently the Age Trial was launched to review the benefit of screening women from 40–50 years. The Swedish Two-County trial has the longest follow up of 29 years and consistently demonstrates a 29% reduction in long-term breast cancer mortality among women invited to screening.[12] A summary of the characteristics of these studies can be found in the Table 2.15.1.1.

The aim of all trials has been to assess the effect of offering screening to women rather than the effect among those who actually underwent screening (i.e. an intention to treat approach). Non-attenders have a greater than average risk of dying from breast cancer. All the studies involved mammography; however, variation in study protocol was observed in the number of views performed, whether films were dual read, the interval timing, and the screening of the control group.

Breast cancer screening in the United Kingdom

In the UK the Forrest Report published in 1986 led to the development of the NHS Breast Screening Programme. Initially women aged 50 to 64 years were invited to screening every 3 years with single craniocaudal view mammography. There has been significant change within the programme including the introduction of two view mammography (craniocaudal and mediolateral oblique) initially within the prevalent round. By 2007 there was extension to nine rounds of screening. From 2011, digital mammography has been introduced. The sensitivity of screening mammography is 83–95% (lower in younger patients and those with dense breast tissue) with a specificity of 90–98%. The risk of a false positive result is 10% within the prevalent round and 13% in subsequent rounds. The positive predictive value is 13.6% in the prevalent round (detection

Table 2.15.1.1 Characteristics of randomized controlled trials to investigate the efficacy of breast cancer screening[12–16]

Study	Age at entry	Randomization	Screening modality	Screening interval	Screening sample	Control sample	Attendance first round	RR node positive cancer	RR mortality
Swedish Two County[12]	40–74	Cluster	MMG (1)	24–33	65518		85%	0.69	
Health Insurance Plan 1963[13]	40–64	Individual	MMG (2) and CBE	12	30239	30756	67%	0.85	.078
WE 1977	40–74	Cluster geographic	MMG (1)	24–33	78085	56782	89%		
Malmo 1976	45–69	Individual	M MG (2)	18–24	21088	21195	74%	0.83	0.78
Stockholm 1981	40–64	Cluster birth cohort	MMG (1)	28	39164	19943	87%	0.82	0.90
Edinburgh 1979[14]	45–64	Cluster GP registers	MMG (2) and CBE	12–24	23226	21904	61%	0.81	0.78
Canada 1[15]	40–49	Individual	MMG (2) and CBE	12	25214	25216	100%		
Gothenburg 1982[16]	40–59	Individual < 50 Cluster > 50	MMG (2)	18	20724	28809	84%	0.80	0.79
NBSS 1 and 2	50–59	Individual	MMG (2) and CBE	12	19711	19694	100%	NBSS 1 1.20 NBSS 2 1.09	NBSS 1 0.97 NBSS 2 1.02
UK Age	40–48	Individual	MMG (2)	12	43709		81%	0.89	0.83

MMG, mammogram; CBE, clinical breast examination; RR, relative risk.

Source: data from Tabar L *et al.*, Swedish Two county trial: Impact of mammographic screening in breast cancer during 3 decades, *Radiology*, Volume 260, pp. 658–63, Copyright © 2011 (12); Shapiro S *et al.*, Periodic screening for Breast cancer: The Health Insurance Plan project and its sequelae 1963–1986, The John Hopkins University Press, Maryland, USA, Copyright © 1988 (13); Alexander FE *et al.*, The Edinburgh randomized trial of breast cancer screening: results after 10 years of follow-up, *British Journal of Cancer*, Volume 70, pp. 547–8, Copyright © 1994 (14); Miller AB *et al.*, The Canadian National Breast Screening Study: update on breast cancer mortality, *Monographs of the National Cancer Institute*, Volume 22, pp. 37–41, Copyright © 1997 (15); and Bjurstam N *et al.*, The Gothenburg Breast Screening Trial: the first result on mortality, incidence and mode of detection for women ages 39–49 years at randomization, *Cancer*, Volume 80, pp. 2091–9, Copyright © 1997 (16).

rate 10.1 per 1000 population screened) and 15% in subsequent rounds (detection rate 5.4 per 1000 population screened).[17]

International breast cancer screening programmes

There is considerable variation in international breast screening practice which is summarized within Table 2.15.1.2.[18]

Controversies in breast cancer screening

There are a number of clear benefits to breast cancer screening, most obviously the reduction in breast cancer mortality and an increase in breast conserving surgery. These benefits however must be viewed in light of the drawbacks of the screening programme:

1. Patients spend more years as a cancer patient, with the psychological morbidity associated with this.

2. There are both false positive and false negative rates. The false positive rate is approximately 0.7–6.6% in the first round of screening and 0.5–5.2 % in subsequent rounds. It is not feasible to directly measure false negative rates, however a surrogate marker is the interval cancer rate which stands at 24%.

3. Given that there is currently no way to determine which *in situ* carcinoma will progress during a patient's lifetime, there is a potential to 'overtreat' carcinoma *in situ*.[19] However, screen-detected ductal carcinoma *in situ* managed by wide local excision is associated with a 10% 10-year risk for the development of invasive breast cancer.

4. Low-dose radiation exposure associated with annual screening from 50 years of age induces 15/100 000 cases of breast cancer for every 1500 lives saved.

5. The age of 50 is an arbitrary pseudo-marker of menopause and does not reflect the physiological changes in breast density or the apparent mortality reduction for women screened in a younger age group.[20]

Screening for colorectal cancer

Colorectal cancer is the second most common cause of cancer-related death in the UK, with more than 15 700 deaths per annum in the UK alone. The overall 5-year survival is 55%; however, detection of the disease at its earliest stage (Dukes A) is associated with a 5-year survival of greater than 90%.[4] A number of bowel cancer screening programmes have been developed, including in the USA, UK, Germany, and the Netherlands.[21–23]

UK national bowel cancer screening programme

The UK bowel cancer screening programme was introduced in 2006 and was fully operational by 2010.[21] The programme utilizes faecal occult blood testing in participants from the age of 60 onwards to identify those at higher risk of intestinal polyps and malignancy with a view to selective endoscopic investigation with colonoscopy. The aim of this screening programme is twofold: Firstly it aims to identify and manage adenomatous polyps with a view to reducing colorectal cancer incidence. Secondly it should identify those patients with colorectal cancer at an early stage of the disease to allow curative treatment, thus reducing cancer deaths.

Initial results of UK screening

After over 1 million screening tests uptake was in the order of 53%, with abnormal faecal occult blood detected in 2% of participants.

Table 2.15.1.2 International breast screening programmes

Country	Year commenced	Detection method used	Age groups	Interval of mammography 40–49	50+	Number screened	Participation
Australia	1991	MM/DM	40–75+	2 yrs	2 yrs		
Canada	1988	MM/DM/CBE	50–69	1 yr	2 yrs	196 187	47.3%
China	2009	MM/CBE/USS	40–59	3 yrs	3 yrs	1 200 000	
Denmark	1991	DM	50–59		2 yrs	275 000	73%
Finland	1987	DM	50–64		2 yrs		85%
France	1989	MM/DM/CBE	50–74		2 yrs	2 34 980	52.3%
Iceland	1987	DM/CBE	40–69	2 yrs	2 yrs	20 517	60%
Israel	1997	MM/DM	50–74		2 yrs	220 000	72%
Italy	2002	MM/DM	50–69		2 yrs	1 340 311	60.5%
Japan	1977	MM/DM/CBE	40–75+	2 yrs	2 yrs	2 492 868	19%
Korea	1999	MM/DM	40–75+	2 yrs	2 yrs	2 602 928	39.3%
Luxembourg	1992	DM	50–69		2 yrs	14 586	64%
Netherlands	1989	MM/DM	50–74		2 yrs	961 766	80.7%
New Zealand	1998	MM/DM	45–69	2 yrs	2 yrs	211 922	67.5%
Norway	1996	DM	50–69		2 yrs	199 818	67%
Poland	2006	MM/DM	50–69		2 yrs	985 364	39%
Portugal Central	1990	DM	45–69	2 yrs	2 yrs	100 348	63%
Portugal Alentejo	1997	DM	45–69	2 yrs	2 yrs	7298	58.4%
Saudi Arabia	2007		40–64			6200	19%
Spain Catalonia	1995	MM/DM	50–69		2 yrs	527 000	65%
Spain Navarra	1990	DM	45–69	2 yrs	2 yrs	40 016	87.3%
Sweden	1986	MM/DM	40–74	18 mths	2 yrs	1414 000	70%
Switzerland	1999	MM/DM	50–69		2 yrs	60 700	48.2%
UK	1988	MM/DM	50–69		3 yrs	1 957 124	73.3%
Uruguay	1995	MM/DM/CBE	40–75+	1–2 yrs	1–2 yrs	416 000	66.5%
	1990	MM/CBE/U/BSE	40–69	2 yrs	1 yr	352 000	

BSE, breast self-examination; CBE, clinical breast examination; DM, digital mammography; MM, screen-film mammography; mths, months; USS, ultrasound scan; yrs, years.

Source: data from Breast Cancer Surveillance Consortium, International Cancer Screening Network, Copyright © 2012, available from http://breastscreening.cancer.gov/.

Just over 80% of these individuals attended the offered screening colonoscopy. At colonoscopy 12% of men and 6.2% of women had adenomatous polyps, and 11.6% of men and 7.8% of women had colorectal cancers. Men were less likely to take up the offer of faecal occult blood tests, despite a higher chance of a positive test and both adenomatous polyps and colorectal cancers.[21] Patients identified with malignancy via the screening programme were at an earlier stage of the disease with just 3% having evidence of metastatic spread.[21]

Impact of screening on the patient population

Early results of the screening programme are promising, but the impact on our patient population remains unclear. The expectation is that screening will lead to a 16% reduction in overall colorectal cancer mortality.[21] There are conflicting reports on the current and expected incidence of colorectal cancer, which is in part

attributable to screening programmes. The American guidelines on colorectal cancer screening report that incidence and prevalence in the United States is falling, with this attributed to their own screening programme of colonoscopies in patients over the age of 50.[22] This is at odds with much of the published literature that is predicting an increase in cancer incidence as a result of increasing population age and screening.[23,24]

Further difficulties in predicting the impact of screening on patients with advanced disease pertain to the wide variations in the rate of uptake of the test. Patients from areas of greater socioecomic deprivation are less likely to participate in bowel cancer screening despite evidence suggesting they have a poorer survival.[21,25] Even if we accept that screening will result in large numbers of patients presenting with less advanced disease, the effect of this on the incidence and prevalence of potentially resectable metastases (liver and lung) is uncertain. Currently more than 50% of patients have evidence of local nodal metastases or systemic metastases at presentation.[26] In addition, a significant proportion of patients presenting with non-metastatic disease go on to develop hepatic metastases.[27] It is therefore probably overly optimistic to assume that the bowel cancer screening programme will result in any meaningful fall in the numbers of patients presenting with resectable hepatic metastases.

Conclusion

Cancer screening is now commonplace in most healthcare systems. Their inception is based on the concept that early detection leads to better survival, although the evidence for this in parts is lacking. All screening tests should follow the direction of the World Health Organization, who published clear guidelines in 1968.[1] Screening for cervical cancer, breast cancer, and colorectal cancer is widespread, and there is a clear movement towards screening in other malignancies such as prostate cancer.[28]

References

1. Wilson J. *Principles and Practice of Screening for Disease*. Public Health Papers Number 34. Geneva: The World Health Organization, 1968.
2. Arbyn M, Castellsagué X, de Sanjosé S, *et al*. Worldwide burden of cervical cancer in 2008. *Ann Oncol* 2011; 22(12): 2675–86.
3. Van der Aa MA, Pukkala E Coebergh JW, *et al*. Mass screening programmes and trends in cervical cancer in Finland and the Netherlands. *Int J Cancer* 2008; 122: 1854–8.
4. National Cancer Intelligence Network UK Cancer Information Service. Available from http://www.ncin.org.uk/home (accessed 14 August 2014).
5. Sasieni PD, Cuzick J, Lynch-Farmery E. Estimating the efficacy of screening by auditing smear histories of women with and without cervical cancer. The National Co-ordinating Network for Cervical Screening Working Group. *Br J Cancer* 1996; 73. 1001–5.
6. Kulasingham SL, Havrilesky L, Ghebre R, *et al. Screening for Cervical Cancer: A Decision Analysis for the US Preventive Services Task Force*. AHRQ Publication No. 11-05157 EF-1. Rockville, MD: Agency for Healthcare Research and Quality, 2011.
7. Sasieni P, Castañón A, Cuzick J. Effectiveness of cervical screening with age: population based case-control study of prospectively recorded data. *BMJ* 2009; 339: b2968.
8. Siebers AG, Klinkhamer PJ, Grefte JM, *et al*. Comparison of liquid based cytology with conventional cytology for detection of cervical cancer precursors: a randomized controlled trial (NETHCON). *JAMA* 2009; 302: 1757–64.
9. Peto J, Gillham C, Deacon J, *et al*. Cervical HPV infection and neoplasia in a large population-based prospective study: the Manchester cohort. *Br J Cancer* 2004; 91 (5): 942–53.
10. Kitchener HC, Gilham C, Sargent A, *et al*. A comparison of HPV DNA testing and liquid based cytology over three rounds of primary cervical screening: extended follow up in the ARTISTIC trial. *Eur J Cancer* 2011; 47(6): 864–71.
11. Virnig BA, Turtle TM, Shamlyan T, *et al*. DCIS of the breast: a systematic review of incidence, treatment and outcomes. *J Natl Cancer Inst* 2010; 102(3): 170–8.
12. Tabar L, Vitak B, Chen THH, *et al*. Swedish Two-county trial: Impact of mammographic screening in breast cancer during 3 decades. *Radiology* 2011; 260: 658–63.
13. Shapiro S, Venet W, Strax P, *et al. Periodic Screening for Breast Cancer. The Health Insurance Plan Project and its Sequelae 1963–1986*. Baltimore, MD: The John Hopkins University Press, 1988.
14. Alexander FE, Anderson TJ, Brown HK, *et al*. The Edinburgh randomized trial of breast cancer screening: results after 10 years of follow-up. *Br J Cancer* 1994; 70: 542–8.
15. Miller AB, To T, Baines CJ, Wall C. The Canadian National Breast Screening Study: update on breast cancer mortality. *Mon Natl Cancer Instit* 1997; 22: 37–41.
16. Bjurstam N, Björneld L, Duffy SW, et al. The Gothenberg Breast Screening Trial: the first result on mortality, incidence and mode of detection for women ages 39–49 years at randomization. *Cancer* 1997; 80; 2091–9.
17. NHS Breast Screening Statistics 2012 http://www.cancerscreening.nhs.uk/breastscreen/statistics.html (accessed 14 August 2014).
18. Breast Cancer Surveillance Consortium International Cancer Screening Network 2012 http://breastscreening.cancer.gov/ (accessed 14 August 2014).
19. Welsh HG, Black WC. Overdiagnosis in cancer. *J Natl Cancer Inst* 2010; 102(9); 605–13.
20. Hellquist BN, Duffy SW, Abdsaleh S, *et al*. Effectiveness of population-based service screening with mammography for women ages 40–49 years. *Cancer* 2011; 117: 714–22.
21. Logan RFA, Patnick J, Nickerson C, *et al*. Outcomes of the Bowel Cancer Screening Programme (BCSP) in England after the first 1 million tests. *Gut* 2012; 61(10): 1439–46.
22. Smith RA, Brooks D, Cokkinides V, *et al*. Cancer screening in the United States, 2013: A review of current American Cancer Society guidelines, current issues in cancer screening, and new guidance on cervical cancer screening and lung cancer screening. *CA Cancer J Clin* 2013; 63(2): 88–105.
23. Neerincx M, Buffart TE, Mulder CJJ, *et al*. The future of colorectal cancer: implications of screening. *Gut* 2013; 62(10): 1387–9.
24. Anaya DA, Becker NS, Abraham NS. Global graying, colorectal cancer and liver metastasis: new implications for surgical management. *Crit Rev Oncol Hematol* 2011; 77(2): 100–8.
25. Mansouri D, McMillan DC, Grant Y, *et al*. The impact of age, sex and socioeconomic deprivation on outcomes in a colorectal cancer screening programme. *PLoS One* 2013; 8(6): e66063.
26. Morris EJA, Forman D, Thomas JD, *et al*. Surgical management and outcomes of colorectal cancer liver metastases. *Br J Surg* 2010; 97(7): 1110–8.
27. Haddad AJ, Bani Hani M, Pawlik TM, *et al*. Colorectal liver metastases. *Int J Surg Oncol* 2011; 2011: 285840.
28. Lee YJ, Park JE, Jeon BR, *et al*. Is prostate-specific antigen effective for population screening of prostate cancer? A systematic review. *Ann Lab Med* 2013; 33(4): 233–41.

Principles of surgical oncology

Dhanny Gomez, Hassan Z. Malik,
Stephen Fenwick, and Graeme J. Poston

Introduction

The management of cancer patients has evolved significantly over the last two decades, with the majority of patients with solid tumours now having an opportunity to undergo potentially curative procedures, so increasing survival rates. With advances in diagnostic, anaesthetic, and surgical techniques, the morbidity and mortality of major oncological surgery is greatly outweighed by the potential of cure or palliation of symptoms. Advances in surgery are not the sole reason for improved outcomes. The increased use of neo-adjuvant therapy, the application of multimodal therapy, and the earlier detection of underlying malignancy through screening have all contributed to the improved overall outcomes for cancer patients.

In general, patients presenting with suspicion of (or histologically proven) cancer will undergo a management pathway that consists of preoperative diagnosis and staging, primary therapy with or without neo-adjuvant therapy, adjuvant therapy, and surveillance and treatment for recurrent disease. This management pathway (Figure 2.15.2.1) is crucial as it allows accurate diagnosis and staging of cancers with subsequent operative removal of loco-regional disease. Following this, as seen in most malignant disease processes, the addition of adjuvant therapy may increase the overall survival rates of cancer patients by decreasing recurrence rates.

The role of surgery has changed with the expansion of the multidisciplinary approach to cancer. Besides its well-established role as potentially curative therapy, surgery also plays a role in obtaining tissue for diagnosis and further management, as a debulking procedure, and to palliate symptoms in incurable patients. Hence, it is important to adhere to the general principles of surgical oncology as described below.

Preoperative diagnosis and staging

History, examination and laboratory tests

Some authorities argue that the preoperative staging is the most crucial stage in the management of cancer patients, as it determines their subsequent treatment and outcome. Following a complete history and physical examination, laboratory testing and radiological imaging is performed depending on the site of interest. In general, alarming symptoms include anorexia, weight loss, nausea, night sweats, and malaise. Symptoms corresponding to the anatomic site involved include: melena or haematemesis for patients with gastrointestinal cancer; persistent cough and haemoptysis for patients with lung cancer; haematuria for renal tract cancer patients; and

enlarging mass in the breast or blood-stained discharge from the nipple. Of note, the duration of symptoms may indicate the aggressiveness of the underlying cancer. In addition, it is also important to elucidate possible aetiological environmental factors such as smoking, alcohol intake, asbestos exposure, and radiation exposure that could be related to organ-specific sites of tumour development. Asbestos exposure leads to mesothelioma, lung cancer, asbestosis, and plural plaques.[1] Similarly, smoking has a strong association with the development of a variety of cancers such as oral, lung,[2] and pancreatic cancers.[3]

Routine blood tests include a full blood count, coagulation profile, and serum biochemistry profile. Anaemia should be regarded as a sinister sign, and a gastrointestinal tumour should be considered as the most likely diagnosis until proven otherwise. Besides these routine laboratory tests, serum tumour markers may also be helpful in establishing a diagnosis (Table 2.15.2.1). In general, serum tumour markers have been most useful in following the patient's response to therapy. However, tumour markers can also be useful in assisting clinicians in making a diagnosis, especially in indeterminate cases. Serum tumour markers such as carcinoembryonic antigen (CEA), thyroglobulin and α-fetoprotein (AFP) are useful in the management of patients with specific tumours. For example, CEA is useful in the follow-up protocols of patients who have had surgery for colorectal cancer and liver resection for colorectal liver metastases. An increase in CEA levels above the normal reference range may indicate recurrent disease. A high CEA level pre-liver resection for colorectal liver metastases has been shown to be associated with poorer disease-free survival.[4] With respect to hepatocellular cancer, AFP is used to achieve diagnosis in tandem with cross-sectional imaging as well as in follow-up protocols post-liver resection. Studies have also shown that a high AFP level is associated with poorer disease-free and overall survival in patients with hepatocellular cancer.[5] With respect to ovarian cancer, the National Institute for Health and Care Excellence has recently recommended that women with symptoms that could be related to underlying ovarian malignancy should be offered a CA-125 blood test.[6] Serum CA-125 levels are also useful in monitoring a patient's response to treatment, as studies have observed that the duration of disease-free survival correlates with the rate of reduction of CA-125 levels. Persistently elevated CA-125 levels during therapy are associated with poorer overall survival. In addition, an increase in CA-125 levels following surgery is a predictor of recurrent disease.[7] Hence tumour markers are a useful adjunct in the management of cancer patients, not only in assisting in making a diagnosis, but also used in monitoring patients during the follow-up period following treatment.

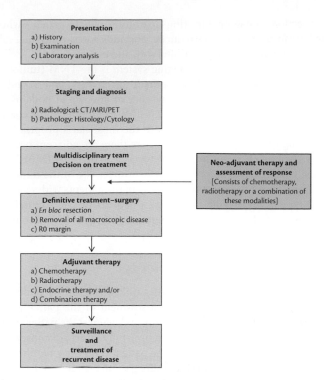

Fig. 2.15.2.1 Management algorithm of cancer patients.

Fitness for surgery

Another key aspect that is important in the clinical assessment is the patient's operative risk. Modern cancer treatments can be extremely demanding on both the physical and psychological resources of the patient. Major oncological surgery can be associated with high morbidity and mortality, and hence patients have to be assessed with respect to their fitness for surgery and their subsequent reserves to deal with postoperative complications. Therefore, all patients being considered for major cancer surgery are required to have an assessment of their clinical status, in particular their cardiac and pulmonary function. A history of prior cardiac events

should be noted, in particular, ischaemic heart disease, hypertension, congestive cardiac failure, or valvular disease. The severity of these conditions can have an impact on myocardial performance and most anaesthetists recommend further cardiac assessment in patients with a background history of underlying cardiac disease. Common investigations include an electrocardiogram, chest X-ray, and echocardiogram.

With respect to pulmonary function, it is important to recognize patients with co-morbidities such as chronic bronchitis, chronic obstructive pulmonary disease, and previous pulmonary embolism. In addition, chronic use of tobacco should be noted, and it is advisable to encourage complete smoking cessation in cancer patients prior to major surgery. In general, a chest X-ray and pulmonary function tests, including spirometry, are used to assess patients' pulmonary function.

More recently some centres have started using cardiopulmonary exercise testing (CPET) to assess patients' fitness for surgery. CPET is a type of exercise stress test that measures both cardiac and pulmonary function as a combined unit. A recent study assessing survival following abdominal aortic aneurysm surgery demonstrated that preoperative CPET identified patients less likely to survive in the mid-term, even after successful abdominal aortic aneurysm repair.[8] Preoperative CPET prior to liver resection has also been shown to predict postoperative complication.[9] Although CPET provides useful prognostic information, its clinical role in surgical decision making is less clear. Older patients with good CPET performance may gain reassurance of a relatively better prognosis and operative risk. High-risk patients performing poorly on CPET are likely to have an unpredictable response to surgery and may have an increased risk of developing postoperative complications, but these patients will be better informed about their perioperative risk. Thus, the clinical value of CPET in cancer surgery may lie in providing additional prognostic information to assist in the decision-making process, rather than in being an absolute or relative contraindication to surgery.

Modern surgical oncology requires precision and accuracy when appropriately resecting tumours, performed with minimal

Table 2.15.2.1 Serum tumour markers

Tumour site	Tumour marker	Clinical relevance
Colorectal	CEA	Used in follow-up following resection of the colon/rectum and also liver metastases
Pancreas	CA 19.9	Used to assist diagnosis. Some institutions will perform a staging laparoscopy if CA19.9 levels are elevated prior to pancreatic resection Used in follow-up protocols following pancreatic resection
Prostate	PSA	Used in post-treatment follow-up: more accurate following surgery rather than radiation therapy
Liver	α-FP	Used to assist diagnosis and in follow-up protocols following liver resection
Ovary	CA-125	Used to assist diagnosis and in follow-up protocols
Thyroid	Thyroglobulin	Used in follow-up for papillary and follicular cancer following thyroidectomy
	Calcitonin	Used in follow-up for medullary cancer (this type of thyroid cancer can be part of the MEN-2 syndrome)
Carcinoid tumours	5-HIAA	Used to assist diagnosis. An elevation of urinary 5-HIAA levels indicates underlying carcinoid tumour with liver metastases
Myeloma	Bence-Jones immunoglobulins	Used to assist diagnosis

CEA, carcinoembryonic antigen; CA, cancer antigen; PSA, prostate-specific antigen; α-FP, alpha-fetoprotein; 5-HIAA, 5-hydroxyindole acetic acid.

morbidity and mortality. Preoperative testing of the patient's physical status is crucial to obtain good postoperative results and survival outcomes following major cancer surgery.

Radiological imaging and staging

Accurate staging of the extent of disease is crucial in formulating a management plan for all cancer patients. Surgeons rely heavily on detailed and accurate preoperative imaging when diagnosing, staging, and planning the type of surgery that is appropriate. At present, nearly all patients are usually staged with a computer tomography (CT) scan. Over the last decade, CT scans have become more accurate and are the first-line investigation of choice with respect to detecting metastatic disease. Subsequent cross-sectional imaging is usually dependent on the site of tumour. For example, in cases of rectal tumours, patients usually undergo a colonoscopy to obtain tissue diagnosis and have a CT scan of the thorax, abdomen, and pelvis to detect metastatic disease, mainly in the liver and lung. In addition, these patients also require magnetic resonance imaging of the pelvis to determine T stage and whether the tumour has invaded surrounding pelvic structures.[10] Cross-sectional imaging is important to stage patients to enable consideration of the use of neo-adjuvant therapies. In patients receiving neo-adjuvant therapy, cross-sectional imaging is required to assess response to treatment. This imaging also enables the choice of postoperative chemotherapy regimen if there is no or little response to the neo-adjuvant strategy. Chemoresponders are likely to be treated with a similar regimen during their adjuvant therapy.

Besides cross-sectional imaging, preoperative endoscopic assessment plays an important role in staging oesophageal, gastric, and pancreatic tumours. Endoscopic ultrasound obtains images of the internal organs in the chest and abdomen. It can be used to visualize the walls of these organs, as well as assess adjacent structures. With the combination of Doppler imaging, surrounding vascular structures can also be evaluated. For example, in cases of cancer in the head of the pancreas, following CT scan of the thorax, abdomen, and pelvis, endoscopic ultrasound can be used to confirm the presence of vascular invasion by the tumour as well as the benefit of obtaining cytology through fine-needle aspiration.

More recently, positron emission tomography (PET) scanning has emerged as an important imaging modality. PET scanning tends to complement other diagnostic modalities especially in cases of lung, melanoma, and gastrointestinal cancers. Although this modality is not widely in use, its use is growing and recent studies have showed that the utilization of PET scanning altered patient management in 15–44% of patients with colorectal cancer, lung cancer, and melanoma.[11]

Although the sensitivity and specificity of cross-sectional imaging has improved, in certain intra-abdominal cancers, laparoscopy is an added staging method that enables the detection of low-volume peritoneal disease. Laparoscopy is an effective method for determining the resectability of intra-abdominal malignancies with low cure rates, such as gastric cancer, hilar cholangiocarcinoma, and gallbladder cancer. In addition to direct visualization of solid organs and the peritoneal cavity, direct organ ultrasound, tissue biopsy, and peritoneal cytology can also be performed. Around 40% of patients with cancer of the stomach, oesophagus, and liver benefit from laparoscopy with the avoidance of a futile laparotomy. To date, surgeons are still reliant on diagnostic laparoscopy to detect small (1–5 mm) hepatic or peritoneal metastasis not visualized by cross-sectional imaging. Limiting laparotomy only to patients who may benefit from resection reduces morbidity rates, time interval for other therapy, length of hospital stay, and overall cost.

The most commonly used staging system is the TNM (tumour, nodes and metastases) system. Suffixes to the T, N, and M indicate the size of the tumour and presence or absence of nodal disease or metastases. For example, T2 N1 M0 carcinoma of the colon indicates the tumour has spread into the muscularis propria but not through the wall of the colon where there are adjacent lymph nodes involved (N1) but no distant metastases detected (M0). The staging system varies according to the primary site of the tumour. Therefore following appropriate staging of the patients with respect to the type of underlying malignancy, patients can be counselled with regards to the appropriate operative strategy if the tumour is resectable.

Surgical therapy

Following the preoperative diagnosis and staging of the underlying malignancy, as well as fitness assessment of the patient, the next stage is to determine resectability and counsel the patient and their family regarding surgery. Obtaining fully informed consent is essential and important for both the patients and their families to understand the benefits and risk of surgery. Intra-abdominal malignancy usually requires major surgery and is associated with significant morbidity and mortality even in the high volume institutions.

Principles of surgery

The main principle of curative surgery is to remove *en-bloc* all macroscopically visible malignant tissue, which in certain cases may involve multi-organ resection. The *en-bloc* technique states that the tumour is to be resected intact with the incorporation of structures involved by or near the tumour, without violation of tissue planes contiguous to the tumour or of tissues interposed between the structures to be resected.[12] In certain cases, frozen section of the resection margin is analyzed intraoperatively to determine that the resection margin is clear of tumour. This practice is aimed at obtaining complete local control to prevent recurrence at the resection site. Nevertheless, the adequate resection margin varies depending on the type of cancer. Traditionally, it was always assumed that the wider the resection margin, the less chance for local recurrence to occur and this would translate into improved overall survival. Published randomized control trials have proven that this concept is incorrect. Although breast cancer patients who were treated with radical mastectomy achieved a good local control rate of more than 90% compared to simple excision of the tumour, their overall survival was still poor.[13] This observation was related to the fact that these patients already had distant metastases that were not detected at time of presentation. Since then, large multicentre trials have shown that wide local excision achieves equivalent results to radical mastectomy and survival has improved due to the addition of multimodal therapy including radiotherapy to control local disease, and chemotherapy and/or endocrine therapy to control systemic disease.[13]

In some cases, the tumour may be adherent or fixed to normal adjacent structures. For such cases, *en-bloc* resection of the tumour is required, and any attachment should be considered malignant in nature. Any breach of the tumour leads to malignant cell spillage and implantation that ultimately increases the recurrence rate either at the resection site or nearby structures. For example, resection of colonic cancer involves obtaining adequate margin of normal colon proximally and distally. If other structures are involved with the tumour, such as small bowel or the bladder, then *en-bloc* resection of the segment of small bowel or bladder with the colon is required to obtain oncological clearance. Adhering to these surgical principles is crucial to give cancer patients their best possible survival outcome following surgery.

Resection of regional lymph nodes

Tumour-draining regional lymph nodes are the most prevalent site of metastasis for most tumours, and the presence of metastasis in these nodes represents an important prognostic factor in the staging of the cancer patient. Hence, to obtain adequate oncological clearance, the regional lymph nodes are resected at the time of resection of the primary tumour. Current understanding suggests that lymphadenectomy provides regional control of the disease and decreases the chance of recurrent disease. For example, following wide local excision of breast cancer with no axillary lymph nodes palpable clinically, axillary node sampling is performed to stage the disease. More recently, sentinel lymph node biopsy is increasingly being performed to enable breast surgeons to remove the first lymph node that drains the tumour.[14] This lymph node is one of the most likely sites to contain micrometastasis, if present. Similar procedures are also performed in cases of malignant melanoma. In intra-abdominal malignancy, comparable lymphadenectomy is also performed. For example, patients with a caecal tumour usually undergo a right hemi-colectomy that removes the lymph nodes in the mesentery of the ileocolic and right colic pedicles.

Due to the radical nature of oncological surgery, in difficult or borderline cases, intraoperative decision is crucial. For example, performing an extended hemi-hepatectomy for a large hepatocellular carcinoma in an elderly patient. A risk versus benefit ratio for the potential of the operation to be curative or palliative must be considered when the morbidity and mortality associated with such surgery are significant.

The role of neo-adjuvant therapy

Over the last decade, many studies have demonstrated the benefits of neo-adjuvant (preoperative) therapy prior to potentially curative surgery. This is a major shift from previous traditional practices where patients were given adjuvant therapy following surgery. The aim behind the neo-adjuvant approach is to reduce tumour burden and increase the chances of curative resection, with the overall end result to improve survival.

Neo-adjuvant chemotherapy and/or radiotherapy are being used increasingly in the management of large, locally invasive or node-positive rectal cancer, followed by total mesorectal excision, rather than postoperative radiotherapy. A recent review of 12 randomized control trials involving 9410 patients treated preoperatively with either short-course radiotherapy and long-course chemoradiation showed a relative risk reduction of 50% in local recurrence in appropriately selected patients with stage II and III rectal cancer.[15] Nevertheless, this oncological benefit comes at the cost of a 50% relative risk increase in both acute treatment-related toxicity and long-term anorectal dysfunction. Hence, it is crucial that these patients are staged accurately, counselled appropriately and only selected patients are entered into this neo-adjuvant therapy pathway.

Gastric adenocarcinoma is another cancer where neo-adjuvant therapy has become an important part of the management pathway. The milestone study by Cunningham *et al.*[16] found that perioperative chemotherapy significantly improved progression-free and overall survival in patients with operable gastric, gastro-oesophageal junction, and lower oesophageal lesions compared to patients who underwent surgery alone.[16] Others have since published similar findings.[17]

Although the application of neo-adjuvant therapy is increasing, it must be used in a selected patient group, where its benefits are likely to be observed long-term. This form of therapy is not suitable for all patients, in particular early stage disease, and its administration is not without adverse effects (see Chapter 2.15.5).

The role of adjuvant therapy

Traditionally, following apparently curative surgery, cancer patients used to be monitored in the clinic for possible recurrent disease. However, studies demonstrated that following potentially curative surgery, the addition of adjuvant therapy reduced the risk of recurrent disease, and increased overall survival. This observation was well demonstrated in cases of colonic and breast cancer.

In cases of breast cancer, various studies have shown the benefits of adjuvant therapy, including endocrine therapy, radiotherapy, and chemotherapy, or a combination of these treatment modalities. From a surgical perspective, there has been a shift towards organ preservation surgery with the addition of adjuvant therapy, rather than radical surgery alone. This is partly due to increased understanding of tumour biology and its means of dissemination. Tumour progression does not necessarily follow lymphatic channels to local regional nodes, but may directly spread to distant sites through haematogenous dissemination. Therefore, vascular spread may bypass regional lymphatic channels, rendering radical surgery with *en-bloc* resection of the primary tumour and lymph nodes futile. With the use of adjuvant therapy, more conservative surgery may achieve similar oncological results to radical surgery, and is more beneficial with respect to resecting the primary tumour while preserving organ function and reducing morbidity. For example, a small breast tumour is usually treated with wide local excision with lymph node sampling or excision followed by postoperative radiotherapy, chemotherapy, and endocrine therapy. The decision on the type of adjuvant therapy is based on the tumour size, lymph node status, vascular invasion, the presence of oestrogen and/or progesterone receptors, and gene expression. Studies have shown that the addition of radiotherapy reduces local disease recurrence. Chemotherapy is usually given to younger patients and patients with lymph node involvement, with published studies showing better overall survival in patients who received chemotherapy, especially patients with tumours that were negative for oestrogen and progesterone receptors.[18] Following this, patients are usually started on endocrine therapy (such as tamoxifen or androgen inhibitors) for approximately 5 years to reduce the risk of disease recurrence.[18] This treatment pathway is an example of the progress made in clinical oncology to improve patient outcome with multimodal therapy.

With regard to pancreatic cancer, randomized trials have shown the benefits of adjuvant chemotherapy in improving overall survival following potentially curative surgery. The ESPAC-1 trial demonstrated a significant survival benefit for patients who received chemotherapy compared to patients who did not, irrespective of whether the patients were randomized to receive chemoradiotherapy.[19] Subsequent ESPAC studies have also demonstrated improved overall survival with the addition of adjuvant chemotherapy following resection for pancreatic adenocarcinoma.[20] Following pancreatic resection for pancreatic cancer, all patients should be offered adjuvant chemotherapy to improve long-term outcomes, as at present, there is no convincing evidence showing benefit for the use of neo-adjuvant chemotherapy or chemoradiotherapy.

Surgery for synchronous primary and metastatic disease

In the majority of cancers, the presence of metastatic disease renders patients incurable and so they are treated with palliative chemotherapy and/or supportive therapy. However, hepatic resection has become the treatment modality of choice for resectable colorectal liver metastases and is associated with long-term survival in these patients with 5-year survival rates up to 58% being reported.[21,22] Approximately 25% of patients have synchronous liver metastases at the time of presentation and a further 20% subsequently develop metachronous liver disease, usually within 2 years following resection of the primary tumour.[23] In addition, resection of pulmonary colorectal metastases has been associated with improved long-term survival, in particular cases with solitary metastasis that were suitable for anatomical resection.[24] Hence, there is a subgroup of colorectal cancer patients that present with synchronous or metachronous liver disease that should be considered for aggressive treatment with liver resection, with or without down-staging chemotherapy. Synchronous resection of colorectal primary and liver disease have shown good results. In addition, 'liver-first' resection, following by rectal cancer resection has also shown promising results.[25] Recently, studies have shown that patients with liver metastasis from colorectal cancer are considered cured following liver resection if they remain disease-free for 10 years or longer after hepatectomy.[26] Hence, in this group of patients with metastatic disease, aggressive multimodal therapy that includes liver resection and chemotherapy, improves the overall survival and can be potentially curative.

Follow-up and treatment of recurrence

Follow-up of cancer patients is important following their surgery and adjuvant therapy. This stage of the management pathway may not been seen as crucial, but it is pointless investing effort in the preoperative and operative stage management of cancer patients and then neglecting them at follow-up. Although recurrent disease may not be treated by surgery, other treatment modalities can be offered that will influence their overall outcome.

For example, patients with disease recurrence following resection for colorectal liver metastases were considered to have a poor prognosis and very few were offered repeat liver resections. However, with more hepatobiliary centres adopting a more aggressive surgical approach towards hepatic and/or extra-hepatic recurrences following curative resection for colorectal liver metastasis, an intensive surveillance programme designed to detect recurrences for which surgical intervention can alter survival outcome is crucial.[27] The benefits of surveillance following resection of colorectal liver metastases have been exemplified by studies that have reported up to 40% survival at 5-years following repeat liver resection for liver

recurrence, with acceptable morbidity and mortality rates.[28–31] Furthermore, lung metastases from colorectal cancer can be cured by radical surgery.[24] These results are directly related to surveillance protocols adopted by these hepatobiliary centres. Detection of recurrence through these programmes enables the earlier treatment of recurrent disease through re-resection.

With respect to hepatocellular carcinoma, liver resection is considered the treatment of choice for single lesions arising in non-cirrhotic livers, and in patients with Childs Pugh grade A cirrhosis who have well-preserved liver function. The literature would suggest that 80–90% of recurrences are seen within the liver remnant following hepatic resection for hepatocellular carcinoma.[32] Therefore due to the high risk of recurrence, these patients should be entered into a surveillance programme to detect early recurrence. Recurrent disease could be treated with further liver resection, liver transplantation, radiofrequency ablation, or transarterial chemoembolization.

Conclusion

With the constantly evolving pathways in cancer management, clinicians are duty bound to keep up to date with the latest evidence and change their practice appropriately for the benefit of their patients. By adhering to the general principles of surgical oncology, improved outcomes can be achieved in cancer patients, especially with the application of multimodal therapy, and advances in modern chemotherapy regimens.

It is important to stage and diagnose cancer patients appropriately in order to deliver the most appropriate treatment. In cases where surgery is indicated, the role of neo-adjuvant or adjuvant therapy should be considered. Following treatment, all patients should be entered into active surveillance programmes to detect treatable recurrent disease. Although surgery has a well-established role as a form of curative therapy, the multidisciplinary approach to cancer is the best way forward to improve patient outcomes.

References

1. Liu G, Cheresh P, Kamp DW. Molecular basis of asbestos-induced lung disease. *Annu Rev Pathol* 2013; 8: 161–87.
2. Mordant P, Grand B, Cazes A, *et al*. Adenosquamous carcinoma of the lung: Surgical management, pathologic characteristics, and prognostic implications. *Ann Thorac Surg*. 2013; 95(4): 1189–95.
3. Yeo TP, Lowenfels AB. Demographics and epidemiology of pancreatic cancer. *Cancer J* 2012; 18(6): 477–84.
4. Spelt L, Andersson B, Nilsson J, *et al*. Prognostic models for outcome following liver resection for colorectal cancer metastases: A systematic review. *Eur J Surg Oncol* 2012; 38(1): 16–24.
5. Wu CC, Cheng SB, Ho WM, *et al*. Liver resection for hepatocellular carcinoma in patients with cirrhosis. *Br J Surg* 2005; 92(3): 348–55.
6. Sturgeon CM, Duffy MJ, Walker G. The National Institute for Health and Clinical Excellence (NICE) guidelines for early detection of ovarian cancer: the pivotal role of the clinical laboratory. *Ann Clin Biochem* 2011; 48(Pt 4): 295–9.
7. Santillan A, Garg R, Zahurak ML, *et al*. Risk of epithelial ovarian cancer recurrence in patients with rising serum CA-125 levels within the normal range. *J Clin Oncol* 2005; 23(36): 9338–43.
8. Carlisle J, Swart M. Mid-term survival after abdominal aortic aneurysm surgery predicted by cardiopulmonary exercise testing. *Br J Surg* 2007; 94(8): 966–9.
9. Junejo MA, Mason JM, Sheen AJ, *et al*. Cardiopulmonary exercise testing for preoperative risk assessment before hepatic resection. *Br J Surg* 2012; 99(8): 1097–104.

10. Cellini F, Valentini V. Current perspectives on preoperative integrated treatments for locally advanced rectal cancer: a review of agreement and controversies. *Oncology (Williston Park)* 2012; 26(8): 730–5, 741.

11. Krause BJ, Schwarzenbock S, Souvatzoglou M. FDG PET and PET/CT. *Recent Results Cancer Res* 2013; 187: 351–69.

12. Enker WE, Pilipshen SJ, Heilweil ML, *et al.* En bloc pelvic lymphadenectomy and sphincter preservation in the surgical management of rectal cancer. *Ann Surg* 1986; 203(4): 426–33.

13. Fisher B, Redmond C, Fisher ER, *et al.* Ten-year results of a randomized clinical trial comparing radical mastectomy and total mastectomy with or without radiation. *N Engl J Med* 1985; 312(11): 674–81.

14. Moody LC, Wen X, McKnight T, *et al.* Indications for sentinel lymph node biopsy in multifocal and multicentric breast cancer. *Surgery* 2012; 152(3): 389–96.

15. Fleming FJ, Pahlman L, Monson JR. Neoadjuvant therapy in rectal cancer. *Dis Colon Rectum* 2012; 54(7): 901–12.

16. Cunningham D, Allum WH, Stenning SP, *et al*, Participants MT. Perioperative chemotherapy versus surgery alone for resectable gastroesophageal cancer. *N Engl J Med* 2006; 355(1): 11–20.

17. Ajani JA, Mansfield PF, Janjan N, *et al.* Multi-institutional trial of preoperative chemoradiotherapy in patients with potentially resectable gastric carcinoma. *J Clin Oncol* 2004; 22(14): 2774–80.

18. Cardoso F, Loibl S, Pagani O, *et al.* The European Society of Breast Cancer Specialists recommendations for the management of young women with breast cancer. *Eur J Cancer* 2012; 48(18): 3355–77.

19. Neoptolemos JP, Stocken DD, *et al.* Influence of resection margins on survival for patients with pancreatic cancer treated by adjuvant chemoradiation and/or chemotherapy in the ESPAC-1 randomized controlled trial. *Ann Surg* 2001; 234(6): 758–68.

20. Neoptolemos JP, Moore MJ, Cox TF, *et al.* Effect of adjuvant chemotherapy with fluorouracil plus folinic acid or gemcitabine vs observation on survival in patients with resected periampullary adenocarcinoma: the ESPAC-3 periampullary cancer randomized trial. *JAMA* 2012; 308(2): 147–56.

21. Pawlik TM, Scoggins CR, Zorzi D, *et al.* Effect of surgical margin status on survival and site of recurrence after hepatic resection for colorectal metastases. *Ann Surg* 2005; 241(5): 715–22, discussion 722–14.

22. Fernandez FG, Drebin JA, Linehan DC, *et al.* Five-year survival after resection of hepatic metastases from colorectal cancer in patients screened by positron emission tomography with F-18 fluorodeoxyglucose (FDG-PET). *Ann Surg* 2004; 240(3): 438–47; discussion 447–50.

23. Choti MA, Sitzmann JV, Tiburi MF, *et al.* Trends in long-term survival following liver resection for hepatic colorectal metastases. *Ann Surg* 2002; 235(6): 759–66.

24. Yedibela S, Klein P, Feuchter K, Hoffmann M, *et al.* Surgical management of pulmonary metastases from colorectal cancer in 153 patients. *Ann Surg Oncol* 2006; 13(11): 1538–44.

25. De Rosa A, Gomez D, Brooks A, *et al.* 'Liver-first' approach for synchronous colorectal liver metastases: is this a justifiable approach? *J Hepatobiliary Pancreat Sci* 2013; 20(3): 263–70.

26. Tomlinson JS, Jarnagin WR, DeMatteo RP, *et al.* Actual 10-year survival after resection of colorectal liver metastases defines cure. *J Clin Oncol* 2007; 25(29): 4575–80.

27. Gomez D, Sangha VK, Morris-Stiff G, *et al.* Outcomes of intensive surveillance after resection of hepatic colorectal metastases. *Br J Surg* 2010; **97**(10): 1552–60.

28. Muratore A, Polastri R, Bouzari H, *et al.* Repeat hepatectomy for colorectal liver metastases: A worthwhile operation? *J Surg Oncol* 2001; 76(2): 127–32.

29. Suzuki S, Sakaguchi T, Yokoi Y, *et al.* Impact of repeat hepatectomy on recurrent colorectal liver metastases. *Surgery* 2001; 129(4): 421–8.

30. Yamada H, Katoh H, Kondo S, *et al.* Repeat hepatectomy for recurrent hepatic metastases from colorectal cancer. *Hepatogastroenterology* 2001; 48(39): 828–30.

31. Nishio H, Hamady ZZ, Malik HZ, *et al.* Outcome following repeat liver resection for colorectal liver metastases. *Eur J Surg Oncol* 2007; 33(6): 729–34.

32. Morris-Stiff G, Gomez D, de Liguori Carino N, *et al.* Surgical management of hepatocellular carcinoma: is the jury still out? *Surg Oncol* 2009; 18(4): 298–321.

CHAPTER 2.15.3

Principles of chemotherapy

Robert P. Jones, Derek McWhirter, and Graeme J. Poston

Introduction

An understanding of the concepts surrounding the use of systemic chemotherapy is essential for surgeons interested in the management of malignant disease. Sixty per cent of patients cured of cancer are cured by surgery alone. Traditionally, these have been patients presenting with early localized tumours. However, the use of appropriate chemotherapy alongside surgery has improved the outcome for patients with more advanced disease that was previously considered incurable. The last decade has seen enormous advances in the chemotherapeutic treatment of malignancies. As well as non-specific cytotoxic agents, modern treatment regimens include targeted biological and small molecule targeted agents. This chapter will provide a summary of the key concepts surrounding chemotherapy for solid organ cancers.

Goals of chemotherapy

Chemotherapy may be given with curative or palliative intent (Table 2.15.3.1).

Curative chemotherapy

Neo-adjuvant chemotherapy

Neo-adjuvant chemotherapy is treatment administered before surgery with the aim of reducing tumour size, resulting in downstaging or reduction in tumour size (downsizing), allowing easier surgical removal, or a more limited surgical resection (e.g. a malignant breast lesion treated with neo-adjuvant therapy may become amenable to wide local excision as opposed to mastectomy).

Survival after neo-adjuvant chemotherapy before surgery has been shown to be superior to surgery alone in a number of cancers[1,2] and response to neo-adjuvant therapy can also guide treatment after surgery. For example, the likely chemoresponsiveness of recurrent disease after surgery may be predicted from response to earlier neo-adjuvant therapy. Also the extent of tumour necrosis following prior neo-adjuvant therapy in resected specimens has also been identified as an independent predictor of long-term survival in patients with colorectal liver metastases resected following neo-adjuvant therapy.[3] Patients with extensive viable tumours may therefore be considered candidates for adjuvant (postoperative) therapy.

Neo-adjuvant chemotherapy is often given in combination with radiation therapy to enhance reduction of tumour size. In rectal cancer, neo-adjuvant chemoradiotherapy is used when preoperative imaging suggests threatened resection margins (T3b, T4, suspected lymphovascular invasion, etc.).[4] Post-resection analysis of cancers treated with neo-adjuvant chemoradiotherapy has identified a proportion of patients in whom treatment has resulted in complete tumour disappearance, referred to as complete pathological response. However, accurately identifying these patients on preoperative imaging is difficult, and pathological complete response can only be accurately identified after resection. Surgery therefore remains the gold standard for these patients.

Adjuvant chemotherapy

Adjuvant therapy is given after surgery in an attempt to reduce recurrence through the destruction of unidentified micrometastatic disease that may still remain after resection, especially at distant sites. Adjuvant chemotherapy is now considered routine for high-risk stage II and all stage III colorectal cancer;[5] stage I, II, and III breast cancer;[6] high-risk ovarian cancer;[7] and pancreatic cancer.[8] It is important to note that neo-adjuvant therapy is often better tolerated than adjuvant therapy, and the appropriate oncosurgical strategy should therefore be defined at the earliest opportunity in a multidisciplinary team by oncologists, surgeons, and radiotherapists involved in the patient's treatment.

Palliative chemotherapy

Many patients with irresectable tumours are offered palliative chemotherapy. These patients are likely to benefit most from a sequential step-wise approach to chemotherapy, with the aim of prolonging long-term overall survival, while minimizing toxicity. However, there is growing recognition that for certain subgroups of patients with initially irresectable metastatic disease, systemic chemotherapy can reduce tumour burden allowing subsequent potentially curative surgical resection. For example, patients with irresectable liver-limited metastatic colorectal cancer may respond so well to chemotherapy that their lesions become amenable to liver

Table 2.15.3.1 Terminology used to describe intent of chemotherapy

Neo-adjuvant	Chemotherapy given in the preoperative period to resectable disease with the aim of reducing tumour size allowing easier resection or less radical surgery
Adjuvant	A short course of chemotherapy given to a patient with no evidence of residual cancer after surgery with the intent of destroying unidentified micrometastases
Palliative	Chemotherapy given to control symptoms or prolong life for patients in whom cure is unlikely
Induction	High-dose, usually combination, chemotherapy given with the intent of inducing sufficient reduction in tumour size to allow surgical resection
Salvage	A potentially curative, high-dose, usually combination, regimen given in a patient who has failed or recurred following a different induction regimen

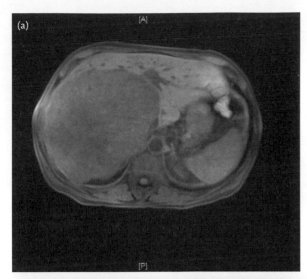

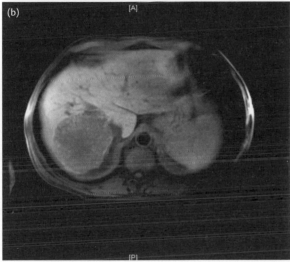

Fig. 2.15.3.1 (a) MRI scan of a patient with a large irresectable colorectal liver metastasis. (b) After six cycles of systemic induction chemotherapy, the lesion had shrunk sufficiently to allow curative resection.

resection (Figure 2.15.3.1). Approximately 40% of these initially irresectable patients are alive 5 years after such surgery.[9] For these patients, a more aggressive (and potentially toxic) first-line therapy may be adopted to maximize the potential of conversion to curative intent surgery. This approach is often referred to as induction chemotherapy, in an attempt to clarify the difference between this approach and both truly palliative therapy and true neo-adjuvant chemotherapy for already resectable disease. In patients who have shown a partial response but remain irresectable, second-line (or salvage) therapy may be adopted.

Tumour kinetics

The rate at which a tumour grows depends on the number of cells that are actively dividing (the growth fraction), the length of the cell cycle (doubling time), and the rate of cell loss. These three factors are responsible for the differing rates of tumour growth seen between tumour types, as well as between metastatic and primary tumours with the same underlying histology. In the early 1970s, it

was recognized that leukaemia cells divided rapidly in a logarithmic fashion, as virtually all cells were undergoing active division and should therefore be susceptible to chemotherapy. However, single agent cytotoxic chemotherapy did not result in cure. This understanding led to the development of combination chemotherapy, with increasing effectiveness via a fractional kill approach (e.g. a single agent destroys 90% of cancer cells, whereas a double agent destroys 99%).[10] However, it was also recognized that solid tumours do not grow in a linear fashion (their growth following a sigmoid, or Gompertzian, growth curve), as not all cells are actively dividing simultaneously. Smaller tumours were found to grow faster than large tumours, as increasing lesion size resulted in feedback inhibition and outgrowth of arterial blood supply. As a result, small tumours have the highest proportion of proliferating cells, making them more susceptible to chemotherapy.[11]

Chemotherapeutic agents are therefore rarely given individually, and a number of principles have been established to guide drug selection in combination regimens.

- Drugs known to be active as single agents should be selected for combinations.
- Drugs with different mechanisms of action should be combined in order to allow for additive or synergistic effects on the tumour.
- Drugs with differing dose-limiting toxicities should be combined to allow each drug to be given at full or nearly full therapeutic doses with tolerable toxicity profile.
- Drugs should be given at consistent intervals. The treatment-free interval between cycles should be the shortest possible time for recovery of the most sensitive normal tissue.
- Drugs with different patterns of resistance should be combined to minimize cross-resistance.

Chemotherapeutic agents

Cytotoxic agents

Traditional cytotoxic chemotherapeutic agents can be classified according to whether they target a specific part of the cell cycle (phase specific) or the whole of the cell cycle (cycle specific). For example, anti-metabolites such as 5-fluorouracil, gemcitabine, and methotrexate are more active against the S phase of the cell cycle (phase specific), whereas doxycycline and irinotecan cause double-stranded DNA breaks throughout the cell cycle (cycle specific). Table 2.15.3.2 lists some commonly used cytotoxic chemotherapy drugs, their mechanism of action and common indications.

Biological agents

Monoclonal antibody therapy

With increased understanding of tumour biology, newer targeted therapies aimed at specific defects in cancer cell behaviour have been developed. One of the key developments of the last decade has been the development of antibody therapy against these specific targets. It is now recognized that only tumours expressing the target protein will respond to these therapies, offering potentially predictive biomarker for positive tumour response.

Trastuzumab, a humanized monoclonal antibody targeted against the HER2 protein, was the first of these biological agent to be developed. It has proven effective in the treatment of HER2-positive breast cancer[12] and gastric cancer.[13]

Table 2.15.3.2 Commonly used cytotoxic chemotherapeutic agents

Drug	Mechanism of action	Indications
Bleomycin	Inhibition of DNA synthesis	Head and neck, testicular and cervical cancer
Carboplatin	DNA cross linking Cycle specific	Ovarian cancer
Cisplatin	DNA cross linking, inhibition of DNA synthesis and transcription	Testicular, ovarian, bladder and gastric cancer
Cyclophosphamide	DNA crosslinking	Breast, ovarian cancer
Docetaxel	Mitotic arrest	Breast, gastric cancer
Doxorubicin	Topoisomerase II inhibitor, inhibiting DNA repair	Breast, bladder and gastric cancer, sarcoma
Epirubicin	Topoisomerase II inhibitor	Breast cancer
5-Fluorouracil	Inhibition of DNA and RNA synthesis	Colorectal, breast, gastric, and pancreatic cancer
Gemcitabine	Inhibition of DNA synthesis	Pancreatic, breast, ovarian cancer
Irinotecan	Topoisomerase I inhibitor, preventing DNA repair	Colorectal cancer
Oxaliplatin	DNA crosslinking	Colorectal cancer
Paclitaxel	Mitotic arrest	Breast, ovarian cancer
Vinblastine	Microtubule depolymerization	Testicular, breast cancer

Cetuximab is a recombinant human/mouse chimeric antibody that binds specifically to the extracellular domain of the human endothelial growth factor receptor, inhibiting this pathway. Panitumumab is a fully human monoclonal antibody with a similar method of action. It is now recognized that patients who have a mutation in the downstream *KRAS* proto-oncogene are resistant to cetuximab and panitumumab therapy, and so *KRAS* testing is routinely performed prior to commencing treatment[14].

Vascular endothelial growth factor is one of the most important regulators of the dynamic balance between proangiogenic and antiangiogenic factors that are crucial for tumour growth and metastasis, with signalling leading to angiogenic proliferation and increased microvascular permeability. Bevacizumab is a humanized monoclonal antibody directed against vascular endothelial growth factor receptors. Proposed mechanisms of action include inhibition of vessel development, regression of aberrant tumour vasculature, and normalization of tumour perfusion.[15] Table 2.15.3.3 lists commonly used monoclonal antibodies used in solid tumours, mechanisms of action, and common indications.

Small molecule targeted agents

Most recently, refined antineoplastic agents have been developed that target proteins specific to tumour cells. Table 2.15.3.3 lists some commonly used small molecule targeted agents.

Approximately 80–85% of gastrointestinal stromal tumours harbour an activating mutation in the proto-oncogene *c-KIT* that encodes a tyrosine kinase. Imatinib is a tyrosine kinase inhibitor

Table 2.15.3.3 Commonly used biological therapies

Drug	Type	Mechanism of action	Indication
Monoclonal antibody agents			
Trastuzumab	Humanized monoclonal antibody	Binds to HER2 protein, inhibiting tumour cell growth	HER2 positive breast and gastric cancer
Bevacizumab	Humanized monoclonal antibody	Binds to VEGF, inhibiting formation of new blood vessels	Colorectal cancer, non-small cell lung cancer
Cetuximab	Chimeric monoclonal antibody	Binds to EGFR, blocking receptor kinases	Colorectal cancer, head and neck cancer
Panitumumab	Human monoclonal antibody	Binds EGFR and inhibits binding of ligands for EGFR	Colorectal cancer
Small molecule targeted agents			
Erlotininb	Tyrosine kinase inhibitor	Inhibition of phosphorylation of tyrosine kinase associated with EGFR	Pancreatic cancer, non-small cell lung cancer
Imatinib	Tyrosine kinase inhibitor	Inhibition of c-Kit	GIST
Sunitinib	Tyrosine kinase inhibitor	Inhibition of tumour cell proliferation and angiogenesis	GIST, renal cell cancer
Sorafenib	Multikinase inhibitor	Blocks Raf kinase, VEGF receptors	Renal cell carcinoma, hepatocellular carcinoma

EGFR, endothelial growth factor receptor; GIST, gastrointestinal stromal tumours; VEGF, vascular endothelial growth factor.

Table 2.15.3.4 Common toxicities seen after systemic cytotoxic therapy

Acute complications	Chronic complications
Nausea and vomiting	Carcinogenesis (especially alkylating agents which can cause leukaemias)
Diarrhoea	Pulmonary fibrosis
Mucositis	Infertility
Alopecia	
Bone marrow suppression	
Renal and cardiac toxicity	

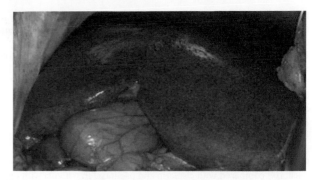

Fig. 2.15.3.3 A liver showing the characteristic 'yellow liver' of steatohepatitis caused by irinotecan therapy for colorectal liver metastases.

that has been shown to produce impressive response rates in gastrointestinal stromal tumours,[16] a tumour-type previously thought to be chemoresistant.

Sorafenib is a small molecule that inhibits tumour cell proliferation and tumour angiogenesis and increases the rate of apoptosis in a variety of tumour models. It has a number of actions, primarily through the inhibition of intracellular kinase. A large phase III trial demonstrated much improved survival in patients with hepatocellular carcinoma treated with sorafenib.[17]

Toxicity from chemotherapy

Unsurprisingly, the administration of non-targeted cytotoxic therapies can also affect normal tissues leading to systemic toxicity (Table 2.15.3.4).

As well as systemic toxicity, there is a growing recognition that neo-adjuvant chemotherapy can cause tissue damage resulting in increased morbidity and mortality after surgery Figure 2.15.3.2 and Figure 2.15.3.3.[18]

Methods of drug delivery

The majority of chemotherapy is administered systemically, usually via an oral or intravenous route. However, there are instances where regional chemotherapy can be used. For example, in patients with colorectal liver metastases the unique blood supply of the liver, with portal blood exclusively supplying the healthy hepatic parenchyma and arterial blood supplying both parenchyma and metastases, led to the concept of delivering transarterial chemotherapy in an effort to increase metastatic exposure to the agent, while reducing systemic dose and off-target side effects. Hepatic arterial infusion involves a catheter inserted at laparotomy into the hepatic artery (along with cholecystectomy to avoid chemical cholecystitis), through which a portable pump delivers an infusion of chemotherapeutic agent. Floxuridine, a chemotherapy agent commonly given by this route, undergoes first-pass metabolism limiting systemic exposure. However, this approach is limited by high rates of technical complications.[19] Transcatheter arterial chemoembolization is another modality that takes advantage of the dual blood supply of the liver.[20] Chemotherapeutic agents are delivered along with embolic agents, combining chemotherapeutic exposure with reduced drug washout and increased local toxicity, along with tumour ischaemia. Commonly used agents include doxorubicin, cisplatin, and irinotecan. This therapy is routinely used for the management of hepatocellular carcinoma.[21]

Intravesical therapy with mitomycin and biological agents such as *Bacillus* Calmette-Guerin have been used successfully in superficial bladder cancers,[22] and isolated limb perfusion with melphalan and tumour necrosis factor-α has also proven effective in unresectable limb melanoma and isolated soft tissue sarcoma of the limb.[23]

Conclusion

Chemotherapy for cancer has advanced considerably over the past few decades. Increased understanding of tumour biology has led to the development of targeted agents, minimizing toxicity. The development of novel predictive biomarkers has led to the identification of patients who will respond to treatment, further improving the personalization of treatment. Novel drug administration techniques have also led to improved response and reduced toxicity to existing agents.

References

1. Neoadjuvant cisplatin, methotrexate, and vinblastine chemotherapy for muscle-invasive bladder cancer: a randomised controlled trial. International collaboration of trialists. *Lancet* 1999; 354(9178): 533–40.
2. Cunningham D, Allum WH, Stenning SP, *et al*. Perioperative chemotherapy versus surgery alone for resectable gastroesophageal cancer. *N Engl J Med* 2006; 355(1): 11–20.

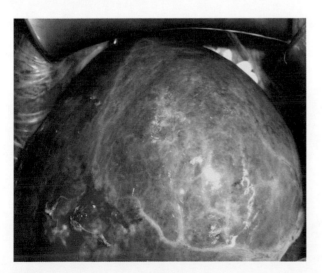

Fig. 2.15.3.2 A liver showing the characteristic 'blue liver' of sinusoidal obstruction syndrome caused by oxaliplatin therapy for colorectal liver metastases.

3. Blazer DG, Kishi Y, Maru DM, *et al.* Pathologic response to preoperative chemotherapy: a new outcome end point after resection of hepatic colorectal metastases. *J Clin Oncol* 2008; 26(33): 5344–51.

4. Poston J, Tait D, O'Connell S, *et al.* Diagnosis and management of colorectal cancer: summary of NICE guidance. *BMJ* 2011; 343(2): d6751.

5. Gill S, Loprinzi CL, Sargent DJ, *et al.* Pooled analysis of fluorouracil-based adjuvant therapy for stage II and III colon cancer: who benefits and by how much? *J Clin Oncol* 2004;22(10): 1797–806.

6. Joensuu H, Kellokumpu-Lehtinen PL, Bono P, *et al.* Adjuvant docetaxel or vinorelbine with or without trastuzumab for breast cancer. *N Engl J Med* 2006; 354(8): 809–20.

7. Ozols RF, Bundy BN, Greer BE, *et al.* Phase III trial of carboplatin and paclitaxel compared with cisplatin and paclitaxel in patients with optimally resected stage III ovarian cancer: a Gynecologic Oncology Group study. *J Clin Oncol* 2003; 21(17): 3194–200.

8. Neoptolemos JP, Dunn JA, Stocken DD, *et al.* Adjuvant chemoradiotherapy and chemotherapy in resectable pancreatic cancer: a randomised controlled trial. *Lancet* 2001; 358(9293): 1576–85.

9. Lam VW, Spiro C, Laurence JM, *et al.* A systematic review of clinical response and survival outcomes of downsizing systemic chemotherapy and rescue liver surgery in patients with initially unresectable colorectal liver metastases. *Ann Surg Oncol* 2012; 19(4): 1292–301.

10. Skipper HE, Schabel FM, Wilcox WS. Experimental evaluation of potential anticancer agents. XIV. Further study of certain basic concepts underlying chemotherapy of leukemia. *Cancer Chemother Rep* 1965; 45: 5–28.

11. Norton L, Simon R. Tumor size, sensitivity to therapy, and design of treatment schedules. *Cancer Treat Rep* 1977; 61(7): 1307–17.

12. Slamon DJ, Leyland-Jones B, Shak S, *et al.* Use of chemotherapy plus a monoclonal antibody against HER2 for metastatic breast cancer that overexpresses HER2. *N Engl J Med* 2001; 344(11): 783–92.

13. Bang YJ, Van Cutsem E, Feyereislova A, *et al.* Trastuzumab in combination with chemotherapy versus chemotherapy alone for treatment of HER2-positive advanced gastric or gastro-oesophageal junction cancer (ToGA): a phase 3, open-label, randomised controlled trial. *Lancet* 2010; 376(9742): 687–97.

14. Van Cutsem E, Köhne C-H, Hitre E, *et al.* Cetuximab and chemotherapy as initial treatment for metastatic colorectal cancer. *N Engl J Med* 2009; 360(14): 1408–17.

15. Ellis LM. Mechanisms of action of bevacizumab as a component of therapy for metastatic colorectal cancer. *Semin Oncol* 2006; 33(5 Suppl 10): S1–7.

16. Demetri GD, von Mehren M, Blanke CD, *et al.* Efficacy and safety of imatinib mesylate in advanced gastrointestinal stromal tumors. *N Engl J Med* 2002; 347(7): 472–80.

17. Llovet JM, Ricci S, Mazzaferro V, *et al.* Sorafenib in advanced hepatocellular carcinoma [Internet]. *N Engl J Med* 2008; 359(4): 378–90.

18. Vauthey JN, Pawlik TM, Ribero D, *et al.* Chemotherapy regimen predicts steatohepatitis and an increase in 90-day mortality after surgery for hepatic colorectal metastases. *J Clin Oncol* 2006; 24(13): 2065–72.

19. Allen PJ, Nissan A, Picon AI, *et al.* Technical complications and durability of hepatic artery infusion pumps for unresectable colorectal liver metastases: an institutional experience of 544 consecutive cases. *J Am Coll Surg* 2005; 201(1): 57–65.

20. Jones RP, Dunne D, Sutton P, *et al.* Segmental and lobar administration of drug-eluting beads delivering irinotecan leads to tumour destruction: a case-control series. *HPB (Oxford)* 2013; 15(1): 71–7.

21. Pawlik TM, Reyes DK, Cosgrove D, *et al.* Phase II trial of sorafenib combined with concurrent transarterial chemoembolization with drug-eluting beads for hepatocellular carcinoma. *J Clin Oncol* 2011; 29(30): 3960–7.

22. Brassell SA, Kamat AM. Contemporary intravesical treatment options for urothelial carcinoma of the bladder. *J Natl Compr Canc Netw* 2006; 4(10): 1027–36.

23. Noorda EM, Vrouenraets BC, Nieweg OE, *et al.* Isolated limb perfusion: what is the evidence for its use? *Ann Surg Oncol* 2004; 11(9): 837–45.

CHAPTER 2.15.4

General principles of radiation oncology

Chris D. Lee, Marcel Den Dulk, and Arthur Sun Myint

Introduction

Radiation therapy is one of the modalities for treatment of cancer where ionizing radiation is use to kill cancer cells to achieve a cure or control of cancer.

Types of radiation therapy

External beam radiotherapy

Radiation is delivered using X-rays (photons) away from the patient by a linear accelerator. A radiation beam targets the tumour (gross tumour volume [GTV]) precisely with a margin to include its possible local spread into the surrounding tissues (clinical target volume [CTV]). The radiation beams also include the possible lymphatic spread. Finally, the radiation treatment volume is planned to account for the systematic errors in the treatment set up and possible daily variations (planning target volume [PTV]).[3] Multiple radiation treatment beams are used to cover the primary tumour with possible local and regional lymphatic spread. The dose of radiation is concentrated around the PTV and multiple beams help to spare the normal surrounding tissue (Figure 2.15.4.1). The tolerance of normal surrounding tissues limits the dose of radiation that can be delivered to the PTV without causing serious complications.

Radiation dose

The dose of radiotherapy given is measured in Gray (Gy). This is the amount energy per unit mass delivered to the tumour and is given as a daily fractionated dose from Monday to Friday. Daily treatments with weekend breaks allows normal tissue to recover between treatments while the tumour cells are destroyed within each fraction of radiotherapy. The total dose delivered depends on the radio sensitivity of the tumour and the intent of the treatment. To cure lymphomas for example, radiation doses in the range between 20 Gy and 40 Gy are necessary, whereas for a solid epithelial-type tumour much higher doses of 60–80 Gy will be required. A highly specialized delivery method of radiation treatment is intensity-modulated radiation therapy (IMRT), which is used to deliver much higher doses (if necessary). However, much lower doses of 40–50 Gy are required if given as postoperative treatment (adjuvant) following surgical excision to eradicate the residual microscopic tumour cells, e.g. postoperative radiation for breast cancer following lumpectomy.[4]

Intensity-modulated radiation therapy

Modern radiotherapy machines (Figure 2.15.4.2) can deliver IMRT which allows the sparing of normal tissues (e.g. skin, eye or spinal cord). It also enables the dose distribution to conform to the tumour shape (e.g. tumours that wrap around the spinal cord or major radiosensitive organs). Advances in technology permit computers to tailor the radiation dose to specific areas within the tumour region. The dose is conformed to the three-dimensional shape of the tumour. This is achieved by controlling or modulating the radiation beam intensity increasing the dose of radiation to

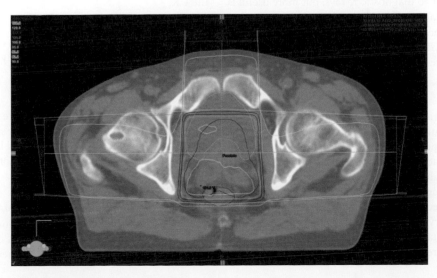

Fig. 2.15.4.1 Three field plan for prostate radiotherapy with lateral wedges.

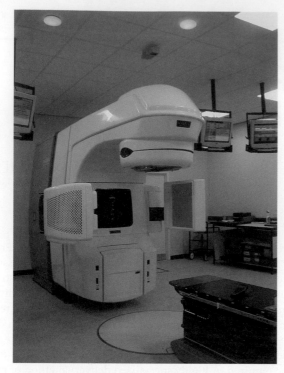

Fig. 2.15.4.2 High-energy linear accelerator with on-board imaging for image-guided radiation therapy.

tumour (e.g. lung) while at the same time minimizing the dose to the normal surrounding tissues (e.g. spinal cord) (Figure 2.15.4.3).[5]

Image-guided radiation therapy

This new technology is designed to track tumour movements and changes in tumour contour during treatment by using four-dimensional (4D) technology. It can be done by implanting a small detectable device or fiducial marker into, or close to, the tumour. Image-guided radiation therapy (IGRT) improves the precision of radiation delivery as changes to the tumour volume can occur during the long course of radiation or as a result of delays in starting the radiation course. This alteration in shape and size can be compensated by IGRT, which can adjust the radiation field to cover the changes in tumour contour over time. This is done using kilovoltage (kV) radiation similar to diagnostic X-rays, but more useful is cone-beam computed tomography (CT) imaging, which is used to produce a three-dimensional dataset for comparison with the original planning CT scan. IGRT improves the precision of radiation delivery and several studies have shown better outcomes for different tumour sites.[6,7]

Stereotactic radiation

This is a special type of radiation therapy that focuses the radiation beam to target the tumour using sophisticated imaging techniques. There are two types of stereotactic radiation: stereotactic radiosurgery and stereotactic body radiation therapy. Stereotactic radio surgery where a high dose of radiation is delivered precisely to a small tumour in a single fraction (e.g. a brain tumour). A stereotactic head frame is necessary to immobilize the patient, as the treatment margins are very small (1–2 mm). The other use of stereotactic radiation is stereotactic body radiation therapy where multiple beams of radiation are used to deliver a high dose of radiation

in a small number of multiple fractions (three to five) to the tumour in the body (e.g. lung cancer).[8]

Types of External beam radiation

1. Photons (X-rays), which are most commonly used.
2. Electrons (negatively charged particles): superficial skin tumours.
3. Protons (particle therapy): occular and childhood cancers.
4. Heavy ion particles (carbon ions): experimental research.
5. Other (gamma rays from cobalt sources).

Photons and electrons

Electrons, required for X-ray production in both a kV tube and a linear accelerator, are generated by passing an electrical current through a wire filament (cathode) in a vacuum. These electrons are accelerated and brought to rest in a high atomic number target (anode) producing X-rays. In a kV tube, the electron acceleration is provided by applying an electrical potential difference between the cathode and anode. For much higher photon energies as in a linear accelerator, an electromagnetic wave from a magnetron is fed into a waveguide where the electrons are accelerated before striking a target to produce X-rays.

Protons

Protons are positively charged particles that can be produced by bombarding hydrogen gas with low-energy electrons in a cyclotron. These are then focused and accelerated by electric and magnetic fields to generate a treatment beam. Protons are attractive clinically due to their depth-dose characteristics. As the relatively heavy particles (approximately 1840 times heavier than electrons) move through tissue, they slow down, gradually lose their energy and increase the dose deposited. It is not until they come to the end of their range that there is a sudden increase in dose deposition. This remarkable phenomenon of the *Bragg peak* means that the protons travel a fixed distance (depending on their energy) and come to an abrupt halt (in <1 mm). A single portal beam can be used and this limits the amount of normal tissues irradiated. Protons are used for treating paediatric tumours in the spine or brain and also used for occular melanomas. However, proton therapy is expensive and is available only in a few specialist centres in the UK.

Heavy ion particles

These are used mainly for experimental research at present and are also expensive to produce commercially with the currently available technology.

Others

Gamma rays from cobalt sources have been the main mode of treatment for megavoltage radiotherapy since the early 1950s. They are still used in many parts of the world but have been replaced by linear accelerators in most if not all radiotherapy centres in the UK.

Radiobiology

Radiotherapy causes damage to the DNA of the cancer cells. This underpins the principle of how radiation works in the treatment of cancer. There are two ways that DNA can be damaged. It can be achieved by either direct or indirect mechanisms. Direct damage

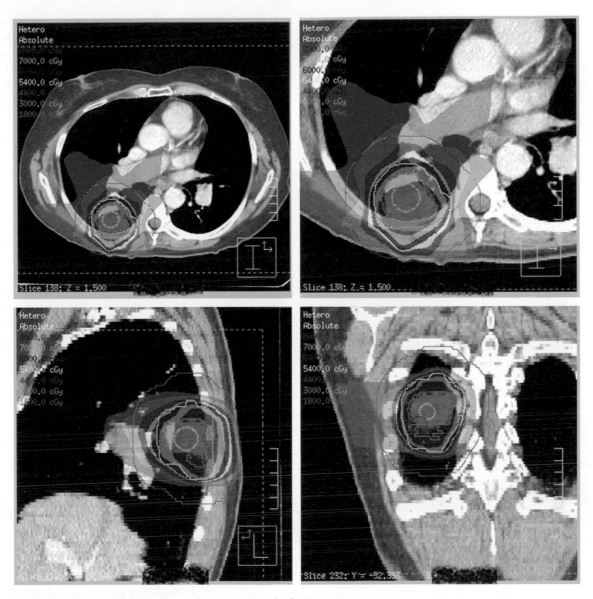

Fig. 2.15.4.3 Radiotherapy intensity-modulated radiation therapy treatment plan for lung cancer.

destroys the DNA strand and indirect damage is caused by ioni-zation of water releasing free radicals (hydroxyl radicals). These damage the atoms that make up the DNA chain of the cancer cells. In photon therapy most of the damage is caused by the indirect mechanism.[1]

Two types of events occur when radiation is delivered to the tumour tissue. A single hit with a double-stranded DNA break, where repair of the damage is not possible, and a sub-lethal hit with a single-stranded DNA break where repair is possible. Sub-lethal damage usually recovers after a period of time, but two sub-lethal hits to the DNA can induce programmed cell death through a process known as 'apoptosis'. Cells have the ability to repair single strand damage over time (sub-lethal damage), but double-stranded DNA damage is irreparable leading to cell death. Protons and other heavy particles with high linear energy transfer can, however, cause direct cell kill by a single hit damaging both DNA strands as these particles have a much larger mass than the smaller and lighter electrons.[9]

Radiotherapy is based on the concept that the tumour cells have less ability to repair the sub-lethal damage whereas the normal cells can repair this radiation damage allowing them to recover during the period between each radiation treatment fraction. Therefore, in radiosensitive tumours (e.g. lymphomas), after completion of the treatment the tumour cells are destroyed before they can recover. However, in less radiosensitive tumours (e.g. adenocarcinoma), there is a residual tumour at the end of radiation therapy that needs to be removed surgically to achieve cure (e.g. rectal cancer).[2]

Brachytherapy

Introduction to brachytherapy

Brachytherapy (*Greek*), meaning 'short distance' or 'near treatment', was one of the earliest forms of radiation therapy developed soon after the discovery of radioactivity by Henri Becquerel in 1896. Two years later in 1898, from work carried out by Marie and Pierre Curie, radium was discovered in its salt form. By the 1950s, brachy-therapy was being carried out all over the world.

Afterloaders

These were introduced to improve radiation protection. From the 1960s, the radiation protection problems associated with radium were becoming apparent and 'safer' artificially manufactured radioisotopes such as caesium-137, iridium-192, and iodine-125 were gradually replacing the source. In addition to new sources, the concept of afterloading was developing. This was the idea that non-radioactive templates, needles, or catheters are inserted into the treatment site defining the geometry of the implant, and are then subsequently loaded with radioactive sources by appropriately trained members of staff. In the modern era, this form of manual afterloading has been replaced with remote afterloading in which the source is mechanically driven into the applicator using a machine under computer control where the remote method of source deployment completely eliminates the dose received by members of staff. Early remote afterloaders used cobalt-60 or caesium-137 but the newer machines use iridium-192 and produce a much higher dose rate.

Common brachytherapy sources:

Caesium-137 (Cs-137):

- became available in the 1960's and replaced radium-226
- used in manual and remote afterloading. Now largely obsolete.

Iridium-192 (Ir-192):

- Common in two forms:
  - wire that needs to be cut to the desired length by the user (less common and expensive)
  - as small source typically 3.4 mm long and 0.9 mm diameter. This has a high activity and is used in an afterloader.

Iodine-125 (I-125):

- principally used for prostate brachytherapy
- available in strands of ten or as loose seeds
- each seed is 4.5 mm long and 0.8 mm diameter.

Common treatment sites

Cervix treatments

The Manchester dosimetry system[10] was developed for gynaecological intracavitary brachytherapy treatments in the 1930s using radium-226 tubes. Clinical applicator systems were designed based on this system or similar, consisting of an intrauterine tube and two vaginal ovoid source carriers. Similar applicators had been developed for the iridium-192 remote afterloader units, though these have a smaller diameter.

The prescription point for dosimetric calculations was defined as point A. This point is 2 cm lateral to the centre of the uterine canal and 2 cm superior to the mucous membrane of the lateral fornix along the line of the uterine canal. This point was chosen to be representative of the minimum dose of the most malignant tissue in cervix cancer treatment.

Over the last 10 years, with developments in imaging techniques and computer planning hardware and software, more complex planning techniques are possible with image fusion, dose optimization, and three-dimensional dose evaluation. Along with this development came the need for applicators to be redesigned such that they could be imaged safely using different imaging modalities. CT/

MR compatible applicators made from plastic or non-ferrous materials are now commercially available. Treatments can be delivered using standard source loadings but the flexibility to control both dwell times and positions with an afterloading stepping source such as a high-dose rate iridium-192 source, coupled with good imaging, permits treatment optimization shaping the dose around the tumour and away from radiation sensitive normal tissue such as the rectum and bladder.

These three-dimensional concepts have been detailed in the GEC-ESTRO recommendations,[11] and the Royal College of Radiologists[12] have published guidelines for the implementation in the UK.

Endometrial and vaginal treatments

There are a range of applicators to treat both the endometrium and vaginal vault. A single line source can be used which has cylindrical spacers of varying diameter to fit the patient to allow for a lower surface dose is used for the endometrium. The dose is prescribed to 5 mm from the applicator surface.

Prostate brachytherapy

The prostate organ is ideally suited for brachytherapy techniques for early stage prostate cancer where the target volume is located close to critical structures such as the bladder, anterior rectal wall, and urethra. External beam radiotherapy could damage these critical structures whereas brachytherapy would minimize the radiation damage. Both permanent seed and temporary high-dose rate (HDR) brachytherapy are now accepted as routine treatments. Accurate source/catheter placement via the perineum is achieved using a template guided method together with real-time transrectal ultrasound imaging (Figure 2.15.4.4). This imaging is linked directly to the treatment planning computer, allowing for continuous feedback of source/catheter position and dynamic, real-time dose calculation (Figure 2.15.4.5). Suitable low-risk patients for brachytherapy are selected depending on: the stage, prostate-specific antigen , Gleason score, urinary flow, and prostate volume.

Permanent seed prostate brachytherapy

In the UK, tiny iodine-125 seeds are used. The seeds used are 4.5 mm long and 0.8 mm diameter and remain permanently implanted in the prostate (Figure 2.15.4.6). The dose delivered slowly decays

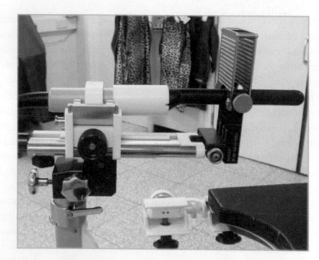

Fig. 2.15.4.4 Trans-rectal ultrasound probe mounted on stepper unit with needle grid.

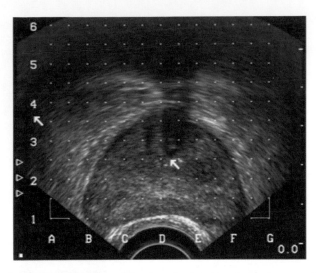

Fig. 2.15.4.5 Image showing section through prostate, urethra, and rectum with the position of the needle grid shown superimposed.

with time, with most of the radiation dose being given within the first few months. It has fewer side effects compared to surgery.

Temporary high-dose rate remote afterloading prostate brachytherapy

This type of brachytherapy is used for more advanced bulky prostate cancers. There are similarities between low-dose rate (LDR) and HDR prostate brachytherapy. The imaging is trans-rectal ultrasound and the catheters are inserted into the perineum via a grid template system. However, with HDR prostate brachytherapy, all the catheters are initially inserted and then a plan is computed. The ability of the remote afterloading unit to dwell the source at different positions for different lengths of time allows for the dose distribution to be optimized to a much greater extent than for iodine seed implants.

Breast brachytherapy

Brachytherapy to the breast is most commonly delivered as a boost following a course of external beam radiotherapy. Due to

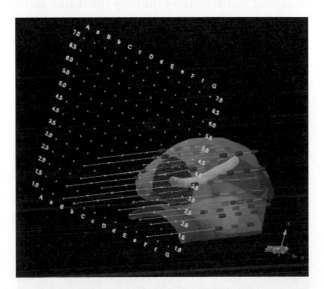

Fig. 2.15.4.6 Planning system visualization of prostate, urethra, rectum: seeds and grid.

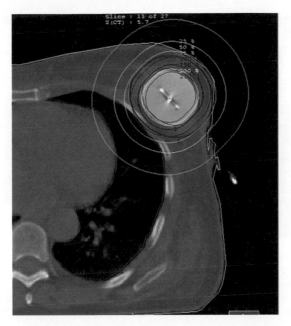

Fig. 2.15.4.7 Isodose distribution for intraoperative brachytherapy for breast cancer using MammoSite applicator.

the physics of brachytherapy, regions close to the source receive a very high dose while the dose to more distant tissues is significantly lower. For the case of breast brachytherapy, the implanted tumour will receive a very high dose and critical structures such as the skin, heart, lungs and ribs will be spared.

There are primarily three methods for treatment delivery:

1. Using a multi-catheter interstitial implant:
   - Can be used for both boost and monotherapy treatments.
   - A bridge supporting two templates is positioned over the breast.
   - The templates have a series of holes to allow the passage of rigid needles.
   - The holes are arranged so as to conform to the Paris dosimetry system (parallel rows of squares or triangles) in 2 or 3 planes with a typical spacing of 10-15mm.
   - The treatment lengths between the plates for each catheter can be determined from accurate measurement during the theatre procedure ensuring 5mm of skin sparing.
   - For this rigid bridge technique, radiographic catheter reconstruction is not necessary and the implant can be reconstructed via simple geometric methods.

2. Using a balloon catheter such as the MammoSite®:
   - The MammoSite® is a balloon catheter with two ports; one to allow inflation of the balloon with a mixture of sterile water and contrast and the other for the HDR source (Figure 2.15.4.7).
   - This catheter is used mainly for monotherapy but can be used to deliver a boost.

3. Electronic intraoperative brachytherapy:
   - One of the machines for this treatment technique uses a miniature 50 kV X-ray source mounted at the end of an articulated gantry stand (Figure 2.15.4.8).

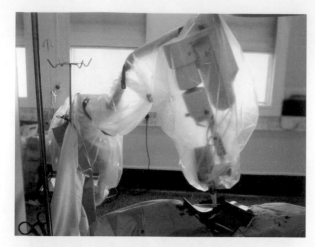

Fig. 2.15.4.8 Machine for intraoperative breast brachytherapy.
Reprinted from *The Lancet*, Volume 376, Number 9735, Jayant S. VaidyaTargeted *et al.*, intraoperative radiotherapy versus whole breast radiotherapy for breast cancer (TARGIT-A trial): an international, prospective, randomised, non-inferiority phase 3 trial, pp. 91–102, Copyright © 2010 Elsevier Ltd., http://www.sciencedirect.com/science/journal/01406736.

- After the surgery and during the same procedure, a suitable spherical applicator is secured to the end of the X--ray tube. This is then positioned within the surgical cavity and the required dose delivered (Figure 2.15.4.9).

High-dose rate rectal brachytherapy

HDR brachytherapy can be carried out preoperatively to downstage the tumour. For those patients who are unsuitable for surgery, rectal brachytherapy can also be given in addition to other forms of non-invasive treatment.

The treatment applicator used is cylindrical in shape and can have single or multiple channels (Figures 2.15.4.10 and 2.15.4.11). A multiple channel applicator enables the delivered dose distribution to be conformally planned, whereas a single channel applicator only allows circularly symmetric dose distributions.

Head and neck brachytherapy

The traditional technique for treating head and neck cancer with brachytherapy was using LDR iridium-192 wire manually afterloaded into catheters that had been geometrically positioned

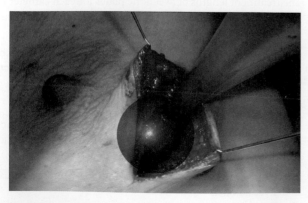

Fig. 2.15.4.9 Intraoperative breast brachytherapy applicator.
Reprinted from *The Lancet*, Volume 376, Number 9735, Jayant S. Vaidya Targeted *et al.*, intraoperative radiotherapy versus whole breast radiotherapy for breast cancer (TARGIT-A trial): an international, prospective, randomised, non-inferiority phase 3 trial, pp. 91–102, Copyright © 2010 Elsevier Ltd., http://www.sciencedirect.com/science/journal/01406736.

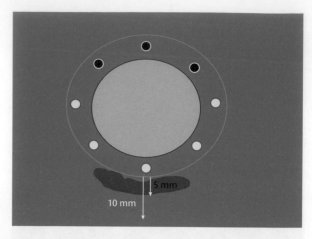

Fig. 2.15.4.10 Rectal brachytherapy applicator showing multiple treatment channels.

during a surgical procedure. At the present time, iridium-192 wire is very difficult to resource and is very expensive. An alternative is using the remote HDR afterloader. The catheters are positioned in the same way as for the LDR case described above and these are subsequently connected to the HDR unit and the dose delivered.

1.3 Surface moulds

Surface moulds are designed for treating superficial skin lesions. They contain a series of catheters running parallel at a fixed distance (10–20 mm) from the skin surface. The choice of stand-off distance will depend on the depth required for treatment and acceptable skin dose. The inverse square law applies, i.e. the closer the source to the skin, the higher the dose and the steeper the dose gradient.

1.4 Quality assurance

In order to ensure the clinical intent is achieved as accurately and as safely as possible it is necessary to have in place, a quality assurance programme. As part of this quality assurance programme regular checks and measurements are carried out with suitably tight tolerances to ensure a high level of accuracy.

1.5 Systemic radio-isotope therapy (unsealed source)

This type of therapy is a form of targeted radiotherapy. It can be delivered as an infusion intravenously (e.g. Strontium-89 therapy

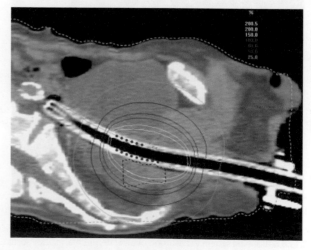

Fig. 2.15.4.11 Showing rectal applicator insitu for brachytherapy treatment.

for bony metastases) or as an oral therapy (e.g. radioactive iodine therapy for thyroid cancer). Another form of systemic radio-isotope therapy is to label glass spheres or resin spheres with Yttrium-90 which can be injected into the hepatic artery to radio-embolize primary liver tumours or hepatic metastases that are inoperable. More recently, radio-immunotherapy using CD20 monoclonal antibodies conjugated to Yttrium-90 (e.g. ibritumomab tiuxetan [Zevalin®]) or radioactive iodine (tositumomab/iodine I-131®) have been used to treat refractory non-Hodgkin's lymphoma.

Indications for radiotherapy

Preoperative radiotherapy

This type of radiation is used to improve local control (e.g. preoperative radiotherapy for operable rectal cancer). There have been at least three large randomized trials over three decades. All except the initial Swedish trial have shown improved local control but no improvement in survival. The Swedish trial was criticised for poor results in the surgical alone arm (local recurrence 27% versus 11%).[13] As a result, TME (total mesorectal excision) surgical training was mandatory in the next trial. However, the mature Dutch trial showed that despite adequate surgical training the local recurrence was high in the surgical arm (11% versus 5.5%).[14] The MRC CR07 trial in the UK showed similar results with improved local control for radiotherapy even for patients who had an optimal surgical plane of resection.[15]

Intraoperative radiotherapy

Intraoperative radiotherapy following lumpectomy was first used in Milan using electrons. This was followed by 50 KV X-rays used in the TARGIT trial.[16] An update of the randomized trial showed equipoise local control if the radiation was used immediately after local excision. The TARGIT B trial will evaluate the role of intraoperative radiotherapy using 50 KV X-rays as a boost following lumpectomy.

Postoperative radiotherapy

Local recurrence is high in patients with involved resection margins following surgery. Therefore, postoperative radiotherapy is used to improve local control (e.g. head and neck, oral, sarcomas, and brain tumours), where further surgical resection is not possible or appropriate.

Combined modalities with radiation

Radiation alone is not always effective, especially in bulky cancers that are not radiosensitive (e.g. rectal, cervical, and lung cancers). Therefore, chemotherapy can be added to make the radiation more effective. The exact mechanism of how chemotherapy helps radiation is not fully understood, but radiosensitization is thought to be significant here. The drawback is higher side effects from combined treatment.

Side effects of radiotherapy

Side effects vary from patient to patient, but most side effects from radiation are predictable. It is important to explain to the patient that these are expected and that they usually settle after a period of time. Radiotherapy is painless and the side effects are confined to the treated area but gradually build up during the course of treatment and usually last for 4 to 6 weeks following treatment. Acute side effects occur within a few days to a few weeks and late side effects occur after a few months. The intensity of the side effects depends on the dose of radiation, fractionation, the area treated, the volume treated, and whether chemotherapy is used concurrently. Palliative radiotherapy should cause very few side effects as the radiation dose used is low. Radical radiotherapy on the other hand may cause significant side effects, although these usually settle after a few weeks following treatment.

Acute side effects (up to 12 weeks)

Acute side effects occur within a few days to a few weeks and usually settle down after about 4 to 6 weeks.

Skin and mucosa: Damage to epithelial surfaces depends on the area treated (e.g. skin, oral mucosa, pharynx, small bowel, bladder, urethra, and anus). The skin becomes erythematous after about a week and gradually becomes dry and desquamates. The treated area then ulcerates, leading to moist desquamation. It is worse in areas where there is skin friction (e.g. the groin). It can be uncomfortable for a few weeks but recovers very quickly without many long-term squealae (e.g. anal cancer treatment).[17]

◆ Gastrointestinal: The mouth can become sore if the head and neck areas are treated. The throat can become sore and swallowing may become painful. Hydration and maintaining nutrition during treatment is important. Small bore nasogastric feeding can help to maintain the fluid and nutritional needs. Simple local analgesics and lozenges can also help.

Frequent or loose motions follow pelvic radiotherapy and can start a week or two into radiation treatment. This is due to radiation enteritis of the small bowel. The height of the reaction is towards the end of the treatment and can continue for 2 to 4 weeks after completion. Dietary advice to avoid a high fibre intake is given and simple antidiarrhoeals such as loperamide (2 mg) can help. Nausea and vomiting are not common and are usually mild. It can be controlled with oral domperidone (10 mg) or cyclizine (50 mg).

◆ Bladder and prostate: Frequency of micturation can occur, which can be painful. Urine culture is necessary to exclude infection, which can aggravate symptoms.

◆ Hair loss occurs a few weeks following brain irradiation. The amount of hair regrowth varies but may not be complete.

◆ A cough, which is usually unproductive due to acute pneumonitis, can be troublesome. Sputum should be sent for culture (if productive) to exclude infection.

◆ Tiredness may follow a few weeks after radiotherapy and can be troublesome. The mechanism is poorly understood. Supportive treatment can be given if an obvious cause is found e.g. blood transfusion for anaemia.

Late side effects (from 12 weeks to years)

Late radiation side effects occur months to years after treatment and usually affect the area or organ treated. It can affect the quality of life and modern radiation techniques are focused on reducing both acute and long-term side effects. Patients who are affected severely may need referral to specialist clinics if symptoms are severe e.g. lymphoedema clinic, late radiation effect clinic for children.

- Skin: Radiation dermatitis can cause altered pigmentation, deformity due to scarring, dryness of skin, loss of elasticity due to subcutaneous fibrosis, and telangiectasia (rare). Radiation can cause delay in wound healing after surgery.

- Hair loss (epilation) can occur after radiotherapy. The extent of hair loss depends on dose of radiation and the area treated.

- Dry mouth can occur due to reduced salivation from radiation damage to the salivary gland following radical head and neck radiotherapy.

- Cataracts may occur a few months to years after radiation near the eye. Dry eye with cornea damage can result due to late radiation effect on the lachrymal glands.

- Rectum: radiation proctitis can cause bleeding, tennesmus, and pain. Anastomotic leakage can occur and defunctioning stoma is usually necessary to reduce this risk after preoperative radiotherapy.

- Bladder: radiation cystitis can cause haematuria, dysuria, and frequency of micturation due to reduced bladder capacity.

- Vagina: Radiation can cause dryness, dyspareunia, and stenosis. Sexual counselling may be necessary. Lubricants during intercourse and vaginal dilators can help. Rectovaginal fistula is a rare complication but when it occurs, it is serious and may require corrective surgery.

- Fertility: the gonads (ovary and testis) are both sensitive to radiation and infertility can occur following radiation. Banking of sperm or ovum is not always successful and careful counselling is necessary in treating patients in their reproductive age.

- Brain: radiation can cause varying degrees of brain damage and special care and consideration is necessary in treating brain tumours in children. Long-term memory and cognitive function can be affected.

- Secondary cancers: radiation can cause secondary haematological malignancies within 5 years and solid tumours within 10 to 20 years. The risk of secondary malignancies is usually small, occurring in less than 1/1000. The risk of second malignancies is much higher in children and protons are the preferred method of radiation in children to reduce this risk.

Future of radiotherapy

Technology has advanced in the past decade and radiotherapy has improved enabling safe and effective delivery of radiation treatment with fewer side effects. This improves the outcome in many tumour sites. Dose escalation is possible through IMRT with the addition of dose painting to increase the dose of radiation where it is most needed. Micro multi-leaf collimators in modern radiotherapy machines can shape the radiation beam accurately, which improves the shielding of normal structures around the tumour. IGRT enables a more precise delivery of the radiation beam by tracking the tumour shape and position during treatment and tighter radiation treatment margins can be applied resulting in fewer side effects (e.g. lung cancer treatment using stereotactic body radiation therapy). Advances in brachytherapy enable interstitial, intraluminal, and intracavitary HDR afterloading. HDR is more convenient for the patient as treatment times are considerably shorter than the equivalent low-dose rate techniques where prolonged inpatient stays were necessary. Combined multimodality radiation with newer chemotherapeutic agents allow oral medication to be used (e.g. capecitabine instead of infusional 5-fluorouracil-based chemotherapy for gastrointestinal malignancies such as oesophagus, anus, and rectum). It is hoped that advances in translational research may identify predictive markers to offer personalized multimodality treatments to tailor to patient needs. Radiation can either be omitted or used depending on tumour radiosensitivity. This will avoid radiation where it is not needed and its use where appropriate. In future, newer targeted radiation will allow organ preservation treatments for early cancer and avoid extirpative surgery, which will be reserved for more advanced radio-resistant cancers (e.g. contact radiotherapy for early rectal cancer). Multidisciplinary team meetings will be crucial for the pivotal decisions to select the use of radiation where indicated. Referral for second opinion may be necessary for difficult and complicated cases.

Further reading

Bomford CK, Kunkler IH, Sherrif SB (eds). *Walter and Miller's Textbook of Radiotherapy: Radiation Physics, Therapy and Oncology*. London: Churchill Livingstone, 2003
Hoskin P (ed.). *Radiotherapy in Practice: External Beam radiotherapy*. Oxford: Oxford University Press, 2012.
Hoskin P, Coyle C (eds). *Radiotherapy in Practice: Brachytherapy*. Oxford: Oxford University Press, 2011.
Mayles P, Rosenwald JC, Nahum A. *Handbook of Radiation Therapy Physics: Theory and Practice*. London: Taylor & Francis, 2007.

References

1. Hall E. *Radiobiology for Radiologist*. Philadelphia: Lippincott Williams & Wilkins, 2006.
2. Thariat J, Hannoun-Levi J-M, Sun Myint A, et al. Past, Present and Future of radiotherapy for the benefit of patients. *Nat Rev Clin Oncol* 2013; 10(1): 52–60.
3. Dobbs J, Barrett A (eds). *Practical Radiotherapy Planning*. London: Edward Arnold, 2009.
4. Clark RM, McCulloch PB, Levine MN, et al. Randomized clinical trial to assess the effectiveness of breast irradiation following lumpectomy and axillary dissection for node-negative breast cancer. *J Natl Cancer Inst* 1992; 84: 683–9.
5. MacKay RI, Staffurth J, Poynter A, et al. UK guidelines for the safe delivery of intensity-modulated radiotherapy. *Clin Oncol* 2010; 22(8): 629–35.
6. Sharpe MB, Craig T, Moseley DJ. Image guidance: treatment target localization systems. In Meyer JL (ed) *IMRT-IGRT-SBRT: Advances in the treatment planning and delivery of radiotherapy. Frontiers in Radiation Therapy Oncology* 2007; 40: 72–93. Madison, WI: Karger.
7. Dawson, LA; Sharpe, MB. Image-guided radiotherapy: rationale, benefits, and limitations. *Lancet Oncol.* 2006; 7(10): 848–58.
8. Chang JY, Liu H, Balter P, et al. Clinical outcome and predictors of survival and pneumonitis after stereotactic ablative radiotherapy for stage I non-small cell lung cancer. *Radiat Oncol* 2012; 7: 152.
9. Hall EJ. What will molecular biology contribute to our understanding of radiation-induced cell killing and carcinogenesis? *Int J Radiat Biol* 1997; 71: 667–74.
10. Tod M, Meredith W. Treatment of cancer of the cervix uteri: A revised 'Manchester method'. *Br J Radiol* 1953; 26: 252–7.

11. Haie-Meder C, Potter R, Van Limbergen E, et.al. Gynaecological (GYN) GEC-ESTRO Working Group. Recommendations from Gynaecological (GYN) GEC-ESTRO Working Group (I): concepts and terms in 3D image based 3D treatment planning in cervix cancer brachytherapy with emphasis on MRI assessment of GTV and CTV. *Radiother Oncol* 2005; 74: 235–45.

12. Royal College of Radiologists. *Implementing Image-Guided Brachytherapy for Cervix Cancer in the UK*. London: The Royal College of Radiologists, 2009.

13. Swedish Rectal Cancer Trial. Improved survival with preoperative radiotherapy in resectable rectal cancer. *N Engl. J Med* 1997; 336: 980–7.

14. Kapiteijn E, Marijnen CA, Nagtegaal ID, *et al* for the Dutch Colorectal Cancer Group. Pre-operative radiotherapy combined with total mesorectal excision for resectable rectal cancer. *N Engl J Med* 2001; 345: 638–46.

15. Sebag-Montefiore D, Stephens R, Steele R, et.al. Pre-operative radiotherapy versus selective postoperative chemoradiotherapy in patients with rectal cancer (MRC CR07 and NCIC-CTG C016): a multicentre, randomised trial. *Lancet* 2009; 373(9666): 811–20.

16. Vaidya JS, Joseph DJ, Tobias JS, *et al*. Targeted intraoperative radiotherapy versus whole breast radiotherapy for breast cancer (TARGIT-A trial): an international, prospective, randomised, non-inferiority phase 3 trial. *Lancet* 2010; 376(9735): 91–102.

17. Sun Myint A. Follow up. ACPGBI Position Statement for Management of Anal Cancer. *Colorectal Dis* 2011; 13: 39–43.

Hormonal therapy in cancer

Declan Dunne, Derek McWhirter, and Graeme J. Poston

Introduction

Cancer cells arising from hormonally active tissue frequently over-express hormone receptors. Their growth and function is often dependent on hormone availability and activity. As a result of this phenomenon, hormonal cancer therapy has been developed to treat a number of cancers. The most common cancers managed either entirely or in part with hormonal therapy include breast cancer, prostate cancer, and neuroendocrine tumours. In this chapter we discuss the main hormonal agents in each of these conditions, including their indications and side effects.

Hormonal treatment of breast cancer

The effects of oestrogen and progesterone are key factors in the development of the majority of cases of breast cancer. While surgical resection remains the gold-standard treatment of breast cancer, the use of hormonal therapy has been shown to be associated with improved outcome in patients whose tumour is hormone-receptor positive. Hormonal therapy is also relatively safe when compared to the chemotherapy regimens frequently employed for other forms of cancer.

Selective oestrogen modulators

Mode of action

A range of selective oestrogen modulators exist, with actions ranging from full agonistic activity in all tissues, such as naturally occurring oestrogen, to full antagonistic activity in all tissues. The most common drug in use for treating cancer is tamoxifen, which has mixed antagonistic/agonistic activity. It acts as an antagonist in breast tissue but as a partial agonist in the uterus. Tamoxifen is activated in the liver to form its active agent 4-hydroxy-tamoxifen. This activated form then acts in breast tissue to block the oestrogen receptor (ER) and prevent transcription of oestrogen-dependent genes, and consequently inhibit cell growth and division.

Uses

Selective oestrogen receptor modulators (SERM) are used in the treatment of oestrogen receptor (ER-positive) breast cancer. A number of clinical indications have been considered for their use.

Prevention of breast cancer

The use of SERMs in the prevention of cancer in women at high risk has been suggested following the finding that adjuvant treatment with tamoxifen reduced the incidence of cancers in the contralateral breast. The Breast Cancer Preventional Trial (P-1) in the United States demonstrated that treatment with tamoxifen for a 5-year period led to a risk reduction of over 50%.[1] There were associated increased risks of developing endometrial cancer as a result of its agonist effect on endometrial proliferation, but despite this observation, it has been approved for use in prevention for high-risk patients.

Adjuvant treatment of early stage cancer

SERMs have been used in the adjuvant setting for over 30 years. They are used after surgical resection alongside other adjuvant modalities including radiotherapy and chemotherapy. Length of therapy has varied from 5 to 10 years and in some cases as long as 15 years. A recent meta-analysis has shown that 5 years of therapy with tamoxifen reduces the 15-year risk of disease recurrence and mortality. The greatest benefit is seen in the first 5 years (RR 0.53), then 5-9 years (RR 0.68), after which the benefit appears to be lost.[2] A number of recent trials looking at different hormonal therapies have led to a number of different regimens being used. In some cases women switch to an aromatase inhibitor (AI) after 2 to 3 years of tamoxifen, to a total of 5 years of hormone therapy, while others offer further treatment with an AI after 5 full years of tamoxifen. Tamoxifen is predominately used in premenopausal women, who usually have too much aromatase for an AI to work effectively.

Treatment of metastatic breast cancer

Tamoxifen has been shown to be effective and equivalent to ovarian ablation in premenopausal women with metastatic ER-positive cancer. In postmenopausal women, AIs can be used when the tumour progresses despite treatment with tamoxifen.

Primary endocrine management

In elderly women with significant medical co-morbidities, where the risks preclude surgery and/or chemotherapy, treatment of ER-positive cancer can be primarily with tamoxifen ± AIs to slow disease progression.

Side effects of selective oestrogen modulators

The partial agonistic effect of tamoxifen on uterus and bone is associated with significant side effects. In the uterus it leads to endometrial proliferation and increases the risk of developing endometrial cancer. In bone, it can prevent osteoporosis by inhibition of osteoclasts, but in premenopausal women it can reduce bone mineral density. As a consequence, assessment of bone density and preventative therapy with a bisphosphonate is often undertaken. Tamoxifen is also associated with an increased risk of deep vein thrombosis, pulmonary embolism, and stroke.

Aromatase inhibitors

Mode of action

AIs are drugs that block the production of oestrogen by inhibiting the key enzyme aromatase. Commonly used AIs include letrozole

(Femara) and anastrazole (Arimadex), which temporarily inhibit the enzyme, and exemestane (Aromasin), which permanently inactivates the enzyme.

Uses

AIs are predominately used in postmenopausal women, because premenopausal women often have too much aromatase for the inhibitors to effectively block.

Prevention of breast cancer

Exemestane has been shown to reduce the risk of developing breast cancer in high-risk postmenopausal women.[3] Longer follow-up studies are required and at present its use in the prevention of breast cancer remains controversial.

Adjuvant treatment of breast cancer

Letrozole, anastrazole and exemestane are all established for use in the adjuvant treatment of ER-positive tumours in postmenopausal women. It can also be used in patients previously treated with tamoxifen. A 10-year follow-up of the ATAC study[4] has shown that anastrazole has superior efficacy and safety over tamoxifen in postmenopausal women.

Metastatic breast cancer

Letrozole and anastrazole can be used in the primary management of metastatic breast cancer. Phase III studies have shown a superiority over tamoxifen in reducing progression, but not in overall survival.[5]

Side effects of aromatase inhibitors

Inhibition of oestrogen leads to reduced bone mineral density and development of osteoporosis. Dietary and, if necessary, medical therapies are needed to reduce the risk of fracture. The use of AIs is also associated with increased cardiovascular risk in the form of myocardial infarction, angina, heart failure and hypercholesterolemia.

Hormonal treatment of prostate cancer

Hormonal therapy forms the mainstay of treatment for prostate cancer in older men. It is also a key component in therapy in younger men where the disease may be more biologically aggressive; this can be either in resectable local disease or metastatic disease. The key aim of hormonal therapy in prostate cancer is to eliminate androgen dependant growth and progression.

Anti-androgens

Anti-androgens prevent androgens expressing their biological effects on androgen-sensitive tissues. These agents are predominantly used in the treatment of prostate cancer. The aim of therapy in this setting is to induce medical castration, and this is often achieved in combination therapy with other agents. Anti-androgens are classified as either steroidal or non-steroidal. Non-steroidal anti-androgens include bicalutamide,

The major androgen acting on the prostate is dihydrotestosterone (DHT), which is produced from circulating testosterone by the actions of 5α-reductase enzymes.

Mode of action

Steroidal anti-androgens, including cytopterone, competitively inhibit DHT and testosterone to androgen receptors. They bind to progesterone receptors inhibiting luteinizing hormone (LH) release within the pituitary and production of testosterone by the testis.[6]

Non-steroidal anti-androgens such as bicalutamide and flutamide act to competitively block androgen receptors preventing the activity of both testosterone and DHT. They also lead to increased LH secretion and testosterone production.

Uses in prostate cancer

Anti-androgens are used to achieve the goal of androgen deprivation therapy. A number of trials examined the role of dual therapy with anti-androgen and gonadotropin-releasing hormone (GnRH) agonists, to achieve combined androgen blockage. A recent meta-analysis assessing the therapy found only minimal survival benefit in a very limited cohort of patients with the best prognostic features.

In combination with surgery

Androgen deprivation therapy (ADT) has been examined in the neo-adjuvant and adjuvant setting, in combination with radical prostatectomy. In the neo-adjuvant setting there has been evidence that 3 months of neo-adjuvant ADT can reduce the size of prostate, and so reduce the incidence of positive margins following surgery for T2b tumours. Despite this observation, no difference has been shown in disease recurrence rates, overall survival, or complications following surgery.[7]

There is no evidence to support the use of adjuvant ADT, except if there is failure to reduce prostate-specific antigen to an undetectable level, or confirmed lymph node metastasis. In this setting there is a high incidence of undetected metastatic disease.[8, 9]

In combination with radiotherapy

When combined with radiotherapy, ADT is aimed at reducing the size of the prostate, thereby decreasing the radiation field and consequently dose related radiation injury to other organs (in particular, the rectum). There is also evidence to support an additive effect of ADT with radiation.[10]

As primary hormone treatment

Anti-androgens are often used as monotherapy, or in combination with other agents instead of surgery to treat prostate cancer. Early initiation of this therapy has been shown to delay the development of metastasis, and the associated complications of urethral obstruction, pathological fractures, and cord compression. However, these benefits are at a cost of increased hospital attendance, and higher economic costs.[11] There is evidence supporting the use of ADT to slow progression in metastatic disease.[12]

Intermittent androgen deprivation therapy

Given the negative health and quality of life effects associated with ADT, there have been moves to investigate the feasibility of intermittent ADT. Early evidence suggests this may be a viable alternative management strategy.[13]

Side effects of anti-androgens

Steroidal anti-androgens have similar side effects to surgical castration, including loss of libido, erectile dysfunction, hot flushes, anaemia, obesity, decrease in muscle strength, and development of female sexual characteristics such as gynaecomastia. Mood changes such as depression are common, and there is concern about the potential cardiovascular risks of treatment. Long-term treatment induces osteoporosis, and this must be monitored when considering therapy.

Non-steroidal anti-androgens do not cause the side effects of chemical castration, but can be associated with nausea, vomiting, and in rare cases liver toxicity. Monitoring of liver function tests is advised in all patients taking these drugs.[12]

Gonadotropin-releasing hormone analogues

Mode of action

GnRH agonists bind to the GnRH receptor in the pituitary causing release of follicle-stimulating hormone (FSH) and LH. Unlike their endogenous counterparts, they do not quickly dissociate from the receptor. This results in an initial 'flare effect' or surge of FSH and LH, with subsequent profound decrease in circulating FSH and LH.

GnRH antagonists block the GnRH receptor in the pituitary, which serves to block the release of LH and FSH. This leads to a rapid drop in testosterone production, bringing levels down to those seen after castration.

Uses

Primarily GnRH analogues are used in the treatment of prostate cancer to induce chemical castration. This may be in isolation, or in conjunction with anti-androgens to achieve ADT. These actions are described in the anti-androgen section.

Side effects of gonadotropin-releasing hormone analogues

The surge associated with introduction of GnRH agonists can induce an initial increased activity in metastases, and in the case of spinal bone metastases can lead to severe pain and cord compression. GnRH analogues are injected medicines, and as such can be associated with injection site complications. Other side effects of GnRH therapy are typical of the deprivation of androgens as mentioned earlier.

Hormonal treatment of neuroendocrine tumours

Gastrointestinal neuroendocrine tumours are a rare group of malignancies, which are often diagnosed late when they are already metastatic. They often overexpress somatostatin hormone receptors in comparison to the rest of the gastrointestinal tract, and as such hormonal manipulation of this pathway has been developed to aid in their management.

Somatostatin analogues

Somatostatins are naturally occurring peptide hormones that inhibit the release of many hormones and other secretory proteins, motility and cell growth. Most neuroendocrine tumours occurring within the gastrointestinal tract overexpress somatization receptors.

Mode of action

Octreotide and lanreotide are long-acting analogues of natural somatostatin that, unlike naturally occurring somatostatin with a circulation half-life of just a few minutes, are not rapidly degraded. They bind to somatostatin receptors on tumours, inhibiting their secretory functions and in some cases cell division and tumour growth.

Uses

Somatostatin analogues are primarily used in the treatment of symptomatic secretory gastrointestinal and pancreatic neuroendocrine tumours, although they are also used in some rare paraneoplastic syndromes to manage the consequences of ectopic adrenocorticotrophic hormone, GnRH, and parathyroid hormone production.

Management of hormone-producing neuroendocrine tumours

Somatostatin analogues are established in the treatment of functioning hormone-producing neuroendocrine tumours, with mean response rates in excess of 70%. These therapies serve to minimize the symptoms associated with hormone-producing neuroendocrine tumours, while slowing tumour progression.[14] They should be considered for all patients expressing symptoms of functionally active tumours and in patients with tumour progression, even in the absence of symptoms relating to the functional activity.

Prevention of carcinoid crisis

Carcinoid crisis is a rare but life-threatening complication seen during surgery and anaesthetic induction in patients with carcinoid syndrome. Treatment with somatostatin analogues prior to such interventions can protect against this life-threatening complication.[15]

Prevention of long-term complications of carcinoid syndrome

Cardiac disease was responsible for the deaths of around 30% of patients with carcinoid syndrome prior to the introduction of somatostatin analogues. Treatment with somatostatin analogues has reduced this complication to less than 4%.[14]

In non-hormone-producing neuroendocrine tumours

The use of somatostatin analogues in this setting is controversial,[14,15] but evidence suggests that the administration of high doses of somatostatin analogues can slow progression in such tumours.[16]

Side effects of somatostatin analogues

Common side effects of somatostatin therapy include abdominal pain, diarrhoea, nausea, and complications relating to the injection site. Less frequent effects include the development of gallstones, gastric atony, and disorders of glucose metabolism. Some surgeons advocate prophylactic cholecystectomy when resecting any functioning symptomatic neuroendocrine tumours, even for cure.[15]

References

1. Fisher B, Costantino JP, Wickerham DL, et al. Tamoxifen for prevention of breast cancer: report of the National Surgical Adjuvant Breast and Bowel Project P-1 Study. *J Natl Cancer Inst* 1998; 90(18): 1371–88.
2. Davies C, Godwin J, Gray R, et al. Relevance of breast cancer hormone receptors and other factors to the efficacy of adjuvant tamoxifen: patient-level meta-analysis of randomised trials. *Lancet* 2011; 378(9793): 771–84.
3. Goss PE, Ingle JN, Alés-Martínez JE, et al. Exemestane for breast-cancer prevention in postmenopausal women. *N Engl J Med* 2011; 364(25): 2381–91.
4. Cuzick J, Sestak I, Baum M, et al. Effect of anastrozole and tamoxifen as adjuvant treatment for early-stage breast cancer: 10-year analysis of the {ATAC} trial [Internet]. *Lancet Oncol* 2010; 11(12): 1135–41.
5. Mouridsen H, Gershanovich M, Sun Y, et al. Phase III study of letrozole versus tamoxifen as first-line therapy of advanced breast cancer in postmenopausal women: analysis of survival and update of efficacy from the International Letrozole Breast Cancer Group. *J Clin Oncol* 2003; 21(11): 2101–9.

6. Varenhorst E, Wallentin L, Carlström K. The effects of orchidectomy, estrogens, and cyproterone acetate on plasma testosterone, LH, and FSH concentrations in patients with carcinoma of the prostate. *Scand J Urol Nephrol* 1982; 16(1): 31–6.

7. Scolieri MJ, Altman A, Resnick MI. Neoadjuvant hormonal ablative therapy before radical prostatectomy: a review. Is it indicated? *J Urol* 2000; 164(5): 1465–72.

8. Messing EM, Manola J, Yao J, *et al*. Immediate versus deferred androgen deprivation treatment in patients with node-positive prostate cancer after radical prostatectomy and pelvic lymphadenectomy. *Lancet Oncol* 2006; 7(6): 472–9.

9. Trapasso JG, deKernion JB, Smith RB, *et al*. The incidence and significance of detectable levels of serum prostate specific antigen after radical prostatectomy. *J Urol* 1994; 152(5 Pt 2): 1821–5.

10. Bolla M, Laramas M, and Association of Radiotherapy and Oncology of the Mediterranean arEa (AROME). Combined hormone therapy and radiation therapy for locally advanced prostate cancer. *Crit Rev Oncol Hematol* 2012; 84(Suppl 1): e30–4.

11. Nair B, Wilt T, MacDonald R, *et al*. Early versus deferred androgen suppression in the treatment of advanced prostatic cancer. *Cochrane Database Syst Rev* 2002; 1: CD003506.

12. Tammela TL. Endocrine prevention and treatment of prostate cancer. *Mol Cell Endocrinol* 2012; 360(1–2): 59–67.

13. Sciarra A, Abrahamsson PA, Brausi M, *et al*. Intermittent androgen-deprivation therapy in prostate cancer: A critical review focused on phase 3 trials. *Eur Urol* 2013; 64(5): 722–30.

14. Oberg KE, Reubi JC, Kwekkeboom DJ, *et al*. Role of somatostatins in gastroenteropancreatic neuroendocrine tumor development and therapy. *Gastroenterology* 2010; 139(3): 742–53, 753.e1.

15. Oberg K, Kvols L, Caplin M, *et al*. Consensus report on the use of somatostatin analogs for the management of neuroendocrine tumors of the gastroenteropancreatic system. *Ann Oncol* 2004; 15(6): 966–73.

16. Welin SV, Janson ET, Sundin A, *et al*. High-dose treatment with a long-acting somatostatin analogue in patients with advanced midgut carcinoid tumours. *Eur J Endocrinol* 2004; 151(1): 107–12.

Basic surgical skills

Section editor: Jonathan Beard

CHAPTER 3.1

Principles of safe surgery

Amitabh Mishra and Peter McCulloch

Preoperative preparation

Identification and consent

The patient's identity should be confirmed preoperatively by the surgeon and the anaesthetist. This provides an opportunity for the patient to confirm his/her perception of the procedure, and a check as to whether there has not been any change in the patient's condition. Informed consent should be obtained by a person who is capable of performing the procedure themselves, or who has received training in advising patients about the procedure. Consent involves a brief explanation of the procedure, where possible avoiding medical jargon, and the anaesthetic to be used. The process should include a discussion of the risks and benefits of the procedure, alternative methods of management, and risks and benefits of not undertaking any treatment. All this must be documented.

Essential documentation

All effort must be made to ensure that all relevant documentation pertaining to the operation is available. This includes the clinical notes, correspondence, and results of investigations. Transfusion requirements should also be checked: no requirement, group and save, or crossmatched blood? The indications for antibiotic prophylaxis and thromboprophylaxis should be considered according to protocol.

In the case of site/side-specific surgery, this should be checked with the patient's expectation, imaging and records, and the site and side marked by the operating surgeon. Any discordance is an indication for postponement until clarification is achieved.

Nursing checklist

A nursing checklist is conducted prior to transfer to theatre. The purpose of this standard operating procedure (SOP) is to confirm the patient's name, that two independent means of confirming identity have been allocated, that the patient is aware of the procedure being undertaken, and that a surgical consent form has been completed, including (where required) the site or side of surgery. This and other steps later in the pathway illustrate the value of redundancy as a key principle of safe systems (See Box 3.1.1). Wrong-site surgery is a devastating problem that affects both the patient and surgeon and may result from poor preoperative planning, a lack of institutional controls, failure of surgical care, or a communication error between patient and the surgeon. The incidence of wrong-site surgery may be as low as 1 out of 27 686 cases,[1] but it is recognized to be a preventable medical error providing certain steps are taken and SOPs are implemented in the perioperative setting.

Box 3.1.1 The steps necessary for identifying and maintaining safe practice in surgery

- Understanding the system
- Standardization of system
  - Checklists
  - Standard operating procedures
  - Teamwork training
- Maintaining situational awareness
  - SBAR (situation, background, assessment, and recommendation) and formal communications methods
  - Checklists
- Cooperation and mutual support
  - Flat hierarchy
  - Briefing and debriefing
  - Team building
- Redundancy
  - Repetition of key checks
  - Different approaches from different team members
- Audit and improvement
  - Recording performance to identify error
  - Analysis and discussion
  - Plan formulation
  - PDCA (plan/do/check/act) rapid tests of change until perfected
  - Remeasuring

Team briefing

Communication between the members of the theatre team is essential before the working day begins, and before each case. This serves to ensure that all team members share the same 'mental model' of what is happening, and can communicate any problems or discuss any differences in understanding. This is a key element in maintaining shared situational awareness in the team—one of the most important barriers to error. The inclusion of checklists within standard procedures minimizes reliance on memory and should reduce errors of omission. Checklists should include no more than five to nine items, and take less than 90 seconds to complete, as psychological research shows that short-term memory and attention begin to fail beyond these points. The key elements that could cause most

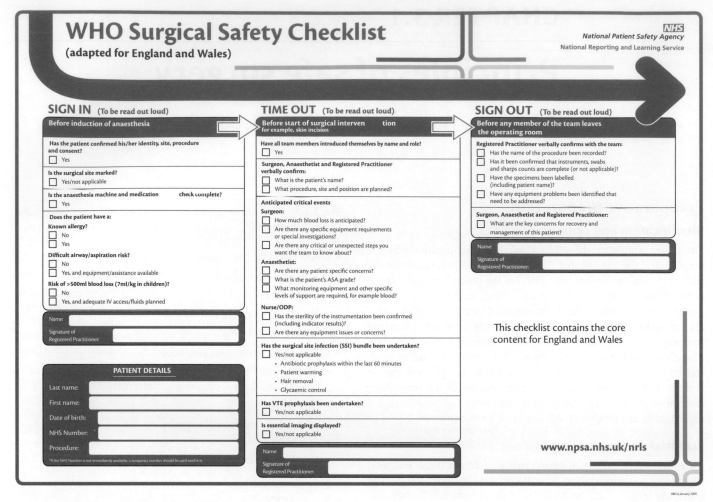

Fig. 3.1.1 World Health Organization surgical safety checklist.

Reproduced with permission from *WHO Surgical Safety Checklist,* Copyright © World Health Organization 2009. All rights reserved. Available from http://whqlibdoc.who.int/publications/2009/9789241598590_eng_Checklist.pdf.

harm if missed should be included, and language should be simple and precise. In current UK practice the World Health Organization (WHO) Surgical Safety Checklist (Figure 3.1.1) is used as the standard framework for this communication. The WHO surgical checklist is designed in three parts. The 'Sign In' part reviews key actions before induction of anaesthesia. The coordinator confirms with the anaesthetist and if possible the patient that his/her identity has been verified, and that the procedure and site are correct and that consent has been obtained. The anaesthetist must be asked about any concerns regarding airway difficulties, allergies, medications, and anaesthetic machines. The surgeon must be asked about anticipated blood loss, patient-specific complicating factors, and any particular instrument requirements.

In the operating theatre prior to incision

The surgeon and anaesthetist should supervise the transfer and positioning of the patient, taking care to avoid risks of injury due to pressure or traction during transfer or surgery. A series of measures are now taken to protect against specific risks of surgery. Stockings or compression sleeves (Flowtrons) may be applied to the legs for protection against deep vein thrombosis. Warming air-blankets are applied to avoid hypothermia, which increases the risk of organ

dysfunction and infection. Antibiotics are administered intravenously, where indicated. Monitoring normally includes electrocardiogram and photoplethysmography plus a central line, and arterial line for more major procedures. Finally, a sterile operating environment is ensured by skin preparation and draping of the patient, and scrubbing up, gowning, and gloving of the surgical team.

Infection has been the greatest risk to surgical patients since antiquity, and remains a potent threat today. Surgical operations are routinely associated with elaborate and standardized routines to avoid bacterial contamination of wounds and to minimize the risks of infection in other areas (chest and urinary tract especially). Operating theatre sterile technique represents an early example of the 'bundle' approach to achieving this important goal. It is difficult to demonstrate definitive benefits for many components of the sterile protocol, but abandonment of all components is known to lead to much higher infection rates. Therefore the safe approach is to maintain a standardized and disciplined approach to all components. This illustrates two more important principles of clinical safety. Standardization of routines is important to make sure that all components occur reliably. Set routines also have an important role in instilling a culture of safety in all who work in the environment involved.

Scrubbing up is a typical example of a formalized or ritualized procedure that is carried out in a standardized fashion to minimize the opportunity for error. The preparations commonly used are 2% chlorhexidine and 7.5% povidone-iodine. A typical routine is as follows:

A sterile scrubbing brush and nail cleaner are used for 90–120 seconds to remove dirt from the nails and deep skin crease. The hands are then washed palm to palm, right palm over left dorsum and then left palm over right dorsum. This is followed by palm to palm, fingers interlaced, then backs of fingers to opposing palms with fingers interlocked. Rotational rubbing of right thumb clasped in left palm and vice versa. And finally rotational rubbing backwards and forwards with clasped fingers of right hand in left palm and vice versa. The arms are then washed from hand to elbow, with elbows flexed. Following the final rinse, the hands are kept aloft at face level. The hands and arms are then dried with a sterile towel on each side, starting from the hands working up the arm.

A folded gown is picked up firmly from the neckline, allowed to unravel completely, with the inside facing the wearer. The wearer's arms are simultaneously inserted, keeping the hands inside the cuffs. The gown is secured by another operating personnel at the neck and at the waist. The closed glove technique is the preferred method. The wearer's hands remain inside the sleeves. The folded cuff of the left glove is grasped with the right hand, and the top edge of the cuff is held in the left hand above the palm. The palm of the glove is placed against the palm of the left hand, while the glove fingers point up the forearm. The back of the cuff is grasped in the right hand and turned over the open end of the left sleeve and hand, while holding the top of the left glove and underlying gown sleeve with the covered right hand. The glove is then pulled over the extended left fingers onto the wrist by pushing the hand through the glove, until it completely covers the cuff of the glove. The right hand is then gloved in a vice versa manner.

In the WHO Checklist framework, this pre-incision phase is the occasion for the second and most elaborate episode of formal team communication—the 'Time Out' procedure (see Figure 3.1.1). During this the patient, site, and procedure are checked again, and the specific elements of prophylactic care are also checked. In addition, introductions are carried out because the management of high-risk situations is more effective when all team members know the identity of each member and their role and capabilities. Following confirmation of the name of the patient using the wristband, checks are repeated to avoid operating on the wrong patient, wrong site, or wrong side by checking reliable documentation and imaging. Anticipated critical events risks are used to highlight important patient issues, allow risk assessment, and rehearse plans to deal with potential difficulties.

The surgeon will lead a discussion of critical or unexpected steps that might involve risks of rapid blood loss, injury, or other major morbidity. The availability of specific instruments should be confirmed at this juncture (e.g. harmonic scalpel). The anaesthetist will discuss the patient's co-morbidities and risk of significant blood loss and confirm that appropriate monitoring equipment and other supportive measures are available (e.g. cellsaver). The nursing staff will confirm sterilization of instruments, availability of staff, and raise any concerns.

Attention is then given to the surgical site infection bundle, to confirm the administration of appropriate antibiotics, maintenance of normothermia, need for hair removal, and maintenance of glycaemic control. Hyperglycaemia in the perioperative period has been linked to postoperative wound infection in patients undergoing major cardiac surgery, and tight glycaemic control has been shown to reduce mortality in critically ill patients. Venous thromboembolic prophylaxis is checked as are final reviews of imaging.

The operation

During the operation the actions of the surgeon and assistant become the focus for all activity in the operating theatre, although of course the performance of the anaesthetic and nursing teams is critical to their success. The tools of surgery are inherently dangerous, and a clear set of principles are therefore needed to use them safely.

Diathermy

Prior to incision, a diathermy plate is applied. It must be confirmed that the patient is not touching any earthed objects, and that there is good contact between the patient and the plate over an area of sufficient muscle mass. All connections to the generator should be checked prior to switching it on. Burns can result from pooling of flammable alcohol based skin preparation, an erroneously placed patient plate electrode, retained heat in electrode, poorly insulated diathermy lead, and inadvertent use. Pacemakers may inadvertently be reprogrammed and conduct current to the heart causing myocardial burns, and so, where possible, bipolar diathermy should be used. Especially in laparoscopic surgery, it should be remembered that insulation failures in ports, and touching of other instruments can cause inadvertent damage to tissue far from the site the surgeon is focusing on.

Sharps

Cuts or needle sticks may occur up in as many as 15% of surgical operations.[2] Surgeons and surgical assistants are at the highest risk for injury, suffering up to 60% of the injuries in the operating theatre. Individuals performing the role of the first scrub assistant sustain the second highest number of injuries. Suture needles are involved in almost 80% of injuries. Up to 16% of injuries occur while passing sharp instruments on a hand-to-hand basis and the body part most commonly injured is the non-dominant hand. A third of devices that cause injuries to healthcare workers, subsequently come into contact with the patient. This therefore increases the risk of disease transmission to the patient. Double gloving reduces the risk of exposure to patient blood by as much as 87% when the outer glove is punctured. The volume of blood on a contaminated solid suture needle is reduced by as much as 95% if it passed through both gloves.

Thus it is recommended that protective gloves be worn in double layers, instruments should not be passed between surgeons and their assistants, instruments should be transferred in a bowl or tray for safe placement, and only one sharp should be handed in one carrier at a time. If two surgeons are operating simultaneously, they should be provided with separate sharp dishes.

Situational awareness and perceptions

All surgeons are aware of and fear the possibility of perceptual errors during surgery, leading to division of vital structures such as the common bile duct or ureter or accidental ingress into major vascular structures. The principal safety mechanisms guarding against this are training and experience, a thorough knowledge of the relevant anatomy, and a shared 'mental model' in which surgeon and assistant are able to exchange perceptions and information freely. The importance of communication of perceptions between at least two skilled operators to maintain situational awareness and avoid critical errors of perception is well recognized in aviation and other high-risk industries.

Completion of the procedure

As the procedure nears completion, a final series of tasks are required to ensure safety. An instrument and swab check is performed, wounds are closed, cleaned and dressed, and the anaesthetic reversal process is begun. Specimens are labelled, notes are made, and the theatre cleaned. The final part of the WHO safety checklist provides a template for reminders at this stage (see Figure 3.1.1).[3] The true incidence of retained foreign bodies after surgery has been difficult to determine but estimated to be 1 in 1000–1500 cases, and the associated morbidity is significant, estimated at 50%, with 10% mortality in the case of retained instruments.[4] This is most likely to occur in three scenarios: during an emergency operation; following an unexpected change in operative procedure; and in obese patients.

The postoperative note should be composed by the primary operating surgeon, who should ensure that the name, hospital number, and date of birth are correct. The date of the operation should be recorded, including the start and finish times. The name of the operation should be accompanied by the names of all the surgeons, anaesthetists, type of anaesthetic (general/regional), and patient position. If the patient was catheterized, this should be documented, along with any antibiotics and the use of thromboembolic prophylaxis. For limb surgery, tourniquet times should be listed.

The indication for the operation should be noted. Operative details should be described, along the headings: incision, findings, procedure, and closure. Within the procedure section, a stepwise documentation of the operation should be noted including the approach taken, identifying any major structures preserved, specific techniques used, and whether any specimens were taken. Diagrams should be used in complex operations. Any intraoperative complications should be stated and any prosthesis used should have an accompanying label applied to the notes.

Postoperative instructions should dictate any observations required and their frequency; continuation of antibiotic and/or thromboprophylaxis; removal of drains and/or sutures as well as information regarding discharge and follow up arrangements, particularly for day case procedures.

Debriefing

Although the aim is to prevent adverse events, it is essential to learn from any mistakes. Debriefing following a procedure allows discussion of individual and team-level performance, recognition of errors made, identification of failures and successes, and construction of plans to improve subsequent performances. From a training point of view, the consensus is that feedback is most constructively received if performed at the end of an operation rather than during it. In the context of the team, it requires the involvement of all team members to be effective, and can be a powerful tool in creating unity and awareness, as well as reducing errors.

Teamwork and communication

Observational studies have demonstrated an association between teamwork and performance in surgery. The complex theatre environment is a forum for unclear communication, clashing motives, and poor interpersonal skills resulting in errors. Errors are increased by mental overload, tiredness, excessive workload, inadequate communication, poor decision making, and inferior evaluation and action regarding information available.[5] The accumulation of small apparently inconsequential errors makes violations of technical procedures more likely.

Experience of development of error management strategies from high-risk industries such as aviation has found the teaching of certain behaviours and attitudes can be used to prevent or mitigate error. Communication protocols such as the read-back of commands, improve comprehension and help reduce communication errors. In aviation, 'Black box' recordings allow assessment of aviation performance, policies, and processes after accidents and near misses. The development of open-error reporting systems, with a degree of immunity from disciplinary action, has evolved from these fields.

Open-error reporting systems are quite different from the blame culture of traditional medical apprenticeship, and surgical training is characterized by a steep professional hierarchy. Aviation has clearly shown that flattening this hierarchy is essential for safe, effective team performance. Teamwork and communication have been deemed potential areas for improvement.

Four main dimensions of non-technical skills are recognized as fundamental to teamwork in the operating theatre:

- leadership and management, which is effective when authority and assertiveness provide and maintain standards
- teamwork and cooperation, maintaining team function, considering others' skills sets and resolving inter-personnel conflicts
- problem solving and decision making: defining a problem, generating options to solve it, assessing their risks and option
- situation awareness: system awareness, environmental awareness, awareness of time and anticipation of future events.

These dimensions are not mutually exclusive, and good communication is essential to all. The most critical teamwork skill is perhaps situation awareness. When assessed quantitatively, greater situation awareness has been shown to be associated with fewer technical operative errors[6] (Figure 3.1.2).

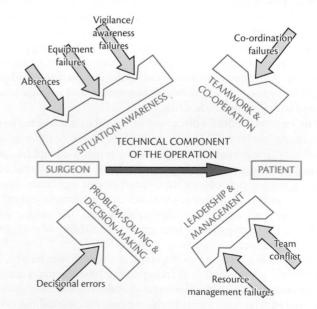

Fig. 3.1.2 Depiction of how teamwork skills may be useful in protecting from factors hindering operative performance.

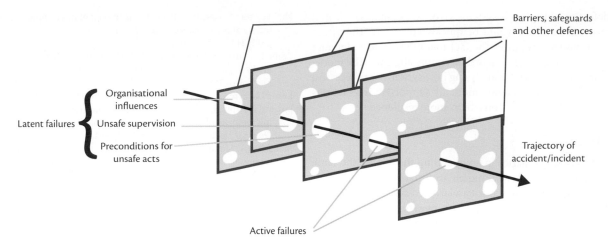

Fig. 3.1.3 Modification of James Reason's Swiss cheese model. 'Holes' in the defence mechanisms can line up, resulting in an adverse event.
Adapted with permission from Reason J., Human error: models and management, *British Medical Journal*, Volume 320, Issue 7237, pp. 768–770, Copyright © 2000, British Medical Journal Publishing Group.

Teamwork training

Teamwork training programmes have been developed in medicine, based on principles derived from aviation. Training programmes are evaluated in terms of effectiveness at four levels:

◆ response judged by feedback

◆ attitude as evaluated by questionnaire

◆ behaviour i.e. teamwork and communication as assessed by behavioural marker systems

◆ effect on outcomes as measured by operative technical error rates and complications.

Teamwork training can improve response, attitude, and behaviour, and to an extent technical error rates, but small sample sizes have limited the ability to show an improvement in error rates and complications in most studies.[7]

Safe technology

Surgical technology is constantly evolving. Rigorous evaluation of new technology is required, together with safe integration with existing devices, maintenance of existing technology and training in their use. Technology, working optimally and appropriately deployed, is influential in the quality and safety of the service provided.

Models and theory

Several theoretical models of organizational risk and safety have been developed that help to understand error and harm in surgery. Evidence from high-risk industries suggest that by adopting a systems approach, errors can be predicted, and developing proactive methods of preventing these are more effective than identifying individuals to blame following an event. Two forms of system failures have been identified:

◆ active failures that are immediate errors at the point of interaction between human and system

◆ latent conditions, which arise from areas such as the organization and its culture, staff training and competence, and control and monitoring of practice.

Swiss cheese model

Most adverse events occur due to an accumulation of latent conditions. Barriers to accidents or errors may be thought of as multi-layered; some dependent on hardware, some dependent on people, and some on procedures and management. However, these layers have holes, which represent the latent conditions. Reason developed this illustrative model, pointing out that when the holes in all the barrier layers line up, the result will be an adverse event (Figure 3.1.3).[8] These latent conditions may remain inactive for long periods and include error-prone conditions in the workplace such as pressure of time, understaffing, and inadequate equipment, and common but apparently innocuous failures in everyday practice which appear unnoticed.

Three-dimensional model of safety

A model of healthcare safety at the 'microsystem' (i.e. operating theatre level) has been proposed, which looks at risk and error in terms of three causative dimensions: system, culture, and technology.[9] This model (Figure 3.1.4) elaborates on the Swiss cheese theory of error, by recognizing that the three dimensions are interdependent, so that changes in one dimension have important effects on other dimensions, which may augment or decrease safety risks or modify them in a variety of other ways. As an example, a

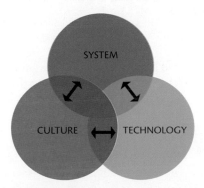

Fig. 3.1.4 Three-dimensional systems model. Interactions between dimensions of systems, technology and culture may be negative or positive, unidirectional or bidirectional, and may take multiple forms.

culture defect might allow a systems error to persist, which in a more appropriate culture would be quickly corrected. The three-dimensional model recognizes the fact that safety defects interact with each other more dynamically than simply aligning. The model also provides a framework for analysing how systems are successful at preventing error, by arranging mutually supportive interactions between two or more dimensions to promote resilience.

Conclusions

The principles of safe practice in an operating theatre are the same as for any other high-risk working environments. The key issues are to have a carefully thought out standardized system of work and a team that communicates clearly and supports each other, using appropriate technology for which proper training and maintenance are available. Systems of work often migrate, drift, or degrade through time, and it is important to understand what actually happens rather than what is supposed to happen when considering risks. Standardization is aided by checklists and SOPs, but also by an informal team culture, by which new members quickly learn how the team functions. Leadership and training can help to set and maintain standards of team behaviour, which should allow any member to speak up if concerned, and should encourage proactive mutual cooperation and support to anticipate and avoid problems. It is particularly important to avoid communication barriers caused by negative attitudes associated with hierarchy or inter-group rivalry. Redundancy is a key principle in organizational safety, as seen in the multiple checks on identity and procedure in the WHO safety checklist system. Finally, maintenance of good performance requires an attitude of continuous improvement through debriefing, audit and analysis of errors, and the use of rapid tests of change to troubleshoot solutions.

Further reading

Brennan TA, Leape LL, Laird NM, et al. Incidence of adverse events and negligence in hospitalized patients: results of the Harvard Medical Practice Study I 1991. *Qual Saf Health Care* 2004; 13(2): 145–51.

Christian CK, Gustafson ML, Roth EM, et al. A prospective study of patient safety in the operating room. *Surgery* 2006; 139(2): 159–73.

Gawande AA, Thomas EJ, Zinner MJ, et al. The incidence and nature of surgical adverse events in Colorado and Utah in 1992. *Surgery* 1999; 126(1): 66–75.

Gawande AA, Zinner MJ, Studdert DM, et al. Analysis of errors reported by surgeons at three teaching hospitals. *Surgery* 2003; 133(6): 614–21.

Helmreich RL. On error management: lessons from aviation. *BMJ* 2000; 320(7237): 781–5.

Hull L, Arora S, Aggarwal R, et al. The impact of nontechnical skills on technical performance in surgery: a systematic review. *J Am Coll Surg* 2012; 214(2): 214–30.

Leape LL, Brennan TA, Laird N, et al. The nature of adverse events in hospitalized patients: results of the Harvard Medical Practice Study II. *N Engl J Med* 1991; 324(6): 377–384.

Leape LL. Errors in medicine. *Clin Chim Acta* 2009; 404(1): 2–5.

Lingard L, Espin S, Whyte S, et al. Communication failures in the operating room: an observational classification of recurrent types and effects. *Qual Saf Health Care* 2004; 13(5): 330–4.

Makary MA, Mukherjee A, Sexton JB, et al. Operating room briefings and wrongsite surgery. *J Am Coll Surg* 2007; 204(2): 236–43.

Makary MA, Sexton JB, Freischlag JA, et al. Patient safety in surgery. *Ann Surg* 2006; 243(5): 628–32.

Reason JT. *Human Error*. Cambridge, MA: Cambridge University Press; 1990.

Panesar SS, Carson-Stevens A, Fitzgerald JE, et al. The WHO surgical safety checklist—junior doctors as agents for change. *Int J Surg* 2010; 8(6): 414–6.

Symons NR, Almoudaris AM, Nagpal K, et al. An observational study of the frequency, severity, and etiology of failures in postoperative care after major elective general surgery. *Ann Surg* 2013; 257(1): 1–5.

Vincent C, Neale G, Woloshynowych M. Adverse events in British hospitals: preliminary retrospective record review. *BMJ* 2001; 322(7285): 517–9.

References

1. Meinberg EG, Stern PJ. Incidence of wrong-site surgery among hand surgeons. *J Bone Joint Surg Am* 2003; 85-A(2): 193–97.
2. Berguer R, Heller PJ. Preventing sharps injuries in the operating room. *J Am Coll Surg* 2004; 199(3): 462–67.
3. Gonzalez-Ojeda A, Rodriguez-Alcantar DA, Tenas-Marquez H, et al. Retained foreign bodies following intra-abdominal surgery. *Hepatogastroenterology* 1999; 46(26): 808–12.
4. Byrne AJ, Oliver M, Bodger O, et al. Novel method of measuring the mental workload of anaesthetists during clinical practice. *Br J Anaesth* 2010; 105(6): 767–71.
5. Mishra A, Catchpole K, Dale T, et al. The influence of non-technical performance on technical outcome in laparoscopic cholecystectomy. *Surg Endosc* 2008; 22(1): 68–73.
6. McCulloch P, Rathbone J, Catchpole K. Interventions to improve teamwork and communications among healthcare staff. *Br J Surg* 2011; 98(4): 469–79.
7. Haynes AB, Weiser TG, Berry WR, et al. A surgical safety checklist to reduce morbidity and mortality in a global population. *N Engl J Med* 2009; 360(5): 491–99.
8. Reason J. Human error: models and management. *BMJ* 2000; 320(7237): 768–70.
9. McCulloch P, Catchpole K. A three-dimensional model of error and safety in surgical health care microsystems. Rationale, development and initial testing. *BMC Surg* 2011; 11: 23.

CHAPTER 3.2

Anaesthetic techniques

Daniele Bryden and Stephen Wilson

Introduction

The development of anaesthetic techniques has helped revolutionize surgical practice. Techniques have progressed enormously since the fairground use of nitrous oxide for dental extraction in the early 19th century.

This chapter provides an overview of the three main types of anaesthetic techniques used in the UK today: local anaesthesia, regional anaesthesia, and general anaesthesia. Discussion of local and regional techniques will be based on the pharmacology of local anaesthetics and the importance of a knowledge of applied anatomy, whereas that of general anaesthesia will be based on outlining the nature and risks of general anaesthesia so that surgeons are better able to understand risk assessment and the contribution anaesthesia can make to patient outcome.

Local anaesthetics

In 1884 Koller, an ophthalmologist, recognized that topical cocaine produced localized insensitivity of the conjunctiva to touch and injury. Within a year of this discovery, Knapp had injected cocaine behind the eye to perform an enucleation.

Modern local anaesthetic agents are safer than their predecessors. However, systemic toxicity remains a real danger. Therefore the safe use of these drugs requires a thorough understanding of the agents used, in particular, dose and concentration required, speed of onset, and duration of action. An ability to recognize and manage systemic toxicity is essential.

Mode of action

Local anaesthetics reversibly block transmission of peripheral nerve impulses. They act by diffusing across nerve membranes and then reversibly binding to voltage-gated sodium channels from inside the nerve cell. Binding of the local anaesthetic to the inside of the sodium channel results in their blockade and if sufficient channels are blocked, the conduction of electrical impulses will stop (Figure 3.2.1). Characteristics of the individual nerves determine how susceptible they are to being blocked by a local anaesthetic. In general, small nerve fibres are more sensitive to local anaesthetics than large nerve fibres. Moreover, myelinated fibres are blocked before non-myelinated fibres of the same diameter. Autonomic fibres, small unmyelinated C fibres (mediating pain), and small myelinated A-delta fibres (mediating pain and temperature sensation) are therefore blocked before larger myelinated A-gamma, A-beta, or A-alpha fibres (mediating touch, pressure, muscle and postural inputs). Clinically, the loss of nerve function proceeds as loss of pain, temperature, touch, proprioception, and then skeletal muscle tone, in that order. Therefore, by titrating the dose, it is possible to selectively block pain while preserving other nerve function.

Types of local anaesthetics

The molecular structure of local anaesthetic agents consists of a lipophilic aromatic ring and a hydrophilic amine group that are joined either by an ester or an amide linkage (Figure 3.2.2). This linkage classifies local anaesthetics into either ester or amide types. Esters include cocaine, procaine, and benzocaine, and amides include lidocaine, bupivacaine, prilocaine, and ropivacaine. The varying structure of the different local anaesthetics gives them different physiochemical properties, such as lipid solubility, degree of ionization (pK_a), protein binding, and speed of metabolism (see Table 3.2.1). These properties determine how a local anaesthetic acts.

Lipid solubility

The more lipid soluble the local anaesthetic is, the easier it passes through the lipid membrane of the nerve fibre to reach its site of

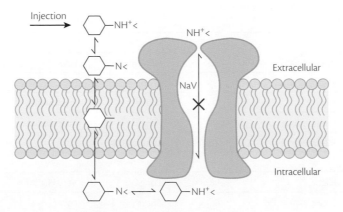

Fig. 3.2.1 Access path of local anaesthetics to sodium channel. NaV, voltage-gated sodium channel.

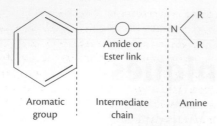

Fig. 3.2.2 Local anaesthetic structure.

action. Therefore lower concentrations of the more lipid soluble local anaesthetics are required.

Degree of ionization

In solution local anaesthetics exist as either a cationic ion or a neutral base. The proportion of each state depends on the drug's dissociation constant (pK_a). As local anaesthetics have a pK_a greater than physiological pH (7.4) a greater proportion exists as a cationic ion. However, as only the neutral base can cross the nerve cell membrane to reach its target of action, drugs with a lower pK_a have a greater speed of onset. This explains why in infected and inflamed tissues (that have a lower pH), the speed of onset of local anaesthetic is slower.

Protein binding

Local anaesthetics bind to plasma proteins; the extent to which they bind has a positive correlation to their duration of action. Plasma concentrations can rapidly rise, with a risk of toxicity when plasma protein binding sites become saturated, or when plasma pH falls causing local anaesthetics to dissociate from the protein.

Vasoconstrictors

Local anaesthetics have a mild vasoconstrictor effect, and epinephrine may be added to prolong the duration, improve quality or speed of onset of the block, and reduce the risk of toxicity. Epinephrine achieves this by causing further local vessel vasoconstriction and reducing the quantity of local anaesthetic absorbed into the bloodstream. It should not be used in concentrations greater than 1:200 000 and is contraindicated in any form of ring block or intravenous regional anaesthesia due to the risk of causing tissue ischaemia.

Dosage, toxicity and side effects

Calculations of doses and 'safe dose' ranges

Local anaesthetics have the same effect on myocardial cells and the brain as they do on nerves. If high plasma concentrations occur the effect on these organs brings about signs and symptoms of systemic toxicity. High plasma concentrations can result if local anaesthetic is accidentally injected into a blood vessel, injected in high concentration near to a blood vessel (e.g. intercostal nerve blockade), or the safe dose range is exceeded by administering repeated doses.

Systemic toxicity: signs and treatment

Patients will often report central nervous system-type symptoms such as tongue or mouth numbness, dizziness, tinnitus, or anxiety. These should always be treated seriously and any further injection stopped immediately. Other symptoms may include slurred speech, drowsiness, loss of consciousness and convulsions. Occasionally some local anaesthetics (e.g. bupivacaine) may have a direct myocardial effect before a central nervous system one, producing cardiac dysrhythmias and, in severe cases, cardiovascular collapse.

Any patient showing signs and symptoms of systemic toxicity should be assessed and resuscitated using an 'ABCDE' type approach, including calling for expert anaesthetic assistance. Specific treatments available for cardiovascular collapse from toxicity include the use of Intralipid 20%.[1]

Methods of administration

Local anaesthetics can be administered by local infiltration (e.g. when suturing a wound), as blockade of a peripheral nerve (e.g. femoral nerve block), or by means of central nerve blockade. They can be used as a sole means of anaesthesia to perform surgery (e.g. peribulbar blocks for eye surgery) or as an adjunct to a general anaesthetic technique for analgesia in the perioperative period. Factors that influence choice of technique include patient preference, co-morbidities and medication, the site and duration of the proposed surgery, as well as operator preference related to familiarity with techniques and facilities available. Therefore when planning any procedure, surgeon and anaesthetist must communicate well with each other and with the patient prior to starting the procedure in order to produce the best outcome.

Table 3.2.1 Characteristics and suggested maximal doses for commonly used local anaesthetic agents

Agent	pK_a	Speed of onset	Potency	Protein binding (%)	Duration	Toxicity	Maximum dose–plain (mg/kg)	Maximum dose– with vasoconstrictor (mg/kg)
Amide agents								
Lidocaine	7.7	Fast	Intermediate	64	Intermediate	Low	5	7
Bupivacaine	8.1	Slow	High	95	Long	High	2	3
Levobupivacaine	8.1	Slow	High	96	Long	Intermediate	2.5	3
Ropivacaine	8.1	Slow	Intermediate	94	Long	Intermediate	2.5	4
Prilocaine	7.9	Fast	Intermediate	55	Intermediate	Low	5	8
Ester agents								
Cocaine	8.7	Slow	High	98	Long	Very High	1.5	
Procaine	8.9	Slow	Low	6	Short	Low	8	10

Learning point

Surgeons using local anaesthetics must understand the mode of action and safety profile of the agents they use. An ability to recognize toxicity and manage the side effects is essential.

Regional anaesthesia

Peripheral nerve blocks

Prior to performing any local anaesthetic block, the patient must be suitably prepared with an adequate explanation of the proposed procedure, and all equipment needed must be checked.[2] Resuscitation equipment should always be available. Short-bevel, single-use needles are used for performing peripheral nerve blocks. Peripheral nerve blockade was traditionally performed using a combined anatomical landmark technique and a nerve stimulator to identify the nerve using a local electrical current to produce muscular contractions. However, with the greater availability of portable ultrasound machines, the majority of peripheral nerve blockades are now done under ultrasound guidance. This has enabled a greater use of nerve blocks to facilitate postoperative analgesia (e.g. the use of transversus abdominis plane blocks after abdominal surgery for infraumbilical incisions).

Formal testing of local anaesthetic blocks may not always be possible and sometimes other indicators (e.g. absence of pain in a fractured limb) may indicate that the block is successful. Alternatively, use of an ethyl chloride spray or ice cube may be a useful guide to the success of the block by testing loss of sensation to cold in the skin supplied by the same nerves as the area blocked, although this is not 100% reliable.

Central neuraxial blocks

These are the most common forms of blocks likely to be encountered by surgeons in UK practice. Spinal and/or epidural anaesthetic blocks are performed to provide anaesthesia for surgery whereas epidural blockade may also be used for postoperative analgesia. Caudal blockade is a form of epidural anaesthesia, used to provide analgesia for procedures in the sacral nerve root distribution, but is rarely reliable enough to be used alone to facilitate surgery. The addition of a small quantity of opiate to the local anaesthetic is becoming common practice, as this can improve the quality of the analgesia, but at the risk of causing respiratory depression. A technique combining a spinal anaesthetic for surgery combined with an epidural for postoperative analgesia can be used, as this combines the advantages of both techniques while minimizing the disadvantages.

Cardiovascular depression and hypotension are the most common side effects of spinal and epidural anaesthesia. They occur due to the blockade of the sympathetic chain by the local anaesthetic that produces vasodilation, and if the thoracic sympathetic chain is involved, then bradycardia and a drop in cardiac output may be result. All patients having central nerve blocks therefore require intravenous access prior to administering the block. Vasoconstrictor agents (e.g. ephedrine) may also be used. Due to this frequent and occasionally significant complication, central neuraxial blocks may be undesirable in patients who have a degree of pre-existing hypovolaemia (e.g. those who are already actively bleeding even if apparently haemodynamically stable).

A subdural or epidural haematoma is one of the most feared complications of central nerve blocks, as it can result in permanent paralysis. The risk is increased in patients on anticoagulants and antiplatelet agents. Warfarin should be stopped or reversed and subcutaneous heparin not given for 12 hours. Ideally, clopidogrel needs to be stopped for 5 days. A recent national audit has highlighted the risk of permanent nerve damage from central neuraxial blocks to be between 1:25 000 and 1:50 000 depending on the type of injury.[3]

Regional anaesthesia has no proven advantage in terms of medium- and long-term mortality or morbidity after surgery (>3 months), so use of the technique in surgery is based on patient choice, team preference, and early potential benefits to the patient or surgical outcomes.[4]

Spinal anaesthesia

Spinal anaesthesia involves the injection of a small dose of local anaesthetic (typically 2–3 mL) into the subarachnoid space below the termination of the spinal cord (2nd–3rd lumbar vertebra or below). It can be used to provide anaesthesia for surgery in the pelvis/lower abdomen (below the level of the umbilicus) and lower limbs. A 'single-shot spinal anaesthetic' will usually produce surgical anaesthesia for around 2 hours, and can be the technique of choice for patients where avoiding the side effects of general anaesthesia is desirable (e.g. fractured neck of femur surgery). Although it can be used in patients having surgery as a day case procedure, it may not be the technique of choice as it can delay patient discharge due to the development of side effects.

Table 3.2.2 lists the common side effects and theoretical advantages of spinal anaesthesia. While many complications are rare, some such as total spinal anaesthesia can result in loss of consciousness, cardiovascular collapse, and death.

Epidural anaesthesia

Epidural blockade can be used for intraoperative anaesthesia as the sole technique or in addition to a general anaesthetic for intraoperative and postoperative analgesia. Although it can be inserted after induction of general anaesthesia, most anaesthetists would choose to site an epidural with the patient awake in order to assess the patient during insertion and hopefully more reliably detect any complications that may be related to insertion. A Tuohy needle, with a curved tip, is used to insert a catheter into the epidural space, which allows local anaesthetic to be infused into the epidural fat and to block the nerve roots. The concentration and volume of local

Table 3.2.2 Side effects and advantages of spinal anaesthesia

Side effects	Advantages
Cardiovascular compromise	Reduced blood loss
Headache (post dural puncture headache)	Delayed stress response
Urinary retention (slow return of sacral autonomic fibres after blockade)	Reduced deep vein thrombosis risk (only for duration of blockade)
Neurological complications	Reduced early morbidity and mortality compared to general anaesthesia (e.g. chest infection)
Risk of haematoma or abscess formation	

Table 3.2.3 Side effects/complications of epidural anaesthesia/analgesia

Side effect	Reason	Comparison to spinal anaesthesia
Hypotension	Vasodilation	Usually less rapid onset with epidural anaesthesia
Headache	Dural puncture	Larger diameter of needle, so higher risk of headache if dura punctured
Urinary retention	Blockade of sacral autonomic fibres	Common: therefore urinary catheter usually required if epidural infusion being used
Infection	Lowered patient immunity, presence of epidural catheter, traumatic insertion all increase risk of infection	Higher with epidural anaesthesia: risk 1:24 000 Risk lower if catheter removed after 48 hours
Haematoma	Epidural vessel puncture by needle or catheter. Worse if traumatic insertion or patient on medication affecting coagulation	Lower risk with spinal anaesthesia as single shot and smaller needle
Nerve injury	Physical injury from needle or catheter	Rare but greater risk with epidural
Wrong route administration	Either operator error or catheter migration into a blood vessel	Rare with spinal anaesthesia as single shot
Spinal cord infarction	Severe hypotension, intraoperative positioning in extreme extension also implicated	Less common but can occur

anaesthetic can be varied to produce surgical anaesthesia or analgesia, and the catheter can be left *in situ* for 2 to 3 days, if necessary, to provide postoperative analgesia and facilitate physiotherapy, etc.

Epidurals can be used for major abdominal/pelvic surgery, lower limb procedures and also provide excellent postoperative analgesia after thoracic and upper abdominal surgery. Although local anaesthetic injection can be performed via a needle as a 'single shot' into the epidural space, this technique is usually undesirable due to the risk of inadvertent dural puncture and the risks of producing total spinal anaesthesia. Table 3.2.3 lists the common side effects and advantages of epidurals.

Caudal anaesthesia

Caudal anaesthesia is a form of epidural blockade using the sacral approach. It can be used to provide supplementary analgesia for procedures on the anus, rectum, perineum, penis, urethra, and cervix. A needle is inserted through the sacral hiatus to gain access to the sacral canal. Due to the high risk of infection it must be performed in a sterile fashion and use of a catheter is contraindicated. There are many anatomical variations of the sacral hiatus so access may not always be possible or blockade may be unreliable as leakage of local anaesthetic occurs through the sacral foramina to an unpredictable extent.

General anaesthesia

Stages of anaesthesia

The exact mechanisms underlying why different forms of general anaesthesia are effective have still not been fully delineated. Original theories concentrated on the disruption of brain cell lipid membranes affecting consciousness and memory, but recent research work suggests that general anaesthetic agents effectively target central nervous system proteins.[5]

General anaesthetic agents are either volatile gases based on halogenated hydrocarbons or a diverse group of intravenous agents of which propofol, midazolam, and thiopentone are the most well known in the UK. All effective general anaesthetic agents alter the activity of many of the proteins involved in chemical transmission in the nerve synapse, either augmenting inhibitory signals or inhibiting an excitatory signal: $GABA_A$ receptors appear to be particularly important.

When anaesthesia was first being developed and researched, several stages of anaesthesia were described, based on patients having inhaled induction of anaesthesia (Table 3.2.4). Modern intravenous induction agents produce a smoother anaesthetic by reducing the time a patient spends in the potentially dangerous excitement stage of anaesthesia. Knowledge of the stages of anaesthesia is important, particularly in relation to an understanding of the safe administration of sedative agents. The definition of sedation requires maintenance of verbal contact with the patient throughout. Loss of this means the patient has progressed to a stage of hypnosis or anaesthesia with added risks (e.g. vomiting and loss of a patient's ability to maintain their own airway). Any anaesthetic carries the risk of the patient vomiting and aspirating. Therefore current recommendations for adults undergoing elective surgery are starvation for 6 hours for solids prior to surgery, with clear liquids permissible for up to 2 hours beforehand.[6]

Components of balanced anaesthesia

A classic general anaesthetic consists of three components:

- hypnosis (anaesthesia): e.g. volatile agents or TIVA (total intravenous anaesthesia)

- analgesia: e.g. opiates, peripheral nerve blocks, central neuraxial blockade

- muscle relaxation: e.g. muscle relaxants, deep general anaesthesia/TIVA, central neuraxial blockade, peripheral nerve block.

Table 3.2.4 Stages of anaesthesia

Stage	Signs
1: Analgesia	Loss of consciousness/verbal contact
2: Excitement	Struggling, breath holding, vomiting, coughing, swallowing. Loss of eyelash reflex, lacrimation
3: Surgical anaesthesia	Development of muscle weakness, change to diaphragmatic respiration, central pupillary gaze, constricted pupils
4: Overdosage	All reflex activity lost, widely dilated pupils, can lead to death

Table 3.2.5 Overview of general anaesthetic techniques

Technique	Advantages	Disadvantages
Spontaneous ventilation	Avoids intubation problems, good for quick procedures, potential loss of airway	No airway protection, unable to control ventilation with risk of excessive respiratory depression, often requires more anaesthetic agents to facilitate surgery
Controlled ventilation	Avoids problems of spontaneous ventilation, better physiological control and less use of anaesthetic agents for frail patients, better patient position for surgery	Risks of failed intubation, morbidity from intubation and use of additional drugs eg muscle relaxants, potential risks of patient awareness
Inhaled anaesthesia	Easy to measure concentrations of agents and less risk of awareness, Simple to administer.	Greater risk of nausea and vomiting, environmental exposure to gases, risk of malignant hyperpyrexia
Total intravenous anaesthesia (TIVA)	Possible reduction in nausea and vomting,	Reliance on maintenance of secure iv access, calculated drug levels so potential for awareness

Each component can therefore be provided by different methods and the choice depends on patient co-morbidities/preference, anaesthetist preference, and surgical requirement/preference. Hence, every anaesthetic is tailored to the needs of the patients and the requirements of the procedure. Table 3.2.5 gives an overview of general anaesthetic techniques.

A general anaesthetic is involves in three separate stages:

1. *Induction*: This takes the patient from consciousness to the surgical plane of anaesthesia. During this period, the patient's airway is secured, additional cardiovascular monitoring may be inserted, and the patient stabilized prior to any further physiological insult from the surgery. Induction can be gaseous (usually small children) but is most often intravenous in the UK.

2. *Maintenance*: This is the period of surgery during which balanced anaesthesia is maintained and any physiological responses to the surgery are predicted, monitored, and acted upon.

3. *Emergence*: After completion of surgery, the patient is taken from the unconscious to the conscious state. This is a potentially dangerous period, and in unstable patients it may be decided to continue a period of postoperative ventilation to allow a slower emergence and ensure cardiovascular stability prior to this occurring.

Side effects of general anaesthesia

Side effects can be considered in relation to each specific component of the anaesthetic (e.g. residual muscle paralysis from use of any muscle relaxant) and also general in relation to the provision of a general anaesthetic. Although choice of agents/techniques will attempt to balance these side effects for each patient, there is a morbidity (and mortality) attached to the administration of every anaesthetic.

Cardiorespiratory complications are common and can occur after 5–10% of procedures, particularly in the elderly where their incidence may be considerably higher. Other commonly quoted anaesthetic-related complications include oral/dental trauma (5%), sore throat (up to 40%), nausea and vomiting (up to 33%), shivering (25%), confusion, awareness, nerve/tissue injuries from poor positioning, anaphylaxis, and trauma to tissues and surrounding structures from associated procedures (e.g. central line insertion). Death directly resulting from anaesthesia has an incidence of 1 per 100 000 cases, although the risk is considerably higher for many groups of patients and procedures.

Preoperative preparation and postoperative management

Although the overall risks of death in hospital from surgery are low (<1%), for many groups of patients and types of surgery, these risks are considerably higher. Each component can therefore be provided by different methods and the choice depends on patient co-morbidities/preference, anaesthetist preference, and surgical requirement/preference. Patients who are deemed 'high risk' have a hospital mortality rate of 10–15% and between 1 in 10 and 1 in 20 surgical patients can be considered to be high risk.

Preoperative assessment

Patients undergoing elective and urgent surgery should now undergo a formalized preoperative assessment in an outpatient setting. The purpose of the assessment is to identify the factors that increase perioperative risk, categorize those risks appropriately, and consider whether any additional investigations or therapies are required to minimize the risks.[7] Patient-related factors that increase surgical risk are listed in Table 3.2.6.

Additional patient-related risk factors such as diabetes mellitus, chronic respiratory and cardiovascular disease, anaemia, obesity, and chronic renal disease are considered in many of the scoring systems and often are reflected in frailty assessments. The physiological and operative severity score for the enumeration of mortality and morbidity (POSSUM) assesses global perioperative risk and includes both patient and operative risk factors. It can provide

Table 3.2.6 Patient and surgical factors increasing surgical risks

Factor	Explanation
Age >70 years Approximately 70% of perioperative deaths but 25% of operations	Generally reduced physiological reserve, increasing co-morbidities. Frailty may also increase with age
Frailty	Frailty phenotype independently linked to morbidity and mortality
High-risk score (e.g. ASA, Goldman, POSSUM)	Partially identifies patients with poor organ functional capacity and cardiorespiratory reserve
Length of surgery, type of operation	More physiological disturbance and tissue damage

Table 3.2.7 The American Society of Anesthesiologists grading system

Grade	Definition	Mortality (%)
1	Healthy person	0.05
2	Mild systemic disease, no limits on activity	0.4
3	Systemic disease limiting activity but not incapacitating	4.5
4	Incapacitating disease, life-threatening	25
5	Moribund, not expected to survive beyond 24 hours with/without surgery	50

Based on the Physical Status Classification System of the American Society of Anesthesiologists. A copy of the full text can be obtained from ASA, 1061 American Lane, Schaumburg, Illinois 60173. Reproduced with permission.

an expected mortality figure, but it can only be calculated after surgery and was designed to compare the death rate predicted for a population and not for an individual patient. The American Society of Anesthesiologists (ASA) grading system (Table 3.2.7) is used by anaesthetists during preoperative assessment. Although simple and easy to apply with some linkage to perioperative mortality, it is a crude assessment tool and subject to a degree of subjectivity. No one single scoring system has sufficient sensitivity and specificity to identify patients at high risk or to quantify individual patient risk. Combinations of static assessment/scoring tools (e.g. ASA grade, Goldman Risk Index, Lee Score, etc.), are used to help identify patients who may warrant further dynamic assessment of cardiorespiratory reserve (e.g. by performing cardiopulmonary exercise testing). Assessments of a patient's functional capacity with these dynamic tests do carry a prognostic value and can be used to determine whether a patient is suitable for surgery.

High-risk patients requiring elective surgery may benefit from preoperative cardiorespiratory optimization. This includes a spectrum from smoking cessation through to coronary revascularization. Currently there is considerable anaesthetic research interest in identifying whether patients who are identified as high risk can be improved by a period of preoperative cardiorespiratory training.[8] Patients undergoing emergency surgery need to be assessed by an anaesthetist to determine the balance of risks, plan the conduct of the anaesthetic and to determine if any added investigations or perioperative optimization is needed to facilitate the surgery.

Perioperative management

Surgery produces a biphasic metabolic and physiological response. The first 24 to 48 hours following surgery produces a neuroendocrine response to fluid shifts and tissue injury, followed by a flow phase of increased metabolic rate and energy consumption. Survivors from surgery appear to be able to mount a good physiological response to these stresses whereas those that do poorly have a greater oxygen debt with longer tissue hypoxia. Anaesthetic management in the perioperative period is directed at minimizing this oxygen debt by means of ensuring optimal fluid status and

cardiovascular functioning with pressors and inotropes as necessary during the surgery, and carrying this on into the postoperative period for 24 to 72 hours depending on the type of surgery and patient requirements.[9]

Acute coronary syndromes are estimated to occur in 1–5% of patients having non-cardiac surgery and result in significantly increased mortality. The only cardiac medications shown to reduce the risk of perioperative morbidity are beta blockers, and these should always be continued in the perioperative period.[10]

Further reading

Boyd O, Jackson N. Clinical review: How is risk defined in high-risk surgical patient management? *Crit Care* 2005, 9: 390–6.

National Confidential Enquiry into Patient Outcome and Death. *Perioperative Care: Knowing the Risk*, 2011. Available from http://www.ncepod.org.uk/reports.htm (accessed 1 February 2016).

National Confidential Enquiry into Patient Outcome and Death. *Elective & Emergency Surgery in the Elderly: An Age Old Problem*, 2010.

Poeze M, Greve JWM, Ramsay G. Meta-analysis of hemodynamic optimization: relationship to methodological quality. *Crit Care* 2005, 9: R771–R779.

Prytherch DR, Whiteley MS, Higgins B, et al. POSSUM and Portsmouth POSSUM for predicting mortality. Physiological and Operative Severity Score for the enUmeration of Mortality and morbidity. *Br J Surg* 1998 85(9): 1217–20.

Williams GD, Rhodes A. Pre-operative care of the high-risk surgical patient. *Cont Educ Anaesth Crit Care Pain* 2002; 2(6): 178.

References

1. Association of Anaesthetists of Great Britain and Ireland. *Management of Local Anaesthetic Toxicity*, AAGBI Guideline. Further reading at www.lipidrescue.org and www.aagbi.org

2. Association of Anaesthetists of Great Britain and Ireland. *Standards of Monitoring During Anaesthesia and Recovery 4*. AAGBI, March 2007. Available from. http://www.aagbi.org/sites/default/files/standardsof-monitoring07.pdf (accessed 1 February 2016).

3. Cook TM, Counsell D, Wildsmith JAW. Major complications of central neuraxial block: report on the Third National Audit of The Royal College of Anaesthetists. *Br J Anaesth* 2009;102: 179–90

4. Kettner SC, Willschke H, Marhofer P. Does Regional Anaesthesia really improve outcome? *Br J Anaesth* 2011: 107(suppl 1): i90–i95.

5. Weir CJ. The molecular mechanisms of general anaestheisa: dissecting the GABA$_A$ receptor. *Cont Educ Anaesth Crit Care Pain* 2006; 6(2); 49–53

6. Royal College of Nursing. *Perioperative Fasting in Adults and Children: An RCN guideline for the multidisciplinary team*. London: RCN, 2005

7. Association of Anaesthetists of Great Britain and Ireland. *Pre-operative Assessment and Patient Preparation: The Role of the Anaesthetist*. AAGBI, January 2010,. Available from https://www.aagbi.org/sites/default/files/preop2010.pdf (accessed 1 February 2016).

8. Donati A, Loggi S, Preiser J-C, et al. Goal-directed intraoperative therapy reduces morbidity and length of hospital stay in high-risk surgical patients. *Chest* 2007, 132: 1817–24.

9. Wilson J, Woods I, Fawcett J, et al. Reducing the risk of major elective surgery: randomised controlled trial of preoperative optimisation of oxygen delivery. *BMJ* 1999, 318: 1099–103

10. Scott, T, Swanevelder J. Perioperative myocardial protection. *Cont Educ Anaesth Crit Care Pain* 2009; 9: 97–101.

Basic surgical techniques

David Smith and Jamie Young

Knot Tying

Introduction to knot tying

Knot tying is a basic skill that every aspiring surgeon needs to master. This requires many hours of practice, but a skills laboratory is not required: the arm of any chair will do! A fluid accurate motion is required, ensuring good tissue approximation or ligation. The resulting knot should be safe, secure, and use the minimum of suture material. The most basic is the reef knot, and an understanding of how the knot works and how to throw it is essential. The three knots to be discussed are the:

◆ reef knot

◆ surgeons knot (by hand or by instrument)

◆ slip knot.

The reef knot

The reef knot has two components: a forehand or index finger throw and a backhand or middle finger throw.

Forehand or index finger throw

How you pick up the thread is important; stretch out the tying hand in a supinated position; pick up the thread with the TIPS of the thumb and middle finger. You may wish to use your non-dominant hand so that you can continue to hold an instrument or needle holder in your dominant hand. Using the tips of the fingers ensures that you do not get confused with which fingers are involved with the actual tying. Pass the index finger under the thread (Figure 3.3.1). Bring the suture up to the middle (midpoint) while at the same time the non-tying hand brings up the other end of the suture to the midpoint (Figure 3.3.2). The two movements help with the flow of crossing the threads. With the two parts of the suture at the midpoint, the distal phalanx of the index finger is flexed to trap the thread of the tying hand and pass it under the thread held in the other hand (Figure 3.3.3), and the hands then pass to the side away from where they started, that is crossing the threads, and then snug the throw down securely (Figure 3.3.4).

The backhand or middle finger throw

The thread is now held in the tips of the thumb and index finger and the hand rotated to a pronated position, with the thread on top of the hand (Figure 3.3.5); the thread from the opposite side is then drawn over the middle and ring finger thus crossing the hands again (Figure 3.3.6). The tip of the middle finger then flexes over the non-tying end of the suture and 'flicks' the suture into the loop and is picked up again (Figure 3.3.7), with the hands passing to the side away from where they started.

The two loops of the reef knot pull into each other and tighten, making the knot secure (Figure 3.3. 8). In practice this step is essentially irreversible and it is almost impossible to undo the knot. To tie a reef knot, the threads MUST cross when tying; if the threads do not cross then the loops of the reef knot do not form and you end up with a 'granny' knot, which is not a secure knot. Some surgeons advocate that you should tie with your non-dominant hand, in order to allow the needle holder to remain in your dominant hand while tying. The occasions as to when this is required are few and the surgeon should tie with whichever hand they feel will make the most secure knot, dominant or non-dominant. In practice, you should be able to tie with both your dominant and non-dominant hand.

In general terms three throws (i.e. one-and-a-half reef knot throws) is the minimum number for a braided suture and five or six throws for a monofilament suture, which is required because of its intrinsic memory and monofilament surface, which is more prone to knot slippage. You should ensure that the knot does not move when tying, as this could allow the vessel being ligated to tear and bleed. Keep the tension on the knot with the non-tying hand while the tying hand exerts tension in an equal and opposite direction, so that the net result is no force being exerted on the vessel. This is particularly important when tying at depth and should be practised on a knotting trainer.

Surgeons knot

Tissues that are under tension can open during the tying process (e.g. skin) as there is not enough friction in a single throw to hold the two sides together, especially if a monofilament suture material is being used. In this instance a surgeons knot is used, with the initial throw having two loops on it in order to increase the friction. To form a surgeons knot, hold the suture material in the standard manner but then cast the forehand throw twice so that there is a 'double loop' on the first throw. The knot is then completed by a standard single throw backhand, with a reef knot formed on top of this. Vice versa you can start with a backhand double throw and then a single forehand throw, with a reef knot on top. This is a very secure knot.

Instrument tie

When tying at the skin surface, some surgeons prefer to tie with the needle holder rather than by hand, in order to get more ties per suture length. Usually a surgeons knot is required, as the skin edges can spring apart with the small monofilament suture that is normally used to approximate the skin edges. The needle holder is placed between the two ends of the suture, parallel to the wound. The long end (with needle) is wrapped twice around the needle

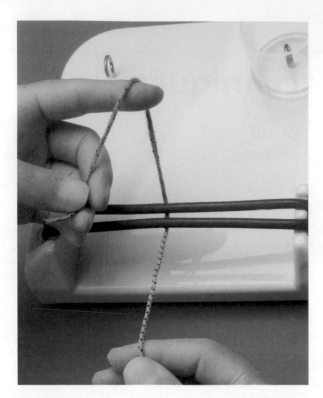

Fig. 3.3.1 Starting position for index finger knot.

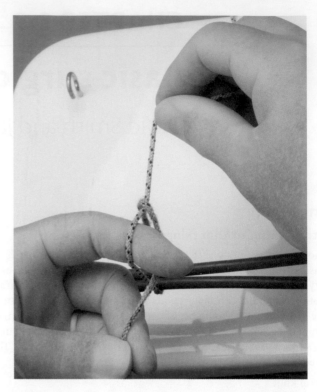

Fig. 3.3.3 Tip of index finger used to pass distal thread under proximal thread thus forming first throw.

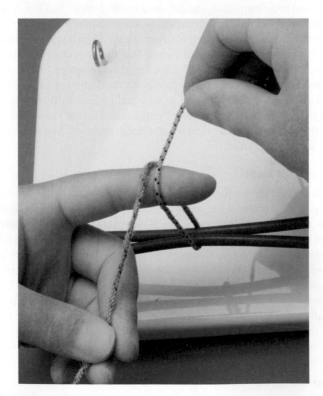

Fig. 3.3.2 Forming loop for index finger throw.

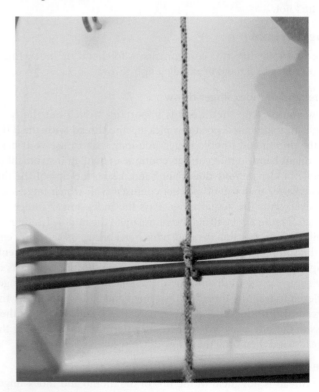

Fig. 3.3.4 Completion of index finger throw.

holder and the needle holder then grasps the tip of the short end of the suture. The ends are then crossed over the wound, forming the first part of the surgeons knot. It is then useful to jam the knot on the short-end side of the wound. Do not pull on the short end of the suture as this only wastes suture length when it comes to cutting

the sutures—keep the short end adjacent to the wound. This helps with the tension of the knot and also keeps the knot away from the wound itself. The needle holder is replaced in between the suture ends, again parallel to the wound, and a further two separate throws performed, crossing the thread ends each time to form a reef knot.

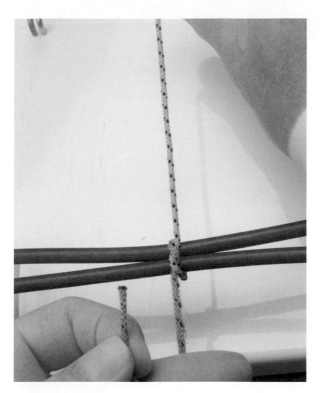

Fig. 3.3.5 Position of hand for middle finger throw.

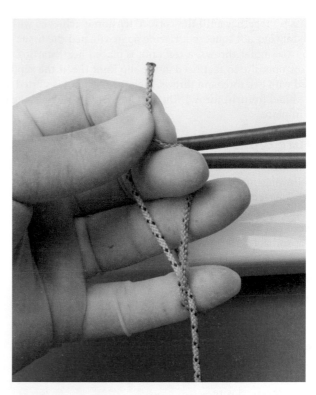

Fig. 3.3.7 Flex distal phalanx of middle finger used to pass proximal thread under distal thread.

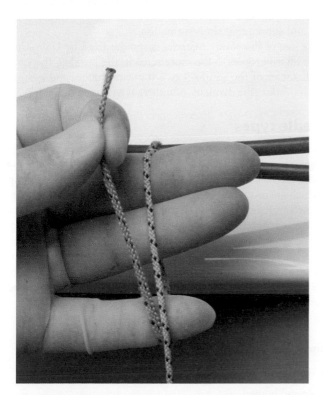

Fig. 3.3.6 Draw distal thread over middle and ring fingers.

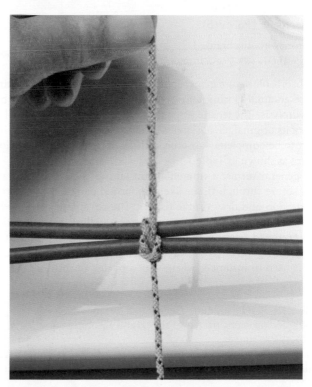

Fig. 3.3.8 Snug down firmly to complete reef knot.

In practice a monofilament suture is commonly used on the skin, and so it will require five or six throws using the instrument.

Slip knot

While a reef knot offers security, it is unable to be slipped into position and tightened once the two loops are formed. A slip knot may therefore be useful when approximating two tissues together (e.g. in a bowel anastomoses). Tie a throw with either a forehand or backhand and bring the throw down to the surface but not tightly; then repeat the same throw (i.e. two forehands or two backhands) and bring the second throw down to the surface. Then with the index finger adjacent to the throw, approximate the two tissues together until the 'correct' tension is achieved with the ends snug but not squeezed. Having approximated the tissue with these two similar throws, a reef knot is placed next; starting with a throw opposite to that used in the slip knot (i.e. if the slip knot started with two forehand throws, then the reef knot is started with a backhand [return] throw). The reef knot serves to 'lock' the slip knot in place.

Suture types

A wide variety of suture materials are available, but all should have the following important characteristics: there should be no or minimal tissue reaction, good knot security, the suture should be easy to handle, and should not promote infection of the wound. Suture material can be divided into four different groups: absorbable and non-absorbable, and monofilament and multifilament (braided). Examples are given below:

- absorbable monofilament
  - polydiaxone (PDS)
  - polyglyconate (Maxon)
  - polyglecaprone (Monocryl)
- non-absorbable monofilament
  - nylon (Ethilon)
  - polypropylene (e.g. Prolene or Surgipro)
  - stainless steel wire
- absorbable braided
  - polyglactin (Vicryl)
  - lactomer (Polysorb)
- non-absorbable braided
  - synthetic silk (e.g. Nuralon).

An absorbable suture gives support to a wound for a period of time before gradually losing tensile strength and then being absorbed by hydrolysis. The tensile strength period is that time taken to lose 50% of its original tensile strength, and absorption time is the time taken to be completely absorbed. These periods differ for various sutures as shown in Table 3.3.1.

In general terms, a monofilament suture is used when passing a suture through tissue like skin, bowel or vessels, as there is less friction and drag on the tissues. The advantage of a braided suture is that it has less memory (better handling characteristics) and improved friction (knotting security) which are important for secure ligatures (e.g. a vascular pedicle). Absorbable sutures can be used in instances when, after a period of time, the wound

Table 3.3.1 Tensile strength (as measured by time (days) taken for 50% decline in original tensile ability) and absorption time (days) for absorbable sutures

Suture	Tensile strength	Absorption time
Vicryl (Polyglactin)	21	56–70
Vicryl rapide	5	42
PDS (Polydiaxone)	42	183–238
Polysorb	14–21	56-70
Maxon	28	180
Monocryl	7	91–119

Table 3.3.2 Suture size by United States Pharmacopeia (USP) and diameter

UPS	Diameter
2	0.6 mm
1	0.5 mm
0	0.4 mm
2/0	0.35 mm
3/0	0.3 mm
4/0	0.2 mm
5/0	0.15 mm
6/0	0.1 mm
10/0	0.02 mm

is well healed and there is no ongoing requirement for any tensile strength from the suture. For example, bladder wall heals very quickly (5 to 7 days) and needs no further support after this period and so an absorbable suture with a shorter tensile strength and absorption period can be used (e.g. polyglactin). Aponeuroses (e.g. the linea alba), tendons and bone require a much longer period of support with prolonged tensile strength, and so either a non-absorbable suture (e.g. nylon or wire) or a long lasting absorbable suture (e.g. polydiaxone) is used. The use of non-absorbable sutures may result in local irritation by the knot and subsequent sinus formation.

The size of the suture material is standardized by USP (United States Pharmacopeia)—the more zeros in the number, the smaller the diameter of the suture (e.g. 5-0 means 00000, and is smaller than 3-0, etc.). The diameter of sutures is as shown in Table 3.3.2.

Needle types

A needle has three components: the tip, the body, and the swage end. Swaging is the factory process involved in attaching the suture to the needle. Needles have a variety of sizes, profile, and shapes, examples of which are given in Box 3.3.1 and Figure 3.3.9. Pliable tissue, such as bowel wall, only requires a round body needle that separates the tissue causing minimal local trauma. Other tissues such as skin or atherosclerotic vessel wall require a cutting needle to penetrate the tissue. Blunt tip needles may also be used (e.g. in abdominal wall closure). This helps to prevent injury to underlying bowel or surgeons hands! Most needles designed for instrument use have a square body to prevent rotation of the needle in the jaws of the needle holder.

Box 3.3.1 Needle sizes, profiles, and shapes
- Cutting: reverse or standard
- Round bodied
- Dolphin nosed blunt tip
- 1/2–3/8 circumference
- Round bodied
- Cutting/reverse cutting
- Blunt tip

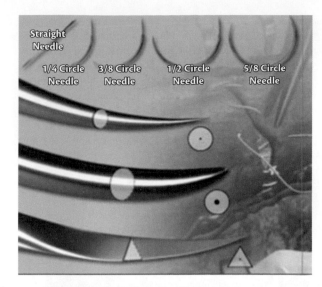

Fig. 3.3.9 A selection of the needle types available.
Image courtesy of Ethicon US, LLC.

Suturing

Suturing is an essential skill to master. The accurate placing of stitches in tissue is imperative to allow good apposition for healing but must not be so tight as to impede blood supply, be it skin, bowel, blood vessel, or muscle. Sutures in general are placed by mounting a needle into a needle holder and using the curve of the needle to pass through the tissues. A common mistake is to mount the needle too far away from the tip. This increases the difficulty in directing the needle in the correct direction. For less delicate work a number of larger hand-held needles in straight and curved varieties are available and maybe suitable for skin or drain suturing. However these are now being used less for fear of needle stick injuries.

The most common stitch is the *simple interrupted stitch*. A single stitch is placed by inserting the needle at 90 degrees to the tissue and rotating the wrist allowing the curve of needle to pass through the tissues on one side of the wound, crossing the gap, and then exiting on the other side at an equal distance from the wound edge. The trailing thread is then tied into a knot at the appropriate tension and the thread cut. Further stitch placement is based on tissue type and location with the distance between each suture generally equal to the distance from the suture to the wound edge. This is repeated until the tissue edges are opposed along the length (see Figure 3.3.10).

Horizontal and *vertical mattress stitches* are interrupted stitches, but the stitch passes more than once across the defect in equal planes (horizontal) or deep and superficial planes (vertical). This allows good distribution of tension and accurate eversion of skin edges.

Figure-of-8, Z stitch and *box stitches* are used for haemostasis and are interrupted sutures placed in the named fashion.

Purse strings are circular sutures where multiple small bites are taken to ultimately form a circle. It may be used to bury an appendix stump or to hold the anvil of a stapler in place.

Continuous suture techniques are quicker to perform and more haemostatic, but risk failure of the whole length of the wound if a single bite fails, cuts out, or if any part is divided. It is essential for each bite to be placed accurately an equal distance from the wound edge and from the adjacent bite. Jenkins's rule states that the length of suture material used should be four times the length of the

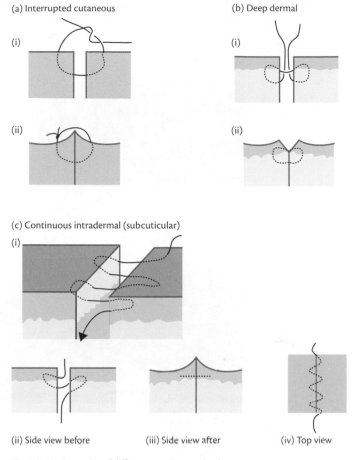

(a) Interrupted cutaneous
(i)
(ii)

(b) Deep dermal
(i)
(ii)

(c) Continuous intradermal (subcuticular)
(i)

(ii) Side view before   (iii) Side view after   (iv) Top view

Fig. 3.3.10 Examples of different suturing methods.
Reproduced with from Henk Giele and Oliver Cassell, *Oxford Specialist Handbook of Plastic and Reconstructive Surgery*, Oxford University Press, Oxford, UK, Copyright © 2008, with permission from Oxford University Press.

wound. It is also important that the suture is not pulled too tight, otherwise the tissue within the suture will be rendered ischaemic.

Continuous subcuticular suturing is used for skin closure and leaves a wound with no visible stitches. If a braided absorbable suture is used, an anchoring knot is placed at one end of the wound, the needle is then passed into the subcuticular plane (junction of dermis and epidermis) before the wound is closed taking multiple bites in the subcuticular tissue parallel to the wound edges until the opposite end of the wound is reached. The stitch may then be tied using the Aberdeen knot or by continuing suturing beyond the corner with abrupt angle changes. A non-absorbable monofilament suture may also be used in this technique, which is subsequently removed. In this case no knotting is undertaken at the ends of the wound and the ends may be secured by a bead or small adhesive dressing.

Glue (e.g. cyanoacrylate) may also be used to join skin edges and for skin grafts in situations where there is no tension.

Instruments

It is important that any worker knows their tools and how to use them. A surgeon should know the names (which may vary depending on individual hospital inventory), their uses and limitations, and be able to apply and remove clips or cut sutures using both dominant and non-dominant hands.

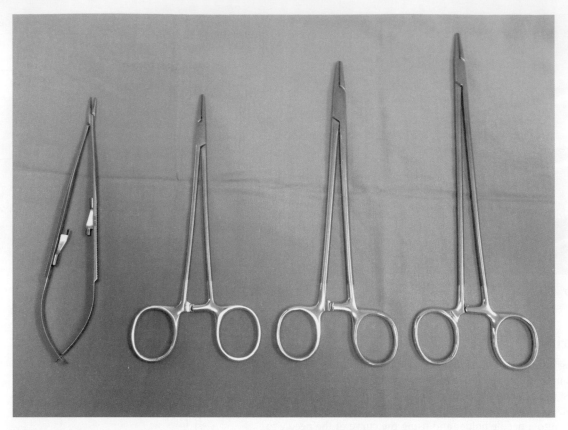

Fig. 3.3.11 Different needle holders. Castro-Viejo to left, standard needle holders in increasing sizes.

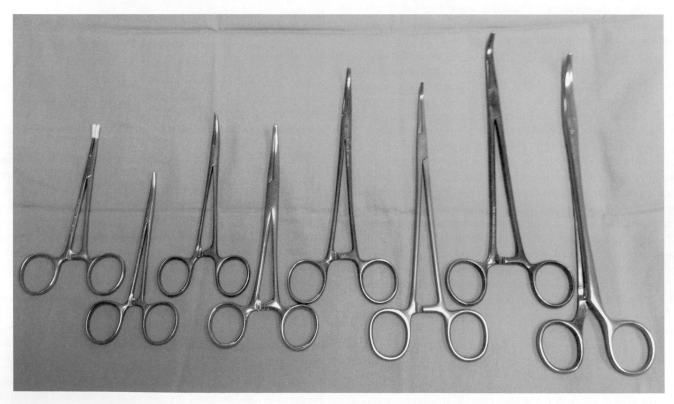

Fig. 3.3.12 Clips including a rubber shod mosquito, mosquito, Crile, Mayo, Spencer Wells, right angles (fine and broad Mixter) and O'Shaughnessy.

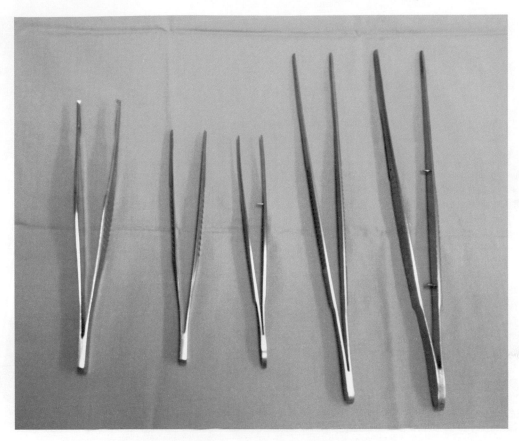

Fig. 3.3.13 A variety of tissue dissecting forceps, toothed and non-toothed - note that there is horizontal milling of the McIndoes while there is vertical milling on the DeBakey forceps.

Needle holders or drivers

Needle holders or drivers are used to perform suturing (see Figure 3.3.11). They are usually straight and it is important to use the correct size in weight and length for the needle size. Needle holders are held using the thumb and ring finger but with practice may be held free in the palm, allowing improved rotation. A number of specialist needle holders are also available such as the Castro-Viejo for microsurgery using a 4-0 suture or smaller, and curved needle holders for deep in the pelvis.

Haemostats or clips

Haemostats or clips are used widely and named according to size and straight or curved configuration. The smallest are Mosquito's and run through Crile's, Spencer Wells, Mayo, and Kelly (see Figure 3.3.12). Haemostats cause a crushing injury and render tissue non-viable. They will also damage sutures, and must only be applied to the part of a suture that will be retained if protected by silicone sleeves (shod clip, yellow in the picture).

Dissecting forceps

Dissecting forceps (see Figure 3.3.13) come in a number of lengths and weights, but the important distinction is between toothed and non-toothed varieties. Toothed forceps, such as Adsons or Lanes, are used for holding skin as the teeth prevent crushing of the skin.

Toothed forceps are also useful for holding bone and tendon. Non-toothed forceps, such as DeBakey or McIndoes, are used for holding other soft tissues. The milling in the jaws at the end of each instrument also varies depending on its usage.

Scissors

Scissors come in two main groups and are divided into delicate tissue scissors such as Metzenbaum or McIndoe scissors and heavier suture cutting such as Mayo scissors that may be straight or curved (see Figure 3.3.14). It is important not to use tissue scissors to cut sutures as this causes premature blunting. Specialist scissors include Potts scissors for vascular work.

Bowel clamps

Bowel clamps come in crushing and non-crushing varieties. The crushing clamp, such as the Schumacher clamp, securely occludes the bowel lumen but damages tissue and is used on the end of the specimen to be resected (see Figure 3.3.15). Non-crushing clamps, such as the Doyen, provide a less secure seal but do not completely close and thus they do not cause damage to the bowel or blood supply but stop spillage of contents and are used on the bowel end that is to remain in the body. Vascular clamps, such as those designed by DeBakey, are designed to occlude blood vessels without crushing, while gripping the vessel firmly.

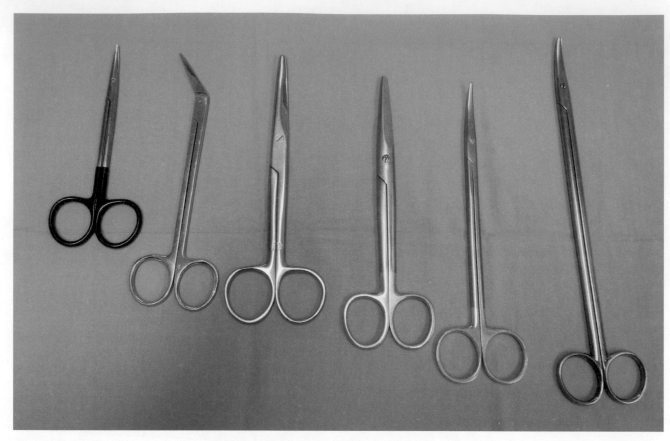

Fig. 3.3.14 Strabismus, Potts, Mayo (curved and straight), Metzenbaum (short and long) scissors.

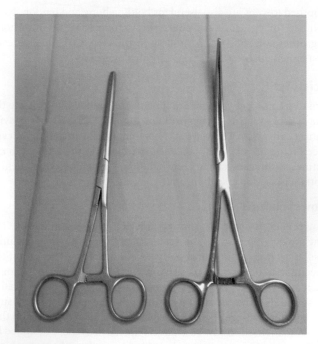

Fig. 3.3.15 Schumacher and Doyen clamps. Notice the crushing and non-crushing jaws.

Tissue-holding forceps

Tissue-holding forceps are available in a number of forms and lengths and all trade security of grasp against damage to the held tissue. These include Rampley, Duval, Allis, and Babcock (see Figure 3.3.16).

Retractors

Retractors may be hand-held, self-retaining, or part of a system. Hand-held retractors include the smaller skin hooks or cats paws for skin edges, Langenbeck for superficial wounds, and for intra-abdominal work the larger Deaver which is curved and the Morris which is straight but with a lip (Figure 3.3.17). A specialist St Marks retractor is available for pelvic work. Self-retainers come in a variety of sizes such as the Travers for soft tissue retraction and the Balfour for intra-abdominal retraction. Other systems utilize either a ring with apposing retractors, or a post fixed to the operation table with a series of bars and retractors attached to this (e.g. Omnitract).

Scalpel holders

Scalpel holders come in a range of sizes and lengths for holding a blade (see Figure 3.3.18). Blades should be carefully mounted pointing away and downwards using a needle holder.

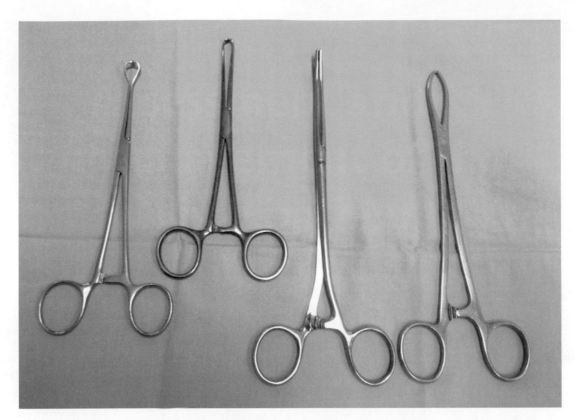

Fig. 3.3.16 Babcock, Allis, Duval, and Littlewoods tissue-holding forceps.

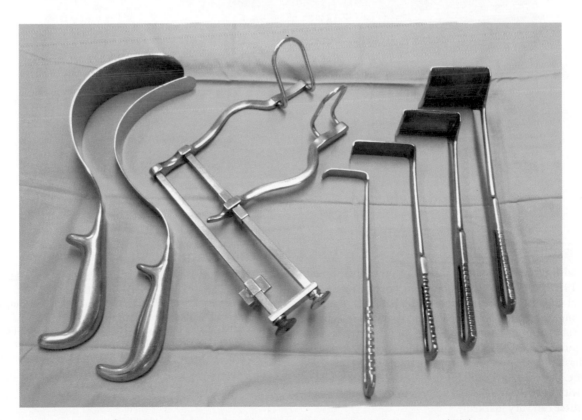

Fig. 3.3.17 Deaver hand-held retractors (left), Balfour self-retaining clamp (centre), and Langenbeck and Morris retractors (right).

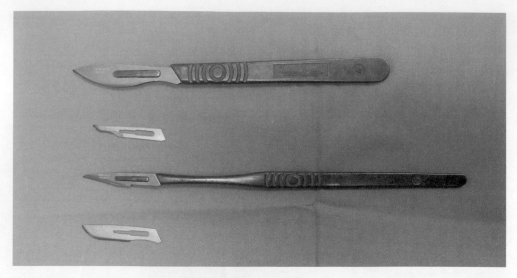

Fig. 3.3.18 Scalpel holders and different blades. Premounted disposable versions are available.

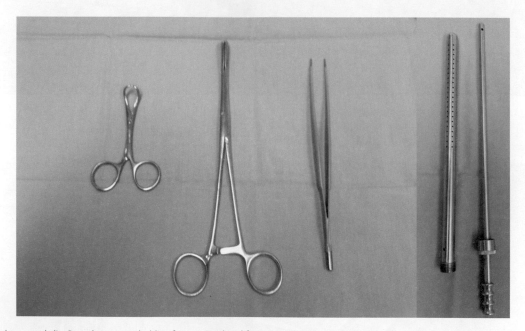

Fig. 3.3.19 Items such as towel clip, Rampley sponge-holding forceps, insulated forceps, and Poole sucker are often found on trays.

Others

Many surgical trays also contain a variety of other instruments (Figure 3.3.19). These vary greatly between hospitals and may include towel clips (not to be clipped to the patient!), Rampley sponge-holding forceps for skin preparation, insulated forceps for diathermy, and a sump sucker.

The need for practice with knotting techniques and suturing cannot be emphasized enough. Time spent practising will be rewarded with further experience in theatre for the adept. It is important to be familiar with the instruments and sutures in the hospital where working as these can vary markedly.

Further reading

Intercollegiate Basic Surgical Skills Course Handbook, 5th edition. London: Royal College of Surgeons of England, 2012.

Kirk RM (Ed). *Basic Surgical Techniques*, 6th edition, Edinburgh: Churchill Livingstone, 2010.

Thomas WEG. Basic surgical skills and anastomoses. In Williams N, Bulstrode C, O'Connell PR (eds) *Bailey and Love's Short Practice of Surgery*, 26th edition. London: CRC Press, 2013, pp. 33–49.

Surgical wounds

James N. Crinnion

Physiology of wound healing

A basic understanding of the physiology of wound healing helps to reinforce good surgical technique.[1-4] Following primary closure of a surgical incision the wound heals in three well-characterized stages:

- inflammatory (preparative) phase (0–4 days)
- proliferative phase (4–30 days)
- maturation (remodelling) phase (1 month to 1year)

The initial acute inflammatory reaction occurs in response to the local tissue injury and is manifest as swelling, erythema, and pain. The purpose is to achieve haemostasis, breakdown any dead or devitalized tissue, and to attract fibroblasts to the wound margins. The cellular elements critical for this phase are platelets, polymorphonuclear cells (neutrophils), and macrophages. Platelets and macrophages release growth factors that include platelet-derived growth factor and transforming growth factor beta. These cellular-derived proteins attract fibroblasts into the deeper layers of the wound, and it is these cells that produce the immature type III collagen matrix that is the hallmark of the proliferative phase. The rapid production of collagen occurs for the first month often producing a hard red scar. The wound then enters the final and protracted maturation phase in which type III collagen is replaced by type I collagen fibres that become aligned in the direction of the local tension across the wound. Over 12 months there is a gradual restoration of tensile strength with the production of a supple, flat, and pale scar.

This normal healing process can only occur if epithelial cover is maintained until the proliferative phase is established, and sufficient tensile strength is restored to prevent distraction of the wound edges.[4] Until this occurs sutures must support the wound. If the surgical incision breaks down as a result of ischaemia, haematoma, or infection, this will produce an open wound. In such wounds there is a prolongation of the inflammatory phase, and the wound will then heal by the process of wound contraction and the formation of granulation tissue (known as healing by granulation or secondary intention). The proliferative phase cannot begin properly until epithelial cover is restored, leading to a significant delay in wound healing. Furthermore, healing by secondary intention produces excessive collagen deposition and an unsatisfactory scar. Many of the factors that lead to the early breakdown of a closed surgical incision are directly related to poor surgical technique and can be avoided (Table 3.4.1). To minimize complications the surgeon must adopt a meticulous approach when opening and closing a surgical incision.

Surgical incisions

Lines of cleavage (Langer's lines)

Within the skin dermis, collagen fibres usually lie in parallel strands that produce natural lines of cleavage corresponding to visible skin creases (Fig 3.4.1). Incisions made along these lines typically heal with minimal scarring, while those made across Langer's lines often leave thickened and ugly scars. This is particularly the case if an incision is made across the natural skin crease in the popliteal and antecubital fossae that may impair joint mobility. Access to these areas is typically made with an 'S'-shaped incision with the horizontal component in the line of the skin crease. All surgeons must be aware of and respect Langer's lines when siting their proposed incision.

Incising the skin and subcutaneous tissue

When using a scalpel to incise the skin, firm tension must be applied across the wound to facilitate a clean perpendicular cut. This must be done deliberately but with care, avoiding any tendency to make a tangential cut. Undermined skin edges may become ischaemic. Until relatively recently a scalpel or surgical scissors were invariably used to incise the skin and deeper layers of the wound, and any bleeding encountered was controlled with either ligatures or diathermy. Now many surgeons prefer to use a hand-held or pencil diathermy. This instrument has been specifically designed to incise through the tissues while simultaneously sealing the small vessels. Thus, incisions may be made rapidly while maintaining a dry surgical field. The hand-held cautery usually has cutting and coagulation settings with the former setting providing a rapid cut but limited haemostasis, and the latter setting incising the tissues more slowly but without any bleeding. Initially the skin is usually partially incised with a scalpel down to the dermis, and then the deeper layers of the skin may be opened with the diathermy 'scalpel' using the cutting mode. The subcutaneous tissue layers of the wound can then be incised using the coagulation setting (Figure 3.4.2).

Preparation of the wound prior to closure

Before suturing begins, the vascularity of the wound must be assessed. Most wounds, especially those on the head and neck, trunk, and upper limbs have a rich blood supply that will support rapid healing. However, surgical wounds on the lower limbs of patients' suffering from peripheral vascular disease and diabetes are frequently ischaemic. These incisions must be closed very gently and without any tension if primary healing is to be expected.

Table 3.4.1 Technical errors that predispose to wound breakdown and infection of surgical incisions

Technical error	Potential effect
Undermining of the skin and/or subcutaneous tissue	Ischaemic necrosis of the skin edges leading to separation of wound and predisposing to secondary infection
Injury to the skin edges due to instruments or cautery	Necrosis of the skin
Inadequate haemostasis	Wound haematoma predisposing to wound separation, infection and abscess formation
Closure of the skin and subcutaneous tissue using large bites and under tension	Ischaemia and necrosis of the skin and subcutaneous tissue
Inversion of the skin	Poor healing and a portal for infection

Any active bleeding from the wound edges must be stopped to prevent a wound haematoma. This should be performed accurately, and bipolar diathermy is very helpful in this regard as it causes little collateral damage to adjacent healthy tissue. Cautery should be used with care near the skin surface as excessive inaccurate use may lead to small areas of necrosis that predispose to secondary infection. Any loose and potentially non-viable subcutaneous tissue should be excised to prevent it becoming a focus for infection. This is particularly relevant following major amputations when loose pieces of muscle and soft tissue should be excised. Any contaminated incisions (e.g. gastrointestinal, urological surgery) will benefit from a thorough irrigation with saline or an antiseptic solution. Once the wound is clean and dry it may be closed.

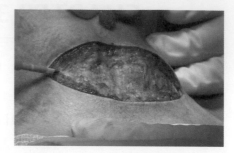

Fig. 3.4.2 The use of hand-held cautery to divide the skin and superficial layers of the neck producing a bloodless thyroidectomy incision.

Wound closure

Closure of fascia and subcutaneous tissue

When closing abdominal or thoracic incisions, careful suture of the muscle and fascial layers is paramount to provide support until the wound is healed and adequate tensile strength is restored (about 2 months). The connective tissue layers are typically closed using a continuous suture technique with either non-absorbable material or longer-lasting absorbable sutures. When closing a midline abdominal incision frequent generous bites (>1 cm) of the linea alba are taken on each side of the wound using a thick nylon, polydioxanone (PDS II®) or polyglyconate (Maxon®) suture. When this repair is performed accurately the risk of wound dehiscence is minimal.

In many incisions several layers of muscle or connective tissue are divided and it is good practice to close each layer individually with a continuous absorbable suture. This principle also applies to the subcutaneous fat. The incised subcutaneous fat is a potential dead space that may predispose to a wound haematoma or seroma. In addition to being haemostatic, suturing the fat layer reduces the amount of tension required from the skin sutures. Interrupted sutures are often helpful to close the subcutaneous fat as they accurately align the skin edges. To ensure the knots are adequately covered they should be buried deeply. To achieve accurate alignment of a long or curved incision it is helpful to initially insert stay sutures at each end of the wound. Pulling on each suture in the opposite direction will accurately align the skin edges and enable precise placement of the subsequent stiches (Figure 3.4.3).

Basic principles of skin closure

The principles of skin suturing are summarized in Box 3.4.1. Slight eversion of the skin edges ensures apposition of the dermis that is

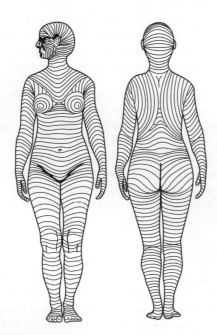

Fig. 3.4.1 Langer's lines.
Reprinted from Chummy S. Sinnatamby, *Last's Anatomy: Regional and Applied*, Eleventh Edition, Figure 1.2, p. 3, . Churchill Livingstone, Elsevier, Copyright © 2006 Elsevier Ltd, with permission from Elsevier.

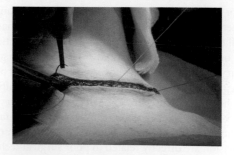

Fig. 3.4.3 The placement of interrupted subcutaneous sutures relieves the tension on the skin layer and helps to obliterate any dead space. The use of stay sutures enables accurate placement of subsequent stiches and alignment of the skin edges.

Box 3.4.1 Closure of the skin (basic principles)

1. Accurately align the wound edges.
2. Handle the skin gently.
3. Use curved cutting needles with a suture of appropriate gauge.
4. Evert the skin edges to facilitate apposition of the dermis.
5. Avoid closing the skin too tightly.
6. Adopt a no-touch technique to avoid needle-stick injury.

vital for wound healing. Inversion of the skin edges must be avoided as this will delay healing and predispose to infection. Although there should be no gaps in the wound, the sutures must be tied gently to accommodate the inflammatory swelling that follows wound closure. Very tight sutures may cause necrosis of the wound edges, which is particularly prone to occur in areas of poor tissue perfusion. The skin is closed using cutting needles that may be curved or straight. However, curved needles are preferred, as they may be grasped by forceps to facilitate a safe no-touch technique.[5]

Simple suture

Skin closure with interrupted non-absorbable sutures is the most simple and versatile method that may be used at any site. The suture should be inserted perpendicular to the skin on one side of the wound and exit on the other side directly opposite and equidistant from the wound edge. Similarly, an equal depth of skin and subcutaneous tissue should be taken on each side of the incision. The skin must be handled gently and, as the knots are tightened, they should be placed to one side of the suture line. This helps to evert the skin edges and assists suture removal. The distance that each suture is placed from the wound edge is dependent upon the site with 3–4 mm bites being optimal for most areas of the body. On the face 1–2 mm bites are required to produce a good cosmetic result.[5] Non-absorbable sutures are removed when the wound has healed sufficiently to hold the skin edges together. Typically, they are removed from the face and neck after 4 to 5 days and from most other areas after 7 to 10 days. The exceptions are the feet and lower limbs where sutures are removed after 10 to 14 days. Sutures must not be left in place for too long as this may lead to unsightly crosshatching of the skin and the suture material becoming buried (Figure 3.4.4).

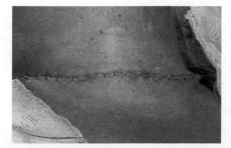

Fig. 3.4.4 Closure of a long curved cervical incision using interrupted 4/0 prolene sutures. Each suture is placed 3–4 mm from the skin edge. This technique will provide excellent results but the sutures must be removed after 4 to 5 days to prevent crosshatching of the skin.

Vertical mattress suture

This type of suture is used to close the deep layers of the incision and the skin simultaneously. The needle is inserted about 1.5 cm from the wound edge and passes through the base of the wound to exit at a similar distance on the opposite side. It is then reinserted on the same side but closer to the wound edge (about 5 mm) and this bite typically only involves the skin edge. The needle exits a similar distance from the edge on the other side where the suture was started. Mattress sutures are often used in areas of skin tension, particularly on the limbs and trunk after an elliptical excision and also to close incisions involving the skin and subcutaneous fat. It provides excellent apposition and eversion of the skin edges, and will eliminate the dead space in the subcutaneous fat layer. However, because the suture is often tied under tension and must be left in place for about 10 days it frequently results in a poor cosmetic result.[5]

Subcuticular suture

This has become the most popular technique of skin closure for relatively straight wounds. The technique places little tension on the wound edges and is thus an ideal method to use to close wounds that may have a precarious blood supply such as following lower limb amputations. Subcuticular sutures are placed intradermally either individually or more commonly as a running suture. The needle is placed horizontally in the dermis about 2 mm from the skin edge. When performing a continuous suture the needle enters the wound at the apex and then an intradermal bite of about 5–10 mm in length is taken along one edge of the wound. The needle is then grasped and the next bite is taken on the opposite side. To produce a very neat result the bites on each side should be of equal length and of equal depth from the skin surface. Suture bites of unequal depth will invert the wound edges and may impair healing. When the suture is tightened it should be done slowly to gently appose the wound edges. If pulled too tight it tends to shorten the wound producing a tethered appearance. Either non-absorbable or absorbable suture material may be used with the former being removed after a few days. The ends of absorbable sutures may either be knotted and buried at each end of the wound or brought out through the skin to be trimmed later. The latter method avoids the skin puckering that may occur at the ends of the wound where the knots are buried (Figure 3.4.5).

Choice of surgical needles

Most wounds are closed with curved needles held in a needle holder or hand-held straight needles. The body of a curved needle may vary from a quarter to five-eighths of a circle. Occasionally a 'J'-shaped needle (a half curve at the end of a straight segment) is useful. This can be inserted into a small skin incision to enable accurate deep fascial closure, and is particularly helpful in closing laparoscopic port sites.

To close the subcutaneous tissue a taper cut or round-bodied needle is used as they produce minimal tearing when passed through soft tissue. To suture the skin a conventional cutting or reverse-cutting needle is necessary. The passage of a reverse-cutting needle is thought to be less likely to injure the tissue during suturing. A three-eighths or half circle reverse-cutting needle is ideal for most skin wounds. Although a straight needle is employed by many surgeons to perform a subcuticular suture, this increases the risk of a needle-stick injury. The use of a curved needle and a no-touch technique is

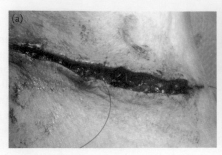 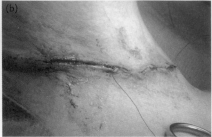

Fig. 3.4.5 Skin closure using a non-absorbable subcuticular suture. Each stitch is placed parallel to the skin edge within the dermis. Each new bite is placed on the opposite side of the incision at the exit point of the previous stich. (a) Several bites may be inserted loosely to enable accurate placement and then (b) the suture is gently tightened to appose the skin edges.

much safer and should be the preferred method. In this regard blunt tipped needles provide additional protection for the surgeon when closing the musculofascial layer of the abdomen.[5,6]

Choice of suture materials

When closing a wound the surgeon must select the most appropriate suture material and diameter (gauge). The surgeon should select the finest suture that will hold the wound together securely until it has healed.

2/0 Polyglactin (Vicryl®) is the most commonly used material for closing subcutaneous tissues and is a very versatile suture. It handles comfortably and knots can be tied easily and securely and is absorbable. 0 or 1 Polyglyconate (Maxon®) and polydioxanone (PDS II®) retain sufficient tensile strength to be routinely used for closure of midline abdominal incisions and muscle layers.

When closing the skin on the face, 5/0 or 6/0 sutures are appropriate and for most other sites 3/0 or 4/0 sutures should be used. Occasionally a 2/0 suture may be needed in areas of thick skin under tension such as on the back.

When closing the skin with interrupted or mattress sutures, polypropylene or nylon are the most appropriate materials. Silk sutures handle nicely but elicit a florid inflammatory response and should be reserved for short-term use such as securing surgical drains. Synthetic absorbable materials are ideal for subcuticular skin closure as their removal is unnecessary and they produce neat scars. They should be placed in the deep dermis to minimize the inevitable mild tissue reaction. Vicryl rapide® is a braided undyed suture specially designed for skin closure. This suture produces a minimal inflammatory reaction and is completely absorbed in 6 weeks. Poliglecaprone 25(Monocryl®) and Glycomer 631 (Biosyn®) are alternative monofilament synthetic absorbable sutures suitable for subcuticular closure that run smoothly through the tissues. Any of these sutures will produce excellent clinical results.

Alternative methods of skin closure

Surgical clips (skin staples)

These provide a quick and convenient method of skin closure that will result in neat wounds. However, they must be inserted with care to avoid inversion of the skin edges. Furthermore, they can be uncomfortable to remove and if left in place too long will produce

a local inflammatory response. For these reasons suture closure is preferred in most instances, unless the wound is very long.

Steri-strips or butterfly stiches

These adhesive strips provide an excellent method to close small skin wounds (<1 cm) and cause less scarring than sutures or staples. They are applied across the wound to gently pull the skin on either side of the incision together. Because they are paper based they must be kept dry to maintain their durability and the application of an overlying waterproof dressing will achieve this aim. Steri-strips can also be used to support a wound allowing early removal of sutures.

Topical skin adhesive ('tissue glue')

The active ingredient 2-octyl cyanoacrylate (Dermabond®) is packaged as sterile viscous liquid. The skin edges of the incision are held apposed and the adhesive is applied in several layers. It rapidly polymerizes to bond together the skin in 1 to 2 minutes. Tissue glue may be used as the primary method of closing small wounds or as an adjunct to subcuticular closure for larger incisions. Studies have demonstrated that application of Dermabond® acts as a barrier preventing the infiltration of bacteria into the healing wound. However, randomized trials have not demonstrated improved primary healing or reduced rates of infection when compared to conventional methods of wound closure. The only consistent benefit is that a skin adhesive can be applied quicker than a suture repair. It is also of value for simple traumatic incisions in children as local anaesthetic may not be required.

Wound complications

Risk of wound infection

The risk of developing a wound infection is related to the likelihood of bacterial contamination. Wounds may be classified as one of four categories, ranging from clean wounds that have a minimal risk of infection to dirty or infected wounds that have a risk of infection approaching 40%[7,8] (Table 3.4.2).

Surgical site infection

This is defined as an incisional or organ space infection occurring within 30 days after an operation or within 1 year if an implant is present.[7,9] Incisional surgical site infection (SSI) may be subdivided into superficial SSI that only involves the skin and subcutaneous

Table 3.4.2 Classification of surgical wounds

Class	Description	Infection rate (%)
I (clean)	Non-infected operative wound	<2
	No inflammation	
	No penetration of viscus	
II (clean-contaminated)	Viscus opened with minimal spillage	<10
	No major break in aseptic technique	
III (contaminated)	Non-purulent inflammation present	15–20
	Gross spillage from open viscus during surgery	
	Major break in aseptic technique	
IV (dirty or infected)	Incision into an abscess	30–40
	Preoperative perforated viscus	

tissue and deep SSI that involves the muscle and fascia.[7,9] SSI is responsible for significant morbidity and prolonged hospital stay and strict perioperative precautions must be taken to minimize the incidence.

Avoiding surgical site infection

Preoperative measures

In elective surgery the length of hospital stay should be kept to a minimum to reduce the risk of contracting a hospital acquired infection particularly methicillin-resistant *Staphylococcus aureus* (MRSA). Most hospitals now screen patients preoperatively for MRSA before elective surgery and those who are carriers should have a course of eradication therapy, whenever possible. Preoperative shaving of the wound is not helpful in reducing SSI. If absolutely necessary then this should occur immediately before the operation, and preferably with electric clippers that are associated with a lower risk of wound infection than shaving the skin. The theatre team must all undergo a thorough surgical scrub using antiseptics and this should include the nails. The theatre must be thoroughly washed between cases and the clean procedures must be performed before the more contaminated operations.[7,9]

Prophylactic antibiotics

A prophylactic antibiotic should be used only when clearly indicated. There is irrefutable evidence that prophylactic antibiotics are effective in reducing SSI in clean-contaminated and contaminated operations, but in clean surgery their use provides no benefit unless a prosthetic implant is used. Antibiotics should be given intravenously at the induction of anaesthesia, and the choice should be based upon the expected pathogens and local guidelines. A commonly used regime for abdominal surgery would be co-amoxiclav 1.2g by slow IV injection at induction and two further doses at

8 and 16 hours. Glycopeptides (e.g. vancomycin or teicoplanin) are used for patients who are MRSA positive.[7,9]

Operative measures

Good theatre discipline is important with regular surveillance of theatre ventilation, sterilization protocols, and aseptic technique. An alcohol- or iodine-based antiseptic should be used to prepare the incision site as this provides optimal and prolonged antibacterial activity.

The surgeon must handle the tissues gently, secure haemostasis, close subcutaneous dead space, and avoid overzealous cautery. The use of suction drains is controversial, but when there is a significant dead space they will help prevent the accumulation of blood and tissue fluid. They may have a beneficial role in extensive soft tissue operations particularly breast, thyroid, and vascular procedures. However, there are no randomized trials that prove their benefit.

Bacterial colonization of suture material is a known risk factor for SSI. In an attempt to prevent this occurring, sutures impregnated with antibacterial activity have been developed. One such broad-spectrum antiseptic is triclosan, which has been used to coat a range of absorbable sutures (e.g. triclosan-coated polyglactin 910 [Vicryl Plus®]). A recently published systematic review and meta-analysis has concluded that the use of triclosan-coated sutures does reduce the risk of SSI.[10] In light of this evidence the use of antiseptic-impregnated sutures should be considered in infection prone wounds.

Following wound closure an occlusive waterproof dressing is applied to prevent postoperative contamination. In grossly contaminated abdominal operations there is an increasing trend to leave the wound open as a laparostomy, with one of the aims being to prevent an abdominal abscess or deep wound infection that frequently occur following primary closure.

SSI must be continuously audited in all surgical units and the likely aetiology and pathogen responsible for each case should be determined. The incidence of SSI should be compared to benchmarked data for the case-mix of operations and is used as a quality outcome measure. Outbreaks of MRSA infection in orthopaedic and vascular wards can have catastrophic consequences, and strict hygiene and isolation protocols must be followed to prevent cross contamination.[7,9]

Pathological scarring

Most surgical wounds will eventually heal to produce thin, soft, and flat scars. However, some patients will develop abnormal scars that can be divided in to three categories namely atrophic, hypertrophic or keloid scars.[11]

Atrophic scars

These are depressed below the skin surface and occur as a result of decreased collagen synthesis or increased collagen degradation. They are prevalent in patients suffering with collagen disorders and those taking steroids.

Hypertrophic scars

These start to develop within a few weeks of an operation and are evident as a red, raised, and often itchy scar that is confined to the border of the original surgical incision. They may increase rapidly for a few months and then after a static phase begin to regress. There then follows a prolonged maturation phase with the eventual development of a wide but flat and symptom-free scar. Hypertrophic scars are more prone to occur following a wound infection or if the incision has been closed under excess tension. Certain anatomical locations (shoulders, neck, sternum, knees, and ankle) will naturally place the wound under tension and predispose to hypertrophic scarring.

Keloid scars

These present as raised pink, red, or purple thickened scars that extend beyond the confines of the surgical incision. They are well demarcated but have an irregular border with a shiny thin epithelial surface. They may not become evident until many months after the wound has healed and are often painful and tender. Unlike hypertrophic scars they do not naturally regress and if excised tend to recur. Anatomical areas prone to keloid scarring include the anterior chest, shoulders, earlobes, upper arms, and cheeks. Keloid scars may occur in all races but they are more prevalent in African patients. Improving the appearance of a keloid scar can be very challenging and cases should be referred to a plastic surgeon. Nonoperative therapeutic measures include pressure therapy, massage, steroid injections, lasers, radiotherapy, and many more. Various operative strategies that include shave excision, Z-plasty, W-plasty, and dermabrasion can be helpful in improving the appearance of keloid scars.

Conclusion

Surgical wounds should be opened and closed with precision and care. If the tissues are handled gently, and the wound is closed accurately without tension, then complications following clean operations are rare. The surgeon must ensure that all precautions are taken to prevent SSI and be a champion of infection prevention measures both on the wards and within the operating theatre.

References

1. Mohan H, Mundi I. Pathology of wound healing. In Sarabahi S, VK Tiwari (eds) *Principles and Practice of Wound Care*. New Delhi: JP Medical Ltd, 2012, pp 11–8.
2. Babu M, Babu RJ, Shanmuganathan S. Recent advances in wound healing. In Sarabahi S, VK Tiwari (eds) *Principles and Practice of Wound Care*. New Delhi: JP Medical Ltd, 2012, pp. 19–26.
3. Early MJ. Wounds, tissue repair and scars. In Williams NS, Bulstrode CJK, O'Connell PR (eds) *Bailey & Love's Short Practice of Surgery*, 25th edition. London: Edward Arnold, 2008, pp 24–31.
4. Talboy GE, Copeland AW. Wounds and wound healing. In Lawrence PF (ed.) *Essentials of General Surgery*, 4th edition. Baltimore, MD: Lippincott Williams and Wilkins, 2006, pp. 147–57.
5. Tiwari VK, Mishra A. Surgical closure of wounds. In Sarabahi S, VK Tiwari (eds) *Principles and Practice of Wound Care*. New Delhi: JP Medical Ltd, 2012, pp. 86–97.
6. Leaper DJ. Basic surgical skills and anastomoses. In Williams NS, Bulstrode CJK, O'Connell PR (eds) *Bailey & Love's Short Practice of Surgery*, 25th edition. London: Edward Arnold, 2008, pp 234–44.
7. Leaper DJ. Surgical infection. In Williams NS, Bulstrode CJK, O'Connell PR (eds) *Bailey & Love's Short Practice of Surgery*, 25th edition. London: Edward Arnold, 2008, pp 32–48.
8. Mohil RS. Classification of wounds. In Sarabahi S, VK Tiwari (eds) *Principles and Practice of Wound Care*. New Delhi: JP Medical Ltd, 2012, pp. 42–9.
9. Malik VK, Dey A. Surgical site infection: Preventive strategies. In Sarabahi S, VK Tiwari (eds) *Principles and Practice of Wound Care*. New Delhi: JP Medical Ltd, 2012, pp. 98–101.
10. Wang ZX, CP Jiang, Cao Y, Ding YT. Systematic review and meta-analysis of triclosan-coated sutures for the prevention of surgical-site infection. *Br J Surg* 2013; 100(4): 465–73.
11. Sarabahi S, Duggirala P. Scars following wound healing. In Sarabahi S, VK Tiwari (eds) *Principles and Practice of Wound Care*. New Delhi: JP Medical Ltd, 2012, pp. 27–41.

CHAPTER 3.5

Surgical haemostasis

Yassar A. Qureshi and Nigel R. M. Tai

Introduction

Surgical haemostasis is an essential component in achieving successful operative outcomes. It is crucial to minimize blood loss intraoperatively, not only to maintain the patient's physiology, but also to enable the surgeon to preserve a clear operative field. A degree of haemorrhage is a normal part of most surgical interventions, but to manage unanticipated or uncontrolled bleeding is a vital skill for a surgeon to acquire, so that haemostatic manoeuvres become second nature.

Primary bleeding may arise during an operation or as a consequence of non-iatrogenic traumatic injury. Bleeding following surgery is classified as either reactionary (up to 48 hours) or secondary (days after).[1] Reactionary haemorrhage may be due to failure to identify a potential source of bleeding during the operation that becomes obvious once the blood pressure returns to normal, a slipped ligature, or disruption of an anastomosis. Secondary bleeding is usually due to infection. The threshold for suspecting bleeding as a cause of a surgical patient's postoperative deterioration should be low.

A thorough understanding of the principles underlying all methods of haemostasis, in conjunction with other facets of operative surgery, should enable the surgeon to be better equipped to manage all eventualities from a minor bleed to a major haemorrhage.

General approach

Prior to performing any operation, it is essential that the patient is fully assessed by the operating surgeon including laboratory tests and scans. This will allow potential issues such as deranged clotting or aberrant blood vessels in the operative field to be identified. Anticipation of such problems allows revision of the operative plan, including the correction of clotting anomalies, requesting of blood products, and notification to the anaesthetist and other members of the surgical team. If necessary, the operation may be deferred altogether if the risks of haemorrhage are deemed to outweigh the clinical urgency of the intervention.

The ideal manner in which to maintain haemostasis during an operation is to identify vessels that lie in the plane of the operative approach prior to inadvertent division, and if appropriate to identify, ligate, and then divide them. This can involve applying haemostatic clips proximally and distally, and transecting the portion of vessel between the haemostats. Ligatures of an appropriate size can then be used to ligate the vessel ends prior to release of the controlling haemostat. A better technique for delicate or large vessels is to apply ligatures while the vessel is in continuity and then divide it. The gap between the ligatures should be twice the width of the vessel. Failure to identify vessels, careless dissection, and poor surgical

technique can result in brisk haemorrhage, but even in ideal circumstances inadvertent vascular or tissue injury is an ever-present threat.

In the event of unanticipated bleeding, a few basic steps should always be followed. Foremost, the surgeon should ensure that he or she controls (1) themselves, (2) the operative field, (3) the available equipment, and (4) the operative team. An abrupt sense of panic can be mitigated by deliberate application of effective digital pressure to the bleeding area, augmented via a gauze swab if necessary. Suction should be utilized to ensure that pressure is applied to the right area, but once digital control is achieved the immediate urgency of the situation is lessened. The surgeon should use the opportunity to regain the initiative by considering the steps required to effect definitive control. Firstly, all theatre team members should be alerted to the haemorrhage, in particular the anaesthetist who may need to orchestrate the transfusion of blood products. If necessary, help from seniors or colleagues should be sought sooner rather than later. Lighting should be adjusted to obtain ideal views of the operative field, and the scrub nurse should be instructed to obtain and have ready any necessary and specific instruments, suture material, or other adjuncts that are required. Pressure should be maintained while these arrangements are completed—firm, direct pressure will often produce definitive haemostasis by itself given sufficient time.

While the experienced surgeon can usually control bleeding with one hand (whether mediated via direct digital control or via a pair of forceps) and suture the bleeding point with the other, in other situations it may pay dividends for the surgeon to have an assistant maintain pressure over the bleeding area (guiding their hand to the correct position). This allows the surgeon to extend the wound and increase exposure of the tissue bed, and use suction and forceps to examine and locate the bleeding point. Further dissection is often required to delineate the bleeding point properly such that clips, clamps or sutures can be applied. Naturally, the type of control is dependent on the volume of blood loss and the type of vessel or tissue affected.

It is essential to remember that the vast majority of haemorrhages can be controlled and curtailed with simple measures, and catastrophic haemorrhage is quite rare (Box 3.5.1). However, hasty application of clamps or hurried dissection in a bloody field may well convert a containable bleed in to a catastrophic one through further iatrogenic damage.

Ligature and suture techniques

The most definitive method of arresting haemorrhage is to ligate the vessel. All vessels may be ligated, although, depending on the end organ, the consequences may be lethal or profoundly life-altering. In these cases vascular repair or temporary shunting is

> **Box 3.5.1** Ligature and surgical haemostasis
>
> ◆ Bleeding should be anticipated, and vessels ligated prior to transection
>
> ◆ Most bleeding can be readily controlled by manual pressure
>
> ◆ A thorough assessment of the bleeding area is vital, making the incision longer if necessary
>
> ◆ Team members must be fully updated
>
> ◆ Simple measures such as clipping and tying, transfixion, or oversewing bleeding tissue will in most cases control bleeding

usually advised. In general, ligation of veins is safer than ligation of arteries, because venous collaterals are more abundant.

Once access is acceptable, a detailed assessment must be made. It is infinitely better to clearly identify the bleeding vessel or tissue rather than blindly suture or use diathermy. This will often make bleeding worse. If it is a vessel, then one should ascertain what type of vessel it is—a vein or an artery. Veins are thin walled, and haemorrhage from veins is less likely to spontaneously arrest than that from muscular arteries, and is hence often more persistent and troublesome. It is also important to remember that a completely transected vessel or tissue bridge will bleed from two ends, and both ends need to be addressed. Proximal and then distal control will need to be established and this may require further dissection. If bleeding is from a named major artery, such as the popliteal artery or the superior mesenteric artery, a repair will almost always need to be undertaken by a specialist vascular surgeon.

The most fundamental skill in haemostasis is that of being able to accurately identify the bleeding source, control it via tissue forceps, and apply a haemostatic clip or diathermy to the area under direct vision. Smaller areas and vessels may be readily diathermied assuming the risks of heat damage to neighbouring structures are not excessive. For larger vessels, once a haemostat has been applied to the vessel end, a ligature can be placed around the tissue beneath the opposed limbs of the clip, encompassing the vessel prior to snug and controlled 'tie-down' and knot completion. It is worthwhile familiarizing oneself with the different sizes and types of artery forceps and surgical clips available, which range from small 'Mosquito' haemostats to large 'Roberts'-type artery forceps (see Chapter 3.3, Basic surgical techniques). If the bleeding is over a larger or less well-defined tissue bed, then it is often better to use a haemostat to gain purchase on the area and apply gentle traction. A second

clip is then applied across the base of the tissue wedge to entrap the bleeding vessel. Vessels that are larger should be double-ligated to provide extra reassurance of haemostasis should one ligature fail. Metal staples can also be applied across cut vessel ends as a form of ligature.

Suture transfixion—as opposed to simple ligation—of divided vessel ends or large tissue stumps is an approach used for additional security in circumstances where a failed ligature would prove calamitous. A suture needle is passed through the bleeding tissue or vessel with a single throw knot at one side, and then the suture material is passed circumferentially around the perimeter of the vessel end and securely knotted (Figure 3.5.1). In situations where it is not possible to identify a discrete bleeding point a suture may be used to under-run the vessel 'in situ' within its tissue bed by using the 'figure-of-8' stitch. This is an especially helpful technique where bleeding is at depth or where access precludes the placement of a haemostatic clip (Figure 3.5.2). Where there is diffuse bleeding from a surface, where haemostatic clips cannot be readily applied, or where a 'figure-of-8' stitch will not suffice, the tissue can be oversewn with continuous suturing. This scenario may be encountered in highly vascular tissue, such as the stomach, a bleeding ulcer or inflamed tissue (Figure 3.5.3).

The type of suture material used will depend on the nature of the tissue and size of vessel. For most scenarios, an absorbable braided suture such as polyglactin (e.g. Vicryl) is used, with the size varying from 3.0 to 0. For larger vessels, which are being transfixed or repaired, a non-absorbable polyprolene (e.g. Prolene) suture is often used, as the lower friction reduces the risk of further vessel injury.

Surgical diathermy: principles and safety

In surgery, diathermy is the use of heat generated by high-frequency electric current for coagulation or cutting of biological tissue. This revolutionary technique was first used in an operation in 1926 by Harvey Cushing. Generally, there are two types of diathermy (monopolar and bipolar), although the principles of heat generation, collateral effects, and safety concerns are similar. Both exploit the impedance presented by the patient's tissue to passage of a high frequency (at least 100 000 Hz and up to 5 MHz) alternating electric current - electrical energy is then converted to heat energy within a localized portion of tissue. The degree of heat energy liberated is influenced by the density of current within the tissue—itself a function of the volume of tissue carrying the current. The high-frequency current minimizes the risk of uncontrolled tissue damage to the patient ('electric shock') which would be seen with

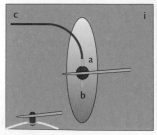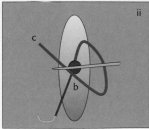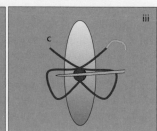

Fig. 3.5.1 Transfixion stitch. i: A needle is passed through the vessel below the clip (inset) at point **a** and exits at point **b**. ii: The loose end of the suture **c** is placed below the clip and a knot tied at point **b**. The loose end **c** is then placed around the clip again. iii: The needle end of the suture is also placed around the clip in the opposing direction to **c** and a final knot is secured at point **a**, prior to removing the clip.

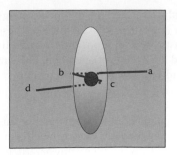

Fig. 3.5.2 Figure-of-8 stitch. A needle passes through tissue at point **a** and out at **b**. Then the needle is passed again through tissue at point at **c** and out at **d**, thus encompassing the bleeding point. Finally, the two suture ends are tied (**a** and **d**), to close off the bleeding point.

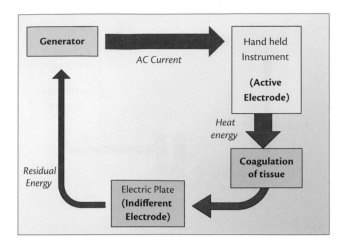

Fig. 3.5.4 A monopolar circuit. Current passes from the generator to the instrument, where current is converted into heat energy, causing the desired coagulation. The residual energy is transferred through the body back to the generator, via the electric plate.

application of domestic alternating current of 50 Hz. The high frequency current is generated by a power source (the 'generator', or Bovie machine in reference to its inventor William Bovie[2]). The generator allows the surgeon to control the strength or the function of the diathermy by controlling the current supply. The current passes through conducting cables from the generator to the hand-held diathermy instrument used by the surgeon. The current is discharged to the patient, being concentrated in a defined area, with heating of water molecules within tissue, evaporation and tissue coagulation—in effect burning.[3,4]

Monopolar diathermy

In monopolar diathermy, the hand-held device is the 'active electrode'; a grounding electric plate placed on the patient is the 'indifferent electrode' and serves to collect the current and return it to the generator (Figure 3.5.4).

The grounding diathermy plate (indifferent electrode) must be placed over a large, clean, dry, hairless area, normally the upper lateral thigh. A good contact between plate and skin is essential to ensure a low current density over the plate; poor contact will concentrate the energy in certain parts and can cause burns and electric shock. It is also necessary to ensure no contact between any metal work and the patient, as energy conducted through metal in contact with the patient will cause damage. The plate must be placed away from internal metal work (e.g. knee or hip replacements) to avoid selective conduction. It is important that alcoholic skin prep is not allowed to come into contact with the plate, or soak the adjacent drapes as this may result in severe burns.

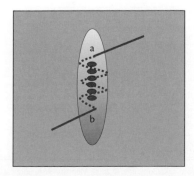

Fig. 3.5.3 Oversewing. A bite of tissue is taken at one end of the bleeding surface and a knot tied (**a**). The tissue is then sewn over with large bites along the whole surface and the suture tied off at the end **b**.

Settings on the generator can be adjusted to effect cutting or coagulation modes. In cutting mode, a higher energy, continuous sine wave current is used, which heats all water in the tissue with such power that a non-conductive vapour forms, thus preventing a disseminating coagulopathic effect. The increased localization of such energy produces the cutting effect. In coagulation mode, the power is lower and the sine wave current is intermittently applied, with the result that the energy is not sufficient to immediately vaporize all water molecules, hence conduction persists for longer and a more congealing effect is obtained. The cutting mode is especially useful for incising tough tissue, such as making skin incisions, or around avascular tissue, as its haemostatic effect is less effective. The coagulation mode is far more haemostatic, and is used for most diathermy dissection.

There are other settings that may occasionally be utilized. Fulguration mode is where an arc is allowed to develop between the instrument tip and tissue by not making direct contact between the two. The energy in this arc will generate a coagulation effect over a wider area, and will remain superficial. This is especially useful when dealing with capsular organs (such as hepatic and splenic trauma), or when minimizing blood loss from oozing surfaces. In desiccation mode higher energy, akin to cutting, is used but again an arc is allowed to form, thus giving a superficial spreading effect. The heat produces an area of parched, dead tissue, and is primarily used to ablate small nodules (e.g. on the skin or on the liver surface), rather than excising them.[1,4]

It is important to remember that the energy generated in the hand-held instrument will burn where it touches tissue, so movements should be very precise, and under clear vision, with only the tip of the instrument being used. A bloody operative field will not aid the use of diathermy as conduction will be weak and untargeted. The tissue may be cauterized through direct application of the diathermy tip or indirectly via contact between the tip and the forceps grasping the bleeding tissue pedicle (the latter is more controlled).

Bipolar diathermy

In bipolar diathermy, the generator produces current that flows through to one limb of a pair of forceps, through the chosen and

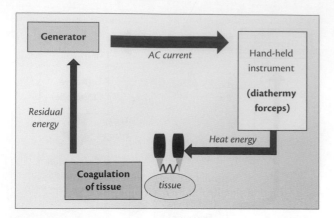

Fig. 3.5.5 A bipolar circuit. Current flows from the generator to the diathermy instrument (forceps), where heat is generated between the tips of the two limbs of the forceps. Residual energy then returns directly back to the generator.

grasped tissue pedicle, and back up through the other limb where residual energy is returned to the generator (Figure 3.5.5). Current is limited to the tissue directly between the forceps and the rest of the patient's body is not part of the circuit—an electric plate is therefore not required. However, the coagulopathic effect of bipolar diathermy is not as strong as monopolar. Bipolar diathermy has many uses and in some instances is preferred. It utilizes less energy and is thus inherently safer. The radius of tissue heat effect generated by monopolar diathermy can range between 5 mm and 10 mm, but is rarely more than 2 mm with bipolar, making it more preferable for controlling haemorrhage when dissecting around vital nerves or other structures that must be preserved. The coagulopathic effect is achieved by a persistent supply of low energy, with reduced collateral injury to surrounding tissue, and the risk of distant burn or shock injury is low making this type of diathermy far more suitable for patients with pacemakers or defibrillators. Monopolar diathermy involves dissipated current that may alter the settings, or worse still, spark an activation of these devices.

A more recently developed use of bipolar energy has yielded the *Ligasure* system (Covidien, USA), which utilizes energy to cause collagen and elastin denaturation, and thus effective vessel sealing. It can be utilized in any type of operation, but is most useful when dissecting around vessel rich tissue and organs.[5]

Safety

Safety is paramount to both the patient and the surgeon. Diathermy involves the use of high-energy current, and the heat energy generated exceeds 400°C. Thus, it is inherently hazardous, and it is the surgeon's responsibility to make all the necessary checks before using it. Table 3.5.1 summarizes key safety issues in the use of diathermy.[1,4–6]

Other energy sources

Ultrasound has been used as a haemostatic technique for many decades. A common example of such a device is the *Harmonic Scalpel* (Ethicon, USA). It utilizes energy gained from ultrasound waves to dissect, coagulate and cut tissue. The basic structure comprises a generator that supplies energy to a hand-held instrument comprising a dissecting tool and a piezoelectric transducer. Current is delivered to the transducer, where small crystals are activated to vibrate, reaching around 55 000 Hz. This ultrasonic frequency is sufficient, when applied to tissue, to coagulate and cut simultaneously. The coagulopathic effect is achieved by the vibrations causing critical protein denaturation in the applied tissue, which the ultrasound waves then cut.[1,7] The advantage of this system is that it utilizes less energy, and vibration rather than heat energy is the chief output. The lateral thermal spread is far less than that of conventional diathermy. It is particularly useful when operating around vascular tissue, and its use has been driven by parallel advances in minimal access surgery.

The use of laser in surgery is also well established. It is able to provide a precise source of heat energy and can be utilized for a cutting, coagulopathic, or ablative effect. For example, a carbon dioxide-based laser is especially utilized to treat skin lesions such as melanoma. Hepatic and ophthalmic surgeons often employ argon

Table 3.5.1 Potential safety concerns relating to the use of diathermy

Safety concern	Potential effects
Faulty generator or instruments	Can cause electric shock, or inappropriate discharge of current
Poor insulation of instruments	Can cause coupling (energy release at non-insulated segments rather than at tip of instrument)
Risk of explosion when in contact with flammable gases	Explosion and severe burns
Poor placement of electric plate	Burns Shock
External metal in contact with patient/staff	Burns
Electric plate close to internal metal prosthesis	Selective conduction through metal causing internal injuries
Monopolar discharges lateral heat at site of coagulation	Collateral damage to surrounding tissue
Monopolar use contraindicated in patients with heart devices	Can trigger malfunction of device
Smoke generated from heating of tissue (containing nitriles, aldehydes and amines)	May be toxic/harmful

Source: data from Cuschieri A et al., *Essential Surgical Practice, Fourth Edition*, Butterworth-Heinemann Publishing, Oxford, UK, Copyright © 2000; Memnon MA, Surgical diathermy, *British Journal of Hospital Medicine*, Volume 52, Number 8, pp. 403–408, Copyright © 1994; Spivak H et al., The use of bipolar cautery, laparosonic coagulating shears, and vascular clips for haemostasis of small and medium-sized vessels, *Surgical Endoscopy* Volume 12, Issue 2, pp. 183–185, Copyright © 1998; and Fitzgerald JEF et al., A single blind controlled study of electrocautery and ultrasonic scalpel smoke plumes in laparoscopic surgery, *Surgical Endoscopy*, Volume 26, Issue 2, pp. 337–342, Copyright © 2012.

Table 3.5.2 Commonly used topical adjuncts to surgical haemostasis

Topical haemostatic agent	Mode of action	Commonly used example
Collagen	Vasoconstriction, platelet aggregation	*Instat MCH* (Ethicon, USA)
Bone Wax	Direct pressure (useful in bleeding from bone/marrow)	
Oxidized Regenerated Cellulose	Vasoconstriction, platelet aggregation	*Surgicel, Fibrillar* (Ethicon, USA)
Gelatin	Vasoconstriction, matrix for platelet aggregation	*Floseal* (Baxter, UK)
Thrombin	Activates plasminogen	*Evithrom* (Ethicon, USA)
Fibrin Sealant	Activates plasminogen	*Tisseel* (Baxter UK)
Synthetic Sealant	Physical barrier, matrix for platelet aggregation	*CoSeal* (Baxter, UK) *Omnex* (Ethicon, USA)

laser. An energy source delivers current to a lasing medium that ionizes atomic particles. These are then transmitted to a vacuum resonator that emits photons as a laser beam. This beam is applied directly to tissue. The safety concerns with laser are critical, and this limits its use. Similarly, radio waves can be utilized for thermal ablation, as in radiofrequency ablation. An electrode is directly placed into tissue, and energy passed through it. The ionization this causes to local tissue results in friction: this is the source of the heat, which is sufficient to destroy surrounding tissue. It is used in cardiology to treat arrhythmias and in hepatic surgery to treat small metastases. Radiofrequency ablation is advancing both experimentally and in practice, and may be useful as an alternative to diathermy in certain settings for purposes of haemorrhage control.

Haemostatic agents

By far the most commonly used haemostatic agent is surgical gauze. It has no inherent haemostatic properties *per se*, but it allows pressure to be applied directly to bleeding tissue. In a laparotomy following abdominal trauma, for example, the surgeon may see only blood. Systematically placing large gauze in each quadrant will allow direct pressure to be applied to all bleeding tissue over large surface areas. If it is not readily controllable at this stage, then the gauze can be left *in situ*, and the peritoneal cavity temporarily closed or contained through application of an appropriate dressing (laparostomy). Following restoration of the patient's physiology, and once coagulation is normalized, the packs are removed.

Commercial haemostatic agents and dressings, although a valuable adjunct to haemorrhage control, are not a substitute to sound operative haemostasis. One common group of such agents are oxidized regenerated cellulose polymers, first used in 1947. A well-known example is *Surgicel* (Ethicon, USA). It is placed directly over a mildly bleeding surface, such as a capsule tear or oozing inflamed

tissue, and exerts its effect through its low pH by stimulating vasoconstriction and platelet plug formation.[8] Another group of such agents are collagen or gelatin based, and these again are placed topically. They work by a combination of vasoconstriction, raising local tissue concentrations of thrombin, and by providing a framework for platelet aggregation. Gelatins contain animal or human thrombin, and are potent in stimulating clot formation directly, with a much used example being *Floseal* (Baxter, UK). Topical thrombin, derived from animal or human plasma, can be applied directly as a spray or bound to bio-absorbable dressing-type materials. Individual use is dependent on the nature of bleeding, anatomical site, and the nature of surgery, and varies with surgeon preference. Table 3.5.2 summarizes the use and mechanism of these adjuncts.

Various intravenous products are available to aid surgical haemostasis and keeping the patient warm is also essential. Identification of patients who have a bleeding tendency prior to an operation is ideal, but not always feasible. The haemostatic cover for such patients should be discussed with a haematologist. The options include well-established drugs such as vitamin K, calcium, fresh frozen plasma, platelets, and cryoprecipitate. Newer agents that include individual clotting factors and thrombin should be used judiciously, as they do carry risks akin to a blood transfusion and will only aid in correcting coagulopathy. They are no substitute for finding and controlling a surgical bleed.

Further reading

Martin MJ, Beekley AC. *Frontline Surgery: A Practical Approach*. New York: Springer 2010.
Monson J, Duthie G, O'Malley K. *Surgical Emergencies*. Oxford: Wiley-Blackwell Ltd 1999.
Picknik, R. *Suture and Surgical Haemostasis: A Pocket Guide*. Philadelphia: Saunders Elsevier 2006.
Russell RCG, Bulstrode CJK, Williams NS, et al (eds). *Bailey and Love's Short Practise of Surgery*, 23rd edition. London: CRC Press 2000.

References

1. Cuschieri A, Steele RJC, Moossa AR. *Essential Surgical Practice*, 4th edition Oxford: Butterworth-Heinemann Publishing, 2000.
2. Bovie WT, Cushing, H. Electrosurgey as an aid to the removal of intracranial tumors with a preliminary note on a new surgical-current generator. *Surg Gynecol Obstetr* 1928; 47: 751–84
3. Pollack SV, Carruthers A, Grekin RC. The history of electrosurgery. *Dermatol Surg* 2000; 26(10): 904–8
4. Memnon MA. Surgical diathermy. *Br J Hosp Med* 1994; 52: 403–8.
5. Spivak H, Richardson WS, Hunter JG. The use of bipolar cautery, laparosonic coagulating shears, and vascular clips for haemostasis of small and medium-sized vessels. *Surg Endosc* 1998; 12: 183–5.
6. Fitzgerald JEF, Malik M, Ahmed I. A single blind controlled study of electrocautery and ultrasonic scalpel smoke plumes in laparoscopic surgery. *Surg Endosc* 2012; 26(2): 337–42.
7. Msika S, Deroide G, Kianmanesh R, et al. Harmonic scalpel in laparoscopic colorectal surgery. *Dis Colon Rectum* 2001; 44(3): 432–36.
8. Spangler D, Rothenburger S, Nguyen K, et al. In vitro antimicrobial activity of oxidized regenerated cellulose against antibiotic-resistant microorganisms. *Surg Infect* 2003; 4(3): 255–62.

CHAPTER 3.6

Anastomoses, stomas, and drains

Dermot Burke

Anastomoses

The word anastomosis derives from the Greek words for mouth, *stoma* and against, *ana*. Anastomosis therefore means 'against mouth' or 'mouth to mouth' in modern parlance. It applies, therefore, to the apposition of two hollow organs and joining them together. This often applies to organs of the digestive tract (e.g. stomach to jejunum, ileum to colon), but also applies to the urinary tract (e.g. ureter to bladder) as well as to blood vessels (e.g. vein graft to artery) and artificial grafts such as Dacron graft to aorta.

Principles of anastomoses

The aim of an anastomotic technique is to make a secure, healthy join between the two parts involved. If this is not achieved, then the anastomosis may leak or disrupt resulting in severe bleeding (vascular anastomosis) or peritonitis (intestinal anastomosis).

Traditionally the three factors that are thought to be important are:

◆ a good surgical technique
◆ a good blood supply to the parts
◆ a lack of tension at the anastomosis.

A good surgical technique

This is something that must be practiced at all times. There are many different forms of anastomotic technique, some of which will be discussed in this chapter. Different techniques may be observed and practiced, but obsessive attention to detail, careful use of sutures/staplers, and meticulous checking will pay dividends and are strongly advised.

A good blood supply

It seems obvious that organs should have a good blood supply. However, this is particularly important in the case of an anastomosis. Tissue repair requires an increase in local oxygen and substrate levels, greater than that required for standard function. It is easy to damage local blood supply during surgery. Gentle dissection, careful inspection of tissues, and accurate technique all play a role in ensuring a good local blood supply.

A lack of tension at the anastomosis

This is vital. Tension between the elements to be joined will naturally distract the anastomosed parts, no matter how good the surgical technique. In addition, it is thought that such tension reduces local blood supply, further increasing the risk of a failure of the join. The parts to be joined must be fully mobilized so that they approximate readily. If there is a risk of tension, further dissection and mobilization should be performed before the anastomosis is constructed.

There are a very large number of anastomoses possible within the human body. In addition, there are a great number of techniques available for each of these. It is not within the scope of this chapter to describe every one of these. Rather, the basic approach to common examples will be outlined.

Gastrointestinal anastomoses

Excision of part of the intestinal tract and subsequent anastomosis is a very common procedure. From lips to anus, there is a huge variety. Common operations include: oesophageal excision with oesophago-gastric anastomosis; partial gastrectomy with gastrojejunal anastomosis; small bowel excision with small bowel anastomosis; and partial colonic excision with ileocolonic, colocolonic or colorectal anastomosis.

Configuration

The configuration of these anastomoses is usually one of three types: end-to-end; end-to-side; side-to-side. A typical end-to-end anastomosis occurs within a left hemicolectomy, where the distal end of the colon is directly anastomosed to the proximal end of the rectum. A typical end-to-side anastomosis occurs following excision of the pancreas, where the end of the common bile duct is anastomosed to the side of the jejunum. A typical side-to-side anastomosis follows a partial gastrectomy when the side of the body of the stomach is anastomosed to the side of a jejunal loop. Traditionally, surgeons perform end-to-end anastomoses where possible. Many of the 'side' anastomoses arise from necessity due to discrepancy in size, rather than preference. However, there are some data to suggest that the side of an organ has a better local blood supply than the cut end.[1] This seems logical. Additionally, use of the side suggests that there is less likely to be tension, as the organs will be close together. There has therefore been an increase in the use of end-to-side and side-to-side anastomoses over the last 20 years. A good example of this change of practice is that of right hemicolectomy, where the ileum is anastomosed to the transverse colon.

Materials

There are a wide variety of materials available to perform the anastomosis. Often the choice is dictated by personal preference. Firstly the surgeon must choose between staples and sutures and then must choose which staples or which sutures. Studies suggest that stapled anastomoses perform better than sutured.[2]

Staples

These usually come colour coded to aid the surgeon. The colour of the removable cartridge reflects the height of the staples, with larger staples typically used for thicker tissues. The *green* cartridge is used for thicker tissues (e.g. stomach), whereas the *blue* cartridge

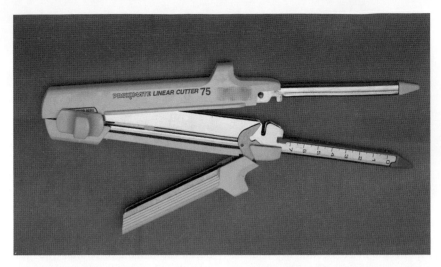

Figure 3.6.1 A linear stapler in the open position, prior to insertion into the intestine to perform a side-to-side anastomosis.

is used for the thinner small and large intestine (*aide-memoire:* green = gastric, blue = bowel). Staplers are available in many sizes and shapes. The stapler usually inserts a double row of staples while simultaneously dividing the intervening tissue. There are two basic types: the linear cutting stapler (Figure 3.6.1) used to form a side-to-side anastomosis, and the circular stapler (Figures 3.6.2) used to from an end-to-side or end-to-end anastomosis in the chest (oesophageal resection) or pelvis (anterior resection of the rectum).

Sutures

A wide variety of different types of sutures is available. An absorbable suture is usually used for intestinal anastomoses. Commonly used materials include vicryl and PDS (polydioxanone suture). A 2/0 or 3/0 gauge suture is usually used, depending on individual preference. There are a large number of techniques used to suture the intestine. These include the interrupted extramucosal technique (as taught on the Intercollegiate Basic Surgical Skills Course), an interrupted mattress technique, a continuous suture technique, or a double layer (interrupted and continuous) technique. Provided that the tissues are handled carefully, that blood loss is kept to a minimum, that the sutures are tied securely without undue tension, all are suitable.

Urological anastomoses

Most urological anastomoses will be end-to-end (e.g. ureteroureteric), but they may be end-to-side (e.g. ureterocystic). As urine may easily leak out, specially designed impervious stents are available

to leave across the anastomosis while it heals. These stents are made from silicone and are therefore inert. They have holes at both ends that allow urine to reach its destination (e.g. from kidney to bladder). The stents come in different lengths (e.g. 22–30 cm) and different gauges (e.g. 6-7). The stent is removed once the surgeon is assured that the anastomosis has healed. This is usually a few weeks later, following radiological assessment. Although uncommon, stents may suffer from complications such as dislocation, encrustation, and infection. A urinary catheter is usually left in the bladder after an anastomosis that involves the bladder to reduce the risk of leakage.

Materials

Urological anastomoses are usually made with interrupted absorbable sutures (e.g. vicryl and PDS). The gauge of suture varies according to the organ involved (e.g. ureter 4/0, bladder 2/0). The sutures are passed through the entire thickness of the wall of the ureter/bladder involved, as there is not the opportunity to perform an extramucosal technique, as with the intestine. Knots are tied on the outside of the lumen, so that they do not act as a focus for encrustation and the development of calculi. In the case of the ureter, the ends are first spatulated both proximally and distally, so as to avoid anastomotic stricture.

Vascular anastomoses

Blood vessels are very demanding structures. This is because the vessel wall is made up of three delicate layers that are easily damaged. The damage is most dangerous in the innermost layer, the

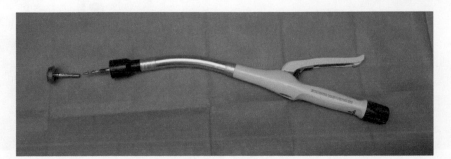

Figure 3.6.2 A circular stapler in the open position. The head of the anvil (the mushroom shaped object on the left) is placed into proximal intestine. The device is closed and placed in the distal intestine. The device is then opened, which advances the trocar to poke through the end of the distal intestine.

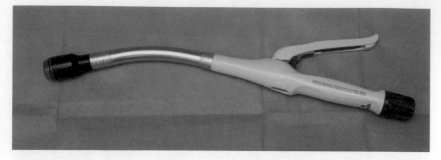

Figure 3.6.3 A circular stapler in the closed position. When the anastomosis is to be performed, the trocar is placed within the anvil and the device is closed, bringing the two parts of the intestine together.

intima, as it is below this layer that atheromatous disease occurs. Such disease, which is a common reason for the surgery, makes damage more likely and this may result in a dissection flap or distal embolization, both of which can occlude the artery. The atheroma and wall of the artery may also be calcified, which can make suturing difficult or sometimes impossible.

Configuration

Vascular anastomoses are usually either end-to-end (e.g. aortic inlay graft) or end-to-side (e.g. femoropopliteal bypass graft). Sound surgical technique, including eversion of the adventitia, avoidance of narrowing and intimal flaps, and lack of tension on the anastomosis are all vital.

Materials

For all vessels, a synthetic, non-absorbable, monofilament suture on an atraumatic needle is used. The sutures are designed to pass easily through the wall of the vessel, so that minimal trauma is caused. The needles used in vascular surgery are gently curved. This design is deliberate, in order that the smallest hole possible is created in the vessel wall. This reduces the risk of bleeding. However, it is important that the needle is placed perpendicular to the vessel wall to achieve this. As a general rule, sutures should be passed from inside the vessel lumen to the outside. This technique is used so that the intima layer is applied to the media layer, so reducing the likelihood of the intimal layer acting as a flap leading to dissection, once blood

flow is restored. Knots are tied on the outer surface of the vessel. For a similar reason, a particular technique is applied to passage of the needle through the vessel wall. The suture is passed through the vessel wall with a series of short advances of the needle by the surgeon. It is important that the main shaft of the needle, rather than the tip, is grasped at all times, as grasping the tip will cause it to blunt, with subsequent damage to the vessel wall. Additionally, short, gentle advances ensuring rotation of the needle will keep the holes small, rather than shearing the vessel wall with a rapid, vigorous technique.

Specially designed vascular clamps are applied to the vessel wall while it is sutured to prevent blood flow, so enabling the suturing to take place. However, it is also important that the clamp is maintained while tying knots, as this will ensure that they are not tied loosely. The clamp should be removed temporarily before the last suture is tied to ensure no clot passes distally, and then again once the anastomosis is complete, to determine whether there is any bleeding. If there is, the site should be reinforced with an interrupted suture after temporary re-application of the clamp.

The gauge of suture to be used on the various vessels is shown in Table 3.6.1.

Complications of Anastomoses

Leakage or disruption

Whatever the nature of the anastomosis, the most feared complication is leakage of the contents through the join. This may be due to a

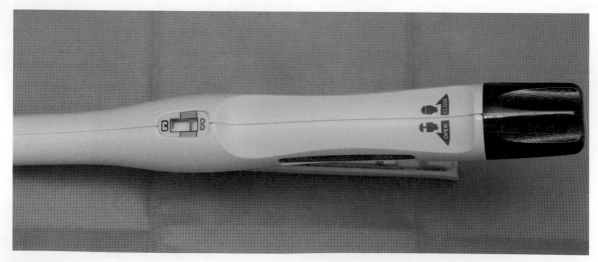

Figure 3.6.4 The red line within the green range (on the handle of the shaft) indicates that the tissues are together and it is now appropriate to fire the gun and anastomose the tissues.

Table 3.6.1 A guide to the gauge of suture to be used depending upon the size of vessel

Artery	Gauge of suture
Aorta	2/0 to 3/0
Iliac	3/0 to 4/0
Femoral	4/0 to 5/0
Popliteal and carotid	5/0 to 6/0
Visceral and tibial	6/0 to 7/0

gap between sutures, infection, and ischaemia, which may be due to sutures that were too tight or tension on the anastomosis. Leakage may occur at any time, but is usually evident within a week. The signs of a leak may be bleeding from a vascular anastomosis, and peritonitis from an intestinal anastomosis. Both of these are serious complications that need to be addressed rapidly with re-operation, additional sutures or revision. A vascular leak may require an interposition graft and an intestinal leak may require the formation of a stoma.

Stenosis

This is usually a late complication of an anastomosis, occurring months or weeks afterwards. In the case of urological and intestinal anastomoses, a stricture is thought to result from ischaemia. With a vascular anastomosis, it is more likely to be due to technical error or recurrent disease. In either case, the anastomosis may need to be dilated from the inside (with a balloon or stent), or may need to be refashioned.

Stomas

Most stomas are gastrointestinal. A urological stoma (a urostomy) is usually formed because the bladder has been removed. Stomas may be classified according to Table 3.6.2.

Organ

A colostomy is formed from the colon and is made flush with the skin. It produces normal stool. An ileostomy is formed from the ileum and has a spout, approximately 2 cm in length, which projects from the skin. This is fashioned in this way so that contents fall directly into the stoma bag, and not onto the skin. As the contents are from the small bowel, they contain digestive enzymes that would otherwise damage the skin. Stomas can also be formed from other parts of the gastrointestinal tract (e.g. jejunostomy, gastrostomy).

Purpose

Most stomas are functional (i.e. they produce effluent). A mucus fistula is the name given to a stoma when the distal non-functioning

Table 3.6.2 Classification of stomas

Organ	Bowel	Ureter
Purpose	Functional	Mucus fistula
Duration	Permanent	Temporary
Configuration	End	Loop

part of bowel is also brought out onto the abdominal wall. It discharges only mucus, not intestinal contents. A good example of this is when a patient has ischaemic bowel, which is resected and the healthy ends are brought to the surface as two stomas: one a functioning stoma, and the other a mucus fistula.

Duration

A stoma may be permanent. A good example is an end colostomy after the anus has been excised during an abdomino-perineal excision of the anorectum Figure 3.6.5. The anal sphincter is removed during this procedure, the perineum is sutured closed, so there is no chance of closing the stoma. A urostomy after excision of the bladder is also permanent. However, some stomas may be temporary - for example, following resection of ischaemic small intestine, the intention is to join the intestine together when possible. Another good example is a loop ileostomy. This is a stoma above an anastomosis (e.g. a colorectal anastomosis, an ileal pouch anal anastomosis), which is designed to defunction the distal bowel and divert the faecal stream away from the anastomosis until the anastomosis has healed. Once the surgeon is assured that the anastomosis has healed satisfactorily, the ileostomy is closed (reversed).

Configuration

A loop stoma is created with a view to future closure, such as a loop ileostomy, although any part of the intestine can form a loop stoma. The term loop indicates that the posterior part of the intestinal wall is not divided, but remains in continuity throughout. The anterior part of the wall is divided to form the stoma. The reason for this is that subsequent closure of the stoma is much easier than if the two parts were separated. There is no need to go looking for both parts of intestine, as they are adjacent, as part of the loop. All that is needed to close the stoma is for both sides to be freed from the skin and the anterior wall sutured, before the entire intestine is replaced into the abdominal cavity.

Complications

There are a number of complications that can arise from stomas:

Retraction

This occurs early, when the intestine has not been sufficiently mobilized. Provided that the intestine does not retract into the peritoneal cavity, the situation can usually be managed with careful application of stoma bags. However, occasionally surgical revision is necessary.

Necrosis

This is an early complication, usually within a week. It is due to ischaemia. This may result from not having mobilized the intestine sufficiently to reach the skin, or may result from the original disease process. In some cases, the surface of the stoma looks dusky, but not frankly necrotic. In these cases, the stoma should be carefully examined, with a light source and a scope if necessary, to see whether the mucosa is viable deeper within the intestine. Should the stoma become necrotic it will need to be surgically revised.

Stenosis

This is a late complication that results from either long-term retraction or from chronic ischaemia. It may result in difficulty in evacuation and, in extreme cases, intestinal obstruction. It can usually be

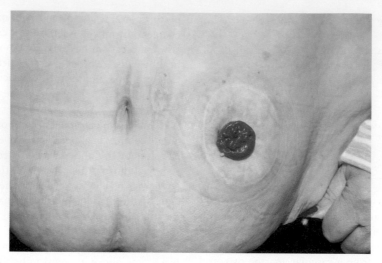

Fig. 3.6.5 Formation of an end colostomy.

managed conservatively with enemas, laxatives, and dilators, but surgical revision may be necessary.

Prolapse

This is a late complication, when the intestine prolapses through the stomal defect. The stoma usually continues to function satisfactorily, but the prolapsed intestine may make it difficult to apply the stoma bag adequately. Surgical revision may be necessary.

Hernia

This is a late complication. Most people with a parastomal hernia are content to live with it, but sometimes surgical repair is necessary. The long-term results from repair, however, are not good, although the use of mesh has improved the outcome of repair.

Surgical drains

Drains are common in surgical practice. They serve a number of purposes. Firstly, they are employed prospectively to remove material (e.g. blood, serous fluid) that would otherwise accumulate at the site of surgery Secondly, they provide a path of least resistance so that harmful fluids can be removed from a particular site (e.g. drain placed into an abscess cavity).

Types of drain

A wide variety of drains and methods are available depending upon the function required. Most are simple tubes in various sizes, made of silicone or rubber. The flat, corrugated drain is a variation that is often used to drain infection. Its design allows drainage from a wider area than that of a tube drain, and is less likely to block. Placement of a drain is usually straightforward, but they must be sutured firmly in place, with a non-absorbable suture, otherwise they will fall out (or in!) easily.

Drains may be placed at the time of surgery or with the assistance of imaging. Computed tomography-guided drainage is a commonly utilized method for drainage of an abscess following a small postoperative leak from an intestinal anastomosis. This can improve the patient's clinical situation, without recourse to a second operation.

Open drainage

This is when a soft drain is placed into a space to be drained, such as the drainage of an abscess cavity. The drain is removed when the surgeon is sure that the track for drainage has been established (usually 7 to 10 days). Another good example is a seton. This is a small drain, often made of rubber, that is placed inside a fistula-in-ano and then tied on the outside. It enables drainage of pus.

Closed drainage

A closed system is when a tube drain is placed into a viscus to drain fluid contents into a collecting bag. This allows drainage of fluid, but prevents contamination of the fluid from outside. A T-tube, placed within the common bile duct is a good example of this. Chest drains may be considered as closed drainage, but require an underwater seal to prevent further air entering the pleural cavity.

Closed suction drain

These drains are usually used after clean elective surgery in order to remove fluid from the site of surgery and so prevent a collection with subsequent infection. A good example of this is after the use of skin flaps in reconstructive surgery (e.g. breast reconstruction). The negative atmospheric pressure generated within the system, effectively sucks fluid out of the area.

Complications

Complications from drains are uncommon. They may fall out early if not adequately sutured or, rarely, a drain may erode into a vessel and cause haemorrhage. Drains can also introduce infection. It is important to document both the amount and the type of fluid that drains out. This fluid may be sent to the laboratory for further analysis (e.g. microbiological, enzymes).

Removal

Drains are removed when they are no longer required, usually when the amount of fluid that is draining has reduced sufficiently. This is a clinical decision. Drains are removed by simply cutting the suture that holds them in place and removing the drain from the patient.

With suction drains, it may be wise to remove the suction, or negative pressure, before removing the drain. In some cases, drains are left in place long enough for a track to form so that drainage can continue, even after the drain has been removed.

Further reading

Bafford AC, Irani JL. Management and complications of stomas. *Surg Clin North Am* 2013; 93: 145–66.

Fichera A, Zoccali M, Kono T. Antimesenteric functional end-to-end hand-sewn (Kono-S) anastomosis. *J Gastrointest Surg* 2012; 16: 1412–6.

Formijne Jonkers HA, Draaisma WA, Roskott AM, *et al.* Early complications after stoma formation: a prospective cohort study in 100 patients with 1-year follow-up. *Int J Colorectal Dis* 2012; 27: 1095–9.

Gurusamy KS, Allen VB, Samraj K. Wound drains after incisional hernia repair. *Cochrane Database Syst Rev* 2012; 2: CD005570.

Gustavsson K. Gunnarsson U, Jestin P. Postoperative complications after closure of a diverting ileostoma—differences according to closure technique. *Int J Colorectal Dis* 2012; 27: 55–8.

Hubner M, Larson DW, Wolff BG. 'How I do it'—radical right colectomy with side-to-side stapled ileo-colonic anastomosis. *J Gastrointest Surg* 2012; 16: 1605–9.

Leichtle SW, Mouawad NJ, Welch KB, *et al.* Risk factors for anastomotic leakage after colectomy. *Dis Colon Rectum* 2012; 55: 569–75.

Martin ST, Vogel JD. Intestinal stomas: indications, management, and complications. *Adv Surg* 2012; 46: 19–49.

Neutzling CB, Lustosa SA, Proenca IM, *et al.* Stapled versus handsewn methods for colorectal anastomosis surgery. *Cochrane Database Syst Rev* 2012; 2: CD003144.

Olson TP, Becker YT, McDonald R, *et al.* A simulation-based curriculum can be used to teach open intestinal anastomosis. *J Surg Res* 2012; 172: 53–8.

Park J, Fuzesi S, Temple LK, *et al.* Rectal cancer patients' quality of life with a temporary stoma: shifting perspectives. *Dis Colon Rectum* 2012; 55: 1117–24.

Person B, Ifargan R, Lachter J, *et al.* The impact of preoperative stoma site marking on the incidence of complications, quality of life, and patient's independence. *Dis Colon Rectum* 2012; 55: 783–7.

Phan TQ, Xu W, Spilker G, *et al.* Technique and indication of distal arterial-to-proximal venous anastomosis at an amputated distal phalanx. *Hand Surg* 2012; 17: 135–7.

Picchio M, De Angelis F, Zazza S, *et al.* Drain after elective laparoscopic cholecystectomy. A randomized multicentre controlled trial. *Surg Endosc* 2012; 26: 2817–22.

Polese L, Vecchiato M, Frigo AC, *et al.* Risk factors for colorectal anastomotic stenoses and their impact on quality of life: what are the lessons to learn? *Colorectal Dis* 2012; 14: e124–8.

Sjodahl R, Schulz C, Myrelid P, *et al.* Long-term quality of life in patients with permanent sigmoid colostomy. *Colorectal Dis* 2012; 14: e335–8.

Wang R, Wood DPJr, Hollenbeck BK, *et al.* Risk factors and quality of life for post-prostatectomy vesicourethral anastomotic stenoses. *Urology* 2012, 79: 449–57.

References

1. Hallböök O, Johansson K, Siödahl R. Laser Doppler blood flow measurement in rectal resection for carcinoma--comparison between the straight and colonic J pouch reconstruction. *Br J Surg* 1996; 83: 389–92.
2. Choy PY, Bissett IP, Docherty JG, *et al.* Cochrane Database Syst Rev. 2011 Sep 7;(9):CD004320.

Principles of surgical endoscopy and minimal access surgery

Katie Schwab, Deepak Singh-Ranger, and Timothy Rockall

Surgical endoscopy: introduction and history

Endoscopy, derived from the Greek words '*éndon*—within/inside' and '*skopía*—watching/looking at', refers to the ability to look inside a body cavity or through a natural orifice to observe what is hidden to the naked eye. Records date back to ancient civilizations, where early forms of speculae were used, limited by the ability to illuminate.[1,2]

After the invention of the electric light bulb, urologists such as Nitze and Newman pioneered further advances with more complex endoscopes that included separate channels for light, vision, and instrumentation.[3] The 20th century progressed further with the invention of semi- and fully flexible instruments.

Laparoscopy was first pioneered by a German physician called Kelling. He performed what he termed celioscopy on dogs and also described the use of CO_2 as the gas for pneumoperitoneum.[2,3] Human laparoscopy was first reported by a Swedish doctor called Jacobaeus in 1910, and by the 1930s it was utilized for minor interventional procedures such as adhesiolysis and biopsy. The subsequent development of fibre optics and the Hopkins's rod lens system allowed the technique to become more established, especially in gynaecology. In the 1980s, with the development of the video chip camera systems, more complex procedures were undertaken and Kurt Semm, one of the fathers of minimal access surgery (MAS), documented the first laparoscopic appendicectomy as well as developing laparoscopic haemostasis techniques and automatic insufflators.[4]

Minimal access surgery: fundamentals

The key points of MAS are:

- reduced complications associated with access
- reduced postoperative pain
- reduced hospital stay
- improved surgical view
- improved patient satisfaction
- equivalent oncological outcomes[5,6]
- longer learning curve and training requirements.

MAS uses small incisions that result in reduced trauma from surgery. In the immediate perioperative period, there is reduced pain and consequently a more rapid recovery, earlier mobilization, and reduced length of hospital stay (and its associated complications such as deep vein thrombosis/pulmonary embolism and pneumonia).[7,8] However, at times these advantages can be offset by a significantly longer operation time. Wound complications such as infection, dehiscence, and incisional hernia are also reduced.[9] Longer-term outcomes have demonstrated faster return to normal activities, greater patient satisfaction, and better cosmesis.[10,11]

Cancer outcomes have been shown to be equivocal compared to open surgery, and initial concerns regarding port site metastases have been disproven in randomized controlled trials.[5,6] Cost-effectiveness studies are generally in favour of MAS, as initial set-up, maintenance and instrumentation costs are offset by reduced hospital stay, a greater shift to day case surgery, and reduced complications.

Disadvantages relate to the surgical learning curve and increased operating time. MAS is a highly skilled operative technique where loss of tactile feedback, depth perception, and limited movement need to be overcome.[12] Consequently, operating time can be longer, especially in early training, and risk of iatrogenic injury can be higher. Sophisticated virtual reality training systems and simulations can assist in training programmes, but in spite of well-regulated training there is still a close correlation between numbers of cases and the potential for complications. In certain complex laparoscopic surgery the learning curve is steep and long.

Minimal access surgery equipment and set-up

Visual technology

Visual technology (equipment needed to visualize the operating field internally) is combined together in a 'stack' for ease of use, transfer, and to prevent cables trailing throughout an operating theatre. The component parts consist of the following:

- Telescope:
  - rigid scope consisting of rod lenses between objective lens and eyepiece, in different diameters (3 mm, 5 mm, 10 mm)
  - objective lens available in different degrees of angulation (0°, 30°, 45°). Variable angulation and flexible tip scopes also available.
- Camera:
  - microchip video camera containing one or three (higher resolution) silicon charge-coupled devices or 'chips'

- video camera attaches to eyepiece of the scope with locking mechanism
- focus and illumination can be adjusted.
- Light source:
  - fibre optic light lead transmits white light from a source to scope with virtually no loss of intensity
  - light sources tend to use xenon lamps (300 W) or halogen systems (150–200 W).
- Monitor:
  - high-quality image projection
  - video recording and picture capturing/printing systems.
- Insufflator:
  - CO_2 insufflation for establishment and maintenance of pneumoperitoneum
  - pressurized release, at set flow rates; feedback to allow set pressure to be achieved and maintained
  - alarms signal over-pressure, occlusion, and low tank gas-levels.

Laparoscopic instrumentation

Laparoscopic tools (see Table 3.7.1), are ergonomically designed for easy manipulation by the surgeon extra corporally, and can be disposable or reusable.

Other specialized tools include:

- needle holders
- suction/irrigation devices
- specimen bags
- retractors
- pre-formed knot loops
- stapling devices
- clip applicators.

Patient safety/risk management

Positioning

Operating tables can be manipulated to allow optimum patient position for height and angulation during MAS: Trendelenburg (head down) for pelvic surgery or Reverse Trendelenburg (head up)

Table 3.7.1 Component parts of a laparoscopic instrument

Component	Details
Handle	Ergonomic grip
	Can have 'bow' handles for open/close of jaws
	± Ratchet
Rotator knob	360° rotation of tip with operators finger
Diathermy connector	Connection of monopolar or bipolar circuitry
Shaft	Long and slim to pass through access ports
	Can be extra long (bariatric surgery)
	Insulated
Tip	Various
	Scissors, hook, scalpel
	Dissectors: blunt, pointed, dolphin nosed
	Graspers: toothed, atraumatic

for upper abdominal surgery. Tilting the patient improves exposure by allowing mobile organs such as small bowel to move and stay out of the operating field. When tilting is required, measures to guarantee the safety of the patient such as placement on a non-slip surface and deploying shoulder and lateral supports, should be used. Legs can be placed in leg supports for movement and access to perineum. Arms should be wrapped and pressure points padded to prevent injury.

Equipment placement

The stack should be positioned near the patient for easy reach of leads and tubing. The monitor(s) need to be opposite the surgeon to allow ergonomic operating and a view for assistants. Energy sources need to be accessibly placed and all cabling should be secured, protected, and easily visible.

Patient adjuncts

Urinary catheters (important for pelvic surgery) will decompress the bladder, reducing risk of trocar injury. If not being used, ensuring the patient has voided urine preoperatively is a sensible precaution.

Nasogastric or orogastric tubes should be considered intraoperatively in the presence of gastric distension that interferes with surgery.

Pneumatic compression devices reduce deep vein thrombosis risk, and warming blankets help maintain temperature without surgeon hindrance. Enhanced recovery protocols may include the use of cardiac monitoring, such as oesophageal Doppler, and allowing goal-directed fluid replacement.

Techniques of minimal access surgery

Access

- Open or 'Hasson':
  - described by Hasson 1974
  - direct dissection through peritoneum before inserting blunt primary trocar
  - port secured in place by stay sutures.
- Blind or 'Veress needle'
  - uses spring-loaded needle to puncture and inflate pneumoperitoneum
  - was developed by Veress in 1932 for creating pneumothoraces in tuberculosis
  - initial access port is placed once pneumoperitoneum established
  - particular care should be taken in the presence of previous surgery or suspected adhesions
  - optical trocars (laparoscope is placed within the primary trocar) can be used to visualize entry of further instruments/ports into the inflated peritoneal cavity.

Establishing the pneumoperitoneum

- Ensure insufflator is on and correct pressure settings entered before commencing.
- Begin with slow flow, and observe:
  - patient for even distension of the abdomen

- insufflator to ensure correct pressure readings (rapid high pressure may imply incorrect position of trocar or Veress needle, for example extraperitoneal or intravisceral)
- anaesthetic monitoring as pneumoperitoneum can cause profound bradycardia, difficulties in mechanical ventilation, pneumothorax, or (rarely) gas embolus. It may be necessary to stop and release insufflation, or reduce the set pressure.

Port placement

- Ports can be:
  - reusable, part reusable, or disposable
  - blunt, sharp, bladed, retractable bladed, or dilating tip
  - blunt primary ports may have a conical device or a balloon system to secure and maintain a gas seal; others may have a ribbed shaft to hold the port in position
  - at least one port requires a gas tap for insufflation
  - variety of sizes (3, 5, 10, 11, 12, or15 mm diameter).
- Port size and positioning varies with the operation and surgeon preference. The concept of triangulation (instruments meet at the apex of a triangle) is most ergonomic.
- Secondary ports are placed under direct vision to avoid iatrogenic injury, and observed on removal to ensure no port site bleeding is overlooked.

Recognizing and managing complications

If there is suspicion of visceral injury, inspect everything thoroughly, including 'walking through' the bowel with atraumatic graspers. Obvious injury (evident contamination) may require thorough lavage and suturing or resection to repair the injury.

Vascular injury is likely to be apparent. Minor vascular injury may be controlled with calm organized steps including:

- pressure (using small swabs)
- isolation and identification of source
- haemostasis with diathermy or chemical agents in sprays, gels or sheets
- haemostasis with clips or sutures.

If the vascular injury is more significant, it may require open conversion to definitively solve, while liaising with the theatre team to ensure awareness of the problem and always consider seeking more senior/specialist input. NEVER blindly clip or diathermy anything.

While operating, the surgeon should ensure that methodical steps are followed and progress is made. If there are concerns or a failure to progress, the surgeon should consider seeking more experienced input as well as converting to open procedure.

During surgery, there should be close liaison with the anaesthetic team—the maintenance of the CO_2 pneumoperitoneum produces physiological changes that differ to those during open surgery:

- CO_2 absorbed into blood stream results in hypercapnia and acidosis
- Increasing tidal volume to excrete CO_2 is not always feasible due to mechanical limitations imposed by a distended abdomen, leaving bases under ventilated and oxygen perfusion reduced

- Reduced venous return from abdominal pressure reduces cardiac output, oxygen perfusion, and renal perfusion (stimulating renin-angiotensin-aldosterone loop and production of antidiuretic hormone)
- If there are anaesthetic concerns, consider reducing the pneumoperitoneum working pressure, correcting any tilt of patient or releasing the pneumoperitoneum for a while.

Postoperatively

There should be a low threshold for returning to theatre for laparoscopy if the patient is unwell in the first 48 hours—persistent pain, vomiting, tachycardia, and/or respiratory distress may indicate occult complications.

Radiological imaging has a limited role, because plain X-rays will not exclude perforation due to the retained pneumoperitoneum. Ultrasound has limited specificity or sensitivity when looking for blood or contamination and computed tomography may initially give false reassurance.

In the long term, wound infections and incisional hernias may occur. Efforts to prevent their occurrence should occur perioperatively:

- close the sheath/fascial layer in port sites ≥10 mm
- ensure good asepsis at beginning and end of surgery
- antibiotic prophylaxis as per local guidelines perioperatively
- avoid direct skin contamination with intra-abdominal viscera—use bags to remove specimens or wound protectors for extracorporeal bowel handling.

Advances in technology
Robotic surgery

Robots like the 'da Vinci Surgical System' place a computer interface between the operating surgeon and the surgical tools and camera, with the proposed benefit of improving dexterity, image quality, and image control. The da Vinci comprises a four-armed robot allowing 'docking' of three instrument arms and one camera arm into patient ports. A surgeon sits at a console using finger-tip manipulators for fine tool control and foot pedals for controlling the image, changing position, and operating energy sources. The robotic instruments are wristed at the tips, allowing more degrees of freedom of movement, and tremor is abolished, resulting in greater precision. The camera system provides a binocular view that allows a high-definition three-dimensional (3D) view of the surgical field.

Three-dimensional technology

One of the most striking benefits afforded by the robot is the 3D endoscopic view. A stereoptic view removes the limits of depth perception that accompanies normal MAS, consequently improving precision. Early 3D systems generated a poor quality image and often resulted in headaches and nausea for the surgeon. Newer passive polarizing displays create a high-definition 3D view, which is comfortable for prolonged viewing. The 3D view is made possible by the endoscope containing two lenses—a left eye and a right eye. These two views are processed and projected together on a 3D screen, which is then separated for each individual eye to see. Passive polarizing systems require the surgeon to wear polarizing glasses.

Advances in minimal access

Single-port surgery

The first documented single-port laparoscopic cholecystectomy was performed in 1997, and since then a variety of procedures have been performed through one access incision. The surgery relies on all tools going through one adapted port or multiple ports through a single incision. The theoretical advantages are less trauma and better cosmesis for the patient and possibly less postoperative pain due to one small incision, although this is mostly unproven. Restrictions result from poor triangulation of tools and poor ergonomics of operating and viewing in a straight line. Curved and flexible tools and adapted endoscopes have been developed to try and overcome these difficulties.

Natural orifice transluminal endoscopic surgery

Access is through a natural orifice, most commonly the stomach (via the mouth), vagina, or rectum. While a number of operative procedures have been described (appendicectomy, cholecystectomy), there remain considerable obstacles to overcome, including limitations of operating with flexible scopes, stability of the operating platform, limited instrumentation, and closure of the access site. Most operations performed are hybrid techniques utilizing natural orifice access or specimen removal and some transabdominal instrumentation. These techniques have not yet entered routine practice.

Summary

MAS is utilized by every surgical specialty because of the reduced perioperative complications, more rapid recovery, and greater patient satisfaction. As technology continues to evolve, advances in equipment, access, and visualization broaden the spectrum of operations amenable to MAS and improves quality of surgery and outcomes for patients. Key principles of operating equipment, theatre, and patient set-up, and surgical technique need to be understood and adhered to in order to ensure successful MAS.

Further reading

Ballantyne GH, Marescaus J, Giulianotti PC. *Primer of Robotic & Telerobotic Surgery*, 4th edition. Philadelphia: Lippincott Williams & Wilkins, 2004.

Hotta T, Takifuji K, Yokoyama S, *et al*. Literature review of the energy sources for performing laparoscopic colorectal surgery. *World J Gastrointest Surg* 2012; 4(1): 1–8.

Kalloo AN, Marescaux J, Zorron R. Natural Orifice Translumenal Endoscopic Surgery: Textbook and Video Atlas. Oxford: John Wiley & Sons, 2012.

Mishra RK. *Textbook of Practical Laparoscopic Surgery*, 2nd edition. New Delhi: Jaypee Brothers Medical Publishing, 2009.

National Institute of Health and Care Excellence. NICE Guidelines TA105: *Laparoscopic surgery for colorectal cancer* (issue date August 2006). London: NICE.

Philips PA, Amaral JF. Abdominal access complications in laparoscopic surgery. *J Am Col Surg* 2001; 192(4): 525–36.

Scott-Conner CEH. *The SAGES Manual: Fundamentals of Laparoscopy, Thoracoscopy and GI Endoscopy*, 2nd edition. New York: Springer, 2006.

Soper N, Swanstrom L, Eubanks W. *Mastery of Endoscopic and Laparoscopic Surgery*, 3rd edition. Philadelphia: Lippincott Williams & Wilkins, 2008.

www.websurg.com. The e-surgical reference of Laparoscopic surgery

References

1. Lau WY, Leow CK, Li AK. History of endoscopic and laparoscopic surgery. *World J Surg* 1997; 21(4): 444–53.
2. Spaner SJ, Warnock GL. A brief history of endoscopy, laparoscopy, and laparoscopic surgery. *J Laparoendosc Adv Surg Tech A* 1997; 7(6): 369–73.
3. Berci G, Forde KA. History of endoscopy: what lessons have we learned from the past? *Surg Endosc* 2000; 14(1): 5–15.
4. Litynski GS. Kurt Semm and the fight against skepticism: endoscopic hemostasis, laparoscopic appendectomy, and Semm's impact on the 'laparoscopic revolution'. *JSLS* 1998; 2(3): 309–13.
5. Veldkamp R, Kuhry E, Hop WC, *et al*. Laparoscopic surgery versus open surgery for colon cancer: short-term outcomes of a randomised trial. *Lancet Oncol* 2005; 6(7): 477–84.
6. Kuhry E, Schwenk WF, Gaupset R, *et al*. Long-term results of laparoscopic colorectal cancer resection. *Cochrane Database Syst Rev* 2008; (2): CD003432.
7. Chapman AE, Levitt MD, Hewett P, *et al*. Laparoscopic-assisted resection of colorectal malignancies: a systematic review. *Ann Surg* 2001; 234: 590–606.
8. Braga M, Vignali A, Gianotti L, *et al*. Laparoscopic versus open colorectal surgery: a randomized trial on short-term outcome. *Ann Surg* 2002; 236: 759–766.
9. Schwenk W, Haase O, Neudecker J, *et al*. Short term benefits for laparoscopic colorectal resection. *Cochrane Database Syst Rev* 2005; (3): CD003145,
10. Eshuis EJ, Polle SW, Slors JF, *et al*. Long-term surgical recurrence, morbidity, quality of life, and body image of laparoscopic-assisted vs. open ileocolic resection for Crohn's disease: a comparative study. *Dis Colon Rectum* 2008; 51(6): 858–67.
11. Liem MS, van der Graaf Y, Zwart RC, *et al*. A randomized comparison of physical performance following laparoscopic and open inguinal hernia repair. The Coala Trial Group. *Br J Surg* 1997; 84(1): 64–7.
12. Berguer R, Smith WD, Chung YH. Performing laparoscopic surgery is significantly more stressful for the surgeon than open surgery. *Surg Endosc* 2001; 15(10): 1204–7.

CHAPTER 3.8

Simulation and assessment

Pramudith Sirimanna, Grace Lee,
Sonal Arora, and Rajesh Aggarwal

Introduction

Becoming a surgeon is a significant and costly undertaking and the most effective way to train has not been identified. Traditionally, surgical training used an apprenticeship model. By way of 'see one, do one, teach one,' young surgeons learnt how to operate through sheer volume and experience. As the landscape of rules governing training evolved and ethics came to the fore, it became obvious that this model was both unsafe and inefficient. While clinical experience as documented by logbooks remains vital, there is a trend towards competency-based curricula that also require proficiency be demonstrated. The increasing pressure from regulatory bodies to reduce work hours, minimize patient harm, and be cognizant of the cost of training, has resulted in many training institutions developing a significant interest in simulation as an adjunct to clinical experience.

One definition of simulation from the Society for Simulation in Healthcare is: 'the imitation or representation of one act or system by another. Healthcare simulations can be said to have four main purposes—*education, assessment, research, and health system integration* in facilitating patient safety'.[1] Ideally, simulation in surgery should help reduce the learning curve of surgical procedures so that more clinical time can be spent focusing on intraoperative decisions rather than refining technical skills.[2] Simulation can also introduce trainees and the rest of the team to management of rare situations, both intraoperatively and involving patient care.[3] On a larger scope, simulation can affect healthcare delivery systems by unearthing pitfalls and inefficiencies of current systems. Other high-risk industries, such as the airline and nuclear industries, have already integrated simulation as a mandatory part of training. The healthcare industry, while making great strides, has yet to embrace simulation to that degree. The purpose of this chapter is to review and understand the development of surgical simulation and assessment of surgical skills.

Modes of simulation

Models for simulation in surgical training can be broadly categorized as inorganic and organic. Inorganic models can comprise of synthetic materials as well as computerized virtual reality (VR) simulators, whereas organic models include the use of animal and human tissue. Within each model there lies a spectrum of fidelity (i.e. an inherent level of realism). In addition, a surgical simulator must demonstrate its validity as a training tool, which itself consists of a number of components (Figure 3.8.1). A summary of this hierarchy is displayed in Table 3.8.1.

Simulation of technical skills

Whether it is tying knots or becoming familiar with different ports for minimally invasive surgery, surgery lends itself to simulation. Rather than learning technical skills during an operation, trainees can practice these skills in a safe environment. Basic surgical skills were the impetus for the first modes of simulation. Knot-tying boards are widely available for practice at home, and suturing can be practiced on latex models or on cadaveric animal tissue (Figure 3.8.2). In addition, models were created to perform parts of procedures such as fracture fixation and enteric anastomoses. Such models have been incorporated into formal training courses such as the Basic Surgical Skills Course organized by the Royal College of Surgeons.[4]

Within the minimally invasive surgery domain, box trainers have been developed consisting of synthetic models within a plastic box, which are manipulated using actual laparoscopic instruments and optical systems. These low-fidelity models allow training of hand–eye coordination, depth perception, and technical skills inherent to laparoscopic surgery using exercises such as peg transfers and intracorporeal knot tying. Box trainers have been incorporated into training programs such as the Fundamentals of Laparoscopic Surgery (FLS) educational program designed by the Society of American Gastrointestinal and Endoscopic Surgeons (Figure 3.8.3). As simulation continued to develop, it became clear that modes of simulation should evolve to encompass whole procedures. Higher fidelity dry laboratory simulators made from synthetic materials were created to replicate full operations, such as an inguinal hernia repair kit that allows practice from incision to skin closure.

Technological advances have made VR simulation increasingly popular as a pedagogical technique. Its ability to allow training of basic skills as well as full procedures in a risk-free, standardized, reproducible environment, and provide immediate objective feedback makes VR simulation an attractive proposition for surgical education. A variety of VR surgical simulation trainers exist with varying degrees of fidelity. The MIST-VR laparoscopic simulator (Mentice, Gothenburg, Sweden) is a low-fidelity VR simulator that utilizes abstract tasks, such as the grasping or manipulating various targets, to train basic laparoscopic skills. Higher fidelity VR simulators, which incorporate more realistic animation as well as haptic feedback, have been developed that allow practice of full procedures. The LapSim® (Surgical Science, Gothenburg, Sweden) and LapMentor™ laparoscopic simulator (Simbionix, Cleveland, Ohio, USA) are examples of such high-fidelity VR simulators

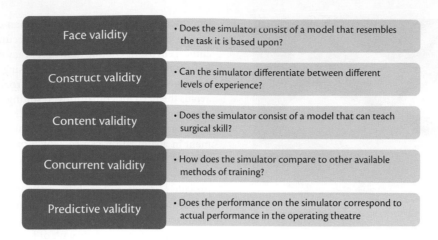

Fig. 3.8.1 Constituents of validity.

Table 3.8.1 The hierarchy of simulation-based training methods

Mode of simulation	Models	Example	Pros	Cons
Inorganic: synthetic	Skill-based models	Knot tying and suturing models	Teaches basic skills applicable to a variety of procedures and specialties	Low fidelity
		FLS box trainer	Wide validity for laparoscopic skills training Transferability of skills learnt to OT demonstrated	Low fidelity Cannot practice full procedures
	Procedural models	Laparoscopic inguinal hernia repair model	Higher fidelity than FLS Ability to practice full procedures Training has been shown to improve patient outcomes	High associated costs on replacement parts as each model can only be used once
	Patient simulation	SimMan, TraumaMan	High fidelity for laparoscopic skills training Can simulate a variety of crisis scenarios Can allow team training	High cost
Inorganic: computer-based	Skills-based models	MIST-VR simulator	Widely validated Transferability of skills learnt to OT demonstrated Development of proficiency-based curriculum Immediate feedback	Low fidelity Cannot practice full procedures Lack of evidence regarding patient outcomes
	Procedural models	LapSim and LapMentor VR simulator	High fidelity Widely validated Transferability of skills learnt to OT demonstrated Development of proficiency-based curriculum Immediate feedback	High cost Lack of evidence regarding patient outcomes
	Patient simulation	Virtual worlds (Second Life)	High fidelity Able to train non-technical skills Able to practice scenarios multiple times in trainees' own time	Time-consuming to develop virtual world and patient scenarios
Organic: animal tissue	Cadaveric animal tissue	Porcine laparoscopic cholecystectomy models	High fidelity Able to practice full procedures on real tissues	High cost Ethical issues Differing anatomy to humans
Organic: human	Patient simulation with actors	Simulated ward rounds	High fidelity Validated method to train non-technical skills	High cost to pay for actors
	Human cadavers	Laparoscopic and open surgery	High fidelity Anatomically accurate Able to practice full procedures on real tissues	High cost Lack of supply

FLS, Fundamentals of Laparoscopic Surgery; OT, operating theatre; VR, virtual reality.

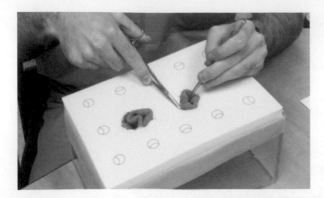

Fig. 3.8.2 Low-fidelity synthetic model to simulate stoma formation.

(Figure 3.8.4). Not only do they allow training of basic laparoscopic skills through abstract tasks, but these validated simulators also allow practice of full operations such as laparoscopic cholecystectomy, appendectomy, nephrectomy, sigmoidectomy, and bariatric surgery, as well as various laparoscopic gynaecological procedures. Furthermore, with the advent of robotic surgery, VR simulators have been developed and validated that utilize the Da Vinci Robot console to allow training and practice of skills required for robotic surgery, in a virtual environment.[5,6]

Cadaveric animal or human tissue models enable high-fidelity simulation for practice of entire procedures. Cadaveric animal tissue can be used to practice fundamental basic surgical skills and even entire procedures. The use of porcine trotters and bowel as models for tendon repair and enteric anastomosis is a key aspect of the Basic Surgical Skills course run by the Royal College of Surgeons. Within laparoscopic skills training, cadaveric animal tissue can be placed within box trainers to allow trainees to rehearse full procedures (e.g. a porcine gallbladder and liver model for

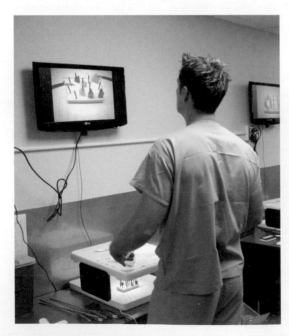

Fig. 3.8.3 Fundamentals of Laparoscopic Surgery box trainer surgical simulator. It comprises synthetic models within a box trainer to train laparoscopic skills using tasks such as peg transfers and intracorporeal knot tying.

laparoscopic cholecystectomy). Human cadavers provide a high-fidelity simulation model that most accurately replicates the actual clinical environment due to the accuracy of anatomy and the ability to operate on real tissues. An increasing number of skills centres now have the facility to store 'fresh frozen' human cadavers. This avoids the need for embalming, resulting in realistic tissue handling once the cadaver has been thawed. These wet laboratory simulations can also be utilized in an actual operating theatre environment in a simulation centre, which provides practice with the full effect of operating theatre pressures and distractions.[2]

Many simulators have been used to create training curricula to provide a structure for skill acquisition. Initially these curricula focused on a time and repetition-based paradigm of training.[7,8] However, as rates of learning may vary between trainees, these curricula resulted in surgeons with differing skill levels. As a result, the development of proficiency-based training curricula, which utilized expert benchmarks of skill as performance goals, allowed each trainee to complete training on simulators with a standardized, proficient level of competency. Such proficiency-based training curricula have been developed for laparoscopy and endoscopy. [9–11]

Simulation beyond technical skills

While the development of technical skills is an obvious focal point for simulation in surgery, an operation involves a team that must work together for successful completion of the procedure. Thus, simulation of entire operating theatres has developed to encourage team-building skills. Operating theatre simulations teach team members to anticipate and troubleshoot situations such as faulty equipment or rare but significant events that affect patient outcomes. Situations such as power failure, loss of airway, and uncontrolled bleeding during an operation can be simulated and reviewed.[12]

Beyond the operating theatre, there are additional opportunities for simulation in surgery. Care for the post-surgical patient is a critical part of patient care and post-surgical crises can be simulated.[13] *In situ* training in the recovery room or on the ward can be performed to improve entire hospital systems.[14] Systems errors such as equipment availability and communications barriers are unearthed through simulation exercises and can be addressed immediately.

Benefits of simulation

Validation and determination of benefit

It is not surprising that simulation was initially met with scepticism because of the lack of evidence demonstrating its cost-effectiveness, as well as a significant benefit on patient outcomes. However, a systematic review has identified 609 studies involving 35,226 individuals that definitively demonstrate a significant benefit of healthcare simulation when compared to no intervention.[15] The effects of simulation significantly improved both knowledge acquisition and technical skills. Surgical simulation training is no exception, and multiple studies demonstrate significant and unique benefits for many modes of simulation. Importantly, a Cochrane review illustrated that VR training reduces operation time and errors, as well as increases accuracy while performing laparoscopic surgery.[16]

Benefits in minimally invasive surgery

Many studies have demonstrated a significant reduction in the learning curve for laparoscopic surgery using simulation. A recent

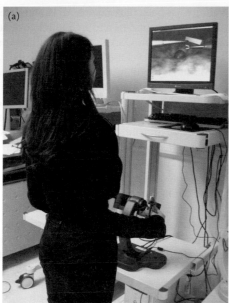 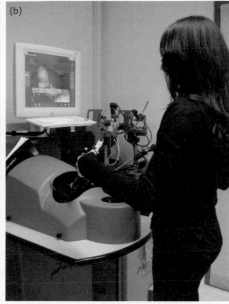

Fig. 3.8.4 High-fidelity virtual reality (VR) laparoscopic simulators allow simulation of basic tasks as well as full procedures. (a) LapSim VR laparoscopic simulator. (b) LapMentor VR laparoscopic simulator.

systematic review of simulation in laparoscopic surgery demonstrated that use of simulation improved knowledge acquisition, time for task completion, overall performance on a simulator task, and quality of the task performed.[17] These benefits were seen in simulation using low-fidelity box trainers as well as in VR simulation trainers. Thus, simulation would ideally be used to create a 'pre-trained novice'.[18] This type of beginner would be familiar with laparoscopic tools and their challenges through simulation exercises. The initial portion of the learning curve for laparoscopic surgery will therefore be overcome sooner, allowing the trainee to move onward to more advanced laparoscopic procedures and operative decision making.

The benefits of simulation in minimally invasive surgery extend beyond laparoscopic surgery. Within gynaecology, VR simulation training has been shown to improve technical skills during laparoscopic salpingectomy for ectopic pregnancy.[19] Additionally, training using a VR colonoscopy simulator was demonstrated to possess excellent construct validity and allow trainees to develop endoscopic skills to proficiency.[11] The development of endovascular VR simulators has not only been demonstrated to differentiate between experience level and improve technical skills during endovascular procedures such as carotid artery stenting, but by uploading three-dimensional reconstructions of actual patients' vascular anatomy using computerized tomography carotid angiogram scans into these simulators, trainees can rehearse carotid artery stenting prior to performance on the actual patient.[20–22] An increasing number of educational bodies and regulators are now requiring trainees and senior surgeons to demonstrate proficiency on a simulator before performing a procedure on a patient. For instance, the Food and Drug Administration requires physicians in the USA to train on a simulator before performing carotid stenting.

Transferring skills to the operating theatre

There is increasing interest in knowing whether the ability to perform a simulated procedure translates into improved operative technique on a real patient, as this is the real test of its effectiveness. Since its development, the FLS proficiency-based box trainer curriculum has not only been widely demonstrated as a valid and effective training tool, but has also been established as a prerequisite for all surgical trainees prior to Board Certification by the American Board of Surgeons.[23,24] Furthermore, training to proficiency using the FLS simulator curriculum has been shown to improve actual performance in the operating theatre.[25] Additionally, a recent study using the Guildford Minimal Access Therapy Technique Unit totally extraperitoneal inguinal hernia task trainer (Limbs and Things, Ltd. Bristol, UK) demonstrated improved trainee performance, decreased operating time, and decreased intraoperative and postoperative complications as well as overnight stays after actual operating theatre laparoscopic totally extraperitoneal inguinal hernia repair.[26]

Indeed, training to proficiency using such laparoscopic VR simulator-training curricula has been shown to reduce the learning curve of surgical trainees during real operating theatre laparoscopic cholecystectomies by improving operative performance, as well as reducing errors and operating time compared to conventionally trained colleagues.[27,28] A comparison of proficiency-based training using a VR or box trainer model demonstrated that, while both significantly improved skills and reduced the learning curve in the actual operating theatre, VR training was more efficient than box training, although box training was the more cost-effective option.[29]

Assessment of surgical skill

The theoretical benefits of simulation seem clear. If one has the opportunity to practice a particular skill repetitively, then surely one's ability will improve in comparison to those without such additional training? This qualitative reasoning is not enough to justify the incorporation of simulation into surgical training. A more rigorous, objective, and validated assessment of skill acquisition is required with the ability to quantify performance gains and ensure that each simulator is valid as a training tool. Furthermore, this assessment tool should ideally of itself be valid, reliable, and applicable to both simulated and actual operative environments such that transfer of skill can be accurately inferred. Multiple studies have also looked at the effect of feedback on performance. Both the quality of task performance and technical markers of skill were improved with feedback. In a systematic review of simulation in laparoscopic surgery, feedback was highlighted as a factor affecting technical skills resulting in improved performance.[17] A number of methods of assessment and feedback have been developed, some of which are discussed below.

Motion analysis systems

The Imperial College Surgical Assessment Device (ICSAD) utilizes sensors placed on the dorsum of the surgeon's hands coupled with an electromagnetic tracking system that track the motion of the sensors through space.[30] This allows a number of dexterity parameters to be measured such as procedure time taken and measures of economy of movement (path length and number of hand movements).[30] ICSAD has been demonstrated as a validated objective assessment tool for both simple tasks and full procedures by its ability to distinguish between varying skill levels, and has been successfully used to assess psychomotor skill acquisition of trainees during laparoscopic training courses.[31-34] The use of these motion tracking systems within the actual operating theatre can allow correlation of dexterity skills learnt in the simulated environment with actual performance.

Virtual reality simulators as assessment tools

A key feature of VR simulators is their intrinsic ability to generate immediate objective measures of psychomotor skill and performance in a repeatable manner without the requirement of an observer. This real-time feedback includes time taken, number and path length of movements, and errors made during task completion allowing trainees to monitor their performance independently. Numerous studies have confirmed the role of VR simulators as valid assessment devices by demonstrating the ability of several VR simulator-derived metrics to distinguish between varying experience levels.[5,9,10,35-37] Using these validated metrics to measure the baseline skill level of experienced surgeons has generated performance goals that trainees can aim for within proficiency-based training curricula.[9-11]

Direct observational assessment

This method of assessment focuses on the use of rating scales to assess a quantitative measure of procedural performance via direct observation by an observer. Two broad categories of rating scales exist; those that are generic to any operation, and those that are specific to a particular procedure. These rating scales are developed by deconstructing an operation into key steps/skills, and then further subdividing these into mini-steps/skills. Quality of performance of each mini-step/skill is scored on a Likert scale to generate an overall score of procedural performance. In order for a rating scale to be useful, it must demonstrate construct validity as well as test–retest and inter-rater reliability (i.e. results for the test must be the same on two separate occasions and between two independent raters).

The most extensively validated rating scale is the Objective Structured Assessment of Technical Skill (OSATS) global rating scale.[38] Its reliability, construct, concurrent, and predictive validity has been illustrated both in simulated and actual operating theatre environments and in a number of surgical specialties.[39-45] Furthermore, an OSATS scale modified for laparoscopic surgery has also been developed and validated.[39]

Although useful, generic rating scales provide little feedback on performance of a specific procedure. As such, procedure-specific rating scales have been developed and validated for a number of laparoscopic procedures, including laparoscopic cholecystectomy, gastric bypass, and colorectal surgery, as well as for other surgical domains (e.g. ear, nose, and throat surgery).[46-51] In the UK, procedure-based assessments (PBAs) have allowed structured, competency-based assessment of clinical skills within the workplace. Comprising of a checklist of key generic and task-specific competencies, as well as a global summary score, the feasibility, validity, and reliability of PBA for assessing surgical skill has been previously demonstrated, as PBA scores correlated positively with surgical experience and were reviewed positively by both supervisors and trainees.[52]

Comparison of assessment tools

VR simulators and motion tracking systems provide a non-biased immediate objective assessment of dexterity without the need of an expert observer. However, the metrics produced may not give an indication of the quality of procedural performance. In addition to both having high initial associated costs, motion analysis systems require an expert to set up the system, and its use in the actual operating theatre has been limited. By comparison, observational assessment tools allow appraisal of actual procedural performances, where trainees can be evaluated immediately post-procedure by their mentor, allowing trainees to observe which aspects of the procedure require further training. However, this process may be prone to subjectivity. To overcome this, research studies have used at least two blinded observers to assess videotaped recordings of procedures with these tools, but this is time-consuming, not practical *in vivo*, and would not permit immediate feedback.

Beyond technical skills training

It is becoming increasingly clear that other human factors affect operative performance beyond technical skills. Generally termed 'non-technical skills' (NTS), this group of skills includes items such as communication, decision making, situational awareness, leadership, fatigue, and coping with stress. Although good technical skills are vital, nearly two-thirds of serious medical errors are associated with errors in communication.[53]

A recent systematic review of the literature has attempted to define the impact of specific NTS on technical skills.[54] Highlighted in the review are the effects of coping skills and feedback. While research on the effect of stress in surgery is a burgeoning field, it is established that stress does have an effect on operative performance. Excessive stress negatively affects technical skill performance while effective coping mechanisms positively affect performance.

Structured feedback of NTS provides a difficult challenge. For the most part, assessment of NTS has focused on the use of observational rating scales. Examples of such instruments include the Surgical NOTECHS (adapted from the NOn-TECHnical Skills aviation instrument) and the Observational Teamwork Assessment for Surgery.[55,56] While these tools have demonstrated validity and reliability with good inter-rate agreement, both focus on the NTS performance of the entire surgical team.[55–58]

The Non-Technical Skills for Surgeons (NOTSS) rating scale concentrates on individual surgeon's intraoperative non-technical skills assessment.[59,60] Within this tool, NTS are classified into four categories; situation awareness, decision making, leadership, and communication and teamwork. Subdivisions of these elements are evaluated using a 4-point scale to give an objective score of NTS. Although this technique has been demonstrated to have good construct validity and internal reliability, a comparison of NOTSS scores as rated by novice and experienced assessors revealed only moderate agreement with some discordance, suggesting that additional formalized training of raters is required.[61,62] However, a further study in a real-world setting illustrated that NOTSS scores were procedure-independent and achieved good reliability when several assessors evaluated one case each.[63] In addition, NOTSS was deemed by assessors to be a valid and feasible method of NTS assessment and feedback, without adding too much time to operating theatre lists.[63] Interestingly, trainees' NOTSS scores positively correlated with assessment of technical skills on PBA and OSATS, as well as surgical experience, adding to the evidence for its validity.[63]

Providing care for the surgical patient extends beyond the operation. Postoperative care plays a crucial role in patient outcomes. In fact, the majority of preventable adverse events in the perioperative stay occur outside of the operating theatre.[64] Given this finding and recent interest in extending simulation outside the operating theatre, virtual and actor patient simulation scenarios within the simulated emergency department and ward have been developed to allow teaching and assessment of NTS, such as communication and decision making, which are vital for effective preoperative and postoperative patient management. Simulated ward rounds would highlight necessary routine components of postoperative care as well as develop the ability to recognize complications before they become adverse events.[65] These simulated ward environments have recently been demonstrated to be valid and realistic as senior trainees performed better with less adverse events than their more junior colleagues during simulated ward rounds.[66] Another innovative application of computer-based simulation is the use of online three-dimensional virtual worlds, such as Second Life, to create virtual surgical patients incorporated into a variety of clinical scenarios and environments (e.g. emergency room, ward, and high-dependency unit).[67,68] Through the use of an avatar, surgical trainees can navigate through these virtual clinical environments to interact with, assess, and manage the virtual patients, and subsequently gain immediate feedback on their performance.[68] This mode of simulation has been demonstrated to be a feasible training tool with high face, content and construct validity.[68]

Conclusion

As a result of the new pressures and expectations of medical care in the 21st century, simulation in surgery is generating interest in experts and trainees alike, and is a growing field. Simulation is not meant to replace clinical practice but rather be an adjunct to aid the training process by providing a safe place for practice and exposure to rare or difficult situations. Indeed, training using simulation has been shown to facilitate development of the skills critical to the practice of surgery.

Research in simulation is evolving rapidly. Future research will delineate which modes of simulation are most effective for specific tasks. Additionally, further work is required with regards to curricular development and incorporation of simulation into surgical residency training. Striking an optimal balance between patient encounters and simulation is another important question.

Simulation may also help to restructure training by focusing on competency-based advancement versus a time-based curriculum. Trainees who meet milestones faster may advance in their training sooner than those who require more time at certain stages before being certified to safely continue independently. Likewise, senior surgeons who are already certified for certain procedures may be re-credentialed using simulations.

The formalized incorporation of such competency-based simulation training into national surgical training programs is scarce, with the mandatory FLS training curriculum in the US being a notable exception. The difficulties incurred with its adoption stems from questions regarding the cost-effectiveness of simulation training, as well as a lack of literature on its effect on patient outcomes. Future studies must address these important issues.

Simulation training must not be looked upon as a magic bullet to cope with all the challenges facing surgical training. It cannot replace extensive real-world clinical experience. Yet, by providing a risk-free, standardized, and reproducible environment that allows judicious deliberate practice, simulation training can act as an adjunct to actual clinical experience to enhance surgical expertise and most importantly patient safety.

Further reading

Levine AI, Bryson EO, De Maria S, Schwartz AD. The Comprehensive Textbook of Healthcare Simulation. London: Springer publications, 2013, pp. 111–20.

References

1. Society for Simulation in Healthcare. What is simulation? 2013 March 31. Ref Type: Internet Communication. Retrieved at http://ssih.org/about-simulation.
2. Aggarwal R, Grantcharov TP, Darzi A. Framework for systematic training and assessment of technical skills. *J Am Coll Surg* 2007; 204(4): 697–705.
3. Aggarwal R, Mytton OT, Derbrew M, *et al.* Training and simulation for patient safety. *Qual Saf Health Care.* 2010; 19(Suppl 2): i34–43.
4. Sarker SK, Patel B. Simulation and surgical training. *Int J Clin Pract* 2007; 61: 2120–5.
5. Hung AJ, Zehnder P, Patil MB. Face, content and construct validity of a novel robotic surgery simulator. *Urology* 2011; 186(3): 1019–24.
6. Hung AJ, Patil MB, Zehnder P. Concurrent and predictive validation of a novel robotic surgery simulator: a prospective, randomized study *J Urol* 2012; 187: 630–37.
7. Grantcharov TP, Kristiansen VB, Bendix J, *et al.* Randomized clinical trial of virtual reality simulation for laparoscopic skills training. *Br J Surg* 2004; 91(2): 146–50.
8. Ahlberg G. Does training in a virtual reality simulator improve surgical performance? *Surg Endosc* 2002; 16(1): 126.
9. Aggarwal R, Crochet P, Dias A, *et al.* Development of a virtual reality training curriculum for laparoscopic cholecystectomy. *Br J Surg* 2009; 96: 1086–93.
10. Aggarwal R, Grantcharov TP, Eriksen JR, *et al.* An evidence-based virtual reality training program for novice laparoscopic surgeons. *Ann Surg* 2006; 244(2): 310–4.
11. Sugden C, Aggarwal R, Banerjee A, *et al.* The development of a virtual reality training curriculum for colonoscopy. *Ann Surg* 2012; 256: 188–92.

12. Awtrey CS, Fobert DV, Jones, DB. The Simulation and Skills Center at Beth Israel Deaconess Medical Center. *J Surg Educ* 2010; 67(4): 255–7.

13. Pucher PH, Darzi A, Aggarwal R. Simulation for ward processes of surgical care. *Am J Surg* 2013; 206(1): 96–102.

14. Hunt EA, Heine M, Hohenhaus SM, *et al*. Simulated pediatric trauma team management: assessment of an educational intervention. *Pediatr Emerg Care* 2007; 23(11): 796–804.

15. Cook DA, Hatala R, Brydges R, *et al*. Technology-enhanced simulation for health professions education: A systematic review and meta-analysis. *JAMA* 2011; 306(9): 978–88.

16. Gurusamy K, Aggarwal R, Palanivelu L, *et al*. Systematic review of randomized controlled trials on the effectiveness of virtual reality training for laparoscopic surgery. *Br J Surg* 2008; 95(9): 1088–97.

17. Zendejas B, Brydges R, Hamstra SJ, *et al*. State of the evidence on simulation-based training for laparoscopic surgery: a systematic review. *Ann Surg* 2013; 257(4): 586–93.

18. Gallagher AG, Ritter EM, Champion H, *et al*. Virtual reality simulation for the operating room: proficiency-based training as a paradigm shift in surgical skills training. *Ann Surg* 2005; 241(2): 364–72.

19. Aggarwal R, Tully A, Grantcharov T, *et al*. Virtual reality simulation training can improve technical skills during laparoscopic salpingectomy for ectopic pregnancy. *Br J Obs Gynae* 2006; 113: 1382–7.

20. Van Herzeele I, Aggarwal R, Choong A, *et al*. Virtual reality simulation objectively differentiates level of carotid stent experience in experienced interventionalists. *J Vasc Surg* 2007; 46(5): 855–63.

21. Van Herzeele I, Aggarwal R, Malik I, *et al*. Validation of video-based skill assessment in carotid artery stenting. *Eur J Vasc Endovasc Surg* 2009; 38(1): 1–9.

22. Willaert WI, Aggarwal R, Van Herzeele I, *et al*. Role of patient-specific virtual reality rehearsal in carotid artery stenting. *Br J Surg* 2012; 99: 1304–1313.

23. Peters JH, Fried GM, Swanstrom LL, *et al*. Development and validation of a comprehensive program of education and assessment of the basic fundamentals of laparoscopic surgery. *Surgery* 2004; 135: 21–7.

24. Okrainec A, Soper NJ. Trends and results of the first 5 years of Fundamentals of Laparoscopic Surgery (FLS) certification testing. *Surg Endosc* 2011; 25: 1192–8.

25. Sroka G, Feldman LS, Vassiliou MC, *et al*. Fundamentals of laparoscopic surgery simulator training to proficiency improves laparoscopic performance in the operating room-a randomized controlled trial. *Am J Surg* 2010; 199: 115–20.

26. Zendejas B, Cook DA, Bingener J, *et al*. Simulation-based mastery learning improves patient outcomes in laparoscopic inguinal hernia repair: a randomized controlled trial. *Ann Surg* 2011; 254: 9: 115–20.

27. Ahlberg G, Enochsson L, Gallagher AG, *et al*. Proficiency-based virtual reality training significantly reduces the error rate for residents during their first 10 laparoscopic cholecystectomies. *Am J Surg* 2007; 193: 797–804.

28. Palter V, Orzech N, Reznick R, *et al*. Validation of a structured training and assessment curriculum for technical skill acquisition in minimally invasive surgery. A randomized controlled trial. *Ann Surg* 2013; 257: 224–30.

29. Orzech N, Palter V, Reznick R, *et al*. A Comparison of 2 ex vivo training curricula for advanced laparoscopic skills. A randomized controlled trial. *Ann Surg* 2012; 255: 833–9.

30. Aggarwal R, Moorthy K, Darzi A. Laparoscopic skills training and assessment. *Br J Surg* 2004; 91: 1549–58.

31. Torkington J, Smith SG, Rees BI, *et al*. Skill transfer from virtual reality to a real laparoscopic task. *Surg Endosc* 2001; 15: 1076–9.

32. Smith SG, Torkington J, Brown TJ, *et al*. Motion analysis. *Surg Endosc* 2002; 16: 640–5.

33. Aggarwal R, Hance J, Moorthy K, *et al*. Assessment of psychomotor skills acquisition during laparoscopic cholecystectomy courses. *Br J Surg* 2004; 91(Suppl 1): 66.

34. Moorthy K, Munz Y, Chang A, *et al*. Objective evaluation of the skills acquired by participants during a surgical skills course. *Br J Surg* 2003; 90(Suppl 1): 90.

35. Seymour NE, Gallagher AG, Roman SA, *et al*: Virtual reality training improves operating room performance: Results of a randomized, double-blinded study. *Ann Surg* 2002; 236: 458–63.

36. Gallagher AG, Richie K, McClure N, *et al*. Objective psychomotor skills assessment of experienced, junior, and novice laparoscopists with virtual reality. *World J Surg* 2001; 25: 1478–83.

37. Gallagher AG, Smith CD, Bowers SP, *et al*. Psychomotor skills assessment in practicing surgeons experienced in performing advanced laparoscopic procedures. *J Am Coll Surg* 2003; 197: 479–88.

38. Martin JA, Regehr G, Reznick R, *et al*. Objective structured assessment of technical skill (OSATS) for surgical residents. *Br J Surg* 1997; 84(2): 273–8.

39. Aggarwal R, Grantcharov T, Moorthy K, *et al*. Toward feasible, valid, and reliable videobased assessments of technical surgical skills in the operating room. *Ann Surg* 2008; 247(2): 372–9.

40. Faulkner H, Regehr G, Martin J, *et al*. Validation of an objective structured assessment of technical skill for surgical residents. *Acad Med* 1996; 71(12): 1363–5.

41. Goff BA, Lentz GM, Lee D, *et al*. Development of an objective structured assessment of technical skills for obstetric and gynecology residents. *Obstet Gynecol* 2000; 96(1): 146–50.

42. Datta V, Bann S, Beard J, *et al*. Comparison of bench test evaluations of surgical skill with live operating performance assessments. *J Am Coll Surg* 2004; 199(4): 603–6.

43. Anastakis DJ, Regehr G, Reznick RK, *et al*. Assessment of technical skills transfer from the bench-training model to the human model. *Am J Surg* 1999; 177(2): 167–70.

44. Hance J, Aggarwal R, Stanbridge R, *et al*. Objective assessment of technical skills in cardiac surgery. *Eur J Cardiothorac Surg* 2005; 28(1): 157–62.

45. Beard JD, Choksy S, Khan S. Assessment of operative competence during carotid endarterectomy. *Br J Surg* 2007; 94(6): 726–30.

46. Sarker SK, Chang A, Vincent C, *et al*. Development of assessing generic and specific technical skills in laparoscopic surgery. *Am J Surg* 2006; 191(2): 238–44.

47. Aggarwal R, Boza C, Hance J, *et al*. Skills acquisition for laparoscopic gastric bypass in the training laboratory: an innovative approach. *Obes Surg* 2007; 17(1): 19–27.

48. Sarker SK, Kumar I, Delaney C. Assessing operative performance in advanced laparoscopic colorectal surgery. *World J Surg* 2010; 34(7): 1594–603.

49. Palter VN, MacRae HM, Grantcharov TP. Development of an objective evaluation tool to assess technical skill in laparoscopic colorectal surgery: a Delphi methodology. *Am J Surg* 2011; 201(2): 251–9.

50. Laeeq K, Bhatti NI, Carey JP, *et al*. Pilot testing of an assessment tool for competency in mastoidectomy. *Laryngoscope* 2009; 119(12): 2402–10.

51. Francis HW, Masood H, Chaudhry KN, *et al*. Objective assessment of mastoidectomy skills in the operating room. *Otol Neurotol* 2010; 31(5): 759–65.

52. Marriott J, Purdie H, Crossley J, *et al*. Evaluation of procedure-based assessment for assessing trainees' skills in the operating theatre. *Br J Surg* 2011; 98: 450–7

53. Joint Commission International Center for Patient Safety. Communication: a critical component in delivering quality care. Joint Commission International, Oak Brook, IL, USA, 2009.

54. Hull L, Arora S, Aggarwal R, *et al*. The impact of nontechnical skills on technical performance in surgery: a systematic review. *J Am Coll Surg* 2012; 214(2): 214–30.

55. Mishra A, Catchpole K, McCulloch P. The Oxford NOTECHS System: reliability and validity of a tool for measuring teamwork behaviour in the operating theatre. *Qual Saf Health Care* 2009; 18: 109–115.

56. Healey A, Undre S, Vincent C. Developing observational measures of performance in surgical teams. *Qual Saf Health Care* 2004; 13(Suppl 1): i33–i40.

57. Sevdalis N, Lyons M,Healey AN, *et al.* Observational teamwork assessment for surgery: construct validation with expert versus novice raters. *Ann Surg* 2009; 249: 1047–51.

58. Sharma B, Mishra A, Aggarwal R, *et al.* Non-technical skills assessment in surgery. *Surg Oncol* 2011; 20: 169–77.

59. Yule S, Flin R, Paterson-Brown S, *et al.* Development of a rating system for surgeons' non-technical skills. *Med Educ* 2006; 40: 1098–104.

60. Yule S, Flin R, Maran N, *et al.* Development and evaluation of the NOTSS behaviour rating system for intraoperative surgery. In Flin R, Mitchell L (eds) *Safer Surgery: Analysing Behaviour in the Operating Theatre.* Ashgate: Farnham, 2009, pp. 7–25.

61. Yule S, Flin R, Maran N, *et al.* Surgeons' non-technical skills in the operating room: reliability testing of the NOTSS behaviour rating system. *World J Surg* 2008; 32: 548–56.

62. Yule S, Rowley DR, Flin R, *et al.* Experience matters: comparing novice and expert ratings of non-technical skills using the NOTSS system. *ANZ J Surg* 2009; 79(3): 154–60.

63. Crossley J, Marriott J, Purdie H, *et al.* Prospective observational study to evaluate NOTSS (Non-Technical Skills for Surgeons) for assessing trainees' non-technical performance in the operating theatre. *Br J Surg* 2011; 98: 1010–20.

64. Neale G, Woloshynowych M, Vincent C. Exploring the causes of adverse events in NHS hospital practice. *J R Soc Med* 2001; 94(7): 322–30.

65. Pucher PH, Darzi A, Aggarwal R. Simulation for ward processes of surgical care. *Am J Surg* 2013 March; pii: S0002-9610(13)00135-9. doi: 10.1016/j.amjsurg.2012.08.013. [Epub ahead of print].

66. Pucher PH, Aggarwal R, Srisatkunam T, *et al.* Validation of the simulated ward environment for assessment of ward-based surgical care. *Ann Surg* 2013; 206(1): 96–102.

67. Patel V, Aggarwal R, Taylor D, *et al.* Implementation of virtual online patient simulation. *Stud Health Technol Inform.* 2011; 163: 440–6.

68. Patel V, Aggarwal R, Vishal Patel, *et al.* Implementation of an interactive virtual-world simulation for structured surgeon assessment of clinical scenarios. *J Am Coll Surg* 2013; 217(2): 270–9.

Assessment and management of the surgical patient

Section editor: Malcolm W. R. Reed

History taking and information gathering

Michelle Marshall, Caroline Woodley, and Malcolm W. R. Reed

Introduction

History taking is one of the most fundamental aspects of clinical medicine and is pivotal to making a correct diagnosis. Many diagnoses can be made on the basis of history alone, with the results of physical examination and laboratory investigations merely reinforcing your initial clinical impression. The weight attributed to physical examination findings and to the results of investigations will also greatly depend on the information gained during the clinical history.

When patients have a good relationship with their doctor and feel that they are being taken seriously and being listened too, the quality of information obtained during the history is likely to be greater, with more relevant detail and accuracy. Doctors who communicate well with their patients know how to raise and discuss sensitive issues in a way that no judgement is inferred; they respond to cues, detect patients' concerns, and encourage patients to share openly matters that relate to their condition. Ultimately, a good doctor–patient relationship is key to achieving the best outcome for the patient by working in partnership.

Therefore, when taking a history there are two essential components to be considered: the *content* of the history, to ensure that the relevant information is obtained, and the *process* skills needed to collect this information in a way that ensures that the patient feels that they have been listened to and that their concerns and expectations have been taken seriously.

At the beginning of a consultation, both the patient and the doctor will have prior experiences and expectations that will influence the establishment of the new doctor–patient relationship.

Some patients will have a long history of problems, whereas for others the history will be relatively short. They may have been experiencing pain and discomfort and there will almost certainly have been a period of uncertainty while waiting for investigations, results, referrals, appointments, etc. They may be feeling anxious or concerned about what happens next. They will probably have seen other doctors and healthcare professionals and those experiences may have been positive or not so positive.

Many patients will already have an idea about what is causing their symptoms. They may have spoken with family and friends, or may have looked up their symptoms on the internet. Often, they want to share their ideas with the clinician. All of these factors shape and influence the patient's expectations of the consultation.

It is not only the patients who have a 'history'—doctors do too. Before attending the outpatient clinic or seeing patients on the ward, the doctor will have been engaged in other activities (e.g. operating, stabilizing a deteriorating patient, or reviewing an acute admission). Long shifts and lack of breaks for lunch or coffee can impact on performance. Management or leadership responsibilities can also cause distractions.

In order to develop an effective doctor–patient relationship it is essential that good communication is established to ensure that the patient is listened to and consulted with, rather than talked at. The success of the therapeutic relationship will impact on the quality of information gained during the history-taking process. The nature of the therapeutic relationship between the doctor and patient will vary from person to person; some patients will want the doctor to take the lead in the decision-making process, whereas others will want to take control. The doctor will need to adapt their communication to meet the needs of the patient and work in partnership with them (Figure 4.1.1).

Content

The 'content' of the history should follow the traditional framework outlined below. This systematic approach is essential to provide a structure for the consultation and to avoid important information being missed.

The purpose of this framework has traditionally been to identify the facts relating to the pathological basis of the patient's illness. However, more recently emphasis has been placed on understanding the needs and perspectives of the patient. It is well recognized that the real concern experienced by the patient may differ from that which is voiced during the consultation.

Furthermore, the patient may have arrived at the consultation with an expectation of what the outcome should be and would like to participate in a process of shared decision making with you. Current models of history taking now routinely include consideration of the patient's perspective of their illness in the form of their ideas, concerns, and expectations and this has been included in the model discussed here.

What follows is a generalized model for history taking, which can be used for any scenario that may be encountered during clinical practice:

Presenting complaint

Identify the patient's main problem in their own words. For example, ask 'What is the problem causing you concern?' or 'Can you tell me what the problem is?' Always start with an open question even when you have already been given some information about the patients concern. For example, 'Your doctor tells me you have been

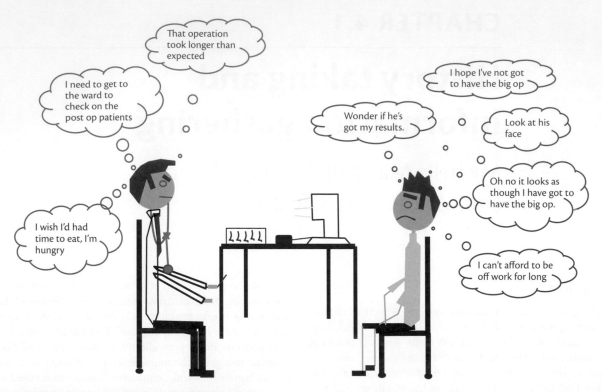

Fig. 4.1.1 Hidden thoughts that can occur during a consultation.

suffering from headaches—could you tell me what is troubling you?' Listen fully to the response and then follow with a further open question. For example, 'Can you tell me anything more about this problem?' before asking more detailed closed questions. It is important to summarize back to the patient to check that their concerns have been captured accurately and that they have been given ample opportunity to advise you of all their concerns. Then move on to a more detailed exploration of the main complaint or concern.

History of presenting complaint

Obtain a detailed chronological description of the problem.

For instance, if the patient complains of pain, obtain a full description of the pain. The SOCRATES mnemonic maybe helpful: *s*ite, *o*nset, *c*haracter, *r*adiation, *a*ssociated symptoms, *t*iming, *e*xacerbating and relieving factors, *s*everity. As information about the presenting complaint is obtained, a differential diagnosis needs to be developed. Consider the most likely diagnoses and ask questions to establish whether the patient is likely to be suffering from one of these conditions.

Obtain full descriptions of any other symptoms that the patient has.

Ensure a full history is taken relating to the relevant body system (e.g. in a patient presenting with a midline neck lump, all of the relevant symptoms of thyroid dysfunction must be considered).

Enquire about specific risk factors, where relevant (e.g. risk factors for atherosclerosis in a patient experiencing leg pain during exertion)

Ask about any treatment the patient has already had and their response to this treatment.

At the completion of the history of the presenting complaint it is helpful to summarize back to the patient and check that an accurate picture of the problem has been obtained.

On completion of each aspect of the history, explain to the patient what comes next. For example, 'I don't have any further questions at this stage about your main problem so I am now going to ask you about your background health and also about your family history.

This can help us work out what is causing the problem'. Linking statements such as this are very helpful to the patient and improve their experience during the consultation. In an examination setting, this also demonstrates a full understanding of the history-taking process.

Previous medical history

Obtain a detailed health record:

Ask about significant illnesses.

Ask about previous operations and other procedures e.g. angioplasty, stenting.

Ask about mental health.

There is no need to ask directly about specific illnesses (e.g. tuberculosis, diabetes) unless they directly link or predispose to any of the differential diagnoses you are considering.

Drugs

Obtain a detailed record of prescribed, over-the-counter and/or complementary therapies. Ask about any reactions to these. Is the patient compliant?

Allergies

Allergies to drugs, food, Elastoplast, latex, etc.

What reaction does the patient have: itch, rash, swelling, anaphylaxis or just a normal side effect?

Family history

Ask about first-degree relatives, their age, and their state of health or cause of death.

Ask about specific familial diseases that may be relevant to the presenting complaint. For example, in a patient who is describing symptoms of coeliac disease, ask about a family history of coeliac disease ('wheat intolerance') and also about other common autoimmune diseases such as type 1 diabetes, vitiligo, and pernicious anaemia.

Social history

Adapt this according to the age of the patient and their medical problem:

Ask whether the patient lives with anyone and if so, whom?

Do they drink alcohol? If so, how much and how often? How many units a week? If problem drinking is suspected, perform a CAGE questionnaire.

Do they smoke/have they ever smoked/when did they stop? Calculate the number of pack years (20 cigarettes = 1 pack; 1 pack per day for 1 year = 1 pack year).

Ask about diet and recreational drugs if relevant.

Does the patient have any dependents (e.g. young children, carer for their spouse/parent)?

What sort of accommodation do they live in (e.g. house, bungalow, tenth-floor flat)?

Do they go out at all?

Are they able to carry out their activities of daily living (e.g. who does their cooking, cleaning, shopping, personal hygiene)?

Do they have social services support?

Are they working? What jobs have they had in the past? Have they been exposed to any occupational risks e.g. asbestos, coal dust?

Have they had any recent overseas travel?

What are their hobbies?

Do they have any pets?

Review of systems

Ask a series of screening questions for each of the main body systems (Table 4.1.1). The questions will be dependent on the patient's age and also on their presenting complaint. Do not repeat the information that you have already gained in the history of presenting complaint.

If the patient describes a symptom not previously elicited in the history of presenting complaint, then explore this in greater depth. At the end of the review ask 'Is there anything else you think I should know?'

At this stage, again summarize the patient's history back to the patient and ask them if anything has been left out.

Next establish the patient's 'ideas, concerns and expectations', as follows:

Ideas: Ask the patient 'What do you think might be happening?' or 'Do you have any ideas about it yourself?'

Concerns: Many patients have an underlying fear that they have cancer, or that their condition is terminal. They probably will not volunteer this information unless asked. For example, 'What are you concerned that it might be?' or even 'What was the worst thing you were thinking it might be?'

Expectations: A patient will enter a medical consultation with an expectation about the outcome. This may be a referral to a specialist, a series of diagnostic tests, a prescription or even an operation. Find out what the patient's expectation is by asking 'What were you hoping we might be able to do for this?' and then discuss with them whether this is an appropriate course of action.

Table 4.1.1 Examples of a structured systematic enquiry

Cardiovascular	Respiratory
Chest pain	Cough
Shortness of breath, at rest or on exertion	Sputum
Breathlessness on lying flat and how many pillows they use	Shortness of breath
	Wheeze
Breathlessness at night	
Palpitations	
Ankle swelling	

Gastrointestinal	Neurological
Change in appetite and/or weight	Headaches
Problems swallowing	Visual disturbance
Indigestion	Faints, fits, blackouts
Change in bowel habit	Weakness
Constipation, diarrhoea	Memory impairment
Blood/mucus/slime per rectum	

Genitourinary	Musculoskeletal
Incontinence	Joint pain, stiffness, swelling
Frequency, dysuria, nocturia	
Hesitancy, dribbling	
Blood in urine	
Menstrual cycle, possibility of pregnancy	

During early clinical training, when taking a history of the patient's presenting complaint a memorized list of questions to ask may be useful. For example, when taking a gastrointestinal history, enquire about:

- pain
- abdominal distension
- nausea and vomiting
- dysphagia (difficulty swallowing)
- dyspepsia (indigestion/heartburn), hiatus hernia, and peptic ulceration
- history of gallstones or previous pancreatitis
- jaundice
- altered bowel habit (diarrhoea, constipation or alternating diarrhoea and constipation)
- blood loss (haematemesis or rectal bleeding)
- mucus or slime per rectum
- appetite
- weight change
- incontinence.

If a patient has one of these symptoms, then bring a further checklist into action. For example, with a patient complaining of altered bowel habit, ask:

- How has the habit altered? Diarrhoea, constipation or both?
- Frequency of stools?
- Any associated abdominal discomfort or urgency?
- Incontinence?

- Appearance of stool? Consistency (formed or unformed)? Does it float in the pan?

- Associated blood, pus or mucus (slime)? Is the blood mixed with the stool, or separate from it? Is it fresh blood or dark, altered blood?

- Associated vomiting?

- Foreign travel?

- Medications, including over-the-counter remedies?

In a patient who has been vomiting, ask:

- How frequent is the vomiting?

- What time of day does it occur?

- Taste, colour, smell, and quantity?

- Is there any blood in the vomit (haematemesis)? Is it fresh blood or altered blood (like coffee grounds)?

If the patient has dysphagia, ask:

- Is it continuous or intermittent?

- How long does it last for?

- Where does the food stick?

- Is it solids, liquids, or both?

- Does it occur between meals? (This may suggest globus hystericus, a psychogenic condition.)

- Do you suffer from acid reflux or dyspepsia?

- Do you suffer from coughing or shortness of breath during the night? (This may be secondary to regurgitation and aspiration.)

Also enquire about the risk factors for oesophageal carcinoma: smoking, alcohol, obesity, and diet lacking in fruit and vegetables.

In a patient with jaundice, depending on the patient and the clinical scenario, ask:

- Have you noticed any changes in the colour of your urine or stools? (To differentiate haemolytic from obstructive jaundice.)

- Do you have any pain? If so, you should establish the full details of the pain using the SOCRATES mnemonic. This may be very useful diagnostically. For example, the pain of pancreatic carcinoma is usually felt in the back, exacerbated by lying flat, and eased by sitting forward.

- Have you ever been diagnosed with gallstones? Have you received any treatment for them?

- Have you had a high temperature or episodes of shivering (rigors)?

- Have you experienced any itching?

- How much alcohol do you usually drink in a week?

- Are you taking any medicines? Have you been taking any medicines that you have purchased over-the-counter or from the internet? Have you ever used recreational drugs?

- Have you travelled abroad recently? Have you ever had a blood transfusion or a tattoo abroad?

- Have you engaged in unprotected sexual intercourse?

These checklists are an essential component of clinical practice and help ensure that all of the needed information is gathered. However, do not become over-reliant on checklists in history taking as patients will sometimes present with symptoms for which there is no pre-prepared list. Also the use of a regimented checklist approach can turn a history-taking interaction into something closer to an interrogation! Questions should focus as much as possible on the patient's response to previous questions rather than moving on to the next item on the checklist. For example, 'You mentioned that the pain has been less severe recently—have you made any changes that you think may have helped?' For cases with less routine presentations, it is necessary to work out the information that is needed from first principles, based on knowledge of the basic medical sciences and understanding of the pathophysiology of disease.

As experience is gained, checklists and frameworks become more subconscious and automatic. More reliance is placed on pattern recognition and questions are framed to determine whether the patient's symptoms fit or refute any diagnosis in mind (hypothetico-deductive reasoning). Some patients, however, will present with a cluster of symptoms that do not fit any recognizable pattern and there will be a need to revert to the basic model outlined above and take a fully comprehensive history, including a systematic enquiry, to determine the likely basis of the patient's problem and the next course of action.

Process

In addition to considering the content of the history, the process by which the information is obtained from the patient must be considered.

For this purpose, the consultation should be considered in four distinct phases: before the consultation, the initial greeting, the main discussion, and the ending.

Before the consultation

Before meeting the patient, the clinician must be prepared mentally by focusing attention on the forthcoming consultation and putting any distractions aside. It is crucial to know the patient's name and be familiarized with the reason for their visit by reading through the notes and referral letters. By undertaking this basic preparation, the consultation can begin as soon as the patient is met, demonstrating that the discussion is focused on them and that they have the clinician's full attention, rather than the alternative of the patient walking into the room while the doctor is still reading the notes. This impacts on communication, immediately sending out the message that the doctor is not prepared and this is open to interpretation by the patient (that the doctor is not paying attention/not interested/has more important things to do than see them). Consider the seating arrangements; a desk can provide a barrier if it is placed between clinician and patient.

Initial greeting

On meeting the patient for the first time, aim to make them feel at ease. The way in which the consultation begins will shape the rest of the discussion. Greet the patient by their name and shake their hand if appropriate (be led by them) and invite them to sit down. Full introductions should be given including your name and title. Much of this is common courtesy, but it is very easy to forget when time is pressured.

The main discussion

During this part of the consultation, the aim is to gather useful and relevant information that will assist in developing a differential diagnosis. The quality of information gathered will be greatly improved if the patient feels that they are being listened to and are given the opportunity to speak. When time is pressured it is easy to slip into using closed questions to explore a line of enquiry, but from the patient perspective, this can sometimes feel like an interrogation. They may feel like they are not being listened to and may not fully engage, resulting in more closed questions and even less engagement—a negative downwards spiral.

There are a number of techniques that can be used to assist engagement and show that the patient is being listened to.

Eye contact

Maintaining eye contact indicates the doctor is listening. When writing in notes or using a computer screen to look up results or enter information, it is easy to focus on that task and forget to make eye contact with the patient.

Open and closed questions

Open questions are much better at the beginning of a line of enquiry, for example: 'Tell me about your pain'. Subsequently one can move on to more specific closed questions. Probing questions are useful for obtaining more depth and clarity, for example 'What do you mean by that?' or 'What makes you think that?'

Structure and signposting

The content of the questions asked may make little sense from the patient's perspective. For example, a patient who has come to see you because they have a breast lump might fail to make the connection when asked about bowel function. Therefore simple signposting can help to provide a logical flow for the patient. For example, 'I am now going to ask you some questions about your daily activities'. Similarly, if a patient goes off-track and introduces another symptom before the current one is adequately explored, say 'I would like to ask you more about that but I hope that you don't mind if I continue asking you about the pain first and then come back to it'. This is much more acceptable than ignoring the point and continuing with the former questions.

Non-verbal communication

Awareness of non-verbal communication is important as it is estimated that approximately 90% of any message is communicated through body language. Attention should be paid to posture; sitting upright and learning forward slightly is more engaging than sitting back in a chair.

The use of head nods, eye contact, and silence can be very facilitative and encourage patients to continue speaking. The use of silence can sometimes feel quite difficult, often resulting in being overcome with an urge to speak, but while it might feel uncomfortable to remain silent, it allows the patient thinking time, which may be followed by them volunteering more information.

Listening

While busy making notes and developing a differential diagnosis, it can become very easy to stop listening, or to convey such a message to the patient. When one considers the earlier point about how note taking or the use of the computer can impact on communication, then it is not surprising that patients often think that the doctor is not listening to them. It is also very distracting for the doctor to have to write notes when they are trying to listen to what the patient is saying. Listening effectively requires effort and concentration.

Listening can be indicated in a number of ways. Summarizing the patient's history clearly indicates to them that the doctor has been listening, whereas repeatedly asking them the same questions suggests the opposite. Patients will not always be explicit with information and detail, sometimes it is necessary to pick up on cues to explore further and gain deeper insight.

Cues can be both verbal and non-verbal and actively listening will help to 'tune in' to them. For example, when enquiring about pain, the patient may describe their pain and then comment that they are worried about work. At this point in the history, the doctor will more likely be focused on the pain but should not ignore the cue about work. They could ask 'What is it that is worrying you about work?' and listen to what the patient has to say, or if it is decided to continue with the current line of enquiry at that time, may respond by saying 'You said that you are worried about work and we should talk about that once we have explored your pain in more detail'. By taking this line of action, the patient's concern is acknowledged and lets them know that the doctor is listening, but keeps to the topic under discussion so as not to miss any other key information.

Non-verbal cues can take a number of forms (e.g. the avoidance of eye contact, a facial expression, or use of gestures). Picking up on these cues by responding 'I can see that this is difficult for you to talk about' will help to facilitate further discussion.

A number of other skills can also assist with active listening, leading to a better quality of information. Facilitation skills encourage a patient to give more information (e.g. 'Please go on' or 'Tell me more about your pain') or seeking clarification (e.g. 'What do you mean by uncomfortable?').

Summarizing can be helpful for both doctor and patient. Summarizing at the end of each section, or if the train of thought is lost, provides the opportunity to check a full understanding of the history and the accuracy of the information elicited. From a patient perspective it demonstrates that the doctor has been listening and provides them an opportunity to fill in any gaps.

Empathy

Patients needing surgery have a diverse range of worries and concerns and it is essential to acknowledge these. They might be worried about the actual surgery itself, the outcome of the surgery, future diagnosis, prognosis, recovery, missing work, leaving their family, etc. People often describe empathy as putting yourself in the other person's shoes, but is it ever really possible to do this? Even if one has been through the same surgical procedure, one's experience of it will still be different, so it is doubtful one can ever truly know what another person is experiencing. However, what one can do is to make a connection between what the patient is feeling through what is said and expressed non verbally. While it cannot truly be said 'I know what you are going through', one can say 'I can see that this is really difficult for you' or 'I can hear from what you are saying that this is really worrying you'.

Care should also be taken when wanting to reassure patients about their surgery. While a comment like 'You will be fine' will be all the reassurance needed for some patients, this can come across as quite dismissive or patronising to someone who is genuinely very anxious. It is easy to forget that while a consultation is routine for the clinician, it is not for the patient. A more appropriate response would be 'While I haven't been through this myself, I have performed this procedure on many patients and in my experience …'.

Language

The use of language is an important element of communication. When working in a specialized clinical area, its own sub-language of terminology, abbreviations, etc., is developed that assists and speeds up communication between clinicians. However, never forget that such sub-language is 'jargon' to others. Ensure that the language that is used when talking to patients is simple and straightforward English with the avoidance of any jargon. The level of language used should also mirror the patient's own level to assist understanding. Many doctors have strong regional accents, and by being aware of this and slowing one's speech it is possible to make it easier for others to understand. Just as specialists have their own language, regional language can also have its nuances. Colloquialisms are often used by patients and it is important for the doctor to ask for clarification if they do not understand what the patient means e.g. 'I don't understand what you mean by that, could you explain further'. Where there is a foreign language problem, it is important to have an experienced interpreter available, and summarizing the history is even more important to ensure that you have fully understood what the patient is seeking to communicate to you.

Ending the consultation

It is useful to signpost that the end of the consultation is approaching so that the patient is aware and the consultation does not end abruptly. If questions or treatment options are still being discussed, an indication can be given by saying 'We have almost finished now'. End by summarizing, but be sure to focus on the key points or take away messages about what will happen next, as recall declines with time. Finally ask the patient if they have any final questions.

Developing communication skills

Clinical communication skills are skills that can be developed. Reading about communication skills is a helpful starting point but it is essential that they are then put into practice. There are a number of strategies that can be useful for practising and developing communication skills and style.

Observation

Requesting colleagues to observe consultations with patients and providing feedback is invaluable. If time is limited, concentrate on one particular aspect of the consultation. There are guides available that can provide helpful prompts for the observer.

Filming

Recording consultations can be useful as it provides the opportunity for self-assessment (subject to the patient giving their consent). Such recordings may also be used as part of a teaching session with students or more junior staff.

Feedback

It is essential that feedback is provided from a wide range of sources. Nursing staff and other colleagues can often provide unique insights that will assist in developing consultation skills. Patients may also be asked for their feedback, either face-to-face or by questionnaire.

Calgary Cambridge communication guides

These guides provide a useful framework for combining both the content and process skills discussed above. Additionally they provide a clear structure for organizing the different sections of the history.

Conclusion

History taking is one of the most important elements of clinical practice. Content and process skills are integral to a good clinical history and should not be thought of as separate entities. The effectiveness of a clinical consultation does not just depend on whether the correct diagnosis was made. Effective doctor–patient communication, and an understanding of the needs and perspectives of the patient, significantly improves the accuracy of the information gained, the therapeutic relationship between patient and doctor, and the health outcome for the patient.

Further reading

Browse NL, Black J, Burnard KG, *et al. Browse's Introduction to the Symptoms and Signs of Surgical Disease*, 4th edition. London: Hodder Arnold, 2005.
Mayfield D, McLeod G, Hall P (1974). *The CAGE questionnaire: validation of a new alcoholism screening instrument.* Am J Psychiatry 131(10):1121–3
Silverman J, Kurtz S, Draper J. *Skills for Communicating with Patients*, 2nd edition. Oxford: Radcliffe Medical Press, 2005.
Silverman J, Kurtz S, Draper J. *Teaching and Learning Communication Skills in Medicine* 2nd edition. Oxford: Radcliffe Medical Press, 2005.

CHAPTER 4.2

The physical examination

Caroline Woodley and Malcolm W. R. Reed

Introduction

The systematic approach described concentrates on the examination of the normal human body and may differ from methods that experienced clinicians with years of experience employ in routine clinical practice. However, it is essential that a thorough examination is employed routinely otherwise diagnoses will be missed.

Frequent repetition is the key to developing sound skills in physical examination, and it may be useful to have a checklist to refer to when needed. It is advisable to adhere to the traditional schemes of 'inspection, palpation, percussion, and auscultation' when examining organ systems and 'look, feel, move' when examining joints.

In the same way that a learner driver stops thinking 'mirror, signal, manoeuvre' and starts concentrating on the road ahead, eventually the examination sequence will become subconscious for the experienced clinician who will learn to concentrate on interpreting the physical signs detected. Time spent examining normal subjects is never wasted and being familiar with the variations of what is normal will make the abnormal stand out more clearly.

It requires repeated practice to communicate the clinical findings concisely and accurately at the end of the examination, describing the key positive and negative findings, in a logical sequence. This is an essential skill, not just in physical examination, but also when discussing clinical cases with colleagues.

Constructing a differential diagnosis

The experienced clinician usually thinks in terms of 'clinical patterns' (i.e. the typical symptoms and signs of each disease), considering such factors as the patient's age, the incidence of various diseases within the population, and the time course of the patient's illness.[1] This process requires significant knowledge and experience and is often performed rapidly and subconsciously.

Initially an inexperienced clinician may lack sufficient knowledge of surgical conditions and clinical experience to work in this way, although with time these skills will develop. The following methods may therefore prove helpful when constructing the differential diagnoses.[2]

Systems-based method

The first method to consider is to construct a systems-based differential. For example, when determining the possible causes of abdominal pain, these may be divided into upper gastrointestinal; lower gastrointestinal; liver, pancreas, and biliary tract; kidneys and urinary tract; reproductive organs; cardiovascular; respiratory; etc. Each category would then be populated with possible diagnoses and these are then narrowed down based on the information gathered from the history and physical examination. Judicious use of closed questions while taking a history will assist in this process.

A variation of this anatomically based method is particularly useful for considering the causes of failure of specific organs (e.g. jaundice [pre-hepatic, hepatic, post-hepatic], renal failure [pre-renal, renal, post-renal]).

The surgical sieve

The surgical sieve provides input as to the possible aetiology of the patient's symptoms. There are many variations on this theme, all of which are based on mnemonics to assist recall. However, a commonly used surgical sieve is shown in Box 4.2.1, which has been populated with some causes of abdominal pain.

The disadvantage of such approaches is the lack of reference to the individual case. Hence, they should be used to ensure possible causes have not been overlooked rather than as a structure for presenting the differential diagnosis.

Once an initial differential diagnosis has been arrived at, additional factors will need to be considered including:

- patient's age
- onset and progression of the illness
- geographic location (including recent foreign travel)
- incidence/prevalence of disease in the local population
- past medical history
- family history (especially relevant for diseases with familial bias)
- occupation
- social history, etc.

Having concluded the patient's history, physical examination, and consideration of the additional factors listed above, the clinician should be left with just a small number of viable differential diagnoses. Judicious use of investigations such as X-rays and blood tests will often establish or refute each of these diagnoses. It is essential that each diagnostic test is requested with a specific question in mind and that a scatter-gun approach is avoided.

As experience is gained, the process of constructing a differential diagnosis will become subconscious and pattern recognition will begin to dominate. However, even experienced clinicians will be faced on occasion with problems with which they are unfamiliar and will need to revert to a systematic approach to reach a diagnosis. It is vital therefore that these basic skills are understood and adopted throughout a clinician's career.

> **Box 4.2.1** An example of a surgical sieve used to develop a differential diagnosis for abdominal pain
>
> This list is illustrative and therefore is not intended to be exhaustive.
>
> ◆ Congenital: hypertrophic pyloric stenosis, Meckel's diverticulum
>
> ◆ Acquired (mnemonic: VITAMIN DEF)
>
> - *Vascular*: mesenteric ischaemia, ruptured abdominal aortic aneurysm
> - *Infective*: (bacterial, viral, fungal) e.g. viral mesenteric adenitis, gastroenteritis, cholecystitis, appendicitis, hepatitis
> - *Inflammatory*: Ulcerative colitis, Crohn's disease
> - *Traumatic*: blunt or penetrating abdominal trauma
> - *Autoimmune*: coeliac disease
> - *Metabolic and endocrine*: hypercalcaemia, diabetic ketoacidosis, porphyria
> - *Mechanical obstruction*
> - *Idiopathic or iatrogenic*: drug side effects
> - *Neoplastic*: primary or secondary intra-abdominal malignancies
> - *Degenerative*: osteoarthritis of the spine
> - *Environmental*: heavy metal poisoning
> - *Functional*: irritable bowel syndrome

General considerations

Thorough hand washing must be undertaken before and after seeing every patient. Gloves must be worn during all patient-care activities that may involve exposure to blood and other body fluids, including contact with mucous membranes and non-intact skin.[3]

Ensure that a chaperone is present during any intimate examination. This applies regardless of the gender of the doctor or the patient. The chaperone does not need to be medically qualified but should be respectful of the patient's dignity and confidentiality and should be familiar with the procedures involved in a routine intimate examination.[4] In most cases another doctor, a member of the nursing staff, or a healthcare assistant should act as a chaperone, and their presence and identity should be recorded in the clinical notes. If the patient does not want a chaperone to be present, it should be recorded that the offer of a chaperone was made and declined.

Examination of a lump

The process of examining any lump is divided into 'look, feel, move, specific tests, and examination of the regional lymphatic drainage'. The following scheme will encourage examination and description of a lump to be undertaken in a logical and well-structured manner.

1. Look (inspection):

   - Location/position, measured from a landmark.
   - Contour (if visible by inspection): Regular or irregular.
   - Colour of the overlying skin, (e.g. erythematous, pigmented).
   - Abnormalities in the overlying skin (e.g. *peau d'orange*).
   - Abnormal vessels/telangiectasia.

2. Feel (palpation):

   - Surface (e.g. smooth, rough, irregular).
   - Shape.
   - Size: Use a tape measure.
   - Tenderness.
   - Temperature: Palpate with the back of the hand.
   - Cough impulse?
   - Consistency (soft, firm, hard, bony hard, rubbery, uniform, varied, lobulated).
   - Compressible?
   - Fluctuant?
   - Pulsatile (high blood flow) or expansile (aneurysmal)? Is there a palpable thrill?

3. Move:

   - Skin tethering: Attempt to pick up a fold of skin over the swelling and compare the degree of tethering with a similar area.
   - Tethering to deeper structures: Attempt to move the swelling in different planes relative to the surrounding tissues.
   - Tethering to muscles and tendons: Palpate the swelling while asking the patient to tense the relevant muscle.

4. Specific tests:

   - Transillumination: If it is suspected that a mass is filled with clear fluid (e.g. a hydrocoele), attempt to shine a pen torch through it.
   - Auscultation for bruits or bowel sounds.

5. Regional lymph nodes:

   - Be aware of the main routes of lymphatic drainage and examine the relevant regional lymph nodes.

Examination of an ulcer

When describing an ulcer, the same scheme of look, feel, move, special tests, and examination of the regional lymphatic drainage should be applied.

1. Look (inspection):

   - Number of lesions: Single or multiple. Multiple ulcers are commonly seen in arterial disease.
   - Site: For example, varicose ulcers are typically vertically oval and are located over the medial malleolus.
   - Size: Use a tape measure to measure the ulcer. Estimate the depth in millimetres.
   - Shape: Malignant ulcers are typically irregular in shape.
   - Margin: The junction between normal and abnormal skin.
   - Edge: The tissue between the margin and the floor of the ulcer (e.g. sloping, punched out, undermined, raised, rolled, everted). Note whether the marginal epithelium is attempting to grow over the surface.

- Floor: The ulcer floor may comprise healthy or unhealthy granulation tissue, slough, scab, fat, muscle, tendon, periosteum or bone.
- Discharge: Wound discharge may be serous (watery), sanguinous (bloodstained), purulent or green (which usually indicates *Pseudomonas* colonization/infection).
- Surrounding skin: Look for hyperpigmentation, oedema, and erythema.
- General area: For example, look for signs of venous and arterial insufficiency and neurological disease in the whole limb.

2. Feel (palpation):
- Tenderness.
- Temperature, using the back of the hand.
- Induration, which is a feature of chronic benign ulcers and of malignant ulcers.
- Bleeding on gentle touch is often a feature of malignancy.

3. Move:
- Fixation to deeper structures may be suggestive of malignancy.

4. Examine the regional lymphatic drainage.

5. Special tests:
- Palpate the peripheral pulses.
- Examine light-touch and pressure sensation.
- If there is evidence of bony involvement, examine the nearby joints and obtain an X-ray of the involved bone.

Abdominal examination

Commence with a general inspection of the patient to assess how well or unwell they look, whether they are in pain, and whether they have jaundice, pallor or wasting. For emergency admissions, it is necessary to make a rapid assessment of their airway, breathing, circulation, and conscious level.

After gaining the patient's consent, adequately expose their abdomen from xiphisternum to pubic tubercles. Later in the examination it will be necessary to expose the patient's inguinal regions and perineum but these should remain covered with a sheet until the appropriate stage of the examination.

After performing a general inspection from the foot of the bed:

1. Examine the hands for:
- Colour: Pallor of the palmar creases suggests anaemia; palmar erythema suggests liver disease.
- Temperature.
- Clubbing: Gastrointestinal causes include hepatic cirrhosis, ulcerative colitis, Crohn's disease, and coeliac disease.
- Leukonychia: Whitening of the entire nail in hypoalbuminaemia (e.g. nephrotic syndrome, liver failure).
- Koilonychia, seen in chronic iron deficiency.
- Dupuytren's contracture: Fibrosis and shortening of the palmar aponeurosis. Usually idiopathic or familial but there is a possible association with trauma, diabetes, epilepsy, alcoholism and liver disease.

- Asterixis (liver flap). Ask the patient to hyperextend their wrists and maintain the position for 15 seconds. A coarse flapping tremor suggests liver failure. However, asterixis can also be seen in renal failure and in respiratory failure with CO_2 retention.

2. Check the patient's pulse and blood pressure.

3. Examine for scratches suggestive of pruritis, which may occur due to bile salt deposition in cholestatic jaundice.

4. Spider naevi occur in 15–20% of healthy individuals but multiple spider naevi may suggest underlying liver disease.

5. Examine the eyes for:
- Jaundice.
- Subconjunctival pallor, suggesting anaemia.
- Xanthelasma, suggesting hyperlipidaemia.
- Corneal arcus which is common in the elderly but may indicate hyperlipidaemia in a younger person.
- Kayser-Fleischer rings, resulting from copper deposition in Wilson's disease.

6. Examine the face for telangiectasia. Hereditary haemorrhagic telangiectasia affects the face, oral mucosa, gastrointestinal tract, lungs, liver, and brain, resulting in recurrent haemorrhage.

7. Examine the mouth for:
- Telangiectasia.
- Pigmentation: Hyperpigmented macules on the lips and oral mucosa occur in Peutz-Jegher syndrome.
- Angular stomatitis, which may be caused by deficiency of Vitamin B_6, B_{12}, folate or iron.
- Glossitis, an abnormal smooth red appearance of the tongue. Painful glossitis is seen in Vitamin B_{12} or folate deficiency whereas glossitis due to iron deficiency tends to be painless.
- Dehydration.
- Halitosis (e.g. fetor hepaticus in portal hypertension).
- Dental caries.
- Aphthous ulcers, which are usually idiopathic but are rarely associated with Vitamin B_{12} deficiency, iron deficiency and Crohn's disease.

8. Examine the chest wall for:
- Spider naevi.
- Gynaecomastia (male breast development), which may be due to increased circulating oestrogens in liver failure.

9. Palpate the lymph nodes in the neck and axillae. Troisier's sign is an enlarged left supraclavicular lymph node (Virchow's node) due to a metastasis from a gastric carcinoma or other upper gastrointestinal tract malignancy.

10. Ask the patient to lie flat with one pillow, arms by their sides. Inspect the abdomen for:
- Scars.
- Skin changes.

- Shape and symmetry. A distended abdomen may be due to fluid (ascites), faeces (constipation), flatus, fetus, or fat. Localized swellings may be due to enlargement of an abdominal or pelvic organ.

- Movement during breathing: diaphragmatic ventilation usually ceases with peritonitis.

- Visible swellings and masses.

- Visible peristalsis may indicate small bowel obstruction, but may also be a normal finding in thin people.

- Visible aortic pulsation. This may indicate the presence of an abdominal aortic aneurysm. In thin people it may be normal.

- Distended veins (e.g. caput medusa due to portal hypertension; distended veins flowing cephalad due to inferior vena cava obstruction from tumour, thrombosis or compression by tense ascites).

11. Palpate the nine regions of the abdominal wall gently and systematically, while observing the patient's face. Use a flat hand with fully extended fingers, flexing slightly at the metacarpophalangeal joints. Assess for areas of tenderness, guarding, rigidity, etc.

12. Repeat, using deeper palpation. Assess for any masses. Determine whether masses are intra-abdominal by asking the patient to raise their head and shoulders off the pillow. Masses within the abdominal wall become more prominent when the recti are contracted, whereas intra-abdominal masses become less prominent. Assess size, surface, shape, edge, consistency, and tenderness of any masses.

13. Proceed to palpation of specific organs:

- Liver: Palpation for the liver should commence in the right iliac fossa. The patient should be asked to take a deep breath while the examining hand palpates deeply to feel the descending edge of the liver being pushed down by the diaphragm. While the patient breathes out, the examining hand should be withdrawn and repositioned slightly nearer the costal margin, whereupon the process should be repeated. The liver can normally be palpated up to 1 cm below the right costal margin on deep inspiration. The gallbladder is not usually palpable unless enlarged.

- Spleen: This is not normally palpable unless enlarged. Palpation should begin in the right iliac fossa and advance towards the left costal margin, while the patient takes deep breaths. As the right hand advances towards the left costal margin to palpate for splenomegaly, the left hand is placed posteriorly, rolling the patient slightly forwards. This *may* bring the tip of a moderately enlarged spleen closer to the palpating fingers and increase the chance of detection. Splenomegaly only becomes palpable once the spleen has enlarged to two to three times its normal size.

- Kidneys: The kidneys should be examined by ballottement. The anterior hand should press deeply, lateral to the margin of the rectus muscle in the upper quadrant of the abdomen. The posterior hand should be placed in the costovertebral (renal) angle and should be used to lift the kidney up against the anterior hand repeatedly. An enlarged kidney should be detectable by the anterior examining hand. The lower pole of the right kidney may be palpable in thin normal people. The left kidney is rarely palpable. To distinguish a palpable kidney from a spleen, attempt to insert the right hand between the upper pole of the kidney and the costal margin, which can be done if the mass is renal but not if it is the spleen. Also, the spleen has a notch which may be palpable; the spleen is not ballotteable.

- Full bladder: Palpate the suprapubic region for a full bladder. If the bladder is full, it will be impossible to feel the lower border of the mass behind the pubis and pressure on the bladder will make the patient want to urinate.

- Aorta and femoral pulses: The normal aortic palpation may be felt, especially in a thin person. However, if the aorta is expansile, this suggests aneurysmal dilatation.

- Palpate the inguinal nodes.

14. Percuss the abdomen:

- Liver (percuss from resonant to dull, from below and above): When percussing, consider the normal surface markings of the superior border of the liver (sixth rib in mid-inspiration). This can be displaced downwards in respiratory diseases such as emphysema giving a false impression of hepatomegaly.

- Spleen (Castell's method): With the patient in full inspiration and then full expiration, percuss the area of the lowest intercostal space (eighth or ninth) in the left anterior axillary line. If the note changes from resonant on full expiration to dull on full inspiration, the sign is regarded as positive. The resonant note heard upon full expiration is likely to be due to the air-filled stomach or splenic flexure of the colon. When the patient inspires, the spleen moves inferiorly along the posterolateral abdominal wall. If the spleen is enlarged and the inferior pole reaches the eighth or ninth intercostal space, a dull percussion note will be heard, indicating splenomegaly.[5]

- Bladder: A full bladder has a dull percussion note.

- If ascites is suspected, test for shifting dullness. Percuss from the centre towards the left flank. If a dull note is heard, keep the finger in position and roll the patient onto their right side. Wait 10 seconds for the fluid to redistribute. If the note becomes resonant, percuss back towards the umbilicus until the note becomes dull i.e. shifting dullness.

15. Auscultate the abdomen: Bowel sounds may be present and normal, present but abnormal (e.g. constant and tinkling in small intestinal obstruction), or absent (paralytic ileus e.g. in peritonitis). Listen for 3 minutes before declaring that bowel sounds are absent. Also listen for aortic and femoral bruits.

16. The 'end-pieces' are recalled by the mnemonic SHRUG:

- Stools: examine the stools if clinically indicated.

- Hernial orifices: femoral and inguinal.

- Rectal examination.

- Urine: perform urinalysis if clinically indicated.

- Genitalia. Always examine the male external genitalia. A vaginal examination may be indicated in parous or sexually active females (only when clinically indicated and always with a chaperone).

In a simulated examination situation (e.g. an OSCE), simply state the need for these 'end-pieces'. In clinical practice, they should always be performed, otherwise the correct diagnosis may be missed.

Examination of the hernial orifices

1. With the patient standing, inspect for a swelling in the groin. Ask the patient to cough (this may make an occult hernia visible).

2. If a swelling is seen, ask the patient to repeat the cough while palpating the swelling. Feel for a cough impulse. Always examine the hernia standing on the same side of the patient as the swelling and using the left hand for left-sided hernias and the right hand for right-sided hernias.

3. Examine the scrotum (see Scrotal examination section). It is impossible to get 'above' an inguinal hernia, whereas the upper extent of lumps originating in the scrotum can be palpated.

4. Ask the patient to lie flat.

5. Identify the pubic tubercle. Identify its relationship to the neck of the hernial sac. Inguinal hernias enter the scrotum via the superficial inguinal ring, above and medial to the pubic tubercle. Femoral hernias pass under the inguinal ligament to enter the thigh, below and lateral to the pubic tubercle.

6. Attempt to reduce the hernia by gentle sustained pressure (or ask the patient to do this—many patients can reduce their own hernia). Once reduced, an indirect inguinal hernia may be controlled by finger-pressure over the deep inguinal ring at the midpoint of the inguinal ligament, midway between the pubic tubercle and the anterior superior iliac spine. A direct hernia will bulge through the abdominal wall medial to this and cannot be controlled by pressure on the deep ring. Be aware that distinguishing clinically between direct and indirect inguinal hernias by this technique is notoriously unreliable and often the correct diagnosis is only established during surgery.[6]

Scrotal examination

Examination of the scrotum should be performed routinely as part of any examination of the abdomen as well as a specific examination in patients presenting with a scrotal swelling.

To determine the nature of a scrotal swelling, four aspects need to be assessed:

♦ Can you palpate 'above' the swelling?

♦ Can the testis and epididymis be identified separately?

♦ Does the swelling transilluminate?

♦ Is the swelling tender?

Firstly, it needs to be confirmed that the swelling originates within the scrotum and is not an inguinoscrotal hernia. A hernia may be reducible, may have a cough impulse, the testis should be palpable separately, and it is not possible to palpate 'above' a hernia. It is also not possible to palpate above an infantile hydrocoele, which is due to a patent processus vaginalis. However, this is irreducible, has no cough impulse, and the testis is impalpable.

The differential diagnosis of lumps arising within the scrotum can be predicted by listing the structures within the scrotum.

1. Testis:
   • Testicular tumours: The testis and epididymis are definable, the lump originates within the testis, and the testis is non-tender.
   • Orchitis: The testis and epididymis are definable and the testis is tender on palpation.
   • Torsion of the testis: This typically affects adolescent boys, and usually presents with acute scrotal pain but occasionally with abdominal pain.
   • Torsion of the testicular appendix (hydatid of Morgagni) presents with acute but less severe scrotal pain than testicular torsion. There is a tender spot at upper pole of testis and a hydrocoele is often present.

2. Processus vaginalis remnants:
   • Hydrocoele: This is a fluid-filled sac that surrounds the testis anteriorly. Note that a hydrocoele can obscure a testicular tumour. The testis and epididymis are non-palpable and the sac transilluminates.
   • Haematocoele: as with a hydrocoele but containing blood (e.g. after testicular trauma or haemorrhage from a testicular tumour). The testis and epididymis are non-palpable and the sac does not transilluminate.

3. Epididymis:
   • Epididymal cyst: The testis and epididymis are definable, and the lump is within the epididymis. The testis and epididymis are non-tender and the lump may transilluminate.
   • Epididymitis: The testis and epididymis are definable, and the swelling is within the epididymis, which is tender on palpation.

4. Pampiniform venous plexus:
   • Varicocoele: Varicose enlargement of the venous plexus. This may be less noticeable when the patient lies flat due to drainage of the venous plexus; 98% of varicocoeles are left-sided.

5. Examine the inguinal and para-aortic nodes.

Examination of the acute abdomen

When examining the acute abdomen, the sequence of examination closely mirrors that described for examination of the non-acute abdomen (see 'Abdominal examination'). However, there are some important considerations to note and some additional tests to perform.

The general appearance of the acute surgical patient may give a significant clue to their underlying pathology. For example, they may be lying still with their hips and knees flexed and may be only able to change position in the bed with pain and difficulty, suggesting generalized peritonitis; alternatively they may have just the right knee flexed, suggesting an appendix or psoas abscess. Patients who are restless and constantly moving around may have ureteric colic and patients who appear comfortable one minute and 'doubled-up' the next, may have intestinal or biliary colic.

On examination of the pulse rate, tachycardia suggests the possibility of hypovolaemia (due to a gastrointestinal bleed) or sepsis. Patients in atrial fibrillation are at increased risk of mesenteric thromboemboli and intestinal ischaemia.

The respiratory rate of patients with shock is likely to be rapid and shallow. Patients with upper abdominal peritonitis may display predominantly thoracic breathing and splint their diaphragm and abdominal musculature.

Before examining the patient it is essential to establish whether the patient is in pain, and if so, palpation should be commenced at the point furthest away from the painful area, which should be examined last. Assist the patient to relax the abdominal musculature by flexing the hips. If necessary, ask an assistant to support the patients flexed knees. Abdominal tenderness is a sign that the peritoneum underneath the tender area is inflamed. The tenderness may be localized, as in early appendicitis, or generalized. Ask the patient to cough or take a deep breath; inability to do so indicates significant tenderness, and palpation will need to commence very gently to avoid unnecessary pain and distress.

In the acute situation, the patient may require treatment (e.g. analgesia, fluids) before a definitive diagnosis has been reached and analgesia should never be withheld from a patient due to concerns about masking their clinical signs.

When palpating the abdomen superficially, look for guarding (i.e. the reflex contraction of the abdominal muscles) which occurs when inflamed parietal peritoneum is stretched during palpation. It is important to examine the patient gently and explain what is going to happen beforehand, so that you can distinguish voluntary guarding due to anxiety from involuntary guarding due to peritonism. In generalized peritonitis, the patient may demonstrate 'board-like' rigidity, whereby they are unable to relax their abdominal musculature and even light percussion on the abdominal wall elicits pain. Patients with perforated gastric and duodenal ulcers tend to exhibit marked rigidity, whereas blood in the abdominal cavity may produce surprisingly little guarding.

The absence of rigidity should be interpreted with caution as it can be misleading. Very poor abdominal musculature may make rigidity difficult to detect, especially if the patient has a thick layer of subcutaneous fat, and rigidity may also be less apparent in patients who are immunosuppressed.

Rebound tenderness can be tested for by pressing firmly and steadily on a patient's abdomen and then releasing the hand suddenly. If the patient finds this agonizingly painful, the sign is considered positive. Remember that this test is very painful and it should never be used if peritonism has already been confirmed by other methods (e.g. light percussion). It is most useful diagnostically when pressure applied in one place causes rebound pain in another. For example, if the release of pressure from the left lower quadrant causes pain in the right lower quadrant, this suggests appendicitis (Rovsing's sign).

Inflammation in the pelvic cavity often does not result in guarding or rigidity of the abdominal wall and hence can be difficult to detect. Inflammation in the rectovesical (male) or rectouterine (female) pouch may be best detected by rectal examination.

The inflamed gallbladder of acute cholecystitis may be detected by Murphy's sign. Ask the patient to breathe out and then gently place your hand over the gallbladder, below the right costal margin in the mid-clavicular line. If inspiration is prevented by the inflamed gallbladder coming into contact with the examiners fingers, the test is considered positive. A positive test also requires no pain on performing the manoeuvre on the patient's left hand side.

Palpation and percussion of the costovertebral angle may reveal tenderness in a patient with pyelonephritis. Bimanual palpation of the kidney may detect a pyonephros or hydronephros.

Palpation of the hernial orifices is particularly important in the patient presenting with an acute abdomen. The inguinal and femoral sites, umbilicus, and any scars should be palpated. Femoral hernias may be small and are easily missed, especially in obese patients. A hernia does not have to be tense, tender, or painful to be obstructed. A patient who has recently reduced their own hernia may have obstruction from 'reduction *en masse*'.

Resonance to percussion over the normal area of hepatic dullness (provided the abdomen is not distended and the liver is not atrophic) is likely to indicate free gas in the peritoneal cavity.

Auscultation of the acute abdomen is also likely to yield some important clues. Decreased or absent bowel sounds may indicate peritonitis or an ileus. A rush of high-pitched tinkling bowel sounds, coinciding with worsening of the patient's abdominal pain, suggests a mechanical obstruction.

Never forget to examine the rectum of a patient presenting with acute abdominal pain. A well-lubricated gloved finger should be inserted as far up the anal canal as it will go and feel for tenderness in all directions. Palpate anteriorly, in a male for an enlarged prostate, a distended bladder, or enlarged seminal vesicles; and in a female for a collection or mass in the rectouterine pouch or displacement of the uterus. Palpate superiorly for a stricture, the ballooning of the anal canal below an obstruction, the apex of an intussusception, or the bulging of an abscess against the rectal wall. Palpate laterally for the tenderness of an inflamed swollen appendix and palpate bimanually for a pelvic tumour or swelling, or for any fullness in the rectouterine or rectovesical pouch. Inspect the glove for blood or mucus.

Finally, not all patients presenting with abdominal pain have intra-abdominal pathology. Basal pneumonia, spinal column pathology, and diabetic ketoacidosis, for example, can all cause acute abdominal pain and should be considered in the differential diagnosis.

Further reading

Browse NL, Black J, Burnard KG, et al. (2005) *Browse's Introduction to the Symptoms and Signs of Surgical Disease*, 4th edition. London: Hodder Arnold, 2005.

Roper TE. *Clinical Skills*, 2nd edition. Oxford: Oxford University Press; 2013.

References

1. Barrows HS, Norman GR, Feightner JW, *et al*. The clinical reasoning of randomly selected physicians in general medical practice. *Clin Invest Med* 1982; 5: 49–55.
2. Fulop M. Teaching differential diagnosis to beginning clinical students. *Am J Med* 1985; 79: 745–9.
3. World Health Organization: Glove Use Information Leaflet (August 2009) http://www.who.int/gpsc/5may/Glove_Use_Information_Leaflet.pdf
4. General Medical Council: Maintaining Boundaries (November 2006). http://www.gmc-uk.org/guidance/ethical_guidance/maintaining_boundaries.asp
5. Yang JC, Rickman LS, Bosser SK. The clinical diagnosis of splenomegaly. *West J Med* 1991; 155(1): 47–52.
6. Ralphs DN, Brain AJ, Grundy DJ, *et al*. How accurately can direct and indirect inguinal hernias be distinguished? *BMJ* 1980; 280(6220): 1039–40.

CHAPTER 4.3

Physical examination of body systems

Caroline Woodley and Malcolm W. R. Reed

Introduction

Examination of the heart and respiratory system form an essential part of the preoperative assessment and the postoperative care of surgical patients. Increasing numbers of older people are undergoing elective and emergency surgery. They often have reduced physiological reserve and multiple co-morbidities, placing them at increased risk of an adverse postoperative outcome (e.g. acute myocardial infarction, pneumonia, cerebrovascular accident). Surgeons therefore need to be skilled at examination of the heart, lungs, and nervous system in order to detect and diagnose such complications expediently.

In this chapter, we therefore present structured examinations of the heart and respiratory system, neurological examination of the limbs, and examination of the cranial nerves. The latter examination also forms an essential component of the assessment and management of patients after head injury or neurosurgical intervention. We also present structured examinations of the neck, thyroid gland, and breast.

Examination of the heart—the 'full cardiac examination'

The full cardiac examination involves a specific examination of the precordium and a more general examination of the patient to detect the peripheral signs of cardiac disease. The scheme to be employed is as follows:

1. Inspect the immediate environment for clues (e.g. GTN spray) and, from the foot of the bed, inspect the general appearance of the patient (colour, breathing, comfort, position, build).

2. Examine the patient's hands for tar staining, vasodilatation/constriction, temperature, pallor of palmar creases, peripheral cyanosis, clubbing, splinter haemorrhages.

3. Check the presence of both radial pulses simultaneously. Assess rate and rhythm in one radial pulse (usually the right).

4. Assess the character and volume of the brachial pulse (normal, slow rising, collapsing/waterhammer pulse).

5. Assess the character and volume of the carotid pulse (one side at a time).

6. Look for cardiac signs in the eyes (e.g. subconjunctival pallor, corneal arcus, xanthelasmata), in the face (e.g. malar flush [mitral stenosis]), and in the mouth/lips (e.g. central cyanosis [under tongue or on mucous membranes inside lips]).

7. Position the patient at 45° and identify the height of the jugular venous pressure (JVP) above a fixed bony landmark (normal = 2–4 cm above sternal angle) (Figure 4.3.1). Check for low JVP using hepatojugular reflux by compressing the liver and observing the JVP (which will rise). Check for high JVP by sitting patient upright and looking near the ear lobes for venous pulsation.

8. Expose the patient's chest and inspect the precordium for a sternotomy scar or visible cardiac pulsation.

9. Palpate for the apex beat and parasternal heave (outward displacement of the palpating hand by cardiac contraction, e.g. in left ventricular hypertrophy) and thrills (palpable murmurs).

10. Auscultate the aortic, pulmonary, tricuspid, and mitral valve areas. If extra sounds are heard, palpate the carotid pulse to time them with the first and second heart sounds.

    ◆ Auscultate the left axilla for mitral incompetence.

    ◆ Switch to the bell and auscultate the apex with the patient rolled 45° to the left (for mitral stenosis).

    ◆ Switch back to the diaphragm, sit the patient forward and auscultate at the 4th/5th intercostal space to the left of the sternum on held expiration (aortic regurgitation).

    ◆ If cardiac tamponade is suspected (e.g. with a penetrating chest injury), palpate the radial pulse for pulsus paradoxus while auscultating the heart. Pulsus paradoxus is an exaggeration of the normal decrease in blood pressure that occurs during inspiration. The 'paradox' is that impulses heard on cardiac auscultation during inspiration cannot be palpated at the radial artery due to decreased cardiac output. Pulsus paradoxus is also seen in severe obstructive airways disease.

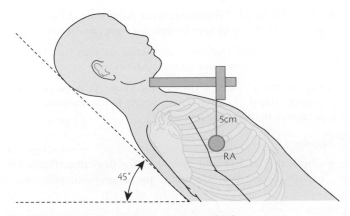

Fig. 4.3.1 Estimating the jugular venous pressure (JVP).

11. Auscultate the lung bases; assess for sacral oedema.

12. Sit the patient back and auscultate the carotids for bruits or a transmitted systolic murmur.

13. Lay the patient flat, if they can tolerate it, and palpate for hepatomegaly. If the liver is enlarged, feel for pulsation (tricuspid regurgitation).

14. Check the femoral pulses. Check synchrony with the radial pulse (radio-femoral delay in coarctation).

15. Check for pitting oedema at the ankles. If present, percuss the abdomen for ascites.

16. The 'end pieces' that should be performed routinely in clinical practice but may be stated in an examination are:

    ◆ Check the blood pressure in both arms and lying and standing in one arm.

    ◆ Obtain a 12-lead electrocardiogram (ECG).

    ◆ Perform ophthalmoscopy for hypertensive retinopathy.

Examination of the respiratory system

The sequence of inspection, palpation, percussion, and auscultation should be applied to the examination of the respiratory system as follows.

1. Inspection

    ◆ Inspect the patient's environment, looking for clues that indicate the presence and nature of the patient's respiratory disease (e.g. inhalers, nebulizer, oxygen mask, sputum pot, peak flow meter).

    ◆ Perform a general inspection of the patient from the foot of the bed, looking at their colour, work of breathing, comfort, position, and nutritional state (obesity may suggest obstructive sleep apnoea).

    ◆ Inspect the hands for clubbing, tar staining, and wasting of the intrinsic muscles (T_1 nerve invasion by an apical lung cancer).

    ◆ Look for tremor (flapping *asterixis* in respiratory failure, fine tremor with beta-agonists, e.g. salbutamol).

    ◆ Assess pulse rate, rhythm, and character (e.g. bounding in CO_2 retention).

    ◆ Assess respiratory rate, rhythm, pattern, and effort.

    ◆ Measure the blood pressure.

    ◆ Check for raised JVP, suggesting cor pulmonale. A raised non-pulsatile JVP may be seen in superior vena cava obstruction.

    ◆ Look for signs of respiratory disease in the eyes and face (e.g. Horner's syndrome) and central cyanosis.

    ◆ Expose the chest and inspect for shape (e.g. barrel chest [hyperinflated in emphysema], severe kyphoscoliosis, use of accessory muscles, and recession).

2. Palpation

    ◆ Check the trachea and apex beat for deviation. Deviation occurs toward the side of the pathology with pulmonary fibrosis or collapse, but away from the pathology with a tension pneumothorax or massive effusion.

    ◆ Assess chest expansion anteriorly at the level of the fourth intercostal space (normal = 3–5 cm). Remember to ask the patient to exhale fully before assessing expansion.

    ◆ Assess tactile vocal fremitus ('say ninety-nine'). Transmission of vibrations is increased in consolidation as sound travels quicker through solids compared to air. Transmission is decreased with an effusion or pneumothorax as the lung tissue becomes separated from the chest wall.

3. Percussion

    ◆ Starting at the apices, percuss from side to side anteriorly. Consider the surface marking of the lungs and their fissures while percussing. Ensure that you have percussed every lobe (including the right middle lobe).

4. Auscultation

    ◆ Starting at the apices, auscultate from side to side anteriorly and laterally with open-mouthed breathing (clavicle to 6th rib, midclavicular line; axilla to 8th rib, midaxillary line). Again, recall the surface markings of the lungs and their lobes while auscultating. Note the presence of vesicular (normal) breath sounds, bronchial breathing, rhonchi (wheezes), crepitations, and pleural rub. Assess for any change in these sounds after coughing (crepitations due to secretions will alter after coughing whereas those in fibrotic conditions will be unchanged).

    ◆ Assess vocal resonance (ask the patient to say 'ninety-nine' while auscultating with the stethoscope). This technique allows discrimination between dullness to percussion from pleural effusion and that from consolidation. Voice sounds, which are created in the larynx, are transmitted more effectively across an area of consolidation. Transmission is reduced across a pleural effusion or pneumothorax.

    ◆ If you suspect an area of consolidation, perform whispering pectoriloquy (whisper 'two-two-two'). Whispers are transmitted more loudly across an area of consolidation.

5. Repeat inspection, palpation, percussion, and auscultation (spine of scapula to 11th rib) on the back with the patient sitting forward.

6. Palpate the cervical lymph nodes.

7. Check the sputum pot (volume, consistency, colour, odour, any haemoptysis?).

8. Assess peak expiratory flow.

Neurological examination of the upper and lower limbs

Neurological examination follows the sequence inspection, tone, power, reflexes, co-ordination, and sensory examination. In clinical practice you will commonly need to perform a full neurological examination, including an assessment of the patient's cranial nerves. However, in an examination situation, due to time constraints, it is common practice to be asked to examine either the upper or lower limbs separately. The lower limb examination should always include an assessment of the patient's gait.

The patient should always be asked if they have any pain before commencing this examination. If they do, adapt the examination and also the interpretation of the results accordingly. For example, muscle power often appears diminished around a stiff or painful joint and this should not be mistakenly interpreted as a primary neurological problem. When examining the upper limbs, first ask the patient whether they are right or left handed, as patients often perform significantly better with their dominant limb.

The sequence of the neurological examination is as follows:

1. Inspection:

   ◆ Note the posture of the limbs at rest.

   ◆ Assess the size, shape, and symmetry of the muscles. Note the presence of atrophy or hypertrophy.

   ◆ Note the presence of any involuntary movements (e.g. tremor, fasciculations).

2. Assess muscular tone by passive movement.

   ◆ Hypotonia (decreased tone) may be seen in lower motor neuron lesions, spinal shock, and some cerebellar lesions. Hypertonia (increased tone) may manifest as either spasticity or rigidity. In extrapyramidal disorders (e.g. Parkinson's disease), patients may have either a cogwheel (stepwise) or lead-pipe (uniform) resistance to passive movement, whereas in pyramidal disorders (e.g. stroke), patients develop clasp-knife rigidity.

   ◆ While assessing tone, also test for wrist and ankle clonus, a series of involuntary, rhythmic, muscular contractions and relaxations, which would suggest an upper motor neuron lesion (e.g. stroke, multiple sclerosis).

3. Assess the power of each muscle group against resistance.

   ◆ Perform a systematic examination of each muscle group in the limb. Ensure adequate stabilization of the joint above the one being tested for muscle power.

   ◆ Report the findings using the Medical Research Council grading system of muscle power, as follows:

     • 5/5 = movement against gravity with full power against resistance.
     • 4/5 = movement against gravity with reduced power against resistance.
     • 3/5 = movement against gravity only without applied resistance.
     • 2/5 = muscle contraction with active movement only when gravity is eliminated.
     • 1/5 = flicker of muscle contraction seen, no movement.
     • 0/5 = no muscle contraction.

   MRC Muscle scale is licensed under the Open Government Licence © Crown Copyright. Used with the permission of the Medical Research Council.

4. Assess the deep tendon reflexes using a tendon hammer. Include the biceps, brachioradialis, triceps, knee, and ankle jerks (Figure 4.3.2). Use reinforcement if necessary.

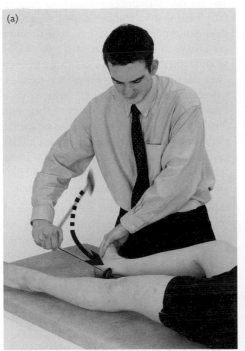 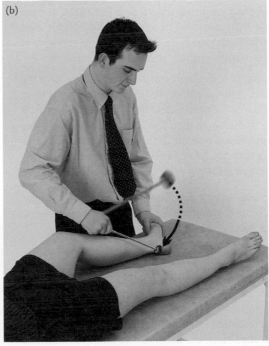

Fig. 4.3.2 (a) Eliciting the right ankle reflex; (b) Eliciting the left ankle reflex.
Reproduced from Roper TE, *Clinical Skills, Second Edition*, Figure 6.70 and 6.71, p. 209, Oxford University Press, Oxford, UK, Copyright © Oxford University Press 2014, by permission of Oxford University Press.

◆ Reflexes are usually described as absent, hypoactive (present only with reinforcement), normal (readily elicited), or brisk. When a reflex is very brisk, clonus is sometimes seen.

◆ Abnormally brisk reflexes are associated with upper motor neuron lesions. However, in addition to neuromuscular pathology, reflexes may be accentuated by stimulants, caffeine, anxiety, or hyperthyroidism, and may be depressed by hypokalaemia, hypomagnesaemia, depression, and hypothyroidism. In hypothyroidism, the reflexes may be both hypoactive and delayed.

5. When examining the lower limb, test the plantar response (Babinski reflex) by running the tip of your thumb firmly up the lateral aspect of the foot from heel to hallux. The normal response is toe flexion. If the toes extend and separate, the test is considered positive and suggests an upper motor neuron lesion.

6. Co-ordination should be tested by evaluating the patient's ability to perform rapidly alternating and point-to-point movements correctly.

◆ Assess rapidly alternating movements by asking the patient to place one hand palm downwards on the outstretched palm of their other hand, and then to turn the palm upwards and back downwards again. Once the patient understands this movement, ask them to repeat it rapidly for approximately 10 seconds. Normally this is possible without difficulty. Dysdiadochokinesia, the inability to perform rapidly alternating movements, is a feature of cerebellar ataxia, most commonly seen in patients with multiple sclerosis.

◆ Ask the patient to extend their index finger and touch their nose, and then touch your outstretched finger with the same finger. Ask the patient to go back and forth between touching their nose and your finger.

◆ Once this has been performed accurately a few times, ask the patient to close their eyes and to touch the tip of their own nose. Dysmetria is the inability to perform point-to-point movements due to over or under projecting one's fingers.

◆ When examining the lower limb, ask the patient to perform the heel-to-shin test. Ask the patient to lie flat and to place their right heel on their left leg just below the knee and then slide it down their leg to the top of their foot. Ask them to repeat this movement as quickly as possible. If the motor and sensory systems (including proprioception) are intact, an abnormal, asymmetric heel-to-shin test suggests an ipsilateral cerebellar lesion.

7. The sensory examination includes testing for the sensations of light touch sensation (cotton wool), pain (pin prick), position sense, vibration, and for stereognosis and graphesthesia (see below).

◆ Test light touch and pain sensation. Initially, demonstrate the stimulus (cotton wool or sharp and blunt ends of a Neurotip™/pin) to the patient over their sternum with their eyes open and check that they can feel it. Ask the patient to close their eyes and apply the stimulus to one of the dermatomes of the limb. Ask the patient to indicate when they can feel the stimulus and, if using a Neurotip™/pin, whether it is the sharp or blunt end that is being applied. Test all of the dermatomes systematically, comparing both limbs, and also test sensation in the peripheral nerve distributions (e.g. anatomical snuffbox for radial nerve). Ask the patient to indicate whether they notice a difference in the strength of the sensation between the two sides of their body.

◆ Test proprioception at either the interphalangeal joint of the thumb or the hallux. Using one hand, stabilize the proximal phalanx. Using the other hand, grasp the distal phalanx. Ask the patient to close their eyes and to report if the tip of their finger or toe is 'up' or 'down' while you move it. Repeat on the opposite limb and compare. Make certain to hold the distal phalanx on its sides, as holding the dorsum or volar/plantar aspect provides the patient with pressure cues which make this test invalid.

◆ Test vibration sense. Apply the base of a vibrating 128 Hz tuning fork to the patient's sternum and check that they can feel the vibration. Stop the fork from vibrating and check that the patient can feel that it has stopped. Ask the patient to close their eyes and apply the base of the vibrating tuning fork to the first metacarpophalangeal joint (MCPJ) / metatarsophalangeal joint (MTPJ). Ask the patient if they can feel the vibration and to tell you when they feel the vibration stop. Stop the fork from vibrating by gently grasping the prongs of the fork. The patient should tell you that the fork is no longer vibrating. If the patient is unable to sense vibration at the MCPJ/MTPJ, move to a more proximal bony prominence and retest.

◆ Test stereognosis by asking the patient to identify an object (coin, key, or pen) that you place in their hand while their eyes are closed. Repeat this for the other hand using a different object. Test graphesthesia by asking the patient to identify a number or letter that you draw on their palm with the back of a pen while their eyes are closed. Repeat on the other hand with a different letter or number. Astereognosis and agraphesthesia suggest a lesion in the sensory cortex of the parietal lobe.

8. Test for pronator drift by asking the patient to hold both arms fully extended in front of them, flexed at the shoulder, with their palms upwards. Ask them to maintain the position. If they are unable to do so the result is positive. Next ask the patient to close their eyes and to continue to maintain the position. They are now reliant on proprioception, as visual clues to the whereabouts of their upper limbs have been extinguished. Finally, tap gently on the palm of their outstretched hands to displace them—the patient should be able to return their limbs to the original position and maintain it. This is a test for upper motor neuron disease. Pronation of a forearm during the test (pronator drift) indicates a contralateral pyramidal tract lesion. Cerebellar lesions produce an upward drift.

9. Gait is evaluated by asking the patient to rise from the chair/couch, walk across the room, turn and return to their original position. Balance, posture, stride length, arm swing, and turning stability should be noted. A decrease in arm swing is a highly sensitive indicator of upper limb weakness and is commonly seen in Parkinson's disease.

If the patient is able to walk normally without too much difficulty, also ask them to walk heel-to-toe (tandem gait), then on their toes only (test for weakness of ankle plantarflexors) and finally on their heels only (test for weakness of ankle dorsiflexors). Abnormalities in tandem gait may be due to alcohol intoxication, weakness, proprioceptive loss, vertigo, and cerebellar lesions. Most elderly patients will find this test difficult due to generalised neuronal loss impairing proprioception, strength, and co-ordination.

10. Finally, perform the Romberg test by asking the patient to stand still with their feet together. Ask them to close their eyes—if they lose their balance on closing their eyes, the test is positive and indicates a failure of proprioception, as per the test for pronator drift above. You must ensure that you are standing near to the patient for safety reasons as you may need to steady them if they start to fall.

Examination of the cranial nerves

Firstly, perform a general inspection of the patient's head and neck, noting any scars, neurofibromas, facial asymmetry, ptosis, proptosis, skew deviation of the eyes or inequality of the pupils.

The twelve cranial nerves should then be examined in order, as follows.

1. Olfactory nerve (I)

   ◆ This is only usually tested if the patient reports an alteration in their sense of smell.

   ◆ If required, either use olfactory testing bottles or easily recognized scents such as soap and coffee. Test each nostril separately, occluding the contralateral nostril by compressing it with your finger.

2. Optic nerve (II)

   ◆ Test visual acuity in each eye separately using a Snellen chart if possible.

   ◆ Test visual fields by confrontation. Sit directly opposite the patient with your eyes at the same level and a gap of approximately 1 m between your chairs. Cover one of your own eyes and ask the patient to cover the eye directly opposite this. Ask the patient to keep staring straight into your other eye. Bring a test object (e.g. a large pin or, if this is unavailable, your index finger), in gradually from a point outside of your own visual field, assuming this is normal, diagonally toward the centre of your visual field. Ask the patient to signal to you when they first see the object. You should repeat this in all four quadrants for each eye. This is a basic test and although not very accurate, it will detect significant discrepancies between your own visual fields and those of the patient.

   ◆ Test direct and consensual light reflexes. Ask the patient to look straight ahead and bring the light source in from the side so that the patient does not focus on it and accommodate. Shine the light into the eye and look for constriction of that pupil (the direct light reflex) and the contralateral pupil (the consensual reflex).

   ◆ Test accommodation. Ask the patient to focus on a distant point and then to focus on your finger, held approximately 30 cm in front of their nose. A normal accommodation response will involve convergence of the eyes and constriction of both pupils.

   ◆ Ophthalmoscopy should be undertaken to complete the assessment.

3. Oculomotor (III), trochlear (IV) and abducens (VI) nerves

   ◆ Ask the patient to keep their head still and to follow your finger with their eyes. Slowly trace a large H shape and a central

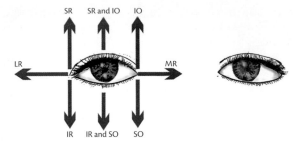

Fig. 4.3.3 Direction of eye movement in response to contraction of the extraocular muscles. MR, medial rectus; LR, lateral rectus; SR, superior rectus; IR, inferior rectus; IO, inferior oblique; SO, superior oblique.
Reproduced from Roper TE, *Clinical Skills, Second Edition*, Figure 6.22, p. 179, Oxford University Press, Oxford, UK, Copyright © Oxford University Press 2014, by permission of Oxford University Press.

I shape with your finger, taking the patients eyes to the limit of their gaze as you do so (Figure 4.3.3). Ask the patient if they experience any diplopia. Observe for dysconjugate eye movements and for nystagmus.

4. Trigeminal nerve (V)

   ◆ Test sensation in the skin supplied by the ophthalmic, maxillary, and mandibular nerves. Initially, demonstrate the stimulus (cotton wool) to the patient over their sternum with their eyes open and check that they can feel it. Ask the patient to close their eyes and apply the stimulus to each of the dermatomes of the trigeminal nerve. Ask the patient to indicate when they can feel the stimulus and whether they notice a difference in the strength of the sensation between the two sides of their body.

   ◆ Test the motor component of the trigeminal nerve by asking the patient to clench their teeth and palpate the contraction of the masseter and temporalis muscles. Next ask the patient to open their mouth against resistance and look for jaw deviation, indicating weakness of the pterygoids.

   ◆ The corneal and jaw jerk reflexes are not routinely performed.

5. Facial nerve (VII)

   ◆ This is the motor supply to the muscles of facial expression. Ask the patient to screw up their eyes and not let them be opened by you, puff out their cheeks, raise their eyebrows, purse their lips and show you their teeth. Remember that muscles of the upper face (frontalis, orbicularis oculi) receive a bilateral upper motor neuron (UMN) supply and therefore may be spared in UMN lesions (e.g. cerebrovascular accident), whereas the muscles of the lower face have a unilateral UMN supply and will be weakened. In a proximal lower motor neuron lesion, the muscles of both the upper and lower face will be affected (Figure 4.3.4).

   ◆ The glabellar reflex and taste sensation do not need to be routinely tested.

6. Vestibulocochlear nerve (VIII)

   ◆ Cover the opposite ear with your hand and whisper a number to the patient. Ask them to repeat it. If an abnormality is suspected, perform Rinnes and Webers tests to determine whether this is a sensory or conductive deficit.

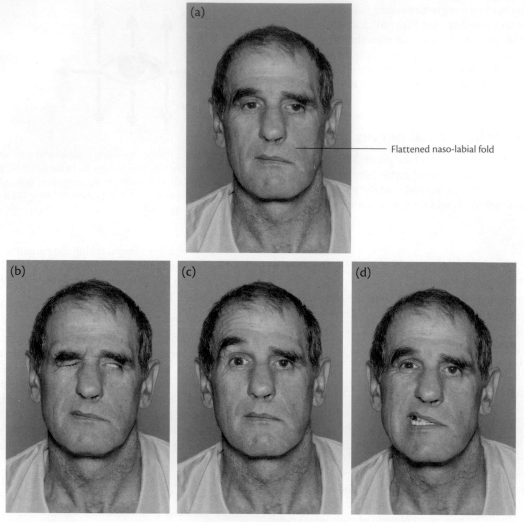

Flattened naso-labial fold

Fig. 4.3.4 A left lower motor neuron (LMN) facial nerve lesion.
(a) The patient at rest. Note the flattened nasolabial fold and drooping of the angle of the mouth on the left. (b) Attempting to close the eyes tightly. (c) Attempting to raise the eyebrows. Note the loss of wrinkling of the forehead due to paralysis of frontalis. This confirms the presence of a LMN lesion. (d) Attempting to show the teeth.
Reproduced from Roper TE, *Clinical Skills, Second Edition*, Figure 6.31, p. 187, Oxford University Press, Oxford, UK, Copyright © Oxford University Press 2014, by permission of Oxford University Press.

- Rinne's test: Hold a vibrating tuning fork (512 Hz) on the mastoid then immediately move it to the external acoustic meatus. If conduction is normal it should sound louder at the external acoustic meatus. If the sound is louder when the tuning fork is on the mastoid, this indicates conductive hearing loss. In sensorineural hearing loss, both air and bone conduction are decreased by a similar amount.

- Weber's test: Hold a vibrating tuning fork against the midline of the forehead. As the distance and the rate of bone conduction is the same to both ears, the vibrations are normally perceived equally in both ears. In conductive hearing loss, the sound appears louder in the abnormal ear than in the normal ear. In sensorineural hearing loss, the sound appears louder in the normal ear.

7. Glossopharyngeal (IX) and vagus (X) nerves

- Ask the patient to open their mouth wide and assess whether the uvula is in the midline at rest. Ask the patient to say 'aah' and note any asymmetry of movement. The uvula will deviate away from the side of a glossopharyngeal nerve palsy.

- Ask whether the patient has any difficulty swallowing. The gag reflex is unpleasant and does not need to be performed routinely.

- Ask the patient to cough. A bovine (non-explosive) cough suggests a vagal palsy.

- Note any hoarseness of the voice.

8. Accessory nerve (XI)

- Test trapezius by asking the patient to shrug their shoulders against resistance. Test the power in the sternomastoids by asking the patient to turn their head against resistance. Palpate the body of the sternomastoid muscle with your free hand while doing so.

9. Hypoglossal nerve (XII)

- Ask the patient to open their mouth and observe their tongue at rest for fasciculation. Ask them to protrude their tongue and note any deviation. Deviation will occur toward the side of a hypoglossal nerve lesion. Ask the patient to push their tongue into their cheek against the resistance of your finger and assess the power in their tongue.

Examination of a neck lump (e.g. cervical lymphadenopathy, salivary gland)

The general approach to the examination of a lump in the neck includes the examination of the mass itself and also the skin of the head and neck, the contents of the anterior and posterior triangles of the neck, and the examination of the ears, nasal and oral cavities, nasopharynx, oropharynx, hypopharynx, and larynx. Specialized equipment is required for the examination of the nasopharynx, hypopharynx, and larynx.

1. Examine the mass itself, following the scheme for the general examination of a lump outlined in Chapter 4.2. The location of the mass will provide an important clue as to the structure of its origin and you should ensure that you are familiar with the anatomy of the anterior and posterior triangles of the neck and the structures within them. You should also recall the anatomical location of congenital masses (e.g. thyroglossal and branchial cysts) and the location of the superficial lymph node groups within the neck. The size, consistency, and mobility of the mass, and the presence or absence of tenderness will provide a number of diagnostic clues. Acute inflammatory masses tend to be soft, mobile, and tender, whereas chronic inflammatory masses are more likely to be non-tender, rubbery in consistency, and fixed to the surrounding tissues. Malignant neoplasms are likely to be non-tender and may be hard in consistency and fixed to the surrounding tissues.

2. Examine the skin of the scalp, face, and neck for primary cutaneous tumours that may have metastasized to the cervical nodes.

3. Examine the nasal cavity, oral cavity, and oropharynx for evidence of neoplasia. In particular, you should inspect the lateral border of the tongue, floor of the mouth, soft palate, and fauces as these are common sites of intraoral malignancy. You should also palpate the soft tissues at the base of the tongue for occult lesions.

4. Palpate the structures of the patient's neck carefully, including bimanual palpation of the submandibular area.

5. Inspect and palpate to determine whether the mass moves with swallowing, and also with tongue protrusion (see examination of the thyroid gland below).

6. Examine the patient's cranial nerves as these may be infiltrated by a malignant neoplasm, providing important diagnostic information.

Examination of the thyroid gland

Seat the patient comfortably in a chair. While introducing yourself to the patient, listen to their voice—a low-pitched or hoarse voice may indicate hypothyroidism.

1. Inspect the general appearance of the patient (build, inappropriate clothing, restlessness, confusion, quality of skin, and hair).

2. Inspect the hands for signs that may indicate thyroid disease, for example, sweating, palmar erythema, clubbing (thyroid acropachy), brittle nails, onycholysis. Feel the temperature of the hands using the dorsum of your own hands.

3. Check for a tremor by asking the patient to hold their hands outstretched and pronated (palms downward) with fingers slightly apart. Place a piece of paper on the dorsum of the outstretched hands and fingers. This will amplify a fine tremor.

4. Check the patient's pulse. Note the presence of bradycardia, tachycardia, or atrial fibrillation.

5. Inspect for muscle wasting.

6. Inspect the eyes for thyroid signs:

- Inspect for exophthalmos (i.e. proptosis [forward displacement of the eye]) occurring in association with hyperthyroidism. Stand behind the patient and look down on their orbit from above. Exophthalmos may lead to inability to close the lids properly and lead to exposure keratopathy.

- Inspect for chemosis (conjunctival oedema), conjunctival injection ('bloodshot' eyes), and periorbital/lid oedema.

- Inspect for lid retraction, which allows the sclera to be seen above the cornea.

- Inspect for lid lag by asking the patient to look up then down. Delayed downward movement of the eyelids on downgaze indicates lid lag.

- Check eye movements in all directions of gaze. There may be a myopathy of the extraocular muscles. Also, diplopia can result from restricted ocular mobility, initially involving the inferior rectus muscles.

- Check visual acuity and perform fundoscopy.

7. Inspect the neck for masses. If a mass is seen:

- Ask the patient to take some water in their mouth then observe the neck while they swallow it. Does the mass move? If so, this indicates a thyroid mass.

- Ask the patient to protrude their tongue. Observe the neck. If the mass moves upwards on tongue protrusion this indicates a thyroglossal cyst.

8. Palpate the trachea. Is it central?

9. From behind, palpate the anterior neck. If there is a mass:

- Determine the size and site.

- Is it diffusely enlarged?

- Is the mass hard or soft on palpation?

- Is the surface smooth or nodular? Is there a single nodule or multiple nodules?

- Are the surrounding tissues mobile over the mass or is the mass fixed to the surrounding tissues?

- Can you palpate above the mass?

- Can you palpate below the mass in the suprasternal notch? If not, it may be a retrosternal goitre.

- Ask the patient to take some water in their mouth then swallow it, while you are palpating. Does it move on swallowing?

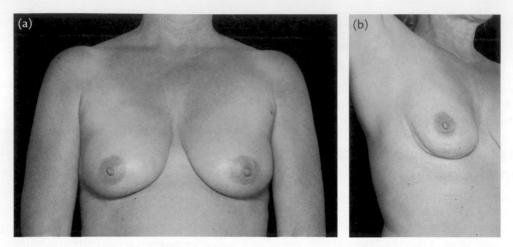

Fig. 4.3.5 Inspection of the breasts. (a) With the arms and chest wall relaxed, the contour of the breast tissue appears normal; (b) Tethering of the skin of the right breast becomes visible when the arms are raised and shoulders externally rotated.

Reproduced from Roper TE, *Clinical Skills, Second Edition*, Figure 10.4A and 10.4B, p. 365, Oxford University Press, Oxford, UK, Copyright © Oxford University Press 2014, by permission of Oxford University Press.

♦ Ask the patient to protrude their tongue? Does the mass move?

10. Palpate the cervical lymph nodes for metastatic spread.

11. Percuss the upper sternum for retrosternal extension of the goitre.

12. Auscultate the thyroid gland for bruits, using the bell of the stethoscope, while the patient is holding their breath.

13. Check the ankle reflexes. Delayed relaxation may occur in hypothyroidism.

14. Inspect for pretibial myxedema.

Examination of the breast

You should have a chaperone present, and the patient should remove all clothing above their waist. Before commencing the examination, ask the patient whether they have any pain.

1. Inspection

   ♦ Position the patient so that they are seated with their arms by their sides.

   ♦ Inspect for symmetry, or abnormalities in the contours of each breast (e.g. tethering or dimpling of the skin).

   ♦ Inspect for visible masses.

   ♦ Inspect for erythema of the skin +/− abnormal scaling or ulceration of the nipple and areolar skin.

   ♦ Inspect for nipple retraction (enquire about its duration as this may be congenital).

   ♦ Ask the patient to raise both arms, put their hands behind their head and push their shoulders back. Inspect the breast tissue while the patient performs this manoeuvre. Look for the appearance or accentuation of skin tethering (Figure 4.3.5).

   ♦ Ask the patient to put their hands on their hips and push inwards. This fixes the pectoralis major and may accentuate lumps tethered to it.

2. Palpation

   ♦ Ask the patient to lie comfortably at 45°. Examination of a large-breasted woman may be easier if their arm is placed above their head.

   ♦ Mentally divide the breast into four quadrants (upper outer, upper inner, lower outer and lower inner), plus the axillary tail and nipple.

   ♦ Palpate each quadrant, the axillary tail, and nipple using the pads of your index, middle, and ring fingers (not your fingertips). Make small circular movements as if you were rolling a marble. Increase the level of pressure to ensure you examine the full thickness of the breast tissue.

   ♦ Palpate the axillary lymph nodes while supporting the patients arm with your free hand (this relaxes the muscles forming the anterior and posterior walls of the axilla and permits easier palpation). Palpate using a rolling action (as above) examining the axillary tissue against the lateral chest wall and superiorly in the axilla. If you identify a lump, determine its characteristics as outlined above.

   ♦ Palpate the nipple and inspect for nipple discharge. It is not necessary to attempt to 'milk' the nipple to determine whether any discharge is present.

   ♦ Examine the supraclavicular fossa for lymphadenopathy.

Further reading

Roper TE. *Clinical Skills 2e*. Oxford: Oxford University Press; 2013

CHAPTER 4.4

Physical examination of the vasculature and joints

Caroline Woodley and Malcolm W. R. Reed

Introduction

In this chapter, we present a structured approach to the examination of the arterial and venous systems of the lower limbs, the musculoskeletal system of the upper and lower limbs and spine, and the examination of the acutely hot, swollen joint.

Examination of the arterial supply of the lower limb

1. Inspect the legs, feet, and toes for symmetry, colour, trophic changes (e.g. loss of hair, shiny skin, wasting of subcutaneous tissues), venous guttering, and ulceration. Inspect the abdomen for a visible aortic pulsation or scars suggesting previous surgery.

2. Feel the temperature in both lower limbs using the dorsum of your hands. A decrease in skin temperature is much more significant if there is a palpable difference in temperature between the two feet than if both feet are equally cold.

3. Palpate the aorta, femoral pulses, popliteal pulses, dorsalis pedis, and posterior tibial pulses. Decide if they are weak, normal, or aneurysmal.

4. Assess light touch sensation and capillary refill in the toes. Press the tip of the nail for 2 seconds then release. Capillary refill time should be <2 seconds.

5. Auscultate the aorta (a bruit can be heard in thin healthy patients) and femoral arteries. Note that there is no bruit over an occluded vessel and severe stenosis can be present without an audible bruit.

6. Perform Buerger's test to assess the adequacy of arterial supply to a limb:

   ◆ With the patient supine, elevate both legs to an angle of 45° and hold for 1–2 minutes. Pallor of the feet indicates ischaemia. The poorer the arterial supply, the less elevation of the limb is required before pallor is observed.

   ◆ Sit the patient up and ask them to hang their legs down over the side of the bed at an angle of 90°. Gravity aids the blood flow and the colour returns to the ischaemic leg. The skin of the leg initially appears blue, as the blood has been deoxygenated during its passage through the ischaemic tissue, and then red, due to reactive hyperaemia from post-hypoxic vasodilatation. Both legs should be examined simultaneously as the colour changes are accentuated when one leg has a normal circulation.

7. Calculate the ankle–brachial pressure index (ABPI) by dividing the highest systolic blood pressure in the arteries at the ankle by the higher of the two systolic blood pressures in the arms. Significant arterial disease is indicated by an ABPI of <0.8 (see Chapter 2.7.1).

Examination of the lower limbs for varicose veins and chronic venous insufficiency

1. With the patient standing, inspect the legs for varicosities, particularly in the distribution of the long saphenous vein (medial thigh and leg) and short saphenous vein (lateral leg), venous eczema, oedema due to venous stasis, lipodermatosclerosis, haemosiderin deposition, venous ulceration (usually in the gaiter area above the medial malleolus), and scars (indicating previous surgery or healed ulceration).

2. Identify the saphenofemoral junction (SFJ). This is located 4 cm lateral and 4 cm inferior to the pubic tubercle. Inspect for a saphenovarix (varicosities at the SFJ).

3. Cough test. Place your finger on the SFJ and ask the patient to cough. Palpate for thrills at the SFJ.

4. Tap test. Place your finger on the SFJ and place a finger of your other hand on any varicosities in the long saphenous vein distribution. Tap on the SFJ and if it is incompetent, you will feel the transmitted percussion wave in the varicosities further down the leg.

5. Trendelenburg test (tourniquet test). Ask the patient to lie flat. Raise the leg to 45° or higher and keep it raised for a few minutes to exsanguinate as much blood as possible. Apply a tourniquet high around the thigh. Ask the patient to stand up and inspect to see whether the varicose veins refill. If not, the problem originates at the SFJ. If the veins do refill, repeat the test at the mid-thigh perforators, the saphenopopliteal junction, and the mid-calf perforators.

6. Perthe's test is used to assess the patency of the deep veins. Ask the patient to lie down. Without exsanguinating the leg, apply a tourniquet around the thigh. Ask the patient to stand and rock up and down onto his tiptoes ten times. If the superficial veins empty, the deep veins must be patent.

7. Perform auscultation using a Doppler probe on the SFJ. Squeeze the thigh. You should hear a single 'whoosh' as the blood is squeezed from the long saphenous vein into the

femoral vein. A second 'whoosh' indicates incompetence of the SFJ as the blood flows back into the long saphenous vein past the incompetent valve.

8. Repeat the Doppler probe auscultation at the saphenopopliteal junction in the popliteal fossa. To enable you to squeeze the calf, the patient will need to relax their calf muscles by transferring most of their weight onto the other limb.

9. Examine the abdomen to exclude an abdominal or pelvic cause of raised venous pressure.

Examination of the hip

Examination of the joints follows the sequence of 'look, feel, move, and special tests'. Always examine the contralateral joint for comparison. Also examine the joint above and below that indicated by the patient in case the pain experienced by the patient originates in a neighbouring joint, or the patient is putting undue stress on the painful joint to compensate for a deformity in a neighbouring joint.

When examining the hip, the patient should be wearing their underpants but should remove their trousers, socks, and shoes.

1. With the patient standing, inspect the patient from the front for pelvic tilt, joint deformities (e.g. fixed flexion), and wasting of the quadriceps muscles; inspect from the side for an exaggerated lumbar lordosis, which may suggest a fixed flexion deformity of the hip; and inspect from behind for wasting of the gluteal muscles and for scoliosis, which may be primary or may be secondary to a pelvic tilt.

2. Position the patient supine on the couch with their hips and knees extended.

   ◆ Inspect the patient's skin for scars in the groin and anterior and lateral thighs. If possible, roll the patient onto each side to inspect the gluteal regions.

   ◆ To measure apparent leg length, use a tape measure to measure from the xiphisternum to the medial malleolus of each leg. This is 'apparent' length as it will be influenced by pelvic tilt as well as the true length of the legs.

   ◆ To measure true leg length, measure from the anterior superior iliac spine to the medial malleolus. If there is a true leg length discrepancy, assess whether this originates in the tibia or the femur, as follows. Position the patient with their knees bent up to a right angle and their heels flat on the bed. Inspect from the side. Place your hand across both tibial tuberosities; if there is femoral shortening, your hand will dip down towards the shortened side. Place your hand across both suprapatellar regions; if there is tibial shortening, your hand will dip down towards the shortened side.

3. Ask the patient whether they have any pain or tenderness. Palpate the greater trochanter for trochanteric bursitis.

4. Check the active range of movement (ROM) of flexion, abduction, adduction, 'internal rotation in extension', and 'external rotation in extension' of each hip. The normal ranges are flexion 115–125°, abduction 40–50°, adduction 15–25°, 'internal rotation in extension' 30–40°, and 'external rotation in extension'

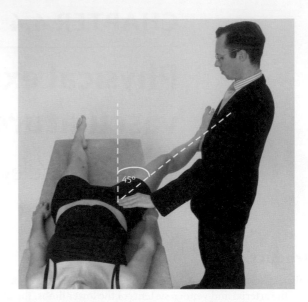

Fig. 4.4.1 Examination of the passive range of hip abduction. You must ensure that the pelvis is stabilized while performing these tests.
Reproduced from Roper TE, *Clinical Skills, Second Edition*, Figure 12.12, p. 423 and Figure 12.13, p. 424, Oxford University Press, Oxford, UK, Copyright © Oxford University Press 2014, by permission of Oxford University Press.

40–50°. Check the passive ROM of each of these movements (Figure 4.4.1).

   ◆ Passively flex the hip and knee up to 90°. Take care when examining a patient who has had a total hip arthroplasty as forced flexion may cause the hip to dislocate. Assess the passive ROM of internal and external rotation *in flexion*. (Normal internal rotation in flexion = 35–50°, external rotation in flexion = 25–40°).

5. Assess the active and passive ROM of extension with the patient lying prone. The normal range is 10–30°.

6. Thomas's test. Assess for a fixed flexion deformity of the *contralateral* hip by flexing the ipsilateral hip fully. Place your hand between the patient's lumbar spine and the bed to check for full correction of the lumbar lordosis then observe the contralateral hip. This manoeuvre will cause the patient with a fixed flexion deformity of the contralateral hip to raise their leg off the bed.

7. Assess the patient's gait. A waddling gait may be associated with hip pain or proximal muscle weakness. An antalgic gait reflects pain on weight bearing.

8. Trendelenburg's test (Figure 4.4.2). Ask the patient to stand on one leg to assess the abductor muscle strength of that hip. In a negative (normal) test, the pelvis remains level or even rises on the contralateral side as the patient contracts their abductors (gluteus medius, gluteus minimus, tensor fascia latae, and sartorius). In a positive test, the pelvis will dip on the contralateral side.

9. You will also need to examine the patient's lumbar spine and the ipsilateral knee joint, and perform a neurological and vascular examination of the patient's lower limb.

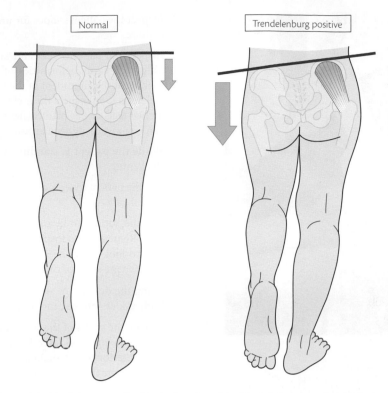

Normal

Trendelenburg positive

Fig. 4.4.2 Trendelenburg's test. Weakness of the hip abductors on the right leads to the pelvis tilting inferiorly towards the left when the left foot is lifted off the ground.

Examination of the knee

This is a basic knee examination to which other specific tests can be added depending on the nature of the patient's complaint.

1. With the patient standing, inspect for swellings in the popliteal fossa (e.g. Baker's cyst), valgus ('knock knees') and varus ('bow legs') deformities, genu recurvatum (knee hyperextension), and flexion deformity.

2. Position the patient supine on the couch with their hips and knees extended. Inspect for symmetry, valgus and varus deformity, skin rashes (e.g. psoriasis), scars, swelling, muscle wasting (particularly in the vastus medialis), displacement of the patella, and flexion deformity.

3. Assess the temperature using the dorsum of your hand in the mid-thigh, over the patella and over the upper tibia. Normally the patellar region feels cooler than the surrounding tissues. Compare both sides.

4. With the knee extended, palpate around the borders of the patella for tenderness. Palpate behind the knee for popliteal swellings or cysts.

5. Assess for an effusion by performing the bulge test or the patellar tap.

   ◆ The bulge test (cross-fluctuation). This test is particularly sensitive in picking up a small effusion. Sweep the hand firmly up the medial fossa, over the suprapatellar pouch, and down the lateral fossa. The medial fossa may refill, producing a bulge of fluid.

   ◆ The patellar tap. With one hand, compress the suprapatellar pouch to empty it then use two fingers of your other hand to 'bounce' the patella against the femur.

6. Flex the knee up to 90° to open the joint line. Palpate the joint line and patellar tendon insertion (tibial tuberosity) for tenderness.

7. Ask the patient to actively flex and extend their knee (normal flexion = 135°, normal extension – 0°).

8. Assess passive movement by placing your hand on the patient's knee and flexing the knee as far as possible. Palpate for crepitus during passive flexion and extension.

9. Assess for posterior cruciate ligament (PCL) damage by performing the posterior sag test. Position the patient with the knee flexed to 90° and the foot flat on the bed. Inspect from the side. A posterior sag of the upper tibia, with a 'step' visible below the patella, is suggestive of PCL damage.

10. Assess for anterior cruciate ligament (ACL) damage by performing Lachman's test (Figure 4.4.3). Flex the knee to 20°. Place one hand behind the tibia with your thumb on the tibial tuberosity. Grasp the patient's thigh with your other hand and pull anteriorly on the tibia. You should feel a firm end-point as the ACL prevents forward translocation of the tibia on the femur. A soft end-point suggests ACL damage. If the patient's thigh is too large or your hand is too small to stabilize the limb adequately, you may perform. Lachman's test with the patients thigh supported by the edge of the examination couch.

    ◆ Lachman's test should be performed in preference to the anterior draw test, due to its higher sensitivity and specificity.

11. Test the integrity of the lateral collateral ligaments (LCL). Flex the knee to 20°. Grasp the patient's heel with one hand while exerting pressure against the inside of the knee with the other

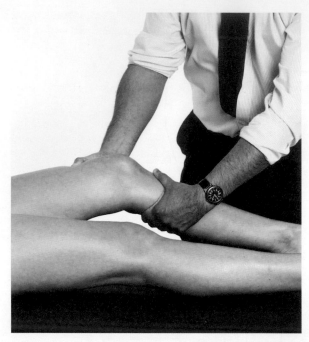

Fig. 4.4.3 Lachman's test.

Reproduced from Michael Hutson and Adam Ward (Eds.), *Oxford Textbook of Musculoskeletal Medicine, Second Edition,* Figure 36.3, Oxford University Press, Oxford, UK, Copyright © Oxford University Press 2015, by permission of Oxford University Press.

hand. The varus stress applied will cause lateral gaping in the laterally unstable knee. A small amount of lateral joint gaping is physiological and it is the asymmetry of the gaping that constitutes the abnormal finding.

12. Test the integrity of the medial collateral ligaments. Proceed as for the LCL above, but apply a valgus stress against the lateral aspect of the knee and assess for medial gaping.

13. If the history is suggestive of a meniscal injury, perform McMurray's test. The test is designed to trap or catch a torn meniscus between the femoral condyle and the tibial plateau. Flex the patient's hip to 90° and maximally flex the knee. Externally rotate the tibia and, maintaining this rotation, move the knee gradually from the fully flexed position to the fully extended position. The test should be repeated with the tibia in internal rotation. An audible, palpable, or painful click over the medial or lateral joint line indicates a meniscal tear. The test has high sensitivity but low specificity and is difficult to perform on an acutely painful knee.

14. Ask the patient to walk and observe the toeing angle – the angle between the orientation of the foot and the direction the patient is walking (normal = 10–15° laterally). Observe for an antalgic (painful) gait.

15. Conclude by examining the ipsilateral hip and ankle, and performing a neurological and vascular examination of the limb.

Examination of the ankle and foot

The basic examination of the ankle includes an assessment of the foot and follows the basic structure 'look, feel, move'. Before commencing, ask the patient if they have any pain in their ankles or feet.

1. Inspect the patient's shoes for uneven wear and the presence of orthoses.

2. Inspect the patient's feet and ankles while they are standing. Valgus or varus deformities of the ankle can be detected by looking at the alignment of the toes relative to those of the contralateral foot. Inspect the arches of the feet for pes cavus (high-arched feet) or pes planus (flat feet). Swelling of the ankle joint can be most easily seen around the malleoli.

3. While the patient is standing, palpate the Achilles tendon for thickening.

4. Ask the patient to walk and observe for a normal heel strike and toe-off gait.

5. Ask the patient to lie on the couch and inspect the nails and skin. Remember to inspect between the toes and also to lift the foot to look at the heel. Check the alignment of the toes and note the presence of calluses, clawing and joint swelling.

6. Using the dorsum of your hands, compare the temperature of both ankles and feet, moving from proximal to distal.

7. Palpate the shafts of the tibia and fibula for tenderness, including the medial and lateral malleoli. To palpate the talus, palpate anterior to the malleoli while everting and inverting the foot. Palpate the ligamentous attachments of the ankle joint and the muscle tendons that cross the ankle joint. Perform a lateral squeeze test on the metatarsophalangeal joints.

8. Assess the active range of dorsiflexion, plantar flexion, inversion, and eversion of the foot. Test muscle power by applying resistance to active movement.

9. Assess the passive ROM with the patient's lower leg supported on the examination couch and their foot unsupported. Stabilize the lower leg against the couch with one hand and use your other hand to assess joint mobility. The normal ranges are passive dorsiflexion 10–15°, plantar flexion 50–70°, inversion 40°, and eversion 10°.

10. Fix the position of the ankle joint with one hand and using your other hand, assess passive inversion and eversion of the midtarsal joints.

11. Test active dorsiflexion of the great toe.

12. Palpate the dorsalis pedis and anterior tibial pulses. If arterial pulsation cannot be detected in the foot, palpate the popliteal pulse.

13. Assess light touch and pressure sensation in the foot, using a 10 G monofilament if available.

Examination of the shoulder

Before commencing your examination, ask the patient whether they have any pain in their arms, shoulders, or neck.

The patient's shoulders, neck, and chest should be exposed, although female patients should retain their bra during this examination.

1. With the patient standing, inspect the patient's shoulders from the front, looking for symmetry, posture, swelling, deformity, bony prominences (sternoclavicular joint; acromioclavicular joint), muscle wasting (deltoid), scars, and any other skin changes (e.g. erythema). From behind, inspect the muscle bulk

in the supraspinatus, infraspinatus, trapezius, and rhomboids. Look for scars, skin changes, and winging of the scapulae.

2. Using the back of your hand, assess the temperature over the shoulder area.

3. Palpate the structures of the shoulder from the front, working from medial to lateral (sternoclavicular joint, clavicle, acromioclavicular joint, acromion process, glenohumeral joint, spine, and body of the scapula). Palpate for increased temperature, joint line tenderness, swelling, and crepitus.

4. Palpate the muscle bulk of the deltoid, supraspinatus, infraspinatus, and trapezius.

5. Before examining the individual movements of the shoulder, perform a screening examination. Firstly, ask the patient to put their hands behind their head and push their elbows back as far as they can (external rotation and abduction). Next, ask the patient to put their hands behind their back (internal rotation and abduction). Inspect for any difficulty, limitation or pain on movement. Note how far the patient can reach up their back.

6. Assess the individual movements of the shoulder actively. If there is a limited active ROM, repeat the test passively.

   - External rotation: Flex the patient's elbow to 90° and tuck it into their side. Ask the patient to rotate their arm outwards.

   - Flexion and extension: Ask the patient to raise their arms in front and behind them.

   - Abduction and adduction: Ask the patient to raise their arm to the side, palm downwards, then lower it again. Normal range of abduction is up to 180°. Observe from both the front and behind for symmetry of scapular movement and pain. Assess glenohumeral movement and scapulothoracic movement. If the patient has rotator cuff pathology, there is often pain from 60–120° (painful arc) that may be alleviated by repeating with the palm facing upwards. Pain only occurring at the end of the movement (120–180°) may indicate acromioclavicular joint (ACJ) arthritis.

There are a number of special tests that may be added to the basic shoulder examination, depending on the patient's history. Here we have included tests for rotator cuff pathology, acromioclavicular joint pathology, and winging of the scapula.

7. To test the power of the muscles of the rotator cuff, perform the following:

   - Resisted active abduction (supraspinatus initiates abduction from 0–15°, deltoid abducts up to 90°, trapezius and serratus anterior cause scapular rotation for abduction beyond 90°).

   - Resisted active external rotation (infraspinatus, teres minor).

   - Resisted active internal rotation—'lift-off' test (subscapularis). Ask the patient to place their hand behind their back with the dorsum of their hand resting over their mid-lumbar spine. The patient should then raise the dorsum of their hand off their back by maintaining or increasing internal rotation of the humerus while extending at the shoulder. To perform this test the patient must have full passive internal rotation so that it is physically possible to place their arm in the desired position. Pain cannot be a limiting factor during the manoeuvre. The ability to actively lift the dorsum of the hand off the back

constitutes a normal lift-off test. Inability to lift the dorsum of the hand off the back indicates an abnormal test due to subscapularis rupture or dysfunction.

8. Test for ACJ pathology by placing the arm into forced adduction across the body at 90° of flexion at the shoulder (the scarf test). Note any pain or tenderness over the ACJ.

9. Test for winging of the scapula by asking the patient to push against a wall, exerting a moderate degree of force, using the palm of their hand. Winging of the scapula is suggestive of weakness of the serratus anterior, which is supplied by the long thoracic nerve.

10. Examine the cervical spine, and perform a neurological and vascular assessment of the upper limb.

Examination of the elbow

Before commencing the examination, ask the patient if they have any pain in the shoulder, elbow, or wrist. The patient's arms should be exposed fully, including their shoulders.

1. Ask the patient to stand with their arms loosely by their sides. Inspect the position of the elbows at rest and note the carrying angle and the presence of a fixed flexion deformity. Inspect the arms, elbows, and forearms closely for scars, swellings, rashes, psoriatic plaques, rheumatoid nodules, and muscle wasting. Remember to inspect the lateral and medial aspects of the elbow joint, the antecubital fossa, and the skin over the extensor surface of the joint.

2. Using the dorsum of your hands, assess the temperature of the skin, moving from proximal to distal and comparing both sides.

3. With the elbow flexed to 90°, palpate the radial head, medial and lateral epicondyles, and the olecranon process for tenderness.

4. Assess the active ROM of flexion, extension, pronation and supination. Repeat passively, while feeling for crepitus.

5. Assess for medial epicondylitis (golfer's elbow). In the supinated position, ask the patient to make a fist and flex their wrist against resistance. Pain will be felt at the medial epicondyle.

6. Assess for lateral epicondylitis (tennis elbow). In the supinated position, ask the patient to extend their wrist against resistance. This will produce pain at the origin of the extensor muscles (lateral epicondyle).

Examination of the hand

The following is a basic hand examination, to which further specific tests are added in clinical practice.

Position the patient seated with their hands supinated and supported on a pillow. Ask the patient of they have any pain or numbness/tingling and take care not to cause the patient excessive discomfort during your examination.

1. Inspect the nails for pitting and ridges (seen in psoriasis), onycholysis, splinter haemorrhages (nail fold infarcts e.g. connective tissue disease / vasculitis), and clubbing.

2. Inspect the fingers, looking for scars and skin changes (e.g. sclerodactyly), colour changes (e.g. Raynaud's phenomenon), and trophic changes (e.g. ulcers, pulp atrophy).

- Look for nodular deformities of the interphalangeal joints (IPJs). Bouchard's nodes occur at the proximal IPJs (PIPJs) and Heberden's nodes occur at the distal IPJs (DIPJs) in osteoarthritis (OA).

- Swan neck and Boutonniere deformities of the IPJs may be seen in rheumatoid arthritis, as may the 'windswept deformity' of ulnar deviation at the metacarpophalangeal joint (MCPJ).

- Identify abnormal posturing suggestive of peripheral nerve injuries (e.g. ulnar claw).

3. Inspect the palm and dorsum of the hand for skin disorders (e.g. psoriasis), scars (suggesting injury or previous surgery), wasting of the interossei (seen dorsally), wasting of the thenar and hypothenar muscles (seen on the palmar aspect), and Dupuytren's contracture.

   Note the presence of swelling of the wrists which may indicate synovitis and look for ganglia. Inspect the elbows for rheumatoid nodules and psoriatic plaques.

4. Assess the temperature of the hands using the dorsum of your own hands.

5. Systematically palpate the bones and soft tissues of the hand and wrist.

   - Palpate the volar and dorsal, radial and ulnar aspects of the wrist. Assess for tenderness.

   - Palpate along the dorsum and volar aspect of the metacarpals and phalanges (squeeze gently using your thumb on the palmar surface and index finger on the dorsum) feeling for tenderness, swelling, and bony deformities.

   - Assess for MCPJ tenderness by performing a lateral squeeze of the row of four MCPJs together. If the squeeze test is painful, localise the disease by palpating each MCPJ individually.

   - Palpate along the radial and ulnar aspects of the phalanges. Assess for swelling and areas of tenderness.

6. Perform a neurovascular examination of the hand.

   - Assess light touch sensation in the dermatomal (C6,7,8) and peripheral nerve (median, ulnar, radial) distributions.

   - Assess the capillary refill. Depending on the clinical case, you may also wish to palpate the ulnar and radial pulses to perform an Allen's test: Compress the ulnar and radial arteries at the wrist. Ask the patient to make a tight fist then release it. Release one of the arteries and observe blood flow back into the hand. Repeat but release the other artery. Check that both arteries perfuse the hand fully and there is no discontinuity of the palmar arches.

7. Test active movement first. If a limited ROM exists, you will need to repeat the movement passively. Take care not to cause the patient excessive discomfort.

   - Ask the patient to 'make a full fist'. If this is not possible you will need to examine flexion of each MCPJ, PIPJ, and DIPJ separately.

   - Ask the patient to 'extend and spread their fingers'. Test the power of their dorsal interossei (abduction) by applying resistance.

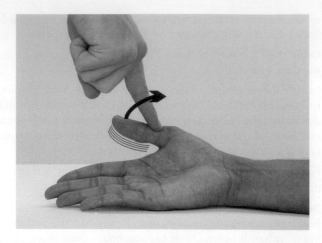

Fig. 4.4.4 Testing palmar abduction of the thumb. The arrow represents the direction of the force generated by the patient.
Reproduced from Roper TE, *Clinical Skills, Second Edition*, Figure 6.54, p. 203, Oxford University Press, Oxford, UK, Copyright © Oxford University Press 2014, by permission of Oxford University Press.

- Test the individual movements of the thumb (abduction, adduction, flexion, extension, palmar abduction (Figure 4.4.4), and opposition).

- Ask the patient to perform the prayer and reverse prayer signs (Figure 4.4.5) to test the range of dorsiflexion and palmar flexion of their wrists. You will need to demonstrate to the patient what you are asking them to do.

8. Assess the patient's grip strength.

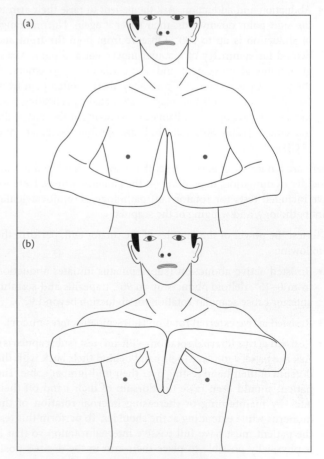

Fig. 4.4.5 (a) Forward prayer sign; (b) Reverse prayer sign.

- Assess power grip by asking the patient to hold a pen in their clenched fist and to stop you pulling it out. (If not available, ask them to grip your fingers.)

- Assess lateral pinch grip (key grip) by asking the patient to hold a key or a pen normally.

- Assess precision by asking the patient to pick up a small object such as coin, button or pin. Ask them if they can do up their buttons when dressing.

9. The following tests are not performed routinely but should be added to the basic hand examination if indicated by the clinical history.

- Test for carpal tunnel syndrome.

  - Tinel's test: Tap strongly over the median nerve as it crosses under the flexor retinaculum via the carpal tunnel. Reproduction of pain, numbness or tingling in the cutaneous distribution of the median nerve is a positive test.
  - Phalen's test: Hold both of the patient's wrists in palmar flexion for 1 minute. Simultaneously apply carpal compression using your thumbs over the median nerve at the flexor retinaculum. Reproduction of pain, numbness or tingling in the cutaneous distribution of the median nerve is a positive test.

- Test ulnar nerve function. Ask the patient to cross their index and middle fingers. Alternatively, ask the patient to grip a piece of paper between the side of their thumb and index finger (using adductor pollicis). Flexion of the IPJ indicates an ulnar nerve lesion (Froment's sign, Figure 4.4.6) as flexor pollicis longus (median nerve) is being used to grip the paper. Finally, test sensation in the ulnar nerve distribution.

- Test median nerve function. Test palmar abduction against resistance (with the patient's palm supinated and held out flat, ask them to point their thumb vertically up to the ceiling. Apply resistance by pushing the thumb back towards the palm with your own thumb). Alternatively, test opposition against resistance (ask the patient to oppose their thumb to their little

finger; do the same yourself, hooking your finger and thumb around the patients', and attempt to pull patient's grip apart). Finally, test sensation in the median nerve distribution.

- Test radial nerve function. Test wrist dorsiflexion against resistance and test sensation in the anatomical snuffbox and dorsum of the first webspace.

Examination of the acutely painful swollen joint

Here we describe the approach to examining a patient presenting with an acutely painful swollen joint, who has no history of trauma.

The most commonly affected joint is the knee (38%), with the knee, wrist, hip, ankle, and elbow together accounting for 87% of clinical presentations. Although there are a number of other diagnostic possibilities, including gout, bursitis, rheumatoid arthritis, psoriatic arthropathy, and reactive arthritis, it is essential to diagnose and treat all cases of septic arthritis urgently. If left untreated, the sequelae include permanent joint damage in up to 30% of patients, and a mortality rate of up to 11%. Septic arthritis may occur due to direct inoculation of the joint with micro-organisms (e.g. via a puncture wound) or may be a consequence of haematogenous spread from a remote focus.

After taking a thorough history, you will need to perform a physical examination.

1. Consider the general appearance of the patient and note whether they are pyrexial. The absence of pyrexia does not exclude the possibility of septic arthritis.

2. Inspect the skin overlying the affected joint carefully for small puncture wounds, lacerations, and insect bites that the patient may not be aware of.

3. Inspect the affected joint for swelling, erythema, and deformity. Swelling may be due to an effusion in the joint or to oedema of the overlying tissues. Swelling over a bursa or tendon is likely to indicate inflammation of that structure. Erythema overlying a joint is relatively uncommon and should raise the suspicion of septic arthritis or gout. If erythema develops in a patient with known inflammatory arthritis, sepsis should be excluded.

4. Assess the temperature of the affected joint using the dorsum of your hand. Compare with the contralateral side.

5. Palpate the joint and surrounding tissues, assessing for tenderness. Point-tenderness suggests inflammation of a peri-articular tissue (e.g. bursitis, inflammation of a ligamentous insertion) rather than of the joint itself.

6. Determine whether there is an effusion using the patellar tap and bulge tests described above.

- If a significant effusion is present, aspiration of the joint may be required. Take care not to aspirate over an area of local cellulitis as to do so may introduce micro-organisms into the knee joint and precipitate septic arthritis. Send the joint aspirate for polarizing microscopy (for crystals) and for an urgent Gram stain, followed by culture and antimicrobial sensitivities. Note that a negative Gram stain and a negative synovial fluid culture do not exclude the diagnosis of septic arthritis. If the clinical suspicion is high, antibiotics should be commenced.

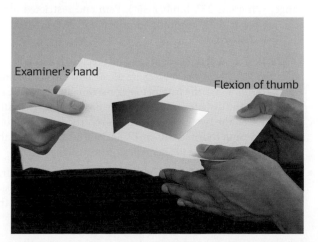

Fig. 4.4.6 Froment's sign is positive on the right.

Reproduced from Roper TE, *Clinical Skills, Second Edition*, Figure 6.56, p. 203, Oxford University Press, Oxford, UK, Copyright © Oxford University Press 2014, by permission of Oxford University Press.

7. Examine the active and passive ROM of the affected joint. It is often very difficult to assess the ROM of an acutely painful joint due to involuntary muscle contraction; adequate analgesia should be provided and the patient should be encouraged to relax as much as possible.

8. Test the stability of the joint by stressing the collateral ligaments.

9. Examine the patient for evidence of joint swelling elsewhere. While doing so, inspect for associated signs of rheumatological disease such as rheumatoid nodules or gouty tophi.

Examination of the spine

1. Inspect the patient from in front, from the side, and from behind. Adequate exposure of the spine is essential and the patient should therefore be dressed in their bra and pants only.

   - Inspect the patient's skin, looking for café-au-lait spots, which may suggest neurofibromatosis, a sacral dimple, naevus, or hairy patch suggestive of spina bifida occulta, or scarring suggestive of a previous thoracotomy or spinal surgery.

   - Inspect the cervical spine for deformity (e.g. cervical spondylosis, acute torticollis). An abnormal head posture may be due to disease in the cervical spine or neck but you should also consider other causes (e.g. extraocular muscle palsy). Look for asymmetry of the clavicles, scapulae, and shoulders.

   - Inspect the thoracolumbar spine for kyphosis (anterior curvature) and lordosis (posterior curvature).

     - If kyphosis is seen, ask the patient to extend their lower back as a postural kyphosis will resolve whereas a fixed kyphosis will not. Causes of a fixed regular kyphosis include senile kyphosis (secondary to osteoporosis or osteomalacia), Scheuermann's disease (abnormally shaped vertebrae), and ankylosing spondylitis. Common causes of a fixed angular kyphosis, with a gibbus or prominent vertebral spine, include a vertebral fracture, spinal tuberculosis and congenital vertebral anomalies.

     - Loss or reversal of the normal lumbar lordosis may be secondary to a prolapsed intervertebral disc, osteoarthritis of the spine or ankylosing spondylitis. Increased lumbar lordosis may be due to spondylolisthesis, or may be secondary to an increased thoracic curvature or a flexion deformity of the hip.

   - Inspect the thoracolumbar spine for scoliosis (lateral curvature of the spine). Idiopathic scoliosis leads to short stature with shortening of the trunk relative to the limbs. Ask the patient to bend forward as postural scoliosis will resolve on forward flexion whereas structural scoliosis will remain. Disappearance of a scoliosis on sitting suggests that the scoliosis may be secondary to shortening of a leg.

2. Palpate for tenderness over the spine and soft tissues.

   - Palpate the cervical spine and neck posteriorly in the midline, laterally, and anteriorly, including thyroid examination. Examine the supraclavicular fossae for masses (e.g. cervical rib, lymph glands, tumours) and the paraspinal muscles for tenderness.

   - Palpate the thoracolumbar spine and sacrum for tenderness. Tenderness between the spines of the lumbar vertebrae, at the lumbosacral junction, and over the lumbar muscles may occur with a prolapsed intervertebral disc and with mechanical back pain.

   - A palpable step at the lumbosacral junction may indicate spondylolisthesis.

   - Palpate for tenderness over the sacroiliac joints (e.g. ankylosing spondylitis).

3. Assess the active ROM of the cervical spine. Repeat the movements passively, feeling for crepitus while doing so.

   - Flexion: Normal range 80°, chin able to touch sternoclavicular joint.

   - Extension: Normal range 50° (note: flexion and extension primarily involves the atlanto-occipital joint).

   - Lateral flexion: Normal range 45° from midline. Restriction of lateral flexion is common in cervical spondylosis and ankylosing spondylitis.

   - Lateral rotation: Normal range 80° to both sides. Lateral rotation primarily occurs at the atlanto-axial joint. It is restricted and painful in cervical spondylosis.

4. Assess the movement in the thoracic and lumbar spine.

   - Flexion is due to a combination of thoracic, lumbar, and hip movements. The composite movement may be recorded as the distance between the patient's fingers and the ground (normally <7 cm) or the lowest level that the person can reach (e.g. mid-tibia). A modified Schober's test should be used to provide a quantitative evaluation of flexion of the lumbar spine. Mark a 15 cm length of the lumbar spine with the patient in the erect position), measuring 10 cm above and 5 cm below the posterior superior iliac spines (dimples of Venus). Instruct the patient to flex his or her spine maximally. Re-measure the distance between the marks. Normal flexion increases the distance by at least 5 cm.

   - Extension: Ask the patient to arch their back (normal range = thoracic 25°, lumbar 35°). Pain and restricted extension are particularly common in prolapsed intervertebral disc and spondylolysis.

   - Lateral flexion: Ask the patient to stand erect with hands at their sides and feet 30 cm apart. Measure the distance from the finger tips to the floor. Ask the patient to flex maximally to the side and re-measure the distance from the finger tips to floor. The difference between the two measurements is recorded as the amount of lateral flexion (normal >10 cm). The contributions of the thoracic and lumbar spine to lateral flexion are usually equal.

   - Rotation: The patient should be seated, asked to fold their arms across their chest then asked and to twist round to each side. The normal range of rotation is 40° and is almost entirely thoracic. The lumbar contribution is <5°.

5. Ask the patient to bend forward and lightly percuss the spine from the root of the neck to the sacrum. Significant percussion tenderness is a feature of infection, fractures, and neoplasia.

6. Assess the patient's gait.

7. Perform a full neurological examination of the patients upper and lower limbs, looking for fasciculation, wasting, and abnormalities in tone, power, reflexes, and sensation. Remember that cervical spinal cord compression may lead to bladder and bowel disturbance, lower limb neurological dysfunction, and abnormal gait.

8. In a patient presenting with lower back pain, perform an abdominal examination to identify any masses, and consider a rectal examination to check for loss of anal tone and perianal sensation (cauda equina syndrome).

9. Examine the peripheral pulses as vascular claudication in the upper and lower limbs may mimic the symptoms of radiculopathy or canal stenosis.

10. In patients presenting with neck pain, you should also examine the shoulder joints. In patients presenting with lower back pain you should examine the hip joints. Osteoarthritis of the hip may present with predominantly back and buttock pain as well as with pain in the groin.

The following special tests should be performed when indicated by the clinical history:

11. Suspected prolapsed intervertebral disc.

  ◆ Straight leg raise: Ask the patient to lie flat on the couch. Passively flex their hip with their leg extended. If the patient complains of back or leg pain the test is positive (hamstring tightness is not relevant). Paraesthesiae or pain in a nerve root distribution indicates nerve root irritation. Back pain suggests, but is not indicative of, a central disc prolapse, and leg pain suggests a lateral protrusion.

    Lower the leg gradually until the pain disappears then dorsiflex the foot. This increases tension on the nerve roots, aggravating any pain or paraesthesiae (Lasegue's sign).

  ◆ Bowstring test: Perform a straight leg raise. If the patient experiences pain, flex the knee slightly then apply firm pressure with the thumb in the popliteal fossa to stretch the tibial nerve. Radiating pain and paraesthesiae suggest nerve root irritation.

  ◆ Femoral stretch test: With the patient prone and the anterior thigh fixed to the couch, flex each knee in turn. This causes pain in the skin overlying the anterior compartment of the thigh by stretching the femoral nerve roots in L2–L4. The pain produced is normally aggravated by extension of the hip.

12. Suspected ankylosing spondylitis

  ◆ Examine chest expansion at the level of the fourth intercostal space (normal = 3–5 cm). This may be reduced in ankylosing spondylitis.

Further reading

Coakley G, Mathews C, Field M, Jones A, Kingsley G, Walker D, Phillips M, Bradish C, McLachlan A, Mohammed R, Weston V. BSR & BHPR, BOA, RCGP and BSAC guidelines for management of the hot swollen joint in adults. Rheumatology 2006; 45:1039 41.

Roper TE. *Clinical Skills 2e*. Oxford: Oxford University Press; 2013.

Solomon L, Warwick DJ, Nayagam S. Apley's concise system of orthopaedics and fractures, third edition. Abingdon, UK: CRC Press; 2005.

CHAPTER 4.5

Information sharing

Michelle Marshall and Malcolm W. R. Reed

Introduction

Information sharing is an important aspect of medicine and surgeons share information with many people, including patients, relatives, other members of the medical team, and members of the wider healthcare team.

The communication process with patients almost always involves information. This may include information about results, diagnosis, prognosis, further management and treatment, or lifestyle advice. Poor information sharing is one of the most common causes of complaint about the NHS, with specific problems highlighted as use of ambiguous language, contradictory or confusing information, use of clinical terms, and poor communication regarding aspects of care such as discharge. It is therefore essential to pay attention to the ways in which information is shared in order to avoid these problems.

The way that information is shared is important as this will impact on patient understanding. It will also impact on the amount of information that is retained and the detail that the patient is able to recall afterwards or when discussing with family and friends. The way that information is shared will also impact on how the patient feels about their care and possible outcomes; do they feel that they were listened to and that their worries and concerns were taken seriously?

Sharing information with colleagues follows many of the principles of communicating with patients. However, there are a number of specific situations that require further consideration, including communication within the operating theatre environment and sharing information about patients whose condition is deteriorating. In these situations, which are time pressured and often require immediate action, it is important that information is shared in an efficient, accurate and concise manner.

In this chapter we will consider how to share information effectively so that the patient understands their diagnosis and treatment plan and has realistic expectations regarding the plan. We will also consider how to share accurate information with colleagues in an efficient manner in specific situations and how to generally enhance team working. We will then finish by considering written communication, which takes many forms within medicine, including referral letters, emails, entries in patient's notes, and, increasingly, the use of social media.

Sharing information with patients

When considering the sharing of information there are two key perspectives that must be taken into account: the person giving the information and the person receiving it. The person giving the information needs to firstly understand the information that is to be shared. If the information relates to the diagnosis, for instance when test results are available, it is important that the doctor giving this information is aware of the full facts, including interpretation and implications for future management and treatment and prognosis, as the patient will most likely have questions to which they will want answers. It is important to seek all the relevant information before meeting with the patient wherever possible. This will help when conveying information to the patient, as it is important that the information is given in a clear and accurate manner and that questions are immediately answered in order to aid the decision making process.

Ensure an appropriate setting

In addition to ensuring that full knowledge and understanding of all the relevant information is to hand, it is wise to anticipate any reasonable questions the patient may ask, and be fully prepared for sharing important information. In many instances it is appropriate for a Specialist Nurse to be present to support the patient and to ensure the environment is appropriate. For instance, attention should be given to seating, privacy, and the avoidance of interruptions such as telephone calls or bleeps. Patients should be given the opportunity to have a family member or carer with them when receiving important information.

Check the patients starting point

Prior to sharing information with a patient it is important to check their starting point. As discussed in the previous chapter, some patients will already have given some thought to what their results, diagnosis, treatment, or prognosis might be. Most patients will have had consultations with other doctors and will have spoken to family or friends, or have checked the internet. Checking a patient's starting point by asking them what they understand so far, or what they have been told so far, and what they are concerned about, will then enable you to start at the appropriate point. This will help the patient feel that they have been listened to and that their concerns have been taken seriously. It is also important to note that not everyone will want the same amount of information. Some patients may want to know every detail, whereas others may want to know very little. It is important to take guidance from the patient by asking if they would like to go into more detail. Checking the patients starting point will also provide an indication into the level of language and detail that will be most appropriate to use in order to aid the patient's understanding.

Be prepared to respond to questions. If there are any aspects of further treatment or management that you are unsure of, seek clarification before seeing the patient if possible. Remember that honesty is essential if there is uncertainty as to what the outcome, management or treatment plan will be. Patients will be much more accepting of a lack of information if one is honest with them. Any point of uncertainty should be acknowledged with an offer to find out and get back to the patient—which must be followed through.

Receiving information

When receiving information, the recipient needs to be able to concentrate on what is being said and so it is important to ensure a suitable environment where there will be no interruptions. It is also important to allow time for news to be absorbed.

Patients are able to remember information more easily if they are able to link it to existing knowledge. By checking the patient's starting point, you will have some insight into what they already know and this insight can be used to make links to the new information to be shared with them.

It can also help to aid memory if the patient is asked to repeat what has been said. At the end of the discussion, asking the patient to explain what has been discussed, provides an opportunity to check their understanding and to go over any areas of misunderstanding again. Similarly frequent summarizing of the information given will aid understanding and allow the patient a chance to ask for further clarification.

Guidelines for information sharing

Set the agenda

Inform the patient what information is to be shared, whether this is about results and/or diagnosis, management, further investigations, or treatment.

Summarize the current situation

At this point, it is important to summarize any previous information, results, or treatment plans. The meeting with the patient may be for any of the reasons mentioned, but it is important to recap to ensure that both the clinician and the patient are clear about the starting point for further information sharing.

Find out the patient's current understanding

It is important to establish the patient's understanding about their condition. There will almost certainly have been previous discussions, either with you, other members of the team or their GP. For example, if the patient states that they are waiting for the results of the computed tomogram/magnetic resonance imaging scan or a histology result to see if they would need surgery, then use this as the starting point for giving information 'As you said, we were waiting for the results of your recent biopsy before making a decision as to what happens next. Well the results show that the lump is a form of cancer, therefore I would confirm that surgery is recommended. There are a number of things to consider before you make your decision about the type of operation, but before we address those, do you have any questions?'

Provide structure

Structure will help ensure that the necessary information is imparted and will also aid the patient's recall. Prior to meeting with the patient, organize the information and discussion points into a logical order. When thinking about organization and structure, if there is a lot of information to give it can help to give the most important information first because recall decreases with time. Also, if you have provided a lot of information, repeating the main points as a 'recap' can aid recall.

Language

Ensure that the patient can understand the language used. Avoid using jargon and medical terms, but if this is unavoidable, use lay language first and then give the medical term.

Drawings

Drawings can be helpful when conveying information relating to the anatomy and surgical procedures and can help to aid understanding. If there is access to a computer, there are also a number of patient information resources available that include diagrams and pictures for a number of procedures.

Shared decision making

Once the information has been shared, it is important to explore the patient's view so that alternative management options can be discussed and a decision taken about the most appropriate management and treatment plan.

Check understanding

Finally, it is important to check that the patient has fully understood the information that has been shared and also that any decision taken is fully understood by both patient and clinicians. A straightforward way to check for understanding is to ask the patient to repeat back what has been said and what will happen now.

Sharing information with colleagues

Doctors work with medical colleagues with different levels of experience and grade, and from different specialities. In addition, doctors also have to share information with other members of the healthcare team.

Many of the principles of sharing information are the same for both patients and colleagues. However, when sharing information with colleagues, the topic is often more focused and usually relates directly to patient care. There are a number of factors that can influence the information sharing process that need to be considered. Regardless of whether the colleague is the same profession or from a different profession, they will have their own workload to consider and their own set of priorities. The information to be shared might be considered of high importance to you, but other members of the healthcare team might not realize the significance of the information unless it is made clear to them. Therefore the information needs to be clear and presented in a structured manner, using understandable language with action points.

When considering language, it is important to note that each speciality has its own subset of language, which becomes shorthand to aid communication between the team. However, these language subsets are often 'jargon' to others. Therefore, if the information sharing involves doctors from other specialities such as when making a referral, it is important to avoid abbreviations and jargon and to use language that will be understandable to others.

It is also important to check that the information that has been shared has also been understood. A way of ensuring this is to ask for the information to be repeated back to allow for checking and interpretation. It is also good practice to ask if any further clarification is required. Finally, if action is required as a result of the information, then stating this and identifying the salient points will assist the person receiving the information.

A number of tools have been developed that aid the information-sharing process between clinicians when it is imperative that information is communicated in a structured an organized way, to enable priorities to be set, and to ensure action is taken when immediate attention is required.

Handover

Handovers are an area that have received increasing attention in the UK in recent years and this refers to situations when responsibility for patient care is transferred, for example, between shifts, for new admissions, when responsibility for a patient changes (transfer to a different specialist), or when patients are to move wards or departments or go to the operating theatre.

Toolkits[1] provide guidelines and structure to handover mechanisms with recommendations that training in handover should be provided for all staff. How information is shared has a major impact on the information retained and acted upon. Again, structure is of major importance and the checklists include key information to be shared, including the ongoing chain of care, the number of patients handed over and their priority (red, amber, green), and those patients requiring special attention. Sharing information in this way, using a structured approach to sharing information, improves patient safety.

For handover to another speciality or organization, a standardized handover document has now been developed by the Royal College of Physicians.[2]

SBAR: Situation, background, assessment, recognition

The SBAR tool has been developed to aid conversations when immediate action is required. It prompts staff to formulate information in a standardized manner to ensure that information is shared using a concise and focused approach.

The tool includes four sections:

S—Situation

- Identify yourself and the site/unit/ward that you are calling from.
- Identify the patient by name and the reason for your call.
- Describe your concern.

B—Background

- Give the patient's reason for admission.
- Explain significant medical history.
- Give the patient's background (admitting diagnosis, date of admission, prior procedures, current medications, allergies, relevant laboratory results and other diagnostic results).

A—Assessment

- Vital signs.
- Clinical impressions and concerns.

R—Recommendation

- Explain what you need (be specific about request and timeframe).
- Make suggestions.
- Clarify expectations.
- What is your recommendation?

Adapted from the SBAR Toolkit, available from the Institute for Healthcare Improvement at: http://www.ihi.org/knowledge/Pages/Tools/SBARToolkit.aspx. The SBAR Toolkit was originally developed by Michael Leonard, Doug Bonacum, and Suzanne Graham at Kaiser Permanente of Colorado.

This approach is particularly useful for telephone consultations with senior colleagues in urgent situations when it is essential to be comprehensive, clear and concise. This will enable the colleague to make a clear decision and plan of action.

Written communication

Referral letters

An essential component of information sharing is through the written word and this frequently involves writing referral letters, emails, and making entries in patient notes.

It is important to strike a balance between covering all of the essential information and not overloading the reader with detail. Formal referral letters should be structured and organized and include relevant content. The following is a guide to the structure and content of a referral letter but as the content for referrals differs, decisions will need to be made about the exact detail to include depending on the reason for referral.

The patient demographic information should include name, date of birth, address, telephone number, and name and address of GP practice. It should also be clear on the referral letter who the referral is being made too (by name) and who the referrer is.

The next section should include clear information about the reason for referral, including the urgency of the referral, followed by the patient's history (presenting complaint, history of presenting complaint, relevant past medical history, medication and social information), examination findings, and management to date, including investigations and assessments.

The final section of the letter should include an indication of expectations of the referral. A summary of the discussions with the patient and their current understanding and expectations should be provided.

Referral letters should always be written with the view that the patient will see it, regardless of whether this is routine policy or not, and therefore the use of medical language should be avoided wherever possible, or explained to the patient so that they understand the content.

Email

Email correspondence is now a major form of communication within our working lives. Emails tend to be written slightly less formally than letters and often quite informally to people that we know well and, while this is on the whole hugely beneficial, it can also bring with it a number of challenges.

When writing emails we sometimes have a conversation with the person we are writing to in our head and hear the 'tone' of the conversation. However, our 'tone' is not always translated into written word or interpreted in the same way that we intended by the reader and so we need to be conscious of this when constructing an email message.

Email provides a very quick method of communication but there are downsides to this. For example when we receive an email, or someone says something that we are not happy about, the initial temptation is to write an email in response, indicating our dissatisfaction. Very often, after we have reflected on this, we are left with some regret about the tone and content of our message sent 'in the heat of the moment' (sometimes to the whole department). When we are feeling unhappy or dissatisfied, it is advisable to resist pressing the send button for a few hours, during which time you will have had time to calm down and review the situation. At this point you may want to edit the message to give a more reasonable response, while still making your point.

As a result of the speed and convenience of email, most of us receive a large volume of messages. This impacts on how we read our messages, often scanning quickly on our smartphones, rather than at our desks. We therefore need to think about the content of our messages. Messages that are very long with extensive detail can be more difficult to read, with the reader often not fully engaging or switching off. Be sure to keep content to the essential information with key points only.

Social media

The use of social media has increased exponentially in recent years and can provide very useful tools for keeping in touch with colleagues and friends and getting updates from professional organizations with social media profiles. However, there are a number of factors that need to be considered as others can easily access online information. Information published online can also be difficult to remove.

Patient confidentiality should never be compromised. Confidentiality is much more than simply not identifying a patient by name, as the collective information that is available may be enough for someone to identify the patient.

With regard to privacy, you may have protected your profiles, but social media providers do not guarantee to reset the privacy settings you have chosen originally when updating software.

The General Medical Council published the document 'Doctors' use of social media' which provides useful guidance on the use of social media.[3]

Conclusion

Information sharing is a core element of daily work and is something that can lead to dissatisfaction for colleagues and more importantly for patients when we do not get it right. Within this chapter we have considered a number of basic principles for sharing information. Frameworks and structures can be useful when sharing important information, whether with patients or colleagues and whether face to face or in written form. Tools, such as the SBAR tool and handover framework, particularly when we have concerns that a patient's condition may be deteriorating, are incredibly useful for ensuring that information is shared in an efficient and effective way. The increased use of technology with email and social media results in new considerations to ensure that our sharing of information is maintained in an effective way.

References

1. Royal College of Physicians. *Acute care toolkit 1: Handover*. London: Royal College of Physicians, 2011. Available from https://www.rcplondon.ac.uk/resources/acute-care-toolkit-1-handover (accessed 1 February 2016).
2. Royal College of Physicians. *Standards for admission, handover, discharge, outpatient and referral records*. London: Royal College of Physicians, 2013. Available from https://www.rcplondon.ac.uk/resources/standards-admission-handover-discharge-outpatient-and-referral (accesssed 1 February 2016).
3. General Medical Council. *Doctors' use of social media*. London: General Medical Council, 2013. Available from http://www.gmc-uk.org/guidance/ethical_guidance/21186.asp (accessed 1 February 2016).

CHAPTER 4.6

Surgical consent

Robbie Lonsdale

History of consent

The history of consent is the history of the balance of power between the patient and the surgeon. According to Plato,[1] the need for consent depended on the status of the patient, from a slave it was unnecessary, but when treating a free man there was a duty to discuss the nature and proposed treatment of the condition and obtain his permission to undertake the treatment. When treating Kings and Emperors the balance of power was shifted so far towards the patient that not only was consent obtained verbally but the patient had to physically put the scalpel into the hand of the surgeon to indicate his free will for the surgical intervention.[2]

The power of surgeons relative to their patients was perhaps highest during the Victorian era. Prominent surgeons such as Cooper and Liston were famous, wealthy, and had few social equals. The very act of having sought the help of such an eminent man was felt to be sufficient to allow him to do whatever he felt fit. Surgeons were paternalistic and in theory sought to decide what was good for their patient. Any communication that did take place was directed towards reassuring patients of a good outcome.

With the onset of the twentieth century there was a gradual recognition that consent, which had long been established in English common law as a defence against a charge of battery, was needed for surgical practice. This was perhaps most famously enunciated by Justice Cardoza[3] who said in 1914 that 'every adult human being of adult years in sound mind has a right to determine what shall be done with his own body; and a surgeon who performs an operation without his patient's consent commits a battery for which he is liable in damages'. He did not however, stipulate that there was any responsibility on behalf of the surgeon to ensure that the patient was informed.

The Second World War brought profound changes in doctor's relationships with patients and to the practice and understanding on consent. In Europe and its empires the old-fashioned class system, whereby the masses were content to be ruled by a small elite, was swept away bringing a majority Labour government in the United Kingdom and independence for colonies. The common man and woman were determined to have their say in how they were governed and also in how they were medically cared for. The horrors divulged during the German Doctors' Trials broke the spell that doctors were by dint of their profession good, and opened the door to a climate in which it was acceptable to challenge a doctor's thinking and advice. The requirements for consent in medical research were codified at Nuremberg and were followed by the rapid realization that patients were entitled to the same rights when considering involvement in treatment. America now led the way with a number of important cases defining the legal requirements of informed consent.

In Salgo vs Leland Stanford Jr University Board of Trustees 1957[4] the court of appeal in California was asked to consider the case of Martin Salgo who in 1954 had suffered paralysis following a translumbar aortogram. They ruled that the procedure had not been negligently done but that the doctor had negligently failed to inform the patient of the risks of the procedure and therefore did not have valid consent. Justice Bray, borrowing the words of a submission by the American College of Surgeons, said 'A physician violates his duty to his patient and subjects himself to liability if he withholds any facts which are necessary to form the basis of an intelligent consent by the patient to the proposed treatment.' Having produced such clarity, Bray immediately opened up another debate on how much information should be disclosed to a patient.

Here the American and English courts diverged. American courts adopted the standard laid out in Canterbury vs Spence 1972[5] that required a disclosure of information if a reasonable person in the patient's position would be likely to attached significance to the risk. In Sidaway vs Bethlam Royal Hospital Governors 1985[6] English courts adopted the Bolam standard for informed consent which allowed a defence that a surgeon was not required to inform patients of rare complications if a reasonable body of similar surgeons would not do so. While the Law defined the minimum requirements of informed consent, medical bodies and health organizations in many countries were issuing guidance on informed consent which attempted to define ideal practice. In the UK the General Medical Council consent guidance 'Consent, patients and doctors making decisions together' came into effect in June 2008.[7] The guidance provided increasingly suggested that surgeons needed to provide the information required by the patient to make a decision. In this respect the practice recommended for obtaining consent followed the American legal position rather than that of Sidaway. This change in practice and change in the relationship between surgeon and patient was recognized in the United Kingdom Supreme Court in 2015. In a landmark judgement, Lord Reed and Lord Kerr after referring to the GMC consent guidance said "The doctor is therefore under a duty to take reasonable care to ensure that the patient is aware of any material risks involved in any recommended treatment, and of any reasonable alternative or variant treatments."[8]

Information giving

Information giving or sharing is a two-way process of mutual education between surgeon and patient. A surgeon may have detailed knowledge of a patient's condition and the potential treatments but may know nothing of what is important in a patient's life. An individual patient may know much or little of their condition and possible treatments and may have a limited or profound understanding of complex issues such as risk and probability. The process, whereby a surgeon comes to an understanding of a patient's needs and wishes and the patient develops a depth of understanding about their condition, begins at the time of referral and develops through the process of consultation. This process of mutual education may not necessarily be achieved in one consultation and the process of consent may be spread over a number of consultations. Other healthcare professionals and other sources of information such as patient leaflets and on line resources may contribute to the process.

The General Medical Council in its guidance to doctors in the UK has indicated that they have an overriding duty to give information to the patients about:

(a) The diagnosis and prognosis.

(b) Any uncertainties about the diagnosis or prognosis, including options for further investigations.

(c) Options for treating or managing the condition, including the option not to treat.

(d) The purpose of any proposed investigation or treatment and what it will involve.

(e) The potential benefits, risks and burdens, and the likelihood of success for each option; this should include information, if available, about whether the benefits or risks are affected by which organization or doctor is chosen to provide care.

(f) Whether a proposed investigation or treatment is part of a research programme or is an innovative treatment designed specifically for their benefit.

(g) The people who will be mainly responsible for and involved in their care, what their roles are, and to what extent students may be involved.

(h) Their right to refuse to take part in teaching or research.

(i) Their right to seek a second opinion.

(j) Any bills they will have to pay.

(k) Any conflicts of interest that you, or your organization, may have.

(l) Any treatments that you believe have greater potential benefit for the patient than those you or your organization can offer.[7]

Reproduced from General Medical Council, *Consent guidance: Sharing information and discussing treatment options*, Copyright © General Medical Council 2015. All rights reserved. Available from http://www.gmc-uk.org/guidance/ethical_guidance/ consent_guidance_sharing_info_discussing_treatment_options.asp

It is important that the information given to patients is individual to that patient. Any assessment of risk may be informed by a surgeon's overall success rate for that procedure but must also take into account any additional risk stemming from the patient's own individual characteristics and co-morbidities. It is important that a surgeon confirms that a patient has retained and understood the information given.

Level of risk discussed

The likelihood of a particular adverse event occurring as a result of an intervention may vary from certainty (i.e. a probability of one) to an infinitesimally small chance (i.e. a probability of 0.0000001 or less). For example, a patient undergoing a sapheno-femoral ligation, stripping of the long saphenous vein and multiple avulsions for extensive varicose veins will certainly experience some bruising but is most unlikely to suffer an arterial injury resulting in limb loss. A surgeon seeking consent from a patient would certainly explain about postoperative bruising but should he/she discuss the minute

risk of an arterial injury? Prior to 2015 the legal position in the USA was slightly different from that in the UK. In the USA the standard adopted is that the surgeon should explain a risk that a reasonable patient would wish to consider however remote that risk may be. In the United Kingdom a surgeon was only required to explain risks that a reasonable surgeon would explain and it had been suggested that a risk of less than 1% need not be discussed.

Both positions have their problems particularly where patient's understanding of the quantification of risk may be limited. In the USA there is a danger that a patient may be confronted with a long list of terrible possible complications such that the patient may decline to undergo a potentially life-saving procedure that they would otherwise have agreed to. In the UK there is a risk that a surgeon may not explain a rare complication to a patient that unbeknown to the surgeon is of crucial importance to the patient in deciding whether or not to undergo the treatment. In practice the legal positions define the minimum defensible standards and surgeons on both side of the Atlantic aim to apply best practice to provide patients with as much information as they need to develop sufficient understanding of the proposed treatment in order to make an informed decision. This includes exploring with patients the complications that are important to them and their understanding of risk.

It is important to recognize that individual patients may have very different thresholds for accepting particular complications; to one patient a colostomy may be a minor inconvenience whereas to another it may be completely unacceptable. It is also important to recognize that many patients find different levels of risk hard to understand. Some patients will understand risk in terms of numerical chance, whereas others will have a better understanding if risk is described in comparative terms such as the risk of travelling 100 miles in a car.

Capacity

If a patient is to give informed consent they must have 'capacity' to do so. 'Capacity' is the ability of a patient to reach a clear understanding of their condition, the proposed treatment, and the risks and side effects involved. They should also be able to make and communicate a decision as to whether they wish to consent or refuse the medical care proposed. If a patient is unable to reach this clear understanding or to make or communicate a decision they may be said to lack 'capacity'. 'Capacity' is therefore procedure specific and a patient may only be said to lack 'capacity' once every effort has been made to obtain informed consent. A patient cannot be said to lack 'capacity' simply because they make an unwise decision, nor can they be said to lack 'capacity' simply because they are detained for reason of their mental health. Surgeons must be prepared to spend the necessary time and to use all possible methods of communicating with patients to allow a patient to give informed consent.

When patients lack 'capacity'

The management of patients who lack 'capacity' differs between jurisdictions. In England and Wales the Mental Capacity Act of 2005[9] includes provision for advanced directives to refuse treatment, lasting powers of attorney, and an independent mental capacity advocate service that has greatly simplified these issues. Importantly in the UK, although relatives of patients can expect to be consulted, they do not have the right to give consent on behalf of a patient who lacks 'capacity'. In other jurisdictions such as Canada and some States in the USA, arrangements for patients without 'capacity' involve the use of a substitute decision maker with a hierarchy of legal substitutes and family members.

In considering surgery on patients who lack 'capacity' there are a number of generally agreed principles:

Patients should be involved in the decision-making process as much as they are able. Where the patient's prior views are known these should be respected.

Where 'capacity' may return and a procedure is not urgent the procedure should be delayed until 'capacity' has returned.

Any intervention should be in the patient's best interest. This is particularly important where a third party contributing to making a decision on behalf of a patient may have a vested interest in the decision. This may apply to a surgeon who may receive a fee for undertaking an operation or a relative who may stand to gain from an inheritance if the patient does not survive.

In all cases it is sensible to seek the opinion of both medical and other colleagues and it is useful to remember that going to court before the event is likely to be less traumatic than after the event.

Deprivation of Liberty safeguards, introduced into the Mental Capacity Act through the Mental Health Act 2007,[10] additionally allow application to be made to detain a patient who lacks 'capacity' for the purpose of care or treatment.

Coercion

For informed consent to be valid the patient must have made a decision free of outside pressure. Coercion in this context can manifest itself in many ways. The mildest form of coercion, encountered reasonably frequently, is by medical staff or family members who seek to coerce a patient into making a particular decision in the belief it is in the patient's best interest. Coercion may be subtle but may have sinister motives. For example, a surgeon may seek to dissuade a high-risk patient from having an operation by giving an over bleak assessment of the likely outcome when the surgeon's true motive is to avoid damage to his published outcome figures. Similarly, a family member may seek to persuade a patient with a chronic infected leg ulcer to undergo an amputation because the family member finds the smell offensive rather than because of any benefit to the patient. Financial coercion of patients remains a controversial subject. The crudest example has been the 'cash for organs' controversy where the sale of body parts for transplantation has been the subject of much media interest. In the UK and USA altruistic donation of organs between two strangers is legal but donation in return for payment is not. This area of law is, however, difficult to regulate and there is significant evidence that a 'cash for organs' trade goes on in some of the poorest communities in developing countries. The shortage of organs for donation and the evidence that a significant illegal underground trade in organs goes on has led some to question whether the sale of organs should be allowed. This has been considered by the medical ethics committee of the British Medical Association who remain opposed to the practice.[11]

Children

The issue of gaining consent for the treatment of children is complex and the law varies from country to country and sometimes between different states within the same country. In each case the child's age and their capacity are of crucial importance. In general, very young children will not have the 'capacity' to make medical decisions whereas older teenagers will. However, there is no specific age at which 'capacity' can be assumed. As with adults 'capacity' is procedure specific. For example, a young child brought to the emergency department with an asthma attack who has previously had nebulizers may have 'capacity' to give consent to treatment with a nebulizer. However, the same child may not have sufficient understanding to give consent for complex invasive surgery. Where a child does not have 'capacity' to make a decision they should still be involved in the decision-making process as much as possible.

In England and Wales children aged 16 and 17 years would normally be expected to have 'capacity' and therefore the consent process is essentially identical to that in an adult. In these circumstances it would seem reasonable to encourage the child to seek the views of their parents but if the child is disinclined so to do then their confidentially should be respected unless there are specific circumstances in which disclosure should be made to protect the child from harm. Very occasionally the courts have agreed to overrule a competent child's decision not to undergo treatment if the treatment has been considered to be in the child's best interest. Children aged 16 and 17 who lack 'capacity' to take a decision are treated differently from adults who lack 'capacity' in that a parent or more strictly a person with parental responsibility can give consent. The Children's Act 1989[12] sets out who legally has parental responsibility but in some respects the act does not fit in with modern domestic arrangements that may include strong caring relationships without the formality of marriage or, in the case of parents of the same sex, civil partnership. In particular, fathers do not have an automatic legal right to give consent for treatment of their children. Where there is disagreement between parents or where parents refuse consent to treatment that a surgeon considers to be in the child's best interest then it is sensible to involve the courts. The arrangements in Scotland for children aged 16 and 17 years, who lack 'capacity' is different—parents cannot give consent on their behalf but rather they are treated in the same way as adults who lack 'capacity'.

Whereas children of 16 years and older are presumed to have 'capacity', those under 16 years are not. Nevertheless some children under 16 years will have 'capacity' to consent to some procedures. This is sometimes referred to as Gillick competence after the House of Lords ruling in the case of Gillick versus West Norfolk and Wisbeck Area Health Authority 1985.[13] This ruling established that 'the parental right to determine whether or not their minor child below the age of sixteen will have medical treatment terminates if and when the child achieves sufficient understanding and intelligence to understand fully what is proposed.' This ruling has been followed in Australia, Canada, and New Zealand. In practice a surgeon consulted by a child under 16 years must first establish whether the child is competent to give consent for the procedure in question. If the child is found to be competent, the surgeon should discuss with the child whether they wish a parent or other adult to be involved in the decision-making process but if the child does not, their confidentiality must be respected and the child be allowed to make the decision on their own behalf.

If a child under 16 years does not have 'capacity' to give or refuse consent then an adult with parental responsibilities should make the decision on the child's behalf.

Difficulties in obtaining consent for the treatment of children who lack 'capacity'

In the vast majority of cases there is clear agreement between health professionals and parents as to the best treatment for the child. In these cases obtaining consent is straightforward. Difficulties can arise if there is disagreement between the parties or where one or other parent lacks 'capacity'. Where parents disagree with a treatment plan that the surgeon feels is in the child's best interest, for example where blood transfusion is considered in a child whose parents are Jehovah's Witnesses, then it is sensible to seek a second opinion prior to proceeding to involvement of the courts. Occasionally there will be disagreement between parents particularly when parents are estranged. In these cases it is not a legal necessity to obtain the consent of both parents and treatment can be given, if it is in the child's best interest, with the consent of one parent. However, where the child's main carer is the parent objecting, then it is sensible to proceed with caution and perhaps involve the courts anyway. Occasionally one or other parent may not be able to give consent, either because they lack 'capacity' or because the parent is a child themselves. In these cases it is sensible to seek the views of other important carer's of the child, for example grandparents.

Consent for procedures that are not therapeutically beneficial to the child (e.g. bone marrow harvest for donation to a sibling)

The concept of the patient's best interest is fundamental to decision making in patients, including children, who do not have 'capacity'. Where a child lacking in 'capacity' is volunteered as a bone marrow donor by parents who are primarily considering the interests of the recipient child, this concept is tested. It could perhaps be argued that preserving the life of the recipient child is in the best interest of the donor child, but this seems an artificial argument and it could be equally argued that in later life when it comes to dividing an inheritance one more sibling might be a disadvantage. An alternative argument is that we allow parents to make decisions that disadvantage one child in favour of another. Many little sisters freezing on the touchline while an older brother plays football will attest to this. The important issue then becomes the degree of harm done to the donor child. The current view is that bone marrow harvest is perhaps 'no big deal' and therefore permissible, but that a more invasive procedure such as kidney donation would not be.

Similar arguments are used when considering surgical procedures on children that are undertaken primarily because of parent's cultural and religious beliefs. Male circumcision and female genital mutilation fall into this category. The World Health Organization estimates that between 100 million and 140 million women and girls have undergone female genital mutilation.[14] Despite this there is widespread support for the view that it causes unacceptable harm and it is specifically prohibited in the United Kingdom, Sweden, and Belgium and prohibited under more general legislation in many other countries. Male circumcision is more difficult. It is an intrinsic part of two major religions, Islam and Judaism, and is undertaken on millions of young boys globally. In the vast majority of cases the harm done is limited and short lived, but in a small number of cases significant harm is done. Historically, law makers seeking to ban circumcision have largely been motivated by a desire to repress communities of the Jewish or Muslim faith rather than any primary concern for the child's right. However, a body of medical opinion is opposed to circumcision on religious grounds. In 2012 this view was supported by a district court in Cologne, Germany, where a doctor was charged following complications in a 4-year-old boy on whom a circumcision had been performed for religious reasons. The court, while acquitting the doctor, ruled that circumcision that was not medically necessary was an assault and conflicted with the child's right to subsequently decide on their religious beliefs.[15] The case caused considerable concern among the Muslim and Jewish communities worldwide and attracted support from other religious leaders seeking to safeguard religious freedoms. The German government legislated to overturn the ruling in December 2012[16] and religious circumcision therefore remains legal in Germany. In other jurisdictions it remains common practice but untested in law.

Emergency care

In the emergency situation the ability of a surgeon to obtain consent may be limited by the patient's 'capacity' if the patient is seriously ill with significant impairment of consciousness, and may be limited by time if the patient's best interest is served by immediate treatment. In the former case the matter is straight forward and should be dealt with as in any patient lacking 'capacity' excepting the fact that there is limited opportunity for a surgeon to consult others. The latter situation is more difficult. The patient may be fully conscious and have 'capacity' but the need for emergency intervention may limit the clinician's ability to fully inform the patient and to be informed of the patient's wishes. In this situation a pragmatic approach must be adopted using what time is available to explain the patient's options as fully as the time permits while at the same time providing the immediate treatment needed to save life or prevent a serious deterioration in the patient's condition. It is important to be aware that initial treatment of an individual may allow a situation to be stabilized and allow time for fully informed consent to definitive treatment.

Procedures requiring consent

Legally any touching of another human being, whether in a medical or non-medical context, requires consent. In normal life this consent is often implied and we accept a varying degree of contact from others depending on the situation. A rugby player accepts being tackled by his opposite number during the course of a game but would find it unacceptable elsewhere; a passenger entering a crowded train carriage accepts a greater degree of contact with fellow passengers than would otherwise be appropriate. Much of medical contact with patients takes place on the same basis. A doctor asking to take a patient's blood pressure would regard the rolling up of a patients sleeve as implying consent. In all cases the onus rests on the doctor to ensure that the patient fully understands the implications of the procedure and gives their consent free from coercion. The same doctor who asked a patient to give a blood sample and accepted a rolled up sleeve and proffered antecubital fossa as consent, would be falling short of acceptable standards if he/she had not explained to the patient the nature of the test to be undertaken and its possible implication for the patient. On a pragmatic basis the greater the implications of the intervention the greater the care needed in obtaining and recording consent.

Recording consent

Consent to measure a patient's blood pressure would not normally be recorded, and consent to undertake physiotherapy on a patient may be recorded in the patient's notes by the practitioner but not necessarily signed by a patient. Consent for all surgical procedures is always recorded on a specific consent form which documents the nature of the discussion had with the patient and to which the patient adds their signature as a record of their consent. The consent form is a record and, as with any record, it is only valid if it is a true reflection of the discussion and decision making that has taken place. Where patients lack 'capacity' to make the decision a specific consent form exists in which the doctor should record the decision-making process and also who has been consulted in making the decision about treatment.

Further reading

British Medical Association. Consent Toolkit. London: British Medical Association (available from bma.org.uk/practical-support-at-work/ethics/consent-tool-kit).
General Medical Council. 0–18 years: guidance for all doctors. London: General Medical Council, 2007 (available from http://www.gmc-uk.org/guidance/ethical_guidance/children_guidance_index.asp).

References

1. Bury RG. *Plato Laws*. London: Heinemann, 1926:212–3; 238–9; 306–9; 454–7.
2. Ioannes von Ephesos. *Historia ecclesiastica, vol III*. Louvain: EW Brooks, 1964: 91–6.
3. Schloendorff vs Society of New York Hospital, 211 N.Y. 125, 105 N.E. 92 (1914).
4. Salgo vs Leland Stanford Jr. University Board of Trustees. 154 Cal. App. 2d 560, 317 P.2d 170 (1957).
5. Canterbury vs Spence, 464 F.2d 772 (D.C. Cir. 1972).
6. Sidaway vs Bethlam Royal Hospital (1984) All Engl Law Rep. Feb 23; [1984] 1: 1018–36.
7. General Medical Council. Consent: patients and doctors making decisions together. http://www.gmc-uk.org/static/documents/content/GMC_Consent_0513_Revised.pdf (accessed 10th February 2014)
8. Montgomery v Lanarkshire Health Board. UKSC 11 (11 March 2015). https://www.supremecourt.uk/cases/uksc-2013-0136.html (accessed 19th March 2016).
9. UK Mental Capacity Act 2005. http://www.legislation.gov.uk/ukpga/2005/9/contents (accessed 10th February 2014).
10. UK Mental Health Act 2007. http://www.legislation.gov.uk/ukpga/2007/12/section/50 (accessed 10th February 2014).
11. Kidney sale proposal sparks medical ethics debate. *The Guardian*. http://www.theguardian.com/society/2011/aug/03/kidney-sale-proposal-medical-ethics (accessed 10th February 2014)
12. UK Children Act 1989. http://www.legislation.gov.uk/ukpga/1989/41/contents (accessed 10th February 2014).
13. Gillick vs West Norfolk and Wisbeck Area Health Authority. 1984 All Engl Law Rep. 1984 Nov 19-Dec 20 (date of decision); 1985(1): 533–59. http://www.bailii.org/uk/cases/UKHL/1985/7.html (accessed 10th February 2014)
14. World Health Organization. Female genital mutilation and other harmful practices. http://www.who.int/reproductivehealth/topics/fgm/prevalence/en/index.html (accessed 10th February 2014).
15. Zeldin W. Law library of Congress. Germany: Regional court ruling criminalizes circumcision. http://www.loc.gov/lawweb/servlet/lloc_news?disp3_l205403226_text (accessed 10th February 2014).
16. Federal Republic of Germany. Civil Code § 1631d circumcision of the male child. http://dejure.org/gesetze/BGB/1631d.hatml (accessed 10th February 2014).

Perioperative management

Section editor: Jeremy Groves

CHAPTER 5.1

Preoperative assessment

Mireille Berthoud

Introduction

There are three primary goals of preoperative assessment. The first is to assess perioperative risk. This requires a detailed knowledge of the patient's underlying fitness, the level of their functional reserve, and the risks of the surgical and anaesthetic procedure that is planned. The second is to minimize perioperative risk by developing an appropriate care plan, which may include medical or social optimization. The third is to educate the patient about the choices he or she has before, during, and after their procedure, both to relieve anxiety and to enable the patient to give informed consent. To achieve this preassessment needs to be timely, allowing for the possibility of medical optimization prior to surgery.

Secondary aims of preoperative assessment are economic. It allows elective patients to be admitted to hospital on the day of their surgery, fully prepared with a documented perioperative plan that is tailored to their individual needs. It disseminates the information needed to run theatres efficiently, thus minimizing delays and cancellations. It reduces length of stay in hospital and offers opportunities for general health promotion that has lasting effect for patients beyond their immediate surgical need.

Preoperative assessment is a multidisciplinary process. The service is increasingly nurse practitioner led with support from other clinicians. The surgeon's role is vital. An understanding of the patient's perioperative risk will ensure early referral to the preoperative assessment clinic, and will enable frank discussions at every stage of the process with the operating team, the patient, their family, and general practitioner.

The preoperative assessment clinic is aimed at the elective surgical patient. Patients are assessed by a history, physical examination, and investigations. Of these a thorough history is the most informative. Further information gathering is frequently needed and the process can be resource heavy and time consuming. Recently, secure electronic questionnaires have been developed that patients can fill in online. These aim to streamline the process and triage the patients so that the most complex of them are directed to the most senior assessors. For the fittest they may even avoid a hospital visit altogether.

Emergency surgical patients are still assessed and prepared by the admitting surgical team. The same fundamental principles of risk assessment and optimization apply to the emergency surgical patient, but are made much more difficult by time constrains in balancing preoperative preparation against the risk of surgical delay.

Understanding and communicating perioperative risk

Risk is the probability of something harmful happening in the perioperative period and must be balanced against the likely benefit of surgery. Communicating risk to patients is a difficult art. Medical practitioners do not always have an objective understanding of individualized operative risk, and patients often have their own established perceptions of risk and the level they think acceptable. The way that risk is presented to a patient will influence the way they understand it. Risk can be presented in words, in numbers or visually (Figure 5.1.1).[1] Relating probability to everyday events such as winning the lottery can also help. Offering someone a 5% chance of dying sounds very different from offering them a 95% chance of survival.

Scoring systems can help clarify perioperative risk. The most widely used scoring system in anaesthesia is the ASA (American Society of Anesthesiologists) grade. This was first proposed in 1963,[2] and is based on the patient's history and examination. It stratifies risk for mortality and morbidity.[3] British anaesthetists often misinterpret these grades as relating to functional capacity. The ASA grade has a number of problems; its very simplicity makes it subjective, it fails to account for the type and urgency of surgery, and disregards the age of the patient (Table 5.1.1).

Metabolic equivalents (METs) are also widely used to assess functional status in terms of cardiorespiratory reserve. One MET can be defined as the oxygen cost of sitting quietly, and in the average person is equivalent to 3.5 mL/kg/min. Four METs are equivalent to climbing a flight of stairs briskly without stopping. The stress of major surgery has a metabolic cost that can extend for several days postoperatively, and patients who cannot deliver enough oxygen to meet this extra demand will be at higher risk of organ failure, sepsis, and death. Patients who cannot manage four METs have been shown to be at high risk of postoperative complications and death after abdominal surgery.[6] Conversely, when functional capacity is high the prognosis is excellent, even in the presence of stable ischaemic heart disease or other risk factors.

The Physiology and Operative Severity Score for Enumeration of Mortality and Morbidity (POSSUM) is used to predict mortality based on physiological and on operative factors.[3,7] For this reason it cannot be used preoperatively. This score tends to over predict mortality in patients with low scores and in certain surgical specialties. This has led to modifications such as the P POSSUM and CR POSSUM. Links to ready calculators for these and other risk scores can be found at http://www.riskprediction.org.uk and http://www.surgicalriskcalculator.com.

Cardiovascular risk

Major cardiovascular complications (defined as myocardial infarction, cardiogenic pulmonary oedema, or cardiac arrest) are still the leading cause of death within 30 days of surgery. Mortality increases with the severity of surgery and this must be factored into

Numbers	1 person in 10	1 person in 100	1 person in 1000	Up to 1 person in 10000	1 person in 100000
Numbers	10%	1%	0.1%	0.01%	0.001%
Words	Very common	Common	Uncommon	Rare	Very rare
Pictures	Someone in a family 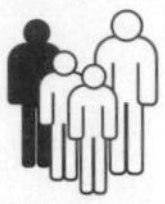	Someone in a street 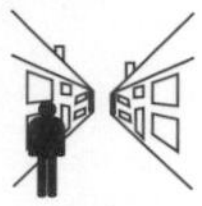	Someone in a village 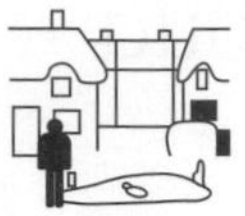	Someone in a small town 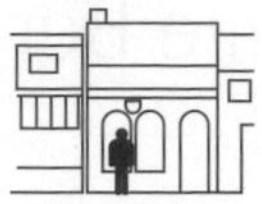	Someone in a large town 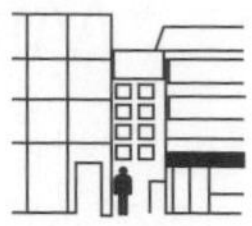
Common examples	The chance of rolling a 6 with a dice	The chance of getting three balls in the UK lottery	The chance of getting four balls in the UK lottery	The chance of dying in a car accident in any one year in the UK	The chance of dying of murder in any one year in the UK

Fig. 5.1.1 Some ways of expressing risk and probability.

Adapted with permission from Dr Mark Withers, Rotherham General Hospital and The Royal College of Anaesthetists, *Risks and Probability*, Copyright © 2003 The Royal College of Anaesthetists (RCA) and The Association of Anaesthetists of Great Britain and Ireland (AAGB), available from http://www.rcoa.ac.uk/node/427

any preoperative risk assessment (Table 5.1.2). The most common co-existing conditions seen in patients requiring surgery are cardiovascular. The American College of Cardiology and American Heart Association (ACC/AHA) have developed guidance to assist with preoperative management of these, updated in 2014.[4,8]

The ACC/AHA stratifies predictors of operative cardiovascular risk into major, intermediate, and minor. Major risk is associated with five conditions: acute (within 1 week) or recent (within 1 month) myocardial infarction (MI); unstable angina (Canadian class 3 or 4); malignant arrhythmias including fast atrial fibrillation; decompensated heart failure; and severe valve abnormalities, especially critical aortic stenosis. Full clinical evaluation of these conditions at preassessment often requires complex or invasive investigations. Patients with major cardiovascular risk need a multidisciplinary approach that includes anaesthetists, surgeons, and cardiologists. Every effort must be made to optimize these patients and, if possible, surgery should be delayed until this is achieved, or even reconsidered. This approach is important for any patient

undergoing general anaesthesia, but is especially so for high-risk surgical procedures. Patients with these conditions will need expert anaesthetic care, invasive monitoring, meticulous goal directed fluid management, and planned critical care postoperatively.

Considering each of these major risk factors in more detail:

◆ The ACC/AHA recommends that elective surgery should be postponed for 6 weeks after an MI, provided a recent stress test does not indicate residual myocardium at risk. Optimization of angina increasingly favours the medical approach.

◆ Revascularization is reserved for those patients in whom it would be independently indicated, for example in left main stem disease or acute coronary syndrome, and where elective surgery can wait for 6 weeks. Coronary bypass surgery itself carries risks, and surgical patients who have coronary stents pose special challenges with regard to the management of their dual antiplatelet agents. Premature discontinuation of antiplatelet therapy after coronary stents, especially drug eluting ones, markedly increases

Table 5.1.1 American Society of Anesthesiologists (ASA) grade and perioperative risk of death in different surgeries and ages

ASA Grade	Definition	Mortality % All surgical Patients[4]	Mortality % Age under 50, major emergency surgery[2,5]	Mortality % Age over 70, major emergency surgery[2,5]	Mortality % Age under 50, major elective surgery[2,5]
1	Normal healthy individual	0.05	1.6		0.3
2	Mild systemic disease that does not limit activity	0.14	4.5	12.9	0.9
3	Severe systemic disease that limits activity but is not incapacitating	0.93	12.4	30.6	2.7
4	Incapacitating systemic disease which is constantly life threatening	6.17	29.6	56.9	7.6
5	Moribund, not expected to survive 24 hours with or without surgery	27.35	Close to 100		

Source: data from Bainbridge D et al., For the Evidence-based Peri-operative Clinical Outcomes Research (EPiCOR) Group. Perioperative and anaesthetic-related mortality in developed and developing countries: a systematic review and meta-analysis, *The Lancet*, Volume 380, Issue 9847, pp. 1075–81, Copyright © 2012; and Donati A et al., A new and feasible model for predicting operative risk, *British Journal of Anaesthesia*, Volume 93, Issue 3, pp. 393–9, Copyright © 2004.

the risk of stent thrombosis, MI, and death, especially at the time of surgery when the associated stress response leads to a hypercoagulable state.

- Arrhythmias must be controlled preoperatively. Atrial fibrillation should be rate controlled, aiming at a resting heart rate below 90 beats per minute. Cardioversion can be considered, but would need to be followed by warfarin therapy for at least six weeks.

- Goldman[9] in his cardiac risk index gave most points to patients with decompensated heart failure; treating this preoperatively is essential.

- Aortic stenosis needs special consideration because it can be critical (defined as a valve area of less than 0.6 cm^2/m^2 body surface area or a peak gradient of more than 65 mmHg) yet asymptomatic. Critical aortic stenosis, of all the above conditions, is associated with the worst cardiac outcome after non-cardiac surgery. Patients with undiagnosed systolic murmurs should be investigated by cardiac echocardiogram (ECHO), especially if they are symptomatic, or have electrocardiogram (ECG) or chest X-ray changes. Patients with known moderate or severe aortic stenosis should have a repeat ECHO at least annually. Aortic valve replacement prior to elective but necessary non-cardiac surgery is recommended in symptomatic patients and in patients with critical aortic stenosis.

Patients should undergo tests only if the results of the investigations are likely to influence management. The decision to investigate becomes more difficult when the potential benefit of the investigation is less clear cut, as in patients with the ACC/AHA guideline's intermediate cardiovascular risk. Intermediate risk has been defined by Lee's Revised Cardiac Risk Index[5,10] and this, together with an

Table 5.1.2 Surgical specific cardiac risk (combined risk of cardiac death and non-fatal MI) stratification: Examples of procedures are given[8]

High risk (cardiac risk > 5%)	Intermediate risk (cardiac risk 1% to 5%)	Low risk (cardiac risk <1%)
Aortic and other major vascular surgery	Intraperitoneal surgery	Body surface surgery
Peripheral vascular surgery	Intrathoracic surgery	Breast surgery
	Carotid endarterectomy	Cataract surgery
	Head and neck surgery	Ambulatory surgery
	Major orthopaedic surgery	
	Prostate surgery	

Reprinted from *Journal of the American College of Cardiology*, Volume 54, Issue 22, Fleischmann *et al.*, 2009 ACCF/AHA Focused Update on Perioperative Beta Blockade, pp. 2102–28, Copyright © 2009, with permission from Elsevier, http://www.sciencedirect.com/science/journal/07351097

assessment of the patient's functional capacity and the surgery specific risk, are used to decide a management strategy (Figure 5.1.2). Lee's risk index was designed for patients undergoing non-cardiac surgery. It has been validated and widely adopted, and includes five independent clinical determinants of risk for major perioperative cardiac events: a history, or ECG evidence, of ischaemic heart disease; compensated or prior heart failure; cerebrovascular disease; diabetes mellitus treated with insulin; and impaired renal function (creatinine > 177 μmol/L). Each factor contributes equally, scoring 1 point, and the incidence of major cardiac complications is estimated

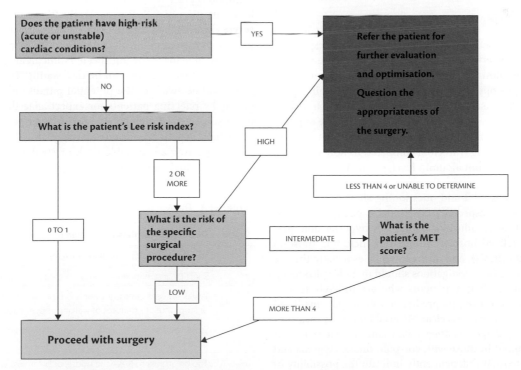

Fig. 5.1.2 Simplified guideline for the preoperative assessment of elective surgical patients with cardiac risk factors.

at 0.4%, 0.9%, 7%, and 11% in patients with an index of 0, 1, 2, and ≥3 points, respectively. It is recommended that patients who are undergoing major surgery, and whose Lee index is 2 or more, should be managed in the same way as those patients with high cardiovascular risk. The approach for patients with a Lee index of 2 or more undergoing intermediate surgery depends on their functional capacity.

Patients who have excellent functional capacity are unlikely to develop serious cardiac complications, even in the presence of pre-existing cardiac disease. The ACC/AHA guidelines recommend that patients with functional capacity greater than or equal to four METs without symptoms should proceed to planned intermediate surgery. If a patient's functional capacity is less than four METs or is difficult to assess, or if they are symptomatic, then a Lee index of 2 or more will indicate the need for further preoperative evaluation. Left ventricular function assessment, cardiac stress testing or cardiopulmonary exercise testing could be considered.

Patients with intermediate risk factors undergoing low-risk surgery can probably proceed for surgery without additional sophisticated cardiac assessment.

Minor cardiovascular risk factors do not require complex cardiac assessment and elective surgery should not be delayed. A common exception is where a patient's hypertension is sustained and above grade 2, or associated with end organ damage such as left ventricular hypertrophy or renal impairment. In such a situation blood pressure control is recommended preoperatively.

Cardiospecific β-blockers, low-dose aspirin, and statins should be considered preoperatively in patients undergoing surgery with high or intermediate cardiovascular risk factors. Patients already taking these agents must continue with them throughout the perioperative period if at all possible.

Respiratory risk

This section considers surgical patients with intrinsic respiratory disease, pulmonary hypertension, sleep apnoea, or a difficult airway.

Postoperative pulmonary complications are the second most common cause of postoperative mortality. Shallow breathing, poor lung expansion, and basal lung collapse are a particular risk in upper abdominal or thoracic surgery, where the incidence of pneumonia is between 10% and 40%. Other factors that contribute to this risk are heavy smoking (threefold compared to non-smokers), alcohol misuse, a low serum albumin level, or an abnormal blood urea nitrogen.

A detailed history is vital and questioning should explore the severity of the disease, especially functional capacity, complications such as right heart failure or pulmonary hypertension, previous respiratory-related hospital admissions including those to intensive care units (ICUs), and all treatments, especially the use of home oxygen. Specific investigations should include spirometry, which can accurately identify patients who are unlikely to survive lung resection; however, its predictive role in patients listed for other types of surgery is less clear. Arterial blood gas measurement should be considered in patients who cannot exercise to four METS, and is required in those with cor-pulmonale. Hypoxia and carbon dioxide retention independently indicate the possibility of postoperative respiratory failure, and patients with abnormal blood gases undergoing general anaesthesia will need a critical care bed postoperativly. A routine chest X-ray is rarely helpful preoperatively, and alters management in only 1–4% of respiratory patients.

Patients with Medical Research Council scale dyspnoea grade 4 or 5 (Table 5.1.3)[11] undergoing major surgery will need expert advice. All elective surgical patients with current lower respiratory tract infection or bronchospasm must be treated fully before surgery. Another preoperative intervention of proven benefit to patients with significant chronic lung disease is pulmonary rehabilitation.[12] This is a complex intervention that includes exercise and training in breathing techniques as well as counselling and education. It is expensive and time consuming for clinic and patient alike, and so expert advice should be sought before recommending it.

Patients with severe pulmonary hypertension (right ventricular/systemic systolic pressure ≥ 0.75) pose a particularly challenging problem as the symptoms are non-specific and the perioperative mortality is very high. The cardinal symptom is dyspnoea; other worrying symptoms are chest pain and syncope. The ECG, chest X-ray, and spirometry may all be normal, although an ECG will show right ventricular hypertrophy in 87%, and right axis deviation in 79% of patients with idiopathic pulmonary hypertension. An ECHO is the non-invasive test of choice to estimate systolic pulmonary artery pressure.

Obstructive sleep apnoea (OSA) is another under diagnosed condition. When unsuspected, it can result in serious perioperative complications following general anaesthesia. These include difficult intubation, hypoxia, pneumonia, MI, pulmonary embolism, cardiac arrhythmias, and unanticipated admission to ICU. The risk increases with severity of OSA, with major or airway surgery, and with the use of opiate analgesia. The ASA task force have validated a questionnaire[13] that may indicate who would benefit most from expert referral before surgery. Sleep studies are diagnostic and are helpful in determining the severity of the condition. The preoperative interventions that have been advocated for OSA patients are continuous positive airway pressure (CPAP) treatment and weight loss. Initiation of CPAP preoperatively should be considered in severe OSA. High-risk patients require postoperative care that can provide oxygen monitoring and respiratory support if needed.

Failure to manage the unexpected difficult airway in anaesthesia is a rare occurrence, but can be devastating. Head and neck surgeons will be aware of the potential pitfalls; others can also help greatly by referring patients for expert anaesthetic assessment if this is suspected. A difficult airway can be suspected from previous anaesthetic experiences or records suggesting this, and from symptoms suggesting an unstable neck or stridor. Clinical signs may include a limited mouth opening, tongue obscuring the view of the

Table 5.1.3 The Medical Research Council breathlessness scale

Grade	Degree of breathlessness related to activities
1	Not troubled by breathlessness except on strenuous exercise
2	Short of breath when hurrying on the level or walking up a slight hill
3	Walks slower than most people on the level, stops after a mile or so, or stops after 15 minutes of walking at own pace
4	Stops for breath after walking about 100 yards or after a few minutes on level ground
5	Too breathless to leave the house, or breathless when undressing

Reproduced from *British Medical Journal*, Significance of Respiratory Symptoms and the Diagnosis of Chronic Bronchitis in a Working Population, Fletcher C *et al.*, 1959 August 29; Volume 2, Issue 5147, pp. 257–266, Copyright © 1959 with permission from BMJ Publishing Group Ltd.

posterior pharyngeal structures (modified Malampatti[14] score of 3 or 4), or restriction in flexion and extension of neck movements and a short thyromental distance (≤6 cm).

Cardiopulmonary exercise testing

Cardiopulmonary exercise testing (CPET), is fast becoming a routine preoperative evaluation for patients undergoing major surgery. CPET is an objective assessment of cardiac, respiratory, and cellular function and differentiates between these systems in any potential cause for an individual being unable to meet their oxygen demands. It is the best test we have for heart failure; it is also able to detect myocardial ischaemia, ventilation and perfusion mismatch, and pulmonary hypertension. There are three important derived measurements in CPET testing: VO_2 max (the maximum possible oxygen consumption, or maximal aerobic capacity of an individual); VO_2 peak (the highest oxygen consumption achieved during the CPET if VO_2 max is not reached); and AT (the anaerobic threshold, or the point at which oxygen debt is being met by anaerobic metabolism in the cell).

Many studies have shown that the risk of developing serious complications after major surgery is closely associated with peak VO_2, and AT.[7,15] Predicted peak VO_2 differs in men and women and falls with increasing age. Increased mortality seems to be associated with VO_2 levels of less than 15 mL/kg/min^{-1}. The AT is often reached before the end of the CPET, and is not determined by the patient's effort, unlike the peak VO_2. It therefore offers a more objective measure of the combined efficiency of the lungs, heart, and circulation. An AT of at least 10–11 mL/kg/min is required to undertake major surgery safely.

In high-risk patients, CPET can suggest early interventions that may improve risk preoperatively and it allows an appropriate perioperative management plan that includes high dependency or intensive care. In very high-risk patients, it informs decisions about the appropriateness of the planned surgery.

CPET takes about 20 minutes to perform. The patients must consent to the test and it is important that any referral include details of the patient's health, as well as any drugs they may be taking. Some patients will need medical supervision during the test. The patient needs to be able to cycle, or walk on a treadmill, and will be connected to a 12-lead ECG, blood pressure cuff, and pulse oximeter. Inspired and expired gases are sampled via a mouthpiece or facemask (Figure 5.1.3). Contraindications to CPET can be found at

http://ajrccm.atsjournals.org/content/167/2/211.full.pdf+html.[16] It has a reported mortality of 2 to 4 in 100 000.

Renal risk

Postoperative acute kidney injury (AKI) is a serious complication, increasing the risk of progressive renal failure, and death in both the short and long term. Patients with AKI who need renal support after surgery have the poorest outcome. By far the most important determinant of postoperative AKI is the baseline renal function. A recent meta-analysis[17] has suggested that estimated glomerular filtration rate (eGFR) is predictive of both AKI and death after surgery, with the risk of 30-day mortality increasing twofold, fourfold, and sixfold in chronic kidney disease stages 3, 4, and 5, respectively, when compared to patients with normal renal function. Quick calculators for eGFR are available online from the Renal Association (http://www.renal.org/egfrcalc).

Kheterpal et al.[18] identified seven independent predictors of AKI in patients with normal preoperative renal function undergoing major non-cardiac surgery: age over 59; peripheral vascular disease; chronic obstructive pulmonary disease needing bronchodilators; liver disease; body mass index over 32 kg/m^2; high-risk surgery; and emergency surgery. They found that the overall incidence of AKI was 0.8%, rising to 4.3% when three or more of these risk factors were present.

Preassessment of surgical patients with existing chronic renal failure needs to review and treat both the causes and complications. It is essential that advice is sought from the patient's renal physician. Electrolyte, acid–base, and fluid balance must be optimized and corrected preoperatively. Fluid overload can lead to pulmonary oedema and pleural effusions. Patients on, or needing, dialysis must have this timed to within 24 hours of surgery. Chronic renal failure is also associated with hypertension, accelerated ischaemic heart disease, and peripheral vascular disease. Anaemia of chronic disease is very common, and patients may have either a bleeding risk though poor platelet function, or an increased clotting risk. Endocrine problems include hyperparathyroidism and diabetes. Venous access may be difficult and cannulation sites must be chosen to preserve arteriovenous fistulas and potential fistula sites.

Preoperative renal risk stratification provides the best opportunity for early planning to minimize renal damage, including operating on high-risk patients where facilities for postoperative renal support are available.

Perioperative management of diabetes

Good perioperative diabetic control is important in reducing surgical complications. The main anxiety for surgeons and patients is the increased incidence of wound and other infections. Postoperative infection and even mortality are associated with poor preoperative diabetic control,[19] irrespective of whether or not the patient is on insulin. The effectiveness of a patient's diabetic control for the preceding three months can be determined by measurement of the HbA1c. Many preoperative assessment units will postpone routine surgery if the HbA1c is above 8.5% (70 mmol/mol), to enable better diabetic stabilization before surgery. Performing this screening test early in the referral pathway will minimize delay. The risk of delaying surgery should always be weighed against the infection risk from poor diabetic control.

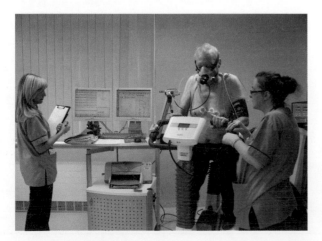

Fig. 5.1.3 Inspired and expired gases are sampled via a mouthpiece or facemask.

Further information is given in the chapter on Metabolic and Endocrine Disorders.

Neuromuscular disorders

Many of these conditions have commonalities when it comes to preassessment (Table 5.1.4). All are associated with respiratory insufficiency to some degree and bulbar dysfunction may also be present. Cardiomyopathy and autonomic dysfunction is sufficiently common that preassessment should fully investigate this possibility. Patients need formal assessment of respiratory reserve, and often echocardiography, especially if major surgery is contemplated. Monitoring must continue into the postoperative period and the requirement for respiratory support be considered.

Malignant hyperpyrexia is a rare life-threatening familial condition of abnormal calcium release from the sarcoplasmic reticulum to specific agents. Volatile anaesthetics and non-depolarizing muscle relaxants are powerful triggers. All patients presenting for anaesthesia, not just those with neuromuscular disorders, must be questioned about previous complications of pyrexia or of ICU admissions following anaesthesia in either themselves or blood relatives. The British Malignant Hyperthermia Association based in Leeds can be contacted for advice and a register of known patients with malignant hyperpyrexia in the UK (http://www.bmha.co.uk/indexpatients.html).

The patient with addiction

Morbidity associated with chronic alcohol misuse is increasingly common and the demographic is becoming younger. Surgical patients who misuse alcohol are two to five times more likely to develop complications, have admissions to ICU, or have a prolonged hospital stay. Every preassessment should explore alcohol use. The CAGE questionnaire[20] (www.uspreventiveservicestaskforce.org/Home/GetFileByID/838) is short and easy to use in clinical practice. It highlights those patients with a score of ≥2, indicating that they may be at risk of alcohol withdrawal syndrome (AWS). Testing the gama gluteryl transferase, mean cell volume , aspartate transaminase will increase sensitivity. AWS commonly occurs 6 to 24 hours after ceasing drinking, and if not treated can be life threatening. Prophylactic treatment with benzodiazepines can prevent AWS in up to 75% of patients and can reduce symptoms in the rest. Thiamine and vitamin B complexes are given to prevent complications that may occur from nutritional deficiencies. Other conditions associated with chronic alcohol use that must be screened for and optimized are malnutrition, liver disease (including cirrhosis), cardiomyopathy, autonomic dysfunction, thrombocytopenia, and polyneuropathy.

Drug misuse is also becoming more common in the surgical population. All patients should be questioned about their use both of prescription medications and other substances. The DAST questionnaire (https://www.drugabuse.gov/sites/default/files/files/DAST-10.pdf)[21]

can provide a more detailed assessment. The perioperative problems associated with drug misuse are withdrawal, co-morbidity especially in intravenous drug users, and planning analgesia for chronic opioid users. Conditions in drug misuse that need to be screened for are malnutrition, difficult venous access, human immunodeficiency virus, hepatitis, and endocarditis.

Patients who are acutely under the influence of drugs or alcohol should not undergo elective surgery.

The elderly

Postoperative mortality increases exponentially with age. In one study[22] of 7696 surgical procedures, in patients aged over 80 the morbidity rate was 51% and the mortality rate 7%, compared with 28% and 2.3% in the cohort as a whole. Much of this is due to pre-existing disease, but age alone is a significant independent risk factor after 80 years. Patients with poor nutrition and patients who are in residential care have more than twice the mortality rate after major surgery when compared with other patients of a similar age.

The physiology of ageing reduces cardiorespiratory, renal, and neurological reserve. A healthy 80-year-old person's systemic vascular resistance will increase by 45% compared to a 25 year old. This increase in after load leads to systolic hypertension, left ventricular wall thickening, and longer systole in an attempt to preserve stroke volume, and a delay in early diastole. These changes make accurate fluid balance essential, as both under filling and overload are very poorly tolerated. Cardiac diseases are less well tolerated, present

Table 5.1.4 Perioperative problems associated with neuromuscular disorders

Associated anaesthetic problem	Multiple sclerosis	Parkinson's disease	Muscular dystrophies	Myotonic syndromes	Myasthenia gravis
Respiratory insufficiency, including aspiration risk	Yes	Yes	Yes	Yes	Yes
Cardiac abnormalities, cardiomyopathy or conduction abnormalities		Rarely	Yes	Yes	
Autonomic dysfunction	Yes	Yes	Yes	Yes	
More sensitive to anaesthetic agents or muscle relaxants	Yes	Yes	Yes	Yes	Yes
Sustained contraction or massive hyperkalaemia with suxamethonium			Yes	Yes	
Malignant hyperpyrexia			Yes[a]		
Essential to continue all specific therapy		Yes			Yes

[a]For hypokalaemic periodic paralysis with abnormal post-junctional Ca++ channel.

differently, and often need a different therapeutic approach. For example, ischaemic heart disease is more likely to present as dyspnoea rather than angina.

The main physiological change in the lungs in old age is an increase in ventilation and perfusion mismatch due to increases in both lung and chest wall compliance allowing airways collapse. Sleep apnoea is common and the cough reflex reduced. The elderly are more likely to suffer postoperative hypoxia, atelectasia and, in up to 25% of patients, pneumonia.

Renal blood flow and the number of nephrons decline with increasing age, but the creatinine may stay normal until 80% function is lost as the muscle mass also declines. Postoperative acute renal failure is more common in the elderly.

There is a progressive loss of neurones, with a decline in grey matter with increasing age. This may not be clinically detected until 80% loss has occurred. Postoperative cognitive dysfunction in the elderly is common and distressing. Detectable preoperative cognitive deficits are associated with especially poor outcomes. Cognitive function should be assessed before surgery.

Concurrent disease in the elderly surgical patient is common and may affect several systems. Preassessment requires methodical examination and optimization of potentially complex disease states. A multidisciplinary approach is often needed, and early input from physicians with an interest in the elderly improves outcome and decreases length of stay after surgery. Anticipation of postoperative complications, with a written management plan in place before surgery, allows early intervention, limits disability is a simple and cost-effective way of saving both lives and resources. The possible requirement for organ support and considerations for future quality of life must be discussed with the patient and their family, and their views observed in any management plan.

Preoperative management of iron-deficient anaemia

Preoperative anaemia affects 24–43% of patients having major non-cardiac surgery, depending on age and type of surgery. Its presence is associated with increased postoperative mortality, morbidity and length of hospital stay. This is a correctable condition that must be addressed, so early identification becomes very important. When identified, further investigations are needed to answer two questions. First, what is the underlying cause of the anaemia; and secondly, will it respond to iron or other medications preoperatively? Follow up tests should include serum iron, ferritin, and transferrin saturation index.

Traditionally, preoperative patients with iron-deficient anaemia are treated in two ways. They are either prescribed oral iron, which is still the preferred method provided time allows it (a 70 kg patient with a chronically low haemoglobin of 90 gms/L would take 2 weeks of treatment for the haemoglobin to start to rise, 2 months for it to reach normal values, and 6 months for the iron stores to fill), or for more urgent surgery patients are treated by blood transfusion. However, allogeneic blood transfusion is independently associated with poorer outcome after surgery, and should be avoided if at all possible. Many recent studies in a variety of surgical specialities have shown that preoperative administration of the newer intravenous iron preparations is a safe alternative, and reduces the need for perioperative blood. Intravenous iron is the best way of guaranteeing delivery of available iron to the bone marrow. It can be given as an outpatient, takes about 15 minutes to administer, and increases haemoglobin by 10.0 ±6.0 gms/L, 2 weeks after the start of treatment.

Preoperative laboratory tests

Preoperative tests should never be routine. Each one must be clinically justified. Investigating patients is costly and unnecessary testing can result in harm and anxiety, for example, where false positive results lead to further or more invasive tests or delays. Conversely, omitting important tests can also result in surgical delay, cancellation, and even in unnecessary surgery. In 2003 the National Institute for Health and Clinical Excellence issued guidance for the common preoperative tests (summary of pre-operative testing guidance https://www.nice.org.uk/guidance/cg3 and full guidance https://www.nice.org.uk/guidance/cg3/chapter/5-Full-guideline). This is based on patients' cardiovascular, respiratory and renal co-morbidity as determined by ASA grade, and on the complexity of the surgery. NICE state that their recommendations 'should be considered only as a guideline. Healthcare professionals involved in pre-, peri- and postoperative care must use their professional knowledge and judgement when applying the recommendations to the management of individual patients'.

Managing patients' medications preoperatively

In general patients should continue their medications as normal before surgery, with some exceptions. This is especially true where acute withdrawal could result in harm, in which case alternative agents or routes of administration must be prescribed where patients may be unable to take or absorb oral medications (Table 5.1.5). Tablets can safely be taken with a sip of water 2 hours before anaesthetic induction. Where patients are advised to stop medications before surgery, they must be given written instructions which include when it is safe to restart them.

Angiotensin-converting enzyme inhibitors and angiotensin II receptor blockers may exaggerate the hypotensive effects of anaesthesia, which can be difficult to control with vasopressors. Stopping them may result in hypertension. A pragmatic approach is to stop them on the day of surgery, except where they are prescribed for poor left ventricular function rather than hypertension. They can be restarted soon after anaesthesia, when the patient is haemodynamically stable.

Stopping low-dose aspirin may cause a rebound prothrombotic state, which will be exaggerated by the stress response to surgery. Many patients are taking aspirin for secondary prevention of cardiac or cerebral thrombosis. Omitting aspirin in this scenario has been shown significantly to increase the risk of major adverse cardiac events post surgery.[23] Patients with cardiac stents, especially drug-eluting stents, are at very high risk of stent thrombosis if antiplatelet therapy is omitted during the first year after revascularization. The perioperative mortality of stent thrombosis is around 50%. Aspirin is associated with increased surgical bleeding, but in many operations this is not clinically significant, especially when compared with the risks due to thrombosis. Mounting evidence suggests that low-dose aspirin should be continued peri-operatively except in those operations where bleeding could be critical, such as during neurosurgery.

Table 5.1.5 Guidance for perioperative management of common medications

Drugs that are more likely to cause harm if stopped	Comments	Drugs that more likely to cause harm if continued	Comments
Aspirin 75 mg daily	Continue UNLESS neurosurgery, middle ear surgery or very high risk of bleeding	Aspirin ≥ 300 mg daily	Omit for 7 days or change to low-dose aspirin. (Seek advice if patients has a coronary stent)
Antidepressants, anxiolytics or anti-epileptics	Potential for withdrawal or precipitate seizures	Clopidogrel	Omit for 7 days. (Seek advice if the patient has a coronary stent)
β-Blockers	Cardio-protective and potential for with drawl	Dipiridamole	Omit for 48 hours
Statins	Cardio-protective and anti-inflammatory	Warfarin	Omit for 5 days: assess need for bridging anticoagulation
Cardiac drugs, especially treatments for heart failure		Newer oral anticoagulants	Seek advice
Clonidine	Withdrawal hypertension	ACE inhibiters and Angiotensin 2 blockers	Omit on the day of surgery UNLESS the treatment is for left ventricular impairment
Asthma treatments	May need to increase these peri-operatively	Non-steroidal anti-inflammatory drugs	Omit 72 hours
Steroids	Increase dose in patients who are on replacement steroids for pituitary or adrenal insufficiency	Herbal medicines	Omit for 7 days
Proton pump inhibiters		HRT	Omit for one month
Oral contraceptive	Will need appropriate DVT prophylaxis	Viagra	Omit 24 hours
Anti-Parkinsonian treatments		Long acting insulins	Omit on the day of surgery
Diuretics	Except K sparing, which should be stopped	Long acting oral hypoglycaemics	Omit on the day of surgery
Opioid analgesia	Potential for withdrawal	Anti-tumour necrosis factor α medications	Omit for two weeks before surgery

References

1. Smith A, Adams A. Principles in raising the standard: Information for patients. In: Lack JA, Rollin A, Thoms G, White L, Williamson C (eds). *Risk Communication and Anaesthesia*. London: The Royal College of Anaesthetists; 2003. Available from http://www.rcoa.ac.uk/document-store/raising-the-standard-information-patients-february-2003.
2. Dripps RD. New classification of physical status. *Anesthesiology* 1963; 24: 111.
3. Wolters U, Wolf T, Stützer H, *et al*. ASA classification and perioperative variables as predictors of post operative outcome. *Br J Anaesth* 1996; 77(2): 217–22.
4. Bainbridge D, Martin J, Arango M, *et al*. Perioperative and anaesthetic-related mortality in developed and developing countries: a systematic review and meta-analysis. *Lancet* 2012; 380(9847): 1075–81.
5. Donati A, Ruzzi M, Adrario E, *et al*. A new and feasible model for predicting operative risk. *Br J Anaesth* 2004 Sep; 93(3): 393–9.
6. Karapandzic VM, Petrovic MZ, Krivokapic ZV, *et al*. Duke Activity Status Index in coronary patients undergoing abdominal nonvascular surgery. *Internet J Cardiol* 2010; 1(9): DOI: 10.5580/16b.
7. Copeland GP, Jones D, Walters M. POSSUM: a scoring system of surgical audit. *Br J Anaesth* 1991; 78(3): 355–60.
8. Fleisher LA, Fleischmann KE, Auerbach AD et al. ACC/AHA guideline on perioperative cardiovascular evaluation and management of patients undergoing noncardiac surgery: executive summary: a report of the American College of Cardiology/American *Circulation*. 2014;130(24):2215–45.
9. Goldman L, Caldera DL, Nussbaum SR, *et al*. multifactorial index of cardiac risk in noncardiac surgical procedures. *New Engl J Med* 1977; 297(160): 845–50.
10. Lee TH, Marcantonio ER, Mangione CM, *et al*. Derivation and prospective validation of a simple index for prediction of cardiac risk of major noncardiac surgery. *Circulation*. 1999; 100: 1043–9.
11. Bestall C, Paul EA, Garrod R, *et al*. Usefulness of the Medical Research Council (MRC) dyspnoea scale as a measure of disability in patients with chronic obstructive pulmonary disease. *Thorax* 1999; 54(7): 581–6.
12. Sekine Y, Chiyo M, Iwata T, *et al*. Perioperative rehabilitation and physiotherapy for lung cancer patients with chronic obstructive pulmonary disease. *Jpn J Thorac Cardiovasc Surg* 2005; 53: 237–43.
13. Gross JB, Bachenberg KL, Benumof JL, *et al*. Practice guidelines for the perioperative management of patients with obstructive sleep apnea: a report by the American Society of Anesthesiologists Task Force on Perioperative Management of patients with obstructive sleep apnea. *Anesthesiology* 20; 104(5):1081–93.
14. Samsoon GL, Young JR. Difficult tracheal intubation: a retrospective study. *Anaesthesia* 1987; 42(5): 487–90.
15. Smith TB, Stonell C, Purkayastha S, *et al*. Cardiopulmonary exercise testing as a risk assessment method in non cardio-pulmonary surgery: a systematic review. *Anaesthesia* 2009; 64(8): 883–93.

16. The American Thoracic Society. ATS/ACCP Statement on Cardiopulmonary Exercise Testing. *Am J Resp Crit Care Med* 2003; 167(2): 211–77.

17. Mooney JF, Ranasinghe I, Chow CK, *et al.* Preoperative estimates of glomerular filtration rate as predictors of outcome after surgery: a systematic review and meta-analysis. *Anesthesiology* 2013; 118(4): 809–24.

18. Kheterpal S, Tremper KK, Englesbe MJ, *et al.* Predictors of postoperative acute renal failure after noncardiac surgery in patients with previously normal renal function. *Anesthesiology* 2007; 107(6): 892–902.

19. Frisch A, Chandra P, Smiley D, *et al.* Prevalence and clinical outcome of hyperglycemia in the perioperative period in noncardiac surgery. *Diabetes Care* 2010; 33(8): 1783–8.

20. Ewing JA. Detecting alcoholism: the CAGE Questionnaire. *JAMA* 1984; 252(14): 1905–7.

21. Skinner, H. The Drug Abuse Screening Test. *Addict Behav* 1982; 7(4): 363–71.

22. Turrentine FE, Wang H, Simpson VB, *et al.* Surgical risk factors, morbidity and mortality in elderly patients. *J Am Coll Surg* 2006; 203(6): 865–77.

23. Oscarsson A, Gupta A, Fredrikson M, *et al.* To continue or discontinue aspirin in the perioperative period: A randomized, controlled clinical trial. *Br J Anaesth* 2010; 104 (3): 305–12.

CHAPTER 5.2

Intraoperative care

David M. Cressey

Prior planning and preparation protects patients

World Health Organization 'Safe Surgery Saves Lives'

In 2008, the World Health Organization (WHO) established the 'Safe Surgery Saves Lives' initiative to reduce the number of unnecessary surgical deaths and complications. The initiative aims to address important safety issues including inadequate safety practices, avoidable surgical site infections, and poor communication among team members. WHO established ten essential objectives for safe surgery:[1]

1. The team will operate on the correct patient at the correct site.

2. The team will use methods known to prevent harm from administration of anaesthetics, while protecting the patient from pain.

3. The team will recognize and effectively prepare for life threatening loss of airway or respiratory function.

4. The team will recognize and effectively prepare for risk of high blood loss.

5. The team will avoid inducing an allergic or adverse drug reaction for which the patient is known to be at significant risk.

6. The team will consistently use methods known to minimize the risk for surgical site infection.

7. The team will prevent inadvertent retention of instruments and sponges in surgical wounds.

8. The team will secure and accurately identify all surgical specimens.

9. The team will effectively communicate and exchange critical information for the safe conduct of the operation.

10. Hospitals and public health systems will establish routine surveillance of surgical capacity, volume and results.

Adapted with permission from *World Health Organization (WHO) Surgical Safety Checklist,* Copyright © WHO 2009, available from http://www.who.int/patientsafety/safesurgery/tools_resources/9789241598552/en/

The WHO surgical checklist and local adaptations of it is a recommended set of standard procedures to follow for every patient undergoing surgery.

This includes the 'sign-in' before induction of anaesthesia, which confirms the correct patient is present and has consented for the agreed procedure, and that the surgical site is correctly marked and allergies and risks of bleeding or difficult intubation have been identified.

The 'time-out' before the start of surgical intervention is a further check that the correct patient is present on the operating table and that all necessary staff are present and equipment available. Any significant surgical or anaesthetic risks are identified at this point and consideration given to aseptic technique, antibiotic, and venous thromboembolism prophylaxis.

The 'sign-out' is for confirmation of an adequate record of the procedure, that all equipment used is accounted for, specimens labelled, and that any concerns for postoperative care have been identified.

Five steps to safer surgery

In December 2010, along with the three steps of the WHO Surgical Check list, the National Patient Safety Agency (NPSA) supported the addition of team brief and debriefing sessions at the beginning and the end of theatre lists to make 'five steps to safer surgery'. These steps aim to promote team performance and safety, with additional benefits of reducing delays, improving communication, and creating a safety climate.[2]

Patient positioning

Another key aspect of intraoperative care is the protection of the patient from inadvertent injury while under anaesthesia. Safe transfer of the patient and positioning on the operating table are vital. Knight and Mahajan have published a concise summary of this aspect of care.[3]

All patients are at risk of injury if attention to positioning is not ensured, but certain patient groups (extremes of age, particularly the older patient, morbid obesity or marked cachexia, those with skin fragility [long-term steroid use]) and certain procedures that require specific patient positioning (e.g. lithotomy) will carry extra risks of inadvertent injury.

The types of potential injury include pressure sores (increased risk in longer operations) and skin injury from adhesive dressings, nerve injury (direct pressure or stretch on susceptible nerves), thermal injury (both hypothermia and burns), corneal abrasions, vascular compromise, and electrical injury associated with diathermy use. Faulty equipment or misuse of equipment pose significant risks.

Pressure sores

Pressure sores are a major source of pain and distress, increasing the length of stay and costs. The process of skin necrosis may begin in the operating theatre. Simple measures, such as pressure relieving mattresses, gel pads for heels or occiput may reduce if not remove the risk.

Extra care when applying and removing adhesive drapes or dressings (electrocardiograph dots and eye tapes included) may reduce the risk of skin loss. Those patients on long-term steroids or those with thin and fragile skin are at increased risk.

Nerve injury

Nerve injury can be profoundly debilitating for the patient and is the second most common class of injury associated with claims in the USA (American Society of Anesthesiologists [ASA] Closed Claims Project database). Likely mechanisms include stretch, compression, and ischaemia of the nerve, although a clear-cut cause is often not identified. Certain co-morbidities such as diabetes (microvascular complications affect nerves) or pre-existing neuropathy may increase incidence, but all patients should be assumed to be at risk of nerve injury.

Brachial plexus injury is most likely to occur if the arm is abducted by more than 90° while the head is rotated away from the abducted arm causing compression against first rib, clavicle, and humerus. In the prone position care must be taken to ensure the chest support does not impinge on and cause compression of the plexus in the axilla.

More than 25% of all intraoperative nerve injuries involve the ulnar nerve. It is vulnerable to stretch and external compression in the ulnar groove at the elbow. Appropriate padding should be applied, especially in the prone position.

In the Lloyd-Davies and lithotomy positions, sciatic and obturator nerve injury can be caused by extreme flexion of the hip joints causing stretch. This may also lead to compression of the femoral nerve under the inguinal ligament. The common peroneal nerve (as it passes the neck of the fibula) and saphenous nerve (as it passes the medial condyle) are also at risk of compression injury. In the lateral position a pillow should be placed between the knees to prevent damage to these nerves.

The lithotomy position can lead to calf compression. The resulting reduction in perfusion pressure may increase the risk of venous thromboembolism and compartment syndrome. The longer the procedure, the higher the risk. If positioning the patient in lithotomy for over 5 hours invasive monitoring of calf pressures may be considered.

Eye injury

Corneal abrasion is the most common type of injury. The application of tape to keep the eyelid gently closed should minimize this risk, but eye ointment does not influence it. Direct pressure to the eyeball has the potential to cause retinal artery occlusion with the risk of loss of vision. During prone positioning a suitable head support that keeps pressure off the eyes must be used and the position of it checked during the course of surgery.

Patient falls

Major injury can arise as a result of a patient falling from the operating table during anaesthesia. Adequate measures should be taken to minimize this risk. This may be in the form of side supports, arm boards, and straps placed around the patient's legs and pelvis. When a patient is being transferred between bed or trolley and operating table it is vital for both patient and staff safety that staff are trained in techniques for transfer.

Physiological compromise from positioning

The supine position, particularly when associated with head-down tilt, increases the pressure applied to the diaphragm by the viscera. This causes reduction in lung volumes and increased atelectasis. Hypotension may arise as a result of venacaval obstruction against the vertebral bodies. Intracranial and intra-ocular pressures rise. There is an increased risk of passive regurgitation and aspiration of gastric contents. These features are magnified in the patient with morbid obesity. With head-up position the reverse applies but the risk of venous air embolism must be considered.

Temperature management

Inadvertent hypothermia

Inadvertent perioperative hypothermia is a common but preventable complication of operative procedures. Heat loss occurs from various physical processes (radiation, evaporation, conduction, and convection). Administration of cold fluids (intravenously or as intraperitoneal lavage) plus impairment of thermoregulatory heat-preserving mechanisms (i.e. peripheral vasoconstriction) caused by general or regional anaesthesia will further exacerbate this. Core temperature can be monitored at a variety of sites including nasopharynx, distal oesophagus, tympanic membrane (beware of errors relating to ear wax occluding the canal), rectum, and bladder.

Hypothermia, as well as being distressing for the patient, is associated with a variety of physiological disturbances, such as increased sympathetic activity, coagulopathy, and immunosuppression. Metabolic demands on the patients in the recovery phase increase due to shivering. Other risks from hypothermia include cardiovascular events, bleeding, delayed wound healing, infection, and increased morbidity. National Institute of Health and Care Excellence clinical guideline 65 addresses these issues.[4]

National Institute of Health and Care Excellence guidance

Hypothermia is defined as a patient's core temperature of below 36.0°C. Elective surgery should not commence if the patient's temperature is below 36.0°C. A variety of methods are available to actively warm patients but according to NICE there is only sufficient evidence to recommend forced air warming.[4]

Patients should be managed as higher risk for perioperative hypothermia if any two of the following apply:

◆ ASA grade II to V (higher the grade, greater the risk)

◆ preoperative temperature below 36.0°C (and preoperative warming not possible because of clinical urgency)

◆ undergoing combined general and regional anaesthesia

◆ undergoing major or intermediate surgery

◆ at risk of cardiovascular complications.

Those at higher risk who are having anaesthesia for less than 30 minutes and all patients for operations lasting longer than 30 minutes should be actively warmed intraoperatively.

All patients should be adequately covered throughout the intraoperative phase to conserve heat, and exposed only during surgical preparation. All intravenous fluids (500 mL or more) and blood products should be warmed to 37°C. All irrigation fluids used intraoperatively should be warmed to 38–40°C.

Monitoring standards during surgery

Basic and advanced techniques

In March 2007 the Association of Anaesthetists of Great Britain and Ireland (AAGBI) produced guidelines on perioperative monitoring standards. Monitoring devices supplement usual clinical observation by qualified medical staff. The minimum standard includes pulse oximeter (SpO2), electrocardiograph, and non-invasive blood pressure with appropriate alarm limits set. Advanced monitoring (CVC, arterial line, cardiac output assessment) may be indicated for specific patient co-morbidities or for certain operations associated with major physiological challenges. The key features of these monitoring modalities are outlined in Box 5.2.1 and 5.2.2.

Universal precautions

'Standard precautions'[5] are the basic level of infection control precautions that are to be used in the care of all patients to minimize the risk of transmission of blood-borne and other pathogens from both recognized and unrecognized sources to or from patients. In addition to hand hygiene, WHO recommends that the use of personal

---

Box 5.2.1 Principles of basic monitoring

Electrocardiography

- Allows interpretation of rate and rhythm, identifies conduction disorders, coronary ischaemia can be detected by ST segment depression
- Prone to artefacts from skin impedance and electromyographic noise
- Three or five electrode combinations can be used. The CM5 (clavicle-manumbrium-V5) lead modification is good for identifying left ventricular ischaemia

Non-invasive blood pressure

- Oscillometry is the most common method. The cuff is inflated above systolic pressure and then slowly deflates. The vibrations of arterial wall are detected. Systolic and diastolic arterial pressure are measured, mean is calculated. The cuff width must be 20% greater than the arm's diameter (too small a cuff will cause over-reading and too large under-reading)
- Arrhythmias and external pressure cause measurement inaccuracies
- Repeated measurements during prolonged surgical cases may cause pressure injuries and ulnar nerve damage

SpO2: Pulse oximetry

- Continuous measurement of arterial blood oxygen saturation, based on the difference in absorption spectra of oxygenated and de-oxygenated haemoglobin at 660 and 940 nm wavelengths
- Inaccuracies can arise due to low perfusion states, motion artefact, ambient light, venous congestion, carboxyhaemoglobin (artefactually high reading) and methaemoglobin (artefactually low reading), signal interference from nail varnish
- Prolonged use maybe associated with localized heat or pressure injury

Source: data from *Recommendations for Standards of Monitoring during Anaesthesia and Recovery, Fourth Edition*, The Association of Anaesthetists of Great Britain and Ireland, London, UK Copyright © 2007, available from http://www.aagbi.org/sites/default/files/standardsofmonitoring07.pdf

---

Box 5.2.2 Principles of advanced monitoring

Arterial line

- Records reliable beat-to-beat variation in blood pressure (important with expected rapid changes in blood pressure: rapid haemorrhage, planned hypotensive-anaesthesia (ear, nose, and throat, craniotomy, etc.))
- During long operations it avoids potential injury caused by repeated blood pressure cuff inflation
- It allows repeated blood gas sampling and analysis
- It may facilitate calculation of cardiac output (PiCCO, LiDCO, pulse pressure variation)
- There is an inherent risk of disconnection and exsanguination, arterial wall damage, thrombosis or vasospasm with distal ischaemia and infection

Central venous catheter

- May assist in the diagnosis of hypovolaemia/cardiac failure. Provides an estimate of right ventricular filing
- Monitors response to fluid volume challenge
- Provides central venous access to administer vasoconstrictors, inotropes and parenteral nutrition, and thrombophlebitic drugs
- Potential sites include jugular (preferred site NICE guidance), subclavian and femoral veins
- Ultrasound guidance with full asepsis for insertion is a NICE recommendation
- Complications include arrhythmias (from wire), vessel damage (including neighbouring artery) and haemorrhage (check for coagulopathy prior to insertion), catheter related infections (increased with femoral site) & thrombosis, pneumothorax, haemothorax, air embolus (use head-down position and occlusive ports for all access points during insertion and use)

Oesophageal Doppler

- Provides an estimate of cardiac output using Doppler principle to measure speed of flow and estimated vessel diameter to calculate volume of flow
- It displays beat-to-beat variation in cardiac output and helps to guide optimization of cardiac function
- Patient tolerance is poor unless under general anaesthesia
- NICE published guidance in 2011 supporting the adoption of ODM and other technologies that can monitor cardiac output and guide intraoperative fluid therapy.

Transoesophageal echocardiography

- Provides real time information and images of cardiovascular anatomy and physiology
- It can be used to assess cardiac status during non-cardiac surgery and to evaluate the effects of surgical intervention on the heart during cardiac surgery

Source: data from *Recommendations for Standards of Monitoring during Anaesthesia and Recovery, Fourth Edition*, The Association of Anaesthetists of Great Britain and Ireland, London, UK Copyright © 2007, available from http://www.aagbi.org/sites/default/files/standardsofmonitoring07.pdf

protective equipment by staff should be guided by risk assessment and the extent of contact anticipated with blood and body fluids, or pathogens. An effective screening programme of high-risk patient groups may facilitate risk assessment but cannot be fool proof. Since, without testing, there may be no way of telling who is infected with a blood-borne virus, most UK organizations recommend staff should practice 'Universal Precautions' for *all* patients in their care.

Personal protective equipment

This comprises, as a minimum, gloves (double-gloving may be appropriate for high-risk circumstances) and a fluid-resistant gown (sterile for most operative procedures otherwise clean but non-sterile) and facemask and eye protection or a face shield.

Gloves should be worn when touching blood, body fluids, secretions, excretions, mucous membranes, and non-intact skin. Facial protection should be worn during any activities that are likely to generate splashes of blood, body fluids, secretions, or excretions. Gowns are worn to protect skin and clothing during similar episodes.

Sharps injury prevention

It is the duty of all healthcare workers to reduce the risk of needle stick injury to themselves, their co-workers, and patients. Institutions can assist in this by the provision of appropriately designed equipment such as non-cutting suture needles and safety cannulae for intravenous access. All used sharps should be discarded immediately into a sharps bin. Never re-sheath, bend, or disconnect needles. Do not overfill sharps bins, seal and replace when three-quarters full.

Actions for needle stick and other contamination injuries

Each institution is likely to provide guidance on procedure to follow in the event of contamination injuries. For eye splash this usually includes profuse irrigation of the eyes with saline. For sharps injuries an immediate attempt to 'bleed' the injury by squeezing is often advised to assist in flushing out pathogens or infected blood, thereafter thorough washing of the area with chlorhexidine or other antimicrobial scrubs is routine. Once these measures have been taken it is essential to assess the risk of infection arising from the injury: the type of injury (superficial or deep), the type of contaminated fluid (is it high risk for viral agents [blood, cerebrospinal fluid, semen, etc.] or low risk [faeces, urine, vomit, etc.]), the potential quantity of inoculation (visibly contaminated implements, in particular hollow needles, etc.), the risk of the 'source' individual from whom the body fluids were contacted. Assessment will usually involve asking the 'source' individual to give a blood sample for viral testing. The person sustaining the contamination injury should have a baseline sample of their blood taken to demonstrate whether they were free from viral infection prior to the injury. This raises ethical issues when patients are unable to consent. Once risk is fully assessed, occupational health or infectious diseases advice should be taken to guide any anti-viral or antibiotic therapy that may be warranted and counselling of affected individuals if indicated.

Precautions for electrical safety for staff and for the patient

Electricity can damage the body by electrocution, burns, or ignition of a flammable material. Damage is dependent upon the current pathway and density, the type (direct or alternating), and the duration of current.

Electrocution

Current pathway and density

The pathway that current takes through the body will determine which tissues are damaged. Current passing through the chest may cause ventricular fibrillation or asphyxia, whereas a current passing vertically through the body may cause loss of consciousness and spinal cord damage.

Current density (the amount of current flowing per unit area) will determine the effect. A 50 Hz alternating current flowing between each hand would cause a tingling sensation at 1 mA but ventricular fibrillation at 75 mA. Theatre staff should wear antistatic shoes with high impedance to reduce any current flowing through the body.

A current flowing directly into the myocardium (or in very close proximity to it) may generate a much higher local current density; theoretically 50 µA at 50Hz could cause ventricular fibrillation. This is known as microshock. Examples of equipment that may facilitate microshock include central venous catheters and intracardiac pacemakers.

Electrical burns

When an electric current passes through any substance having electrical resistance, heat is produced. Whether or not this produces a burn depends on the current density. The patient should never be in contact with an earthed object (operating table, drip stand, etc.) as if this completes an electrical circuit the patient may receive a burn at the site. Burns may also result from poor contact between a diathermy neutral plate and the patient resulting in localized increased current density.

Fires and explosions

Spark proof switches and electrical sockets should be used in theatres to reduce the risk of spark generation, which can ignite flammable vapours. The use of diathermy may also ignite vapours or gases such as alcohol based cleaning solutions or bowel gas.

Surgical diathermy

Surgical diathermy uses the heating effects of high frequency (kHz–MHz) electrical current to coagulate and cut tissues. Accidental electrical burns may be caused by inadvertent depression of the foot switch. Keeping the forceps in a protective quiver and the installation of a buzzer, activated when the switch is depressed, may reduce this risk.

There are two types of diathermy—monopolar and bipolar.

Monopolar diathermy generates electrical energy at 200 kHz to 6 MHz. The energy is applied between two electrodes (neutral and active). The neutral electrode has a large conductive surface area producing a low current density with no measurable heating effect. The active electrode has a very small contact area resulting in a very high current density and high temperature.

Bipolar diathermy operates with a much lower power output. The output is applied between the points of a pair of specially designed forceps producing high local current density. Minimal current passes throughout the rest of the body.

Monopolar diathermy can inhibit or permanently damage pacemakers. If diathermy is essential, the bipolar variety should be used. Bipolar diathermy should be applied well away from the pacemaker and its wiring.

Conclusion

Optimal perioperative care of patients requires careful planning, coordinated team work, and attention to detail. Generic structured pathways of care that highlight common potential pitfalls will reduce risk of errors. Set standards of monitoring and awareness of likely mechanisms of injury enable development of routine practices to minimize risks. A universal approach to maintain these standards for all patients is the goal.

Further reading

Association of Anaesthetists of Great Britain and Ireland (AAGBI). *Recommendations for standards of monitoring during anaesthesia and recovery*, 4th edition. London AAGBI, 2007. Available from http://www.aagbi.org/sites/default/files/standardsofmonitoring07.pdf (accessed 1 February 2016).

Boumphrey S, Langton JA. Electrical safety in the operating theatre. *Br J Anaesth CEPD Rev* 2003; 3(1): 10–14.

National Confidential Enquiry into Patient Outcome and Death (NCEPOD). *Knowing the risk: A review of the peri-operative care of surgical patients*. London: NCEPOD, 2011. Available from http://www.ncepod.org.uk/2011report2/downloads/POC_fullreport.pdf (accessed 1 February 2016).

References

1. World Health Organization. *Safe Surgery Saves Lives*. Available from http://www.who.int/patientsafety/safesurgery/bibliography/en/ (accessed 1 February 2016).
2. National Patient Safety Agency. *Five steps to safer surgery*, December 2010. Available from http://www.nrls.npsa.nhs.uk/resources/?entryid45=92901 (accessed 1 February 2016).
3. Knight D, Mahajan R. Patient positioning in anaesthesia. *Cont Ed Anaesth Crit Care Pain* 2004; 4(5): 160–3.
4. National Institute for Health and Clinical Excellence. *Inadvertent perioperative hypothermia: The management of inadvertent perioperative hypothermia in adults*. National Institute for Health and Care Excellence, 2008. Available from http://www.nice.org.uk/Guidance/CG65 (accessed 1 February 2016).
5. World Health Organization. *Standard precautions in healthcare*. Geneva: World Health Organization, 2007. Available from http://www.who.int/csr/resources/publications/standardprecautions/en/ (accessed 1 February 2016).

CHAPTER 5.3

Postoperative care

Gary H. Mills and Jeremy Groves

Introduction

In the European Surgical Outcomes Study, a 1-week snapshot in 2011 of 46 539 patients across Europe, death during surgery was uncommon but 4% of patients died before discharge.[1] Importantly, 73% of the patients who died were not admitted to critical care. Death may be uncommon but pain after surgery is a fear of many and a barrier for some. The key roles of postoperative care are thus to ensure that mortality and morbidity are minimized and the patient's pain needs are addressed. This requires careful planning, particularly with regard to the location of care, and early identification and treatment of problems.

Phases of recovery

Recovery from a surgical procedure can be divided into three phases.

+ Phase 1 encompasses the period after the end of anaesthesia and prior to the patient awaking.

+ Phase 2 lasts from the end of phase 1 to discharge from hospital.

+ Phase 3, or late recovery, ends when the patient is fully recovered from the procedure.

Immediately following a surgical procedure most patients will spend the first phase of their recovery in a designated area, the Post-Anaesthetic Care Unit or PACU.

Post-anaesthetic care unit

A PACU facilitates the monitoring of the immediate transition from anaesthesia to a state of physiological stability. It should be open for 24 hours in centres performing emergency surgery and staffed by nurses trained in the core competencies for post-anaesthetic care. Competencies include the ability to manage an airway, respond to deteriorating physiological signs, and effective management of pain. The staff should observe admissions on a one-to-one basis until they have regained control of their own airway, have a stable cardiovascular and respiratory system, and are awake, free of surgical complications and able to communicate.[2]

Pressures on critical care facilities mean PACUs are increasingly being used to manage critically ill patients. Where this occurs for surgical admissions, responsibility rests with the critical care and surgical teams.

Day case (ambulatory) surgery

Day case surgery is becoming increasingly popular for a wide range of procedures. This is driven by financial considerations and the benefits to the patient in terms of a reduced hospital stay and faster recovery. Approximately 80% of all surgical procedures are now performed as day cases.[3]

Postoperative care on the day case unit will be directed towards managing immediate surgical complications, pain, and nausea and vomiting. Ideally this will have been facilitated with the administration of analgesic and antiemetic premedication. The majority of patients are encouraged to eat and drink as soon as they feel able, although mandatory intake is not necessary. Voiding is encouraged and, in cases where a patient has had a spinal anaesthetic, essential.

Patients and carers should receive oral and written instructions prior to discharge. This will include advice to avoid alcohol and tasks requiring significant manual or intellectual dexterity for 24 hours. Patients should receive a supply of analgesics, ideally in a pack. In the event of a problem or query the instructions should include a contact, available for at least the first 24 hours, who can provide advice. Telephone follow-up the day after surgery provides useful information for audit purposes and is reassuring for patients.

The British Association of Day Surgery have produced a useful guide[4] and further information can be found on their website.[5]

Inpatient surgery

Though only 20% of surgical cases are managed as inpatients, they represent a heterogeneous group with varying postoperative needs. To clarify the terminology used to describe the level of care for inpatients the Department of Health, in a document entitled 'Comprehensive Critical Care',[6] proposed the classification listed in Table 5.3.1.

Table 5.3.1 Levels of care

Level 0	Patients whose needs can be met through normal ward care in an acute hospital
Level 1	Patients at risk of their condition deteriorating, or those recently relocated from higher levels of care, whose needs can be met on an acute ward with additional advice and support from the critical care team
Level 2	Patients requiring more detailed observation or intervention including support for a single failing organ system or postoperative care and those 'stepping down' from higher levels of care
Level 3	Patients requiring advanced respiratory support alone or basic respiratory support together with support of at least two organ systems. This level includes all complex patients requiring support for multi-organ failure

Reproduced from Department of Health, *Comprehensive Critical Care: A Review of Adult Critical Care Service*, © Crown Copyright 2000 licensed under the Open Government Licence v3.0. Available from http://webarchive.nationalarchives.gov.uk/20130107105354/ http://www.dh.gov.ukprod_consum_dh/groups/dh_digitalassets/@dh/@en/documents/ digitalasset/dh_4082872.pdf

The majority of routine surgery will require level 0 or level 1 care, and more major surgery will require level 2 or 3 care. Though the boundaries may blur, high dependency care usually refers to level 1 and 2, intensive care to level 3. A decision as to the level of postoperative care a patient warrants will depend on patient and surgical factors and the availability of a given resource. Postoperative complications are frequent (30%) in patients selected for level 2 and level 3 care, with most morbidity and mortality occurring in the first 48 hours.

Planning postoperative care

Determining where a patient should be managed after surgery is not an exact science. However, the following factors should be considered:

* **patient factors:** preoperative health, co-morbidity, perioperative deterioration, postoperative complications, epidural anaesthesia

* **surgical factors:** complexity of surgery, intraoperative complications, enhanced recovery pathways

* **resource considerations:** the availability of critical care beds varies widely across Europe, with seven times as many critical care beds in Germany than the UK.[7,8] This leads to frequent pressure on beds and means patients who may benefit are managed in less than optimal surroundings.[9-11]

Risk prediction

Experienced clinicians are very effective in patient selection; however, this can be aided by perioperative risk prediction. This, if incorporated into the planning routine, is important in directing cases to the most appropriate environment.

Physiology and Operative Severity Score for Enumeration of Mortality and Morbidity (POSSUM)

POSSUM and P-POSSUM were developed to estimate the likely frequency of risk of death and morbidity associated with a patient and their procedure. It relies on physiological parameters (age, cardiac signs/symptoms, respiratory, electrocardiogram (ECG) findings, blood pressure, pulse rate, haemoglobin, white cell count, urea, sodium, potassium, Glasgow Coma Scale [GCS]) and features of the operation (complexity, number of procedures, blood loss, peritoneal contamination, malignancy status, elective/urgent/emergency status).[12]

Postoperative ward care (level 0 and level 1)

The majority of inpatient postoperative surgery episodes in the UK will take place in a ward environment. Ensuring these patients are safe and detecting those who encounter problems relies on a team approach. This approach is encapsulated in the *Care of the Critically Ill Surgical Patient* course and follows the standard airway, breathing and circulation methods.[13]

Monitoring on the ward

Frequent monitoring is the key and there should be a seamless continuation from theatre. Basic monitoring such as respiratory rate, temperature, blood pressure, and heart rate and rhythm by palpation or ECG (bearing in mind that fast atrial fibrillation may only be detectable by listening to or monitoring the heart) should

be possible on any ward. Once monitoring detects a deterioration of organ system function, an organized and timely response is needed. Education of ward staff in how to respond and who to call is needed. National Institute for Health and Care Excellence (NICE) clinical guideline 50,[14] describes a graded response strategy and physiological track and trigger systems. This, combined with the development of critical care outreach and medical emergency teams has led to significant improvements in this area.[15]

In 2012 the Royal College of Physicians looked at the elements used in a number of different scoring systems and produced a revised system called the National Early Warning Score (NEWS; Figure 5.3.1). Each physiological parameter attracts a score; the scores are aggregated and a response determined on the total score. In addition to the physiological parameters a weighting score of 2 is added to any patient requiring supplemental oxygen.[16,17]

Complications after surgery

In elective cases complications often have their origins in inadequate preoperative preparation or patient selection. Emergency cases may suffer from late diagnosis, failure to rapidly resuscitate, and promptly move to surgery to provide source control of infected areas. Common complications are summarized in Table 5.3.2.

Airway and breathing: the respiratory system

Failure to maintain an airway after surgery leads to the risk of airway obstruction, hypoventilation, or pulmonary aspiration of gastric contents. Inability to rapidly correct an airway problem may lead to the need for intubation and ventilation.

Atelectasis

Atelectasis (alveolar collapse) is common following anaesthesia. It complicates up to 50% of abdominal surgery cases.[18] The mechanical effect of retractors, insufflation of the abdomen with gas, an extreme head down position, or intra-abdominal compartment syndrome all compress the lungs. Intraoperative PEEP (positive end expiratory pressure) and active inflation of the lung (recruitment) may help reduce the consequent atelectasis. Postoperative continuous positive airway pressure (CPAP) may be beneficial in established cases.[19-21]

Inflammation and pulmonary oedema

Perioperative pulmonary aspiration of gastric contents may lead to infection (aspiration pneumonia) and inflammation of the alveolar epithelium. Pulmonary oedema can occur in fluid overload or left ventricular failure. Sepsis, the systemic inflammatory response syndrome (SIRS), acute respiratory distress syndrome, and transfusion related lung injury can lead to 'leaky lungs' (non-cardiogenic pulmonary oedema). Even relatively short periods of invasive ventilation can cause barotrauma.

Functional considerations

Patients with lung diseases or chest wall deformities such as kyphoscoliosis or neuromuscular diseases may be destabilized by surgery. Perioperative central line insertion may have caused a pneumothorax.

Neuromuscular respiratory issues

Breathing may be impaired by residual neuromuscular block. This typically presents with agitation, anxiety, and rapid jerky attempts at breathing after tracheal extubation.

National Early Warning Score (NEWS)*

PHYSIOLOGICAL PARAMETERS	3	2	1	0	1	2	3
Respiration Rate	≤8		9–11	12–20		21–24	≥25
Oxygen Saturations	≤91	92–93	94–95	≥96			
Any Supplemental Oxygen		Yes		No			
Temperature	≤35.0		35.1–36.0	36.1–38.0	38.1–39.0	≥39.1	
Systolic BP	≤90	91–100	101–110	111–219			≥220
Heart Rate	≤40		41–50	51–90	91–110	111–130	≥131
level of Consciousness				A			V, P, or U

*The NEWS initiative flowed from the Royal College of Physicians' NEWS Development and Implementation Group (NEWSDIG) report, and was jointly developed and funded in collaboration with theRoyal College of Physicians, Royal College of Nursing, National Outreach Forum and NHS Training for Innovation

Fig. 5.3.1 National Early Warning Score.
Reproduced from Royal College of Physicians, *National Early Warning Score (NEWS): Standardising the assessment of acute illness severity in the NHS*, Report of a working party, London: RCP, 2012. Copyright © 2012 Royal College of Physicians. Reproduced with permission.

Table 5.3.2 Common problems in the early postoperative period

Problem	Cause	Action
Not maintaining airway	Too sedated	Wait for recovery. If slow reintubate
	Muscle relaxant still effective	Check train of four and reverse
	Foreign body in airway	Remove
Breathing rapid/shallow	Atelectasis, fluid overload, pneumothorax. Pain	Make diagnosis clinically; consider CXR Atelectasis: CPAP/NIV or reventilate If fluid overload: CPAP and diuretics Pneumothorax: chest drain Pain: top up epidural or titrate pain relief
Breathing frequency is excessively slow	Opiate effect	Keep intubated and support If extubated, consider reintubation or titrated naloxone
Blood pressure low	Hypovolaemia	Examine for clinical signs of poor perfusion, low CVP, low CVP, low SpO$_2$, poor urine output. Bolus fluids, consider ongoing bleeding and need for transfusion or clotting correction and surgical reopening
Blood pressure low	Over dilated by epidural	Check block level, look for bradycardia Stop or slow rate. Exclude other causes May need low-dose norepinephrine
Blood pressure low	Sepsis	Source control, culture blood urine and source then antibiotics. Central access, start norepinephrine
Blood pressure low	Possible cardiac cause	12-lead ECG, low CVP, low SpO$_2$, monitor CVP, maintain perfusion. May need reventilation or CPAP. CXR, ECHO: consider MI, heart failure, tamponade, pulmonary embolism. Avoid overload. Cardiology referral. May need CTPA
Arrhythmias	Ischaemic heart disease, MI, Electrolyte disturbance	12-lead ECG, check ABG and U&E, Ca, Mg. Look for indicators of pre-existing tachy or bradyarrythmia tendency. Treat or cardiology referral
Urine output poor	Hypovolaemia or low BP	Ensure adequately filled. BP sufficient compared to preoperataive. CVP useful to avoid overload, CVP O$_2$ saturations

ABG, arterial blood gas; BP, blood pressure; Ca, calcium; CPAP, continuous positive airway pressure; CTPA, computed tomography pulmonary angiography; CVP, central venous pressure; CXR, chest X-ray; ECG, electrocardiogram; ECHO, echocardiogram; Mg, magnesium; MI, myocardial infarction; NIV, non-invasive ventilation; U&E, urea and electrolytes.

Other

Patients who are acidotic, cold, or unstable may be returned from theatre ventilated. Every effort should be made to stabilize these patients as soon as possible to allow early successful extubation.

Circulation: cardiovascular complications

Hypotension

The most common cause is hypovolaemia. It is often easy to underestimate blood and evaporative fluid loss. Leaky cellular membranes and vasodilatation in the critically ill also lead to hypovolaemia.

Cardiogenic shock

This is less common, but a serious complication in the perioperative period. It is catastrophic if associated with septic shock because the heart cannot compensate for the vasodilatation.

Cardiac arrhythmias

These, whether slow or fast, should be aggressively managed. Paroxysmal atrial fibrillation is the most common.

Pulmonary embolism

A cause of major morbidity. Deep vein thrombosis prophylaxis is vital in the postoperative period, together with a timely return to warfarin for those on long-term therapy. It is also important to be aware of the potential for heparin-induced thrombocytopaenia.[22]

Haemorrhage

Any surgical patient has the potential to bleed postoperatively. While modern practice permits tolerance of haemoglobin levels above 70 g/L,[23] when active bleeding occurs or patients have heart disease, a target of 90–100 g/L may be more appropriate.

Neurological disturbance

Delirium

In the elderly, pre-existing cerebrovascular disease predispose to delirium. The combination of anaesthesia, removal from normal residence, disturbance to sleep–wake cycles, and pharmacological intervention aggravate the problem. Other neurological issues are summarized in Table 5.3.3.

Other systems

Gastrointestinal

Ileus is covered in Chapter 5.4.

The stress of surgery leads to an increase in protein catabolism. Basal metabolic rate increases by up to 40% and relative insulin resistance occurs. Enteral feeding reduces hyperglycaemia, maintains gut integrity and reduces stress ulceration. NICE guidelines recommend nutritional support for people who are malnourished and for those who have eaten little or nothing for more than 5 days or are likely to eat little for the next 5 days or have poor absorptive capacity, high nutrient losses, or increased nutritional needs. In terms of calories NICE recommends 25–35 kcal/kg/day and ESPEN (European Society for Clinical Nutrition and Metabolism) recommends 20–25 kcal/kg/day initially and then 25–30 kcal/kg/day in recovery phase.[24] Feeding route will ideally have been determined at surgery, with passage and confirmed positioning of nasogastric or nasojejunal tubes (or percutaneous endoscopic gastrostomy or percutaneous endoscopic jejunostomy, if the oral route is felt to be impaired.

Table 5.3.3 Perioperative neurological disturbance

Dementia	Exacerbated by unfamiliar events and location
Alcoholism	Alcohol withdrawal (or withdrawal of other drugs of addiction)
Psychiatric disorder	Withdrawal of medication due to illness, restricted oral intake or poor perioperative gastric function
Convulsions	May present as confusion rather than tonic clonic fits. May have been provoked by withdrawal of anticonvulsants
Hypoglycaemia	May be on diabetes related or medication or may be a feature of disease such as adrenocortical insufficiency or hepatic failure. May present pre, intra or postoperatively
Cerebral vascular congestion	Excessive head down during surgery
Cerebral event	Ischaemic stroke (including emboli), intracranial bleed (including subarachnoid, subdural or within the brain substance). Sinus venous thrombosis. Consider clotting disorders, hypovolaemia or trauma

Renal

The human kidneys are sensitive to hypotension. Drugs, including radiological contrast media, may cause direct damage. If contrast is required for a computed tomography (CT) scan, protection with a sodium bicarbonate infusion may reduce renal injury.

Hourly measurement of urine output and a comprehensive fluid balance are essential in those who are at risk of renal failure. In hypertensive patients, autoregulation may be compromised with a fall in blood pressure below the patient's usual blood pressure. Appropriate measures to maintain renal perfusion may be required.

Table 5.3.4 A comparison of intensive and high dependency care

Unit	High dependency care	Intensive care
Staff: patient ratios	1:2	1:1
Description	Level 2	Level 3
Type of patient	Single failing organ system	Isolated respiratory failure requiring invasive ventilation. Multiple organ dysfunction
Monitoring	Standard patient monitoring. Usually continuous via a bedside monitor. Will include invasive monitoring of central venous pressure and arterial pressure	As for HDU but also includes monitoring of cardiac output via Doppler or pulse contour methods. Echocardiography becoming routine. Monitoring of respiratory function through ventilator. Cerebral function monitoring
Therapy	Administration of non-invasive ventilation and continuous positive airway pressure. Low-dose inotropic drugs to support the circulation	Invasive ventilation. Complex inotropic and mechanical support of the circulation. Renal support through continuous veno-veno haemofiltration

Critical care

Critical care units admit patients for intensive postoperative monitoring so that developing problems can be rapidly addressed or the more severely ill can receive support for failing organ systems (Table 5.3.4).

Systemic inflammatory response syndrome

SIRS can develop in a multitude of conditions that will be managed by surgeons and require critical care support. The definitions, clarified in Table 5.3.5, enable professionals discussing the critically ill to be clear about the processes they are managing. It is important to note that SIRS can arise from conditions that are not directly related to infection.[25,26]

Sepsis

Sepsis kills more people annually than heart disease or stroke. The principles of management are relatively straightforward and the key to success is rapid diagnosis and early treatment. For patients with shock:

♦ Early protocolized resuscitation: central venous pressure (CVP) 8–12 mmHg, mean arterial pressure > 65 mmHg, urine output ≥ 0.5 mL/kg/hr, central venous oxygen saturation > 70%.

♦ Screening for sepsis in all seriously ill patients.

♦ Diagnosis: cultures and imaging.

♦ Antimicrobial therapy: empirical antibiotics once cultures have been taken and within 1 hour of diagnosis. Daily review and adjustment of antibiotic regimes if necessary.

♦ Source control: this may require surgical or radiological intervention.

The surviving sepsis campaign aims to reduce the burden of sepsis and surgeons have a major role to play in this effort.[27]

Multiple organ dysfunction syndrome (MODS)

Severely ill surgical patients admitted to critical care can develop MODS. This is a syndrome characterized by the presence of altered organ function in the acutely ill patient such that homeostasis cannot be maintained without intervention. Such intervention is likely to necessitate cardiovascular support with inotropic drugs, respiratory support with invasive ventilation, and occasionally renal support. MODS can be primary, when it results directly from an insult, such as trauma, or secondary when it develops as a consequence of the host response (SIRS) as in severe body cavity infection.

Critical care monitoring

Shock is a term that is often used loosely in medicine. It develops as a consequence of a wide variety of conditions and is characterized by impaired tissue oxygenation usually as a result of cardiovascular failure and reduced clearance of tissue metabolites. Monitoring and therapy in critical care aim to reverse it.

Cardiovascular monitoring

Central venous pressure

Traditionally CVP was thought to reflect preload (right atrial filling) and thus to be closely related to cardiac output. However, the relationship varies between individuals and is better for left rather than right atrial filling. As the right atrium fills, the cardiac output increases and eventually plateaus;[28] however, the poor correlation between changes in CVP and changes in cardiac output preclude an easy to follow guide.[29]

CVP measurements considered in terms of a low versus a high value become more valuable, particularly in haemorrhage or renal failure. In haemorrhage a falling CVP is a good guide to further blood loss, and in renal failure a high CVP such as 15–20 mmHg is likely to indicate fluid overload.

CVP is part of the surviving sepsis protocol, aiming for pressure of 8–12 mmHg or 12–15 mmHg during mechanical ventilation.[30] This is to ensure that patients are not at an extreme of vascular over or under filling during sepsis.

Central venous oxygen saturations ($ScvO_2$) provide further information. If cardiac output is normal, the fully saturated arterial blood (SaO_2 97%) will pass to the capillaries where oxygen will be removed, leaving blood with a saturation of 70–75% returning to the right heart. If cardiac output is low, less oxygenated blood will reach the capillaries and a larger proportion of the oxygen will be consumed, leaving lower venous oxygen saturations. If cardiac output is considerably reduced $ScvO_2$ may reach 50%.

CVP monitoring in terms of a target (8–12 mmHg), together with target mean arterial pressure and $ScvO_2$ (>70%) formed a major part of the study by Rivers, who looked at 'early goal-directed therapy' (GDT) in the treatment of septic shock. This resulted in a mortality of 42.3% with GDT compared to 56.8% with standard therapy.[31] Associated therapies included boluses of crystalloid to maintain CVP, blood transfusion, dobutamine as an inotrope, and norepinephrine and other vasopressors.

Cardiac output monitoring

Cardiac output can be determined from the driving pressure and systemic vascular resistance (SVR):

$$Cardiac\ output = (mean\ arterial\ pressure - CVP) / SVR$$

In order to effectively manage shock the intensivist requires information on both CO and SVR. Measuring CO enables SVR to be derived. Cardiac output measurements can be made using the Fick principle

Table 5.3.5 Systemic inflammatory response syndrome

Term	Definition
Systemic Inflammatory Response Syndrome (SIRS)	A syndrome resulting from a variety of insults and characterized by two or more of the following: Temperature: >38°C or <36°C Heart rate: >90 beats/minute Respiratory rate: >20 breaths/minute White cell count: >12 000 mm^3 or <4000 mm^3
Sepsis	SIRS as a result of infection
Severe sepsis	Sepsis with organ dysfunction, hypoperfusion (including lactic acidosis, oliguria and alteration in mental state) or hypotension (systolic blood pressure < 90 mmHg)
Septic Shock	Sepsis induced hypotension despite adequate fluid resuscitation

(dye or thermodilution) with a Swan Ganz catheter (pulmonary artery flotation catheters).[32] Shoemaker believed that patients who had goal-directed increase in cardiac output and hence tissue oxygen delivery were more likely to survive.[33] However GDT employing supramaximal targets in mixed or septic critical care patients subsequently failed to show benefit in studies by Hayes[34] and Gattinoni.[35] In the septic ICU patient, the benefits from the use of the pulmonary artery flotation catheter could not be shown to outweigh the risks. More recently in the context of managing acute lung injury, central venous catheters have produced half as many catheter-related complications as pulmonary artery flotation catheters.[36]

This led to the development of less invasive cardiac output monitors including pulse contour analysis, echocardiography, oesophageal Doppler, and bioimpedance methods. Perioperative surgical management of high-risk cases does seem to benefit from haemodynamic intervention to improve outcome.

Fluid optimization is an important feature of enhanced recovery protocols. Intraoperative oesophageal Doppler monitoring cuts morbidly and length of stay in colonic resections and surgery for fractured neck of femur. Pulse contour analysis may be the simplest way forward in perioperative major surgery, because it relies on intravascular lines that are normally present.

A simpler method of assessing the adequacy of intravascular fluid in ventilated patients is the swing on an arterial trace during mechanical ventilation. Systolic pressure variation or stroke volume variation if high will indicate a relatively empty vascular compartment.

Echocardiography

Echocardiography is increasingly used at the bedside by critical care staff to identify basic cardiac features, including whether the heart is contracting well, whether it is empty or overloaded, and whether the chambers are of normal size.

Respiratory monitoring

Oxygen saturation monitoring is simple and essential; however, it may not function adequately in shut down or hypothermic patients. Counting respiratory rate is a good indicator of potential complications although changes in impedance allow the calculation of respiratory rate from the ECG signal.

Markers of gas exchange and ventilatory problems

The acid–base status including the pH and the bicarbonate and base excess give useful information on the metabolic state of the patient when organ perfusion is poor. Most analyses also provide a lactate level, so anaerobic metabolism can be assessed. The anion gap, which is the difference between the measurable cations (Na and K) and anions (Cl and HCO_3^{2-}), help define the cause of an acidosis.

The PaO_2 enables us to look at the degree of shunt or ventilation/perfusion mismatch, and the $PaCO_2$ measures the respiratory drive and the efficiency of alveolar ventilation. A raised $PaCO_2$ may be normal in an individual with chronic lung disease or may point to over narcotization or the residual effects of anaesthesia in a postoperative patient.

Imaging

Bedside monitoring of more complex respiratory function, other than by mechanical ventilators, is limited to chest X-ray and ultrasound. These can provide guidance on effusions, pneumothoraces, and consolidation. Continuous monitoring is more difficult. In ventilated patients CT scanning of the lung may show areas of collapse, which can be re-expanded during lung recruitment and maintained with PEEP. Unfortunately this requires transport to the CT scanner and involves exposure to ionizing radiation. Magnetic resonance (MR) scanning of the lung is possible, but simple images do not show the gas filled lung well.

Monitoring conscious level

Simple monitoring such as AVPU (*a*wake, *r*esponsive to *v*oice, *p*ain or *u*nconscious) or the GCS are important. A patient with a GCS below 8 or a deteriorating GCS is at increased risk of failing to maintain or protect their airway. Aspiration is a real risk after abdominal surgery, especially if the obtunded patient is lying flat. A falling conscious level as a result of decreasing perfusion is a sign of severe shock and must be urgently corrected.

Low blood sugar or extremely high blood sugar affects conscious level, and if found to be abnormal, will need treatment and monitoring. Hypercarbia may obtund conscious level, though loss of consciousness is unusual below a $PaCO_2$ of 9 KPa.

Delirium is an acute confusional state characterized by disturbed consciousness and cognitive function.[37] It occurs in between 10% and 50% of patients undergoing major surgery. Delirium may be reduced by ensuring good pain control, adequate hydration and nutrition, an appropriate environment with familiar staff and relatives, appropriate drugs, encouraging sleep at night (correction of disordered circadian rhythms that are common in critical illness, which may be helped by suitable lighting, ear plugs, and/or white noise/music), and treatment of infections. Once possible causes or exacerbating factors are corrected, it may be necessary to consider therapy with haloperidol or olanzapine.

Monitoring renal function

Although a reduction in urine output is a feature of the stress response, a urine output of >0.5 mL/kg/hr is an important sign of adequate perfusion and renal function. Changes in serum creatinine occur later. In 2013 NICE commented on renal dysfunction[38] following on from the 2009 NCEPOD (National Confidential Enquiry into Patient Outcome and Death) report.[39] The risk of acute injury before surgery was identified as greatest in emergency operations. Risk factors include sepsis, hypovolaemia, intraperitoneal surgery, chronic kidney disease, diabetes, heart failure, age 65 years or over, liver disease, and use of drugs with nephrotoxic potential, especially non-steroidal anti-inflammatory drugs. The reports highlight the need for monitoring with urine dipstick and ultrasound where infected or obstructed kidneys are suspected.

Early intervention with the aim of preventing renal failure becoming established is important. Forty-seven per cent of patients admitted to critical care who have severe acute renal failure will die before discharge from hospital. Around 15% of those who are treated with renal replacement therapy will become dialysis dependent at hospital discharge.[40]

Post critical care follow-up

After discharge from critical care patients frequently have residual issues consequent on their stay. Critical care outreach teams can use follow-up to provide counselling on psychological or physical problems that have arisen as a consequence of the critical care stay. Physical issues, such as remaining indwelling catheters or tracheostomies, may be dealt with infrequently on the ward and the advice from the critical care team can be beneficial. Providing written information about critical care is well received by patients. Follow-up also provides the opportunity for audit and research.

Postoperative pain control

No patient should be in unnecessary discomfort following surgery. This is not only important from the patient's psychological perspective but also due to the impact of pain on other body systems. Atalectasis for example may result from postoperative hypoventilation caused by pain.

Analgesia techniques

The World Health Organization (WHO) developed a graded response to cancer pain that now finds general application. Known as the WHO analgesia ladder,[41] it allows a stepwise approach to pain relief that combines agents that work in different ways. This simple and relatively cheap approach extends from oral analgesics at the lower end of the ladder to strong opiates at the top. It relies on regular administration of analgesics to be effective.

Analgesia on demand (PRN) often fails as patient's delay asking for analgesics. Patients with pre-existing chronic pain problems may need additional medication. In some situations, drugs such as ketamine are added to achieve pain control.

As a group the opioids are the most important major analgesics. They act on the mu, kappa, and delta opioid receptors in the brain. These receptors are also found in the brainstem periaqueductal grey matter where, by blocking gamma-aminobutyric acid, they have an inhibitory action on pain fibres. However, they also promote respiratory depression by reducing the sensitivity of the chemoreceptors to CO_2 and impair peristalsis. Other adverse effects include central nervous system depression and the production of nausea and vomiting.

Intravenous infusions of opioids provide continuous analgesia but have two major problems. A bolus is needed initially to bring plasma levels up to a satisfactory point and patients with organ dysfunction run the risk of accumulation. Therefore infusions are normally only used in specialized settings, such as in critical care, where monitoring is readily available or in the relief of chronic or terminal pain.

Patient-controlled analgesia

Patient-controlled analgesia (PCA) is a technique that utilizes technology to deliver a bolus dose of an opioid to a patient on demand. PCA is often run in tandem with regular simple analgesics such as paracetamol. It can be combined with a background infusion, but normally is used with bolus doses separated by at least 5 minutes, with an hourly total limit. Patients are protected from overdose by the limits set and by the need for patients to adequately press the demand button. It is well accepted by patients as it gives them control of when and how much analgesia they receive.

Local and regional techniques

Local analgesia can provide safe anaesthesia both intraoperatively and postoperatively. Regional anaesthesia is probably safer than general anaesthesia and is particularly relevant where patients have lung or airway problems. As with all drugs, local anaesthetics are toxic if excessive doses are used. The maximal dose on a mg/kg basis should not be exceeded and intravascular injection, with the exception of Bier's block, avoided.

Ultrasound-guided nerve blocks have expanded the effectiveness of local analgesia for surgical procedures. Occasionally catheters are placed in the wound to allow infusion of local anaesthetic postoperatively, such as the 'bombs' seen in rectus sheath blocks or pleural catheters.

Intra-abdominal, intrathoracic, and major orthopaedic surgery can produce pain lasting several days. Epidural techniques have evolved to manage this and are commonly combined with general anaesthesia for intracavity procedures. They can be used as a sole technique or combined with a spinal block for the lower limb. Epidurals are not without problems. The sympathetic outflow from the spinal cord is blocked and the consequent vasodilatation leads to hypotension. Such hypotension is often more effectively treated with vasoconstrictors, such as norepinephrine, rather than unnecessary fluid boluses. Infection is a risk and patients with coagulopathy or on anticoagulants may develop an epidural haematoma (Table 5.3.6). The incidence of neurological complications following epidurals has been found to be low.[42–45]

Table 5.3.6 Epidural complications

Complication	Detection
Placement of catheter in epidural vein	Blood aspirated, patient feels faint on injection of local anaesthesia test dose or fits, odd taste in mouth. Test dose local plus 1 in 200 000 epinephrine produces tachycardia
Dural tap/catheter in subarachnoid space	Test dose rapidly produces block of lower limbs i.e. a 'spinal anaesthetic'
Block failure because catheter not in epidural space	No block. Analgesia fails. Often suspected intraoperatively. Abdomen remains very tender even if block topped up at end of operation. Re-site if possible
Unilateral block	Catheter may not lie in midline. If catheter long then withdraw so 5cm remains in epidural space
Some block present, but still in pain	Check block with ice and measure extent. Try topping up
Arms or hands weak with or without shortness of breath	Suspect very high block. Stop epidural and check extent of block. Consider whether this could be subarachnoid block
Very dense or progressive block	Stop epidural. If block does not regress consider epidural haematoma. However, also consider coincidental injury such as prolapsed intravertebral disc, which are more common
Hypotension	Exclude other causes. Check block height is not too extensive. Most commonly due to hypovolaemia. Occasionally low-dose vasoconstrictor may be needed. Check for bradycardia or reason for fixed cardiac output
Bradycardia	Consider other causes such as β-blockade or pre-existing cardiac problems. Check height of block. Cardiac sympathetic inflow from T1/T2. Consider high plasma levels of local anaesthetic. Look for heart block

Conclusion

An operation is only one stage in a patient's surgical journey. Postoperative care, whether it be brief (as in ambulatory surgery) or prolonged (as in major surgery) requires detailed planning. The planning needs to chart the most appropriate postoperative course and, when the unexpected arises, ensure complications are managed in a timely fashion in conjunction with the critical care team.

Further reading

Andreae MH, Andreae DA. Regional anaesthesia to prevent chronic pain after surgery: a Cochrane systematic review and meta-analysis. *Br Journal Anaesth* 2013; 111(5): 711–20.

Goddard JK, Janning SW, Gass JS, *et al*. Cefuroxime-induced acute renal failure. *Pharmacotherapy* 1994; 14(4): 488–91.

Hamilton MA, Cecconi M, Rhodes A. A systematic review and meta-analysis on the use of preemptive hemodynamic intervention to improve postoperative outcomes in moderate and high-risk surgical patients. *Anesth Analg* 2011; 112(6): 1392–402.

Khuri SF, Henderson WG, DePalma RG, *et al*. Determinants of long-term survival after major surgery and the adverse effect of postoperative complications. *Ann Surg* 2005; 242(3): 326–41; discussion 41–3.

Kumar A, Haery C, Paladugu B, *et al*. The duration of hypotension before the initiation of antibiotic treatment is a critical determinant of survival in a murine model of Escherichia coli septic shock: association with serum lactate and inflammatory cytokine levels. *J Infect Dis* 2006; 193(2): 251–8.

Kirkpatrick AW, Roberts DJ, De Waele J, *et al*. Intra-abdominal hypertension and the abdominal compartment syndrome: updated consensus definitions and clinical practice guidelines from the World Society of the Abdominal Compartment Syndrome. *Intensive Care Med* 2013; 39(7): 1190–206.

Linton AL, Clark WF, Driedger AA, *et al*. Acute interstitial nephritis due to drugs: Review of the literature with a report of nine cases. *Ann Intern Med* 1980; 93(5): 735–41.

Marshall JC, Cook, DJChristou, *et al*. Multiple organ dysfunction score: a reliable descriptor of a complex clinical outcome. *Crit Care Med* 1995; 23(10): 1638–52.

Pearse R, Dawson D, Fawcett J, *et al*. Early goal-directed therapy after major surgery reduces complications and duration of hospital stay. A randomised, controlled trial [ISRCTN38797445]. *Critical Care* 2005; 9(6): R687–93.

Pearse RM, Belsey JD, Cole JN, *et al*. Effect of dopexamine infusion on mortality following major surgery: individual patient data meta-regression analysis of published clinical trials. *Crit Care Med* 2008; 36(4): 1323–9.

Pronovost PJ, Jenckes MW, Dorman T, *et al*. Organizational characteristics of intensive care units related to outcomes of abdominal aortic surgery. *JAMA* 1999; 281(14):1310–7.

Rhodes A, Cecconi M, Hamilton M, *et al*. Goal-directed therapy in high-risk surgical patients: a 15-year follow-up study. *Intensive Care Med* 2010; 36(8): 1327–32.

References

1. Pearse RM, Moreno RP, Bauer P, et al. Mortality after surgery in Europe: a 7 day cohort study. *Lancet*. 2012; 380(9847): 1059–65.
2. The Association of Anaesthetists of Great Britain and Ireland. AAGBI Safety Guideline: Immediate Post-anaesthesia Recovery 2013. Available from http://www.aagbi.org/sites/default/files/immediate_post-anaesthesia_recovery_2013.pdf (accessed 1 February 2016).
3. http://www.productivity.nhs.uk/Dashboard/For/National/And/25th/Percentile.
4. Verma R, Alladi R, Jackson I, et al. Day case and short stay surgery: 2 *Anaesthesia*, 2011; 66: 417–34.
5. British Association of Day Surgery. Available from http://www.daysurgeryuk.net/en/home/ (accessed 1 February 2016).
6. Department of Health. Comprehensive critical care: a review of adult critical care services. Available from http://webarchive.nationalarchives.gov.uk/+/www.dh.gov.uk/en/Publicationsandstatistics/Publications/PublicationsPolicyAndGuidance/DH_4006585 (accessed 1 February 2016).
7. Rhodes A, Ferdinande P, Flaatten H, et al. The variability of critical care bed numbers in Europe. *Intensive Care Med* 2012; 38(10): 1647–53.
8. Wunsch H, Angus DC, Harrison DA, et al. Variation in critical care services across North America and Western Europe. *Crit Care Med* 2008; 36(10): 2787–93.
9. Findlay G, Goodwin A, Protopappa K, et al. Knowing the risk: a review of the peri-operative care of surgical patients. London: National Confidential Enquiry into Patient Outcome and Death, 2011.
10. Pearse RM, Harrison DA, James P, et al. Identification and characterisation of the high-risk surgical population in the United Kingdom. *Crit Care* 2006; 10(3): R81.
11. Jhanji S, Thomas B, Ely A, et al. Mortality and utilisation of critical care resources amongst high-risk surgical patients in a large NHS trust. *Anaesthesia* 2008; 63(7): 695–700.
12. Smith JP, Tekkis PP. Risk prediction in surgery. Available from http://www.riskprediction.org.uk/pp-index.php (accessed 1 February 2016).
13. Royal College of Surgeons. Care of critically ill surgical patient (CCrISP). Available from http://www.rcseng.ac.uk/courses/course-search/ccrisp.html (accessed 1 February 2016).
14. National Institute of Health and Care Excellence. NICE Clinical Guideline 50: Acutely ill patients in hospital: Recognition of and response to acute illness in adults in hospital. Available from www.nice.org.uk/nicemedia/pdf/CG50FullGuidance.pdf (accessed 1 February 2016).
15. Cuthbertson BH, Boroujerdi M, McKie L, et al. Can physiological variables and early warning scoring systems allow early recognition of the deteriorating surgical patient? *Crit Care Med* 2007;35(2): 402–9.
16. Royal College of Physicians. National Early Warning Score 2012. Available from: http://www.rcplondon.ac.uk/sites/default/files/documents/national-early-warning-score-standardising-assessment-acute-illness-severity-nhs.pdf.
17. Royal College of Physicians. National Early Warning Score (NEWS). Available from http://www.rcplondon.ac.uk/resources/national-early-warning-score-news (accessed 1 February 2016).
18. Arozullah AM, Daley J, Henderson WG, et al. Multifactorial risk index for predicting postoperative respiratory failure in men after major non-cardiac surgery. The National Veterans Administration Surgical Quality Improvement Program. *Ann Surg* 2000; 232(2): 242–53.
19. Squadrone V, Massaia M, Bruno B, et al. Early CPAP prevents evolution of acute lung injury in patients with hematologic malignancy. *Intensive Care Med* 2010; 36(10): 1666–74.
20. Ferreyra GP, Baussano I, Squadrone V, et al. Continuous positive airway pressure for treatment of respiratory complications after abdominal surgery: a systematic review and meta-analysis. *Ann Surg* 2008; 247(4): 617–26.
21. Thompson JS, Baxter BT, Allison JG, et al. Temporal patterns of postoperative complications. *Arch Surg* 2003; 138(6): 596–602.
23. Hebert PC, Wells G, Blajchman MA, et al. A multicenter, randomized, controlled clinical trial of transfusion requirements in critical care. Transfusion requirements in Critical Care Investigators, Canadian Critical Care Trials Group. *New Engl J Med* 1999; 340(6): 409–17.
22. Ahmed I, Majeed A, Powell R. Heparin induced thrombocytopenia: diagnosis and management update. *Postgrad Med J* 2007; 83(983): 575–82.
24. National Institute of Health and Care Excellence. NICE Guidelines 32: Nutrition support for adults: oral nutrition support, enteral tube feeding and parenteral nutrition. Available from http://publications.nice.org.uk/nutrition-support-in-adults-cg32/other-versions-of-this-guideline (accessed 1 February 2016).

25. Bone RC, Balk RA, Cerra FB, et al. Definitions for sepsis and organ failure and guidelines for the use of innovative therapies in sepsis. The ACCP/SCCM Consensus Conference Committee. American College of Chest Physicians/Society of Critical Care Medicine. *Chest.* 1992;101(6):1644–55.

26. Scottish Intensive Care Society. Available from http://www.scottishintensivecare.org.uk/training-education/sics-induction-modules/sepsis/ (accessed 1 February 2016).

27. Surviving Sepsis Campaign. Available from http://www.survivingsepsis.org/Pages/default.aspx (accessed 1 February 2016).

28. Magder S. More respect for the CVP. *Intensive Care Med* 1998;24(7): 651–3.

29. Marik PE, Baram M, Vahid B. Does central venous pressure predict fluid responsiveness? A systematic review of the literature and the tale of seven mares. *Chest* 2008; 134(1): 172–8.

30. Dellinger RP, Levy MM, Carlet JM, et al. Surviving Sepsis Campaign: international guidelines for management of severe sepsis and septic shock: 2008. *Crit Care Med* 2008; 36(1): 296–327.

31. Rivers E, Nguyen B, Havstad S, et al. Early goal-directed therapy in the treatment of severe sepsis and septic shock. *N Engl J Med* 2001; 345(19): 1368–77.

32. Swan HJ, Ganz W, Forrester J, et al. Catheterization of the heart in man with use of a flow-directed balloon-tipped catheter. *N Engl J Med* 1970; 283(9): 447–51.

33. Shoemaker WC, Appel PL, Kram HB, et al. Prospective trial of supranormal values of survivors as therapeutic goals in high-risk surgical patients. *Chest* 1988; 94(6): 1176–86.

34. Hayes MA, Timmins AC, Yau EH, et al. Elevation of systemic oxygen delivery in the treatment of critically ill patients. *N Engl J Med* 1994; 330(24): 1717–22.

35. Gattinoni L, Brazzi L, Pelosi P, et al. A trial of goal-oriented hemodynamic therapy in critically ill patients. SvO2 Collaborative Group. *N Engl J Med* 1995; 333(16): 1025–32.

36. National Heart, Lung, and Blood Institute Acute Respiratory Distress Syndrome (ARDS) Clinical Trials Network, Wheeler AP, Bernard GR, et al. Pulmonary-artery versus central venous catheter to guide treatment of acute lung injury. *N Engl J Med* 2006; 354(21): 2213–24.

37. National Institute for Health and Care Excellence. Delirium: diagnosis, prevention and management 2010. Available from: http://www.nice.org.uk/nicemedia/live/13060/49909/49909.pdf.

38. National Institute of Health and Care Excellence. Acute kidney injury: prevention, detection and management NICE Guidelines https://www.nice.org.uk/guidance/cg169 (accessed 1 February 2016).

39. Stewart J, Findlay G, Smith N, et al. Adding Insult to Injury: A review of the care of patients who died in hospital with a primary diagnosis of acute kidney injury (acute renal failure). National Confidential Enquiry into Patient Outcome and Death, 2009/ Available from http://www.ncepod.org.uk/2009report1/Downloads/AKI_report.pdf (accessed 1 February 2016).

40. Silvester W, Bellomo R, Cole L. Epidemiology, management, and outcome of severe acute renal failure of critical illness in Australia. *Crit Care Med* 2001; 29(10): 1910–5.

41. World Health Organization. WHO's cancer pain ladder for adults. Available from http://www.who.int/cancer/palliative/painladder/en/ (accessed 1 February 2016).

42. Royal College of Anaesthetists. The 3rd National Audit Project of The Royal College of Anaesthetists: Major complications of central neuraxial block in the United Kingdom. Available from http://www.rcoa.ac.uk/system/files/CSQ-NAP3-Full_1.pdf (accessed 1 February 2016).

43. Kuehn BM. Anesthesia-Alzheimer disease link probed. *JAMA* 2007; 297(16):1760.

44. Baranov D, Bickler PE, Crosby GJ, et al. Consensus statement: First International Workshop on Anesthetics and Alzheimer's disease. Anesth Analg 2009; 108(5): 1627–30.

45. Aromaa U, Lahdensuu M, Cozanitis DA. Severe complications associated with epidural and spinal anaesthesias in Finland 1987–1993. A study based on patient insurance claims [see comment]. *Acta Anaesth Scand* 1997; 41(4): 445–52.

Nutritional management of the surgical patient

Mattias Soop and Gordon Carlson

Introduction

The importance of nutrition to health has been recognized since Hippocrates, and his instruction 'Let food be thy medicine and medicine be thy food' remains relevant to surgical outcome today. This chapter will focus on the practical issues of nutritional assessment, the problems of malnutrition, and how to achieve adequate nutrition in the surgical patient. To provide context, essential background physiology will be discussed.

Assessment of nutritional status and screening for nutritional impairment

Macronutrient metabolism in health, starvation, and injury

A healthy sedentary human requires a daily energy intake of approximately 25 kcal/kg ideal body weight and 1 g/kg ideal body weight of protein. Carbohydrate, fat, and protein (macronutrients) are all essential, in addition to micronutrients such as electrolytes, trace elements and vitamins. There is a constant turnover so that normally, anabolism (synthesis) occurs at the same rate as catabolism (breakdown).

During fasting plasma concentrations of insulin fall whereas those of glucagon and catecholamines increase. These changes lead to breakdown of glycogen in liver and muscle, followed by gluconeogenesis (*de novo* production of glucose from amino acids). There is also increased lipolysis from adipose tissue and the resulting fatty acids are used as an energy substrate. Glucose remains the main fuel for the brain and white blood cells during early starvation.

In prolonged starvation overall energy requirements decrease due to falling plasma concentrations of tri-iodothyronine (T3) and weight loss. The liver converts fatty acids to ketone bodies (acetoacetate and beta-hydroxybutyrate). These are used as fuel by many tissues, including the brain, and the consequent reduction in gluconeogenesis decreases protein catabolism by approximately 25%. These changes preserve energy stores and ensure efficient utilization of what little food is available.

Nutritional assessment

It has long been recognized that approximately 50% of surgical patients present with significant weight loss.[1,2] Patients with malignancies and gastrointestinal disease are at particular risk of disease-related malnutrition (for a definition of malnutrition, see Box 5.4.1). The significant detrimental effect of impaired nutritional status on postoperative outcome justifies the inclusion of nutritional assessment in any effective strategy for managing surgical patients. Although perioperative nutritional support may reduce the risks posed by malnutrition (see Perioperative nutrition section), it must first be recognized. All patients undergoing elective and acute operations should therefore be screened for malnutrition prior to surgery so that early nutritional intervention can be instituted where appropriate.

Measuring the nutritional state in surgical patients

Diagnosing malnutrition in the surgical patient is more difficult than it might seem. Malnutrition is likely when body mass index (BMI) is below 18.5 kg/m^2 or there has been unintentional weight loss of 10% or more over 3 to 6 months. Muscle mass and fat stores can be estimated by anthropometry, including mid-arm circumference and triceps skin fold thickness. These assessments are commonly used for malnutrition screening in the community. They are less useful for surgical patients in whom fluids shifts caused by systemic inflammation, liver disease, and iatrogenic fluid overload lead to water retention. The ensuing oedema may result in overestimation of body weight and anthropometric variables. Blood tests are equally unreliable. Proteins such as albumin, transferrin, retinol-binding protein, and pre-albumin have traditionally been thought of as reflecting nutritional state. However, it is now known that simple protein-energy malnutrition does not result in a decrease in serum albumin concentration.

A decreased albumin concentration is a common finding in surgical patients. This is not due to malnutrition *per se*[3] but to redistribution of albumin. This is as a result of increases in capillary permeability, clearance, dilution, and a suppression of production. Albumin and other carrier proteins are therefore said to be *negative acute phase proteins*.

A third approach to assessing nutritional status is to measure muscle and immune function. Voluntary handgrip strength is a

Box 5.4.1 A common definition of malnutrition
Malnutrition: A state of deficiency of energy, protein, or other nutrients, severe enough to cause measurable adverse effects on tissue or body form, composition, function, or clinical outcome.

remarkably accurate gauge of protein malnutrition. Cell-mediated immunity is evaluated by delayed cutaneous hypersensitivity to common recall antigens. These functional tests require specialized equipment and training.

Scoring systems, such as the Subjective Global Assessment and Malnutrition Universal Screening Tool (Figure 5.4.1), combine several measures in order to improve sensitivity and specificity.[4] A weighting for acute illness is often added.

Malnutrition and operative outcome

Causes of malnutrition in the surgical patient

Diseases treated by surgeons predispose to protein-calorie malnutrition by two important mechanisms: impaired dietary intake and net catabolism. Anorexia and nausea are common in malignant disease and cause reduced food intake. A mechanical blockage in the digestive tract will also impair dietary intake. In many disease states and in injury and infection, net catabolism occurs despite provision of apparently adequate nutrition (see Metabolic responses to injury section). Malnutrition in surgical patients is often due to the combination of impaired food intake and net catabolism. Additional factors are sometimes observed, such as reduced absorptive capacity due to proximal stomas or fistulas, and impaired digestion due to pancreatic insufficiency.

Malnutrition and outcomes

Malnutrition has important adverse physiological consequences, including muscle weakness and immunosuppression. Muscle weakness results from net catabolism of skeletal muscle. Even mild degrees of muscle wasting cause a clinically significant decline in the strength and endurance of respiratory and skeletal muscle. Key components of immune function, such as cell-mediated immunity, phagocyte function, secretory immunoglobulin A antibody concentrations, complement activity, and cytokine production are also adversely affected by nutritional impairment. Consequently, malnourished patients have a higher rate of postoperative infection, respiratory complications, and delayed recovery when compared with adequately nourished patients undergoing the same procedures. It remains

unclear whether wound and anastomotic healing is impaired. Importantly, many surgical patients still do not get appropriate nutritional screening or early intervention.[5]

Obesity and surgical outcome

Obesity is also a form of malnutrition. The World Health Organization defines obesity as BMI over 30 kg/m^2, while Japanese and Chinese recommendations have a threshold of 25 and 28, respectively, based on epidemiological data of Asian populations. The World Health Organization estimated in 2008 that more than 10% of the world's population are obese.[6] Operations in body cavities, whether open or endoscopic, are technically more challenging in obesity. In addition, obesity is associated with co-morbidity including insulin resistance and diabetes, hypertension, ischaemic heart disease, and sleep apnoea.[7,8] These (and other comorbidities) lead to a significant increase in surgical morbidity and mortality.[9]

Metabolic responses to injury

Perioperative physiological stressors

Surgery causes a series of coordinated changes in cardiovascular, renal, immunological, and metabolic function known collectively as the 'physiological stress response'. These act to help the body recover from the pathophysiological stress of injury. The most important stressor is tissue damage, but surgery is also associated with pain and, in many cases, bacterial infection. Each of these factors can independently trigger a stress response. Other perioperative stressors include anxiety, hypothermia, immobilization, starvation, and fluid balance derangements. An important concept in contemporary surgery is that these stressors can be attenuated or eliminated altogether. For example, tissue injury is minimized by minimally invasive techniques. Pain, contamination, anxiety, and the other stressors can all be addressed by specific perioperative interventions (see Chapter 3.7 Laparoscopy and Chapter 5.5 Enhanced recovery after surgery).

Mediators of the metabolic responses to injury

Some mediators that appear rapidly in the systemic circulation after surgical injury are released from the surgical wound itself.

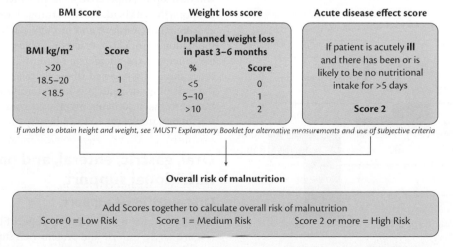

Fig. 5.4.1 Malnutrition Universal Screening Tool ('MUST') categorizes patients at low, medium, or high risk of malnutrition, and guides nutritional interventions.
The Malnutrition Universal Screening Tool ('MUST') is reproduced with the kind permission of BAPEN (British Association for Parenteral and Enteral Nutrition). For further information on 'MUST' please see www.bapen.org.uk, Copyright © BAPEN 2012.

These include prostanoids such as thromboxane A2, and cytokines such as tumour necrosis factor and interleukin-6. Activation of nociceptive afferents, and of autonomic afferents when the peritoneum or pleura are injured, results in tachycardia and tachypnoea. Catecholamines, cortisol, glucagon, and growth hormone (the 'counter-regulatory hormones') are released, whereas the release of anabolic hormones such as insulin is suppressed.

Changes in macronutrient metabolism in injury

Sir David Cuthbertson described two distinct phases in the metabolic response to accidental injury.[10] The initial *ebb* phase is characterized by a reduced energy expenditure and hyperglycaemia. After several hours, the ebb phase merges into the *flow* phase. The flow phase lasts for days or weeks depending on the magnitude of injury and is characterized by two important and linked metabolic derangements: protein catabolism and insulin resistance. Increased nitrogen excretion in the urine come from net catabolism of protein in skeletal muscle. The amino acids thus released are used for gluconeogenesis and protein synthesis. Protein catabolism is little influenced by administration of exogenous amino acids or anabolic hormones. Glucose and fat oxidation increase during the flow phase, resulting in a rise in energy expenditure.

A state of insulin resistance persists for days or weeks after injury, the so-called 'pseudo-diabetes of injury'. Despite a compensatory rise in circulating insulin concentrations, a resistance to the normally powerful anabolic effects of insulin develops. This is associated with net breakdown of fat and protein. Hyperglycaemia results from impaired glucose uptake in insulin-sensitive tissues and accelerated gluconeogenesis.

These responses have developed during evolution and confer a survival benefit in the injured, immobile and starving subject.[11,12] Such a benefit is questionable in the context of contemporary surgical care. Minimizing the stress associated with surgery, using multimodal interventions such as minimally invasive surgical techniques, regional analgesia, and nutritional support is certainly of benefit and results in marked attenuation of the response to injury (Figure 5.4.2).[13,14]

These metabolic responses remain significant in sepsis and severe injury and have important implications for nutritional support. Calorie and protein requirements may increase to up to 35 kcal/kg

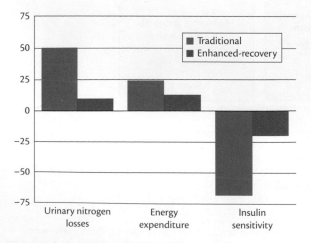

Fig. 5.4.2 Metabolic responses during the flow phase after major abdominal surgery in traditional practice vs enhanced-recovery practice.

and 1.3 g/kg, respectively. Lipids play a more important role as energy substrate as glucose utilization is impaired, and 50% or more of non-protein calories should be provided as lipid.

Perioperative nutrition

Preoperative phase

Malnourished patients requiring elective surgery require a period of preoperative nutritional support. This should be introduced gradually. Sudden and potentially hazardous falls in plasma electrolytes, notably phosphate, potassium, and magnesium, may accompany provision of food in malnutrition (refeeding syndrome). This is due to increased cellular uptake of the electrolytes with the nutrients.[15]

In patients who can tolerate oral liquids, protein-rich nutritional sip feeds are the simplest option. In some patients, preoperative nasogastric or nasojejunal tube feeding may be possible. In the absence of active catabolism 7 to 10 days of parenteral nutrition has been shown to reduce the incidence of postoperative complications by approximately 25%.[16]

Postoperative phase

Unless contraindicated or poorly tolerated, resumption of feeding within 24 hours of surgery will meet nutritional requirements. Early resumption of oral diet is associated with a significant reduction in the rate of infectious complications and more rapid recovery despite an often-observed increase in postoperative nausea and vomiting. It is firmly established that early oral diet is safe in patients with an intestinal anastomosis.[17–19]

A key objective in perioperative care is to actively minimize gastrointestinal paralysis (ileus) by a range of interventions, including minimal surgical trauma, avoiding opioid analgesia, and avoiding fluid overload (see Chapter 5.5 Enhanced recovery after surgery). Using these techniques, a daily oral intake averaging 1500 kcal from the first postoperative day and avoiding significant net catabolism is possible in patients undergoing bowel resection.[20]

Early oral intake may be contraindicated in some patients including those with an oesophageal, gastric, or duodenal anastomosis. Enteral tube feeding with a surgical jejunostomy or parenteral nutrition may be safer. Despite best efforts, some patients will develop postoperative ileus, in which case oral diet should be temporarily withheld. Early warning signs of ileus include nausea, abdominal discomfort, and hiccups. Although routine nasogastric intubation is unnecessary after elective gastrointestinal surgery and may increase the incidence of respiratory infection, nasogastric tubes should be inserted where there is clinical concern regarding the possibility of ileus. It is important to avoid pulmonary aspiration of stomach contents. Significant vomiting should lead to cessation of oral intake for 12 to 24 hours.

Oral, gastric, enteral, and parenteral nutritional support

Oral nutritional support

The simplest form of nutritional support is to supplement the diet (Figure 5.4.3). Calorie and protein-rich supplements are often used before and after major surgery to achieve desired nutritional targets. These sip feeds typically come in 200-mL containers and contain 200–300 kcal and 10–20 g of protein.[21]

Gastric feeding

If swallowing is impaired, nutrients can be administered directly into the stomach via either a fine-bore nasogastric tube, a surgical gastrostomy, or a percutaneous endoscopic gastrostomy (see Figure 5.4.3). Nasogastric nutrition tends to cause troublesome diarrhoea and is also associated with a risk of aspiration pneumonia. A gastrostomy is preferred to a nasogastric tube for periods of greater than 6 weeks.

Enteral feeding

It is generally recommended to bypass the stomach and deliver nutrients directly into the small bowel in patients with an oesophageal, gastric, or duodenal anastomosis (see Figure 5.4.3). This also may be necessary where gastroparesis and acute severe pancreatitis affect gastric motility. The small bowel may be accessed by passing a fine-bore tube through the nose and upper gastrointestinal tract (*nasojejunal feeding*), by an extension to a gastrostomy tube, or by creation of a surgical *tube jejunostomy*. Gastric and enteral feeding is often commenced at a low rate, and then gradually increased over several days to meet requirements. Abdominal distension, pain, vomiting and diarrhoea, and respiratory distress suggest intolerance and are initially managed by reducing the infusion rate.[22-24]

Indications for parenteral nutrition in the perioperative period

Parenteral nutrition is indicated when requirements cannot be met by normal diet or enteral nutrition, usually because of disease or resection of the small intestine. This is a condition termed *intestinal failure*.[25] A multidisciplinary nutrition team is essential for effective management of patients whose nutritional and metabolic problems are complex. Providing nutrition via the gut is physiologically simple and safer, and considerably less expensive than parenteral nutrition. It may be associated with better outcome. The two approaches

are now regarded as complementary and are often combined. Even meeting 10% of requirements via enteral feeding may be associated with beneficial immunological effects.

Intestinal failure can be brief (<28 days) and reversible (type I), more protracted but potentially reversible (type II), or chronic (type III) (Table 5.4.1).[26] Postoperative ileus is the most common cause of type I intestinal failure, and is seen not only in abdominal surgery but also in retroperitoneal and orthopaedic surgery, trauma, and critical illness. This is initially managed by nasogastric drainage and appropriate fluid and electrolyte infusions. Underlying causes, such as electrolyte disorders or intra-abdominal abscess are addressed. Nutritional requirements must be met within 7 days. In the event that the clinical problem has failed to resolve by then, parenteral nutrition is indicated.[27] If the patient is already malnourished it may be appropriate to start parenteral nutrition immediately.[28]

Type II intestinal failure is due to severe abdominal disease or injury causing a prolonged (>28 days) but potentially reversible disruption of gastrointestinal continuity or function. Parenteral nutrition is almost always required, and surgery is often indicated. Enterocutaneous fistulas are the most common cause of type II intestinal failure and typically arise as a result of complications of abdominal surgery. More than half of postoperative enterocutaneous fistulas will close spontaneously and parenteral nutrition is used to maintain nutritional status until enteral feeding can resume or surgery is undertaken.

Type III intestinal failure, often referred to as short bowel syndrome, results from a permanent reduction in functioning gut mass. This condition includes states with small bowel of adequate length but impaired digestive or absorptive capacity, such as in radiation enteritis. The most common cause, however, is small bowel resection due to repeated operations for complications of Crohn's disease. Type III intestinal failure is usually managed by home parenteral nutrition, although intestinal transplantation may be undertaken in selected patients.

Administration of parenteral nutrition in practice

Brief (<10 days) periods of parenteral nutrition can often be provided via peripheral cannulas. 'Peripheral parenteral nutrition' is simpler and less prone to complications than parenteral nutrition delivered via the central venous route.[29] To avoid the phlebitis that results from peripheral nutrient administration ultrafine (22 G)

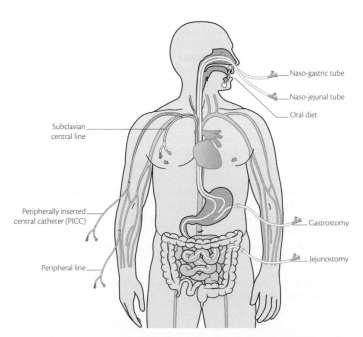

Fig. 5.4.3 Sites for administration of nutrition. Common routes of enteral (green lines) and parenteral (red lines) feeding.

Table 5.4.1 Types of intestinal failure

	Duration	Reversibility	Example
Type I	≤28 days	Yes. Usually spontaneous recovery possible	Postoperative ileus, or acute small bowel obstruction treated in hospital
Type II	>28 days	Yes, but frequently requires surgical treatment	Postoperative enterocutaneous fistula
Type III	Permanent	Not reversible. Small bowel transplantation sometimes possible	Massive small bowel resection, treated with long-term home parenteral nutrition

Source: data from Andrea Kopp Lugli et al., Strategies for perioperative nutrition support in obese, diabetic and geriatric patients, *Clinical Nutrition*, Volume 27, Issue 1, pp. 16–24, Copyright © 2007 Elsevier Ltd and European Society for Clinical Nutrition and Metabolism. All rights reserved.

and long (15 cm) cannulas are used and feeding solutions modified to make them less hypertonic and acidic (by reducing glucose and amino acid content). Cannula insertion requires an aseptic technique. The cannula and insertion site must be changed if signs of inflammation arise.

Most parenteral nutrition is administered via central venous catheters (including peripherally inserted central catheters or peripherally inserted central catheter lines). For long-term home parenteral nutrition, a tunnelled subclavian central line or a *totally implantable venous access system* is a safer and more secure access route. Strict asepsis is essential whenever catheters are inserted or handled. Parenteral nutrition is associated with a significant (but almost completely avoidable) risk of bloodstream infection, thrombosis, and catheter occlusion.

In addition to infection and catheter-related complications, parenteral nutrition is associated with a variety of metabolic complications. Glucose oxidation leads to a high carbon dioxide production, and may precipitate respiratory failure, especially in patients with pre-existing lung disease. Hyperglycaemia is common in parenteral nutrition and needs to be aggressively treated with insulin in surgical patients. Conversely, sudden interruptions may cause hypoglycaemia and weaning is therefore advisable. Hypertriglyceridaemia is common in parenteral nutrition and requires a reduction of the lipid content.

In the longer-term, hepatic steatosis can occur, particularly if there is excessive administration of glucose. This is potentially serious complication characterized by deranged liver function tests. It is difficult to reverse, but lowering the calorie content and changing to fish oil based lipid emulsions may be beneficial.

Conclusion

The nutritional state of the patient is an important determinant of the outcome of surgery. Before surgery, scoring systems should be used to identify patients with malnutrition so that it can be addressed early. With some important exceptions, most surgical patients can resume a normal oral diet soon after surgery. If this is not possible, gastric, enteral, or parenteral feeding should be commenced at an appropriate time. Importantly, such nutrition support should be provided in collaboration with a multidisciplinary nutrition service.

References

1. Burden ST, Hill J, Shaffer JL, *et al*. Nutritional status of preoperative colorectal cancer patients. *J Human Nutr Dietet* 2010; 23(4): 402–7.
2. Stratton RJ, Hackston A, Longmore D, *et al*. Malnutrition in hospital outpatients and inpatients: prevalence, concurrent validity and ease of use of the 'malnutrition universal screening tool' ('MUST') for adults. *Br J Nutr* 2007; 92(5): 799.
3. Smith G, Robinson PH, Fleck A. Serum albumin distribution in early treated anorexia nervosa. *Nutrition* 1996; 12(10): 677–84.
4. Studley HO. Percentage of weight loss. *JAMA* 1936; 106(6): 458–60.
5. Lugli A, Wykes L, Carli F. Strategies for perioperative nutrition support in obese, diabetic and geriatric patients. *Clin Nutr* 2008; 27(1): 16–24.
6. Makino T, Shukla PJ, Rubino F, *et al*. The impact of obesity on perioperative outcomes after laparoscopic colorectal resection. *Ann Surg* 2012; 255(2): 228–36.
7. Donohoe CL, Feeney C, Carey MF, *et al*. Perioperative evaluation of the obese patient. *J Clin Anesth* 2011; 23(7): 575–86.

8. Mullen JT, Moorman DW, Davenport DL. The obesity paradox. *Ann Surg* 2009; 250(1): 166–72.
9. Dindo D, Muller MK, Weber M, *et al*. Obesity in general elective surgery. *Lancet* 2003; 361(9374): 2032–5.
10. Cuthbertson DP. Post-shock metabolic response. *Lancet* 1942; 239(6189): 433–7.
11. Van den Berghe G, Wouters P, Weekers F, *et al*. Intensive insulin therapy in the surgical intensive care unit. *N Engl J Med* 2001; 345(19): 1359–67.
12. Finfer S, Chittock D, Su S, *et al*. Intensive versus conventional glucose control in critically ill patients. *N Engl J Med* 2009; 360(13): 1283–97.
13. Soop M, Carlson GL, Hopkinson J, *et al*. Randomized clinical trial of the effects of immediate enteral nutrition on metabolic responses to major colorectal surgery in an enhanced recovery protocol. *Br J Surg* 2004; 91(9): 1138–45.
14. Soop M, Nygren J, Myrenfors P, *et al*. Preoperative oral carbohydrate treatment attenuates immediate postoperative insulin resistance. *Am J Physiol Endocrinol Metab* 2001; 280(4): E576–83.
15. Mehanna HM, Moledina J, Travis J. Refeeding syndrome: what it is, and how to prevent and treat it. *BMJ* 2008; 336(7659): 1495–8.
16. Klein S, Kinney J, Jeejeebhoy K, *et al*. Nutrition support in clinical practice: review of published data and recommendations for future research directions. National Institutes of Health, American Society for Parenteral and Enteral Nutrition, and American Society for Clinical Nutrition. *JPEN J Parenter Enteral Nutr* 1997; 21(3): 133–56.
17. Lewis S, Andersen H, Thomas S. Early enteral nutrition within 24 h of intestinal surgery versus later commencement of feeding: a systematic review and meta-analysis. *J Gastrointest Surg* 2009; 13(3): 569–75.
18. Lewis SJ, Egger M, Sylvester PA, *et al*. Early enteral feeding versus 'nil by mouth' after gastrointestinal surgery: systematic review and meta-analysis of controlled trials. *BMJ* 2001; 323(7316): 773–6.
19. Lassen K, Kjaeve J, Fetveit T, *et al*. Allowing normal food at will after major upper gastrointestinal surgery does not increase morbidity: a randomized multicenter trial. *Ann Surg* 2008; 247(5): 721–9.
20. Basse L, Madsen JL, Kehlet H. Normal gastrointestinal transit after colonic resection using epidural analgesia, enforced oral nutrition and laxative. *Br J Surg* 2001; 88(11): 1498–500.
21. Keele AM, Bray MJ, Emery PW, *et al*. Two phase randomised controlled clinical trial of postoperative oral dietary supplements in surgical patients. *Gut* 1997; 40(3): 393–9.
22. Weimann A, Braga M, Harsanyi L, *et al*. ESPEN Guidelines on enteral nutrition: Surgery including organ transplantation. *Clin Nutr* 2006; 25(2): 224–44.
23. National Collaborating Centre for Acute Care (UK). Nutrition Support for Adults: Oral Nutrition Support, Enteral Tube Feeding and Parenteral Nutrition. London: National Collaborating Centre for Acute Care (UK); 2006 (available from www.nice.org.uk/CG032; accessed on 10 January 2013).
24. Teubner A, Morrison K, Ravishankar HR, *et al*. Fistuloclysis can successfully replace parenteral feeding in the nutritional support of patients with enterocutaneous fistula. *Br J Surg* 2004; 91(5): 625–31.
25. Carlson GL, Dark P. Acute intestinal failure. *Curr Opin Crit Care* 2010; 16(4): 347–52.
26. Lal S, Teubner A, Shaffer JL. Review article: intestinal failure. *Aliment Pharmacol Ther* 2006; 24(1): 19–31.
27. Braga M, Ljungqvist O, Soeters P, *et al*. ESPEN Guidelines on Parenteral Nutrition: surgery. *Clin Nutr* 2009; 28(4): 378–86.
28. Schricker T, Wykes L, Meterissian S, *et al*. The anabolic effect of perioperative nutrition depends on the patient's catabolic state before surgery. *Ann Surg* 2012; 257(1): 155–9.
29. Anderson A, Palmer D, MacFie J. Peripheral parenteral nutrition. *Br J Surg* 2003; 90(9): 1048–54.

CHAPTER 5.5

Enhanced recovery after surgery

Dileep N. Lobo and Olle Ljungqvist

Enhanced recovery: The philosophy

Many leading centres involved in enhanced recovery after surgery (ERAS) are engaged in the implementation of novel and improved care processes. A key to success lies in this change from traditional management to use of evidence-based best practice (Table 5.5.1), a change that frequently takes time.

Why does enhanced recovery after surgery work?

ERAS protocols are based on the best available evidence in the medical literature.[1-3] Experts in the field perform careful review and grade the evidence for effective perioperative management. Processes shown to have positive effects on outcome are included into a complete perioperative care programme that is then protocolized. Studies show that the more of these evidence-based treatments that the patients receive, the better the outcome.

Based on such work, societies and healthcare organizations (e.g. the International ERAS Society (http://www.erassociety.org) and the United Kingdom's National Health Service) run programs promoting the implementation of ERAS principles (http://www.institute.nhs.uk/quality_and_service_improvement_tools/quality_and_service_improvement_tools/enhanced_recovery_programme.html) One of the key aspects of these programmes is an emphasis on the coordinated training of teams of professionals from all disciplines directly involved in the patient's journey. An important aspect of the training concerns the use of audit. This ensures that, where outcomes do not meet the desired goals, they are reviewed and adjusted accordingly.

An important concept of ERAS is a common approach and a common view of the patient's journey. Silo working, where the patient passes through departments with little communication, leads to a lack of coordinated care. ERAS ensures that a treatment plan is developed that fits the patients' overall needs allowing them to pass seamlessly through the surgical process and achieve the optimal outcome (Figure 5.5.1).

A typical example of how a decision early in the journey can cause problems further down the line is in poor fluid management. The surgeon may prescribe bowel preparation. At the anaesthetic preassessment a standard overnight fast may be ordered. Both these decisions will risk a dehydrated the patient coming to theatre. Once the patient is anaesthetized, hypotension will develop more readily in view of the dehydration. This is likely to cause the attending anaesthetist to infuse intravenous fluid to counteract the hypotension. This may be continued postoperatively, which can lead to over hydration with a significant weight gain due to fluid retention. The fluid accumulating in the gastrointestinal tract can lead to a postoperative ileus delaying recovery. By employing the ERAS approach, this problem could potentially be avoided.

Preoperative considerations

Patient involvement

An important aspect of the ERAS process is patient involvement.[4,5] Tailored and in-depth information is given to the patient and his/her carer/relative. This is ideally given both orally and in writing. A folder or booklet using easy to understand and clear descriptions of the procedure and the perioperative care is helpful. Pictures and lay language are important to make the information understandable. If the patient has serious pathology it is sensible to give the diagnosis at a different interview to the details of any required procedure and care pathway. An emotive diagnosis, such as cancer, will often be a shock to a patient and they will be unlikely to absorb anything else. It is, therefore, wise to plan for a second visit a few days prior to surgery to go over the details.

At the second visit a more in-depth discussion should focus on what the patient can expect while in hospital. Issues such as pain and its management should be addressed. Actions that the patient can perform to enhance their recovery, such as ensuring good nutrition and the advantages of early mobilization, are stressed. It is also an opportunity for the patient to meet some of the professionals they may encounter in hospital such as physiotherapists, dieticians, and stoma nurses. Training in the management of a stoma prior to surgery can facilitate early discharge. The benefits of informing staff early if they have pain or nausea so they can be promptly treated to avoid slowing down recovery must be mentioned. Many institutions use patient diaries with targets outlined for food intake and mobilization. This can be very useful and motivating for patients. Older patients with daily or weekly care at home need to have the care givers involved in preparation for early discharge.

In the preoperative phase it is also important to screen for nutritional status. Any unplanned weight loss, reduction in food intake, and loss of appetite is of concern. It should prompt a full nutritional assessment and liberal use of preoperative oral nutritional supplements to promote caloric and protein intake. Inadequate nutrition will increase the risk of the patient becoming catabolic and also the risk of perioperative complications.

The patient should be advised to stop smoking as it has been shown that even a few weeks of refraining from smoking can improve outcomes substantially.[6,7] Similarly, patients with excessive alcohol intake should consider reducing their intake.[8,9] As both these life style changes are difficult it is often advisable to

Table 5.5.1 ERAS care compared with traditional perioperative care

Traditional care elements	ERAS treatments
Patient information is often short and often unstructured	Specific and detailed information about the entire care process including preoperative, intraoperative, and postoperative care elements with an emphasis on patient involvement. Expectations, including short recovery time and early discharge planning are clearly defined and laid out to the patient and caretakers
No special preparation of patient's physical status	Preoperative assessment of patient condition. Specific optimization to improve preoperative nutritional, medical and functional status
Preoperative bowel cleansing the afternoon before surgery. No food, only clear liquids the afternoon and evening before surgery	No bowel cleansing, normal food the day before surgery
Fasting from midnight, nil by mouth	Intake of clear fluids and specific carbohydrate drinks until 2 hours before surgery
Long-acting sedatives as pre-anaesthetic medication	Avoidance where possible of sedative premedication. Analgesic premedication prior to surgery
No specific prophylaxis for postoperative nausea and vomiting (PONV)	Active screening for risk patients for PONV and liberal use of multimodal PONV prophylaxis
General anaesthesia using opioids and long-acting drugs	General anaesthesia using short-acting substances, avoiding long-acting opioids. Thoracic epidural for open surgery and surgery expected to take several hours or with high conversion rates
No specific temperature control	Maintenance of temperature above 36.5°C using heating blankets and warmed infusions
Open surgery	Laparoscopic and minimally invasive techniques
Crystalloids to control volume status	Strict fluid balance. Use of goal-directed therapy monitoring of stroke volume, using crystalloids (or colloids) and vasopressors to control haemodynamics
Nasogastric tubes until bowel movements	No nasogastric tubes after surgery
Urethral catheters for several days after surgery	Removal of urinary catheters the day after surgery
No oral intake on day of surgery, slow resumption of oral fluids and food	Free intake of fluids immediately after surgery, intake of solids optional day of surgery
Intravenous low caloric glucose for several days	Intravenous fluids discontinued the day after surgery
Slow mobilization	Immediate and active mobilization
Postoperative pain control using opioids	Avoidance of opioids, multimodal pain control based on thoracic epidural, paracetamol and NSAIDs
Slow resumption of food intake	Food and oral nutritional supplements to secure energy and protein intake
Slow in-hospital recovery	Enhanced recovery and early discharge

consult specialist units for support. Prescribed medication should be reviewed and advice given where necessary. There is mounting evidence that even brief periods of physical training in the weeks before surgery can materially improve patient outcome and physical activity should be encouraged. Excessive alcohol intake should be avoided in the weeks preceding surgery and preoperative anaemia should be corrected using iron therapy.

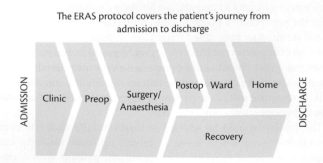

The ERAS protocol covers the patient's journey from admission to discharge

Fig. 5.5.1 The patients' journey through surgical care.
Copyright ©ERAS Society, with permission.

Curtailed fast

Ensuring normal metabolic function in the perioperative period is important. The tradition of starving patients for long periods prior to surgery is unnecessary, lacks evidence, and may be harmful.[10] Overnight fasting has a deleterious effect on preoperative well-being, increasing thirst, hunger, and anxiety. The prolongation of a catabolic state after the operation causes protein and muscle loss hampering mobilization. It also increases insulin resistance, leading to hyperglycaemia.[11,12]

ERAS guidance suggests that a shorter period of starvation for clear carbohydrate drinks and clear fluids permissible up to 2 hours preoperatively.[1-3] Carbohydrate drinks can counteract catabolic effects maintaining nitrogen balance and reducing insulin resistance.[12,13]

Avoidance of bowel preparation

Bowel preparation has been postulated to decrease the risk of spillage of bowel contents and surgical sepsis in the event of anastomotic breakdown. This tradition is being challenged by increasing evidence that avoiding bowel preparation is safe and the consequent reduction in the risk of dehydration advantageous.[14,15]

Intraoperative considerations

Surgical issues

Antibiotic prophylaxis

Wound infection is a significant concern. A single dose of prophylactic antibiotics, given according to local protocol prior to skin incision, can reduce the risk.[16] Ideally antibiotic prophylaxis should be given 30 to 60 minutes before the incision as this may be more beneficial than when given after the incision.

Approach and incision

The surgical approach should be selected to minimize the stress response. In practice this means considering a laparoscopic approach for abdominal procedures. Where this is not possible the incision should be as short as possible and ideally transverse. Recent trials have shown that the combination of minimally invasive techniques and ERAS results in the fastest recovery.

Drains, tubes, and catheters

Drains,[17] nasogastric tubes,[18] and urinary catheters[19] are often uncomfortable, can delay mobility, and are not without risks. A nasogastric tube can impair the integrity of the oesophageal sphincters leading to pulmonary aspiration of gastric contents. There is evidence that they can delay the return of gastric motility. Routine drainage after abdominal procedures is not associated with significant benefit. Urinary catheters should be removed as soon as is practical.

Hypothermia

Surgical patients can lose heat in a number of ways. Transfer to theatre down cold corridors risks heat loss via convection and radiation. An anaesthetized patient lacks the compensatory mechanisms to raise their body temperature. An unheated operating table may increase conductive heat losses. Fluid evaporating from exposed bowel will lead to a drop in temperature, as will the infusion of cold fluid. The ensuing hypothermia can lead to an increased incidence of surgical site infection, impaired coagulopathy, myocardial ischaemia, and arrhythmias. A patient who is cold also risks splanchnic vasoconstriction and the additional oxygen consumption caused by postoperative shivering is not to the patient's benefit.

Patients should reach theatre with a normal body temperature and some preoperative warming may be necessary to achieve this. If surgery is expected to last over 30 minutes measures to warm the patient should be considered. Warming may be passive, using blankets and foil wraps, or active with forced air warming or heated blankets.[20] Fluid should be warmed and the theatre should not be too cold.

Fluid management

ERAS relies on meticulous attention to fluid management. Unfortunately, it is often neglected and frequently left to inexperienced doctors. Poor fluid management causes major disturbances in homeostasis and has been shown to lead to a substantial rise in postoperative complications. Uncontrolled intraoperative fluid management can lead to a 4–6 kg increase in body weight even after removal of large organs such as the colon. The traditional postoperative fluid regime of 2 litres of 0.9% saline and 1 litre of 5% glucose a day often resulted in massive overload of sodium, chloride, and water. The ensuing splanchnic oedema can slow down the return of gut function, by affecting gastric emptying and enteral motility.[21]

It is not only over-use of intravenous fluids that may cause problems. Inadequate fluid replacement will also have adverse effect on outcome. Maintaining the right balance of fluids and electrolytes will achieve the best results.[22]

As discussed, the first stage in fluid management is ensuring the patient is well hydrated at the outset. Provision of clear fluids up to 2 hours prior to induction of anaesthesia and the avoidance of mechanical bowel preparation help ensure that patients are not fluid depleted. Once in theatre the aim of fluid management is to ensure optimal tissue oxygenation. The key components to consider in achieving this are cardiac output, oxygenation, and prevention of anaemia.

Anaemia may occur from blood loss, best avoided by meticulous attention to surgical technique, or from haemodilution by over hydration. Oxygenation is maintained by the anaesthetic team ensuring that the PaO_2 is adequate. There is some evidence that maintaining a supra-normal PaO_2 may be beneficial, although this needs to be balanced against the potential pulmonary risk.

Maintenance of cardiac output is achieved by use of judicious fluid boluses and vasopressors. Modern monitoring has made the process of estimating the cardiac output possible. The two principle techniques used in theatre are oesophageal Doppler and pulse contour analysis. The oesophageal Doppler monitors flow in the descending aorta whereas pulse contour devices analyse the arterial waveform.[23-25]

Oesophageal Doppler

Small fluid boluses (200–250 mL) are given and the resultant change in stroke volume and cardiac output noted. If there is no increase in stroke volume and cardiac output in response to a fluid bolus the heart is at the optimum position on the Starling curve. Further fluids will not increase the output further and vasopressors should be considered if hypotension is affecting end organ perfusion.

Pulse contour analysis

An alternative to oesophageal Doppler is the monitoring of the stroke volume variability. This occurs as a result of the variations in intrathoracic pressure with respiration. Keeping the stroke volume variability below 10% is in keeping with an adequate circulating volume.

Postoperatively over hydration is best avoided by early oral or enteral nutrition and discontinuation of intravenous fluids (see Box 5.5.1).

Postoperative considerations

Analgesia

To move a patient though an enhanced recovery pathway it is necessary to manage pain effectively. While opiates and their analogues are excellent analgesics, avoiding them, except for rescue purposes, is prudent. The side effects of opiates such as nausea, vomiting and ileus can delay recovery. Managing pain starts with the prescription of an analgesic premedicant often combined with an antiemetic. Paracetamol and, where tolerated, a non-steroidal anti-inflammatory drug (e.g. ibuprofen) can be used in combination with an antiemetic drug.[1-3]

A general anaesthetic combined with an epidural allows the benefits of the epidural to be continued in to the postoperative period.[26,27] A dense motor block should be avoided and this is best achieved by combining a low dose of a long-acting local anaesthetic with a short-acting opiate such as fentanyl. Epidurals are not

Box 5.5.1 Suggested algorithm for perioperative fluid therapy

Preoperative

Ensure adequate hydration by letting patients drink clear fluids up to 2 hours before induction of anaesthesia and avoiding mechanical bowel preparation

Patients with ongoing losses (e.g. enterocutaneous fistulae) should have fluid losses replaced adequately before being sent to theatre

Intraoperative

Avoid excess fluid administration (balanced fluid preferable to 0.9% saline)

Optimize stroke volume and cardiac output by administering small boluses of fluid (200-250 mL) in response to data obtained from intraoperative monitoring (e.g. transoesophageal Doppler or pulse contour analysis)

Give blood transfusion when appropriate

Postoperative

Avoid excess fluid administration – try to achieve state of zero fluid balance (most patients do not need more than 2-2.5 L water, 70 mmol sodium/potassium/day)

Discontinue intravenous fluids once oral intake is adequate (achieved in most patients 1 or 2 days postoperatively)

In patients with inadequate oral intake, supplement with intravenous fluids, avoiding excess. Consider enteral nutrition (or parenteral nutrition in cases of intestinal failure)

without risk. Hypotension that may require vasopressors can occur and this may delay mobilization. The epidural should be kept under constant review and, if the postoperative course is proceeding as planned, should be discontinued within 24 hours of surgery. The paracetamol and non-steroidal started as a premedicant should be continued into the early postoperative period.

Ward and social issues

The patient and staff involved in ERAS care should be aware of the recovery process. Recovery begins as soon as the patient is lucid after surgery.

Intravenous fluids

Overzealous administration of intravenous fluid should be avoided and vasopressors may be more appropriate to manage hypotension than fluids particularly in patients with epidurals. Where

Table 5.5.2 Discharge criteria

Factor	
Gut	Gut function back to normal: eating normal food and bowels moving (passing gas and/or moving bowels)
Pain control	Using oral analgesics
Mobilization	Mobile to preoperative levels, managing actions of daily living
No complication	No complication in need of hospital care

intravenous fluid is required it should be kept to a minimum and excess sodium and chloride avoided by the use of Hartmann's solution or other balanced crystalloids.

Nutrition

The patient should be offered oral fluids at an early stage, preferably within hours of surgery, and shortly thereafter an attempt should be made to include solids. Later in the day a light dinner may be appropriate. The information the patient received preoperatively will have appraised them that oral intake is a key target.

Early mobilization

On the day of surgery (providing the operation occurs early enough) a second key target is early mobilization. The patient should be out of bed for at least 2 hours, mobilizing with assistance. A structured plan should be in place with a named physiotherapist to facilitate it.

The patient should move to the ward as soon as he or she is stable. While there is no protocol that fits every patient, most patients will be able to follow a protocol provided the earlier parts have been fulfilled. Intravenous infusions should be discontinued the morning after surgery, and bladder catheters should be removed within a day or two regardless of the presence of an epidural. Intra-abdominal drains are usually removed no later than the day after surgery. These actions will help to liberate the patient from anything hindering a return to normal. It may be necessary to maintain the epidural if pain control remains an issue.

A functional programme will allow most patients to recover from their surgery and fulfil discharge criteria (Table 5.5.2) within a few days even after major surgery.

In most institutions implementing the postoperative aspect of the ERAS care is difficult. There are many reasons for this, the most common being that the preoperative and intraoperative care have not been optimal. The early ERAS protocol elements are critical to facilitate postoperative recovery, since the treatments given during the earlier phases have a marked impact on what it is possible to achieve in the postoperative phase. Intravenous fluids as discussed in the note are one example. A very common mistake in the preoperative phase is the failure to administer antiemetic prophylaxis. Nausea and vomiting result in poor nutritional intake and can also be caused by the use of long-acting sedatives and opioids. Care delivered in accordance with agreed protocols may avoid these pitfalls.

Most patients and carers have some preconceptions about the length of hospital stay from taking to relatives and friends. This is usually at odds with ERAS standards and is another reason why the preoperative preparation, explaining the targets for recovery, is so important.

Upon discharge, the patient and their carers/relatives should receive clear oral and written instructions for the ongoing care. They will receive information on follow-up events including nurse follow-up phone calls, usually within a couple of days after discharge, removal of sutures, and follow-up in clinic. These instructions should also be clear about early signs of potential problems and when to contact the hospital for advice. It is important to realize that some complications, for instance anastomotic leaks, may occur in the later phases of recovery. For this reason it is important to give the patient the ability to contact a surgical ward that has the experience in handling ERAS patients and can provide appropriate advice and enable readmission, if required, without delay.

Further reading

Basse L, Thorbøl JE, Løssl K, et al. Colonic surgery with accelerated rehabilitation or conventional care. Dis Colon Rectum 2004; 47(3): 271–7; discussion 277–8. Erratum in: Dis Colon Rectum 2004; 47(6): 951. Dis Colon Rectum 2005; 48(8): 1673.

Feldman LS, Delaney CP, Ljungqvist O, Carli F (eds.) The SAGES/ERAS® Society Manual of Enhanced Recovery Programs for Gastrointestinal Surgery. Springer: London; 2015.

Francis N, Kennedy RH, Ljungqvist O, Mythen MG (eds.) Manual of Fast Track Recovery for Colorectal Surgery. Springer: London; 2012.

Greco M, Capretti G, Beretta L, Gemma M, Pecorelli N, Braga M. Enhanced recovery program in colorectal surgery: a meta-analysis of randomized controlled trials. World J Surg 2014; 38: 1531–41

Kehlet H, Wilmore DW. Multimodal strategies to improve surgical outcome. Am J Surg 2002; 183: 630–41.

Kehlet H, Wilmore DW. Evidence-based surgical care and the evolution of fast-track surgery. Ann Surg 2008; 248: 189–98.

Ljungqvist O. ERAS-Enhanced Recovery After Surgery: Moving Evidence-Based Perioperative Care to Practice. JPEN J Parenter Enteral Nutr 2014; 38: 559-66.

Lobo DN, Lewington AJP, Allison SP. Basic Concepts of Fluid and Electrolyte Balance. Bibliomed – Medizinische Verlagsgesellschaft mbH: Melsungen; 2013.

NICE Guidelines [CG174] Intravenous Fluid Therapy for Adults in Hospital. London: National Institute for Health and Care Excellence, 2013. Available at http://www.nice.org.uk/guidance/cg174/resources/guidance-intravenous-fluid-therapy-in-adults-in-hospital-pdf (accessed 1 February 2016).

Varadhan KK, Neal KR, Dejong CHC, Fearon KCH, Ljungqvist O, Lobo DN. The enhanced recovery after surgery (ERAS) pathway for patients undergoing major elective open colorectal surgery: A meta-analysis of randomized controlled trials. Clin Nutr 2010; 29: 434–40.

Wilmore DW, Kehlet H. Management of patients in fast track surgery. BMJ 2001; 322: 473–6.

References

1. Gustafsson UO, Scott MJ, Schwenk W, et al. Guidelines for perioperative care in elective colonic surgery: Enhanced Recovery After Surgery (ERAS®) Society recommendations. Clin Nutr 2012; 31: 783–800.
2. Nygren J, Thacker J, Carli F, Fearon KC, et al. Guidelines for perioperative care in elective rectal/pelvic surgery: Enhanced Recovery After Surgery (ERAS®) Society recommendations. Clin Nutr 2012; 31: 801–16.
3. Lassen K, Coolsen MM, Slim K, et al. Guidelines for perioperative care for pancreaticoduodenectomy: Enhanced Recovery After Surgery (ERAS®) Society recommendations. Clin Nutr 2012; 31: 817–30.
4. Stergiopoulou A, Birbas K, Katostaras T, et al. The effect of interactive multimedia on preoperative knowledge and postoperative recovery of patients undergoing laparoscopic cholecystectomy. Methods Inf Med 2007; 46: 406–9.
5. Edward GM, Naald NV, Oort FJ, et al. Information gain in patients using a multimedia website with tailored information on anaesthesia. Br J Anaesth 2011; 106: 319–24.
6. Grønkjær M, Eliasen M, Skov-Ettrup LS, et al. Preoperative smoking status and postoperative complications: A systematic review and meta-analysis. Ann Surg 2013; 259(1): 52–71.
7. Lindstrom D, Sadr AO, Wladis A, et al. Effects of a perioperative smoking cessation intervention on postoperative complications: a randomized trial. Ann Surg 2008; 248: 739–45.
8. Tonnesen H, Kehlet H. Preoperative alcoholism and postoperative morbidity. Br J Surg 1999; 86: 869–74.
9. Tonnesen H, Rosenberg J, Nielsen HJ, et al. Effect of preoperative abstinence on poor postoperative outcome in alcohol misusers: randomised controlled trial. BMJ 1999; 318: 1311–6.
10. Maltby JR. Fasting from midnight—the history behind the dogma. Best Pract Res Clin Anaesthesiol 2006; 20: 363–78.
11. Awad S, Constantin-Teodosiu D, Macdonald IA, et al. Short-term starvation and mitochondrial dysfunction—A possible mechanism leading to postoperative insulin resistance. Clin Nutr 2009; 28: 497–509.
12. Ljungqvist O. Jonathan E. Rhoads lecture 2011: insulin resistance and enhanced recovery after surgery. JPEN J Parenter Enteral Nutr 2012; 36: 389–98.
13. Awad S, Varadhan KK, Ljungqvist O, et al. A meta-analysis of randomized controlled trials on preoperative oral carbohydrate treatment in elective surgery. Clin Nutr 2013; 32: 34–44.
14. Sanders G, Mercer SJ, Saeb-Parsey K, et al. Randomized clinical trial of intravenous fluid replacement during bowel preparation for surgery. Br J Surg 2001; 88: 1363–5.
15. Slim K, Vicaut E, Launay-Savary MV, et al. Updated systematic review and meta-analysis of randomized clinical trials on the role of mechanical bowel preparation before colorectal surgery. Ann Surg 2009; 249: 203–9.
16. Hawn MT, Richman JS, Vick CC, et al. Timing of surgical antibiotic prophylaxis and the risk of surgical site infection. JAMA Surg 2013; 148: 649–57.
17. Catton JA, Lobo DN. Tubes and drains in abdominal surgery. In Taylor I, Johnson CD (eds.) Recent Advances in Surgery 31. London: RSM Press, 2008, pp 13–26.
18. Nelson R, Tse B, Edwards S. Systematic review of prophylactic nasogastric decompression after abdominal operations. Br J Surg 2005; 92: 673–80.
19. McPhail MJ, Abu-Hilal M, Johnson CD. A meta-analysis comparing suprapubic and transurethral catheterization for bladder drainage after abdominal surgery. Br J Surg 2006; 93: 1038–44.
20. Kurz A, Sessler DI, Lenhardt R. Perioperative normothermia to reduce the incidence of surgical-wound infection and shorten hospitalization. Study of Wound Infection and Temperature Group. N Engl J Med 1996; 334: 1209–15.
21. Chowdhury AH, Lobo DN. Fluids and gastrointestinal function. Curr Opin Clin Nutr Metab Care 2011; 14: 469–76.
22. Varadhan KK, Lobo DN. A meta-analysis of randomised controlled trials of intravenous fluid therapy in major elective open abdominal surgery: Getting the balance right. Proc Nutr Soc 2010; 69: 488–98.
23. Grocott MP, Dushianthan A, Hamilton MA, et al. Perioperative increase in global blood flow to explicit defined goals and outcomes after surgery: a Cochrane Systematic Review. Br J Anaesth 2013; 111(4): 535–48.
24. Giglio MT, Marucci M, Testini M, et al. Goal-directed haemodynamic therapy and gastrointestinal complications in major surgery: a meta-analysis of randomized controlled trials. Br J Anaesth 2009; 103: 637–46.
25. Srinivasa S, Taylor MH, Sammour T, et al. Oesophageal Doppler-guided fluid administration in colorectal surgery: critical appraisal of published clinical trials. Acta Anaesthesiol Scand 2011; 55: 4–13.
26. Block BM, Liu SS, Rowlingson AJ, et al. Efficacy of postoperative epidural analgesia: a meta-analysis. JAMA 2003; 290: 2455–63.
27. Werawatganon T, Charuluxanun S. Patient controlled intravenous opioid analgesia versus continuous epidural analgesia for pain after intra-abdominal surgery. Cochrane Database Syst Rev 2005; 3: CD004088.

CHAPTER 5.6

Principles of transfusion and haemostasis

Jeff Garner, Andrew Fletcher, and Jeremy Groves

Introduction

Haemorrhage is an inherent risk in any surgical procedure. It may be the primary presentation as in trauma, upper gastrointestinal bleeding, and ruptured aneurysm, or it may occur as a postoperative complication. Despite the first successful human blood transfusion in 1829, surgical management of these problems was hampered until the recognition of the major blood groups by Landsteiner in 1900. This paved the way for the safe use of donated blood products to combat excessive blood loss. Blood was donated and stored prior to the Battle of Cambrai in 1917, but the first true blood bank opened in Russia in 1930. Advances in the science of haematology have provided ready availability of, albeit expensive, blood products, to allow surgeons to better address the issues of blood loss and coagulopathy in surgical practice. This chapter considers the provision and use of blood products and the processes that underpin the management of haemorrhage in surgery.

Haemorrhage and haemostasis

Haemostasis is the physiological process that stops haemorrhage. It can be considered in three parts. Initially a transected blood vessel will contract. Next the expression of tissue factor on the endothelial cell wall results in primary haemostasis; the stimulation, then aggregation and adherence of platelets lead to the formation of a plug. Finally, secondary haemostasis involves an interaction of platelet and blood factors that ultimately leads to the formation of fibrin and a stable clot. Many facets of this process, such as the surgical adjuncts to haemostasis, are covered elsewhere in this book.

Haemorrhage may be revealed or concealed. It can also be described as 'primary', 'reactionary', or 'secondary'. Primary haemorrhage is the direct result of surgery or injury, whereas reactionary haemorrhage occurs shortly after seemingly successful haemostasis (restoration of blood pressure and failure of surgical ligation are common culprits). Secondary haemorrhage is a result of delayed (7–14 days) sloughing of the vessel, due to things like malignancy, pressure necrosis, or infection).

Coagulation

The comprehensive global model of coagulation, which considers many procoagulant and anticoagulant factors such as proteins C and S, tissue factor plasminogen activator, thrombomodulin, inflammatory cytokines, and fibrinolysis, has replaced the simpler traditional cascade model (Figure 5.6.1). The cascade model, however, remains useful as the standard tests of coagulopathy are related to the extrinsic and intrinsic pathways. Table 5.6.1 highlights derangements in standard clotting tests and likely causes.

Conditions that impair haemostasis

Inherited bleeding disorders

Inherited bleeding disorders are relatively infrequent (Table 5.6.2) but remain an important consideration in surgical practice.

Von Willebrand's disease

Von Willebrand's disease is, in most cases, a relatively mild condition presenting in the form of bleeding from the microvasculature that is seen as cutaneous bruising. The rare autosomal recessive form though manifests with a significant bleeding tendency akin to haemophilia. The bleeding time is usually prolonged reflecting failure of platelet-endothelial adhesion and activated partial thromboplastin time (APTT) may be prolonged due to interference with factor VIII carriage. Desamino-D-arginyl vasopressin (DDAVP) raises circulating von Willebrand factor (vWF) and factor VIII levels. Drugs that interfere with platelet function, such as aspirin and non-steroidal anti-inflammatory drugs, should be avoided for postoperative analgesia.

Haemophilia

Both forms of haemophilia (A and B) are clinically indistinguishable and in their severest form present early in life with haemorrhage into the skin and joints. The APTT is usually >100 seconds but the prothrombin time is normal. Minor surgery can be safely performed with a factor VIII level of 30–50%, but major surgery requires levels >80%. Patients with factor VIII levels below 10% should be managed in specialist haemophilia units if at all possible, but major surgery, provided there is adequate perioperative monitoring, meticulous surgical technique, and timely replacement of clotting factors, rarely leads to significant haemorrhage.[2] It is notable that clots will form after surgery but they are friable and bleeding may restart many days after apparently successful haemostasis. DDAVP will increase release of stored factor VIII and the antifibrinolytic agent, tranexamic acid can help to stabilize friable clots. Inhibitors of factor VIII may be acquired after repeated infusions of

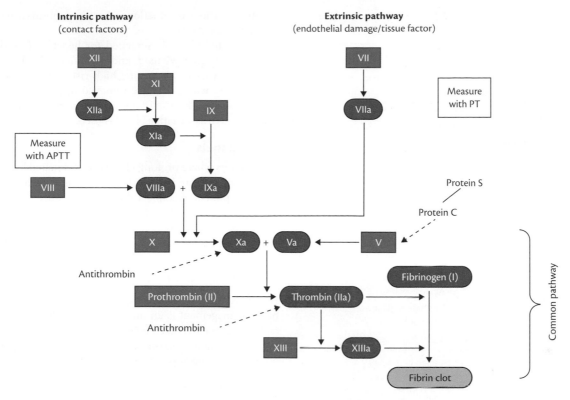

Intrinsic pathway
(contact factors)

Extrinsic pathway
(endothelial damage/tissue factor)

Measure
with PT

Measure
with APTT

Protein S

Protein C

Antithrombin

Antithrombin

Common pathway

Fig. 5.6.1 The coagulation cascade and the tests used to assess it.
Reproduced from Marco Tubaro *et al.* (eds.), *ESC Textbook of Intensive and Acute Cardiac Care*, Oxford University Press, Oxford, UK, Copyright © European society of Cardiology 2011, by permission of Oxford University Press.

factor VIII concentrate and is an indication for the use of recombinant factor VII. Haemophilia B is treated with infusion of specific factor IX concentrate.

Acquired bleeding disorders

All the factors of the coagulation cascade, as well as many other contributors to the global model of coagulation, are synthesized in the liver and thus hepatic impairment can affect most haemostatic pathways. Reduced intake or poor absorption of vitamin K can lead to impaired coagulation by virtue of decreased synthesis of factors II, VII, IX, and X. The anticoagulant warfarin takes advantage of this. Alcohol excess, hypersplenism, and folate deficiency will potentiate these problems by their effects on platelet number and function.

Acute coagulopathy of trauma is detectable on presentation (prior to resuscitation) in one-quarter of severely injured patients. It results from the activation of protein C, a natural anticoagulant, leading to inactivation of factors V and VIII and the inhibition of coagulation. Endothelial damage also releases tissue plasminogen activator, leading to fibrinolysis. The severity increases as the injury severity increases.[3] Major trauma is also associated with a dilutional coagulopathy from crystalloid resuscitation exacerbated by acidosis and hypothermia.

Drugs including antiplatelet agents (aspirin and clopidogrel) and anticoagulants (warfarin, heparins, and the novel anticoagulants) all lead to (deliberately) impaired coagulation and it is important to review all medication prior to surgery in the preoperative assessment process, and consider how these might be reversed.

Blood products

In the UK the blood donation service is administered by National Health Service' Blood and Transplant (NHSBT). Donated whole blood is centrifuged to produce a variety of component products, the standards for which are delivered by the British Committee for Standards in Haematology (BCSH). Similar arrangements are in place in many countries worldwide.

Whole blood

Use of whole blood is uncommon in general surgical practice but has been used by British and American military to good effect[4] and can be used in remote or austere circumstances after activation of a blood donor panel (see Donor panel section).

Packed red cells

The cells are suspended in a small volume of plasma augmented with preservative, either SAG-M (saline, adenine, glucose, and mannitol) or CPD-adenine (citrate, phosphate, dextrose, and adenine). One unit provides approximately 280 mL of volume and will raise the haemoglobin concentration by approximately 10 g/L. It is stored at 2–6°C and has a shelf life of approximately 35 days.

Table 5.6.1 Pattern of laboratory coagulation results and probable causes[1]

Abnormality	Associated results	Possible causes
Prolonged PT	Normal APTT, fibrinogen and platelets	Factor VII deficiency Oral anticoagulation with vitamin K antagonists
Prolonged APTT	Normal PT, fibrinogen and platelets	Factor VIII, IX, XI, XII or contact factor deficiency Von Willebrand disease Coagulation inhibitors (heparin, lupus anticoagulant)
Prolonged PT and APTT	Normal platelets and normal or low fibrinogen	Vitamin K deficiency Oral anticoagulation with vitamin K antagonists Multiple factor deficiency (liver disease)
Prolonged PT and APTT and low fibrinogen	Normal or low platelets	Acute liver disease Disseminated intravascular coagulation Massive transfusion

[1] APTT, activated partial thromboplastin time; PT, prothrombin time.

Adapted from M. Laffan and R. Manning, Investigation of haemostasis, p. 379, in S. Mitchell Lewis and Barbara J. Bain (Eds.), *Dacie and Lewis Practical Haematology, Tenth Edition*, Churchill Livingstone, Philadelphia, USA, Copyright © 2006, with permission from Elsevier.

Platelets

Platelets are pooled from four donations from a single donor and have a volume of approximately 50 mL/unit. They should be ABO compatible and are stored at 22°C for up to 5 days.

Fresh frozen plasma

Plasma is the acellular liquid component of blood and contains all clotting factors. It is stored frozen and then thawed as required (which takes 20 minutes). The thawed product has a life of approximately 2 hours; it should be ABO compatible. One unit is approximately 200 mL of volume.

Cryoprecipitate

Produced by centrifugation of the precipitated residues as fresh frozen plasma is thawed, it is rich in fibrinogen and factors VII, VIII, and IX and vWF. One unit equates to 20 mL. It is normally given in ten-unit infusions in situations where hypofibrinaemia is the main clotting abnormality.

All donated blood is screened for hepatitis B and C, human immunodeficiency virus 1 and 2, human T-cell lymphotropic virus, and syphilis. In specific high-risk circumstances, leukoreduced (stray white cells are removed to prevent alloimmunization), irradiated (for use in the severely immunocompromised), or cytomegalovirus-negative blood is used.

Donor panels

In situations where prolonged storage of donated blood is impractical or where there is a specific indication for whole blood rather than component therapy, a donor panel is useful. Volunteers are pre-screened for all the above diseases and blood grouped; when needed individuals are contacted to donate and the sample is rapidly rescreened and group-typed.

Patient blood management

Blood products are scarce, expensive and not without risk. Patient blood management is an international, evidence-based, multidisciplinary approach taken by transfusion services to ensure rational practice. It divides surgical transfusion into preoperative, perioperative, and postoperative care.

Preoperative patient blood management

Preoperatively, patient blood management aims to optimize the patient's clinical condition, with particular regard to anaemia and coagulopathy.[5] The prevalence of anaemia increases with age, and 11% of men and 10% of women are affected by the age of 65.[6] One-third of elective orthopaedic patients, for example, have haemoglobin levels below 130 g/L.[7] Untreated preoperative anaemia and transfusion with allogenic blood are associated with increased morbidity and mortality[8,9] and worse long-term oncological outcomes.[10,11] Mortality is increased below a haemoglobin of 100 g/L, an effect that is more pronounced in those with cardiovascular disease.[12] A lower haemoglobin on admission for orthopaedic surgery is associated with delayed functional recovery and decreased quality of life.[13,14]

Iron deficiency anaemia identified preoperatively can be addressed by oral iron or, if the urgency of surgery precludes 3 months of oral treatment, intravenous iron will raise the haemoglobin by approximately 20 g/L within 6 weeks.[15] Other causes for anaemia such as haemolysis or chronic renal disease should be sought and, if possible, corrected. Unselected coagulation testing of preoperative patients and subjective

Table 5.6.2 Inherited bleeding disorders

Disorder	Inheritance	Prevalence	Deficiency	Treatment
Von Willebrand's disease	Autosomal dominant	1 in 100 (clinically significant in 1 in 10 000)	Von Willebrand factor (a protein required for platelet adhesion and circulatory carriage of factor VIII)	Desmopressin or factor VIII concentrate
Haemophilia A	X-linked recessive	1 in 5000	Factor VIII	Factor VIII concentrate
Haemophilia B (Christmas disease)	X-linked recessive	1 in 30 000	Factor IX	Factor IX concentrate

assessment of bleeding history is unlikely to identify any significant bleeding risk,[16] as up to 25% of patients describe previous epistaxis, gum bleeding, and postpartum haemorrhage yet have a normal coagulation profile.[16] Structured questioning about family history, procedure or trauma related bleeding, anticoagulants, and antiplatelet drugs is more useful and, if this clinical assessment is positive, should lead to targeted investigation of coagulation.[17]

Perioperative patient blood management

The aim during surgery should be to avoid the need for transfusion. Blood loss leading to a drop in haemoglobin concentration of more than 40 g/L has been shown to increase mortality in those with cardiovascular disease and increase morbidity in those without.[18]

Alternatives to allogenic transfusion

In addition to employing optimal surgical technique to limit blood loss and maintenance of normothermia there are a number of adjuncts that may avoid or limit the need for allogenic blood transfusion.

Normovolaemic haemodilution

Normovolaemic haemodilution is commonly used in major cardiac or orthopaedic procedures. Haemoglobin can be lowered to 50 g/L in healthy volunteers and 60–90 g/L in patients without cardiovascular disease with no adverse effects.[19] Blood (usually one to three units) is withdrawn during surgery and replaced by colloid and crystalloid to maintain circulating volume. The blood is anticoagulated and maintained at room temperature and can be reinfused during or after the procedure.

Preoperative autologous donation

Blood is extracted and stored in the run up to surgery, significantly reducing the risk of haemolytic, allergic, or febrile transfusion reactions. The evidence suggests that transfusion is more likely to be employed when using autologous blood.

Cell salvage

Aspirated blood is anticoagulated, washed, and centrifuged before being pumped into an infusion bag. Modern cell salvage machines can provide 225 mL of red cells suspended in saline with a haematocrit of 50% in 3 minutes. Contraindications are few but include reinfusion of substances potentially harmful to the patient such as clotting agents, catecholamines, and amniotic fluid. Cell salvage with bacterial contamination from abdominal hollow viscus injury does not give rise to clinically significant infective complications.[20]

Antifibrinolytic drugs

Tranexamic acid inhibits the lysine binding site on plasmin-reducing clot breakdown. The CRASH-2 trial assessed more than 20 000 adult patients following trauma and determined that administration of 1 g given over 10 minutes followed by the same dose infused over 8 hours, started within 3 hours of injury significantly reduced all-cause mortality.[21]

Postoperative patient blood management

There is no demonstrable benefit of transfusion at a liberal haemoglobin threshold of 100–120 g/L compared to a more restrictive threshold of 70–90 g/L except for those with cardiovascular disease.[22]

Complications of transfusions

Reactions to transfusions are widespread and may be immunological, infective, biochemical, or volume related.

Acute haemolytic reactions

These are caused by major blood group antigen incompatibility and are usually due to clerical error. A complement-mediated inflammatory response is characterized by hypotension, tachycardia, tachypnoea, shortness of breath, urticaria, flank pain, and pyrexia. Haemolysis yields haemoglobinuria and anaemia.

Non-haemolytic febrile reactions

These are common and usually mild and caused by reaction to leucocyte-related antigens. Patients become pyrexial about 1 hour into the transfusion. Antipyretics such as paracetamol help. Nausea and vomiting, rigors, and high fever herald a severe reaction. The use of leucocyte-depleted transfusions reduces the incidence.

Transfusion-related circulatory overload

Nine deaths in the UK were attributable to transfusion in 2012 with six being related to transfusion-related circulatory overload (TACO).[23] TACO is a risk particularly in the elderly. It can be minimized by adequate pretransfusion assessment, careful fluid balance, and close nursing supervision during the transfusion; some instances occur on the basis of an erroneous haemoglobin result.

Allergic reactions/anaphylaxis

A papular rash, pruritus, and pyrexia represent a histamine-mediated reaction to blood components that usually settles with an antihistamine. Anaphylaxis is accompanied by hypotension, angio-oedema, and bronchospasm.

Transfusion-related lung injury

This presents with clinical features identical to adult respiratory distress syndrome (hypoxaemia, dyspnoea, cyanosis, fever, tachycardia, and hypotension from non-cardiogenic pulmonary oedema) in the context of a transfusion and is an antibody response to donor HLA.

Transfusion-related infections

These may be bacterial or viral. Viral contamination of blood products may occur in the 'conversion window' when a donor is infective but screening tests are not yet positive. Transfusion-transmitted infection is now very rare, but transmission of hepatitis B to two patients in the UK occurred in 2012 and is a reminder that components should only be transfused if necessary with the reasons documented in the case notes.[23]

Others

Transfusion runs the risk of hypocalcaemia (from citrate binding), hyperkalaemia (from leaching from effete red cells), and hypothermia (from inadequate warming of cold transfusion products).

Serious Hazards of Transfusion report

The Serious Hazards of Transfusion (SHOT) report is an analysis of anonymous reports of transfusion incidents within the UK, making annual recommendations to improve patient safety. The authors of the 2012 report analysed 2638 reports (2767 patients), over half (62%) of which were preventable and 37% pathological.[23] The report shows that while transfusion is safe (the estimated risk of death from transfusion is 3.1 per million components issued and major morbidity is 46.5 per million components issued), there are still incidents of avoidable harm.[23]

The key recommendations of the report are:

◆ Correct patient identification is essential. Patients should be positively identified (asked to say their name and date of birth, and not prompted with a question that requires a yes/no answer).

◆ Zero tolerance is recommended for all pathology samples. No sample should be accepted in the laboratory without the standard four identifiers of first name, last name, date of birth, and hospital number or equivalent.

◆ Meticulous attention to detail and communication at handover is essential.

The most common adverse event was an acute transfusion reaction (allergic, hypotensive, or severe febrile); however, the largest category and the most common error remained transfusion of an incorrect blood component. This is a particular problem in patient groups who did not receive components suitable for their particular needs. For example, those with a past history of Hodgkin's lymphoma require irradiated cells and those with sickle cell disease require more specific red cell phenotypes. It is the doctor's responsibility to inform the laboratory of any such diseases.

The majority of incidents are caused by human error, such as misidentification at the time of sampling or failure to perform the bedside checks at the time of transfusion. Labelling a sample away from the bedside leads to 'wrong blood in tube' errors and for each of these which results in a wrong component transfusion there are about 100 'near miss' events. SHOT 'near miss' data analysis show that doctors are the most likely to commit these errors.[23]

Safety of blood components

Blood components remain safe and effective when used appropriately. Errors aside, in 2012 the most common complications were acute transfusion reactions (60% of pathological events), haemolytic transfusion reactions (19% of pathological transfusion reactions), and TACO in 13%. The breakdown for general surgery and orthopaedics and trauma is shown in Figure 5.6.2.

It is the responsibility of doctors who prescribe transfusions to ensure that they are indicated, that the patient has been informed and consented (where possible), that the specific requirements are notified to the transfusion laboratory, that the patient has been appropriately assessed, and that the transfusion is carefully monitored. Patients should be advised to report any adverse reactions, including those that may occur several hours or days after the transfusion.

Special situations

Massive transfusion

Massive transfusion is defined, arbitrarily, as replacement of a patient's total circulating volume within 24 hours or half of the

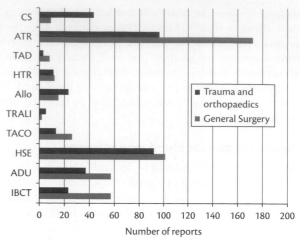

Key.
CS: Cell salvage and autologous transfusion
ATR: Acute transfusion reaction
TAD: Transfusion-associated dyspnoea
HTR: Haemolytic transfusion reaction
ALLO: Alloimmunisation.
TRALI: Transfusion-related acute lung injury
TACO: Transfusion-associated circulatory overload
HSE: Handling & storage errors
ADU: Avoidable, delayed or undertransfusion
IBCT: Incorrect blood component transfused

Fig. 5.6.2 All events reported to the Serious Hazards of Transfusion group for general surgery and orthopaedics and trauma patients 2010–2012.
Source: data from PHB Bolton-Maggs (ed.), D Poles, A Watt, D Thomas and H Cohen on behalf of the Serious Hazards of Transfusion Steering Group, *The 2012 Annual SHOT Report* (2013), Copyright © Serious Hazards of Transfusion 2012, available from http://www.shotuk.org/wp-content/uploads/SHOT-Annual-Report-2012.pdf

blood volume within 4 hours. It aims to restore circulating blood volume, oxygen carrying capacity, coagulation, and biochemistry. Most hospitals now have a dedicated Massive Transfusion Policy that can be activated after trauma, obstetric haemorrhage, or other major bleeds which should be applied concurrently with attempts at surgical arrest of ongoing haemorrhage.

Damage control resuscitation

The recent experience of military doctors has given rise to the concept of damage control resuscitation for seriously injured casualties. It replaces exsanguinated blood with as close a replacement as possible (i.e. packed red cells, fresh frozen plasma and platelets) rather than crystalloid in a ratio of 1:1:1 and improves survival[24] (Figure 5.6.3).

This process is facilitated by point of care testing using rotational thromboelastometry to guide the management of coagulopathy associated with massive haemorrhage. Rotational thromboelastometry measures the speed and strength of clot development, and different traces identify specific deficiencies that allows targeted component therapy (Figure 5.6.4).

Management of those who refuse transfusion

People may refuse to accept blood transfusion for a variety of reasons; Jehovah's Witnesses are likely to be the largest group encountered. The ethical and legal position is that any competent adult is entitled to refuse treatment, even if it is possible the refusal will

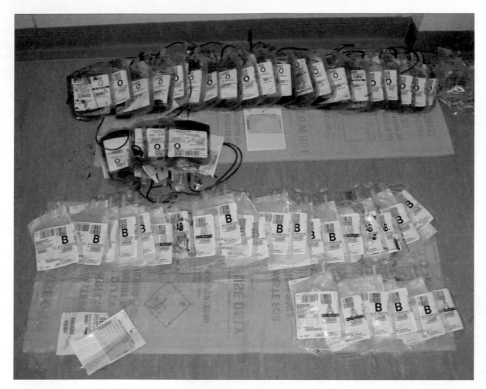

Fig. 5.6.3 The aftermath of massive transfusion following thoracoabdominal gunshot wounding.
Reproduced courtesy of Major Simon Davies QARANC.

result in their own death. It is important to ascertain clearly and in advance if possible, exactly what blood products can or cannot be given and in which circumstances. Cell salvage may be acceptable to some Jehovah's Witnesses if they perceive that the extracted blood remains in contact with the patient through a sealed circuit. It is vital to document these discussions in the medical records. In the elective setting, DDAVP and erythropoietin may be used preoperatively to raise the haemoglobin level and recombinant clotting factors may be used perioperatively.

Acknowledgements
The authors would like to thank Dr Paula Boulton-Magna for her advice on serious hazards of transfusion.

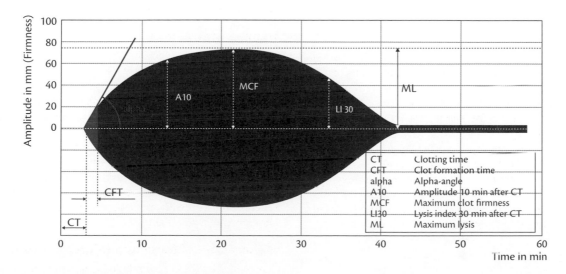

Fig. 5.6.4 Representative rotational thromboelastometry.
Reproduced with permission from Lt Col James McNicholas and JD Henning, Major Military Trauma: Decision Making in the ICU, *Journal of the Royal Army Medical Corps*, Volume 157, Supplement 3, Copyright © 2011 British Medical Journal.

Further reading

Blood Transfusion Further information can be found in many different transfusion guidelines published by the British Committee for Standards in Haematology online at www.bcshguidelines.com and a good e-learning course is available at www.learnbloodtransfusion.org.uk.

Retter A, Wyncoll D, Pearse R, et al. Guidelines on the management of anaemia and red cell transfusion in adult critically ill patients. *Br J Haematol* 2013; 160(4): 445–64.

References

1. Laffan M. Manning R. Investigation of haemostasis. In Bain B, Bates I, Laffan MA, et al. (eds) *Dacie and Lewis Practical Haematology*, 10th edition. Philadelphia: Churchill Livingstone: Philadelphia, 2006, p. 379.
2. Bastounis E, Pikoulis E, Leppäniemi A, et al. General surgery in haemophiliac patients. *Postgraduate Med J* 2000; 76: 494–495
3. Brohi K, Singh J, Heron M, et al. Acute traumatic coagulopathy. *J Trauma* 2003; 54(6): 1127–30.
4. Spinella PC. Warm fresh whole blood transfusion for severe hemorrhage: U.S. military and potential civilian applications. *Crit Care Med* 2008; 36(7 Suppl): S340–5.
5. Goodnough, LT, Maniatis, A, Earnshaw, P, et al., Detection, evaluation, and management of preoperative anaemia in the elective orthopaedic surgical patient: NATA guidelines. *Br J Anaesth* 2011; 106(1): 13–22.
6. Nutritional anaemias. Report of a WHO scientific group. *WHOrgan Tech Rep Ser* 1968; 405: 5–37.
7. Bierbaum BE, Callaghan JJ, Galante JO, et al. An analysis of blood management in patients having a total hip or knee arthroplasty. *J Bone Joint Surg Am* 1999; 81(1): 2–10.
8. Beattie WS, Karkouti K, Wijeysundera DN, et al. Risk associated with preoperative anemia in noncardiac surgery: a single-center cohort study. *Anesthesiology* 2009; 110(3): 574–81.
9. Khanna MP, Hebert PC, Fergusson DA, Review of the clinical practice literature on patient characteristics associated with perioperative allogeneic red blood cell transfusion. *Transfus Med Rev* 2003; 17(2): 110–9.
10. Amato A, Pescatori M. Perioperative blood transfusions and recurrence of colorectal cancer. *Cochrane Database Syst Rev* 2006; 1: CD005033

11. Linder BJ, Frank I, Cheville JC, et al. The impact of perioperative blood transfusion on cancer recurrence and survival following radical cystectomy. *Eur Urol* 2013; 63: 839–45.
12. Carson JL, Duff A, Poses RM, et al. Effect of anaemia and cardiovascular disease on surgical mortality and morbidity. *Lancet* 1996; 348(9034): 1055–60.
13. Gruson, KI, Aharonoff, GB, Egol, KA, et al. The relationship between admission hemoglobin level and outcome after hip fracture. *J Orthop Trauma* 2002; 16(1): 39–44.
14. Halm EA, Wang JJ, Boockvar K, et al., The effect of perioperative anemia on clinical and functional outcomes in patients with hip fracture. *J Orthop Trauma* 2004; 18(6): 369–74.
15. Dillon R, Momoh I, Francis Y, et al. Comparative efficacy of three forms of parenteral iron. *J Blood Transfusion* 2012; 2012: 473514.
16. Chee YL, Crawford JC, Watson HG, et al. Guidelines on the assessment of bleeding risk prior to surgery or invasive procedures. British Committee for Standards in Haematology. *Br J Haematol* 2008; 140(5): 496–504.
17. Sramek A, Eikenboom JC, Briët E, et al. Usefulness of patient interview in bleeding disorders. *Arch Intern Med* 1995; 155(13): 1409–15.
18. Carson JL, Noveck H, Berlin JA, et al. Mortality and morbidity in patients with very low postoperative Hb levels who decline blood transfusion. *Transfusion* 2002; 42(7): 812–8.
19. Weiskopf RB, Viele MK, Feiner J, et al. Human cardiovascular and metabolic response to acute, severe isovolemic anemia. *JAMA* 1998; 279(3): 217–21.
20. Bowley DM, Barker P, Boffard KD. Intraoperative blood salvage in penetrating abdominal trauma: a randomised, controlled trial. *World J Surg* 2006; 30(6): 1074–80.
21. Shakur H, Roberts I, Bautista R, et al. Effects of tranexamic acid on death, vascular occlusive events, and blood transfusion in trauma patients with significant haemorrhage (CRASH-2): a randomised, placebo-controlled trial. *Lancet* 2010; 376(9734): 23–32.
22. Hebert PC, Wells G, Blajchman MA, et al. A multicenter, randomized, controlled clinical trial of transfusion requirements in critical care. Transfusion Requirements in Critical Care Investigators, Canadian Critical Care Trials Group. *N Engl J Med* 1999; 340(6): 409–17.
23. Bolton-Maggs P, Poles D, Watt A, et al. on behalf of the Serious Hazards of Transfusion (SHOT) Steering Group. *The 2012 Annual SHOT Report*. Manchester: Serious Hazards of Transfusion, 2013.
24. Jansen JO, Thomas R, Loudon MA, et al. Damage control resuscitation for patients with major trauma. *BMJ* 2009; 338: b1778.

Venous thromboembolism: deep vein thrombosis and pulmonary embolism

Rhona M. Maclean and Michael Makris

Introduction

Thrombosis is the formation of a clot within a blood vessel preventing the flow of blood. There are distinct differences in the pathophysiology, prevention, and treatment of thrombosis occurring in arteries and veins. Arterial thrombosis takes place in a high-pressure system where platelets are of primary importance and antiplatelet drugs are central to its prevention and treatment. Venous thrombosis, occurring in a low-pressure system and primarily involving the coagulation cascade, is prevented by and treated with anticoagulants. While platelets and coagulation factors are closely interlinked, these differences help explain the presentation and treatment of thrombosis.

Venous thrombosis

The factors leading to venous thrombosis can be divided into three main interrelated categories known as Virchow's triad: changes in the vessel wall, changes in flow of blood, and changes in the constituents of blood (hypercoagulability). A more detailed list of risk factors contributing to venous thrombosis is given in Box 5.7.1. While one risk factor may predominate, there are often multiple, less easily identifiable, risk factors present. If there are no risk factors, the thrombosis is referred to as idiopathic and the recurrence rate is much higher. In a situation where a risk factor is reversible, such as pregnancy or surgery, the risk returns to baseline once the risk factor is no longer present.

Some individuals have inherited abnormalities (e.g. antithrombin deficiency) that increase the risk of thrombosis, the most common of which are listed in Box 5.7.1, and are inherited in an autosomal dominant manner. The most frequent is the factor V Leiden defect that is found in 3–5% of the healthy population. It increases the risk of venous thrombosis fivefold to sevenfold. Because the absolute risk of thrombosis is low, asymptomatic patients should not be screened for thrombophilia unless they have a strong family history of thrombosis.[1] Once an individual has experienced a first episode of thrombosis the risk of recurrence is no higher than in individuals without inherited thrombophilia.

The main type of venous thrombosis is deep vein thrombosis (DVT) of the lower limb. This can lead to pulmonary embolism (PE). PE is invariably due to embolic material breaking up from a DVT and lodging in the lungs even when a DVT cannot be definitively demonstrated with Doppler scanning. Other types of venous thrombosis less commonly encountered include upper limb DVT (often related to central lines), cerebral vein, portal vein, and mesenteric vein thrombosis. As the name implies, superficial vein thrombosis occurs in the superficial veins and may extend to involve the deep venous system. When a superficial vein thrombosis is close to the junction with the deep venous system it should be treated to prevent extension and development of DVT.

Treatment of venous thrombosis is with anticoagulants. The reasons for treatment are threefold: firstly to prevent extension, which would lead to more severe acute symptoms including embolization; secondly to prevent recurrence; and finally to prevent long-term complications such as lower limb post-thrombotic syndrome and pulmonary hypertension.

Venous thromboembolic event risk assessment

The risk of developing a venous thromboembolic event (VTE) is considerably increased by ill-health, admission to hospital and surgical intervention. Patients typically present with a symptomatic VTE 14–28 days after surgery, but remain at significantly increased risk for 12 weeks after discharge.[2] Both medical and surgical patients are at increased risk; one-third of patients presenting with thrombosis will have had surgery in the previous 3 months,[3] and this risk can be significantly reduced by the use of thromboprophylaxis (pharmacological and/or mechanical). It is not possible to identify the specific patient who will go on to develop a VTE, nor the patient who will develop a sudden massive PE. Autopsy studies reported in 2001[4] demonstrated that in patients dying in hospital of PE the diagnosis was not considered in over 70% of patients.

Various risk assessment tools have been developed in an attempt to identify patients at high risk of developing a VTE so that they can be offered prophylaxis.[5,6] These tools typically identify venous thrombosis risk factors that are specifically patient related (e.g. past history of a VTE, obesity, active malignancy) and admission related (e.g. infection, surgical procedure), and guide as to whether thromboprophylaxis should be offered. Some of these tools also identify bleeding risk factors (e.g. active bleeding or thrombocytopenia), recommending caution with pharmacological prophylaxis

> **Box 5.7.1.** Risk factors for venous thromboembolism
>
> **Acquired risk factors**
>
> Older age
> Immobility
> Surgery
> Malignancy
> Obesity
> Pregnancy
> Combined oral contraceptive pill
> Hormone replacement therapy
> Dehydration
> Antiphospholipid syndrome
> Myeloproliferative disorders
>
> **Inherited risk factors**
>
> Antithrombin deficiency
> Protein C deficiency
> Protein S deficiency
> Factor V Leiden
> Prothrombin 20210A variant

if they are present. Many healthcare organizations have introduced systems so that all surgical patients undergo a VTE risk assessment on admission. The UK Department of Health (DoH) has introduced a quality improvement target—the VTE CQUIN (Commissioning for Quality and Innovation). The CQUIN penalises hospitals financially unless 95% of hospital patients have a formal VTE risk assessment (in line with the VTE risk assessment tool published by the DoH in 2010). It is now also routine practice to perform a root cause analysis (RCA) investigation for any patient diagnosed with VTE within 90 days of discharge from hospital. The aim of the RCA is to determine whether the patient had been risk assessed and whether appropriate VTE prophylaxis had been provided.

Thromboprophylaxis: mechanical and pharmacological

Studies investigating the efficacy of VTE prevention strategies (mechanical and pharmacological) utilize imaging (angiography, or more recently duplex ultrasound) to determine whether a lower limb DVT has developed. These studies have demonstrated the strong association between asymptomatic lower limb DVT and symptomatic VTE (proximal DVT and PE).[7] Strategies that reduce these asymptomatic thromboses have been demonstrated to reduce symptomatic VTE and reduce the morbidity and mortality associated with it.

Mobilization and leg exercises

There is no robust evidence to demonstrate that the promotion of increased mobility or the performance of leg exercises reduces the risk of VTE; however, it is well recognized that immobility increases the risk of thrombosis. Enhanced recovery programmes incorporating early mobilization have demonstrated improved patient outcomes; studies have been too small to determine whether the risk of VTE has been significantly reduced. However early mobilization and leg exercises are simple interventions and should be encouraged in all patients.

Mechanical thromboprophylaxis

Mechanical prophylaxis strategies include the application of antiembolic stockings (AES), intermittent pneumatic compression device, and venous foot pumps. These methods are all designed to improve venous blood flow in the lower limb veins, reducing venous stasis.

AES have been designed to apply a graduated compression to the legs, the compression being greatest at the ankle, diminishing towards the knee and the thigh. The intention is to prevent activation of coagulation by reducing venous filling and venous stasis, increasing venous blood flow, and avoiding subendothelial injury. The optimal stocking compression profile was described by Sigel in 1975 (the Sigel profile), with a compression of 18 mmHg at the ankle, 14–15 mmHg mid-calf, and 8 mmHg at the knee.[8] They are simple to apply, do not increase the risk of bleeding, and have been demonstrated to reduce the risk of VTE by up to 68% in surgical patients.[9] AES should not be used in patients with severe peripheral vascular disease or after stroke.

Intermittent pneumatic compression devices typically apply cycles of intermittent low pressure (40 mmHg) to the calf veins. This increases the velocity of venous return, may enhance fibrinolysis and inhibit the activation of coagulation. Intermittent pneumatic compression devices have been demonstrated to reduce the risk of VTE, but as with AES, are more effective when used in combination with pharmacological methods.[10] Compliance is often less than optimal in 'real-life' settings and care must be taken, if used, that they are rigorously applied while the patient is immobile.

Pharmacological methods

Vitamin K antagonists

Prophylactic warfarin significantly reduces the risk of postoperative VTE but is not used routinely because of the risk of haemorrhage and the introduction of newer pharmacological methods.

Aspirin and antiplatelet agents

Aspirin does appear to have some efficacy in the prevention of VTE and in reducing the risk (non-significantly) of recurrence in patients with a history of VTE. There are no robust studies comparing aspirin with other pharmacological agents (such as heparin) and it should not be considered the thromboprophylactic drug of choice.

Heparins and fondaparinux

Low-molecular-weight heparin (LMWH) and fondaparinux have been shown to reduce the risk of VTE in surgical and medical patients by over 66%, with an associate 2% increase in minor bleeding events, an increase in wound haematoma, and a small increase in major bleeding.[7] These medications are excreted in the urine, and the risk of bleeding is greater in those with renal impairment. If patients are given heparin or LMWH for prophylaxis, monitoring for heparin-induced thrombocytopenia should be undertaken in those who have had cardiopulmonary bypass surgery. Risk is low in other populations and routine monitoring is no longer recommended. Fondaparinux has a longer half-life (17 hours, compared with 5–6 hours with LMWH) and is less frequently used; however, it can be used as an alternative in patients with a religious objection to the use of porcine products (LWMHs are of porcine origin). Furthermore, there is no risk of heparin-induced thrombocytopenia associated with fondaparinux.

New oral anticoagulants

Over the last 5 years, dabigatran etexilate (a direct thrombin inhibitor) and rivaroxaban and apixaban (direct Xa inhibitors) have been licensed for use in the prevention of VTE following hip and knee arthroplasty surgery. These agents have considerable advantages over 'traditional' anticoagulants: they are oral medications, given at a fixed dose once or twice daily, with reliable anticoagulant effects. They have been demonstrated to be as effective in the prevention of VTE as LMWH, with similar rates of major bleeding. These agents are now routinely used for extended prophylaxis after orthopaedic arthroplasty surgery.

Duration of thromboprophylaxis

Patients remain at increased risk of VTE for up to 12 weeks after surgery. Studies of extended prophylaxis in specific patient populations (after hip and knee arthroplasty or hip fracture surgery, abdominal or pelvic surgery in patients with cancer) have demonstrated that it reduces the risk of symptomatic VTE. These patients should be offered extended prophylaxis in line with national and international guidelines.[5,6,11,12]

Investigation of deep vein thrombosis

The symptoms and signs of DVT are non-specific; it is not possible to exclude a DVT on the basis of clinical history and examination alone. Patients with DVT may complain of pain, swelling, and redness of the lower leg and be unable to put their foot to the floor. On examination leg swelling, unilateral pitting oedema, erythema, and tenderness of the limb may be seen, but not infrequently many patients with DVT will have few of these clinical signs evident. The differential diagnosis includes a ruptured Baker's cyst, cellulitis, and (rarely) malignancy. Approximately 20% of patients with symptoms of DVT will have that diagnosis confirmed.

Diagnostic algorithms for deep vein thrombosis

Clinical prediction tools use clinical assessment and D-dimer testing, such as the Wells score[13,14] (Table 5.7.1 and Figure 5.7.1). These score patients on the presence or absence of specific characteristics (e.g. cancer, paralysis, recent major surgery) and clinical signs (e.g. entire leg swollen), and categorize patients into 'DVT likely' or 'DVT unlikely'. D-Dimers are produced by the fibrinolysis of cross-linked fibrin, and are increased in patients with VTE following major surgery, in cancer patients, in pregnancy, and in the presence of infection, making their use debatable in the surgical population. Patients who are 'DVT unlikely' and do not have raised D-dimers can be considered to have a DVT excluded, and do not need further imaging performed. Patients who are 'DVT unlikely' with raised D-dimers or 'DVT likely' require further investigation by imaging studies.[15] These scoring systems have not been validated for hospital inpatients developing symptoms of VTE or pregnant patients; such patients should have imaging investigations undertaken.

Most centres use venous ultrasound (duplex ultrasound) to diagnose DVT, and this has high degree of sensitivity and specificity for the diagnosis of symptomatic proximal DVT when compared to contrast venography (the previous gold standard). Sensitivity

Table 5.7.1 The Wells pretest probability deep vein thrombosis score

Clinical feature	Points
Active cancer (treatment ongoing, within 6 months or palliative)	1
Paralysis, paresis or recent plaster immobilization of the lower extremities	1
Recently bedridden for 3 days or more or major surgery within 12 weeks requiring general or regional anaesthesia	1
Localized tenderness along the distribution of the deep venous system	1
Entire leg swollen	1
Calf swelling at least 3cm larger than the asymptomatic side	1
Pitting oedema confined to the symptomatic leg	1
Collateral superficial veins (non-varicose)	1
Previously documented DVT	1
An alternative diagnosis is at least as likely as DVT	−2
Clinical probability score	
DVT **likely**	2 or more points
DVT **unlikely**	1 point or less

DVT, deep vein thrombosis.

Reproduced from National Clinical Guideline Centre (5 May 2015), *Venous thromboembolic diseases: the management of venous thromboembolic diseases and the role of thrombophilia testing (CG144)*, published by the National Clinical Guidelines Centre at The Royal College of Physicians. The National Clinical Guidelines Centre is unable to verify the accuracy of the material presented. Copyright © NCGC. Reproduced by permission.

and specificity for below-knee DVT is considerably less. Recent National Institute of Health and Care Excellence guidelines have acknowledged this and recommended that duplex ultrasound scanning behind the knee (popliteal trifurcation) is undertaken, with repeat scanning performed 1 week later in those who are 'DVT likely' with increased D-dimers (Figure 5.7.1). Computed tomography (CT) and magnetic resonance imaging (MRI) and angiography are not routinely used in imaging for DVT; however, they are useful in the investigation of suspected iliac or inferior vena cava thrombosis. MRI is particularly useful in the investigation of suspected iliac DVT in pregnant women.

Investigation of pulmonary embolism

As with DVT, it is not possible to exclude a diagnosis of PE based on the history and clinical features alone. Patients most commonly present with symptoms of breathlessness, pleuritic chest pain, cough, and haemoptysis.

Diagnostic algorithms for pulmonary embolism

Clinical decision rules have improved the diagnostic process and use D-dimer testing to rule out PE in those considered to be 'PE unlikely'. Patients who are thought unlikely to have a PE using such scoring systems and with low D-dimer levels can have a diagnosis of PE excluded (Table 5.7.2 and Figure 5.7.2).[15] These scoring systems have not been validated in patients already hospitalized or pregnant patients, and these patients should have imaging studies performed if a diagnosis of PE is considered.

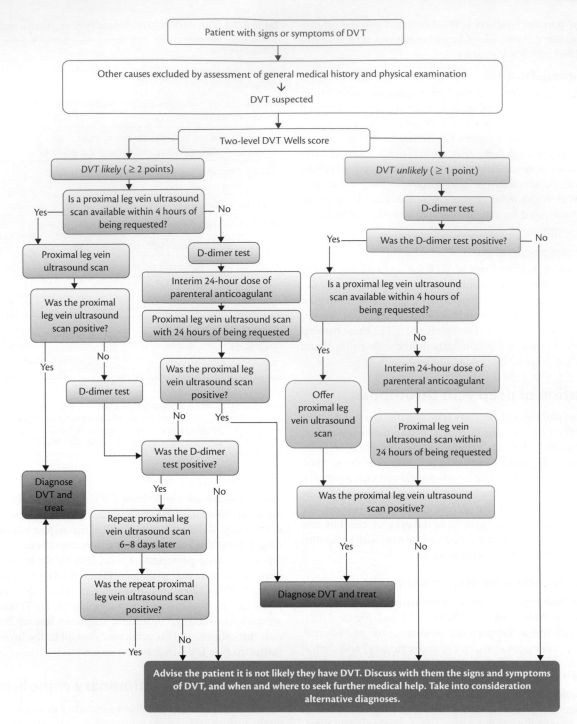

Fig. 5.7.1 Algorithm for the diagnosis of deep vein thrombosis.

Reproduced from National Clinical Guideline Centre (5 May 2015), *Venous thromboembolic diseases: the management of venous thromboembolic* diseases and the role of thrombophilia testing (CG144), published by the National Clinical Guidelines Centre at The Royal College of Physicians, 11 St Andrews Place, Regent's Park, London, NW1 4LE. The National Clinical Guidelines Centre is unable to verify the accuracy of the material presented. Copyright © NCGC. Reproduced by permission.

All patients should have a chest X-ray performed prior to further imaging; while it is frequently normal in PE it will aid in the exclusion of other diagnoses (such as heart failure or infection).

CT pulmonary angiography (CTPA) utilizing a multi-slice scanner is now considered the 'gold standard' for detecting PE (Figure 5.7.2). These allow the pulmonary tree to be visualized in less than 10 seconds, and report sensitivities of 83–100% and specificities of 89–97% in the diagnosis of PE. A good quality negative CTPA on a multidetector scan can be considered to have effectively excluded a PE and anticoagulation can be safely withheld. However, if such patients have symptoms suggestive of DVT, duplex ultrasound must be performed. Ventilation/perfusion scanning is now much less frequently used to diagnose PE; however, it can be used in patients with renal impairment in whom contrast cannot be given for CTPA.

Table 5.7.2 The Wells pretest probability pulmonary embolism score

Clinical feature	Points
Clinical signs and symptoms of DVT (minimum of leg swelling and pain with palpation of the deep veins)	3
An alternative diagnosis is less likely than PE	3
Heart rate >100 beats per minute	1.5
Immobilization for more than 3 days or surgery in the previous 4 weeks	1.5
Previous DVT or PE	1.5
Haemoptysis	1
Malignancy (treatment ongoing, treated in the last 6 months, or palliative	1
Clinical probability score	
PE **likely**	5 points or more

DVT, deep vein thrombosis; PE, pulmonary embolism.

Reproduced from National Clinical Guideline Centre (5 May 2015), *Venous thromboembolic diseases: the management of venous thromboembolic diseases and the role of thrombophilia testing (CG144)*, published by the National Clinical Guidelines Centre at The Royal College of Physicians. The National Clinical Guidelines Centre is unable to verify the accuracy of the material presented. Copyright © NCGC. Reproduced by permission. Source: data from Wells PS et al., Derivation of a simple clinical model to categorize patients' probability of pulmonary embolism: increasing the model's utility with the SimpliRED D-dimer, *Thrombosis and Haemostasis*, Volume 83, Issue 3, pp. 416–20, Copyright © 2001 American College of Physicians–American Society of Internal Medicine.

Some centres use perfusion scanning in pregnant women as a first-line investigation to exclude PE to reduce radiation exposure to the mother; however, with increasing use of breast shields, more centres are using CTPA in pregnant patients in the diagnosis of PE.

Echocardiography can be helpful in unstable patients who cannot be transported to the radiology department. Right ventricular wall hypokinesis and elevated pulmonary pressures are suggestive of PE, and can help differentiate between other clinical conditions such as aortic dissection, myocardial infarction or pericardial effusion or tamponade.

Additional investigations for patients with deep vein thrombosis or pulmonary embolism

It is well recognized that patients with 'idiopathic' VTE are at increased risk of having a malignancy. It remains contentious whether all such patients should be investigated for cancer, but current guidelines recommend that patients over the age of 40 years with idiopathic VTE are considered for further investigation. Such investigations should include bone biochemistry, urinalysis, chest X-ray, abdomen and pelvis CT, and mammography in women.[15] Whether such screening will allow earlier treatment of any malignancy and improved outcomes remains unclear.

Treatment of deep vein thrombosis or pulmonary embolism

The aims of treating DVT and PE are to relieve symptoms, to avoid thrombosis extension and recurrent thromboembolic events, and

reduce the risks of developing the long-term complications of VTE (post-thrombotic syndrome and chronic thromboembolic pulmonary hypertension). Anticoagulation is the mainstay of treatment of VTE.

Anticoagulation should be started as soon as a diagnosis of VTE is made.[15] Baseline blood tests should be requested (full blood count, renal and liver function, coagulation screen), but treatment should be commenced if the clinical situation requires it even if imaging is delayed.

Initial anticoagulation should be given with either LMWH or another immediate-acting anticoagulant (such as unfractionated heparin, fondaparinux, or rivaroxaban depending on the clinical circumstances), followed by oral anticoagulation with a vitamin K antagonist or rivaroxaban. Some patients may benefit from thrombolytic treatment, namely those with PE who are haemodynamically compromised, or have a significant DVT particularly if associated with a painful, blue swollen limb (phlegmasia caerulea dolens).[15,16]

Patients with PE who are haemodynamically compromised should be managed in an appropriate clinical setting such as a coronary care or high dependency unit. Intravenous unfractionated heparin should be used as it exerts its therapeutic effect faster than LMWH and the dose can be adjusted if thrombolysis is required.

The insertion of an inferior vena cava filter can be considered in patients in whom there is a contraindication to anticoagulation or if surgery is required within 1 to 2 months of a significant thromboembolic event, but there is no evidence to support their routine use. Retrievable filters should be used if the indication for the filter is temporary, and should be retrieved within 1 to 3 months of insertion.

Choice of anticoagulant treatment

For many years, heparin (unfractionated and LMWH) and vitamin K antagonists (such as warfarin) were the only anticoagulants available to treat VTE. Rivaroxaban (an oral direct Xa inhibitor) is as effective as LMWH and warfarin in the treatment of DVT and PE. It has a similar time of onset to LMWH and there is no need to give parenteral anticoagulation. It is now licensed in the UK for the treatment and secondary prevention of both DVT and PE. One advantage of rivaroxaban is that no monitoring is required (unlike warfarin). Rivaroxaban should not be used in patients with renal failure or if pregnant or breastfeeding. Other new anticoagulants (dabigatran, apixaban, edoxaban) have been investigated for the treatment of VTE and have been shown to be efficacious, but are not yet licensed for these indications.

Unfractionated heparin should be used for unstable patients, and for initial anticoagulation in those with renal failure (in whom LMWH and rivaroxaban are contraindicated). These patients can later be switched to an oral anticoagulant (warfarin if renal failure, warfarin or rivaroxaban when appropriate in unstable patients).

LMWH is the anticoagulant of choice in pregnant patients (in whom rivaroxaban and warfarin are contraindicated), and in patients with cancer who should usually continue with LMWH anticoagulation.

Hospitals should have in place clear guidelines and treatment protocols for patients with VTE. For the majority of patients either initial treatment with LMWH followed by warfarin, or alternatively oral rivaroxaban would be appropriate treatment regimens. Fondaparinux can be used instead of LMWH in those who decline treatment with porcine LMWH products.

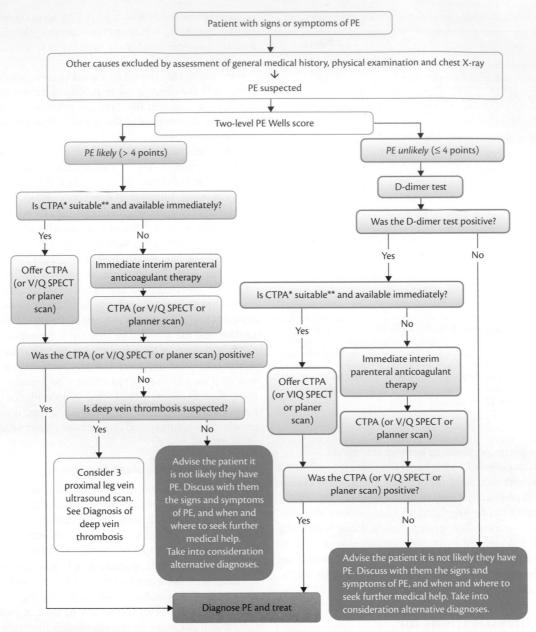

Fig. 5.7.2 Algorithm for the diagnosis of pulmonary embolism.

Reproduced from National Clinical Guideline Centre (5 May 2015), *Venous thromboembolic diseases: the management of venous thromhoembolic diseases and the role of thrombophilia testing* (CG144), published by the National Clinical Guidelines Centre at The Royal College of Physicians, 11 St Andrews Place, Regent's Park, London, NW1 4LE. The National Clinical Guidelines Centre is unable to verify the accuracy of the material presented. Copyright © NCGC. Reproduced by permission.

Many patients presenting with VTE can be managed in an ambulatory fashion, and hospitals will have protocols in place to determine whether patients are suitable for ambulatory care.

Duration of anticoagulation

The optimal duration of anticoagulation after a first VTE event is not definitively known. Short term anticoagulation (less than 3 months) is associated with a higher risk of recurrence compared with longer-term treatment.[17] Patients with a first provoked event (e.g. postoperative proximal DVT or PE) should receive 3 months of anticoagulant treatment. Those with recurrent events, or significant first idiopathic events should be considered for longer-term anticoagulation.[15]

Additional measures

Patients with DVT frequently develop the post-thrombotic syndrome, with leg discomfort, swelling, discolouration, and (not infrequently) ulceration. Wearing class 2 elastic compression hosiery reduces this complication. Patients should be measured for stockings approximately 2 weeks after diagnosis, and should be encouraged to wear them for 2 years (putting them on in the morning, taking them off at night).

Patients should be advised that, as they have had a VTE, they should be offered thromboprophylaxis at times of risk in future. Women should be instructed to avoid the combined oral contraceptive pill (progesterone only pill and mirena coil do not increase the thrombotic risk), and oral hormone replacement therapy (transdermal hormone replacement therapy or tibolone do not increase the thrombotic risk).

References

1. Baglin T, Gray E, Greaves M, *et al.* Clinical guidelines for testing for heritable thrombophilia. *Br J Haematol* 2010; 149: 209–20.

2. Sweetland S, Green J, Liu B, *et al.* Duration and magnitude of the postoperative risk of venous thromboembolism in middle aged women: prospective cohort study. *BMJ* 2009; 339: b4583.

3. Kearon C. Natural history of venous thromboembolism. *Circulation* 2003; 107: I22–30.

4. Pineda LA, Hatahwar VS, Grant BJ. Clinical suspicion of fatal pulmonary embolism. *Chest* 2001; 120: 791–5.

5. Gould MK, Garcia DA, Wren SM, *et al.* Prevention of VTE in Non-orthopedic Surgical Patients: Antithrombotic Therapy and Prevention of Thrombosis, 9th ed: American College of Chest Physicians Evidence-Based Clinical Practice Guidelines. *Chest* 2012; 141: e227S–77S.

6. National Institute of Health and Care Excellence. Venous thromboembolism in adults admitted to hospital: reducing the risk (Clinical Guidelines 92). London: National Institute of Health and Care Excellence, 2010 (available from https://www.nice.org.uk/guidance/cg92).

7. Geerts WH, Bergqvist D, Pineo GF, *et al.* Prevention of venous thromboembolism: the Eighth ACCP Clinical Practice Guidelines. *Chest* 2008; 133(6, Suppl): 318S–453S.

8. Sigel B, Edelstein AL, Savitch L, *et al.* Type of compression for reducing venous stasis: A study of lower extremities during inactive recumbency. *Arch Surg* 1975; 110: 171–5.

9. Wells PS, Lensing AW, Hirsh J. Graduated Compression stockings in the prevention of postoperative venous thromboembolisms. A meta-analysis. *Arch Intern Med* 1994; 154: 67–72.

10. Ho KM, Tan JA. Stratified meta-analysis of intermittent pneumatic compression of the lower limbs to prevent venous thromboembolism in hospitalized patients. *Circulation* 2013; 128: 1003–20.

11. Falck-Ytter Y, Francis CW, Johanson NA, *et al.* Prevention of VTE in orthopaedic surgery patients: antithrombotic therapy and prevention of thrombosis 9th ed: American College of Chest Physicians Evidence-Based Clinical Practice Guidelines. *Chest* 2012; 141: e278S–325S.

12. Scottish Intercollegiate Guidelines Network. Prevention and management of venous thromboembolism (SIGN Guideline 122) Edinburgh: Scottish Intercollegiate Guidelines Network (available from http://www.sign.ac.uk/guidelines/fulltext/122/).

13. Wells PS, Anderson DR, Rodger M, *et al.* Derivation of a simple clinical model to categorise patients' probability of pulmonary embolism: increasing the model's utility with the SimpliRED D-Dimer. *Thromb Haemost* 2000; 83: 416–20.

14. Wells PS, Anderson DR, Rodger M, *et al.* Evaluation of D-dimer in the diagnosis of suspected deep-vein thrombosis. *N Engl J Med* 2003; 349: 1227–35.

15. National Institute of Health and Care Excellence. NICE Guidelines 144: Venous thromboembolic diseases: diagnosis, management and thrombophilia testing. Available from https://www.nice.org.uk/guidance/cg144 (accessed 2 February 2016).

16. Torbicki A, Perrier A, Konstantinides S, *et al.* Guidelines on the diagnosis and management of acute pulmonary embolism: the Task Force for the Diagnosis and Management of Acute Pulmonary Embolism of the European Society of Cardiology (ESC). *Eur Heart J* 2008; 29: 2276–315.

17. Keeling D, Baglin T, Tait C, *et al.* Guidelines on oral anticoagulation with warfarin—fourth edition. *Br J Haematol* 2011; 154: 311–24.

Metabolic and endocrine disorders in the perioperative period

Robert Robinson, David Chadwick, and Leanne Hunt

Complications of glucose metabolism

Diabetes mellitus is common and has two classic presentations:

- Type 1 diabetes results from autoimmune destruction of pancreatic beta-cells. Individuals affected need lifelong insulin.

- Type 2 diabetes is a heterogeneous condition that develops in genetically predisposed individuals exposed to environmental risk factors. Treatment progresses through diet and lifestyle to tablets and insulin.

Diabetes can be an independent risk factor for major cardiac complications after surgery,[1] and this finding has been further validated.[2] However, others have failed to demonstrate that diabetes is an independent risk factor in major non-cardiac surgery,[3] and it seems likely that the risk may not be due to the diabetes itself, but to the end organ damage it causes. End organ damage in diabetes can be thought of as due either to microvascular disease (neuropathy including autonomic neuropathy, retinopathy, and nephropathy) or to macrovascular disorders (ischaemic heart disease, peripheral vascular disease, and cerebrovascular disease).

Preoperative considerations

Preoperative assessment and risk evaluation

Preoperative assessment determines the presence and degree of complications of diabetes, and tries to improve any unstable condition. All patients between the age of 40 and 74 attending hospital should be risk assessed for diabetes and, if at risk, tested.[4] National guidelines recommend that a surgical patient's long-term blood marker of glycaemic control, namely the HBA1c, should be below 8.5% or 70 mmol/mol.[5] If the level is above this, many preassessment units will postpone elective surgery.

Surgery induces a state of insulin resistance. The body's response to the 'stress' of surgery leads to increased secretion of cortisol and catecholamines. The resultant decrease in insulin sensitivity[6] and insulin secretion contribute to a catabolic state, with enhanced breakdown of protein and fat and increased hepatic glucose production. The ensuing hyperglycaemia may predispose to perioperative fluid and electrolyte disturbance and infection. Good glycaemic control prior to surgery helps reduce risks of infection,[7] impaired wound healing,[8] and glycaemic instability.

It is important to recognize that many people with diabetes are expert in self-management. Increasingly patients with type 1 diabetes are managed with multiple daily injection regimens, adjusting pre-meal insulin for the food they are eating. Preoperative counselling should therefore include detailed discussions with patients about their diabetes and should respect the patient's experience and expertise. Joint care planning with the patient enables optimization of glycaemic control. Well-managed diabetes is not a contraindication to day case surgery.

Perioperative glycaemic control

National guidelines[5] recommend maintaining tight blood glucose control throughout surgery and recovery. Target blood glucose should be 6–10 mmol/L (acceptable levels 4–12 mmol/ L). To achieve this target it is necessary, in any regimen, to take into account the duration of perioperative starvation. Enhanced recovery principles can help to minimize the duration of fasting. Whatever the regime it should be emphasized that insulin should never be omitted in type 1 diabetes as this will lead to ketoacidosis.

- If starvation is short (no more than one missed meal) the patient can be managed without additional intravenous insulin according to the principles in the next section. Advice about adjustment of medication will be required; full information on this can be obtained from the online guideline.[5]

- Longer periods of starvation (more than one missed meal) require intravenous insulin as a variable rate intravenous insulin infusion (VRIII) for both type 1 and 2 diabetes.

Variable rate intravenous insulin infusion or sliding scale

A VRIII usually consists of a syringe driver with a solution of insulin at a standard concentration, commonly 1 unit/mL. This is run concurrently with a solution of 0.45% saline with 5% glucose and 0.15% potassium chloride. The rate of the infusion is titrated to the patient's blood glucose according to a standard regime. In general patients on long acting insulin analogues (e.g. Levemir or Lantus) should continue them in the perioperative period. Local guidance should be followed as to the infusion rate in relation to the blood glucose. It is important to maintain good control and blood sugars should be monitored every 1 to 2 hours to maintain blood glucose at the desired 6–10 mmol/L.

Table 5.8.1 Causes of hyponatraemia

Hypovolaemic hyponatraemia		Euvolaemic hyponatraemia		Hypervolaemic hyponatraemia	
NaU (urinary sodium) < 20 mmol/L (non-renal losses)	NaU (urinary sodium) > 20 mmol/L (renal losses)	NaU (urinary sodium) < 20 mmol/L	NaU (urinary sodium) > 20 mmol/L Serum osmolality < 270 mOsm/kg Urine osmolality > 100 mOsm/kg	NaU (urinary sodium) < 20 mmol/L	NaU (urinary sodium) > 20 mmol/L
Gastrointestinal loss (vomiting, diarrhoea)	Diuretics	Psychogenic polydipsia	SIADH	Cirrhosis with ascites	Renal failure
Burns	Addison's disease	Hypothyroidism	Glucocorticoid insufficiency	Nephrotic syndrome	
Fluid sequestration (e.g. pancreatitis, bowel obstruction, peritonitis)	Salt losing nephropathies	Decreased solute intake e.g. Beer potomania		Congestive cardiac failure	

SIADH, syndrome of inappropriate antidiuretic hormone.

Once a patient can eat and drink the change from VRIII to subcutaneous insulin can be made. This should occur when the next subcutaneous insulin dose is due. Local guidance from the diabetic team will be available to the ward staff to manage this change, but it is vital to note that if long acting insulins were discontinued they must be restarted prior to stopping VRIII.

Guidelines for managing hyperglycaemia and hypoglycaemia for a short starvation period

Hyperglycaemia

In those with type 1 diabetes a blood sugar of more than 12 mmol/L should prompt a check for ketones. If capillary ketones are greater than 3 mmol/L or urinary ketones greater than 1 ++, non-urgent surgery should be postponed and the medical team contacted. If blood sugar is above 12 mmol/L without significant blood or urinary ketones, subcutaneous insulin can be given, and doses repeated after 2 hours. One unit will lower glucose by approximately 3 mmol/L in those with type 1 diabetes, and 0.1 units per kg will have a similar effect in those with type 2 diabetes. Full guidance can be obtained from 'Management of adults with diabetes undergoing surgery and elective procedures: improving standards'.[5] If blood glucose is not improving, a VRIII should be commenced.

Hypoglycaemia

Hypoglycaemia should ideally be avoided, but if detected promptly treated, as inpatient mortality is increased even if there is only one episode.[9] If the blood glucose is 4–6 mmol/L and the patient symptomatic, give 50–100 mL of 10% dextrose as an intravenous bolus and recheck glucose after 15 minutes. A blood glucose concentration of less than 4 mmol/L requires administration of 80–100 mL of 20% glucose and a repeat blood glucose. Avoid stopping VRIII in type 1 diabetic patients. If this is unavoidable, restart it when the blood glucose is above 5 mmol/L.

Adrenal and electrolyte disorders

Hyponatraemia

Hyponatraemia is common especially amongst patients taking thiazide diuretics. The causes are given in Table 5.8.1. In the surgical population iatrogenic hyponatraemia, especially from over use of hypotonic intravenous fluids such as 5% glucose, should

be avoided. Hyponatraemia due to the syndrome of inappropriate antidiuretic hormone secretion (SIADH) is associated with a variety of conditions (Table 5.8.2).

Symptoms and signs depend on the degree of hyponatraemia and the rate of change of sodium level, and include headache, nausea, vomiting, and weakness. Late symptoms include confusion, reduced consciousness, and fits. History should focus on medications, past history (cardiac failure, liver failure, renal disease, pituitary disease, or Addison's disease) and gastrointestinal losses or skin burns. Examination should be tailored to assessing the patient's volume status.

Investigations should include urinary sodium, paired urinary and serum osmolality, thyroid function tests to exclude hypothyroidism, renal and liver function tests, and serum cortisol.

Treatment of hyponatraemia

Treatment should be aimed at the underlying cause. If the patient is volume depleted, start an intravenous infusion of normal saline. Monitor fluid output and volume status, and if the patient is not volume depleted restrict fluid to 500–700ml/24 hours.

Symptomatic hyponatraemia, with features such as seizures or coma, requires management in a critical care environment. The aim is to increase serum sodium levels by 0.5 mmol/L per hour or less. Care is required as too rapid correction of sodium levels can lead to

Table 5.8.2 Causes of syndrome of inappropriate antidiuretic hormone (SIADH)

Central nervous system disorders	Trauma, haemorrhage, infection, and tumours
Pulmonary disease	Small cell lung cancer, mesothelioma, tuberculosis, pneumonia, empyema, assisted ventilation, asthma, pneumothorax
Malignancy	Lymphoma, leukaemia, sarcoma, thymoma, and pancreatic
Drugs	Psychiatric drugs, SSRIs, chemotherapeutic agents, carbamezapine, ACE-inhibitors, proton pump inhibitors, opiates, non-steroidal anti-inflammatory drugs
Metabolic	Hypothyroidism, glucocorticoid deficiency, acute intermittent porphyria

ACE, angiotensin converting enzyme; SSRI, selective serotonin reuptake inhibitor.

central pontine myelinolysis. The reader is directed to Verbalis and colleagues[10] and Adrogué[11] for further reading.

Causes of steroid (adrenal) insufficiency

Adrenal insufficiency (AI) results from inadequate adrenocortical function. Primary AI (Addison's disease) is due to destruction of the adrenal cortex, most commonly by autoantibodies. Congenital adrenal hyperplasia is caused by deficient adrenal corticosteroid biosynthesis. Rare causes of primary AI include tuberculosis or metastases. Secondary AI is due to pituitary and hypothalamic dysfunction, most commonly as a result of long-term exogenous glucocorticoids. Other causes include pituitary tumours, craniopharyngiomas, pituitary surgery or radiotherapy, inflammatory conditions, and trauma.

Treatment of adrenal insufficiency

Whatever the cause of AI, patients require daily glucocorticoid replacement. The usual daily dose is equivalent to approximately 20 mg hydrocortisone with doses split three times daily.[12] Individuals with primary adrenal insufficiency also need the mineralocorticoid fludrocortisone whereas those with secondary AI do not.

Intercurrent illness and stress (i.e. surgery, illness, and trauma) increase an individual's cortisol requirements. In the perioperative and postoperative period, doses of glucocorticoid need to be increased and given parenterally. If not then surgery is likely to precipitate an Addisonian crisis. Table 5.8.3 shows suggested glucocorticoid replacement during and after surgery. Doses are given

intramuscularly as advised by the Addison's Clinical Advisory panel as this gives more stable blood concentrations of hydrocortisone.[13]

Addisonian crisis

Addisonian crisis is a life-threatening emergency in a patient with primary or secondary AI at first presentation or when inadequately treated. The patients may present with cardiovascular collapse unresponsive to inotropes. Other features include abdominal pain, anorexia, nausea and vomiting, dehydration, and fever. Pigmentation is present in primary AI.

Investigations should not delay starting treatment. Urea and electrolytes classically show hyponatraemia, hyperkalaemia, and a high urea to creatinine ratio. Random glucose may reveal hypoglycaemia. Other tests include full blood count, arterial blood gases, lactate, and septic screen. Serum cortisol and adrenocorticotrophic hormone should be sent if no prior history of AI.

Large volumes of 0.9% saline are needed to reverse sodium depletion and volume loss. Inject intravenous hydrocortisone immediately and every 6 hours, until the patient is stable and can take oral medication. Intravenous glucose should be given if the patient is hypoglycaemic.

Diabetes insipidus

Diabetes insipidus (DI) is characterized by the production of large volumes of hypotonic urine. The two main types are central (where there is an inability to secrete vasopressin) and nephrogenic (where there is an inappropriate renal response to vasopressin). Individuals with central DI are usually on treatment with vasopressin, taken

Table 5.8.3 Glucocorticoid medication guidelines for surgery

Procedure	Preoperative and operative needs	Postoperative needs
Lengthy, major surgery with long recovery time e.g. open heart surgery, major bowel surgery, procedures requiring ITU	100 mg hydrocortisone i/m just before anaesthesia	Continue 100 mg hydrocortisone i/m every 6 hours until able to eat and drink normally (discharged from ITU). Then double oral dose for 48+ hours. Then taper the return to normal dose
Major surgery with rapid recovery time e.g. caesarean section, joint replacement	100 mg hydrocortisone i/m just before anaesthesia	Continue 100 mg hydrocortisone i/m every 6 hours for 24–48 hours (or until able to eat and drink normally). Then double oral dose for 24–48 hours. Then return to normal dose
Minor surgery e.g. cataract surgery, hernia repairs, laparoscopy with local anaesthetic	100 mg hydrocortisone i/m just before anaesthesia	Double dose oral medication for 24 hours. Then return to normal dose
Invasive bowel procedures requiring laxatives e.g. colonoscopy, barium enema	Hospital admission overnight with i/v fluids and 100 mg hydrocortisone i/m during preparation. 100mg hydrocortisone i/m just before commencing	Double dose oral medication for 24 hours. Then return to normal dose

Notes:

1. For any nil-by-mouth regimen, please arrange an intravenous saline infusion to prevent dehydration and maintain mineralocorticoid stability, e.g. 1000 mL every 8 hours if >50 kg.

2. Intramuscular hydrocortisone is preferable to intravenous administration as it gives more sustained, stable cover. It may alternatively be given by infusion pump, e.g. hydrocortisone 25 mg bolus then 5 mg per hour

3. Please administer bolus hydrocortisone over a minimum of 10 minutes to prevent vascular damage.

4. Note that hydrocortisone acetate cannot be used due to its slow-release, microcrystalline formulation. Please use hydrocortisone sodium phosphate or hydrocortisone sodium succinate, 100 mg.

5. If any postoperative complications arise, e.g. fever, delay the return to normal dose.

i/m, intramuscular; ITU, intensive therapy unit; i/v, intravenous.

Reproduced with kind permission of Addison's Clinical Advisory Panel (ACAP) 2006 and 2012, Copyright © ADSHG, available from http://www.addisons.org.uk/publications

either as a nasal spray or in tablet form. Most patients with DI have intact thirst and drink sufficient fluid to maintain normal fluid balance. Goals of therapy are to reduce polyuria and thirst to an acceptable level. Fluid balance needs to be closely monitored during surgery and anaesthesia. For those unable to take usual replacement vasopressin, subcutaneous vasopressin should be prescribed. Close liaison with the endocrine team should be sought.

Complications of corticosteroid therapy

Treatment of pituitary–adrenal insufficiency aims to mimic endogenous steroid production. However, steroids are common treatments for inflammatory conditions in supra-physiological doses. Side effects of such treatment relevant for the surgeon include poor wound healing, thin skin and easy bruising, and impairment of the immune response.

Pathophysiology of excess and deficiency of thyroxine

Actions of thyroxine

The actions of thyroxine are largely mediated by its conversion to triiodothyronine, the effects of which include:

- increased metabolic rate, with consequent effects on temperature regulation
- effects on growth, protein synthesis and tissue maturation
- potentiation of sympathetic nervous system effects.

In thyrotoxicosis the effects on metabolic rate and sympathetic nervous activity predominate. This leads to weight loss, heat intolerance, palpitations, sweating, agitation, and tremor. In hypothyroidism, metabolic and central nervous system (CNS) effects cause weight gain, skin changes, and CNS depression.

The principal concerns in the perioperative period are the possibility of thyrotoxic or hypothyroid crises (thyroid 'storm' and myxoedema coma). These are rare but life-threatening complications. Nowadays, it is unthinkable that patients having thyroid surgery would develop either condition, since thyroid status would be known. It is patients with undiagnosed thyroid disease who are most at risk, often when undergoing emergency surgery for an unrelated condition.

A goitre, if present, can present a significant risk to the airway. Close liaison with the anaesthetic team and imaging of the upper airway are important in the safe management of such patients. Figure 5.8.1 illustrates a large retrosternal goitre causing significant tracheal compression (Figure 5.8.1).

Thyrotoxic crisis (thyroid storm)

Thyroid storm is a poorly defined but life-threatening clinical syndrome characterized by florid features of thyrotoxicosis. Commonly, there may be hyper-pyrexia, tachycardia, tachyarrhythmias, extreme agitation or confusional states, nausea, vomiting, and diarrhoea.

Precipitants of thyroid storm include surgery, infection, trauma, and administration of iodinated contrast media (hence its importance in 'surgical' patients), in addition to medical conditions such as diabetic ketoacidosis and cerebrovascular accidents.

Prevention is feasible in patients presenting for elective surgery if thyroid disease is known or suspected preoperatively and thyroid function tests performed. If thyrotoxicosis is detected, surgery can usually be deferred until it is controlled. Rapid control can be achieved with full 'blocking' doses of carbimazole or propylthiouracil and, once adequate control is achieved, either titrating the dose to a lower maintenance level, or adding thyroxine. Beta-blockade may be added to facilitate more rapid symptom control and earlier surgery, or occasionally in place of anti-thyroid drugs. The agent of choice is propranolol as it has a specific anti-thyroid effect by reducing peripheral conversion of thyroxine to triiodothyronine. High doses may be needed in thyrotoxic patients, and use should continue postoperatively, as the risk of thyroid storm persists for several days after surgery.

Postoperatively, thyroid storm may be suspected from the clinical features. However, these may overlap with other potential postoperative complications, particularly infection. A high index of suspicion should therefore be maintained, especially in patients with presumed sepsis who do not respond as anticipated. Treatment should commence before receipt of confirmatory blood tests, and includes anti-thyroid drugs (carbimazole/PTU ± Lugol's iodine orally or intravenous sodium ipodate), management of hyperpyrexia (peripheral cooling, paracetamol, small doses of chlorpromazine), adrenergic suppression (propranolol or short-acting intravenous β-blockers e.g. esmolol), and steroid cover.

Hypothyroid crisis

Myxoedema coma is extremely rare after surgery. Patients with undiagnosed hypothyroidism may display milder manifestations, which can complicate recovery. As with thyroid storm, precipitants include surgery, infection and trauma.

Features of relevance in the surgical patient include decreased CNS function with confusion, lethargy, and hypoventilation, plus increased sensitivity to sedatives and anaesthetics, hypothermia, cardiac decompensation, particularly if there is pre-existing heart disease, hyponatraemia, and hypoglycaemia.

If hypothyroidism is detected before elective surgery, it will usually be appropriate to start thyroxine replacement. Surgery may be delayed depending upon the severity and duration of hypothyroidism, urgency of the surgery, and the patient's age/past medical history. In otherwise fit adults, oral thyroxine can be rapidly initiated. In elderly patients, those with pre-existing ischaemic heart disease, or where a long duration of undiagnosed hypothyroidism is suspected clinically, replacement should be instituted more gradually.

Frank myxoedema coma is treated with intravenous triiodothyronine, replaced with thyroxine once clinically improved, in addition to supportive measures aimed at correcting hypothermia, electrolyte abnormalities, and cardiac function. As with thyroid storm, established myxoedema coma has a high mortality.

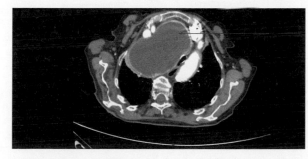

Fig. 5.8.1 A computed tomogram scan of a retrosternal goitre.

Causes and effects of hypercalcaemia and hypocalcaemia

Hypercalcaemia

Hypercalcaemia is a common metabolic abnormality. The potential causes are listed in Table 5.8.4, although primary hyperparathyroidism and malignancy account for most cases. The availability of an accurate assay for parathyroid hormone has greatly simplified diagnosis, separating causes into those associated with suppressed and those with unsuppressed parathyroid hormone (high or mid-upper 'normal range', i.e. inappropriate in the presence of hypercalcaemia).

Clinical features of hypercalcaemia vary depending on the cause and the rate of change in serum calcium. In malignant hypercalcaemia, serum calcium may have increased rapidly, and nausea, vomiting, anorexia, and CNS effects (lethargy, confusion and stupor) predominate.

In primary hyperparathyroidism, calcium levels have often crept up over years and patients may have few symptoms, even at relatively high levels of serum calcium. When symptoms do occur they include neuromuscular complaints (weakness, myalgia), CNS effects (lethargy, low mood, poor concentration), abdominal pain, constipation, and bone pain, in addition to those from long-term effects (osteoporosis, renal stones).

Hypercalcaemia interferes with renal tubular reabsorption of water, so that osmotic symptoms (polyuria, polydipsia) and extracellular fluid depletion may result. Furthermore, renal tubular excretion of excess calcium depends on adequate glomerular filtration and sodium excretion. Therefore serum calcium can rise rapidly in dehydrated patients and fluids are the cornerstone of acute treatment.

Perioperative management depends on the cause and severity of hypercalcaemia and the nature of surgery. Emergency surgery may need to proceed before full investigation and correction of hypercalcaemia, but should be accompanied by effective fluid resuscitation, and subsequent postoperative fluid input to maintain diuresis/natriuresis.

Most elective surgery can be deferred until the cause is established and the patient rehydrated. In primary hyperparathyroidism, hypercalcaemia may not require further treatment before surgery, unless serum calcium is very high (e.g. corrected total calcium > 3.0 mmol/L, following adequate fluid replacement). Consideration should also be given to parathyroid surgery either before or simultaneously with the originally planned operation.

In all cases, correction of hypercalcaemia before surgery may be achieved with fluid replacement, bisphosphonates (oral or intravenous), corticosteroids (in malignancy or sarcoidosis), or calcitonin (where rapid correction is desired). Specific therapy for other malignancies may take precedence over the planned surgery, and ameliorate hypercalcaemia.

Hypocalcaemia

The causes of hypocalcaemia are listed in Box 5.8.1. In surgical patients, the most common causes presenting acutely are hypoparathyroidism after thyroid or parathyroid surgery, acute pancreatitis, and hypomagnesaemia from intestinal failure or prolonged parenteral nutrition.

The clinical features of hypocalcaemia result from neuronal hyperexcitability, and correlate with the magnitude and rapidity of the fall in ionized calcium level. They include tingling/'pins-and-needles' (particularly perioral and in fingers/toes), muscle cramps, tetany, laryngospasm, anxiety or irritability, nausea, prolonged QT interval, arrhythmias (ventricular fibrillation), and convulsions. Severe symptoms rarely arise unless serum corrected calcium falls below 2.0 mmol/L (or ionized calcium < 1.0 mmol/L). Following thyroidectomy/parathyroidectomy, hypocalcaemia is often transient and may not require treatment.

Treatment

Mild hypocalcaemia (corrected calcium 2.0-2.2 mmol/L with mild symptoms or <2.0 mmol/L, asymptomatic) is treated with oral calcium supplements. Consider oral vitamin D if serum calcium not maintained.

Table 5.8.4 Causes of hypercalcaemia

	PTH unsuppressed	PTH suppressed
Common	Primary hyperparathyroidism: Sporadic Familial: MEN, FHPT Lithium-induced	Malignancy: Skeletal metastases Humoral hypercalcaemia of malignancy (lung, breast, squamous carcinomas, myeloma, lymphoma, renal cancer)
Infrequent	Familial hypocalciuric hypercalcaemia 'Tertiary' hyperparathyroidism	Excess 1,25 dihydroxy-vitamin D: Granulomatous disease: sarcoidosis, TB Exogenous vitamin D Transient after immobilization or dehydration Thiazide diuretics
Rare	Malignancy with true ectopic PTH secretion	Milk-alkali syndrome Thyrotoxicosis Adrenal insufficiency

FHPT, familial hyperparathyroidism; MEN, multiple endocrine neoplasia syndromes, PTH, parathyroid hormone; TB, tuberculosis.

Box 5.8.1 Causes of hypocalcaemia

Hypoparathyroidism
  Postsurgical (thyroid, parathyroid, laryngectomy)
  Autoimmune
  Parathyroid infiltration e.g. metastatic malignancy, Wilson's disease
Hypomagnesaemia
  Alcoholism
  Long-term total parenteral nutrition
  Intestinal failure
Acute pancreatitis
Chronic renal failure (inadequate 1α-hydroxylation of vitamin D)
Vitamin D deficiency
Drugs
  Bisphosphonates
  Chelating agents e.g. EDTA, citrate (massive blood transfusion)
  Phenytoin
  Cisplatin
Pseudo-hypoparathyroidism (parathyroid hormone-receptor defects)

Severe hypocalcaemia (severe symptoms or serum corrected calcium < 1.85 mmol/L) should be managed with 10 mL intravenous calcium gluconate 10% (= 2.20 mmol) in 100 mL normal saline over 30 minutes, or as a bolus over 5 minutes with electrocardiogram monitoring. This may be followed by an infusion of 10% calcium gluconate followed by oral supplements as above.

Phaeochromocytoma

Catecholamine-secreting neoplasms of chromaffin cells may arise in the adrenal glands (phaeochromocytoma) or in the postsynaptic ganglia of the sympathetic nervous system (paragangliomas). They are rare, but, in relation to surgery or investigational procedures, may be associated with serious complications (adrenergic/hypertensive crisis, sudden death).

Presentation in surgical patients may be with hypertension plus suggestive symptoms. The classic triad is headache, palpitations, and sweating. There may be intermittent pallor, anxiety, panic attacks, or tremor. Alternatively, there may be coincidental findings of an adrenal or retroperitoneal mass on imaging.

If the diagnosis is suspected preoperatively, invasive tests or surgery should be deferred pending confirmation with serial 24-hour urinary catecholamines. Where they are positive, medical stabilization should precede any further intervention. This is usually achieved with alpha-adrenergic blockade (e.g. oral phenoxybenzamine, doxazosin) or calcium-channel blockers (e.g. nifedipine), under the supervision of an experienced medical or surgical endocrinologist. Definitive surgical treatment of the phaeochromocytoma will usually take precedence over the original surgical pathology, and should be performed in specialist centres with appropriate expertise in managing this rare disease.

Insulinoma

These tumours of the pancreatic β-cells are rare (estimated incidence one to four cases per million population per year). Symptoms arise from hypoglycaemia due to inappropriate secretion of insulin, and are identical to those experienced by diabetic patients as a 'hypo'.

Due to its rarity and non-specific symptomatology, diagnosis is often delayed, but may be confirmed by a 72-hour fast, with inappropriate levels of insulin/pro-insulin/C-peptide observed during hypoglycaemia.

Perioperative management of the patient with an insulinoma involves preventing hypoglycaemia by regular monitoring of blood glucose, avoidance of prolonged fasting, intravenous glucose infusion where necessary. Specific therapy such as diazoxide or octreotide may be necessary if hypoglycaemic attacks are frequent or prior to definitive surgical treatment.

Acknowledgements

The authors would like to thank Dr M Bertoud for additional material on diabetes.

Further reading

Klubo-Gwiezdzinska J. Wartofsky L. Thyroid emergencies. *Med Clin N Am* 2012; 96, 385–403.

Sturgeon C, Duh Q-Y. Phaeochromocytoma., In: Linos D, van Heerden JA (eds) *Adrenal Glands: Diagnostic Aspects and Surgical Therapy.* New York: Springer, 2005, pp. 175–88.

Swan JW, Stevenson JC. The medical management of hypercalcaemia In: Lynn J, Bloom SR (eds) *Surgical Endocrinology.* Oxford: Butterworth-Heinemann, 1993, pp. 341–50.

References

1. Lee TH, Marcantonio ER, Mangione CM, *et al.* Derivation and prospective validation of a simple index for prediction of cardiac risk of major noncardiac surgery. *Circulation* 1999; 100: 1043–9.

2. Boersma E, Kertl D, Schouten O, *et al.* Peri-operative cardiovascular mortality in non-cardiac surgery: validation of the Lee cardiac risk index. *Am J Med* 2005; 118(10): 1134–41.

3. Wilson RJT, Davies S, Yates D, *et al.* Impaired functional capacity is associated with all-cause mortality after major elective intra-abdominal surgery. *Br J Anaesth* 2010; 105(3): 297–303.

4. National Institute for Health and Clinical Excellence. Preventing type 2 diabetes: risk identification and interventions for individuals at high risk: guidance. July 2012. Available from https://www.nice.org.uk/guidance/ph38 (accessed 30 October 2015).

5. Dhatariya K, Flanagan D, Hilton L, *et al.* Management of adults with diabetes undergoing surgery and elective procedures: improving standards NHS Diabetes, 2011. Available from https://www.diabetes.org.uk/About_us/What-we-say/Specialist-care-for-children-and-adults-and-complications/Management-of-adults-with-diabetes-undergoing-surgery-and-elective-procedures-improving-standards/ (accessed 30 October 2015).

6. Frayn KN. Hormonal control of metabolism in trauma and sepsis. *Clin Endocrinol* 1986; 24: 577–99.

7. Malone DL, Genuit T, Tracy JK, *et al.* Surgical site infections: reanalysis of risk factors. *J Surg Res* 2002; 103: 89.

8. Stadelmann WK, Digenis AG, Tobin GR. Impediments to wound healing. *Am J Surg* 1998; 176(2): 39S–47S.

9. Turchin A, Matheny ME, Shubina M, *et al.* Hypoglycaemia and clinical outcomes in patients with diabetes hospitalized in the general ward. *Diabetes Care* 2009; 32: 1153–7.

10. Verbalis JG, Goldsmith SR, Greenberg A, *et al.* Hyponatraemia treatment guidelines 2007: expert panel recommendations. *Am J Med* 2007; 120: S1.

11. Adrogué HJ, Madias NE. Hyponatraemia. *N Engl J Med* 2000; 342: 1581.

12. Mah PM, Jenkins RC, Rostami-Hodjegan A, *et al.* Weight-related dosing, timing and monitoring hydrocortisone replacement therapy in patients with adrenal insufficiency. *Clin Endocrinol* 2004; 61: 367–75.

13. Addison's Disease Self Help Group. Available from https://www.addisons.org.uk/system/aboutacap.html (accessed 30 October 2015).

SECTION 6

Assessment and management of patients with major trauma

Section editor: Chris Oliver

CHAPTER 6.1

Assessment of the multiply injured patient

Scott Middleton and Matthew Moran

Introduction

Trauma is one of the leading causes of death and disability in the population. This is particularly the case in younger patients, before the rise in prevalence of cardiovascular disease and cancer in later life. Some trauma patients are killed at the scene from unsurvive-able injuries. Many patients survive the initial trauma and the careful management of these patients in the early phase following injury (hours and days) will increase their chance of surviving their injuries and also markedly reduce the morbidity that they suffer as a result. Simple interventions, such as maintaining adequate oxygenation and preventing hypothermia can make a great difference to the patient's outcome.

In the United Kingdom and throughout the world, there has been a move to the creation of major trauma centres, which concentrate expertise and resources in a single centre to deliver the highest standard of care to a patient as soon as possible. However, a well-trained team in a small hospital with limited resources can provide much of the immediate care needed for a traumatized patient and make a real difference to the patients chance of a surviving their injuries with minimal morbidity.

ABCDE of Advanced Trauma Life Support

Advanced Trauma Life Support (ATLS) is a system that allows the identification and treatment of life- and limb-threatening injuries in an ordered sequence. Since its inception in the 1970s, over a million physicians have been trained in these principles and it is now the most widely used system of immediate evaluation of the traumatized patient in the world. ATLS emphasizes the safety of the patient and treating team and is underpinned by mechanisms to prevent further harm to the patient. ATLS is designed for resuscitation by a single doctor and nurse. However, in real life many of the processes happen simultaneously as more staff are available, with a team leader directing events.

Purpose of ABC approach

The A to E assessment of the multiply injured patient is referred to as the primary survey. The ABC approach identifies and treats injuries in the order in which they would kill the patient. In addition to clinical examination of the patient, the traumatologist relies on a number of simple adjuncts to aid diagnosis. Throughout the assessment and treatment of the patient, the physician must ensure that they do not allow further harm to come to their patient. This may be due to the omission of simple medicines (e.g. oxygen) or due to direct actions of the physician, for example over enthusiastic examination for pelvic stability.

All patients admitted to the resuscitation room should undergo the following assessment.

Initial assessment

Universal precautions

All staff should wear gowns, gloves, and visors for their own personal safety.

Introduce yourself

Staff should introduce themselves and ask the patient their name and what has happened. This helps with the assessment of the patient's airway, along with their breathing and state of shock. It should be noted if they can they speak coherently in sentences.

An AMPLE history of any *a*llergies, *m*edications, and *p*ast medical history should be taken, and it should be determined when they *l*ast ate and *e*xactly what happened.

Secure the cervical spine

This is done with a hard collar, blocks, and tape/straps to prevent further harm.

Assess and clear the airway

Burns, facial fractures, and loose teeth should be identified. Obstructed breathing (snoring/stridor) should be listened for and high-flow oxygen delivered via a non-rebreath mask.

Clearing an obstructed airway allows oxygen to pass to the lungs. Foreign bodies should be removed from the mouth and a chin lift and simple airway adjuncts may be required.

An anaesthetist may be required especially if there is a deteriorating airway (e.g. secondary to burns).

Assess breathing and ventilation

Look for the respiratory rate, symmetrical chest movements and external signs of trauma. Feel that the trachea is central and percuss the chest. Listen for breath and heart sounds and interpret the findings (Table 6.1.1).

Adjuncts to care include pulse oximetry, electrocardiogram and blood pressure monitoring, arterial blood gases, and a chest X-Ray.

These steps are important to identify common life-threatening problems (Table 6.1.2).

Table 6.1.1 Interpretation of examination findings in breathing and ventilation

Examination	Finding	Diagnosis
Trachea position	Deviated	Tension pneumothorax on contalateral side?
Chest movements	Paradoxical segment	Flail chest
	Hemithorax not moving	Pathology on ipsilateral side
Respiratory rate	Raised	Hypoxia, pain, shock
	None	Airway problem: recheck? Artificial ventilation?
Percuss chest	Dull	Haemothorax
	Hyper resonant	Pneumothorax (any)
Breath sounds	Absent	Pneumothorax or Haemothorax? Not breathing?
Heart Sounds	Muffled	Cardiac tamponade

Less common diagnoses such as aortic dissection, tracheobronchial fistula, cardiac tamponade, and diaphragmatic rupture should not be forgotten.

Assess the patient's circulation: stop the bleeding!

Look at the peripheral and central perfusion and identify external injuries and the respiratory rate. Feel the extremities and assess if they are cold and clammy. Check for long bone and pelvic fractures. Listen for the confused or obtunded patient. Adjuncts to assessment of the circulatory system include the measurement of heart rate, blood pressure, and urine output. The pelvis may require splinting and a pelvic X-Ray, FAST Scan (focused assessment with sonography for trauma) or surgical opinion may be needed.

In the traumatized patient, the cause of shock should initially be treated as haemorrhagic. Direct pressure is applied to external bleeding, deformed limbs are repositioned and splinted, and a pelvic binder can be applied. Two large bore cannulae should be inserted and blood sent for haemoglobin, clotting, and urea and electrolyte analysis. Balanced fluid resuscitation should be initiated and blood products transfused according to the major haemorrhage protocols. Surgical help should be requested. Whilst shock in the traumatized patient is assumed to be haemorrhagic, it is important to consider non-haemorrhagic causes of shock.

Assess the patient's disability (neurological evaluation)

Look at the pupillary response and the conscious level, and check that the patient is moving all four limbs. Listen to ascertain if the patient is confused or making inappropriate noises. The Glasgow Coma Score (Table 6.1.3) should be calculated and the 3 individual component scores (Eyes, Verbal and Motor scores) documented.

Head trauma can result in rapid deterioration and needs to be identified during the primary survey. Accurate and repeated recording of the Glasgow Coma Score is helpful. The neurologically injured patient must have their spine protected and neurogenic shock should be identified and managed. The patient should be supported with adequate resuscitation and the urinary bladder catheterized. A neurosurgical consult should be sought at an early stage if neurological compromise is suspected. Intensive therapy unit physicians need to be contacted early in case inoptopic support is required.

Table 6.1.2 Common life-threatening chest injuries and the method of treatment

Diagnosis	Pathology	Treatment
Massive haemothorax[a]	1500 mL total OR >200 ml/hour for 2 to 4 hours	ICD + surgery. Consider autotransfusion
Tension pneumothorax[a]	Air in pleural space, under pressure compressing mediastinal structures	Needle decompression followed by ICD
Open pneumothorax /sucking chest wound[a]	Air enters chest via open wound rather than down trachea	Dressing taped on three sides (flutter valve effect) + ICD
Flail chest[a]	Two or more ribs each broken in two or more places	ICD + supportive care (ICU)
Cardiac tamponade[a]	Blood in the pericardial space	Needle decompression + Surgery
Diaphragmatic rupture	More commonly left sided	Surgery
Oesophageal rupture	Blunt or penetrating	ICD and mediastinal drainage, surgery
Simple pneumothorax	Air in the pleural space	ICD
Tracheobronchial fistula	Major airway injury	One or more ICD Surgery
Aortic disruption	Partial rupture, contained by adventitial layer	Surgery
Pulmonary contusion	Haemorrhage within the substance of the lung	Supportive. Early intubation and ventilation
Blunt cardiac injury	Myocardial contusion, chamber or valve rupture, coronary artery dissection	Monitoring, cardiac support. Sometimes surgery
Haemothorax	Blood in the pleural space	ICD

[a]These conditions should be identified and treated in the primary survey.
ICD, intercostal chest drain; ICU, intensive care unit.

Table 6.1.3 The Glasgow Coma Score

Criterion	Rating	Score
Eye opening		
Open before stimulus	Spontenous	4
After spoken or shouted request	To sound	3
After fingertip stimulus	To pressure	2
No opening at any time, no interfering factor	None	1
Closed by local factor	Non-testable	NT
Verbal response		
Correctly gives name, place and date	Orientated	5
Not orientated but communication coherently	Confused	4
Intelligible single words	Words	3
Only moans/groans	Sounds	2
No audible response, no interfering factor	None	1
Factor interfering with communication	Non-testable	NT
Best motor response		
Obey two-part request	Obeys commands	6
Brings hand above clavicle to stimulus on neck	Localizing	5
Bends arm at elbow rapidly but features not predominantly abnormal	Normal flexion	4
Bends arm at elbow, features clearly predominantly abnormal	Abnormal flexion	3
Extends arm at elbow	Extension	2
No movement in arms/legs, no interfering factor	None	1
Paralysed or other limiting factor	Non-testable	NT

Reproduced with permission from Sir Graham Teasdale. The Structured Aid to Assessment of the Glasgow Coma Scale was developed with support from the Muriel Cooke bequest to the University of Glasgow.

It is important not to cause further harm to the patient and identify neurological deterioration and loss of airway at an early stage. Transfer to specialist care should not be delayed.

Assess exposure and environment

It is important to protect the patient from hypothermia. The patient should be undressed completely and logrolled to inspect their dorsal aspect. Patients cool down rapidly following injury and this should be recognized and treated.

Triage

The word triage is derived from the French 'to sort'. In trauma care, triage is the process by which patients ('casualties') are sorted according to their immediate medical needs. The process of triage is attributed to Baron Domonique Larrey, Surgeon in Chief to Napoleon and it, therefore, has its origins in battlefield medicine.

Triage is most useful in a 'mass' casualty situation, where the medical facilities immediately available are unable to treat all patients at once (contrast this with 'multiple' casualties where the medical system is not overwhelmed). To be effective, triage needs

Box 6.1.1 Commonly used variables for triage systems

Ability to walk
Respiratory rate
Breathing
Radial pulse
Capillary refill
Ability to obey commands
Glasgow Coma Score
AVPU
Motor response

to be a rapid and based on a few well-defined criteria, usually examination findings or basic observations (Box 6.1.1). The triage process must accurately sort patients ensuring that those with the most immediately life-threatening injuries (that are treatable) are prioritized. Patients with non-survivable injuries and those with injuries that are not life threatening are given a lower priority.

The system needs to be applicable to different scenarios, be it a fire, explosion, car crash, or mass shooting. It is important to remember that, once triaged, the condition of a casualty may change. Re-evaluation of those casualties given a lower priority is necessary to ensure that casualties with a rapidly deteriorating condition are detected early. In addition, the available resources to treat patients can rapidly alter as more (or less) casualties present. It may be necessary to re-focus efforts on a smaller cross section of the injured population as resources become more stretched. The mechanism of the disaster can have a profound influence on the time it takes for a mass casualty situation to develop. In a sudden 'big bang' disaster, the casualties will present rapidly. However, in a 'rising tide' there may be a very substantial number of casualties that present hours or days later as the disaster evolves.

Tissue response to injury

There is a trimodal distribution of death following trauma. The first peak (45% of patients) occurs within seconds or minutes of the injury. This is due to severe brain or high spinal cord injuries, or rupture of the heart or great vessels. The second peak is smaller (10%) and represents early deaths during the first 24 hours, usually due to hypoxia, hypovolaemia, or intracranial injuries.

The third peak (45%) occurs days or weeks after the initial injury, commonly in the intensive care unit, and represents the consequences of the tissue response to injury. There is a mismatch between proinflammatory and anti-inflammatory mediators, leading to an uncontrolled immunoinflammatory response that is thought to be responsible for this third peak in deaths after trauma (Figure 6.1.1). This systemic inflammatory response syndrome (SIRS) can lead to tissue destruction in organs not originally affected by the initial trauma. These patients most commonly die secondary to acute respiratory distress syndrome (ARDS) and multiple organ dysfunction syndrome. 'Second hits' such as infections or operations can further exacerbate this exaggerated immune response, and form the basis for the arguments surrounding damage control orthopaedics (Figure 6.1.2).

Trauma causes activation of nearly all components of the immune system. The normal physiological responses to injury are therefore manifestations of complex cellular and molecular events (Box 6.1.2). In addition to these proinflammatory substances,

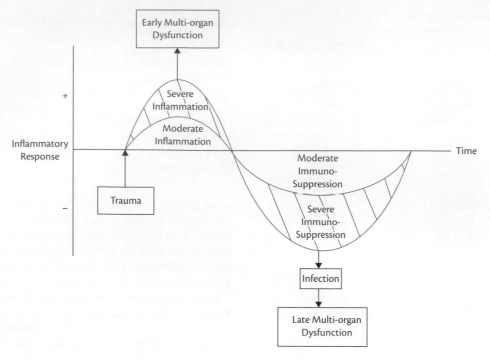

Fig. 6.1.1 Immune response following trauma.

Reprinted from *Surgical Clinics of North America*, Volume 75, Issue 2, Moore FA and Moore EE, Evolving concepts in the pathogenesis of postinjury multiple organ failure, pp. 257–77, Copyright © Elsevier 1995, available from http://www.sciencedirect.com/science/journal/00396109

anti-inflammatory mediators are also released. An overwhelming anti-inflammatory response seems to be responsible for post-traumatic immunosuppression, with a high susceptibility to infections and septic complications. The body aims to create a balance between SIRS and the anti-inflammatory reaction to trauma and in order to allow reparative mechanisms and reduce entry of microorganisms in addition to avoiding destructive inflammation. An imbalance in this dichotomy is thought to be responsible for the subsequent state of immunodeficiency following trauma once the initial SIRS has resolved (Figure 6.1.2).

Shock

Definition of shock

Shock is defined as tissue perfusion that is inadequate to meet metabolic requirements. There is no single laboratory test or clinical finding to define shock; rather, it is a syndrome that requires clinical diagnosis based on a number of clinical signs and simple observations. It is a life-threatening physiological state and rapid identification must be

---

followed by immediate resuscitation to prevent or minimize its inevitable sequelae if it is left undertreated or unrecognized. Shock has been described as a 'momentary pause in the act of death'.

Identification of shock

Shock must be rapidly identified. Reliance on systolic blood pressure alone will result in delay in its recognition and management. Clinically, the shocked patient may appear pale and anxious, with cool peripheries, tachycardia, tachypnea, and a reduced urine output. Only in the latter stages, where there is more severe blood loss and loss of compensatory mechanisms, will the systolic blood pressure drop. Compensatory mechanisms, which include peripheral vasoconstriction, can mask the reduction in intravascular volume until there is a loss of up to 30% of the patient's blood volume.

In the multiply injured patient, the most common type of shock is haemorrhagic shock. The source of the haemorrhage must be identified early: this is covered in the 'C' stage (circulation and haemorrhage control) of an ATLS-based assessment. There are four sites that should be considered as the potential sources of haemorrhage. These are the chest, abdomen, pelvis, and long bones. It is important to remember that substantial blood loss may have occurred at the scene of the accident or *en route* to hospital (Table 6.1.4).

Useful adjuncts in the identification of the cause of shock include chest and pelvic radiographs and a FAST scan. It is no longer considered good practice to attempt to 'spring' or stress the pelvis, which may disrupt a clot that has formed. While a log roll can be useful in the identification of posterior penetrating wounds, in the presence of a pelvic fracture there is a risk of moving pelvic fracture fragments and again disrupting newly formed clot.

With regards to laboratory tests, it is important to understand the context of the full blood count in acute trauma. In this setting,

---

> **Box 6.1.2** Systemic response to trauma
>
> Sympathetic nervous system activation
> Endocrine 'stress response'
>   Pituitary hormone secretion
>   Insulin resistance
> Immunological and inflammatory changes
>   Cytokine production
>   Acute phase reaction
>   Neutrophil leucocytosis
>   Lymphocyte proliferation

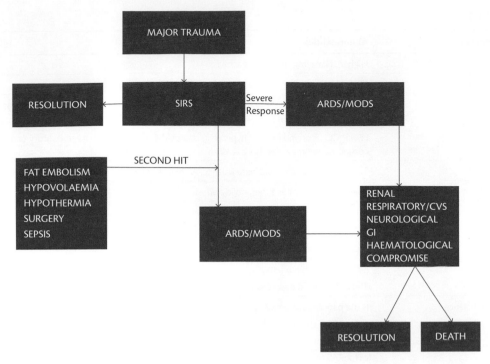

Fig. 6.1.2 The 'two-hit hypothesis'.

the body will lose red blood cells at the same rate as plasma and there will be little or no initial change in haemoglobin or haematocrit until redistribution of interstitial fluid into the blood plasma occurs. Many of the derangements that eventually occur are a result of replacing a large volume of lost blood with crystalloids and colloids. Therefore reliance upon the full blood count is inappropriate as a diagnostic tool, although it can be used to monitor a patient's response to treatment. A baseline clotting screen is sent with initial blood tests.

The lactate level is especially useful in determining the severity of shock. Repeated measurements can guide resuscitation and surgical management. It is easily measured from a venous or arterial blood gas sample (Table 6.1.5).

Types of shock

In the multiply injured patient, shock is presumed to be due to blood loss (haemorrhagic) until proven otherwise. Haemorrhagic shock is by far the most common cause of shock in the traumatized patient. Potential causes of non-haemorrhagic shock in a trauma patient include neurogenic shock, cardiogenic shock, and septic shock.

Outwith the field of trauma, four main types of shock are recognized. These are named in such a way as to identify the underlying aetiology: hypovolaemic, obstructive, distributive, and cardiogenic. Each type of shock has several possible causes (Table 6.1.6).

Table 6.1.4 Potential blood loss from major orthopaedic injuries

Site of bony injury	Potential blood loss
Pelvis	3 litres +
Femur	1.5 litres
Tibia/humerus	0.5–1 litre

Head injury alone is rarely a cause of hypotension and is never the cause of massive blood loss unless there is massive external bleeding from scalp wounds.

Neurogenic shock leads to disruption of the sympathetic pathways in the spinal cord with resultant uncontrolled peripheral vasodilation, a decrease in peripheral vascular resistance, and a profound reduction in blood pressure. Depending on the level of spinal cord injury, there may also be a loss of sympathetic cardiac innervation with a resultant bradycardia. These features allow differentiation from hypovolaemic shock where the patient will appear peripherally shut down and tachycardic. Do not forget that both causes of shock may co-exist.

The term 'spinal shock' refers to the complete loss of all neurological activity (motor, sensory, reflex, and autonomic) below the level of spinal cord injury. Following a variable time period, from several days up to 6 weeks, spinal reflexes return and eventually become exaggerated as the syndrome of spasticity develops. This is not the same as neurogenic shock.

The following formula underpins the pathophysiology of neurogenic shock. As systemic vascular resistance drops, so does the patient's blood pressure:

blood pressure = cardiac output × systemic vascular resistance.

Classification of severity

Shock may also be classified into four groups, depending on simple clinical signs, observations, and investigations. Table 6.1.7 provides a guide to possible clinical presentations of different classes of haemorrhagic shock.

Treatment/differential diagnosis

The most common type of shock in the multiply injured patient is haemorrhagic shock. The principle of treatment is to replace the lost blood and stop further bleeding.

Table 6.1.5 Arterial blood gas interpretation

	Normal value	Abnormalities
pH	7.35–7.45	High in alkalaemia, low in acidaemia
H^+	35–45 nmol/L	Opposite to pH i.e. high in acidaemia and low in alkalaemia
P_aO_2	11–13 kPa	Low P_aO_2 is an indicator of respiratory failure, subtypes of which include type 1 (normal or low P_aCO_2) or type 2 (raised P_aCO_2)
P_aCO_2	4.7–6 kPa	Low P_aCO_2 is an indicator of hyperventilation, either due to a primary respiratory condition e.g. PE, or as compensation for a metabolic acidosis
Base excess	−2 to +2	This is an indicator of acid/base balance. An excess of base (> +2) implies a metabolic alkalosis
HCO_3^-	22 28 mmol/L	Low HCO_3^- indicates a metabolic acidosis. High HCO_3^- indicates a metabolic alkalosis
Lactate	0.5–1.6 mmol/L	A raised lactate is an indicator of inadequate organ perfusion and a potentially unwell patient
1. How is the patient?		This will provide valuable clues to help with interpretation of the results
		This will also help detect when a sample is venous with a P_aO_2 result out of context with the clinical picture
2. Assess oxygenation		Is the patient hypoxaemic?
		The P_aO_2 should be >10 kPa on air and about 10 kPa less than the % inspired concentration
3. Determine the acid base balance		Is the patient acidaemic?
		pH < 7.35 (H^+ > 45 nmol/L)
		Is the patient alkalaemic?
		pH > 7.45 (H^+ < 35 nmol/L)
4. Determine the respiratory component		P_aCO_2 > 6.0 kPa = respiratory acidosis (or respiratory compensation for a metabolic alkalosis)
		P_aCO_2 < 4.7 kPa = respiratory alkalosis (or respiratory compensation for a metabolic acidosis)
5. Determine the metabolic component		HCO_3^- < 22 mmol/L = metabolic acidosis (or renal compensation for a respiratory alkalosis)
		HCO_3^- > 28 mmol/L = metabolic alkalosis (or renal compensation for a respiratory acidosis)

In the primary survey, haemorrhage is controlled through prompt recognition of the bleeding source and pressure on any external sources of exsanguination. Any injured patient who has haemodynamic compromise must be placed in a pelvic binder as early as possible as doing so will protect and promote clot formation and only rarely affect interpretation of pelvic radiographs. Long bone fractures are splinted. If there is any suspicion of intra-abdominal or intrathoracic haemorrhage, the respective surgical teams must be contacted immediately as these patients may require surgical intervention to control the source of haemorrhage.

Fluid therapy must be rapid both in its initiation and rate of flow. Large bore intravenous cannulae should be cited in each antecubital fossa. The Hagen–Poiseuille equation (Figure 6.1.3) states that flow is directly proportional to the pressure difference, and to the fourth power of the radius. It also states that flow is inversely proportional to viscosity and length. Thus, the ideal cannula is short and of large calibre.

In addition to providing an estimate to the degree of blood loss, the classification system for haemorrhage (Table 6.1.7) is useful for determining initial fluid therapy and the response to treatment.

Warmed crystalloid solutions (0.9% sodium chloride, Hartmann's solution) are used for initial resuscitation. In the adult patient with suspected haemorrhagic shock, a warmed fluid bolus of 1 to 2 litres is administered. Blood samples are sent for type-specific and fully cross matched blood. O negative blood may be used *in extremis*. Further fluid resuscitation should be with blood products. Initially this is with red cells; however, it is important to remember that the patient will become rapidly deficient in clotting products and platelets and plasma should also be given. The exact ratio is variable but a typical regime would a 1:1:1 ratio of platelets:plasma:red cells. Two recent developments in the management of haemorrhagic shock are the earlier use of blood products and balanced resuscitation.

Crystalloid is rapidly distributed throughout the intravascular, interstitial, and intracellular fluid compartments and its use is therefore limited in the bleeding patient (Figure 6.1.4).

In the context of haemorrhagic shock, there has been a trend towards 'low-volume resuscitation' and 'hypotensive resuscitation'.

Table 6.1.6 Different categories of shock and their possible causes

Type of shock	Possible causes
Hypovolaemic	Blood loss (haemorrhagic shock), dehydration (secondary to diarrhoea, vomiting, high stoma output), burns
Obstructive	Massive pulmonary embolism, cardiac tamponade, tension pneumothorax
Distributive	Neurogenic shock, anaphylaxis, sepsis
Cardiogenic	Myocardial infarction, arrhythmias

$$\text{Flow rate} = \frac{\Pi(\text{Pressure difference})(\text{Radius})^4}{8(\text{Viscosity})(\text{Length})}$$

Fig. 6.1.3 The Hagen-Poiseuille equation.

Table 6.1.7 Clinical signs and examination findings depending on percentage blood loss

	Class I	Class II	Class III	Class IV
Blood loss (mL)[a]	Up to 750	750–1500	1500–2000	>2000
Blood loss (% blood volume)	Up to 15%	15–30%	30–40%	>40%
Blood pressure	Normal (pulse pressure[b] may increase)	Normal (pulse pressure may decrease)	Decreased	Decreased
Pulse rate	<100	100–120	120–140	>140
Respiratory rate	14–20	20–30	30–40	>35
Urine output (ml/hour)	>30	20–30	5–15	<5
Mental status	Normal	Anxious	Confused	Lethargic/obtunded

[a]The blood loss volumes are based on a 70 kg adult male, where the estimated blood volume is approximately 5 litres.
[b]Pulse pressure is the difference between the systolic and the diastolic blood pressure.

Fluid resuscitation may trigger coagulopathy by diluting coagulation factors and favouring hypothermia. Furthermore, restoration of a 'normal' blood pressure may result in an increased rate of blood loss. There is a paucity of evidence for these approaches, and most trauma units have protocols in place for such scenarios. Despite variations in fluid resuscitation, there is agreement that, in a bleeding patient, the most important intervention is definitive control of haemorrhage. Tranexamic Acid is increasingly used in trauma situations, to reduce blood loss.

In all patients it is critical to frequently reassess the patient's response to treatment (Table 6.1.8) and also to consider the additional consequences of trauma in the elderly and athletes, and in pregnancy and the obese (Table 6.1.9).

Priorities of care

The care of the traumatized patient begins before they arrive in the emergency department. The patient will often have received early management of their injuries by pre-hospital personnel. It is vital to liaise with the pre-hospital team to determine the mechanism of the injury, condition of the patient and the interventions undertaken so far. The department should be prepared for the patient(s) arrival with appropriate personnel ready to receive as soon as they arrive. In a mass casualty situation the casualties are triaged.

Evaluation follows the ATLS principles given above. During the initial assessment, the physician in charge of the trauma team must make an assessment as to whether the patient will require transfer to another hospital for definitive care. The timing of transfer depends on the patient's condition, local expertise, and the nature of the problem requiring transfer. Adequate communication between the referring and receiving team is vital for safe transfer of the patient. Time-consuming investigations that are not immediately necessary should not delay the patient's transfer. The possible deterioration of the patient during transfer should be anticipated prior to transfer taking place.

Prior to transfer or proceeding to the secondary survey, the patients ABC's should be re-evaluated. A detailed secondary survey is then carried out. This may be days following the initial trauma, for example if the patient has been ventilated on ICU. It may be necessary to repeat the secondary survey several times to ensure that no injuries are missed. The secondary survey is a detailed history and examination (and investigation as indicated) from head to toe.

Acute respiratory distress syndrome

Definition of acute respiratory distress syndrome

ARDS is a rare but life-threatening sequela of trauma with dyspnoea, tachypnea, and hypoxaemia resistant to oxygen therapy. A blunt injury initiates an exaggerated inflammatory cascade known as SIRS with subsequent pulmonary complications.

The incidence following blunt trauma is 0.5%, with an incidence as high as 10% where three or more anatomical regions have been injured. Patients with long bone fractures, particularly of the lower limb, following trauma are also at an increased risk of ARDS.

Pathophysiology of acute respiratory distress syndrome

The pathophysiology of ARDS is complex and remains poorly understood. There is an overwhelming and exaggerated inflammatory response leading to alveolar epithelial and vascular endothelial injury. The release of cytokines and other inflammatory mediators leads to increased permeability of pulmonary microvasculature with resultant leakage of fluid across the alveolar-capillary membrane. Furthermore, there is disruption of surfactant secondary to inflammation. Both of these mechanisms lead to severe disruption of the gas exchanging qualities of the lung with subsequent

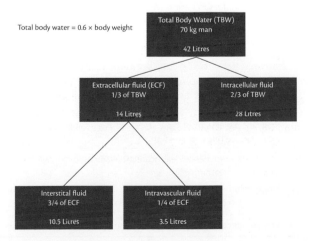

Fig. 6.1.4 Distribution of total body water in a 70 kg man.

Table 6.1.8 The three groups of responders to an intravenous fluid challenge[a]

	Rapid responder	Transient responder	Minimal or no response
Observations	Return to normal	Transient improvement, recurrence of decreased blood pressure and increased heart rate	Remain abnormal
Estimated blood loss	Minimal (10–20%)	Moderate and ongoing (20–40%)	Severe (>40%)
Need for more crystalloid	Low	Low to moderate	Moderate as a bridge to transfusion
Need for blood	Low	Moderate to high	Immediate
Blood replacement	Typed and cross matched	Type-specific	Emergency blood release
Need for operative intervention	Possible	Likely	Highly likely
Early surgical review	Yes	Yes	Yes

[a]Isotonic crystalloid solution, 2000 mL in adults; 20 mL/kg in children.
Reproduced with permission from *Advanced Trauma Life Support (ATLS) Students Manual, Ninth Edition*, American College of Surgeons, Copyright © 2012.

hypoxaemia. This may be one manifestation of a more generalized disruption of endothelium associated with SIRS.

Causes of acute respiratory distress syndrome

The causes of ARDS can be broadly categorized by their aetiology into direct lung injuries and indirect lung injuries (Table 6.1.10).

Identification and treatment

The early signs of ARDS can be subtle and easily missed. Identification requires a high index of suspicion in patients at risk. ARDS is part of a more systemic inflammatory disorder and therefore it is important to identify concurrent medical complications including multiple organ failure and coagulation cascade abnormalities. The most recent criteria for diagnosis include:

◆ Lung injury of acute onset, within 1 week of an apparent clinical insult and with progression of respiratory symptoms.

◆ Bilateral opacities on chest imaging not explained by other pulmonary pathology (e.g. pleural effusions, lung collapse, or nodules).

◆ Respiratory failure not explained by heart failure or volume overload.

◆ Arterial P_aO_2/FiO_2* < 300 mmHg (<40 kPa) (*Arterial oxygen tension/fraction of inspired oxygen).

An arterial blood gas performed in the early stages will demonstrate type 1 respiratory failure.

Additionally, in cases of fat embolism syndrome, patients may display neurological signs in the form delirium and a petechial rash present on the upper chest/back. This is particularly common following fractures of long bones.

The mainstay of treatment for patients with ARDS remains that of general supportive care as with any critically ill patient, including

Table 6.1.9 Additional considerations in trauma of the elderly and obese, and in pregnancy and obesity

Group of patients	Additional considerations	Consequences in trauma
Elderly	Reduced sensitivity to catecholamines	Hypotension is poorly tolerated in this group
	Reduced cardiac function	Failure to mount a tachycardic response due to medications or pacemakers
	Beta-blockers, rate-limiting calcium channel antagonist medications or pacemakers	Potential for fluid overload and pulmonary oedema with over-vigorous fluid resuscitation. More invasive monitoring should be considered to measure fluid balance
Athletes	Increased blood volume	Late to display signs of hypovolaemia
	Increased cardiac output	
	Resting bradycardia	
Pregnant	Increased blood volume	Increased blood loss is required to before displaying signs of hypovolaemia
	Potential for IVC compression when supine	Pregnant patients must be resuscitated in a position with left lateral tilt to reduce IVC compression
Obese	Airway problems secondary to reduced pulmonary compliance, increased chest wall resistance and difficult intubation	Requires an experience healthcare professional to manage the airway and breathing
	Increased risk of aspiration	Blood volume estimates should be made using ideal body weight in order to avoid significant overestimations
	Frequently suffer from numerous co-morbidities	
Children	A multitude of anatomical and physiological differences	Require specialist paediatric resuscitation protocols and expertise

IVC, inferior vena cava.

Table 6.1.10 Causes of acute respiratory distress syndrome

Indirect lung injuries	Direct lung injuries
Trauma	Pneumonia
Sepsis[a]	Aspiration of gastric contents
Acute pancreatitis	Fat embolism syndrome
Blood transfusion	Inhalation injury
Severe burns	

[a]Most common cause of acute respiratory distress syndrome.

infection control, early enteral nutrition, stress ulcer prophylaxis, and thromboprophylaxis, with treatment of the underlying cause if possible. Patients should be managed in an intensive care setting, with positive pressure mechanical ventilation to maintain an acceptable level of oxygenation. Although numerous pharmacological therapies have shown promising results in animal models, these have positive results have failed to translate to human studies.

In the context of trauma, there is a paucity of evidence surrounding the controversial subject of timing of long bone stabilization and the effect this has on survival and respiratory complications. This discussion surrounding 'damage control orthopaedics' is beyond the scope of this chapter.

Prognosis: mortality and morbidity of acute respiratory distress syndrome

The overall mortality from ARDS is approximately 40%, however, this varies according to the aetiology, with trauma patients displaying a lower mortality rate (25%) compared to sepsis. The most prevalent cause of demise in patients with ARDS is multiple organ failure, as opposed to respiratory failure itself. Although lung function parameters tend to recover well in ARDS patients, physical limitations and a poor quality of life are common long term sequelae.

Conclusion

The expert management of the polytraumatized patient in the early period following trauma is a well-structured process of care. There are many pitfalls for the unwary; however, by following simple principles with timely re-evaluation and treatment these may be avoided. The adequate resuscitation (but not over-resuscitation) and stabilization of the patient reduce the risk of the patient developing later complications such as adult respiratory distress syndrome and an exaggerated and deleterious response to injury.

The team that cares for a trauma patient in the initial phase of management must be aware of their own and their institutional limitations to manage the patient(s) ongoing problems. Early transfer of a patient or patients whose needs exceed the capacity of the receiving hospital is required. Activation of an institutions plans for the management of multiple casualties or major haemorrhage protocols may be necessary.

Further reading

It is recommended that all surgical trainees attend an Advanced Life. Support Course and maintain their accreditation throughout their career.
Advanced Trauma Life Support Student Manual, 9th edition. Chicago: American College of Surgeons, 2012.

Bernard GR, Artigas A, Brigham BL, *et al*. The American-European Consensus Conference on ARDS. Definitions, mechanisms, relevant outcomes, and clinical trial coordination. *Am J Respir Crit Care Med* 1994; 149: 818–24.

Dushianthan A, Grocott MPW, Postle AD, *et al*. Acute respiratory distress syndrome and acute lung injury. *Postgrad Med J* 2011; 87: 612–22.

Foex B. A Systemic response to trauma. *Br Med Bull* 1999; 76: 352–4.

White TO, Jenkins PJ, Smith RD, *et al*. The epidemiology of post traumatic adult respiratory distress syndrome. *J Bone Joint Surg Am* 2004; 86: 2366–76.

White TO, Watts AC. Systemic complications. In: Bucholz W, Court-Brown C, Heckman JD, *et al*. (eds). *Rockwood and Green's Fractures in Adults*, 7th edition. Philadelphia, PA: Lippincott Williams & Wilkins, 2010, p590–601.

CHAPTER 6.2

Skin loss

Nada Al-Hadithy

Introduction

Wounds are classified as open or closed, dependant on skin coverage and are chronic if they fail to close within 3 months.

Wound healing and wound repair

Wound healing has three principal phases: inflammatory, proliferative, and remodelling (Table 6.2.1).

The goal of wound healing is to obtain successful closure of the wound with an intact epithelial layer. Left to their own devices, wounds will heal by second intention (Table 6.2.2). Wound contraction is part of the normal healing process. Fibroblasts in contracting wounds have increased actin microfilaments and are known as myofibroblasts; these orient themselves along lines of tension and pull collagen fibres together. The final strength of the new collagen only reaches 80% of normal pre-wound tensile strength.[1]

Assessment of wounds

Trauma patients should be approached in the same way using the Advanced Trauma Life Support protocol[2] (Chapter 6.1). Assessment should be systematic, careful, and repeated at intervals to check for neurovascular deterioration.

Additional points for the History of the presenting complaint

Different parts of the body will require different areas of focus. For hand injuries, the occupation, hobbies, and handedness of the patient are important. Hand trauma can involve a range of injuries, including lacerations, tendon damage, nerve damage, factures, crush injuries, tissue loss, and loss of digits. Other factors to consider include:

♦ time of/since injury

♦ mechanism of injury; were others involved; outcomes of all parties; action taken

♦ degree of contamination: marine, agricultural or sewage contamination?

♦ loss of function or sensation since the injury

♦ body part injured

♦ likelihood that the wound will be problematic:

• systemic: Ehlers-Danlos syndrome; vitamin C deficiency; sickle cell anaemia; steroid usage; malnutrition; anaemia and extremes of age

• local: contamination, oedema, infection.

Examine the wound

On initial approach of an open wound, retain an algorithm in your head to ensure nothing is missed out (Figure 6.2.1). Open fractures need to be treated urgently, as exposed tissue is vulnerable to infection. If infection sets in at a deep level it can be difficult and complex to treat. Despite the complex and serious nature of open fractures, the best outcomes are achieved by timely specialist surgery, rather than by emergency procedures carried out by less experienced teams. The following should be covered:

1. Soft tissue injury: Open or closed; location, size, and depth of wound; edges and bed; quality of surrounding skin; cap refill; viability and associated pain.

2. Bone injury: Are there long bone fractures that require stabilization. Have deformities been anatomically reduced?

3. Vascular injury: Check all pulses and review the appendage distal to the injury to ensure that no vascular compromise is ensuing. If any reductions are carried out check vascularity again.

4. Muscle, tendon/ligament, nerve injury.[3]

5. Compartment syndrome.

Table 6.2.1 Three phases of wound healing

	Inflammatory	Proliferative	Remodelling
Time	24–48 hours	2–14 days	2 weeks–2 years
Dominant Cells	Platelets → Growth factors; neutrophils & macrophages	Fibroblasts Keratinocytes	Fibroblasts
Action	Remove necrotic debris and bacteria Production of type III collagen	Produce type I collagen Angiogenesis Epithelialization	Collagen synthesis and degradation reach equilibrium. Type III collagen is replaced by type I collagen to restore the normal dermal collagen composition
Phenotype	Open wound with eschar forming	Pink scar	Narrower paler scar

Table 6.2.2 Types of wound healing

	First intention	Second intention	Third intention
Explanation	Closure of wounds in which the edges can be directly approximated	Promotes spontaneous re-epithelialization of the wound from viable epithelial elements in the wound itself	Allow initial granulation then close the wound surgically by bringing tissue from elsewhere
Example	Surgical wound: closure with sutures, staples, tape, or other means to approximate the wound	Burn wound	Flap or graft

6. Associated infection.

7. Distracting injury.

8. Special areas: vermilion border, eyelid or orbit, over joints, hands or high tension areas, which are more likely to lead to keloid scarring.

Ensure that a secondary survey is carried out when the patient has had some analgesia and other less dramatic injuries can become apparent.

Managing the injury in accident and emergency

Manage the patient according the Advanced Trauma Life Support guidelines. Reduce fractures to anatomical alignment in the emergency department to protect against further injury to the soft tissue and watch for compartment syndrome. Minimize bleeding and manage pain. Neurovascular assessment should always be performed both before and after manipulation and operative intervention. Wound review in the emergency department is necessary to identify the degree of contamination; gross contamination can be removed, but definitive irrigation of open fractures should not be performed. The wound should be photographed following patient consent. Re-lay any de-gloved skin to the anatomical position and then cover the wound with a saline soaked gauze and an impermeable film to prevent desiccation.

Administer intravenous antibiotics if there are any open fractures or gross contamination has occurred within 3 hours of injury.[4] Intravenous co-amoxiclav 1.2 g three times daily up until debridement, when gentamicin is added for first-line treatment.[4]

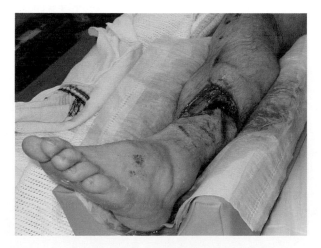

Fig. 6.2.1 An open Gustilo-Anderson grade 3b injury to left leg.

According to current combined British Orthopaedic Association and British Association of Plastic Reconstructive and Aesthetic Surgeons guidelines,[5] if the patient is mildly penicillin allergic, intravenous cefuroxime 1.5 g TDS can be used.

Tetanus immunoglobulin[6] can be administered if required.

Early referral to the definitive management team(s) is essential. Antibiotics should continue until soft tissue closure or 72 hours post injury. Early debridement, with skeletal stabilization and soft tissue reconstruction is now the gold standard.[7,8]

Classification

These injuries can be classified by several systems,[9–13] the most widely accepted of which are the Gustilo-Anderson and the AO classifications. The latter describes contamination, neurovascular status, and soft tissue injury associated with a fracture[14–16] (see Table 2.10.1.1).

The 'reconstructive ladder'

The reconstructive ladder describes the different levels of complex wound management[17] (Figure 6.2.2). Each patient will have different needs; in the hand trauma patient surgery varies according to the nature of the injury sustained. Burns and skin loss, for instance, will require surgical flaps and grafts, whereas the traumatic loss of digits may be treated by microsurgical replantation of the amputated parts. Each procedure has its own indication according to the size and depth of the defect, the structures exposed, and local considerations such as vascular status and availability of regional flaps.

In alliance with the patient and his/her expectations, the surgeon must consider function, co-morbidities, smoking status and rehabilitation time. Finally, donor site morbidity must be considered in context of the patient's degree of function and expectation.[18]

Vacuum-assisted closure

In wounds that are too tight to close directly, or have an inappropriate bed to host a skin graft, vacuum-assisted closure (VAC) can promote healing until definitive closure is achieved. The exact mechanism of VAC management's efficacy in treating wounds is not fully understood. However, it has been shown to remove interstitial fluid,[19] decrease the bacterial colonization, and improve vascularity leading to increased granulation tissue formation.[20]

Skin Grafts

A skin graft is skin transplanted from one location to another *without* its own blood supply. Skin grafts are classified as either split-thickness skin graft (STSG) or full-thickness skin graft (FTSG), depending on the amount of dermis included in the graft (variable for STSG, entire

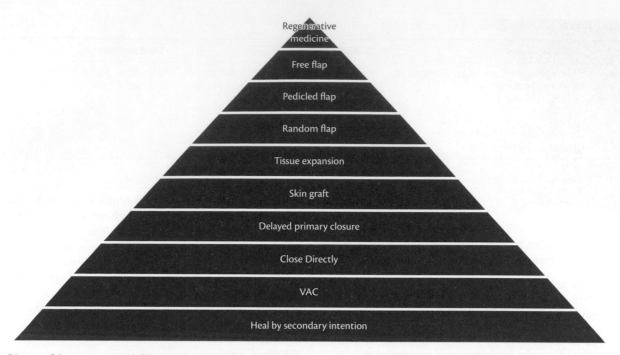

Fig. 6.2.2 Diagram of the reconstructive ladder. VAC, vacuum-assisted closure.
Source: data from Levin LS, The reconstructive ladder: An orthoplastic approach, *Orthopedic Clinics of North America*, Volume 24, Number 3, pp. 393–409, Copyright © 1993.

for FTSG). STSGs are further categorized as thin, intermediate, or thick based on the thickness of graft harvested. The thicker the dermal components, the more the characteristics of normal skin are maintained following grafting. However, thicker grafts require more favourable conditions for survival because of the greater amount of tissue requiring revascularization (Table 6.2.3). The choice between FTSG and STSGs depends on wound condition, location, and size, as well as aesthetic considerations. Of note, STSGs are ultimately hairless,[21] an important consideration when selecting skin from a hair-bearing area or a future hair-bearing area in children.

Graft Harvest

FTSGs are harvested with a scalpel blade and the skin closed with a linear scar. This means that the donor site must have enough laxity

within it to close directly and should be taken in a place where the scar is not too conspicuous.

STSGs can be harvested with a minor skin graft blade on a scalpel or a dermatome (Figure 6.2.3). Graft thickness can be judged by the type of bleeding at the donor site (Figure 6.2.4). Superficial grafts leave many small punctate bleeding points, whereas deep grafts leave fewer bleeding points that bleed more.

Graft Expansion Techniques/Meshing

Because a wound is re-epithelialized from the edges towards the centre, the perimeter of the graft is the only part that contributes to the epithelialization process. Expansion techniques are used to speed up that process. One of the most popular expansion techniques is the mesh graft method, using a mechanical mesher, which cuts multiple slits in the skin graft (Figure 6.2.5). Meshed STSGs are used primarily when insufficient donor skin is available, a highly

Table 6.2.3 Advantages and disadvantages of split-thickness (STSG) and full-thickness skin grafts (FTSG)

	STSG	FTSG
Advantages	Takes more favourably	Less contracture
	Uniform graft	Colour/texture match more similar to normal skin
	Donor site heals quickly	Potential for growth of graft
	Reuse of donor site in 1–2 months	
Disadvantages	Contracture	Requires well-vascularized bed
	Pigmentation	Donor site must be closed/ covered
	Increased susceptibility of trauma and sunburn	Linear scar from donor site

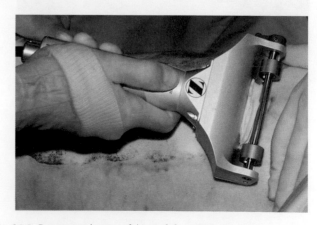

Fig. 6.2.3 Dermatome harvest of skin graft from thigh donor site.

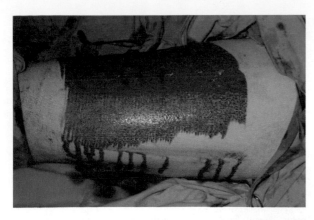

Fig. 6.2.4 Bleeding at thigh donor site after a medium thickness split-thickness skin graft.

convoluted area needs coverage, and/or the recipient bed is less than optimal. The slits in the graft allow sufficient drainage of fluid.

Meshed grafts are contraindicated in cosmetically sensitive body parts such as the face where the unaesthetic mesh pattern should be avoided. Meshed grafts are more prone to contraction, and therefore should be avoided in the neck and dorsum of the hand.

Graft take

Graft take is the adherence and vascularization of the skin graft onto its recipient site. The process starts with fibrin anchoring the graft, and occurs in three phases: plasmatic imbibition, inosculation, and neovascularization.

The quality of the recipient bed is crucial, as skin grafts will not take if there is a limited blood supply, such as on bone, cartilage, tendon, or nerve. Wounds secondary to radiation are also unlikely to support a graft. Skin grafts will survive on periosteum, perichondrium, peritenon, perineurium, dermis, fascia, muscle, and granulation tissue. The wound must also be free of necrotic tissue and relatively uncontaminated by bacteria.

Common causes of graft failure include haematoma or seroma, movement or shear forces, infection, and continued smoking.

Donor site regeneration

In FTSGs, the site does not regenerate and the wound edges are closed with a linear scar. In STSGs, the donor site regenerates from epidermal appendages within the dermis. Cells of the developing

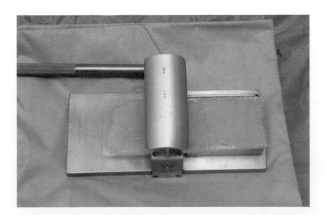

Fig. 6.2.5 A mechanical mesher.

epidermis invade the dermis in the third month of gestation to form intradermal epithelial structures: hair follicles, sebaceous glands, and sweat glands. These epidermal appendages are lined with epithelial cells with the potential for division and differentiation. They are found deep within the dermis and in the subcutaneous fat deep to the dermis. This accounts for the remarkable ability of the skin to re-epithelialize even very deep cutaneous wounds that are nearly full-thickness.

Long-term complications

Wound contraction may present serious functional and cosmetic concerns, depending on location and severity. On the face, it may produce ectropion, retraction of the nasal ala, or distortion of the vermilion border. Over joints it may limit functional range of motion. Contraction probably begins shortly following initial wounding, progressing slowly over 6 to 18 months following grafting. In general, FTSGs contract less than STSGs. Contraction can be ameliorated by splinting or compression devices, such as facial masks or Jobst garments. These devices should be worn as much as tolerated each day for at least the first 6 months' post grafting and often even longer.

Tissue expansion and flaps

Tissue expansion techniques can assist with wound coverage,[22] and are used to distend the overlying tissues to create flaps for reconstructive surgery.

Flaps can also be used and consist of a unit of tissue that is transferred from a donor site to a recipient one while maintaining a continuous blood supply through a vascular pedicle (direct or free).[23]

Further reading

American Society for Surgery of the Hand. History and general examination. In: *The Hand, Examination and Diagnosis*, 2nd edition. New York: Churchill Livingstone, 1983, pp. 3–10.

McGregor AD, McGregor IA. *Fundamental Techniques of Plastic Surgery: And Their Surgical Applications*. London: Churchill Livingstone, 2000.

National Institute of Health and Care Excellence. Pressure ulcers: the management of pressure ulcers in primary and secondary care (Clinical Guideline 29). Available from http://www.nice.org.uk/guidance/cg179 (accessed 17 November 2015)

National Institute of Health and Care Excellence. Surgical site infection: Prevention and treatment of surgical site infection (Clinical Guideline 74). Available from https://www.nice.org.uk/guidance/cg74 (accessed 17 November 2015).

References

1. Levenson SM, Geever EF, Crowley LV, *et al*. Healing of rat skin wounds. *Ann Surg* 1965; 161(2): 293–308.
2. Bouillon B, Kanz KG, Lackner CK, *et al*. The importance of Advanced Trauma Life Support (ATLS) in the emergency room. *Unfallchirurg*. 2004; 107(10): 844–50.
3. Perron AD, Brady WJ, Keats TE, *et al*. Orthopedic pitfalls in the emergency department: closed tendon injuries of the hand. *Am J Emerg Med* 2001; 19: 76–80.
4. Gosselin RA, Roberts I, Gillespie WJ. Antibiotics for preventing infection in open limb fractures. *Cochrane Database Syst Rev* 2004; 1: CD003764.
5. Nanchahal J, Nayagam S, Khan U, *et al. Standards for the Management of Open Fractures of the Lower Limb*. Endorsed by British Association of Plastic Reconstructive and Aesthetic Surgeons and British Orthopaedic Association. Available from http://www.nvpc.nl/uploads/

stand/100NVPC090000DOC-FN-Standards%20for%20Lower%20 Limb.pdf. (accessed 17 November 2015).

6. UK Department of Health. Tetanus. In: *Immunisation against infectious Disease – 'The Green Book'*. London, UK: Department of Health; 2009: 367–84.

7. Godina M. Early microsurgical reconstruction of complex trauma of the extremities. *Plast Reconstr Surg* 1986; 78(3): 285–92.

8. Gopal S, Majumder S, Batchelor A, *et al*. Fix and flap: The radial orthopaedic and plastic treatment of severe open fractures of the tibia. *J Bone Joint Surg Br* 2000; 82: 959–66.

9. Bryd HS, Spicer TE, Cierney G. Management of open tibial fractures. *Plast Reconstr Surg* 1985; 76(5): 719–30.

10. Chiu TW. *Stone's Plastic Surgery Facts and Figures*. Cambridge: Cambridge University Press, 2011.

11. AO Foundation. Principles of management of open fractures. Available from https://www2.aofoundation.org/wps/portal/!ut/p/a1/ jU_JDoIwFPyaXukD4xJvPShxSYjBBXsxJZZCgm3zWiT 69SJnXOY2k5 nJDOU0o1yLe6WEr4wW9Zvzy SVKAOJVCpsk2YfA0kUYH5cAsBt3h vMXA5v-l4cPYPArv6Zc1Sbvp56ZzkczRTnKQqLEoMFOLr23bk6AQ Nu2USBMYRp97Q8GBlUnW0fAGvSiJuAa VBIfQ22lcZ5mgyXU3g7Z cytPLx5X3uM!/dl5/d5/L2dJQSEvUUt3QS80SmlFL1o2XzJPMDBHSV MwS09PVDEwQVNFMUdWRjAwMFE1/?showPage=redfix& bone=Tibia&segment= Shaft&classification=42-Special%20considerat ions&treatment=&method=Special%20considerations&implantstype= Principles%20of%20management%20of%20open%20fractures& approach=&redfix_url=1341318938215. (Access verified 17th November 2015)

12. Martin JS, Marsh JL, Bonar SK, *et al*. Assessment of the AO/ASIF fracture classification for the distal tibia. *J Orthop Trauma* 1997; 11: 477–83.

13. Arnez ZM, Tyler MP, Khan U. Describing severe limb trauma. *Br J Plast Surg* 1999; 52: 280–5.

14. Gustilo, RB. Anderson, JT. Prevention of infection in the treatment of one thousand and twenty-five open fractures of long bones: retrospective and prospective. *J Bone Joint Surg Am* 1976; 58(4): 453–8.

15. Gustilo RB, Mendoza RM, Williams DN. Problems in the management of type III (severe) open fractures: a new classification of type III open fractures. *J Trauma* 1984; 24(8): 742–6.

16. Gustilo RB. Interobserver agreement in the classification of open fractures of the tibia. The results of a survey of two hundred and forty-five orthopaedic surgeons. *J Bone Joint Surg Am* 1995; 77: 1291–2.

17. Levin LS. The reconstructive ladder. An orthoplastic approach. *Orthop Clin North Am* 1993; 24(3): 393–409.

18. Schwabegger AII, Harpf C, Rainer C. Muscle-sparing latissimus dorsi myocutaneous flap with maintenance of muscle innervation, function, and aesthetic appearance of the donor site. *Plast Reconstr Surg* 2003; 111(4): 1407–11.

19. Argenta LC, Morykwas MJ. Vacuum-assisted closure: a new method for wound control and treatment: clinical experience. *Ann Plast Surg* 1997; 38(6): 563–76; discussion 577.

20. Morykwas MJ, David LR, Schneider AM, *et al*. Use of subatmospheric pressure to prevent progression of partial-thickness burns in a swine model. *J Burn Care Rehabil* 1999; 20(1): 15–21.

21. Hierner R, Degreef H, Vranckx JJ, *et al*. Skin grafting and wound healing: The 'dermato-plastic team approach. *Clin Dermatol* 2005; 23: 343–52.

22. Radovan C. Tissue expansion soft tissue reconstruction. *Plast. Reconstr. Surg* 1984; 74: 482.

23. Masquelet AC, Gilbert A. *An Atlas of Flaps of the Musculoskeletal System*. London: Martin Dunitz, 2001.

CHAPTER 6.3

Burns: classification and principles of management

Nada Al-Hadithy

Introduction, epidemiology, and aetiology

About 250 000 people in the UK experience burns annually, and their consequence can be devastating.[1] Over 90% are preventable, yet 1000 patients are admitted each year, half of who are children under the age of 16. Three hundred of these patients die, with the majority aged over 60.[2] Burns are a major component of the trauma workload, and should be considered in healthcare planning and policy.[3]

The aetiology of burns is dependent upon age (Table 6.3.1). Burns victims' health is often compromised by other factors such as alcoholism, epilepsy, or chronic psychiatric or medical illness. Nine per cent of all burn victims in Western countries are caused by self-immolation with suicidal intent.[4]

Burn care

Overview of the seven phases of management

Managing a burns victim is the job of a multidisciplinary team according to the following algorithm.

Rescue

Avoid unnecessary harm to the rescuer. Remove the individual away from the burning source, stop the burning, and provide first aid. Cool small burns (<15% total body surface area [TBSA]) with running water for 20 minutes. Wrap and warm the patient.

Resuscitate

Immediate support for any failing organ system must be provided. This usually involves administering fluid but can also involve supporting cardiac, renal, and respiratory systems.

Retrieve

After initial assessment in the emergency department, retrieval to the site of definitive care is required to promote superior care, especially for complex injuries and conditions.[5,6]

Resurface

All injuries to the skin need to be repaired. This can be done either by wound dressings with appropriate analgesia,[7] or with dermal resurfacing. Sufficiently damaged skin will not heal spontaneously and will warrant early skin grafting.

Rehabilitate

This process starts on the day of admission. The whole burn team's ultimate goal is to return a fully functioning individual to society with unaltered appearance, abilities, and potential.

Reconstruct

Burn scars may require further intervention. This involves removal of troublesome areas of unstable ulcerating areas of skin or skin graft, or release of functionally important areas from contracting scar tissue.

Review

Ensure specialist functional, aesthetic, and psychological rehabilitation with the goal of recovering the individual to the pre-injury state.

Understanding burns

What is a burn injury?

Jackson's 1953 classification system of thermal injury is still the foundation of our burns management model[8] (Figure 6.3.1).

Table 6.3.1 Aetiology and epidemiology of burns

% of burns	Who gets burned	Age (years)	Cause of burn	Sex preponderance
>60%	Working age	15–64	Flame (one-third work related), scald, contact, electrical, chemical, friction	Male
20%	Young children	0–4	Scald (70%), flame, contact, electrical, chemical, sunburn	Male
10%	Older children	5–14	Increasingly flame, scald. Teenagers have a higher proportion of illicit activities: accelerants, petrol	Male
10%	Elderly people	65+	Scalds, contact, flame	Female

Source: data from Forster NA *et al.*, Attempted suicide by self-immolation is a powerful predictive variable for survival of burn injuries, *Journal of Burns Care and Research*, Volume 33, Issue 5, pp. 642–8, Copyright © 2012 The American Burn Association, DOI: 10.1097/BCR.0b013e3182479b28.

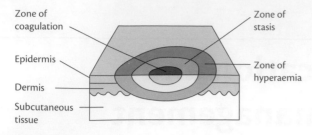

Fig. 6.3.1 Jackson's burn model.
Reproduced from Smith *et al.* (Eds), *Oxford Desk Reference: Major Trauma*, Figure 22.8, Oxford University Press, Oxford, UK, Copyright © 2010, by permission of Oxford University Press.

Temperatures above 50°C will produce tissue necrosis, particularly when the skin is thin as in a child or in the elderly.

How do burns heal?

Superficial burns heal by re-epithelialization from epidermal cells at the periphery of the wound or from those in adnexal structures such as hair follicles and sweat glands.

For deep burns, myoblasts[9] cause wound contraction,[10] which reduces the surface area of the burn and is the basic mechanism for closure. This can result in rigid scar contractures and often a skin graft or flap is required.

Burns assessment: total body surface area

Measurement of the surface area of the burn is expressed as the body surface area percentage or the TBSA. It is the cornerstone of management of patients with burns and is necessary to establish the need for fluid resuscitation and the volume required, and the prognosis and progress. There are three main methods.

Rule of nines

The rule of nines divides the body surface area into areas of 9% or multiples of 9% (Figure 6.3.2). The rule of nines in children has different ratios to account for their larger head.[11]

Lund and Browder chart

This is the most accurate and widely used chart, but it does not take into consideration obesity, breast size, pregnancy, or amputated body parts.[12–14]

Use of hand as 1% of total body surface area

Alternatively, the patient's hand can be used as an estimation of 1% of the TBSA;[15] the palmar surface including the fingers is approximately 0.8% of TBSA.

Burns assessment

Depth

Burn depth can progress and should be reassessed after 48 hours (Table 6.3.2). Understanding the anatomy of the skin can illicit as greater understanding of the clinical features, healing process, and management options for varying burns depths.

Escharotomy

For deep/circumferential burns, the skin cannot stretch and therefore causes a tourniquet effect as burn oedema develops. This may require incising (escharotomy) to relieve pressure or to prevent

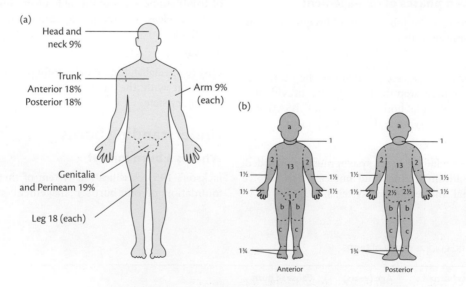

Relative percentage of body surface area (% BSA) affected by growth

Body Part	Age				
	0 yr	1 yr	5 yr	10 yr	15 yr
a = ½ of head	9½	8½	6½	5½	4½
b = ½ of 1 thigh	2¾	3½	4	4¼	2¼
c = ½ of 1 lower leg	2½	2½	2%	3	3¼

Fig. 6.3.2 Wallace's rule of nines for differing age groups.
Reproduced from Crouch *et al.* (Eds), *Oxford Handbook of Emergency Nursing*, Figure 12.1, Oxford University Press, Oxford, UK, Copyright © 2010, by permission of Oxford University Press.

Table 6.3.2 Features of superficial, partial-thickness, and full-thickness burns

Burn depth	Skin level involved	Colour	Presence of pain	Blisters	Capillary refill	Thrombosed vessels
Superficial	Epidermal	Red, may be shiny and wet	Yes	No	<2	No
Partial thickness	Superficial dermal	Pink, may be dry	Yes	Yes	<2	No
	Deep dermal	Blotchy red	Yes	No	>2/fixed staining	Yes
Full thickness	Sub dermal	Thick, white, leathery	Insensate	No	None	Yes

In reality most burns are mixed depth.

respiratory embarrassment. Limb escharotomies should be carried out within 3 hours to prevent irreversible ischaemic damage to the tissues.

Principles of resuscitation

The goal of burn resuscitation is to maintain adequate tissue perfusion and to prevent hypovolaemia. This requires the administration of salt and water during the resuscitation phase. The optimum sodium load is about 0.5 mmol per kg body weight per % TBSA burned. The chosen fluid regimen should produce a moderate hypernatraemia. Children have a higher fluid requirement than adults, due to their higher surface area to body mass ratio. The additional volume approximates to the daily maintenance fluid requirement. This may be given orally in small amounts at frequent intervals or intravenously as 4% dextrose/0.18% saline solution.

Other patients may also require more fluid than the calculation suggests include those with inhalation injury, pre-existing dehydration, electrical burns, and with delay in commencing resuscitation.

Oral fluid replacement

In burns less than 10% TBSA in children or 15% TBSA in adults, balancing fluid loss by increasing oral fluid intake is usually sufficient. However, there is still a requirement for salt and it is highly dangerous to attempt resuscitation by giving extra water as this will lead to hyponatraemia. As water diuresis is rarely possible during the first 12 to 24 hours after injury, even a moderate excess intake of sodium-free water may lead to water intoxication, possibly with fatal consequences. Dextrolyte™ is a suitable oral fluid for infants and sachets of Dioralyte™ can be used to make up a satisfactory solution for older children. For older children and adults, Moyer's solution contains 4 g of sodium chloride and 1.5 g of sodium bicarbonate per litre. This composition can be obtained by mixing 1 L of normal saline (0.9%) with 1 L of tap water and 100 mL of isotonic (1.26%) sodium bicarbonate solution. The quantity of fluid required will obviously vary according to the size of the burn and the weight of the patient but should be about two to three times the maintenance fluid requirement.

Intravenous fluid replacement

The fluid resuscitation formula provides a 'guideline' for fluid resuscitation and is frequently adjusted according to monitored clinical indices.[16] Frequent clinical reassessment is vital for effective resuscitation. Clinical measurements should include heart rate, respiratory rate, blood pressure, and core and peripheral temperature.

Hourly urine output should be used to titrate fluid administration: an output in excess of 1.5 mL/kg/h is due to overtransfusion.[17]

In major or complex burns, direct measurement of blood pressure via an arterial line is essential. This clinical information, plus laboratory investigations such as haematocrit, urea and electrolytes, urine concentration (osmolality), and arterial blood gas analysis, should enable the clinician to assess the adequacy of tissue perfusion and, thus the effectiveness of fluid therapy.

Fluid resuscitation protocol

The most enduring protocol for fluid resuscitation is the Parkland formula:

Fluid for the first 24 hours
= 4 mL of crystalloid × body weight (kg)
× % burned (+ maintenance for children)

Time of injury marks the start of fluid resuscitation and Ringers lactate, Hartmann's solution or 0.9% sodium chloride is the choice of fluid. Half of the calculated fluid is given in the first eight hours; the rest is given over the next 16 hours.

The Clinician and the burn
Initial management of burns: First aid

The burning process should be stopped (remove clothing/jewellery), and the burn cooled with cold running water. In chemical burns, wear a thick plastic apron and rubber gloves. Remove corrosive chemicals by brushing dry powder from the clothes and skin. Use copious amounts of water to dilute the chemical, with special focus to the eyes. Do not try to neutralize the burn with acid or alkali. Send any information regarding the nature of the chemical with the ambulance crew.

Primary survey

In addition to the generic features detailed in Chapter 6.1, the following features specific to the burns casualty must be considered and managed.

Fires kill more people by asphyxiation than by the thermal injury, and any suspicion that airway obstruction may develop should illicit protection of patency of the upper airway, provision of high flow oxygen, and referral to senior anaesthetist and if necessary intubation.

Remember that carbon monoxide binds preferentially to haemoglobin and if there is any possibility of carbon monoxide poisoning the oxygen saturations are unreliable and an arterial blood gas sample should be carried out. Administer humidified oxygen at 12–15 L per minute through a non-re-breathing mask.

Map out the burned areas on a body outline chart and document time of injury, time of assessment, fluid initiation, and volume given. Ensure that this information is available for the receiving unit. If haemorrhage occurs from other injuries replace volume loss with blood.

Catheterize all patients with burns involving >15% TBSA to monitor adequacy of fluid resuscitation and monitor their urine. Ask for observations of electrocardiogram monitoring, pulse, blood pressure, and respiratory rate every 15 minutes.

Expose the patient and logroll for full examination and burn assessment. Take clinical images and temporarily dress any burned area with cling film before covering the patient with blankets for warmth preservation.

Take an AMPLE history from the patient, any witnesses, and the ambulance crew. Note if protective clothing had been worn, if this was soaked in hot liquids, and whether it had been removed and when.

Secondary survey

Examine the patient systematically from head to toe. Consider the possibility of non-accidental injury in children, vulnerable adults, and elderly people in care. Arrange for photography.

Insert further lines such as arterial lines if appropriate or nasogastric tube for larger burns. Carry out further investigations including X-rays and/or CT scans if indicated.

Look for complications of hypovolaemia, impaired renal function, haemochromogenuria and over-transfusion, pulmonary damage, or burn encephalopathy.

Referral

National Burn Care Review Committee NBCRC guidelines state that all complex burn injuries should reach the burn service site within 6 hours of injury across the British Isles and within 4 hours of injury if referred from an urban site.[18]

Continuing burn care

Burn shock

This is the inability of the circulatory system to meet the needs of tissues for oxygen and nutrients and the removal of their metabolites.[19]

Clinical features of shock

These represent reflex and hormonal compensatory mechanisms that serve to maintain the blood flow to the cerebral and coronary vessels until the last possible moment. Restoration of the circulation is essential, and given the predictable time course of greater tissue permeability in the first 8 hours, burns presents an opportunity to address the potential for shock early in its evolution.

Burn oedema

Within minutes of sustaining a burn, oedema will develop. In those tissues affected, but not devitalized by heat, local vasodilatation occurs in an attempt to dissipate the heat and will have an increased capillary permeability. However, the increased filtration of fluids and proteins into the interstitial space exceeds the capacity

of the lymphatic drainage. Without treatment, the patient with an extensive burn (>50% TBSA) will lose one-third of the circulating volume within 3 to 4 hours of the accident and will be in life-threatening shock.

Other complications

Burns patients may also develop systemic inflammatory response syndrome, inhalation injury, renal failure, haemochromogenuria, and increased nutritional requirements during the recovery phase. All must be recognized and managed accordingly.

Prognosis in major burns

The ability of an individual to survive depends on the TBSA and the age of the individual. Survival is also influenced by the presence of an airway injury from smoke, vapours or heat, and the pre-existence of medical conditions affecting the ability of the individual to respond to trauma.

Several prognostication tools are available and the use of probit analysis to calculate lethal area 50 values has been used by numerous authors and is the standard method for reporting and comparing mortality outcome after burn injury.[20] Prognosis can be significantly improved by rapid referral to burns teams[21] and with the establishment of burns networks (see Further reading).

Further reading

Alvarado R, Chung KK, Cancio LC, Wolf SE. Burn resuscitation. Burns 3 5 (2009) 4–14.

Herndon DN. Total Burn Care. Vol 3. Saunders; 2007.

Muir IFK, Barclay TL. Bums and their treatment. Lloyd Luke Ltd., London, 1974.

Munster AM, Smith-Meek. The effect of early surgical intervention on mortality and cost-effectiveness in burn care 1978–1991. Burns 1994; 20: 61–4.

Reiss E, Stirman JA, Artz CP, Davis JH, Anispacher WH. Fluid and electrolyte balance in burns. JAMA, 152: 1309–12, 1953.

WHO Surgical Care at the District Hospital 2003, WHO/EHT/CPR 2004 reformatted.

References

1. Gardner PJ, Knittel-Keren D, Gomez M. The Posttraumatic Stress Disorder Checklist as a screening measure for posttraumatic stress disorder in rehabilitation after burn injuries. *Arch Phys Med Rehabil* 2012; 93(4): 623–8.

2. National Burn Care Review Committee. *Standards and Strategy for Burn Care: A review of burn care in the British Isles.* The International Burn Injury Database, March 2001. Available from http://ibidb.org/downloads/cat_view/14-general-reports (accessed 9 November 2012).

3. Kalson NS, Jenks T, Woodford M, *et al.* Burns represent a significant proportion of the total serious trauma workload in England and Wales. *Burns* 2012; 38(3): 330–9.

4. Forster NA, Nuñez DG, Zingg M, *et al.* Attempted suicide by self-immolation is a powerful predictive variable for survival of burn injuries. *J Burn Care Res* 2012; 33(5): 642–8.

5. Wallace PGM, Ridley SA. ABC of intensive care—transport of critically ill patients. *BMJ* 1999. 319; 368–70.

6. UK Department of Health. *Comprehensive critical care; A review of adult critical care services.* London: Department of Health. Available from http://webarchive.nationalarchives.gov.uk/20130107105354/http://www.dh.gov.uk/prod_consum_dh/groups/dh_digitalassets/@dh/@en/documents/digitalasset/dh_4082872.pdf (accessed 17 November 2015).

7. Judkins K. Pain management in the burned patient. *Pain Rev* 1998; 5: 133–46.

8. Jackson D. The diagnosis of the depth of burning. *Br J Surg* 1953; 40: 588.

9. Gabbiani G, Ryan GB, Majno G: Presence of modified fibroblasts in granulation tissue and their possible role in wound contraction. *Experimentia* 1971, 27: 549–50.

10. Rungger-Brandle E, Gabbiani G. The role of cytoskeletal and cytocontractile elements in pathologic processes. *Am J Pathol* 1983, 110: 359–92.

11. Johnson RM, Richard R. Partial thickness burns: identification and management. *Adv Skin Wound Care* 2003; 16(4): 178–87; quiz 188–9.

12. Knaysi GA, Crikelair GF, Cosman B. The rule of nines: its history and accuracy. *Plast Reconstr Surg* 1968; 41(6): 560–3.

13. Lund CC, Browder NC. The estimation of areas of burns. *Surg Gynecol Obstet* 1944; 79: 352–8.

14. Mercer NS, Price RJ, Maude S, *et al*. The Frenchay Burns Chart. *Burns Incl Therm Inj* 1988; 14(1): 58–9.

15. Sakson JA. Simplified chart for estimating burn areas. *Am J Surg* 1959; 98: 693–4.

16. Nagel TR, Schunk JE Using the hand to estimate the surface area of burn in children. *Pediatr Emerg Care* 1997; 13(4): 254–5.

17. Moncrief JA. Medical progress—burns. *N Engl J Med* 1973; 288: 444–54.

18. Settle JAD. Urine output following severe. *Burns* 1974; 1: 23–42.

19. British Burn Association. Standards and strategy for burn care: A review of burn care in the British Isles. Published February 2001, reviewed 1 March 2003. Available from http://www.britishburnassociation.org/downloads/NBCR2001.pdf (accessed 17 November 2015).

20. Dietzman RH, Lillehei RC. The nature and treatment of shock. *Br J Hosp Med* 1968; 1: 300.

21. Bull JP, Squire JR. A study of mortality in a burns unit; standards for the evaluation of alternative methods of treatment. *Ann Surg* 1949; 130: 160–73.

CHAPTER 6.4

Assessment and management of patients with major trauma, and major and multiple skeletal injuries

John Keating

Introduction

Injury to the skeletal system occurs in 65% of those who suffer blunt trauma. Patients with multiple or major skeletal injuries often present dramatically and prioritization can be challenging. With a clear methodical approach these patients can be managed appropriately and a positive outcome can be achieved in the majority of cases.

The orthopaedic surgeon plays an important role in the management of the multiply injured patient. The responsibility starts immediately and continues beyond the early phase of acute management through to post-injury rehabilitation and late reconstructive surgery. The knowledge, skill set, and attributes required to perform this role are diverse.

The purpose of this chapter is to discuss the acute management of patients with major/multiple skeletal injuries.

Classification

Classification of injury severity

Injury severity scoring is a process by which complex clinical information is used to derive a score, which can be used to understand the severity of the injury. While the intricacies of more elaborate classification systems may be beyond emergency department decision making, the underlying principles provide the foundation for making accurate clinical assessments. The clinician must consider the combined effect of the anatomic injury, the physiologic insult and the extent of patient reserve. This will allow for clinical judgment of:

◆ Whether the patient is in a life-threatening situation.

◆ If there is an immediate threat to a limb.

◆ If there is more simply a skeletal injury that may be treated on a routine basis.

Trauma scoring systems may be based on anatomy, physiological parameters, or a combination of the two.

The Abbreviated Injury Scale (AIS) is an anatomic-based system in which injuries are ranked on a scale of 1 to 6, with 1 being minor, 5 severe, and 6 a non-survivable injury. Tables are available for various anatomical regions, which detail the injury and the corresponding score. The AIS provides the core data, which is used in a number of other scoring systems.

The Injury Severity Score (ISS) is also an anatomic scoring system and provides an overall score for patients with multiple injuries. Each injury is assigned an AIS and is allocated to one of six body regions: (1) head including cervical spine; (2) face; (3) chest including thoracic spine; (4) abdomen including lumbar spine; (5) extremities including bony pelvis; and (6) external. The highest AIS score in each body region is used and the three most severely injured regions have their scores taken, the numbers are squared and then added together to produce the ISS score.

The Revised Trauma Score (RTS) is a physiologic-based score centred on first recorded triage and uses the weighed values of the Glasgow Coma Scale (GCS), respiratory rate (RR), and the systolic blood pressure (SBP) according to the formula RTS = 0.9368 GCS + 0.7326 SBP + 0.2908 RR. Tables are available for rapid use of the information and guide management. A score below 10 mandates immediate treatment (Table 6.4.1).

The Trauma Score–Injury Severity Score (TRISS) methodology uses a combination of the anatomic-based ISS and the physiologic-based RTS. Coefficients derived from the Major Trauma Outcome

Table 6.4.1 Parameters used for calculating the Revised Trauma Score

GCS	SBP	RR	Coded value
13–15	>89	10–29	4
9–12	76–89	>29	3
6–8	50–75	6–9	2
4–5	1–49	1–5	1
3	0	0	0

GCS, Glasgow Coma Scale; SBP, systolic blood pressure; RR, respiratory rate.

Reproduced with permission from Howard Champion *et al.*, A Revision of the Trauma Score, *The Journal of Trauma and Acute Care Surgery*, Volume 29, Issue 5, pp. 623–629, Copyright © 1989 Wolters Kluwer Health, Inc.

Study are used in a formula to arrive at a composite score and the probability of survival.

When assessing a patient in the emergency department, it is necessary to use sound clinical acumen to assess the combined effect of the anatomic injury, the physiologic insult, and the extent of patient reserve. In the acute situation the ISS tends to be used as it is readily calculated on the basis of the anatomic injury in this setting.

Classification of skeletal injury

The most comprehensive skeletal classification system is that developed by the AO (Arbeitsgemeinschaft für Osteosynthesefragen) group. This is a hierarchical alphanumeric system that covers the spectrum of fractures by first describing the location of the fracture and then the morphology. Long bone fracture location is described using two numbers. The first descriptor denotes the effected long bone by a number 1, 2, 3, and 4 representing the humerus, forearm, femur and tibia, respectively. The second descriptor denotes the location within that bone by a number, with 1, 2, or 3 representing proximal, diaphyseal, or distal locations, respectively. Fractures involving parts of the skeleton other than the long bones are also covered in this system. The system is now widely used although it is rather complex for the acute phase of management in skeletal trauma.

Classification of open fractures

Open fractures are described using the Gustilo and Anderson classification system, which categorizes them on the basis of the severity of the associated soft tissue injury. There are three main categories with three subdivisions of grade III injuries:

- Grade I: An open fracture due to low energy trauma with a wound of less than 1 cm in length with no deep contamination.
- Grade II: An open fracture with a wound of between 1 cm and 10 cm in length as a consequence of moderate energy trauma. Some contusion of the wound edge may be present but there is no significant deep contamination or periosteal stripping.
- Grade IIIA: An open fracture with a wound greater than 10 cm in length with some deep soft tissue contamination but no periosteal stripping or bone loss. This grade of injury also applies to

any high-energy trauma irrespective of wound size and any open segmental fracture.

- Grade IIIB: An open fracture with a large wound, deep soft tissue contamination, and periosteal stripping often with some degree of bone loss after debridement. Primary closure of the wound is not possible and flap cover is generally required.
- Grade IIIC: An open fracture with a vascular injury requiring repair.

Some points are worth making about this classification. The final grading is made at the completion of the debridement, as it is only then that the extent of deep soft tissue involvement and the need for bone debridement can be defined. The classification was mainly used for open tibial and femoral shaft fractures but it is commonly applied to other open injuries. The level of interobserver agreement in well-trained trauma surgeons is between 60% and 70%, which is not ideal, but the system has remained in common clinical use in the absence of a superior method of classification.

Pathophysiology

Shock, systemic inflammation, and local tissue damage are the primary pathophysiologic processes to be considered with multiple skeletal injuries. From these processes secondary pathophysiologic pathways arise which may flow into a negative feedback loop, causing systemic inflammatory response syndrome (SIRS), adult respiratory distress syndrome (ARDS) or multiple organ dysfunction syndrome (MODS).

Shock

Four basic types of shock exist, the first being most commonly seen in the multiply injured patient.

1. Hypovolaemic shock is caused by loss of blood. In patients with skeletal trauma it is most frequently encountered in association with long bone fractures and pelvic ring disruptions. Hypovolaemic shock is divided into four classes based on the amount of blood loss. Table 6.4.2 provides values based on the ideal body composition of a 70 kg male.

Table 6.4.2 Classes of hypovolaemic shock[a]

	CLASS I	CLASS II	CLASS III	CLASS IV
Blood loss (mL)	Up to 750	750–1500	1500–2000	>2000
Blood loss (% blood volume)	Up to 15	15–30	30–40	>40
Pulse rate (beats per minute)	<100	100–120	120–140	>140
Systolic blood pressure	Normal	Normal	Decreased	Decreased
Pulse pressure (mmHg)	Normal or increased	Decreased	Decreased	Decreased
Respiratory rate	14–20	20–30	30–40	>35
Urine output (mL/hr)	>30	20–30	5–15	Negligible
CNS/mental status	Slightly anxious	Mildly anxious	Anxious, confused	Confused, lethargic
Initial fluid replacement	Crystalloid	Crystalloid	Crystalloid and blood	Crystalloid and blood

[a]For a 70-kg man.
Reproduced with permission of The American College of Surgeons, *Advanced Trauma Life Support*, Ninth Edition, p. 69, Copyright © 2012 The American College of Surgeons.

2. Neurogenic shock in skeletal trauma is most frequently the result of spinal cord injury and loss of adrenergic stimulation. This results in loss of arterial tissue tension and pooling of the blood, effectively reducing the circulatory volume.

3. Cardiogenic shock is not commonly the result of skeletal trauma. However, patients with pre-existing ischaemic heart disease are at increased risk of myocardial infarction after major trauma and cardiogenic shock may be encountered in this setting.

4. Septic shock as a result of infection is usually seen after the acute phase of injury. It is most common in patients with multiple trauma who may be immunocompromised as a consequence of prolonged ventilation, nutritional impairment, and sources of infection such as open long bone fractures or open pelvic fracture.

Other pathophysiological syndromes in skeletal trauma

In uncomplicated trauma, the systemic inflammatory response is predictable and well balanced between proinflammatory and anti-inflammatory mediators and is a necessary part of healing. In severe trauma, the initial phase may result in an exaggerated pro-inflammatory response, which can cause systemic damage. In the primed state, which occurs after a traumatic event, a second 'hit' that can include surgical trauma or secondary sepsis may result in an exaggerated widespread non-specific response. In severe cases this may manifest as a SIRS, which is a serious clinical condition that may result from multiple aetiologies including hypovolaemic shock and systemic inflammation. Central to the pathogenesis is fibrin deposition, aggregation of platelets, coagulopathy, and uncontrolled inflammatory mediator release. If this process is not controlled, then a clinical picture characterized by MODS may result. The culmination of this may be multi-organ failure, which carries a high mortality.

Fat embolism syndrome

ARDS is a life-threatening lung condition typified by severe dyspnoea, tachypnoea, and resistant hypoxaemia. It may occur in a variety of situations, but in skeletal trauma the precursor is often fat embolism syndrome. Fat emboli occur in 90% of those with severe long bone fractures, but only 1–5% of these cases will be symptomatic. The clinical syndrome is characterized by signs and symptoms typically occurring 24 to 72 hours following trauma and may include dyspnoea, agitation, and petechial rash. A full blood count may reveal anaemia with a thrombocytopenia. The process can result in disseminated intravascular coagulopathy and lead onto SIRS. However, the picture is often dominated by respiratory compromise and in severe cases the clinical manifestations are indistinguishable from ARDS.

Assessment of patients with major/multiple skeletal injuries

Primary survey

The primary assessment of patients with skeletal trauma involves a thorough primary and secondary survey of all systems and that the priority of assessment remain consistent with Advanced Trauma Life Support principles.

The primary survey is intended to identify and simultaneously address life-threatening injuries. Important skeletal considerations during the primary survey include protecting against secondary neurologic damage from unstable spinal column injury, and identifying and controlling bleeding from major skeletal injuries.

Spinal cord injury

Protection of the cervical spine occurs immediately during 'A–Airway Maintenance with Cervical Spine Protection'. This is achieved by initial cervical spine immobilization in a hard collar until the cervical spine is definitively cleared. A screening neurological exam is carried out under the 'D–Disability' section of the primary survey. It must be kept in mind that intact neurologic function does not exclude an unstable spinal column injury.

Blood loss from skeletal injuries

External haemorrhage is identified and managed during 'C–Circulation' of the primary survey. Typically haemostasis is achieved in the first instance with direct manual pressure, but may also be aided by providing preliminary skeletal stabilization to an unstable pelvic fracture with a pelvic binder. Adequate intravenous access with two large bore intravenous lines is mandatory and fluid resuscitation should commence. Administration of tranexamic acid in bleeding trauma patients has been shown to reduce the mortality rate significantly if given early (ideally within 1 hour).

Adjuncts to the primary survey

All patients who have suffered severe blunt trauma should have a plain radiograph of the chest and pelvis. Formerly lateral radiographs of the cervical spine were routinely obtained but these are frequently of inadequate quality to definitively rule out bony injury. The preferred imaging modality is a computed tomography (CT) scan.

Secondary survey

Once the primary survey is complete and treatment of life-threatening injuries has been instituted, a secondary survey is performed to identify other injuries that are not immediately life threatening but are likely to require treatment. This should include a history of the mechanism of injury and the environment in which it occurred. This often provides useful information about the forces imparted on the musculoskeletal system and can give clues as to what injuries are likely to have been sustained.

Road traffic accidents remain the most common cause of patients sustaining multiple skeletal injuries. It is important to know the nature of the collision, location of the patient within the vehicle, the use of safety belts, deployment of airbags, whether a patient was ejected from the vehicle or not, any fatalities at the scene, difficulties with extraction, and exposure to the elements following the incident. This provides important information about the expected severity of injuries and predictable patterns.

Falls from height commonly result in an axial load force vector, which may also result in predictable injuries including calcaneal fractures, tibial plateau fractures, vertical shear pelvic fractures, and spinal column injuries.

The environment in which an injury is sustained is important to consider. Prolonged exposure to cold temperatures will lead to hypothermia. Open wounds sustained in contaminated environments such as farmyards may require more radical surgical debridement and broad antibiotic cover including antibiotics effective for anaerobic organisms.

Physical examination

Examination of the skeletal system must be thorough, systematic, and efficient. Each limb segment must be inspected for open wounds, obvious deformity, abnormal posturing, and neurological and vascular function. In an awake and cooperative patient, assessment of functional movement through major joint complexes is a rapid way of assessing neurological function and integrity of the skeleton. Patients who are uncooperative or with a lowered level of consciousness will be more difficult to examine. All patients will need ongoing re-evaluation and a formal secondary survey should be repeated after 24–72 hours to identify injuries, which may have previously been missed.

Major long bone fractures are generally obvious, but metaphyseal or intra-articular fractures particularly to the hand and foot may not be readily apparent and are easy to overlook in the acute phase of assessment and management. Missing these injuries may result in significant functional disability at a later stage. A high index of suspicion and repeated clinical assessment in the days following admission should lead to detection of other injuries.

Adjuncts to the secondary survey

Further first aid management of skeletal injuries should be undertaken following the secondary survey. Fractures should be provisionally aligned and splinted to provide pain relief and minimize further soft tissue injury. Dislocations, which are causing skin or vascular compromise, must be expeditiously reduced and splinted. Open wounds require a thorough debridement and lavage in a modern operating theatre, and not in less than ideal conditions in an emergency department. Open wounds can be photographed, and sterile dressings applied in preparation for debridement. Antibiotic and tetanus cover for open injuries should be administered and appropriate pain relief administered.

The priority of imaging investigations will vary depending on the severity and pattern of injuries. It is important, where possible, to consider workflow and time management when arranging such investigations. When there is an obvious skeletal injury to a limb, it is often sensible to obtain plain film imaging of this injury before the patient is transferred for CT imaging, as the plain film image will allow for earlier understanding of the injury and permit planning of surgical fracture management and preparation of theatre resources. For most long bone and metaphyseal fractures, plain radiographs will suffice to determine the optimum method of fixation.

Patients with multiple skeletal and other injuries ideally require CT imaging from the occiput to the pubic symphysis, assessing the head, spine, chest, abdominal contents, and the pelvis. CT imaging often requires that the patient be moved from the resuscitation bay and it is therefore essential that the patient has been adequately examined and is haemodynamically stable.

Synthesis of information

By the completion of the primary and secondary surveys it is important to know the extent of insult on the systemic function and the urgency to manage skeletal injuries. This composite assessment allows the clinician to decide if the overall situation constitutes a threat to life, or an immediate threat to a limb in either a physiologically unstable or stable patient, or a skeletal injury, which may be treated on a routine basis.

Principles of managing major/multiple skeletal injuries

General principles of surgical fixation of fractures

Most patients with multiple skeletal injuries require early definitive surgical care of skeletal injuries. The general principles of management of patients with skeletal injuries are:

- long bone fracture reduction and achievement of stable fixation
- reduction of major pelvic disruption with increased pelvic volume and haemorrhage
- wound excision and debridement for open fractures
- anatomic reconstruction of intra-articular fractures
- early mobilization to maintain limb joint function.

The timing and application of these principles have to be adapted to the individual patient, but the following approaches summarize current practice.

Early total care

Evidence form the 1970s and 1980s showed that early stabilization of major long bone fractures could reduce respiratory complications, the duration of time in intensive care unit and the mortality. Therefore, stable reduction and fixation of all skeletal injuries was recommended as soon as possible after admission (early total care).

Damage control orthopaedics

More recently, the universal application of early total care to all multiple trauma patients has been challenged. In particular, there is some evidence to suggest it may be an inappropriate strategy for management of severely injured patients. A small number of patients who are at high risk from surgery are better managed in a staged fashion (Box 6.4.1).

In the presence of complex multiple injury with a very high ISS and evidence of major physiological derangement, it may be in appropriate to subject the patient to prolonged sequential surgical interventions from the time of admission. Damage control orthopaedics (DCO) is the concept of management in which expeditious temporizing surgery is performed. This will include haemorrhage control, debridement of open wounds and temporary, but not definitive, skeletal stabilization of long bone fractures. The aim of this less invasive DCO surgery is to reduce the

---

Box 6.4.1 Conditions in which damage control surgery should be considered

Polytrauma + ISS > 20 and thoracic trauma (AIS > 2)
Polytrauma with severe abdominal/pelvic trauma and haemodynamic shock (SBP < 90 mmHg)
ISS > 40
Bilateral lung contusions
Initial mean pulmonary arterial pressure > 24 mmHg
Pulmonary artery pressure increase > 6 mmHg during long bone IM nailing
Bilateral femoral fractures
AIS, Abbreviated Injury Scale; ISS, Injury Severity Score; SBP, systolic blood pressure.

physiological impact of surgical trauma on the patient's already compromised physiological state and heightened immune response. Systemic function is then optimized and the patient's physiologic and inflammatory responses are allowed to normalize before definitive surgery takes place, commonly 6 to 8 days post injury. DCO principles may be required when the patient is particularly unstable, the expected surgical time exceeds 6 hours, or the skills and resources are not available to deal with the full complement of injuries. In particular it should be considered in patients who on presentation have a combination of hypothermia, acidosis, and are coagulopathic. Patients with these physiological characteristics will withstand prolonged major surgical interventions poorly.

Nevertheless, *the majority* of patients with long bone fractures will not fall into this category and early definitive stabilization remains the treatment of choice in most patients with major long bone fractures.

Pelvic injuries

Unstable pelvic fractures are life-threatening injuries and must be managed decisively. A coordinated multidisciplinary approach is required. Recognition of a patient with an unstable pelvic fracture should occur during the primary survey. Management depends on the combination of haemodynamic and mechanical instability. The main clinical scenarios are:

• stable fracture pattern in a haemodynamically stable patient

• unstable fracture pattern in a haemodynamically stable patient

• unstable fracture pattern in a haemodynamically unstable patient who responds to fluid resuscitation

• unstable fracture pattern in a haemodynamically unstable patient unresponsive to fluid resuscitation.

In the first three settings, urgent treatment of the pelvic disruption is not required. These patients are best investigated by means of a CT scan from the head down to the pubic symphysis. This is the most accurate diagnostic investigation for evaluating the presence of other injuries. Other injuries are frequently present with major pelvic ring injuries. Apart from pelvic vascular injury, there may be intra-abdominal visceral injury, sacral nerve root injury, bladder injury, or urethral disruption. The latter may need a retrograde urethrogram for diagnosis. Once other injuries are determined, a plan can then be made for the definitive management of the pelvic fracture.

Unstable pelvic fracture patterns may be divided into several main categories based on the Young-Burgess classification:

Lateral compression

The pelvis fractures as a result of a lateral force. There are often some other limb fractures such as femur, tibia and humerus, but this pattern of injury does not disrupt the main stabilizing ligaments of the pelvis, and serious pelvic haemorrhage and instability do not commonly occur. Chest and visceral trauma are not uncommon.

Anteroposterior compression

This mechanism of injury results from an anterior force with externally rotates one or both sides of the pelvis producing the well-recognized open book pattern of injury. Intrapelvic haemorrhage is common as is urethral and bladder injury. The anterior pelvic ligaments are disrupted.

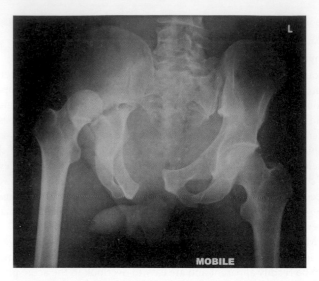

Fig. 6.4.1 Complex combined unstable pelvic and acetabular fracture with right hip dislocation. The patient also had an intraperitoneal bladder rupture and was haemodynamically unstable.

Vertical shear pattern of injury

A vertical shear force separates one hemipelvis (or both) from anterior and posterior attachments. There is anterior and posterior ligamentous disruption involved. This is the most severe pattern of injury. Associated intraperitoneal, genitourinary, and neurological injury are common.

Combined mechanical injury

Combined mechanical injury may produce combinations of the above patterns involving both sides of the pelvis.

In patients with unstable pelvic fractures and haemodynamic instability unresponsive to fluid resuscitation there is often an increase in pelvic volume (Figures 6.4.1, 6.4.2, and 6.4.3). A pelvic binder applied around the greater trochanters is a safe and effective method of reducing the pelvic volume and regaining haemodynamic instability. If the patient remains unresponsive, application of an external fixation and an extraperitoneal approach

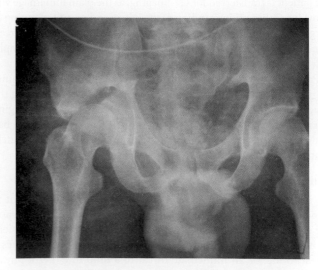

Fig. 6.4.2 The hip dislocation was reduced and a pelvic band has been applied to the trochanters. This assisted restoration of haemodynamic stability.

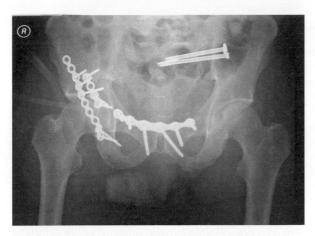

Fig. 6.4.3 Definitive reconstruction of the bony elements of the injury included fixation of the anterior and posterior vertically unstable pelvic disruption, acetabular reconstruction and bladder repair via a lower abdominal laparotomy through which the pubic symphysis was plated.

with pelvic packing may be necessary. The abdominal cavity should not be opened unless there is definite evidence of intraperitoneal blood loss.

Pelvic angiography and embolization may be considered, but it is most useful for 'transient responders', that is, patients who show a temporary response to fluid resuscitation and can have haemodynamic stability maintained for the duration of time the angiography procedure takes.

In the majority of pelvic fractures, the major bleeding is venous in origin. Arterial blood loss amenable to embolization is present in 15–20% of cases. Therefore, operative management is usually the first priority, and arteriography/embolization only performed if there is ongoing blood loss following skeletal stabilization and surgical packing. However, if a bleeding vessel is identified during the contrast phase of a CT scan, arteriography/embolization become the priority.

Definitive skeletal stabilization of pelvic ring disruption is now commonly undertaken. Pelvic ring injuries are characterized by rotational (lateral compression and anteroposterior compression) or vertical patterns of instability. In rotational injuries the main posterior pelvic ligaments remain intact. A good example of this pattern is the open book injury with pubic symphysis disruption. Plate fixation of the anterior ring is the treatment of choice. In vertical instability there is anterior and posterior disruption of the pelvic ring. Both components of the ring disruption need to be addressed. In these injuries the posterior disruption usually comprises a sacroiliac dislocation, a sacral fracture, or a combination of these. Fixation generally entails internal fixation of the anterior and posterior elements of the injury.

Spinal column injuries

Spinal column injuries associated with neurologic compromise are generally managed operatively to decompress the neural elements and confer stability to the zone of injury. Unstable injuries without neurological compromise may also require surgical stabilization if there is significant deformity. Spinal instability is commonly based on the Denis three-column classification:

◆ anterior column: anterior longitudinal ligament and anterior half of vertebral body

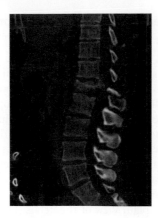

Fig. 6.4.4 Unstable spine fracture of L1. Two-dimensional computed tomogram reconstruction showing three-column involvement.

◆ middle column: posterior half of vertebral body and posterior longitudinal ligament

◆ posterior column: pedicles, facet joints and posterior ligaments.

With modern imaging using CT scanning, occasionally supplemented by MRI, it is possible to define the degree of column involvement. Single column fractures are stable and those with three-column involvement are unstable. Two-column involvement implies a degree of instability, but the extent of deformity has to be taken into account. Two- and three-column fractures should be considered for surgical stabilization even in the absence of neurological involvement (Figures 6.4.4 and 6.4.5).

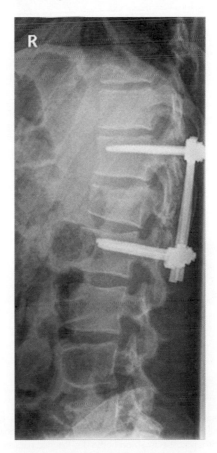

Fig. 6.4.5 Postoperative lateral radiograph after stabilization.

Principles of treating lower limb long bone fractures

Femoral fractures

Early stabilization of femoral fractures in the multiply injured patient has been shown to decrease pulmonary complications, duration of intensive care and overall hospital stay when compared with delayed stabilization (Figure 6.4.6). Anteroposterior and lateral imaging of the entire femur including the hip and knee joint must be obtained to detect additional injuries. These include ipsilateral femoral neck fractures, patellar fractures, and Hoffa fractures (fractures of a femoral condyle in the coronal plane). There is an incidence of posterior hip dislocation and pelvic disruption in association with femoral shaft fractures, but these injuries should be detected on the plain view of the pelvis. Finally, ligamentous injury of the knee and posterior cruciate ligament disruptions in particular are not unusual. These are more difficult to detect in the presence of an unstable femoral shaft fracture, but should be looked for by examination of the knee after fixation of the shaft fracture.

Antegrade reamed locked intramedullary nails are the treatment of choice for most diaphyseal femoral fractures. Retrograde intramedullary nails also have a role for certain femoral fractures (Box 6.4.2). Ipsilateral fractures of the femoral neck and diaphysis fractures should be treated as individual injuries with the neck fracture receiving priority of management.

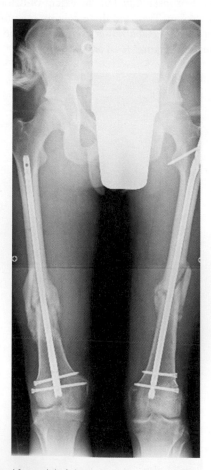

Fig. 6.4.6 Bilateral femoral shaft fractures treated with ante grade reamed locked nail on the left and retrograde nail on the right side. Note abundant callus formation 4 months postoperatively on both sides. Reamed nails are associated with excellent rates of union in femoral shaft fractures.

Box 6.4.2 Indications for retrograde femoral nails

There are no absolute indications, but the following list is a series of clinical scenarios where the technique is particularly applicable.
1. Lower-third diaphyseal/metaphyseal femoral fractures
2. Ipsilateral tibial and femoral shaft fractures
3. Multiple long bone fractures
4. Ipsilateral acetabulum
5. Ipsilateral femoral neck and shaft fracture
6. Hoffa or simple intercondylar fracture with ipsilateral femoral shaft
7. Pregnancy
8. Morbid obesity
9. Previous extensive hip surgery, implants or hip deformity
10. Protrusio acetabulum

Displaced tibial fractures are the most common long bone fracture and 20% are open. The preferred method of treatment is a reamed intramedullary nail. Open fractures require wound excision and debridement at the same time. External fixation is an alternative in open fractures but is associated with an increased risk of malunion and a higher requirement for reoperation. Compartment syndrome is an important early complication to be aware of in these fractures. The overall incidence is low at about 2%, but the incidence increases in higher energy trauma.

Principles of treating lower limb dislocations and periarticular injuries

Hip dislocation requires significant force and concomitant injuries are common. Sciatic nerve palsies are present in 15% of cases, and posterior wall acetabular fractures and femoral head fractures are also common. Following plain film imaging reduction of the hip should proceed urgently to minimize the risk of avascular necrosis of the femoral head. Post-reduction CT scanning is recommended to assess for concentric reduction, presence of femoral head or acetabular fractures, and any entrapped fragments within the joint. Fractures involving more than 25% of the posterior wall of the acetabulum are associated with persistent hip instability and require internal fixation. More complex acetabular fractures are generally treated by open reduction and plate fixation. The main indications are evidence of hip joint instability or incongruency.

Knee dislocations are limb-threatening injuries due to the risk of vascular injury and should be reduced as an emergency. Careful clinical examination of the neurologic and vascular status of the limb is mandatory and close consultation with a vascular service is recommended. CT arteriography is a readily available investigation for imaging the knee and the vasculature. Persistently unstable knees are commonly stabilized with external fixation followed by bony fixation and ligament repair or reconstruction.

Metaphyseal fractures around the knee are treated according to the specific fracture configuration and may involve the use of plates or intramedullary rods. Intra-articular injuries require anatomic reduction of the articular surface and restoration of limb alignment. Coronal and sagittal plane CT reconstructions assist with preoperative planning and fixation. In general, most displaced articular fractures around the knee are treated by open reduction and plate fixation. However, in complex tibial plateau fractures, particularly with soft tissue problems, there is a role for fine wire external fixation.

Distal tibial fractures frequently extend into the ankle joint and high-energy injuries from a vertical load mechanism are often associated with a complex intra-articular fracture configuration. Associated dislocations must be reduced without delay either by qualified paramedic staff or upon presentation to the emergency department. Unstable fractures may require temporary external fixation to permit swelling and soft tissue injury to subside prior to definitive fixation. Open reduction and plate fixation is the preferred method of treatment but soft tissue problems are common in this location. External fixation may be the definitive treatment if the skin condition does not allow for plate fixation to be safely undertaken.

Foot injuries are common in the multiply injured patient and can be easily missed if the surgical team is focused on other injuries. Displaced fractures and dislocations that threaten the soft tissue envelope must be reduced promptly. CT imaging is typically required to complement plane film imaging and further delineate the fracture configuration and plan for management.

Amputation

Occasionally in severe lower limb trauma, the need for amputation may have to be considered. The decision to undertake this is difficult. The main reasons for considering amputation are usually a combination of ischaemia and extensive crushing injuries in the presence of complex open fractures (Figure 6.4.7). Whether or not to amputate is based on a careful clinical evaluation of the patient and the injured limb and the decision should be based on an evaluation by two experienced clinicians. A warm ischaemic time in excess of 6 hours or extensive crushing of the lower leg and foot are associate with a very poor prognosis for limb salvage.

Principles of treating upper limb long bone fractures

Humeral fractures in the setting of the multiply injured patient are typically treated with open reduction and plate fixation. Surgical fixation permits earlier joint movement and patient mobility in the multiply injured patient. Other indications for surgical fixation include open fractures, vascular injury, bilateral humeral shaft fractures, or the presence of an ipsilateral forearm fracture (floating elbow). Intramedullary (IM) fixation can occasionally be used but it is associated with a number of problems in the humerus. Entry

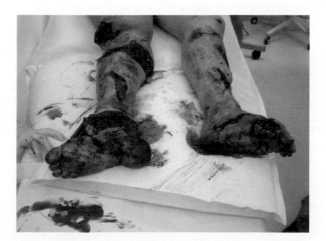

Fig. 6.4.7 Crush injury.

points are not ideal (rotator cuff problems if the shoulder is used and access to the intramedullary canal is difficult just above the elbow). Also the humerus is subjected to a lot of torsional forces and IM nails do not resist these well. IM nails are therefore used in situations where plate fixation may not be technically feasible (i.e. segmental fractures or those with extensive comminution).

Displaced radial and ulna shaft fractures are treated with anatomic reduction and plate fixation aiming to restore forearm biomechanics and permit early mobilization. Restoration of the normal anatomy of the radius is essential to maintain forearm pronation and supination and accurate open reduction and plate fixation is the most reliable way to achieve this.

Principles of treating upper limb dislocations and periarticular injuries

Shoulder girdle injuries in the setting of major trauma commonly herald serious thoracic injury and clinical suspicion of lung, cardiac, and great vessel injury must remain high.

Glenohumeral dislocations are common and most frequently the humerus dislocates anteriorly, but may dislocate posteriorly following electric shocks or seizure activity owing to contraction of the powerful internally rotating muscle group. Posterior shoulder dislocation is a commonly missed diagnosis and adequate imaging is essential.

Periarticular elbow fractures require thorough neurologic and vascular examination. Anatomic reduction with stable fixation is the treatment of choice. Careful soft tissue handling and early mobilization is particularly important to reduce the risk of postoperative stiffness and development of heterotopic ossification.

Intra-articular distal radius fractures are increasingly treated with anatomic reduction and plate fixation to restore wrist anatomy and permit earlier rehabilitation. In very comminuted distal radial fractures this may not be technically feasible and external fixation is commonly used as an alternative.

Compartment syndrome

Compartment syndrome in the multiply injured patient may be difficult to diagnose due to an altered level of consciousness and distracting injuries. The most common sites are the lower leg and the forearm. A high level of clinical suspicion is essential and compartment pressure monitoring is recommended in at risk individuals.

Crush injuries

Crush injury may result in extensive muscle damage either by direct trauma or through ischaemic/reperfusion injury (see Figure 6.4.7). The muscle breakdown results in rhabdomyolysis leading to renal failure. Management may involve renal dialysis and correction of electrolyte and acid/base disturbance. Resection of the crushed muscle is usually necessary to reduce the volume of dead muscle and protect kidney function.

Complications and ongoing care

General considerations

Attention to detail, regular clinical review, chest physiotherapy, providing adequate nutritional support, and monitoring skin pressure areas are necessary to minimize complications following skeletal trauma.

Thromboembolic complications

All patients who sustain multiple skeletal injuries should undergo an individual risk assessment for thromboembolic disease. Those with a specific background or injury risk factors will require more aggressive management. Early mobilization, adequate hydration, and mechanical devices including thromboembolic stockings and foot pumps should be used as much as possible. Optimal chemical prophylaxis of thromboembolism remains controversial, but a low-molecular-weight heparin is appropriate in most cases.

In some multiple trauma patients the use of chemical prophylaxis may be contraindicated. This would apply to patients who may have had life-threatening haemorrhage and a coagulopathy. Thromboprophylaxis may have to be withheld until these patients are stabilized with restoration of normal blood indices. Chemical prophylaxis can then be commenced.

Fat embolism syndrome is most commonly associated with multiple long bone fractures, in particular femoral shaft fractures. Clinical signs should be recognized in the post-injury phase of care with a patient developing respiratory distress with dyspnoea and tachypnoea or systemic manifestations such as agitation or petechial rash. Treatment is generally supportive with oxygen therapy, and antibiotics if infection is associated. Patients may require a period of ventilator support in an intensive care unit in more severe cases.

Specific skeletal complications

Longer term complications originating from multiple skeletal injuries include infection, non-union, malunion, post-traumatic osteoarthrosis, and joint stiffness. A high standard of initial surgical care with good postoperative rehabilitation will reduce the risk of these complications occurring. However, in severely injured patients it is inevitable that the complication rate will be higher than in patients who sustain lower energy isolated fractures.

Determinants of outcome

Patients with complex multiple orthopaedic and other injuries are challenging to treat. There is an accumulating body of evidence to suggest that one of the key determinants of outcome is *time to definitive care*. For many of these patients, this means a level one trauma centre or a major trauma centre staffed by the full range of specialist groups available and equipped with the imaging facilities, interventional radiology, and intensive care unit backup that will be required. Initial treatment in hospitals lacking in these facilities is associated with a high requirement for secondary transfer and higher mortality rates.

Further reading

American College of Surgeons Committee on Trauma. *Advanced Trauma Life Support Program for Doctors*, 7th edition. Chicago: American College of Surgeons, Chicago, 2004.
Baker SP, O'Neill B, Haddon W, *et al*. The injury severity score: a method for describing patients with multiple injuries and evaluating emergency care. *J Trauma* 1974; 14: 187–96.
Bone LB, Anders MJ, Rohrbacher BJ. Treatment of femoral fractures in the multiply injured patient with thoracic injury. *Clin Orthop Relat Res* 1998; 347: 57–61.
Bone LB, Chapman MW. Initial management of the patient with multiple injuries. *Inst Course Lect* 1990; 39: 557–63.
Bosse MJ, Kellam JF. Damage control orthopaedic surgery: A strategy for the orthopaedic care of the critically injured patient. In: Browner BD (ed.) *Skeletal Trauma*, 4th edition. Philadelphia: Saunders, 2008.
Boyd CR, Tolson MA, Copes WS. Evaluating trauma care: the TRISS method. Trauma score and the Injury Severity Score. *J Trauma* 1987; 27: 370–8.
Brautigam RT, Sheppard R, Robinson KJ, *et al*. Evaluation and treatment of the multiple-trauma patient. In: Browner BD (ed.) *Skeletal Trauma*, 4th edition. Philadelphia: Saunders, 2008.
Brundage SI, McGhan R, Jurkovich GJ, *et al*. Timing of femur fracture fixation: Effect on outcome in patients with thoracic and head injuries. *J Trauma* 2002; 52: 299–307.
Champion HB, Copes WS, Sacco WJ, *et al*. The Major Outcome Trauma Study: establishing national norms for trauma care. *J Trauma* 1990; 30: 1356–65.
Court-Brown C, McQueen M, Tornetta P. *Trauma* (Orthopaedic Surgery Essentials Series). Philadelphia: Lippincott Williams & Wilkins.
Crash2 Collaborators, Roberts I, Shakur H, *et al*. The importance of early treatment with tranexamic acid in bleeding trauma patients: an exploratory analysis of the CRASH-2 randomised controlled trial. Lancet 2011; 377(9771): 1096–101.
Ertel W, Keel M, Eid K, *et al*. Control of severe hemorrhage using C-clamp and pelvic packing in multiply injured patients with pelvic ring disruption. *J Orthop Trauma* 2001; 15: 468–74.
Giannoudis PV. Current concepts of the inflammatory response after major trauma: an update. *Injury* 2003; 34: 397–404.
Giannoudis PV, Smith RM, Banks RE, *et al*. Stimulation of inflammatory markers after blunt trauma. *Br J Surg* 1998; 85: 986–90.
Giannoudis PV, Vevsi VT, Pape HC, *et al*. When should we operate on major fractures in patients with severe head injuries? *Am J Surg* 2002; 183: 261–7.
Hooper GJ, Keddell RG, Penny, ID. Conservative management or closed nailing for tibial shaft fractures. A randomised prospective trial. *J Bone Joint Surg Br* 1991; 73(1): 83–5.
Johnson KD, Cadambi A, Seibert GB. Incidence of adult respiratory distress syndrome in patients with multiple musculoskeletal injuries; effect of early operative stabilization of fractures. *J Trauma* 1985; 25: 375–84.
Pape HC, Ciannoudis P, Krettek C. The timing of fracture treatment in polytrauma patients: relevance of damage control orthopedic surgery. *Am J Surg* 2002; 183: 622–9.
Pape HC, Grimme K, van Grievesen M, *et al*. Impact of intramedullary instrumentation versus damage control for femoral fractures on immunoinflammatory parameters: Prospective randomized analysis by the EPOFF study group. *J Trauma* 2003; 55: 7–13.
Riska EB, Myllynen P. Fat embolism in patients with multiple injuries. *J Trauma* 1982; 22: 891–4.
Riska ER, von Bonsdorff H, Hakkinen S, *et al*. Primary operative fixation of long bone fractures in patients with multiple injuries. *J Trauma* 1977; 17: 111–21.
Rüedi TP, Buckley RE, Moran CG. *AO Principles of Fracture Management: Specific Fractures*, 2nd edition. Stuttgart: Theieme, 2007.

CHAPTER 6.5

Trauma in conflict zones

James Singleton and Jon Clasper

Introduction

War and conflict expose both combatants and civilians to a host of serious injury mechanisms seen far less frequently outside of combat zones. However, the increasing threat of acts of terrorism can bring the battlefield to any civilian hospital. Therefore, all surgeons should be aware of the specific challenges posed by 'battlefield injuries', both in their diagnosis and acute management. Battlefield injuries fall into three main groups:

◆ gunshot injury, often referred to as gunshot wounds

◆ blast injuries

◆ other causes (falls, road traffic collisions, etc.).

It is important to mention the latter group, as those providing medical care in conflict zones will also see 'civilian' type injuries. In fact, during military operations not in an active 'warfighting' phase, road traffic collisions are often the main cause of death and serious injury.

Gunshot injuries

Bullets have caused injuries for over 800 years, since the invention of firearms in 12th century China.[1] Gunshot injuries are almost exclusively secondary to penetrating trauma. However, since the adoption of protective body armour in the 1970s, an emerging injury pattern is 'behind armour blunt trauma'.[2] This occurs when the impact of a projectile does not perforate body armour, but transmits a force to the individual wearing it and so causes injury, which in extreme cases can be lethal.

Ballistics and relevant terminology

Ballistics is the science of projectiles. Firearms ballistics falls into three areas:

◆ **Internal ballistics**: The effects of bullet design, weapon design, and projectile materials on the bullet while within the barrel of the weapon.

◆ **External ballistics**: The effect of mass, velocity, drag, and gravity on the projectile from the barrel to the target.

◆ **Terminal or wound ballistics**: The behaviour of the projectile in tissue.

A round is the combination of a bullet mounted on a cartridge case filled with explosive powder (Figure 6.5.1).

On pulling the trigger of a gun, the propellant detonates as a controlled, confined explosion, producing high-pressure expanding gas forcing the bullet out of the cartridge along the barrel and out of the muzzle. The inner diameter of the barrel, known as the calibre, corresponds to the diameter of the bullet. Most gun barrels are 'rifled' with spiral grooves on the interior, imparting spin to the bullet around its longitudinal access and gyroscopically stabilizing it in flight. This takes time to become optimal and imperfections in the bullet, pressure differences in the barrel, or barrel movement may cause the bullet to 'wobble'. This creates 'yaw', a rotation of the bullet tip away from the line of flight. This can be up to 10° in the first 20–30 m of flight, but tends to settle to <3° after this until the bullet strikes its target.[3] Yaw becomes important again in wound ballistics. The cartridge case is ejected from the weapon and forms no part of the projectile.

Gunshot injuries

The single most important factor influencing the potential for a bullet to cause injury is *placement*. The entry point and subsequent path determine the structures affected by the bullet. However, other determinants also affect a bullet's wounding effects:

◆ physical characteristics, most importantly *mass*

◆ flight characteristics, most importantly *velocity*

◆ physical properties of the tissues with which the bullet interacts, most importantly *tissue density*.

The kinetic energy (KE) of a bullet is described by the following equation:

$$KE = 0.5 \times mass \times (velocity)^2$$

Thus, increasing bullet mass causes a linear increase in KE, while greater velocity increases KE exponentially. This has led to gunshot injuries frequently being classified as 'high velocity' (>600 ms⁻¹) or 'low velocity' (<600 ms⁻¹). This is potentially misleading as it misses a crucial aspect of the wounding mechanism. It is the *energy transfer* that is the overriding determinant in creating a wound.

Projectile shape/orientation

The smaller the area of the projectile presented to the tissue, the lower the resistance and the energy transfer. The resistance afforded by the tissue is related to the orientation of the bullet. If the long axis of the bullet is aligned with the direction of travel, less energy is transferred than if the bullet yaws (or tumbles) and presents a greater surface area.[4] Bullets are inherently unstable in tissues, and the resistance of the tissue may be sufficient to cause a bullet to tumble. This will result in greater energy transfer to the tissue and thus greater tissue damage.

This is one reason why entry wounds are often small, whereas exit wounds may be much larger, with torn skin and a ragged or stellate appearance. In addition, any deformation or breaking up

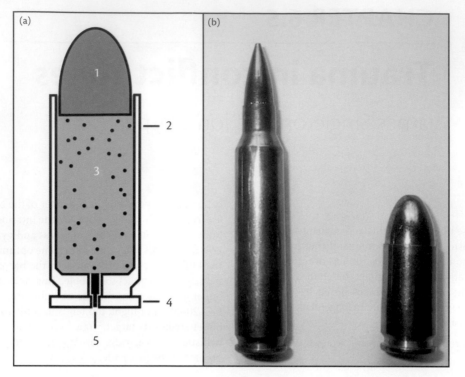

Fig. 6.5.1 (a) Cross section of a modern round of handgun ammunition consists of: 1, the bullet (projectile); 2, the cartridge, which holds all parts together; 3, the propellant; 4, the rim, which provides the extractor on the firearm a place to grip the casing to remove it from the chamber once fired; and 5, the primer, which ignites the propellant. (b) 5.56 mm rifle and 9 mm pistol rounds.
Images copyright © CanStock Photo Inc.

of a bullet will result in greater energy transfer and more extensive wounding. This was the main reason for the development of soft nose, hollow nose, or 'dum-dum' bullets, or the bullet tip being deliberately notched. All these modifications encourage breaking up, to increase the 'stopping power' (injury severity) of a round. Such modifications were made illegal for military use by the Hague Declaration of 1899. These rounds are still used for hunting and by some law enforcement agencies. Despite the use of 'legal' bullets, fragmentation can still occur, particularly if the bullet strikes bone, and this breakup is accompanied by more severe wounding.

Mechanism of gunshot injury

There are two well-accepted mechanisms by which projectile energy transfer may cause tissue damage:

Laceration/crushing

The creation of a permanent cavity/wound tract by the projectile. This is a common mechanism for both high and low velocity bullets.

Temporary cavitation

The formation of a temporary cavity, behind the bullet is the most significant factor in tissue injury from high-energy transfer wounds. As the projectile passes through the tissue, energy is transferred by contact and the tissue is accelerated radially away from the projectile. This results in the formation of a temporary cavity as the inertia of the tissue results in continued displacement even after the projectile has passed through the tissue (Figure 6.5.2).

As well as the obvious injury caused by the compression and shear forces applied to the tissues, the void created by temporary

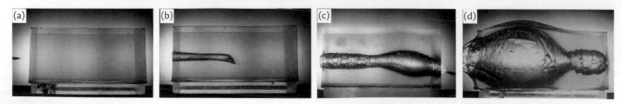

Fig. 6.5.2 A military 7.62 mm rifle bullet (a) about to enter; (b) passing through a gelatin block, starting to tumble; (c) exiting the block (NB facing backwards) with cavitation effects starting; and (d) cavitation continuing after the bullet has exited.

(a–c) Reprinted from Current Orthopaedics, Volume 20, Issue 5, S.A. Stapley and L.B. Cannon, (i) An overview of the pathophysiology of gunshot and blast injury with resuscitation guidelines, 322–32, Copyright © 2006 Elsevier Ltd, with permission from Elsevier, http://www.sciencedirect.com/science/journal/02680890; and (d) Reprinted from Current Orthopaedics, Volume 20, Issue 5, D. Griffiths and J. Clasper, (iii) Military limb injuries/ballistic fractures, 346–53, Copyright © 2006 Elsevier Ltd, with permission from Elsevier, http://www.sciencedirect.com/science/journal/02680890

cavitation generates a transient negative intracavity pressure. This can result in increased contamination of the wound tract by drawing in material such as soil, dirt, or clothing fragments. The size of the cavity, although one determinant of injury severity, is not the most significant; the properties of the tissue energized by the projectile primarily determine the outcome. Muscle is able to withstand the distension produced by the temporary cavity due to its elasticity, and although the tissue may be contused, recovery is possible. Less elastic tissue, particularly if enclosed by a fibrous capsule (e.g. liver), is unable to withstand the distension and severe disruption is possible.[5] Brain is also very susceptible to distension, and the severe trauma resulting from cerebral compression and shearing is usually unrecoverable.

Energy transfer is also affected by the tissue involved in the wound tract, and is related to the density and rigidity of the tissue. Muscle is denser than lung tissue, thus greater energy transfer occurs when a projectile passes through muscle. More rigid tissue such as bone resists deformation, and offers greater resistance, resulting in greater energy transfer. Bone can be fractured, either directly or indirectly by temporary cavitation, and furthermore, can be converted to secondary fragments causing further injury.

The *shockwave* imparted to tissue by a traversing high-velocity bullet may also cause tissue damage,[6] although this is not universally accepted.[7]

Although wounds are often classified as high or low-energy transfer, wounds of 'intermediate energy transfer' can also occur. It is, therefore, wrong to base treatment protocols exclusively on a division of wounds into two types. The temporary cavity is not an all-or-nothing phenomenon, and the size of the cavity is related not only to the energy transfer, but also to the tissue involved. In addition, although the exit wound of a high-energy transfer wound is usually ragged and large, this is not always the case, and smaller entrance and exit wounds may be present despite high-energy transfer.[8]

Behind armour blunt trauma

Body armour is an essential component of protective equipment for military and law enforcement personnel. It has been proven to prevent lethal ballistic injuries from bullets or fragments from explosions. However, while the armour may not be breeched if struck, it will transfer at least some of the energy from the striking projectile to the wearer and if of sufficient magnitude, this can result in behind armour blunt trauma (BABT), or in extreme cases, death.[9] BABT refers to a spectrum of non-penetrating injuries with characteristics of both primary blast injury and blunt trauma.

Mechanism of behind armour blunt trauma

Body armour is designed to absorb the energy from a projectile. However, the rapid deformation involved in retarding the projectile and preventing penetration can result in much of the projectile's energy being propagated through the armour and into the body wall. This occurs via multiple mechanisms:

- Following bullet contact, a shock wave is propagated through the armour and into the body prior to any deformation of the armour or body wall. This is analogous to primary blast injury, and may cause injury, both locally and at distant sites, as well as electrophysiological disturbances.

- Localized deformation of the armour accelerates the thoracic wall. This generates a second shock wave and deflection of the thoracic wall, causing shear injury to tissues immediately underneath the deflection (e.g. cutaneous injury [Figure 6.5.3], pulmonary or myocardial contusions).

- As thoracic wall deflection continues, sternal and or rib fractures may result and displace, causing laceration of underlying tissue (e.g. pneumothorax from torn pleura, hepatic or splenic injuries).

Diagnosis and management of behind armour blunt trauma

A compatible history and cutaneous signs of chest wall trauma make the diagnosis straightforward, but in some cases chest wall injury is not significant. Also, in the heat of battle, an individual might not realize they had been struck by a bullet that did not penetrate their body armour. Therefore, a high index of suspicion is required and following initial examination/resuscitation, a low threshold for further investigation of possible BABT is prudent. The gold standard tests are a computed tomography (CT) angiogram of the chest and an electrocardiogram.

Treatment is mainly supportive, but thoracostomy/otomy may be indicated in cases of suspected aortic injury.

Blast injuries

Explosive munitions encompass a wide variety of devices. Conventional weapon systems include grenades, artillery shells, rockets, mines, and aircraft-delivered ordnance. Non conventional weapons, known as improvised explosive devices, can range from a few grams of explosive in a letter bomb designed to injure a target's hands, to a truck loaded with several hundred kilograms of homemade explosive capable of destroying a large building. The unifying feature of all these munitions is the capacity to cause injury through the multiple 'blast injury' mechanisms.

There are four categories of blast injury (Figure 6.5.4):

- **Primary blast injury**: Shock wave-mediated tissue damage. *Interfaces between tissues/structures of differing densities are most affected.*

- **Secondary blast injury**: Ballistic injury (predominantly penetrating) from fragments thrown out by the explosion. *This occurs at a much greater range from an explosion than primary blast injuries.*

- **Tertiary blast injury**: Blunt trauma from whole-body displacement. *Injury from building collapse after an explosion is also classified as tertiary blast injury.*

- **Quaternary blast injury**: Other mechanisms of injury including burns, exposure to toxic products of detonation, exacerbations of pre-existing medical conditions, and psychological trauma.

Specific blast injuries

Most blast casualties sustain multimodal blast injuries, but up to 90% are due to penetrating fragments (secondary blast injury). Metallic fragments predominate, particularly in terrorist incidents where nuts, bolts, nails, or ball bearings may be packed around the explosive to maximize injury. Fragments can also be non-metallic,

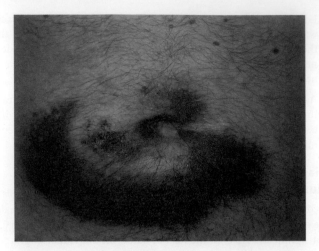

Fig. 6.5.3 Behind armour blunt trauma with periumbilical abrasion and bruising. This casualty was wearing Kevlar™ body armour extending distally to his abdomen and was stuck by a 9 mm bullet.
Reproduced with permission.

such as stones, wood, or other organic matter. This can include human tissue, especially in suicide bombings. Updated guidance on appropriate post-exposure prophylaxis against hepatitis B and C, human immunodeficiency virus, and tetanus is available from the US Centre for Disease Control.[10]

Blast injuries by system

Pulmonary system

The lungs and respiratory system are at increased risk of primary blast injury with their inherent extensive air/tissue interface. Primary blast lung injury (PBLI) resulting from shockwave-induced parenchymal damage, ranges from scattered petechial haemorrhages, parenchymal tears (traumatic pneumatocoeles), and pneumothorax/haemothorax, up to extensive pulmonary contusions and bronchovascular fistulae resulting in arterial air embolism.[11] These can cause stroke, myocardial, and spinal cord infarction and death.

PBLI symptom onset (dyspnoea, cough, haemoptysis, and retrosternal chest pain) is acute in most cases. Signs include tachypnoea, cyanosis, ± signs of tension pneumothorax, which would require immediate medical attention. Mild cases may present later as pulmonary interstitial oedema, as part of the local inflammatory response, further compromises respiratory function.

Investigations for PBLI include arterial blood gas and chest X-ray. Further imaging with CT may be necessary if the plain film is equivocal, and CT is both more sensitive and specific for PBLI diagnosis.

Management is supportive and centres on minimizing further parenchymal damage/barotrauma and avoiding precipitating air emboli. Chest tube thoracostomies are often required and the use of positive pressure ventilation should be minimized. Over-aggressive fluid resuscitation can be problematic, precipitating/exacerbating pulmonary oedema and further worsening respiratory function.

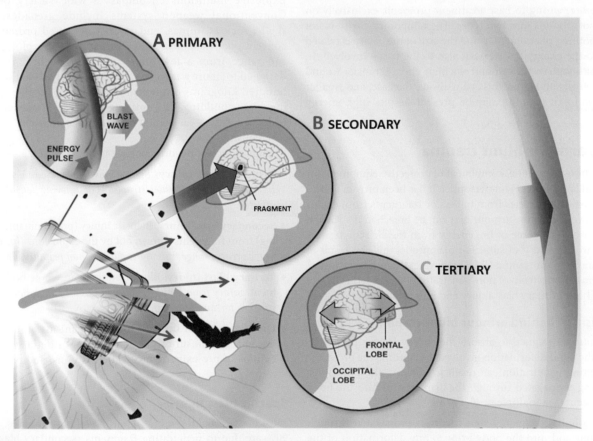

Fig. 6.5.4 Blast injury modalities. Primary blast injury (A): shockwave causing primary blast injury. Secondary blast injury (B): fragments thrown out by the explosion causing (mainly) penetrating secondary blast injury. Tertiary blast injury (C): whole-body displacement from the blast wind causing blunt trauma tertiary blast injury (the multiple mechanisms of quaternary blast injury are not shown here).
Reproduced with permission.

Gastrointestinal system

The air content of the gastrointestinal system renders it vulnerable to primary blast injury, either immediate rupture (e.g. caecum and colon), or delayed perforation. Symptoms include abdominal pain, vomiting, haematemesis, loose bloody stools, or malaena. Guarding, rebound tenderness, and absent bowel sounds are classic examination findings.

Haemodynamically unstable patients with suspected abdominal blast injuries should be resuscitated and undergo a trauma laparotomy. Focused abdominal sonography for trauma (FAST) scanning can detect intraperitoneal fluid, but cannot exclude a non-perforated abdominal primary blast injury. Stable patients benefit from CT as a preoperative planning investigation.

Solid abdominal organ injury is more likely to be due to secondary or tertiary blast injury. Fragments may take oblique, non-linear paths or ricochet internally so entry wounds may be above the diaphragm, distal to the groin/buttocks or hidden in skin creases.

Auditory system

This system is the most frequently injured by primary blast effects and at the lowest relative overpressures. Tympanic membrane (TM) rupture is the most common injury pattern and should be excluded in all blast casualties. In any casualty with likely primary blast exposure, the presence of any respiratory or abdominal symptoms should prompt further investigation regardless of TM integrity.[12]

Other primary blast auditory injuries include sensorineural deafness, tinnitus (both self-limiting), and ossicle disruption (surgical intervention required). TM ruptures involving more than 5% of membrane surface should undergo ear, nose, and throat assessment for surgical management. Smaller tears usually heal spontaneously, although ear, nose, and throat referral is still advised as any keratinized fragments seeded into the middle ear have potential to form cholesteatomae and warrant formal removal.

Central nervous system

Head injuries are most commonly due to secondary and tertiary blast injury. There is also increasing evidence that primary blast can cause traumatic brain injury by acceleration of the head, direct passage of the blast wave via the cranium, and/or by propagation of the blast wave to the brain via the thorax.

A serious central nervous system primary blast injury is cerebral vessel air embolism. This occurs secondary to bronchovascular fistulae following PBLI and, together with coronary air embolism, is considered the principal cause of immediate/early mortality from primary blast.[13] Signs and symptoms of cerebral emboli include headache, vertigo, ataxia, convulsions, altered levels of consciousness, weakness or sensory loss, facial or tongue blanching, and retinal artery air emboli. Suspicion of cerebral emboli requires prompt administration of oxygen. Definitive treatment requires hyperbaric oxygen which reduces the volume of gas bubbles and improves blood flow to hypoperfused tissues.

The eye and orbit

The eyes make up only 0.1% of body surface area, but up to 10% of blast survivors sustain ocular injuries.[14] Most are due to secondary blast injury, as the eye is extremely vulnerable to small fragments causing abrasions or penetrating trauma. The globe is reasonably resistant to primary blast injury, being of relatively uniform density. Pressures sufficient to cause globe rupture or orbital floor blow out fractures are likely to be lethal.

CT is the most useful modality for demonstrating intraocular fragments (magnetic resonance imaging is contraindicated as fragments may be ferrous) and emergent ophthalmic surgical referral is indicated to minimize long term visual disturbance.

Musculoskeletal system

The majority of injuries sustained in conflict zones are to the extremities as helmets and body armour decrease the likelihood of concomitant head or chest injury in this group.[15,16] While protective body armour enables patients to survive larger explosions, they now present with more severe extremity trauma than previously.

Musculoskeletal injuries can be caused by all four blast injury modalities (Figure 6.5.5). Primary blast waves can cause fractures,[17] fragments can cause extensive soft tissue damage, and tertiary blast can cause further fractures, dislocations or gross flailing/traumatic amputation. Proximity to improvised explosive device detonation can also cause thermal injury (quaternary blast injury) through flash burns or setting fire to clothing/equipment.

Extremity blast injuries are often clearly evident, but spinal injuries may not be symptomatic due to distracting injuries or an

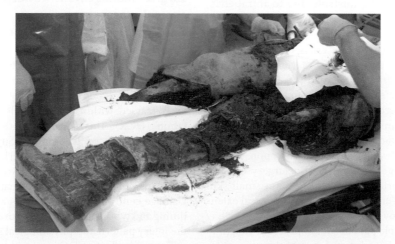

Fig. 6.5.5 Lower limbs of an improvised explosive device casualty showing signs of all modalities of blast injury. Note the soft tissue stripping and scorching of the left femur and right tibia. The left leg has retained some thigh soft tissue continuity but is essentially an above knee traumatic amputation.
Image courtesy of Colonel Paul Parker, L/RAMC.

unconscious patient. Extremity neurovascular status must be carefully assessed. Plain films may suffice for isolated extremity injury imaging, but often the patient are polytraumatized and whole-body CT is a quick and efficient method of providing a comprehensive skeletal assessment in addition to head, chest, abdominal, and pelvic imaging.

Combat/conflict casualty management

Initial management

This refers to management achievable in a well-equipped modern civilian hospital capable of dealing with major trauma. Clearly, these casualties are most frequently seen in very different environments:

- **Deployed military medical facilities**. Equipment, resources, and training should equal or surpass modern trauma centre equivalents. However, the time from point of wounding to arrival at hospital may be extended, depending on the tactical environment.

- **Non-government organization-led facilities** (e.g. International Committee for the Red Cross, Médecins Sans Frontières). Clinicians may have excellent training, but limited resources may constrain the severity or number of casualties able to be managed.

- **Local medical facilities**. These are dependent on local infrastructure and there are highly variable levels of care.

The majority of combat casualties are 'walking wounded'. Many may not require admission and can be adequately managed and discharged by the emergency department. However, there is a cohort of severely injured patients for who rapidly administered medical care can be lifesaving.

Assessment and resuscitation should follow Advanced Trauma Life Support guidelines. However, it should be noted that military medical doctrine utilizes a <C> ABC (catastrophic [i.e. life threatening], bleeding, airway, breathing, circulation) approach, as the main treatable cause of death from battlefield injury is uncontrolled haemorrhage.

Extremity haemorrhage can be controlled with tourniquets. If a patient is haemodynamically unstable due to intrapelvic, abdominal, or thoracic haemorrhage, surgical haemostasis via proximal vascular control is required. This can require thoracotomy in the resuscitation room and cross clamping of the thoracic aorta.

Tetanus prophylaxis and intravenous broad spectrum antibiotics should be given and entry/exit wounds should be noted via a rapid but comprehensive external examination including log roll and digital rectal/vaginal examination. Wounds should be photographed then dressed with betadine or saline-soaked gauze.

It is important to 'treat the wound and not the weapon'. If there is extensive soft tissue damage, an early plastic surgery opinion should be sought. It is important to be aware that a small skin wound sustained from a high-energy projectile may conceal extensive underlying soft tissue/bony damage.

A haemodynamically unstable patient should proceed straight to theatre. Surgical haemostasis is an integral part of their resuscitation. A stable patient provides the opportunity for further investigations beyond the chest and pelvic radiographs and initial blood tests.

Whole-body CT with modern multidetector scanners takes seconds and is an invaluable source of data in conflict casualties. It can clearly demonstrate:

- PBLI including subtle contusions, pneumothorax, and haemothorax not evident on chest X-ray

- retained metallic fragments (wound tracts may not be clear depending on scatter/artefact and tissue restitution)

- skeletal injuries

- visceral injury

- vascular injury (via CT angiography)

In conjunction with clinical assessment and blood tests, any imaging investigations undertaken can help to prioritize cases for surgery or enable non-operative management to be trialled.

Surgery or not?

A civilian patient with an isolated low-energy gunshot or fragment injury may be appropriate for non-operative management. The wounds tend to be clean, and the patient typically arrives at the trauma centre within an hour of the injury. This contrasts markedly with the traditional military experience. For example, the mean time taken from injury to arriving at a British surgical hospital during the first Gulf War of 1991, was 10.2 hours,[18] whereas during the second Gulf War of 2003 with much shorter lines of communication and better casualty evacuation, the mean delay was still 6 hours.[19] More recent operations in Afghanistan have shown shorter evacuation times of 75 minutes,[20] and this may be an emerging trend in more asymmetric conflicts.

What remains constant is the gross contamination of combat wounds, which should be irrigated and debrided, unless they are superficial fragment wounds (<1 cm with no cavity/multiple), where simple cleaning and dressing, leaving the wounds open and a course of antibiotics may suffice.

Not all fragments need to be excised, and can be assessed case by case. One absolute indication for removal is an intra-articular bullet/bullet fragment to prevent a destructive arthropathy – lead can cause profound chondrolysis.

Surgical management: concept of damage control surgery

The initial aim when treating conflict casualties is to identify and treat any life-threatening injuries. In military medicine, however, adjustments have been made to take into account the two main causes of battlefield mortality, namely uncontrolled haemorrhage and central nervous system injury. This begins in the field and is encompassed within the principles of 'damage control resuscitation' (DCR). This is a systematic approach to major trauma, based on Advanced Trauma Life Support principles, but utilizing the <C>ABC paradigm with a series of clinical techniques from point of wounding to definitive treatment in order to minimize blood loss, maintain tissue oxygenation, and optimize outcome.[21] Damage control surgery (DCS) is a component of DCR and the timing and type of surgical procedure performed will be dictated by the injury pattern and physiological state of the patient.

The main effort of DCS is rapid control of bleeding by ligature, suture, or packing. This may involve approach to and control of major vessels. Damaged bowel should be taped or stapled to prevent further contamination. The procedure should not take longer than an hour, and as a rule the abdomen will be left open to prevent intra-abdominal hypertension. Application of a pelvic fixation device where indicated could be part of this process. Debridement of contaminated extremity trauma is required as part of surgical haemostasis and prevention of life-threatening sepsis.

If DCS is necessary, the patient may be severely physiologically compromised or highly likely to become so. Preventing/mitigating this is the underpinning tenet of DCR and requires close coordination between surgeon and anaesthetist. Intraoperative pauses to 'catch-up' with ongoing haemostatic resuscitation may be required, or curtailment of surgery may be necessary to minimize the traumatic insult to the patient and allow physiological optimization in a critical care setting.

After physiological optimization (24 to 48 hours of intensive care), relook surgery is undertaken. Packs are removed, bleeding points secured, damaged viscera removed or repaired, intestinal continuity restored, or stomas fashioned if indicated. Debridement of wounds is completed. It may or may not be possible to close the abdomen at this point.

Overview of conflict extremity wound management

The principles of management of conflict extremity injuries/ballistic fractures are simple.

Resuscitate/haemostase

Haemostatic resuscitation describes the early use of blood and clotting products in proportions similar to whole blood, to minimize risk of developing acute traumatic coagulopathy. However, ongoing haemorrhage must be addressed surgically.

Appropriate antibiotics

Ideally, these should be given within 3 hours of injury. Traditionally, intravenous penicillin is used initially, as it covers Gram-positive *Clostridia* species and anaerobic streptococci.

Antitetanus

A booster may be required as well as tetanus immunoglobulin for the unvaccinated.

Wash

This should be done with non-pulsatile lavage (to avoid seeding bacteria deeper into the wound)[22] and with copious volumes. Nine litres is recommended for the most contaminated wounds, and a preoperative scrub/wash with aqueous iodine solution may be necessary. If sterile, warm saline is not available, potable water can be used as a substitute.

Debride

This is the core principle of conflict injury management. The aim is to remove all foreign material and non-viable tissue from the wound. The '4 Cs' approach is key:

+ **Colour**: dead muscle appears dark/discoloured.
+ **Consistency**: Non-viable tissue has lost its material integrity has a mushy consistency.
+ **Contractility**: Dead muscle will not contract when compressed with forceps or touched with a diathermy probe.
+ **Capillary bleeding**: Appropriate vascularity demonstrates healing potential.

To debride adequately, the wound must be fully visualized. The zone of soft tissue injury will often extend far beyond the wound, so the wound will need to be extended proximally and distally to enable full examination of the injured tissue. Skin is generally very resistant to trauma and has a good capacity to heal. Therefore the wound edges should be excised with care and only enough to leave healthy skin edges, normally 1 mm or less. Bone fragments with no soft tissue attachments are non-viable and should be removed.

Fasciotomize

Surgeons should have a low threshold for fasciotomies in extremity blast or gunshot injury. Clinical symptoms and signs may be lacking due to obtunded/unconscious casualties, there may be multiple casualties (reduced re-assessment opportunity), and the significant volume of traumatized tissue in high-energy extremity conflict wounds increases the likelihood of swelling and development of compartment syndrome.

Pack

Wounds should be lightly packed with sterile gauze, and covered with a bulky dressing to absorb any exudate. Negative pressure wound therapy and specific antimicrobial dressings may have a role in selected cases but research is ongoing in this area.

Stabilize

Stabilization of fractures provides pain relief and helps to prevent further bone and soft tissue injury. Plaster of Paris splintage and skeletal traction both remain appropriate and safe techniques and are available even in basic medical treatment facilities. Casts must never be circumferential acutely.

External fixators are often employed by modern military medical services and are indicated for: extensive bone loss, large soft tissue wounds, vascular injuries requiring repair, fractures associated with burns, multiple injuries, and to facilitate casualty evacuation. However, they carry risks, with pin tract infection and osteomyelitis rates of 35% and 8%, respectively.[23]

Leave: open and alone

This is paramount and primary closure should not be attempted. The International Committee of the Red Cross guidelines recommend a 5 day interval between index debridement and delayed primary closure. Dressings may stain yellow green and smell, but this is the so-called 'good–bad' smell. However, if the patient shows signs of a focus of infection and/or the dressings become extremely offensive with the 'bad–bad' smell of putrefaction, the patient should return to theatre emergently for review.

At the 5-day point the dressings are taken down in theatre, the debridement is completed if necessary, and the wound is closed without tension.

If circumstances allow, a return to theatre for delayed primary closure at 48 hours can be considered. Intra-abdominal or intrathoracic injuries may require re-assessment at 24 to 48 hours and a coordinated management plan including anaesthetics/ITU staff and all required surgical specialties may be required to ensure patients are managed efficiently and within physiological limits conducive to optimal recovery.

Further reading

DiMaio VJM. Gunshot wounds: practical aspects of firearms, ballistics, and forensic techniques: 2nd Edition. CRC Press; 1998.

Elsayed NM, Atkins JL. Explosion and blast-related injuries: effects of explosion and blast from military operations and acts of terrorism: Academic Press; 2008.

Gray R. War wounds: basic surgical management. Geneva: ICRC publications, 1994.

Wolf SJ. Blast injuries. *Lancet*. 2009;374(9687):405–15.

References

1. Chase K. *Firearms: A Global History to 1700*. Cambridge: Cambridge University Press, 2003.

2. Cannon L. Behind armour blunt trauma-an emerging problem. *J R Army Med Corps* 2001; 147(1): 87–96.

3. Knudsen PJT, Sórensen OH. The initial yaw of some commonly encountered military rifle bullets. *Int J Legal Med* 1994; 107(3): 141–6.

4. Kirby NG, Blackburn G, Britain G. *Ministry of Defence Field Surgery Pocket Book*. London: HM Stationery Office, 1981.

5. Ryan J, Rich N, Burris D, *et al*. Biophysics and pathophysiology of penetrating injury. In: Ryan, JM, Rich, NM, Dale, RF, *et al*. (eds) *Ballistic Trauma Clinical Relevance in Peace and War*. London: Arnold, 1997, pp. 31–46.

6. Janzon B, Seeman T. Muscle devitalization in high-energy missile wounds, and its dependence on energy transfer. *J Trauma* 1985; 25(2): 138.

7. Fackler ML. Gunshot wound review. *Ann Emerg Med* 1996; 28(2): 194–203.

8. Clasper J. The interaction of projectiles with tissues and the management of ballistic fractures. *J R Army Med Corps* 2001; 147(1): 52–61.

9. Gryth D, Rocksén D, Persson JK, *et al*. Severe lung contusion and death after high-velocity behind-armor blunt trauma: relation to protection level. *Mil Med* 2007; 172(10): 1110–6.

10. Chapman LE, Sullivent EE, Grohskopf LA, *et al*. Recommendations for postexposure interventions to prevent infection with hepatitis B virus, hepatitis C virus, or human immunodeficiency virus, and tetanus in persons wounded during bombings and other mass-casualty events—United States, 2008: recommendations of the Centers for Disease Control and Prevention (CDC). *MMWR Recomm Rep* 2008; 57(RR-6): 1–21.

11. Avidan V, Hersch M, Armon Y, *et al*. Blast lung injury: clinical manifestations, treatment, and outcome. *Am J Surg* 2005; 190(6): 945–50.

12. Harrison CD, Bebarta VS, Grant GA. Tympanic membrane perforation after combat blast exposure in Iraq: a poor biomarker of primary blast injury. *J Trauma* 2009; 67(1): 210–1.

13. Frykberg ER, Tapas JJ. Terrorist bombings. Lessons learned from Belfast to Beirut. *Ann Surg* 1988; 208(5): 569–76.

14. Horrocks CL. Blast injuries: biophysics, pathophysiology and management principles. *J R Army Med Corps* 2001; 147(1): 28–40.

15. Peleg K, Aharonson-Daniel L, Michael M, *et al*. Patterns of injury in hospitalized terrorist victims. *Am J Emerg Med* 2003; 21(4): 258–62.

16. Griffiths D, Clasper J. (iii) Military limb injuries/ballistic fractures. *Current Orthopaedics* 2006; 20(5): 346–53.

17. Hull JB. Pattern and mechanism of traumatic amputation by explosive blast. *J Trauma* 1996; 40(3S): 198S–205S.

18. Spalding T, Stewart M, Tulloch D, *et al*. Penetrating missile injuries in the Gulf war 1991. *Br J Surg* 2005; 78(9): 1102–4.

19. Hinsley D, Rosell P, Rowlands T, *et al*. Penetrating missile injuries during asymmetric warfare in the 2003 Gulf conflict. *Br J Surg* 2005; 92(5): 637–42.

20. Morrison JJ, Oh J, DuBose JJ, *et al*. En-Route Care Capability From Point of Injury Impacts Mortality After Severe Wartime Injury. *Ann Surg* 2013; 257(2): 330–4.

21. Midwinter M. Damage control surgery in the era of damage control resuscitation. *J R Army Med Corps* 2009; 155(4): 323.

22. Hassinger SM, Harding G, Wongworawat MD. High-pressure pulsatile lavage propagates bacteria into soft tissue. *Clin Orthop* 2005; 439: 27–31.

23. Dubravko H, Zarko R, Tomislav T, *et al*. External fixation in war trauma management of the extremities-experience from the war in Croatia. *J Trauma* 1994; 37(5): 831–4.

Head and neurological injury

Lynn Myles and Paul M. Brennan

Head injury

Head injuries involve the scalp, bone, and brain. They are the leading cause of death and disability before the age of 44 in Europe, and affect approximately 0.2% of the population per year; 15 per 100 000 patients die from their head injury, or from associated injuries sustained at the time of trauma. Head injuries most often arise from motor vehicle accidents or falls. Approximately one-third of motor vehicle accident injuries occur in the context of alcohol excess.

The severity of a head injury should be described in terms of the Glasgow Coma Scale (GCS) (Table 6.6.1). Patients who survive the more serious injuries may be left with significant cognitive or functional deficits. Importantly though, even mild head injuries can be associated with subtle, but persistent, cognitive deficits that can be very disabling. Other long-term consequences of head injury include epilepsy and hypopituitarism, which has been reported in up to 40% of patients and can range from deficiency of a single hormone to total pituitary failure.

Anatomy

The skull is the bony structure of the head and includes both the cranium and the facial bones, other than the mandible. The cranium protects the brain and articulates via its occipital condyles with the first cervical vertebrae. Several immovable fibrous joints called sutures join the bones of the skull. The cranium is covered by the scalp, a highly vascular and sensate structure. Haemorrhage from the scalp can be fatal, especially in children with a small circulating blood volume.

Inside the cranium, the *meninges* surround the brain. They are composed of three layers. The *dura mater* is adherent to the skull and is the outermost layer. It actually consists of two layers that are largely adherent to each other, except where they separate and contain the large venous sinuses. It is firmly adherent to the skull at the sutures. The *pia mater* is the innermost layer that covers the brain. The *arachnoid mater* lies between these two layers and the cerebrospinal fluid (CSF) circulates beneath the arachnoid and above the pia.

Types of head injury

Head injuries can be classified by GCS or as open or closed. A *closed* head injury occurs where the skull and overlying scalp remains intact. The injury is considered *open* if there is a breach in the scalp and underlying cranium. Such fractures may also injure the underlying dura and brain. Penetrating injuries, such as a knife blade, can cause open injuries, but so can blunt trauma. Identification of an open fracture is important, because it is associated with an increased risk of infection and seizures. A skull fracture can occur in the absence of an overlying scalp injury. Fragments of skull depressed into the cranial vault at the site of a fracture may need elevating to improve cosmetic outcome or to reduce the risk of seizures. Antibiotics may be recommended by the neurosurgical team.

Table 6.6.1 The Glasgow Coma Score

Criterion	Rating	Score
Eye opening		
Open before stimulus	Spontenous	4
After spoken or shouted request	To sound	3
After fingertip stimulus	To pressure	2
No opening at any time, no interfering factor	None	1
Closed by local factor	Non-testable	NT
Verbal response		
Correctly gives name, place and date	Orientated	5
Not orientated but communication coherently	Confused	4
Intelligible single words	Words	3
Only moans/groans	Sounds	2
No audible response, no interfering factor	None	1
Factor interfering with communication	Non-testable	NT
Best motor response		
Obey two-part request	Obeys commands	6
Brings hand above clavicle to stimulus on neck	Localizing	5
Bends arm at elbow rapidly but features not predominantly abnormal	Normal flexion	4
Bends arm at elbow, features clearly predominantly abnormal	Abnormal flexion	3
Extends arm at elbow	Extension	2
No movement in arms/legs, no interfering factor	None	1
Paralysed or other limiting factor	Non-testable	NT

Reproduced with permission from Sir Graham Teasdale. The Structured Aid to Assessment of the Glasgow Coma Scale was developed with support from the Muriel Cooke bequest to the University of Glasgow.

Head injuries can also be classified according to the site and type of haemorrhage.

Extradural haematoma

An extradural haematoma (EDH) is located between the outer layer of the dura mater and the inner surface of the skull. EDHs occur in 9% of severe brain injuries. The dura is normally firmly adherent to the skull. A high-pressure arterial bleed is usually responsible for this type of injury, which peels the dura away from the skull as the haematoma enlarges. The classical EDH arises in the temporal–parietal region beneath the pterion, the thinnest part of the skull, although they can occur anywhere. The pterion is formed by the junction of the parietal bone, squamous temporal bone, frontal bone, and the greater wing of the sphenoid. Underlying the pterion is the anterior branch of the middle meningeal artery. This runs in the dura and can be lacerated by the bone fracture.

The classical clinical presentation of an EDH is of a patient who is lucid immediately after a head injury, but who later rapidly drops their conscious level. This clinical picture occurs because EDHs are not associated with significant underlying brain injury at the time of the head injury. Clinical deterioration occurs when the EDH has enlarged to a sufficient size to compress the brain and increase intracranial pressure (ICP) beyond the point that the brain can compensate. The classical computed tomography (CT) appearance of an EDH is of a biconvex or lens-shaped collection of blood. This appearance reflects the fact that the dura cannot be stripped from the skull at the sutures. The sutures therefore limit expansion of the clot.

Subdural haematoma

A subdural haematoma (SDH) is a collection of blood between the dura mater and the arachnoid mater. SDHs are more common than EDHs, occurring in 30% of severe brain injuries. They are thought to develop from tearing of small vessels on the surface of the brain, or of bridging vessels. In the absence of trauma, SDH can result from rupture of a posterior communicating artery aneurysm.

In trauma, SDHs often result from high-speed acceleration/deceleration injuries and are often associated with damage to the underlying brain, causing swelling and resulting in raised ICP and secondary brain injury. Even if the SDH is evacuated surgically, the mortality rate is 60–80%.

Patients with SDHs often present with a reduced conscious level at the time of injury and can deteriorate further as the brain swells or the haematoma expands. The appearance of an acute SDH on CT is of a hyperdense (white) collection of blood. SDHs arise between the dura and the brain and so they are not limited in their extent by the adherence of the dura to the cranial sutures. They are often associated with contusions of the tip of the temporal or frontal lobes.

Chronic SDHs are also found in the subdural space and probably arise from torn bridging veins. Chronic SDHs generally occur in older patients with underlying atrophic brain, or those with a history of alcohol excess. The atrophic brain is thought to place the bridging veins under tension, predisposing them to bleeding, often with only minor, or no, trauma. Antiplatelet and anticoagulant agents may contribute to this risk. The acute bleed in these patients is usually not clinically apparent. As the acute haematoma organizes and liquefies over time, it absorbs water. This increases the size of the haematoma, causing increased mass effect and clinical sequelae such as headache or neurological deficit. CT imaging identifies an isodense or hypodense subdural collection rather than

the hyperdense acute blood seen in acute SDH. The blood clot is often liquefied by the time of presentation.

Intracerebral haematoma and contusion

The brain can be injured at the site of a blow to the head (coup) or on the opposite side (contre-coup). The brain has a soft consistency and is poorly anchored in the skull, so when a force is applied to the head the brain accelerates/decelerates even once the skull has stopped. When the brain subsequently contacts the skull a contusion results. A contusion occurs when multiple small blood vessels are injured, leading to bleeding into the parenchyma of the brain. The haemorrhage causes destruction of brain tissue. The mass of the contusion compresses adjacent tissue.

The distinction between intracerebral haematomas and contusions is rather indistinct. The term intracerebral haematoma is used to describe a larger collection of intraparenchymal blood, whereas the term contusion describes smaller, often multiple, rather indistinct lesions. Contusions are most common and severe where the brain is related to bony ridges of the skull, such as the inferior surface of the frontal lobe and the temporal lobes. These areas of brain injury are associated with oedema and the contusions can coalesce over time to form larger collections, contributing to increasing mass effect and raised ICP, which may continue for 5 to 7 days before improving.

Contusions can underlie a subdural haematoma, and where the two are in continuity this is called a 'burst lobe'. Intracerebral bleeding can also occur into the ventricular system. Blood in the CSF spaces reduces the efficiency of CSF reabsorption at the arachnoid villi, contributing to a communicating hydrocephalus. This may persist after the haematoma and blood admixed with CSF have resolved, necessitating permanent CSF diversion, for example with a ventriculo-peritoneal shunt.

Diffuse axonal injury

Diffuse axonal injury (DAI) results from a shearing injury to axonal tracts, due to a rapid rotational acceleration/deceleration injury. It occurs in half of all severe brain injuries, but also in mild injuries, either alone or with the other injuries described. The consequences of DAI depend on the anatomical location of the injury and range from a brief loss of consciousness to persistent vegetative state. The axonal injury is located in the white matter tracts and multiple small petechiae may be seen on CT. DAI results in a loss of cellular integrity and brain oedema. Magnetic resonance imaging is more sensitive than CT for these subtle changes.

Pathophysiology of head injury

In order to effectively manage the patient with a head injury it is necessary to understand the pathophysiological processes that are involved.

The skull is rigid and non-expansile and so has a fixed volume in which to accommodate the brain, its blood supply, and the CSF. Any increase in the volume of one of these constituents must be compensated by a reduction in the volume of another one, or else the ICP will increase; this is known as the Monroe-Kellie doctrine. In the context of trauma, a haematoma or brain swelling is effectively a fourth mass inside the rigid fixed volume of the skull, which may therefore result in an increased ICP.

In the presence of a haematoma or brain swelling, the ICP initially remains within the normal range through a combination of reduced blood flow to the brain, reduced CSF production, or increased CSF drainage. However, as the haematoma or swelling increases, a critical threshold is eventually reached, the so-called point of decompensation. The pressure inside the skull will then increase exponentially. Before their cranial sutures have fused, babies can tolerate a greater rise in intracranial volume than adults, because the skull volume is not fixed to the same degree. The baby's head can expand. This is why head circumference measurement can be useful in infants.

The normal ICP of a supine adult is 7–15 mm of mercury (mmHg) and becomes negative on standing. Increased ICP compromises cerebral blood flow, reducing oxygen delivery and ultimately causing brain ischaemia. The concept of cerebral perfusion pressure (CPP) describes the actual flow of blood through the brain. CPP is defined as the mean arterial blood pressure (MAP) minus the ICP. CPP is normally constant over a range of MAP between 50–150 mmHg. However, this autoregulatory mechanism can be disrupted in brain injury, impairing the ability of the brain to compensate for changes in CPP. A fall in MAP can result in ischaemia and infarction, whereas an increase in MAP can exacerbate brain swelling. This is why blood pressure control is so important in head injured patients.

As ICP increases, brain tissue will decompress itself into any available space, such as under the falx cerebri, across the tentorium cerebelli, or through the foramen magnum. This brain herniation causes direct damage to brain structures and ultimately death. The brainstem can be compressed as it herniates through the foramen magnum, or by the uncus of the temporal lobe herniating across the tentorium cerebelli. This is manifest clinically as a series of physiological changes referred to as the Cushing reflex or triad: The heart rate slows, the systolic blood pressure increases, and the pulse pressure widens. Irregular respiration also occurs. These clinical signs presage death unless ICP can be reduced. It is therefore important to detect clinical signs of raised ICP as early as possible.

Management of the head injured patient

Primary brain injury is the injury caused directly at the time of trauma. Secondary brain injury results from processes occurring after the trauma such as raised ICP, hypoxia, hypotension, ischaemia, metabolic derangements, and infection. The goal of patient management is to prevent this secondary injury. The principles of Advanced Trauma Life Support guide the assessment and management of the injured patient and prioritize the need to secure a patient's airway, optimize their breathing or ventilation, and control their circulatory function. All this occurs prior to assessment of any head injury, but these procedures also directly benefit the brain. The cervical spine should be protected immediately if the mechanism of injury suggests it is at risk, if the patient has neck pain, focal neurological deficit, or any other reason to suspect a cervical spine injury.

Clinical assessment

For patients who present with mild brain injuries, the priority is to identify whether they will deteriorate and require specialist neurosurgical management. Most patients with minor and moderate severity head injuries will recover uneventfully and can be managed in the hospital where they first present. Both the National Institute of Health and Care Excellence (NICE) and the Scottish Intercollegiate Guidelines Network provide guidelines for the care of all head injured patient so that they receive optimal care. Patients with moderate and severe brain injuries will require discussion with the regional neurosurgical service.

Assessment of the head injured patient

The GCS is the most commonly used assessment of the conscious state of a patient with a head injury (Table 6.6.1). This is scored between 3 and 15 according to the eye, verbal, and motor responses of the patient. Impairment of the motor score is most significant. By standardizing the clinical assessment of consciousness, the GCS facilitates the identification of changes in a patient's conscious level over time, as well as communication of these changes between medical staff. It is important that any impairment of conscious level is not attributed to alcohol or drug intoxication until a significant brain injury has been excluded. A reduction in the GCS may indicate rising ICP.

The pupillary reflex is another important component of the neurological examination in head injury. It is the parasympathetic fibres on the surface of the third cranial nerve that supply vasoconstrictor tone to the pupillary muscles. The third cranial nerve runs from the brainstem along the medial edge of the tentorium cerebelli towards the orbit and is therefore at risk of compression when raised ICP pushes the uncus of the temporal lobe towards the tentorial edge. Compression of the third cranial nerve is manifest clinically as an ipsilateral dilated pupil unreactive to light.

As brain tissue herniates, other cranial nerves will also be at risk of compression and dysfunction. For example, the sixth cranial nerve, that supplies the lateral rectus muscle in the orbit, can be stretched by downward pressure on the brainstem, because of the fixed bony landmarks that it traverses. The laterality of any sixth nerve palsy may not directly relate to the side of injury, because the downward pressure on the brainstem may result from a lesion anywhere in the cranial vault above the tentorium cerebelli. Sixth cranial nerve palsy is therefore sometimes referred to as a false localizing sign.

Investigation of the head injured patients

Identification of reduced GCS in a patient is an important indication for cranial imaging. In addition, in other patients thought to be at risk of deterioration early imaging will reduce the time to detection of life-threatening complications. Cranial CT imaging is the investigation of choice for detecting clinically important brain injuries. Plain skull radiographs are not appropriate. They may have a role in the skeletal survey where non-accidental injury is suspected in children.

The NICE guidelines indicate that all adult patients with a head injury should have immediate CT head imaging if their GCS is less than 13 on initial assessment, less than 15 two hours after the injury, or if they have an open or depressed skull fracture or any sign of basal skull fracture. A scan is also indicated if they have a post-traumatic seizure, or a focal neurological deficit, or more than one episode of vomiting, or amnesia for events more than 30 minutes before the impact.

Patients over 65 years of age or those with a coagulopathy should be imaged if they have any period of loss of consciousness or amnesia because they are at higher risk of significant pathology. Imaging is also indicated if the history suggests a dangerous mechanism of injury, such as falling more than 1m, or being ejected from a motor vehicle.

Children (under 16 years old) should have a CT head scan if they have loss of consciousness lasting more than 5 minutes, amnesia lasting more than 5 minutes, if they are abnormally drowsy, have three or more episodes of vomiting, or if there is clinical suspicion of non-accidental injury. Children who have a post-traumatic seizure with no pre-history of epilepsy and those with a GCS less than 14 should also be imaged. Imaging is also indicated in children if there is suspicion of an open or depressed skull injury.

Babies with a tense fontanelle and children with any sign of basal skull fracture, a focal neurological deficit, or a bruise, swelling or laceration of more than 5cm on the head should have cranial CT imaging.

Depending on the mechanism of injury, the presence of spinal pain and the clinical examination, consideration should be given to imaging the cervical spine at the same time as the head. Where a patient has suffered poly trauma then the whole spinal axis is usually imaged.

If the CT scan shows evidence of significant traumatic brain injury, and/or the patient has reduced GCS, the regional neurosurgical unit should be contacted. If the patient has a reduced conscious level but an apparently normal CT scan then expert advice may still be necessary because some diffuse brain injuries may not be seen on CT.

A patient should be observed for evidence of clinical deterioration and discharged to the care of a responsible adult once their neurological examination is normal and they are unlikely to worsen. The responsible adult should be given written and verbal head injury advice about symptoms (e.g. vomiting or decreasing conscious level) that would precipitate readmission. It is recommended that all patients who have undergone cranial imaging and/ or been admitted to hospital should be followed-up by their general practitioner within 1 week. Even with a normal neurological examination, patients may complain of headache, or nausea or vomiting that requires symptomatic management, sometimes as an inpatient. Most otorrhoea and rhinorrhoea settles spontaneously, but if it persists then specialist advice should be sought as there is a risk of meningitis. Specialists may initially advise not to give prophylactic antibiotics to patients with CSF leak as the evidence suggests this increases the risk of developing meningitis from a more virulent organism. Antibiotics may be required if the CSF leak persists, or for open head injuries. Always ensure that any other injuries are also adequately managed before discharge.

Management of raised intracranial pressure

Patients with low or falling GCS and those with intracranial haematomas may require admission to a specialist neurosurgical unit. However, it will often be the responsibility of non-neurosurgeons to optimize a patient's care before transfer and so an understanding of the management of ICP is useful.

The patient should be nursed head-up to aid venous drainage. This improves CPP. In patients with a GCS less than 9, there should be early and aggressive airway management (intubation). These patients cannot reliably maintain their own airway and may aspirate stomach contents, or obstruct their airway. Unmanaged pain can increase ICP. Consider splinting fractures and catheterization of a full bladder prior to transfer. Suture bleeding scalp wounds prior to transfer. Patients can exsanguinate from the scalp.

The aim should be to maintain a CPP above 60–70 mmHg. It is therefore important to ensure the patient has a good MAP. In the intubated patient in the neurosurgical unit it is also possible to measure ICP by the placement of an intraparenchymal pressure monitor though a burr hole. A falling CPP can be managed by increasing the MAP or reducing the ICP. If the MAP is not responsive to fluid management, then it can be increased using inotropic support. The ICP should be maintained below 20–25 mmHg. Increasing ICP can be managed pharmacologically and with ventilatory control. Hyperventilation reduces the patient's arterial carbon dioxide tension ($PaCO_2$), which results in cerebral vasoconstriction. This reduces the total volume of blood in the head and so in turn reduces the ICP. However, vascoconstriction also reduces the blood supply to the brain tissue and so the benefit of reduced intracranial blood volume should be balanced against the risk of ischaemia. The target $PaCO_2$ is often 3.5–4 kPa.

Pharmacological strategies to reduce ICP include mannitol. This is an osmotic agent that draws fluid out of brain cells into the circulation, so reduces ICP. It can rapidly reduce ICP and should be considered, for example, if a patient's pupil suddenly dilates, suggesting an increase in ICP. However, repeated mannitol treatments dehydrate the brain, which can impair brain function and resistance to secondary brain injury. It also causes a secondary diuresis that can result in low central venous pressure and hypotension. While mannitol remains a useful initial treatment for raised ICP, more prolonged medical therapy usually involves hypertonic saline, which has less side effects. Hypertonic saline may be used with furosemide.

Other, non-pharmacological medical therapies for managing raised ICP include normothermia and barbiturate-induced coma. Barbiturate comas reduce the metabolic demands of the brain, reducing the amount of blood perfusion required, so a lower CPP may be tolerated.

If increases in ICP are resistant to medical therapies, or if an intracranial haematoma is of sufficient size, then the patient may proceed to surgical decompression. Surgery may include removal of contused lobes, which can have profound implications for the neurological function of the surviving patient. Where raised ICP results from a diffuse brain injury then a decompressive craniectomy may be performed.

It is worth noting that in the context of raised ICP seizures can be particularly problematic, because they will increase ICP. Seizures should be treated with an anti-epileptic drug such as phenytoin. There is not good evidence to support the prophylactic use of antiepileptic medication to prevent long-term seizures following head injury.

Spinal injury

Anatomy

The spine is made up of individual vertebra, intervertebral discs, ligaments, joints, and muscles. The spinal column may be injured without any injury to the underlying cord or nerves (Figure 6.6.1).

It is important to know the location of the main spinal tracts in order to be able to diagnose spinal cord injury. The corticospinal tracts lie anterior in the cord and are the main motor supply to the muscles of the extremities. The posterior columns take proprioception and some touch fibres from the limbs to the central nervous system and lie at the back of the cord. The spinothalamic tracts, which take pain and temperature sensation from the periphery to the central nervous system, lie in the centre of the cord and their fibres decussate around the central canal before passing upwards.

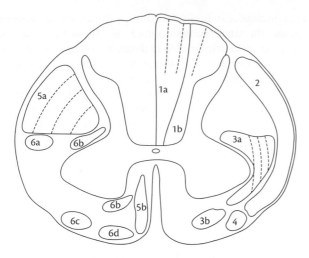

Fig. 6.6.1 Representative anatomy of spinal cord at cervical level. The motor tracts are shown on the left and the sensory tracts on the right. *Sensory tracts* 1: Dorsal columns a, gracilis, b, cuneatus. These are crossed fibres, carrying discriminative touch and conscious proprioception. The medial side carries sacral and lumbar fibres, the lateral thoracic, and cervical. 2: Spinocerebellar tracts (anterior and lateral or posterior). These crossed fibres carry 'unconscious proprioception'. 3: Spinothalamic tracts (a, lateral and b, anterior). These crossed fibres carry crude touch, pain, temperature and pressure. 4: Spino-olivary fibres: these convey proprioceptive information to the cerebellum. *Motor tracts* 5: Pyramidal tracts: the majority of the motor pathways are crossed fibres which run in the lateral corticospinal tract, a. Cervical fibres are medial, sacral are lateral. b, The anterior corticospinal tract, and a small proportion of the lateral corticospinal tract consists of uncrossed fibres which cross at the level at which the spinal nerves exit. 6: Extrapyramidal tracts: these tracts are mainly concerned with maintenance of posture and coordination of movement: a, rubrospinal; b, reticulospinal; c, vestibulospinal, d, olivospinal.
Reproduced from Nathanson M. et al. (eds), *Oxford Specialist Handbook in Neuroanaesthesia*, Figure 2.1, Oxford University Press, Oxford, UK, Copyright © 2011 with permission from Oxford University Press.

Injuries to the spine can affect parts of the spinal cord, leading to various spinal cord syndromes or can cause complete spinal cord injury and paraplegia/quadriplegia.

Spinal cord Injury

Complete injury to the spinal cord will cause complete loss of function below the level of the injury. In the early stages spinal shock will be present and the patient will have flaccid paralysis of the affected limbs. There will be loss of all sensation below the affected level. There may be priapism and other autonomic features such as loss of sweating, loss of vasomotor reflexes, and bradycardia. The blood pressure will be low, because of loss of vasomotor tone and vasodilation. The patient should be kept flat. The stomach may distend and ileus can occur. Bladder and bowel function will be affected.

In high cervical lesions, the diaphragm may be paralyzed and ventilation will be compromised. Even in lower cervical/upper thoracic injuries breathing may be laboured due to paralysis of the intercostal muscles and diaphragmatic breathing will be evident.

After a few weeks, as spinal shock resolves, the patient will develop upper motor neuron signs in the limbs below the level of the injury due to release of spinal reflexes. The tendon reflexes will be brisk and the patient may develop clonus and increased muscle tone.

The immediate management of spinal cord injury follows Advanced Trauma Life Support principles. The airway should be secured, adequate oxygenation ensured, and treatment for any life-threatening blood loss or injuries should be instituted. The blood pressure may be low in patients with spinal shock, but should not be treated with large volumes of intravenous fluid or vasopressors unless renal function or other tissue perfusion is compromised or the systolic pressure is less than 90 mmHg.

Investigations to look for bony spinal column injury should be undertaken and spinal precautions instituted, assuming the spine is unstable until otherwise proven. The bladder should be catheterized and urine output monitored.

There is controversy about the use of early high-dose methyl-prednisolone in acute spinal cord injury and this should be discussed with the local spinal injury unit. It should usually be given within 8 hours of injury or not at all.

Deep vein thrombosis prophylaxis should be started with compression stockings, mechanical compression devices, and subcutaneous heparin. Care should be taken to avoid pressure sores or skin damage. Temperature control may be compromised as a result of autonomic dysfunction and care will have to be taken to maintain normothermia. A nasogastric or orogastric tube should be placed to decompress the stomach. This can be difficult if the head is immobilised.

Referral to the local spinal injuries unit should take place as soon as possible.

Spinal instability

If the spinal column is injured this can lead to instability of the bones which can result in a secondary cord or nerve injury. This must be avoided at all costs.

When trying to decide whether an injury is unstable, it is always wise to assume that instability is present until proved otherwise. The patient should be protected from secondary nerve injury by placing them in a hard cervical collar or spinal board and log-rolling. Advanced Trauma Life Support principles should always be adhered to until spinal injury can be excluded.

It can be difficult even for specialist to decide whether an injury is definitely unstable, and for that reason you may hear terms such as 'potentially unstable' being used until further evaluation can be performed.

Any patient with a head injury must be assumed to have an associated spinal injury until proven otherwise. In an awake patient, the absence of spinal pain, tenderness or deformity and a full range of movement will usually be enough to exclude spinal injury, but in unconscious patients investigations will be required.

The spine can be thought of as having three columns. This model was initially described by Dennis relating to the thoracolumbar spine, but is useful in the cervical spine also. The anterior column consists of the anterior half of the vertebral body, disc, and anterior longitudinal ligament. The middle column consists of the posterior half of the disc and vertebral body and the posterior longitudinal ligament. The posterior column consists of the spines, lamina, facet joints, and associated posterior ligaments.

In general, injuries to one column alone would not be expected to cause acute instability. Injury to two or more columns should be considered to be unstable until proven otherwise. However, there are no absolute rules and if there is any doubt treat the injury as though it is unstable.

Injury to the ligaments can lead to instability even in the absence of bony injury and should always be borne in mind. An anterior column fracture may be associated with rupture of the posterior ligaments leading to instability.

Spinal injuries should always be referred to a specialist for an opinion. Unstable injuries may require a hard collar, Halo vest fixation or surgical internal fixation.

Nerve injury

Anatomy of a peripheral nerve

Peripheral nerves are the nerves that innervate the body and limbs. They are made up of sensory nerves that have their cell bodies in the dorsal root ganglia and lower motor neurones with their cell body in the spinal cord (Figure 6.6.2).

The peripheral nerves are made up of bundles of individual nerve fibres (axons). Axons are supported by Schwann cells and in myelinated axons the Schwann cell forms the myelin sheath. Each axon/Schwann cell unit is surrounded by a basement membrane known as the endoneurium. Bundles of axons are arranged into fascicles. Each fascicle is surrounded by a connective tissue sheath known as the perineurium. Bundles of fascicles are grouped together to form the nerve trunk. The nerve is covered with a connective tissue sheath called the epineurium.

Injury

Injury to peripheral nerves may cause Wallerian degeneration in the nerve. The myelin sheath of axons distal to the injury breaks down and axons degenerate deprived of the influence of the cell body. Schwann cells proliferate and migrate into the endoneurial tubes. The same process occurs in the nerve proximal to the injury. In severe injuries Wallerian degeneration may occur for several centimetres proximal to the injury site and the cell bodies of affected axons may die.

Peripheral nerves can be injured in many ways. Excessive stretch, ischaemia, direct trauma, or compression can cause loss of nerve function. There are many ways to classify nerve injury but the Seddon Classification is the most well known. In this classification there are three types of nerve injury:

- **Neurapraxia:** The axon is injured, usually by compression or stretch, but the nerve is intact with intact endoneurial tubes and Wallerian degeneration does not occur. Full recovery can be expected in 4 to 6 weeks.

- **Axonotmesis:** The axon is completely disrupted with loss of the myelin sheath and endoneurial tubes but the other connective tissues of the nerve remain intact. Wallerian degeneration occurs. Recovery can be expected but it can take many months and may be incomplete or disorganized.

- **Neurotmesis:** The nerve is completely disrupted and may be completely severed. Spontaneous regeneration is impossible. A neuroma may be formed at the proximal stump.

Nerve regeneration

Peripheral nerves will try to regenerate if damaged. If the endoneurial tubes are intact, the Schwann cells migrate from the nerve ends and line the basement membrane. The distal end of the axon sends out a new nerve fibre. This will be guided down the endoneurial

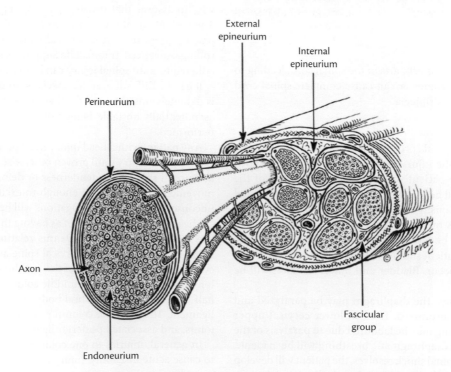

Fig. 6.6.2 The macroscopic organization of a peripheral nerve.

Reproduced with permission from Thomas M. Brushart, *Nerve Repair*, Figure 1.6, Oxford University Press, New York, USA, Copyright © 2011 by Thomas M. Brushart, by permission of Oxford University Press USA.

tube by factors in the basement membrane and Schwann cells, and eventually the axon will make contact with its end organ in the periphery. The myelin sheath will then reform and the nerve will start working again.

If the endoneurial tubes are disrupted, the axons may access the wrong endoneurial tube and be redirected to an incorrect end organ leading to abnormal innervation. The more severe the disruption the less likely the axons are to be able to reach the end organs and more disorganized is the recovery. If there is a significant gap between the nerve ends, regeneration cannot occur and a disorganized bundle of immature nerve fibres and fibrous tissue forms on the end of the proximal nerve end. This is called a neuroma and can cause significant pain.

Treatment

Treatment depends on the cause of injury, type of injury, and the patient's symptoms. Neurapraxias such as seen in a radial nerve palsy caused by pressure on the back of a chair after a night of alcohol excess can be expected to resolve spontaneously after a few weeks and treatment is supportive. Decompressing the nerve surgically can treat compression injuries. Severe traumatic injuries with significant axonotmesis or neurotmesis will require surgical treatment to excise the damaged area of nerve and appose and resuture the nerve fascicles using microsurgical techniques. Nerve grafting may be required to bridge gaps.

Outcomes

Outcome depends on the severity of the injury. Neurapraxias generally have a good outcome and full recovery can be expected. Compression injury can also be relieved in most cases with surgery. The results after treatment of severe nerve injury are still far from perfect and can result in severe disability and chronic nerve pain.

Further reading
Head injury

Advanced Trauma Life Support Student Course Manual, 9th edition. Chicago: American College of Surgeons.

Cooper DJ, Rosenfeld JV, Murray L, et al. Decompressive craniectomy in diffuse traumatic brain injury. N Engl J Med 2011; 364(16): 1493–502.

Kirkham FJ, Newton CRJC, Whitehouse W. Paediatric coma scales. Dev Med Child Neurol 2008; 50: 267–74.

Kokshoorn NE, Wassenaar MJ, Biermasz NR, et al. Hypopituitarism following traumatic brain injury: prevalence is affected by the use of different dynamic tests and different normal values. Eur J Endocrinol 2010; 162(1): 11–18.

National Institute of Health and Care Excellence. Head injury: Triage, assessment, investigation and early management of head injury in children, young people and adults Available from http://www.nice.org.uk/CG176 (accessed 8 October 2015).

Teasdale G, Jennett B. Assessment of coma and impaired consciousness. A practical scale. Lancet 1974; 2: 81–4.

See also http://www.glasgowcomascale.org

Spine injury

Bracken MB, Shepard MJ, Collins WF, et al. A randomized, controlled trial of methylprednisolone or naloxone in the treatment of acute spinal-cord injury. Results of the Second National Acute Spinal Cord Injury Study. N Engl J Med 1990; 322(20): 1405–11.

Dennis F. The three column spine and its significance in the classification of acute thoracolumbar spinal injuries Spine 1983; 8: 817–31.

Raslan AM, Nemecek AN. Controversies in the surgical management of spinal cord injuries. Neurol Res Int 2012; 2012: 417834.

Peripheral nerve injuries

Campbell WW. Evaluation and management of peripheral nerve injury. Clin Neurophysiol 2008; 119(9): 1951–65.

CHAPTER 6.7

Chest injury

Eshan L. Senanayake, Stephen J. Rooney, and Timothy R. Graham

Airway disruption

Pathophysiology of airway disruption

Airway obstruction is a significant injury that can cause death quickly due to asphyxia, intrapulmonary haemorrhage, aspiration of blood, and the risk of causing an air embolus. Transection of the trachea or major bronchi due to either penetrating or blunt trauma is possible. Patients with airway disruption may survive if the surrounding soft tissue seals the disruption. Airway disruption should be suspected in a high-impact injury that causes scapula, clavicular, or upper three rib fractures.

Symptoms and signs of airway disruption

The patient will be acutely short of breath, have stridor due to obstruction or have haemoptysis. Severe surgical emphysema on the neck and thorax will be apparent on examination, with reduced air entry and desaturation. Radiologically, there will be evidence of a significant pneumothorax or presence of haemothorax. On computed tomography (CT) imaging, there will be evidence of pneumomediastinum or pneumopericardium. There may also be pneumoperitoneum. Confirmation is by bronchial endoscopy, but views may be obscured by blood and hence a major airway disruption may be missed. Following placement of a chest drain/drains, there may be evidence of a severe continuous air leak.

Management of airway disruption

A high index of suspicion for airway disruption should prevail in any major high-impact injury. This needs emergency surgical intervention. Endotracheal intubation could be helpful in the short term; in tracheal rupture where the endotracheal tube can be placed across the rupture. An immediate surgical airway may be required if endotracheal intubation is hazardous.

Tension pneumothorax

Pathophysiology of tension pneumothorax

During a tension pneumothorax there is progressive build-up of air within the pleural space between the visceral and parietal pleura such that there is no release of pressure from within this contained space. The air enters the pleural space from either the chest wall or the airway, which acts as a one-way valve.

The progressive build-up of pressure restricts venous return to the heart by displacing the mediastinal contents to the contralateral side. In addition, there is compression of the affected lung and depression of the diaphragm. Eventually cardiac output is diminished, resulting in reduced coronary blood flow, hypotension and hypoperfusion, and cardiac arrest, which may be preceded by respiratory arrest.

However, a tension pneumothorax may be present without any of these clinical and physiological consequences. Tension pneumothorax is a clinical diagnosis and the clinician should not await confirmation radiologically. In a ventilated patient, with positive pressure ventilation, a tension pneumothorax can be exaggerated.

Signs and symptoms of tension pneumothorax

Typically the patient will be breathless and in distress. They may complain of chest pain.

The clinical signs may include; tachycardia, tachypnoea, reduced oxygen saturations, hypotension, weak low volume pulse, hyperexpansion, reduced respiratory movement, reduced air entry and hyper-resonance to percussion on the ipsilateral side and, neck vein distension and tracheal deviation to the contralateral side. There may also be evidence of surgical emphysema.

Management of tension pneumothorax

The emergency management of a tension pneumothorax may require needle decompression, but only to relieve the tension and prevent respiratory or cardiac arrest. However, this should only be considered when a definitive procedure; chest drain placement, cannot be done immediately.

Needle decompression is performed by placing a 14–18G intravenous cannula in the second intercostal space in the midclavicular line. Following this, an intercostal chest drain should be placed within the safe triangle; bordered by the axilla at the apex, lateral border of pectoralis major anteriorly, the anterior border of latissimus dorsi posteriorly and the fifth intercostal space inferiorly.

In the field, unilateral or bilateral thoracostomies may be performed if there is evidence of or high index of suspicion of developing a tension pneumothorax. A thoracostomy is performed ideally in the safe triangle by making a 3–4 cm incision along the rib and entering the intra-pleural space. This allows communication between the intrathoracic space and the atmosphere. This should only be performed if an intercostal drain cannot be inserted. A thoracostomy is not a definitive procedure and subsequent drain placement may be required.

Open pneumothorax

Pathophysiology of open pneumothorax

This is a pneumothorax created by an open wound to the thorax following a penetrating injury. There is disruption to the parietal pleura and hence free passage of air into the pleural space. During inspiration there is negative pressure within the pleural space. Therefore with an open wound, there is preferential flow of air through this space into the pleural cavity, rather than into the lungs via the trachea, resulting in a collapsed lung, particularly when the diameter of the open chest wound is greater than two-thirds the diameter of the trachea. If the wound does not allow air to escape a tension pneumothorax may ensue.

Signs and symptoms open pneumothorax

An open pneumothorax is associated with a large wound to the thorax but may not always be obvious as it could be on the posterior thoracic region. In a multiply injured patient where other injuries (i.e. long bone injuries) are more obvious, careful inspection of the posterior thorax should be made on log-rolling the patient. Other clinical features are consistent with a pneumothorax.

Management open pneumothorax

Initial management should be to inspect the wound and remove any dressings that may prevent air to escape the pleural cavity. An appropriate occlusive dressing should then be placed over the wound to prevent air entry and allow a one-way system for air to escape. A chest drain should then be placed immediately through a different entry site to allow definite management of the pneumothorax. A more formal assessment and closure of the chest defect may be required at a later stage.

Massive haemothorax

Pathophysiology of massive haemothorax

A haemothorax is defined by blood in the pleural cavity. A massive haemothorax is defined by a loss of >1.5 L of blood into the pleural cavity or a drainage of blood at a rate of >200 mL/hr for four hours. This can ensue following injury to any of the intrathoracic vessels, including the great vessels, but commonly following damage to an intercostal or internal thoracic artery. Spillage of blood into the pleural space following cardiac laceration may also result in haemothorax.

Compression of the lung from blood within the pleural space causes reduced ventilation, respiratory compromise, and hypoxia. Furthermore hypovolaemia may become life threatening with ongoing bleeding.

Signs and symptoms of massive haemothorax

The patient may have an obvious penetrating injury. But in blunt trauma, there may be great vessel injury with no obvious external features of injury. In either circumstance the patient will be in hypovolaemic shock. The ipsilateral side will have reduced expansion, be dull to percussion with reduced air entry on auscultation. Vital signs include tachycardia, tachypnoea, and decreased oxygen saturation. Radiologically, if the patient is supine the features of a haemothorax may range from being subtle to complete white-out. In a haemopneumothorax an air-fluid level may be apparent on an erect chest radiograph (Figure 6.7.1).

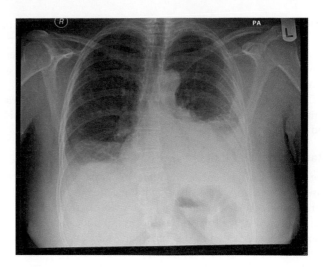

Fig. 6.7.1 Chest radiograph showing a moderate- to large-sized left haemothorax.

Management of massive haemothorax

A large bore >28F chest drain should be inserted and directed towards the costodiaphragmatic recess, to drain the blood within the pleural space allowing lung expansion. Simultaneous resuscitation of the hypovolaemic and hypotensive patient should take place with intravenous access and fluid or blood transfusion. Diagnosis can be confirmed following insertion of the chest drain and measurement of the total drainage from the pleural space.

In the presence of ongoing bleeding, a more definitive surgical intervention maybe required after stabilization and investigations such as contrast CT scan, prior to emergency surgical intervention. However, further investigations should only be performed if there is no delay to treatment, or haemodynamic compromise. Until a major cardiac or vascular injury has been excluded, resuscitation should be managed to allow for permissive hypotension to prevent exsanguination.

Flail chest

Pathophysiology of flail chest

Flail chest is defined by fracture of two or more ribs and/or sternum at two or more places along each rib. This causes a loss of bony continuity with the rest of the thoracic cage and creates an isolated segment of chest wall, which can be of any size. A flail chest may occur with either blunt or penetrating trauma, and the clinician should be suspicious of a flail chest even without external features as muscle splinting with the fractured ribs may mask the features. Following trauma a flail chest is commonly associated with significant underlying lung contusions, although this may not be initially apparent.

The flail segment causes paradoxical movement during the breathing cycle and this may result in respiratory compromise due to increasing pain and worsening lung contusions; with a reduction in tidal volume and functional residual capacity. There may also be an associated pneumothorax or haemothorax, or both.

Signs and symptoms of flail chest

The patient is in pain, which may range from mild to severe. A clinical diagnosis can be made on close inspection by identifying paradoxical movement of the flail segment during the breathing cycle: on inspiration the flail segment is indrawn and on expiration it is pushed out. This is usually a subtle feature. The patient may have a rapid and shallow breathing pattern. There may be evidence of bruising. Vital signs may include desaturation, tachycardia and tachypnoea.

The investigation of choice is a chest CT scan, which may clearly demonstrate the flail segment and any associated lung contusions and is more accurate than chest radiograph.

Management of flail chest

The initial management is adequate analgesia to aid chest wall movement and improve ventilation if the patient is self-ventilating. Intravenous opioids are effective but should be used with caution and in titrated doses to avoid further respiratory depression. The associated hypoxia due to the underlying lung contusions should be treated by adequate supplemental oxygen delivery (i.e. high-flow humidified oxygen). Simultaneous resuscitation of associated hypovolaemia may be necessary.

Subsequent management may include chest drain insertions to manage any associated haemothorax or pneumothorax. The associated pulmonary contusions will need to be monitored by serial radiography and judicious fluid administration should be used to avoid pulmonary oedema in an existing damaged lung susceptible to fluid overload and adult respiratory distress syndrome. Patients may benefit from thoracic epidural analgesia or intercostal blocks. Aggressive physiotherapy following adequate pain control is helpful in lung re-expansion and expectoration to reduce the risk of chest infection.

If the patient cannot sustain self-ventilation, mechanical ventilation with a lung protective ventilator strategy may be necessary to manage hypoxia. Surgical fixation of the flail segment may be required if the extent of the flail segment prevents self-ventilation.

In patients that have been placed on mechanical ventilation, weaning off this support can be prolonged due to the nature and extent of pulmonary injury. In these patients, tracheostomy placement will benefit in weaning sedation and allow the patient to cooperate with rehabilitation while weaning from mechanical respiratory ventilation.

Cardiac tamponade

Pathophysiology of cardiac tamponade

Cardiac tamponade may be associated with penetrating injuries and should be suspected in any trauma to the chest particularly to the thoracic 'shield area' (clavicles to the xiphisternum and from right mid-clavicular line to the left lateral chest wall anteriorly and posteriorly) or in junctional injuries (neck or axilla) until proven otherwise.

A penetrating injury to the heart breaches the pericardium and commonly punctures the anteriorly placed right ventricle, although other mediastinal structures including the great vessels can be injured in isolation or together. This laceration causes bleeding into the pericardial sac that may continue or resolve due to clot formation. However, the pericardial sac can only accommodate a small volume before venous return to the heart is restricted by an increase in intra-pericardial pressure. If the intrapericardial pressure is greater than the central venous pressure, venous return to the heart is restricted (cardiac tamponade). This creates a low cardiac output, leading to reduced coronary blood flow and

myocardial ischaemia, which may result in cardiac arrest. Initially compensatory mechanisms of tachycardia and increased peripheral vascular resistance maintain cardiac output, but if the intrapericardial pressure is not released, these compensatory mechanism fail. Low end organ perfusion and reduced myocardial perfusion leads to metabolic acidosis.

Symptoms and signs of cardiac tamponade

The patient may have an obvious penetrating chest injury within the thoracic shield area. Tachycardia and hypotension may be present, and electrocardiographic evidence of myocardial injury may be present. Classical features of cardiac tamponade include: hypotension, raised jugular venous pressure, or prominent neck veins and muffled heart sounds (Becks' triad). There may be pulsus paradoxus (>10 mmHg fall in pressure during inspiration). However these features are often absent.

Bleeding from the pericardial sac into the pleural space can result in a haemothorax, and there may also be an associated pneumothorax. Radiologically the heart silhouette may be globular in shape. Further investigations (i.e. CT thorax) to confirm clinical suspicion should not be undertaken as this may compromise patient care and clinical deterioration can occur rapidly. In trauma this should be a clinical diagnosis.

Management of cardiac tamponade

The primary aim of management is relief of tamponade by surgical evacuation. During resuscitation in the emergency department, this can be difficult. Ideally surgical evacuation should be performed in theatre based on the clinical urgency.

While preparations are made (i.e. equipment and expertise to formally relieve the tamponade), venous return to the heart can be augmented by raising the patient's legs and by fluid resuscitation. However, aggressive fluid resuscitation can worsen the situation by causing increasing tamponade secondary to more bleeding.

Emergency surgical evacuation in the resuscitation room should only be made if the patient arrests in transfer or in the resuscitation room. Access can be via a left anterior thoracotomy performed by someone who has the expertise to identify the pericardium and relieve the tamponade by expelling blood and clot from the pericardial sac, without causing greater harm. Subsequently a formal procedure to repair the laceration to the heart should be made by a specialist surgical team.

Ideally a median sternotomy would be the preferred approach, judged on the clinical urgency of the intervention. This approach would allow relief of the tamponade and provide adequate exposure to proceed to assess other mediastinal structures and perform a formal repair of the laceration. It also allows the best approach for cardiopulmonary bypass if required. The decision to surgically intervene and the approach taken are based on the expertise, environment, and the equipment available at the time. In theatre trans-oesophageal echocardiography can be used to exclude other intracardica injuries to the valvular and septal structures.

Rib and sternal fractures

Rib fractures are the most common feature in thoracic trauma and mostly occur in the posterior angle (at the weakest point). These can be complicated by life-threatening injuries as described above, or can appear in isolation with or without a simple pneumothorax.

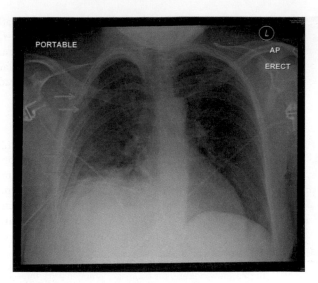

Fig. 6.7.2 Multiple right side rib fractures with a possible flail segment and right intercostal drain directed towards the base. Blue arrows indicate point of rib fractures.

A pneumothorax secondary to trauma should be drained by intercostal drain placement to permit lung re-expansion.

Multiple rib fractures (Figure 6.7.2) are associated underlying lung contusions. Lower rib fractures may be associated with intra-abdominal (liver and splenic) injuries and fractures of the first to third ribs or clavicle implies a high-impact injury.

Rib fractures are associated with severe pain restricting respiration, increasing the risk of chest infections. Patients should be managed with adequate analgesia by way of thoracic epidurals, regional nerve blocks, and/or simple analgesia as required to ensure adequate pain relief. .

If a sternal fracture is noted, further investigation by CT or lateral chest X-ray should be carried out to confirm if this has caused displacement of the sternum. If non-displaced, patients can be managed conservatively. If there is sternal displacement, patients should be managed as a myocardial infarction if there is an increased serum troponin level. Electrocardiography may exclude myocardial ischaemia and identify dysrhythmias. A subsequent transthoracic echocardiogram can exclude regional myocardial wall motion abnormalities and subsequent pericardial effusion.

Myocardial contusions

Myocardial contusions are associated with blunt trauma with high energy transfer and can be difficult to diagnose. The patient may have a period of myocardial stunning and reduced contractility. There might be an associated serum troponin rise in the presence of an abnormal electrocardiogram, although these may be non-specific after trauma. Recognition of a patient at risk of myocardial contusions is important and this would prompt appropriate monitoring and investigations to deal with subsequent arrhythmias and depressed myocardial function. Transthoracic echocardiography may help exclude valvular abnormalities and assess myocardial function.

Oesophageal injury

This is uncommon but can be associated with major morbidity secondary to mediastinitis and empyema formation secondary to oesophageal rupture. The cervical portion of the oesophagus is more prone to injury from penetrating injury and the lower third may be prone to injury from blunt trauma. Radiographically there may be a pneumomediastinum or air-fluid level commonly on the left. Diagnosis can be confirmed with a water-soluble contrast swallow or endoscopy, and will likely need specialist surgical intervention and repair. Surgical access is gained via a posterolateral thoracotomy to provide adequate exposure. Depending on the extent of injury primary repair of the oesophageal injury may be possible. The repair can be further supported, by mobilizing intercostal muscle flaps to cover the primary closure.

Diaphragmatic rupture

This can occur with either blunt or penetrating trauma. The proximity of the injury to the diaphragm can be the only initial clinical feature. With blunt trauma, the most common mechanism is a side impact motor vehicle collision. The right hemidiaphragm is less frequently involved due to the protective effect of the liver. There should always be a high index of suspicion of diaphragmatic injury in the presence of with other intra-abdominal injuries and repair should not be delayed unless contraindicated. Preferably the diaphragm should be repaired at laparotomy; which provides access to deal with other intra-abdominal pathology. A diaphragmatic rupture is difficult to confirm radiographically, but it is suspected by loss of the costodiaphragmatic recess, position of the stomach, and any evidence of a correctly placed nasogastric tube within the chest. A CT chest can confirm the diagnosis although the exact position of the rupture can be difficult to delineate.

Traumatic disruption of the aorta

The most common cause of traumatic disruption of the aorta (TDA) is due to a severe rapid deceleration injury. In blunt trauma rapid deceleration causes traumatic shearing forces of the aorta at fixed points, commonly at the level of the ligamentum arteriosum just beyond the origin of the left subclavian artery; other points include the aortic valve and diaphragmatic hiatus. Typically patients will only survive if there is a partial disruption with localized haematoma contained by the aortic adventitia. TDA should be suspected in any deceleration injury as the clinical findings can range from asymptomatic or transient hypotension to significant cardiac tamponade and/or haemothorax. Therefore if suspected a CT aortogram should confirm or refute the diagnosis following immediate and adequate resuscitation. Figure 6.7.3 shows such a disruption.

Patients should be managed under permissive hypotension to prevent further aortic bleeding/rupture. The term permissive hypotension refers to the accepting lower than normal blood pressure parameters enough to maintain end organ perfusion (i.e. urine output and appropriate cognitive function). This is usually achieved by beta blockade to lower the heart rate and blood pressure, thereby lowering the shear forces exerted on the aorta. Repair of a TDA can be done by either open surgical repair or by thoracic endovascular aortic repair, with stenting. The method used will depend on the site, extent of the disruption, other co-existing injuries and co-morbidities, and the expertise and equipment available at the trauma centre.

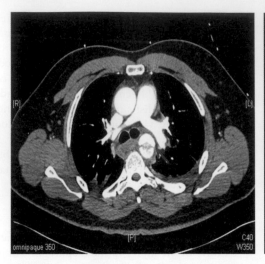
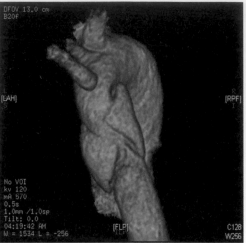

Fig. 6.7.3 Traumatic disruption of the aorta, as evident on an axial slice at the level of the disruption. The red arrow indicates the traumatic disruption (left). Three-dimensional reconstruction of the same computed tomogram, showing a spiral type disruption (right).

Pulmonary contusions and lacerations

Pulmonary contusions are commonly associated with blunt thoracic trauma and can be present in addition to or in the absence of pneumothorax or haemothorax with overlying rib fractures and/or a flail chest. Pulmonary contusions are a progressive condition and

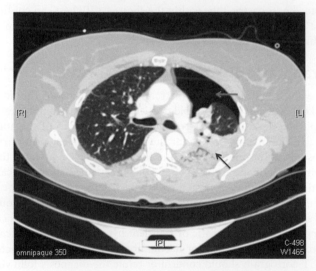

Fig. 6.7.4 Axial computed tomogram image showing a combination of left basal lung contusions (red arrow), pneumothorax (blue arrow) causing collapse of the left lung.

initially are as a result of parenchymal haemorrhage. Following this, the lung parenchyma is more susceptible to oedema and fluid accumulation within the interstitial space. Eventually collapse and consolidation ensue, which causes a ventilation/perfusion mismatch leading to progressive respiratory compromise (lead to acute respiratory distress syndrome).

Pulmonary contusions can initially be detected on chest radiograph and serial chest radiographs can show progression, although a CT chest is more specific and useful in assessing the extent of damage and progression as shown in Figure 6.7.4.

Patients with pulmonary contusions are susceptible to pulmonary oedema and acute respiratory stress syndrome, therefore fluid resuscitation should be judiciously managed following the initial resuscitation. Invasive haemodynamic monitoring and critical care support is helpful in managing these patients.

Further reading

Advanced Trauma Life Support Student Course Manual, 9th addition. Chicago: American College of Surgeons, 2012.

European trauma course—the team approach manual: Edition 6; (July 2013). Available from http://www.europeantrauma.com/the-course/educational-principles.html (accessed 30 November 2015).

Hunt PA, Greaves I, Owens WA. Emergency thoracotomy in thoracic trauma-a review. *Injury* 2006; 37(1): 1–19.

Laws D, Neville E, Duffy J, *et al*. BTS guidelines for the insertion of a chest drain. *Thorax* 2003; 58(Suppl 2): ii53–9.

Trauma.org. Thoracic trauma. Available from http://www.trauma.org/index.php/main/category/C11 (accessed 30 November 2015).

CHAPTER 6.8

Abdominal trauma

Bruce Tulloh

Introduction

Being called to assess a patient with abdominal trauma may seem daunting, but early decision making is straightforward: the only immediately life-threatening abdominal injury is major bleeding, and there is only one therapeutic option (laparotomy). However, less catastrophic injuries can be harder to diagnose and the decision to operate more subtle. Furthermore, for a given injury there may be several therapeutic options to choose from.

If the patient needs immediate exploratory laparotomy, the precise injuries can be diagnosed at operation. If a decision *against* urgent surgery has been made, then the surgeon must diagnose the injuries by other means. Despite the increasing availability of rapid computed tomography (CT) scanning, the major clues to this are still clinical. Many injuries can (and should be) anticipated by considering regional anatomy, the mechanism of injury, and certain well-known injury associations.

Initial assessment

Abdominal examination is normally part of the secondary survey, performed after all life-threatening injuries have been addressed, but if a patient is in hypovolaemic shock then the abdomen will need to be assessed immediately as a potential site of bleeding. If there is no obvious external haemorrhage and the chest is clear, then *immediate laparotomy should be arranged.*

If there is doubt or if the patient is relatively stable, then a more detailed clinical assessment will help determine the appropriate treatment, taking into account the following factors.

Anatomical considerations

A penetrating wound to the upper abdomen may cross the diaphragm and damage intrathoracic structures, and vice versa.

Some of the upper abdominal organs are 'protected' by the rib cage but fractures of the lower few ribs are commonly associated with damage to the liver, spleen, or kidneys.

The pelvic organs are also relatively protected by the iliac crests but may be damaged in penetrating perineal or buttock trauma, and with anterior pelvic fractures. Posterior pelvic fractures are often associated with relentless bleeding from pre-sacral and iliac vessels.

Retroperitoneal organs such as the pancreas, kidneys, duodenum, ascending and descending colon, or rectum may be damaged with penetrating trauma to the back or blunt trauma to the abdomen.

Mechanism of injury

Understanding the mechanism of injury is vital because blunt and penetrating trauma are each associated with different spectra of organ damage.

With blunt trauma, solid organs rupture and bleed, hollow organs may perforate, and the diaphragm may tear. Ribs and pelvic bones may fracture and this will absorb a lot of the energy of the blow but may still result in damage to underlying organs, and also laceration of deeper structures caused by the jagged ends of broken bones. The duodenum, pancreas, and small bowel can be momentarily crushed against the spinal column with ventral blunt trauma, causing the bowel to perforate and/or the pancreas to split.

Penetrating trauma causes lacerations and perforations and these are often multiple. If the trajectory of the knife or bullet is known this may help predict organ damage, but remember that bullets may ricochet inside. It is useful to classify penetrating trauma into three types: stab wounds, low-velocity gunshot wounds (e.g. standard handguns and rifles) and high-velocity gunshot wounds (e.g. military weapons). High-velocity injuries also cause a cavitating shock wave at 90° to the trajectory that can cause extensive tissue damage at some distance from the bullet path.

Some injuries have a mixed component (e.g. common assault, blast injuries or falls onto a sharp object).

Clinical assessment

Primary and secondary survey

Once the airway is secure, the cervical spine controlled, and satisfactory breathing (and ventilation) is established, attention is directed to 'C' for circulation. Major ongoing bleeding should be diagnosed clinically from non-abdominal signs, the most useful of which are skin colour, capillary return, and pulse rate. The response to an initial bolus of intravenous fluid is a very useful early clue: transient responders and non-responders have ongoing bleeding until proven otherwise, and are likely to need surgical intervention. Hypotension is often a late sign and the diagnosis of oliguria takes at least an hour to establish.

An *elevated* jugular venous pressure in a shocked patient, even if supine, tells you that the shock is due to something other than haemorrhage (consider cardiac tamponade or tension pneumothorax).

In the absence of obvious bleeding that would mandate urgent surgery, a more detailed examination follows. The secondary survey must include a careful log-roll to examine the back. Penetrating wounds to the back and buttock may cause intraperitoneal injury and may require a laparotomy.[1] A rectal and vaginal examination is important if pelvic injury is suspected.

The protrusion of intra-abdominal tissue (e.g. omentum or bowel) through a penetrating wound is an indication for laparotomy, although it is not as urgent as a laparotomy for ongoing bleeding.

Tachycardia (>120 beats per minute) is always a concern. It usually indicates ongoing bleeding but may represent early sepsis from organ perforation, or simply inadequately controlled pain.

Perineal bruising may be a sign of ruptured urethra and/or pelvic fracture.

Seat-belt bruising across the lower abdomen should raise the suspicion of small bowel perforation or diaphragmatic rupture.

In patients with spinal injury, signs such as abdominal pain and tenderness may be masked. Repeated clinical examination is a very reliable way to determine the presence or absence of significant intra-abdominal injury. The frequency of re-examination depends on your level of suspicion.

Injury associations

Table 6.8.1 shows some common injury associations. If one is diagnosed, think of the other.

Investigations

If there is no obvious need for urgent laparotomy for either bleeding or evisceration, there is time for investigation. The choice of test depends on the clinical context and thus it is useful to consider blunt and penetrating trauma separately.

Blunt trauma

Ultrasound is quick and can be done at the bedside in an unstable or unconscious patient. This is the 'FAST' scan, for *focused abdominal sonogram in trauma*.[2–4] It is operator dependent but, more importantly, it only answers one question: is there, or is there not, any free fluid within the abdomen? (See Figure 6.8.1.) Free fluid may be blood, urine, bowel content, or bile. Therefore, regardless of the cause, laparotomy is required if the answer is 'yes'.

Thus ultrasound is no more than a tool to aid the decision to operate: free fluid = laparotomy. Be aware that the false-negative

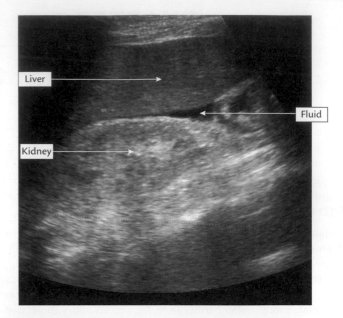

Fig. 6.8.1 Portable abdominal ultrasound scan ('FAST') showing a dark (sonolucent) triangular sliver of free fluid in Morison's pouch, between the liver and the right kidney. The patient proceeded to laparotomy where blood was encountered from a tear in the small bowel mesentery. This was easily controlled with an under-running suture.

rate for FAST scan is significant, so continued clinical observation remains important.[5]

CT scanning gives excellent organ detail and is the investigation of choice in most cases, but *only* if the patient is physiologically stable (see Figure 6.8.2).

Contrast X-ray studies (e.g. oral or urethral) are useful in confirming the suspicion of perforated duodenum or urethra. A urethrogram may be required to confirm that is safe (or otherwise) to insert a urinary catheter. However, modern high-resolution CT scanning demonstrates most of these injuries.

Diagnostic peritoneal lavage, which involves inserting a small catheter into the peritoneal cavity under local anaesthesia, instilling

Table 6.8.1 Common injury associations

If the patient has….	… think of:
# Lower ribs	Liver or spleen trauma
#12th rib	Kidney trauma
Seat-belt bruising	Perforated small bowel / Ruptured diaphragm
Flexion # of lumbar spine (Chance #)	Perforated small bowel
# Transverse process(es)	Ureteric injury
Perineal bruising	Urethral rupture
Anterior pelvic fracture	Bladder or urethral rupture
Posterior pelvic fracture	Bleeding from iliac vessels
Penetrating back wound	Injury to colon, duodenum, pancreas or kidney
Penetrating buttock wound	Perforated rectum (also sciatic nerve injury)
Unexplained bradycardia	Cervical spine injury
Unexplained tachycardia	Ongoing bleeding or bowel perforation

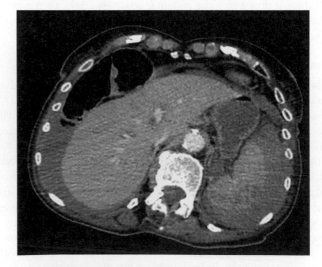

Fig. 6.8.2 Abdominal computed tomography scan showing a ruptured spleen with considerable free fluid surrounding both it and the liver. The splenic perfusion on this arterial-phase image is patchy and it appears that the capsule is deficient posterolaterally.

500 mL of normal saline and then siphoning it out again to look for evidence of bleeding or bowel content, has largely been superseded by CT scanning.

Penetrating trauma

In the UK it is generally recommended that if the peritoneum has been breached, an exploratory laparotomy is required. However, centres that deal with large volumes of gunshot and stab wounds usually develop a more selective approach. There are several ways to confirm a peritoneal breach:

♦ Exploration of the wound under local anaesthesia. This may be difficult particularly in obese patients. It often requires extension of the entry wound and even so, usually only the anterior abdominal wall fascia can be reached.

♦ Plain abdominal X-ray is of limited use. In a supine patient it is moderately reliable in the detection of free gas and may be helpful to locate foreign bodies (e.g. bullets).

♦ Ultrasound will show free fluid, which implies peritoneal breach.

♦ CT will identify intraperitoneal gas to indicate peritoneal breach or bowel perforation and may even show the missile track through the abdominal wall. Free fluid and specific organ injuries are also well seen.

♦ Laparoscopy is an excellent way to look for intraperitoneal bleeding or bowel content,[6,7] although it requires a general anaesthetic. Nevertheless, it may spare someone an unnecessary laparotomy, especially if the peritoneum has been penetrated but there is no significant intra-abdominal injury.

Treatment

Initial resuscitation

As for any trauma patient, initial resuscitation should proceed with attention to the airway with cervical spine control, oxygenation, and administration of intravenous fluids. The response to an initial fluid bolus will help determine whether or not the patient has active, ongoing bleeding and, therefore, whether or not urgent intervention is required.

Nasogastric intubation is a useful early adjunct and relieves the acute gastric dilatation that is often seen after major trauma. However, passage of a nasogastric tube should *not* be attempted if a fracture of the anterior cranial fossa (cribriform plate) is suspected.

Urethral catheterization is also a standard procedure in the management of shocked patients but this is contraindicated when a urethral injury is suspected. Consider suprapubic catheterization instead, or a retrograde urethrogram to rule out urethral damage with involvement of a urologist where possible.

Laparotomy

The two indisputable indications for immediate laparotomy are the presence of ongoing intra-abdominal haemorrhage and a perforated hollow viscus. Establishing that a penetrating wound has passed through the peritoneum is a relative indication but may be over-ridden on clinical grounds, especially in centres where penetrating trauma is common and a more selective approach can be taken.

Technique of trauma laparotomy

Ensure that sufficient compatible blood is available for transfusion and adequate suction, packs, and appropriate surgical equipment (e.g. two suction machines). A midline incision is recommended as it gives optimum exposure to all zones and leaves room for a stoma if necessary, although a transverse incision is often used in children. A systematic approach is required to explore all four quadrants, packing off each in turn to try to isolate the source of bleeding. Examine the entire bowel and mesentery carefully as well as the undersurface of the liver, the gallbladder, and the pelvic organs. The retroperitoneal organs should be examined but the posterior peritoneum should not be opened unnecessarily as this can unleash uncontrollable bleeding that might otherwise have tamponaded itself.

Penetrating wounds through the abdominal wall should be debrided and washed thoroughly as they can be expected to be contaminated over their entire length, in which case delayed primary closure (or no closure at all) may be appropriate initial management with delayed scar revision if necessary.

Damage control

This refers to temporary intervention for life-threatening injury with the plan to return 24 to 48 hours later for definitive repair once other problems such as anaemia, hypothermia, and coagulopathy have been corrected. It typically involves debriding necrotic tissue, clamping or ligating arterial bleeders, packing off the liver and other venous bleeding, or stapling off the ends of resected bowel without anastomosis. Immediate repair of a ruptured diaphragm is usually feasible, and immediate splenectomy is considered part of damage control.

Abdominal closure may not be possible due to the risk of abdominal compartment syndrome. There are a variety of techniques now available to help prevent and overcome abdominal compartment syndrome including simple laparostomy, temporary mesh closure, and vacuum-assisted dressings.[8]

Definitive surgical treatment

Definitive surgical procedures such as partial resection of liver, spleen or kidney, repair, bypass or exclusion of pancreatic and duodenal injuries, or repair of rectal lacerations combined with a proximal diverting stoma require careful planning and expertise. Small and large bowel injuries can often be primarily repaired or resected, but in the presence of gross peritoneal soiling or haemodynamic instability, anastomoses should be avoided in preference for the creation of a double stoma. Oesophageal and gastric lacerations can generally be sutured primarily, although establishment of drainage both inside and outside the lumen is advised to prevent/control a potential leak.

Active monitoring

If a patient is assessed soon after injury, clinical signs and radiological features may not have had time to develop, necessitating close active monitoring and repeated clinical examination, in addition to repeating the CT scan the next day if clinical suspicion for particular injury remains high.

Renal contusion, manifesting as macroscopic haematuria, usually resolves without intervention. Many liver and spleen injuries can also be treated conservatively, especially in children.[9] Rectus sheath haematomas following blunt trauma usually tamponade themselves but may be very painful. Traumatic pancreatitis can be treated as for non-traumatic cases but may be associated with undiagnosed duodenal rupture, or result in pseudocyst formation from pancreatic duct disruption. Subcapsular splenic haematoma may rupture and bleed in the first 7 to 10 days post-injury.

Missed injuries

It is common for perforated small bowel or diaphragmatic injury to become evident several days after trauma, emphasizing the importance of active monitoring and raised awareness depending on the mechanism of injury.

Special cases

Pregnant women have a hyperdynamic circulation and a physiological anaemia, and abdominal examination may be difficult. The splanchnic (uterine) circulation is shut down early in shock, and aggressive resuscitation of the mother is vital to protect the fetus. CT scanning should not be avoided if the mother or child's life is at stake.[10] Early obstetric opinion is advised to monitor the fetus and advise on urgent caesarean section if required.

Patients with spinal injuries are likely to have an impaired perception of pain and tenderness as well as an altered cardiovascular response to fluid loss, resulting in the risk of missing an associated abdominal injury. Fluid resuscitation should be undertaken with care due to the risk of unintended overhydration.

Children have excellent cardiovascular reserve and tend to maintain their blood pressure until very late, although their pulse pressure may narrow. Tachycardia may be difficult to interpret in an injured and frightened child. Ultrasound tends to be used more than CT, to reduce radiation exposure. Fluid and ventilatory requirements must be calculated on a per-kilogram basis.

Summary

- The most important early decision is whether or not the patient needs an immediate laparotomy and this can usually be decided clinically.

- If the patient does not require immediate surgery then there is time for investigation.

- Certain injuries should be suspected from the history and from known injury associations.

- CT scanning is arguably the most useful investigation, but others have their specific indications and repeated clinical examination has an important role.

- Many abdominal injuries can be managed conservatively but if laparotomy is required, consider damage control if the patient is unstable.

- Beware of missed injuries, particularly in patients who cannot communicate and in those who have multisystem injury, especially spinal injury.

- There are two victims in cases of trauma in pregnancy. The circulation in the fetus depends on that of the mother. Involve the obstetricians early.

Further reading

Advanced Trauma Life Support Student Course Manual, 9th addition. Chicago: American College of Surgeons, 2012.

Biffl WL, Moore EE. Management guidelines for penetrating abdominal trauma. *Curr Opin Crit Care* 2010; 16(6): 609–17.

Chiquito PE. Blunt abdominal injuries. Diagnostic peritoneal lavage, ultrasonography and computed tomography scanning. *Injury* 1996; 27(2): 117–24.

Nordenholz KE, Rubin MA, Gularte GG, *et al.* Ultrasound in the evaluation and management of blunt abdominal trauma. *Ann Emerg Med* 1997; 29(3): 357–66.

Petrone P, Talving P, Browder T, *et al.* Abdominal injuries in pregnancy: a 155-month study at two level 1 trauma centers. *Injury* 2011; 42(1): 47–9.

Sivit CJ. Imaging children with abdominal trauma. *Am J Roentgenol* 2009; 192(5): 1179–89.

References

1. Boyle EM Jr, Maier RV, Salazar JD, *et al.* Diagnosis of injuries after stab wounds to the back and flank. *J Trauma* 1997; 42(2): 260–5.

2. Fleming S, Bird R, Ratnasingham K, *et al.* Accuracy of FAST scan in blunt abdominal trauma in a major London trauma centre. *Int J Surg* 2012; 10(9): 470–4.

3. Holmes JF, Harris D, Battistella FD. Performance of abdominal ultrasonography in blunt trauma patients with out-of-hospital or emergency department hypotension. *Ann Emerg Med* 2004; 43(3): 354–61.

4. Natarajan B, Gupta PK, Cemaj S, *et al.* FAST scan: is it worth doing in hemodynamically stable blunt trauma patients? *Surgery* 2010; 148(4): 695–700.

5. Nural MS, Yardan T, Güven H, *et al.* Diagnostic value of ultrasonography in the evaluation of blunt abdominal trauma. *Diagn Interv Radiol* 2005; 11(1): 41–4.

6. Johnson JJ, Garwe T, Raines AR, *et al.* The use of laparoscopy in the diagnosis and treatment of blunt and penetrating abdominal injuries: 10-year experience at a level 1 trauma center. *Am J Surg* 2013; 205(3): 317–21.

7. O'Malley E, Boyle E, O'Callaghan A, *et al.* Role of laparoscopy in penetrating abdominal trauma: a systematic review. *World J Surg* 2013; 37(1): 113–22.

8. Carr JA. Abdominal compartment syndrome: a decade of progress. *J Am Coll Surg* 2013; 216(1): 135–46.

9. Olthof DC, Joosse P, van der Vlies CH, *et al.* Prognostic factors for failure of nonoperative management in adults with blunt splenic injury: A systematic review. *J Trauma Acute Care Surg* 2013; 74(2): 546–57.

10. Sadro C, Bernstein MP, Kanal KM. Imaging of trauma: Part 2, Abdominal trauma and pregnancy—a radiologist's guide to doing what is best for the mother and baby. *Am J Roentgenol* 2012; 199(6): 1207–19.

CHAPTER 6.9

Vascular injury

Zahid Raza

Introduction

The management of patients with vascular trauma is complex in view of the diagnostic difficulties and planning the appropriate management strategy. The initial assessment of the multiply injured patient should focus on resuscitation followed by methodical and systemic assessment of all body systems. A multidisciplinary approach is vital in these circumstances and the vascular specialist should have a clear understanding of the pathophysiology of vascular trauma. The choice of treatment depends upon the nature and extent of the underlying injury and may require expertise ranging from interventional vascular radiology to specialist vascular surgery.

Mechanisms of vascular trauma

Blunt

A vessel can be injured as a result of blunt force applied during a road traffic accident, compression, or as a result of fracture of the adjacent bone. Supracondylar fractures of the humerus can disrupt the brachial artery and similarly knee dislocation or supracondylar fracture of femur can cause popliteal artery injury.[1]

Penetrating

Stab wounds can cause major vascular damage and clinical signs may not be overt at initial evaluation. Gunshot wounds can disrupt vessels either by direct trauma or as a result of cavitational shock wave effects that are much more pronounced in high-velocity firearm injuries as seen in the modern battlefield.[2]

Blast injury

Shock wave from a blast can be severe enough to disrupt blood vessels without external evidence of trauma. Similarly, the shock wave surrounding the trajectory of a high-velocity bullet can cause damage to the vessel in its vicinity.

Iatrogenic

The most common cause of iatrogenic vascular injury is during vascular access for either cardiology or vascular radiology interventions. Iliac arteries and veins can be damaged during pelvic surgery for malignant disease.

Patterns of vascular injury

Incomplete or partial disruption

This results in a pulsatile haematoma with the risk of delayed rupture. It can also lead to thrombosis of the vessel lumen or distal embolization with limb-threatening ischaemia. Formation of a false aneurysm can result in delayed haemorrhage.

Complete transection

A completely transected vessel can lead to intense vasospasm with distal pulse deficit and ischaemia.

Intimal flap and thrombosis

Blunt trauma can disrupt the intimal lining of the vessel leading to intraluminal thrombosis and distal limb ischaemia. These vessels may look normal and intact from outside and exploration is mandatory for correct diagnosis and treatment.

Vascular spasm or stretch

Arterial spasm can be associated with blunt limb trauma and is a rare cause of distal limb ischaemia without concomitant vascular injury. Arterial spasm should only be diagnosed after excluding the vascular injury by either computed tomography (CT) or digital subtraction angiography.

Assessment of patients with suspected vascular trauma

Initial clinical evaluation

A methodical clinical assessment according to the Advanced Trauma Life Support principles. The initial attention to airway, breathing, and circulation should take priority to other systemic injuries. A high index of suspicion is essential for timely diagnosis of vascular injuries, which is based on 'hard' and 'soft' clinical signs as outlined in the Box 6.9.1. However, it should be emphasized that the presence of a distal pulse does not necessarily exclude a major arterial injury.[3,4]

Initial resuscitation and haemorrhage control is vital in unstable patients with limb trauma. In patients with major thoracic or intra-abdominal haemorrhage, an urgent decision for intervention is required to stop ongoing blood loss. However, a non-operative

---

Box 6.9.1 Clinical evaluation of patients with vascular injury

'Hard' signs

- Shock with continued blood loss
- Pale, pulseless, cold limb
- Pulsatile haematoma at site of injury
- Palpable thrill or audible bruit
- Pulsatile bleeding at the time clinical evaluation

'Soft' signs

- History of massive bleeding at the time of injury
- Penetrating trauma in the vicinity of a major vessel
- Non-pulsatile haematoma
- Reduced volume of distal pulse
- Distal neurological impairment

---

management plan would be appropriate in a selected group of patients with limited and stable vascular injury.[5]

Adjuncts to clinical assessment

Pulse oximetry can detect tissue oxygen saturation and serial readings can be helpful for continuous assessment to detect any deterioration from the baseline assessment. Ankle–brachial pressure index (ABPI) using a handheld Doppler can be useful when the injured limb is compared with the non-injured limb. An ABPI <1.0 would be an indication for further investigation. However, in elderly patients, the ABPI may be reduced as a result of atherosclerotic disease and could be misleading. An audible Doppler signal does not necessarily exclude a significant proximal arterial injury.

Diagnostic imaging

Duplex ultrasound is a non-invasive mode that combines the standard b mode ultrasound with pulsed Doppler signals and is a useful test in the majority of extremity vascular injuries. It can detect the disruption of the vessel wall, distal flow, formation of false aneurysm, and arteriovenous fistula. However, the results are operator dependent and further imaging by either CT or digital subtraction angiography is indicated in cases of diagnostic uncertainty.

CT angiography is unsafe in patients with haemodynamic instability and should only be carried out after the vital signs have been stabilized. It is especially helpful for evaluation of vascular injuries in the neck, chest, and abdomen. Digital subtraction angiography is the gold-standard investigation for arterial injuries especially in the extremity injuries and is helpful in defining the precise location and extent of injury in order to plan the treatment strategy.[6] Intraoperative angiography by a C-arm is particularly helpful and is a valuable tool for the operating surgeon.

Principles of treatment in vascular trauma

The following issues should be carefully considered in these high risk patients.

Haemorrhage control

Manual compression of the bleeding point is the safest and most effective way for controlling ongoing blood loss from an extremity injury. Blind application of clamps can aggravate the injury and should be discouraged. Heavy dressings are ineffective, as the site of bleeding is not precisely compressed. Use of temporary balloon catheters before surgical repair can minimize the blood loss. There is good evidence that overzealous resuscitation with transfusion in the presence of uncontrolled bleeding can reduce the survival, and hence there is a need for hypotensive resuscitation until the bleeding site is controlled.

Dissection of injured vessel

The surgical exposure of the injured vessel requires adequate access for both proximal and distal control. Forward and backward bleeding should be confirmed and the intimal lining should be carefully inspected for flaps and dissection. Long saphenous vein from the non-injured leg may need to be harvested for use either as a patch or interposition graft.

Tourniquets

The tourniquet has been a contentious issue for many surgeons. Some advocate them as life savers in vascular trauma, whilst others vilify them.

In trauma, the use of the tourniquet should be limited to the extremities and in situations where bleeding cannot be controlled by direct pressure. Once applied, it should never be covered by bandages and most are brightly covered to alert the recipient doctor that the patient has a tourniquet. During recent wars, correct indication and application of a tourniquet has been responsible for saving countless number of lives. However, this success has been attributed to the timely evacuation of an injured person and transfer to a surgical facility, within the 'golden hour' of trauma.

Techniques of vascular repair

Revascularization of an ischaemic limb during trauma depends on the extent of the injury, any other associated injury, and the timing for vascular surgery (Figure 6.9.1).

Lateral repair with sutures is suitable when one half or less of the vessel circumference is disrupted with the rest of the vessel remaining intact. However, if more than half of the circumference is disrupted with loss of the vessel wall, a patch angioplasty using either the long saphenous vein or a pericardial patch is more appropriate. Primary end-to-end anastomosis is indicated in cases of complete transaction with minimal vessel loss and requires adequate mobilization of the vessel to ensure a tension-free anastomosis.

An interposition graft is indicated with defects of >2 cm, and ideally a vein graft should be used as it is less prone to infection, with better long-term patency compared to synthetic grafts.[7]

Following revascularization, the patient must be observed for any signs of infection, graft thrombosis, and limb swelling. Systemic manifestations of limb reperfusion after a period of ischaemia must also be appreciated as discussed previously.

Role of endovascular treatment

The use of interventional vascular radiology techniques has transformed the management of current clinical practice. Most vascular injuries can be treated by placement of a stent graft across the damaged vessel (e.g. the carotid, subclavian, and axillary arteries). In addition, injuries to the thoracic and abdominal aorta can be effectively treated without the need for a major surgery.[8–10] Embolization of the branches of iliac arteries can be effective in controlling the haemorrhage from pelvic injuries.

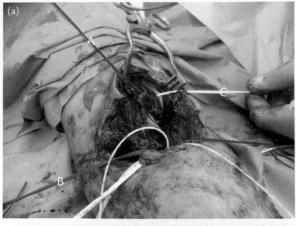

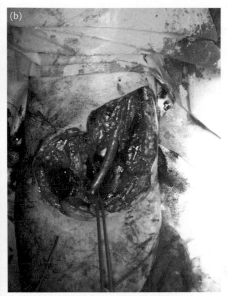

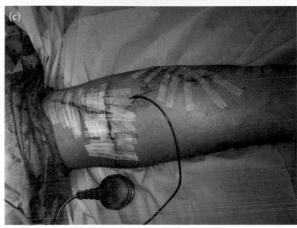

Fig. 6.9.1 (a) Glass injury to the antecubital fossa causing complete transection of the brachial artery which has thrombosed (sling A). The distal brachial artery has retracted (sling B). The median nerve is intact (sling C). (b) The injury has been repaired with an interposition vein graft (V). (c) A suction drain is inserted after irrigation of the wound and the patient placed on intravenous antibiotics post procedure. He made a full and uncomplicated recovery.

Damage control surgery

The principles of damage control surgery should be followed, with an emphasis on the correction of hypothermia, acidosis, and coagulopathy in the multiply injured patient in whom a simple vascular repair cannot be performed within reasonable time. Definitive vascular repair should be delayed in these circumstances until the patient is stabilized.

Ligation of the injured vessel

All isolated major injuries to the arteries and veins should be repaired, provided the patient is in a stable condition. However, in unstable and multiply injured patients, limb arteries can be safely ligated with little risk of limb loss. The risk of critical limb ischaemia is in the order of 10% after ligation of subclavian, axillary, or superficial femoral arteries. Principles of damage control mean that large veins can be ligated in multiple injuries, at the potential cost of limb oedema.

Temporary intraoperative shunting

The use of shunts prior to formal revascularization in traumatic limb injury is a recognized method to allow reperfusion of an ischaemic limb prior to formal surgery to re-establish blood flow.[11] Most vascular trauma is usually repaired at the patient's initial operation. However, in the presence of polytrauma with orthopaedic injury, temporary measures to establish blood flow in the short term may be indicated.[12] This is usually as a result of establishing stability of fractures, allowing orthopaedic surgeons to anatomically reconstruct limb stability. This allows the manipulation of bony fragments and prevent damage to a tenuous vascular reconstruction. Following this, formal vascular repair can be carried out.

Packing

This is especially useful in difficult circumstances as in pelvic bleeding or retrohepatic injuries of the inferior vena cava. Four quadrant packing of the abdomen is useful to control intra-abdominal bleeding when the source has not initially been identified.

Amputation

In some circumstances, amputation of a limb may be the only option in a proportion of trauma victims. Factors that predict favourable limb salvage include early operation, antibiotics, fasciotomy, and vascular reconstruction with adequate tissue coverage. Blunt trauma carries a much higher risk of limb amputation than penetrating trauma. During amputation of a limb, care must be taken that rehabilitation of the patient is taken into account. Healthy tissue must be preserved at all cost and input with advice from the plastic surgeon is essential in order to maintain as much of a functional limb as possible. For obvious reasons, a below-knee amputation is far better for the patient for rehabilitation and ambulation, compared to an above knee amputation. Finally, the long-term outcome for the patient is determined by the multidisciplinary set up

Box 6.9.2 Complications of vascular trauma

- Acute severe haemorrhage, either external or concealed
- Haemorrhagic shock
- Localized haematoma with potential for secondary infection
- Delayed and recurrent bleeding from a missed arterial injury
- Thrombosis with distal ischaemia, either acute or delayed
- Pseudoaneurysm
- Arteriovenous fistula
- Amputation
- Death

by medical personnel to make sure the patient is managed in the optimum way.

Venous injuries

The commonly injured veins include superficial femoral (42%), popliteal (23%), and common femoral vein (14%). Venous injuries should be repaired provided the patient is stable with an isolated venous injury. However, the principles of damage control should apply in unstable and multiply injured patients, with little hesitation to ligate the injured veins.

Paediatric vascular trauma

The management of vascular injuries in children is especially challenging in view of the small size of the vessels and their tendency to go into spasm. Surgical exposure is challenging and the method of repair should take into account any potential effects on subsequent growth and development of the injured part.

Complications of vascular trauma

A prompt diagnosis and timely treatment is vital in preventing complications of vascular trauma. Any delay in either the recognition or treatment of injury can lead to a rapid deterioration of patients with potential of limb loss and high mortality rate. The complications of severe vascular injury are outlined in Box 6.9.2. Poor prognostic signs include a delay in treatment for >6 hours, blunt vascular injuries, and absence of audible Doppler signal at the first presentation. In addition, patients with established critical limb ischaemia and those with multiple musculoskeletal injuries have a higher incidence of limb loss.

Iatrogenic injuries including intravascular drug abuse

Iatrogenic injuries to the vascular system are increasing.[13] The main specialties at risk of producing iatrogenic vascular injuries are interventional radiology, intensive care, cardiology, general surgery, and orthopaedics. Table 6.9.1 shows the common vessels affected during iatrogenic vascular trauma, the effects of which can be catastrophic, resulting in major limb loss or death.

The common femoral artery is the most common vessel damaged during interventional radiology procedures resulting in false aneurysm, arteriovenous fistula, thrombosis, distal embolization, and limb-threatening ischaemia. Small false aneurysms regress with pressure or respond to the injection of fibrin sealant. Larger defects in the vessel wall will require exploration and repair. Angioplasty and stenting of iliac and infrainguinal arteries can disrupt the vessel wall resulting in massive haemorrhage, which can be life threatening. This can be treated either by placing a stent graft across the injured vessel or by open repair. Iatrogenic vascular injuries may also occur during varicose vein surgery and include femoral venous and arterial injuries.[14]

Intra-arterial injection in drug abuse patients is a common problem encountered by a vascular surgeon. Repetitive injection at a site will initially give rise to an abscess, commonly in the groin region. Pulsatile suppuration at this site should be treated with caution as an incision and drainage will result in uncontrollable haemorrhage due to an underlying mycotic femoral artery aneurysm. An abscess over an artery in an intravenous drug addict should ideally be imaged with an ultrasound to determine the involvement of the underlying artery.

Table 6.9.1 Iatrogenic injury: common vessels injured and method of injury

	Femoral	Radial	Brachial	Abdominal vessels	Other vessels
General surgery	Rarely injured	Rarely injured	Rarely Injured	Most common injury is to mesenteric vessels and aorta	Any surgery within the vicinity of a vessel
Anaesthesia and intensive care	During femoral line insertion	During blood gas analysis and arterial line insertion	During brachial arterial line insertion	Rarely injured	Any other vessel cannulation
Cardiology	During cardiac catheterization	During cardiac catheterization	Not common	During advancement of femoral catheter into abdominal vessels	Rarely injured
Interventional radiology	During access to perform intervention	Rarely injured	During access for intervention	Catheter advancement from the femoral artery	Any vessel cannulation
Orthopaedics	During hip surgery the propunda femoris or its branches	Open or closed fracture fixation of radius and ulna	During fixation of supracondylar fractures	Pelvic surgery causing damage to iliac vessels	Any vessel with close association to bones

Treatment is based around anticoagulating the patient to maintain patency of the remaining vessels, steroid injection to stabilize the inflammatory response, and adequate analgesia. Operative intervention should ensure proximal control prior to entering the infected area. In most cases, the artery is very friable and not suitable for reconstruction and the only option is to ligate the vessel. Some surgeons advocate an extra-anatomic bypass such as an ilio-superficial femoral bypass through the obturator foramen to avoid the infected field and prevent the possible needling of a prosthetic graft.

A prolonged period of intense physiotherapy is required, nevertheless, most patients have a significant functional deficit.[15]

Crush injury and compartment syndrome

Crush injury and compartment syndrome are two conditions that are often synonymous with one another. They have differing pathophysiology. Crush injury occurs when there has been significant pressure on large muscles resulting in their disintegration. Compartment syndrome occurs as a result of swelling following crush injury. This may be due to bleeding within the muscular compartments or as a result of a period of reperfusion and swelling of the muscle compartments if there has been a significant length of ischaemia to the crushed muscle.

Crush injury, which results in fractures and vascular compromise, is associated with reduced rates of limb salvage.[16] Vascular injury can be fairly obvious (Figure 6.9.2), but sometimes there is continuity of the vessel with a subintimal tear, usually as a result of a fracture, which has disrupted the adjoining vessel endothelium. This may give rise to detection of blood flow using a Doppler probe, but if left alone, often results in thrombosis and occlusion of the affected artery. This is especially true in injuries involving the brachial and popliteal arteries.

The management of a crush injury depends on initial resuscitation of the patient followed by prioritizing treatment. In cases where there is a severe orthopaedic injury associated with ischaemia of a limb, it is often more helpful to stabilize the fractured limb prior to definitive vascular repair. The warm ischaemia time for limbs is around 6 hours, following which muscle cell death commences. The warm ischaemia time is also directly related to the severity of

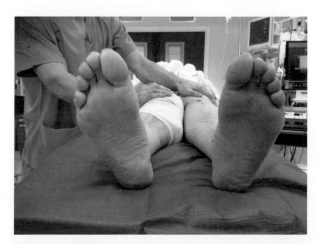

Fig. 6.9.2 A 25-year-old patient following a motorcycle accident resulting in a fracture of his distal right femur and tibial plateau. He sustained a degloving injury of his popliteal fossa and complete transection of his popliteal artery giving rise to an acutely ischaemic limb.

Box 6.9.3 Indications for fasciotomy in patients with vascular injury

- Combined arteriovenous injury
- Crushed soft tissues
- High-velocity missile injury
- Tense leg compartment in blunt trauma
- Following arterial or venous ligation
- Prophylactic, in the absence of above signs

the reperfusion injury. A limb suffering an ischaemic time of over 6 hours will result in a significantly increased reperfusion injury and compartment syndrome.

Treatment of crush injury victims should also involve the judicial use of fluids to maintain perfusion of the kidney by monitoring urine output and the use of osmotic diuretics such as mannitol, correction of the metabolic acidosis, and the associated hyperkalaemia. The patient must be nursed in a high dependency facility with good nursing care.

A decision is usually made at the time of surgery to consider fasciotomy for compartment syndrome. The indications for fasciotomy in patients with vascular trauma are outlined in the Box 6.9.3.

Conclusion

A high index of suspicion is required for the diagnosis of vascular trauma, especially in patients with multiple injuries. Clinical examination for signs of vascular injury is essential. Patients should be adequately resuscitated before further investigations are carried out. However, immediate intervention is indicated in those with active bleeding or rapidly expanding haematoma from an underlying vascular injury. In the absence of hard clinical signs and negative diagnostic imaging, a conservative approach with watchful waiting is justified. Isolated arterial injuries, especially those associated with blunt trauma seen most commonly in current clinical practice can effectively be treated by endovascular stent grafts. Open surgical repair is appropriate in patients with open wounds and requires adequate exposure of proximal and distal segments of the artery. Temporary arterial and venous shunting have been helpful in patients with combined extremity vascular and orthopaedic trauma allowing reperfusion of the distal limb during fixation of fractures before definite vascular repair can be performed. The type of surgical repair depends on the extent of vascular injury, associated injuries, and co-morbid status of the patient. There should be a low threshold to perform fasciotomies in lower limb vascular trauma.

Further reading

Beard JD, Gaines PA. *Vascular and Endovascular Surgery: A companion to Specialist Surgical Practice*, 4th edition. Philadelphia: Saunders, 2009.

Rich NM, Mattox KL, Hirshberg A. *Vascular Trauma*, 2nd edition. Philadelphia: Saunders, 2004.

References

1. Rozycki GS, Tremblay LN, Feliciano DV, *et al*. Blunt vascular trauma in the extremity: diagnosis, management, and outcome. *J Trauma* 2003; 55: 814–24.

2. Fox CJ, Starnes BW. Vascular surgery on the modern battlefield. *Surg Clin N Am* 2007; 87: 1193–211.

3. Barnes CJ, Pietrobon R, Higgins LD. Does the pulse examination in patients with traumatic knee dislocation predict a surgical arterial injury? A meta-analysis. *J Trauma* 2002; 53: 1109–14.

4. Carrillo EH, Spain DA, Miller FB, *et al.* Femoral vessel injuries. *Surg Clin North Am* 2002; 82: 49–65.

5. Dennis JW, Fryberg ER, Veldenz HC, *et al.* Validation of non-operative management of occult vascular injuries and accuracy of physical examination alone in penetrating extremity trauma: 5- to 10-year follow-up. *J Trauma* 1998; 44: 243–53.

6. Gakhal MS, Sartip KA. CT angiography signs of extremity vascular trauma. *Am J of Radiol* 2009; 193: W49–57.

7. Haddock NT, Weichman KE, Reformat DD, *et al.* Lower extremity arterial injury patterns and reconstructive outcomes in patients with severe lower extremity trauma: a 26-year review. *J Am Coll Surg* 2010; 210: 66–72.

8. Brandt MM, Kazanjian S, Wahl WL. The utility of endovascular stents in the treatment of blunt arterial injuries. *J Trauma* 2001; 51: 901–5.

9. Takagi H, Kawai N, Umemoto T, *et al.* A meta-analysis of comparative studies of endovascular versus open repair for blunt thoracic aortic injury. J Thorac Cardiovasc Surg 2008; 135: 1392–4.

10. Reuben BC, Whitten MG, Sarfati M, *et al.* Increasing use of endovascular therapy in acute arterial injuries: analysis of the National Trauma Data Bank. *J Vasc Surg* 2007; 46: 1222–6.

11. Barros D'Sa AA, Harkin DW, Blair PH, *et al.* The Belfast approach to managing complex lower limb vascular injuries. *Eur J Vasc Endovasc Surg* 2006; 32: 246–56.

12. Oliver JC, Gill H, Nicol AJ, *et al.* Temporary vascular shunting in vascular trauma: A 10-year review from a civilian trauma centre. *S Afr J Surg* 2013; 51(1): 6.

13. Giswold ME, Landry GJ, Taylor LM, *et al.* Iatrogenic arterial injury is an increasingly important cause of arterial trauma. *Am J Surg* 1994; 187(5): 590.

14. Rudström H, Björck M, Bergqvist D. Iatrogenic vascular injuries in varicose vein surgery: a systematic review. *World J Surg* 2007; 31: 228–33.

15. Treiman GS, Yellin AE, Weaver FA, *et al.* An effective treatment protocol for intraarterial drug injection. *J Vasc Surg* 1990: 12(4): 456.

16. Odland MD, Gisbert VL, Gustilo RB, *et al.* Combined orthopedic and vascular injury: indications for amputation. *Surgery* 1990; 108(4): 660.

Surgical care of the paediatric patient

Section editor: James A. Morecroft

CHAPTER 7.1

Principles of paediatric surgical care

Nicola R. K. Anders, Laura J. Bowes, and Ross J. Craigie

History and examination of the paediatric patient

Paediatric surgery became a speciality after the recognition of the unique anatomical, physiological, emotional, psychosocial, and surgical conditions that affect infants and children in comparison to the adult population.[1] Centralization of paediatric surgical services as part of the National Service Framework for Children[2] has seen increasing numbers of paediatric surgical patients managed in tertiary centres. Children, however, continue to present at district general hospitals and in those situations they should have immediate access to paediatric medical support and be cared for in an appropriate environment with trained staff.[3]

Differences between the paediatric population and adults mean that their perioperative care should be targeted to the specific conditions that affect them, and a detailed history of their birth, development, immunizations, and medical conditions should form part of the preoperative assessment. As professionals we have a responsibility for the recognition and management of suspected non-accidental injuries.[4] Children may present for emergency surgery as a consequence of non-accidental injury but it is important to be vigilant for signs during unrelated presentations.

History

History of presenting complaint:
  Routine history as for all patients but focusing on specific paediatric conditions and their presentation.

- Pyloric stenosis:
  - male > female
  - first few weeks of life
  - projectile vomiting
  - weight loss
  - dehydration and electrolyte disturbance
  - preoperative nasogastric tube and fluid resuscitation until full correction
  - full blood count (FBC), urea and electrolytes (U&E), capillary blood gases, cross-matched blood.
- Intussusception:
  - 3 months to 3 years, peak incidence at 6 months
  - abdominal pain, vomiting, 'red currant jelly stool'

- severe dehydration and electrolyte disturbance
- may be reduced with barium enema but can require surgery
- preoperative nasogastric tube and fluid resuscitation
- FBC, U&E, cross-matched blood, and 4.5% human albumin solution.
- Appendicectomy:
  - most common cause of acute abdominal pain
  - right iliac fossa tenderness and guarding
  - check FBC and U&E preoperatively
  - intravenous maintenance of fluids preoperatively.
- Testicular torsion:
  - surgical emergency to prevent permanent damage to testis
  - analgesia.
- Adenotonsillectomy:
  - indications: recurrent infections or upper airway obstruction (obstructive sleep apnoea).
- Foreign bodies:
  - aspirated or swallowed
  - 9–24 months years of age
  - wheeze, cough or stridor
  - can cause complete obstruction leading to respiratory arrest.

General review

- Health in general: activity, lively, interactive?
- Normal growth: depending on age review of growth chart in red book (NHS personal child health record).
- Development.
- Appetite/feeding/drinking.
- Changes in personality or behaviour.

Systematic review

- General: fever, rashes (blanching/non-blanching).
- Respiratory: cough (productive/non-productive/duration), wheeze, cyanosis, night sweats, voice changes, shortness of breath, and smokers in the home.

◆ Ear, nose, and throat: recurrent infections, snoring, stridulous breathing, and pauses in breathing at night.

◆ Cardiovascular: murmurs, cyanosis, chest pain, exercise tolerance.

◆ Gastrointestinal: vomiting, diarrhoea/constipation, blood/mucus in faeces, pain, reflux (chronic cough), and weight loss/failure to thrive.

◆ Genitourinary: dysuria, frequency, nocturnal enuresis, wetting, toilet-trained.

◆ Neurological: seizures, headaches, abnormal movements, changes in visual acuity, milestones.

Past medical history

◆ Any antenatal problems identified, maternal obstetric problems.

◆ Mode and events around delivery:
  • gestation
  • birthweight.

◆ Neonatal history:
  • neonatal intensive care unit/SCUBU
  • intubation
  • oxygen therapy
  • light therapy
  • surgical history.

◆ Immunization history.

◆ Congenital abnormalities.

◆ Medical conditions:
  • asthma
  • heart conditions:
    ▪ diagnosis
    ▪ surgery
    ▪ follow-up
    ▪ recent echocardiography/electrocardiography (ECG)
  • epilepsy:
    ▪ type of seizures
    ▪ frequency
    ▪ control
  • renal:
    ▪ dialysis—peritoneal most common in children
    ▪ fluid restriction
    ▪ last dialysis
    ▪ most recent electrolytes
    ▪ anaemia/coagulopathies
    ▪ cardiac failure/hypertension/arrhythmias
  • obstructive sleep apnoea:
    ▪ sleep study
    ▪ evidence of end organ damage secondary to chronic hypoxia—pulmonary hypertension, cor pulmonale and right heart strain (ECG).

◆ Surgical history.

◆ Previous hospital admissions: illness, injury, accident, operations.

Medication

◆ Past and present medication.

◆ Allergies.

Family history

◆ Family tree: consanguinity, positive family history.

◆ Any other family members with same illness.

Social history

◆ Family: parental occupation, housing, relationships, smoking, marital stress, alcohol, poverty, psychiatric illnesses, recent travel.

◆ Is the child happy at home/nursery/school?

Developmental milestones

Failure to achieve developmental milestones may be the first signs of underlying genetic or neurological disorders. Infants and children presenting with failure to meet their milestones initially present to health visitors, general practitioners, or community paediatricians. However, many of these conditions have associations with pathology requiring surgical intervention and knowledge of these associations can assist in the diagnosis and management (see Table 7.1.1).

Clarify with parents any concerns they may have regarding their vision and hearing, reaching of key developmental milestones, bladder and bowel control, temperament and behaviour, sleeping problems, and progress at nursery/school.

Examination

A good rapport with the child and their carers is the first hurdle in a successful examination. Having their cooperation by adapting the examination to suit the child's age and development can improve the information gathered. Examining toddlers and young children requires the doctor to be resourceful and adaptable.

Wash hands before any examination and be sensitive to the child when exposing them for the examination.

All examinations should begin with detailed observation. Signs to aid diagnosis include:

◆ interactions with parents/carers/toys: behaviour and social responsiveness

◆ growth and nutritional status

◆ hygiene and care

◆ position in parents arms/chair/bed

◆ lethargy

◆ pallor or mottling

◆ jaundice

◆ cyanosis: peripheral or central.

Acutely ill children should be recognized quickly and managed rapidly as per Paediatric Advanced Life Support guidelines.[5] After recognizing those children who need further examination, a systematic approach should be used.

Table 7.1.1 Pathology requiring surgical intervention, diagnosis and management

Genetic disorder	Associated surgical pathology	Perioperative considerations
Trisomy 21/Down's Syndrome	Duodenal atresia Hirschsprung's disease ASD/VSD/AVSD/tetralogy of Fallot	Difficult iv access Airway management Risk of hypoglycaemia
VACTERL	Vertebral anomalies—scoliosis Anal atresia/imperforate anus Cardiac/ASD/VSD/Tetralogy of Fallot/truncus arteriosus/transposition of the great arteries Tracheoesophageal fistula Renal agenesis/reflux/obstruction Limb defects	
CHARGE syndrome	Cardiac/ASD/VSD/tetralogy of Fallot Atresia of choanae: unilateral or bilateral Hypospadias/cryptorchidism Scoliosis Exomphalos Swallowing difficulties/aspiration Cleft lip ± palate Oesophageal atresia/trachea-oesophageal fistula	
Cystic fibrosis	Meconium ileus Intussusception Rectal prolapse Nasal polyps	Malabsorption/failure to thrive Chronic respiratory infection/bronchiectasis Diabetes mellitus Pancreatic insufficiency and hyperglycaemia Portal hypertension and oesophageal varices
Duchenne's muscular dystrophy/Becker's muscular dystrophy	Scoliosis Contractures	Respiratory failure Cardiomyopathy Nocturnal hypoxia
Mucopolysaccharidosis: Hunter's, Hurler's	Hepatosplenomegaly Umbilical and inguinal hernias Carpal tunnel syndrome Mitral and aortic valve disease/ASD/PDA Glaucoma Conductive deafness Spinal stenosis Hydrocephalus	Difficult airway management Developmental regression Heart failure/tachyarrhythmias OSA (obstructive sleep apnoea) Restrictive lung disease
Sickle cell anaemia/trait	Splenic autoinfarction	At risk patients should undergo screening using 'Sickledex' test prior to haemoglobin electrophoresis Consider preoperative transfusion if Hb <10 g/dL Hydration and avoidance of hypoxia

ASD, atrial septal defect; AVSD, atrioventricular septal defect; CHARGE, coloboma of the eye, heart defects, atresia of the choanae, retardation of growth and/or development, genital and/or urinary abnormalities, and ear abnormalities and deafness; Hb, haemoglobin; PDA, patent ductus arteriosus; VACTERL, vertebrae, anus, cardiac, tracheesophageal, renal, limb; VSD, ventricular septal defect.

Respiratory system

◆ Respiratory rate: age-dependent (Table 7.1.2).

◆ Work of breathing:
  • nasal flaring
  • expiratory grunting
  • accessory muscles
  • chest wall recession

  • difficulty speaking/feeding

◆ Chest shape:
  • hyperexpansion/barrel chest (e.g. asthma)
  • pectus excavatum or pectus carinatum
  • Harrison's sulcus
  • asymmetry

◆ Stridor or wheeze

Table 7.1.2 Vital signs: variance with age[5]

Age	Respiratory rate (breaths/min)	Heart rate (beats/min)	Systolic blood pressure 5th centile (mmHg)	Systolic blood pressure 50th centile (mmHg)
Under 1 year	30–40	110–160	65–75	80–90
1–2 years	25–35	100–150	70–75	85–95
2–5 years	25–30	95–140	70–80	85–100
5–12 years	20–25	80–120	80–90	90–110
Over 12 years	15–20	60–100	90–105	100–120

Reproduced with permission from M. Samuels and S. Wieteska, Basic Life Support, in *Advanced Paediatric Life Support: The Practical Approach (APLS), Fifth Edition*, John Wiley and Sons, Oxford, UK, Copyright © 2012.

- Cyanosis
- Clubbing
- Palpation:
  - expansion
  - trachea
  - apex displacement due to mediastinal shift
- Auscultation:
  - quality and symmetry of breath sounds
  - stridor
  - wheeze
  - crackles
  - transmitted sounds

Cardiovascular system

- Cyanosis
- Clubbing
- Pulse:
  - rate
  - rhythm
  - volume
- Respiratory distress
- Operative scars: sternotomy or left lateral thoracotomy
- Palpation:
  - apex beat
  - thrill (palpable murmur)
- Auscultation:
  - heart sounds
  - murmurs: systolic/diastolic/continuous
  - radiation
- Hepatomegaly
- Femoral pulses
- Blood pressure

Gastrointestinal system

- Eyes:

- jaundice
- anaemia
- Tongue:
  - colour
  - coating
  - fissures
  - ulcers
- Clubbing
- Abdominal distension:
  - fat
  - fluid (ascites)
  - faeces (constipation)
  - flatus (malabsorption/obstruction)
  - fetus (needs to be excluded in postpubertal females)
- Localized abdominal distension:
  - upper abdomen: pyloric stenosis/hepatomegaly/splenomegaly
  - lower abdomen: bladder/masses/fetus
- Dilated veins/striae
- Operative scars
- Peristalsis (obstruction: pyloric stenosis/intestinal)
- Palpation:
  - organomegaly
  - tenderness/guarding
  - masses
- Auscultation:
  - increased bowel sounds: obstruction/diarrhoea
  - reduced or absent bowel sounds: paralytic ileus/peritonitis

Genitourinary system

Examination of the genital area is routine in young children but tends to only be performed in older children when it is clinically indicated based upon previous history.

- Inguinal region—hernia/undescended testes
- Discharge

- Perineal rash
- Males:
  - normal size penis?
  - well-developed scrotum?
  - palpable testes?
  - scrotal swellings?
- Females:
  - normal external genitalia?

Neurological system

Observing the child play, draw, or write can give important information about the child's development and neurology. Other observations include:

- Walking and coordination
- Inspection of limbs
- Muscle tone
- Power
- Reflexes
- Plantar responses
- Sensation
- Cranial nerves
- Consciousness: Glasgow Coma Scale and Children's Coma Scale.

Blood glucose should not be forgotten as part of any paediatric examination. All children, in particular infants, can become hypoglycaemic when unwell. Glucose should be monitored and corrected.

Paediatric surgery is very much a multidisciplinary speciality involving paediatricians, neonatologists, paediatric surgeons and anaesthetists, nurse specialists, ward nurses and play specialists, and frequently many other individuals. The desired end result is a happy child and family who have felt reassured, supported and well informed throughout the process, starting from the outpatient referral to discharge home postoperatively. Good communication and thorough preparation can achieve this in most situations.

Perioperative care of the paediatric surgical patient

Over the last 20 years there have been tremendous advances in perinatal and neonatal care, resulting in neonates born at the margin of viability who may require surgical interventions. Anaesthetic management of these babies has to take into consideration the immature function of many vital organ systems as well as the effects of the presenting disease and the resulting physiological derangements. Significant disabilities associated with extreme prematurity can be short term (e.g. respiratory distress syndrome, bronchopulmonary dysplasia, persistent patent ductus arteriosus, intraventricular haemorrhage, and necrotizing enterocolitis) or long term (e.g. cerebral palsy, chronic lung disease, and failure to thrive)[6]

Ground-breaking work by Anand and Aynsley-Green in the 1980s demonstrated that neonates are capable of experiencing pain and mounting a stress response that can be blocked by adequate anaesthesia and analgesia.[6] In view of this, neonates deserve the same respect as adults undergoing surgery, and the right to

sufficient anaesthesia with particular attention paid to maintain physiological homeostasis.

Preoperative assessment should include a detailed history, including antenatal details and birth and neonatal history up to and including the presenting complaint. It is important to establish the weight and 'corrected age' in any baby born prematurely. This will influence the risk of apnoeic episodes and the need for elective postoperative respiratory support, active temperature control measures, specific fluid management, etc.

Physical examination should start with a detailed observation of the skin. Signs include:

- lanugo in premature neonates
- dry cracked peeling skin in post-term babies
- pallor or mottling
- peripheral or central cyanosis
- jaundice.

The skull and face should be observed for:

- size, shape symmetry of skull with attention to fontanelles and suture lines
- position of ears
- position of mandible (to anticipate difficult intubation)
- size of tongue
- cleft lip or palate.

Central nervous system:

- level of alertness, pitch/frequency of cry
- posture and tone
- administration of sedative or paralysing drugs.

Respiratory system:

- signs of respiratory distress ('grunting', tachypnoea, nasal flaring, chest wall recession, tracheal tug, cyanosis).

Cardiovascular system

- colour and capillary refill time
- blood pressure and peripheral pulses (all 4 limbs)
- palpation of the apex and auscultation of the heart sounds
- presence of oedema (check sacrum).

Abdomen and genitalia:

- excess saliva (exclude oesophageal atresia)
- scaphoid abdomen (e.g. congenital diaphragmatic hernia), or distended abdomen
- umbilical cord (normally 2 arteries and 1 vein)
- exomphalos or gastroschisis
- hepatomegaly or splenomegaly
- anus (imperforate or abnormally placed anus may be associated with other abnormalities)
- ambiguous genitalia (can be associated with congenital adrenal hyperplasia)
- hypospadias, undescended testes, hydrocele, or hernia.

The presence of one abnormality should always lead to the suspicion of other associated abnormalities, for example, VACTERL association where there are abnormalities in some or all of vertebrae, anus, cardiac, tracheoesophageal, renal, limb, or the presence of a large tongue with exomphalos and hypoglycaemia in Beckwith-Wiedemann syndrome.

Anatomical and physiological differences in a neonate

Airway and respiratory complications are the most common causes of morbidity during general anaesthesia in children. The airway changes in size, shape, and position throughout its development from the neonate to the adult. Firstly neonates have a proportionally larger head and occiput relative to body size. This causes neck flexion and potential airway obstruction when lying supine. The ideal position for the neonatal airway to be kept open is with the head in the neutral position often with some support under the shoulders. Neonates are obligate nasal breathers and if their smaller nasal apertures become obstructed by secretions, blood or oedema, the work of breathing may be significantly increased. This may also contribute to airway difficulties during general anaesthesia. The tongue is relatively large, causing a reduction in the size of the oral cavity and a tendency to contribute to airway obstruction.[7] This is exacerbated by decreased muscle tone.

More distally, the narrowest part of the airway, the cricoid cartilage, is of small calibre and a complete ring, and so the presence of mucosal oedema at this level will severely compromise the airway. If neonates are intubated for prolonged periods of time or on repeated occasions, they are at risk of developing subglottic stenosis in later infancy or childhood.

The thorax is round with horizontal rib orientation that restricts the expansion potential of the chest. The bony elements are softer and more flexible, which tends to cause chest wall collapse during increased efforts at inspiration, and airway collapse at rest. To help overcome this neonates have a rapid respiratory rate with a short expiratory time.

The main inspiratory muscle is the diaphragm. This is relatively flat in the neonatal period. At birth the diaphragm has a relatively high percentage of oxidative fibres (types I, IIa, and IIc) that are fatigue resistant. Over the first 6 months the type I and IIb fibres increase in proportion, whereas type IIa decrease and IIc completely disappear.

Oxygen transport

Fetal erythrocytes contain fetal haemoglobin (HbF) that has a higher oxygen carrying capacity and oxygen affinity than haemoglobin in adults. The purpose of this is to facilitate movement of oxygen from mother to fetus. During the first year of life the proportion of HbF falls from 75% to 7% of total haemoglobin.

The high oxygen affinity of HbF is disadvantageous after birth, and levels of 2,3-DPG rise significantly in the first 5 days to enable the huge increase in oxygen consumption at this time to be met.

Apnoea

Apnoeic attacks are defined as repeated episodes of absence of respiratory movements for >20 seconds or shorter episodes associated with bradycardia and/or colour change. Recurrent apnoeic episodes are very common in premature infants. They may be central or obstructive in origin (or mixed).

Obstructive apnoea occurs when the upper airway becomes totally occluded while the baby is still making regular, increasing respiratory efforts. This may be seen in infants with Pierre-Robin

sequence or trisomy 21 where the tongue falls back to cause airway obstruction.

In central apnoea, both respiratory effort and airflow cease and apnoea occurs at the end of expiration.

Mixed apnoea initially appears like central apnoea; however, the baby then starts to make intermittent respiratory efforts without achieving airflow (indicating airway obstruction). Causes include:

- lung disease and hypoxaemia
- airway obstruction
- cerebral oedema or haemorrhage
- infection
- anaemia
- metabolic disturbance
- rising environmental temperature
- drugs (including post-anaesthesia)
- gastro-oesophageal reflux
- prematurity.

Clinical implications of cardiac adaptation at birth

Structural congenital heart disease occurs in about 0.8% live births. This may be caused by chromosomal abnormality, exposure to maternal infection or drugs, syndromes, maternal disease, or in association with other abnormalities (e.g. VACTERL, exomphalos, etc.)

It may present as:

- heart failure
- collapse
- cyanosis
- asymptomatic.

Signs of neonatal heart failure include:

- poor feeding
- unexpected weight gain
- mottled skin, clammy, poor perfusion
- tachycardia
- hepatomegaly
- respiratory distress, 'head bobbing'
- gallop rhythm
- oedema.

Cardiac conditions presenting with heart failure include heart muscle disease, arrhythmias, arteriovenous malformation, or structural disease (e.g. hypoplastic left heart, coarctation, truncus arteriosus, ventricular septal defect, and transposition of the great arteries).

Collapse may be the presenting feature of arrhythmias or duct-dependent circulation following duct closure.

Cyanosis may be caused by conditions where there is common mixing such as total anomalous pulmonary venous connection or truncus arteriosus. Cyanosis may also be a result of conditions causing right-to-left shunting of blood such as pulmonary atresia, tetralogy of Fallot, or in transposition of the great arteries.

However, other causes such as persistent pulmonary hypertension of the newborn must also be considered, along with respiratory causes of cyanosis.

Murmurs are common in the neonatal period, and are often innocent. However, all babies should have a full examination and if the murmur persists beyond the age of 48 hours they should have a chest X-ray, electrocardiogram, and undergo regular observations of heart rate, respiratory rate, feeding, and daily weight. An infant with an asymptomatic murmur should not be allowed home until it is clear that no form of duct-dependent congenital heart disease is present. This is usually self-evident on clinical grounds, but if there is any doubt, echocardiography is indicated.

Patent ductus arteriosus

Clinically apparent patent ductus arteriosus (PDA) occurs in about 75% infants of birth weight under 1 kg and 10–15% of those 1.5–2kg. The more premature and sick the neonate, the higher the likelihood the PDA will remain open. PDA is associated with high-volume peripheral pulses, systolic murmur radiating to the back, a need for respiratory support, and cardiomegaly with pulmonary plethora on chest X-ray.

It is important that cardiac function is optimized preoperatively. Fluids should be restricted to 75% maintenance, hypoxia should be avoided, and diuretics may be considered, as well as indomethacin or surgical ligation. However closure of the ductus will cause acute deterioration in duct-dependent pulmonary circulations (worsening cyanosis) and systemic circulations (shock and heart failure).

Preoperative investigations

Blood tests should always include a FBC, U&E, and blood glucose.

A ventilated patient should always have a recent blood gas. Other appropriate blood tests include serum bilirubin, liver and bone profiles, C reactive protein, and a coagulation screen.

Imaging investigations should include:

- chest X-ray (in ventilated patient, chronic lung disease, bronchopulmonary dysplasia, to ascertain position of central line, recent chest infection, etc.)
- abdominal X-ray ± contrast/scans (intestinal perforation, malrotation, etc.)
- head scan (ultrasound) in premature neonate at risk of intraventricular haemorrhage.
- ECG/echocardiograph murmurs are common in neonatal period, but if present for longer than 48 hours should be investigated. Any neonate with features of any condition associated with congenital cardiac disease should be investigated preoperatively)

Perioperative nutritional management

Neonates, as with all patients preoperatively, must be fasted.

Guidelines from the Royal College of Anaesthetists state that a patient must be fasted 6 hours for food (including formula milk, fluids with 'thickeners', fruit juice), 4 hours for breast milk, and 2 hours for clear fluids.

However, neonates have inadequate glycogen stores and a tendency to hypoglycaemia, so intravenous access should be established before fasting is commenced and 10% dextrose infusion commenced as maintenance. Additional crystalloid or colloid may also be required to replace losses preoperatively to replace any existing fluid deficit (e.g. as in intestinal obstruction, vomiting,

perforation, or gastroschisis, etc.). A nasogastric tube should be passed in any sick baby or in the presence of intestinal obstruction so nasogastric losses can be accurately replaced with equivalent volumes of appropriate crystalloid (Hartmanns) solution. Neonates have reduced oesophageal motility and there is prolonged gastric emptying in premature and sick babies, so there should be a high index of suspicion that despite fasting according to the guidelines, the stomach may well not be empty.

Signs of dehydration include decreased urine output, decreased skin turgor, sunken anterior fontanelle, sunken eyes, tachypnoea, tachycardia, drowsiness, and irritability. Replacement fluid should be given as isotonic crystalloid (Hartmanns solution) or colloid (usually 4.5% albumin) in aliquots of 10 mL/kg followed by physical assessment and regular blood gas sampling looking for correction of acidosis. This should be in addition to the dextrose maintenance.

Any neonate receiving total parenteral nutrition should have this discontinued preoperatively and a 10% dextrose infusion commenced.

Most neonates will require about 150 mL/kg/day maintenance fluid. It is important to remember situations where this may vary, for example, in the presence of cardiac abnormalities or renal impairment where fluid is restricted, or in the first few days of life when fluids are gradually increased to maintenance, or when there may be an increased fluid requirement such as in prematurity or in a neonate receiving phototherapy for jaundice.

Intraoperative considerations

Positioning

For the vast majority of surgical procedures, the neonate will be positioned supine on the operating table. There are various different types of warming mattresses upon which the baby will lie, or hot air blowing blankets.

The neonate should be lying with the head in the neutral position supported by a gel head ring. Although the baby will almost certainly be intubated, it is important to take great care that the position is as natural as possible. As the environment becomes so warm, the endotracheal tube becomes very prone to kinking and great care must be taken to also support the tube as proximally to the baby as possible.

As much padding as possible should be used to protect vulnerable areas. The skin of a neonate is very delicate and easily damaged by removal of dressings (especially adhesive surgical drapes), ECG electrodes, and pressure areas. Once the baby is prepared for surgery it is of utmost importance that instruments or surgical assistants are not resting on any part of the covered child! Clear drapes are frequently used to cover the head and chest so the upper part of the baby is clearly visible at all times.

For procedures requiring lithotomy position, small rolled towels are often used to support the legs. It is important to make sure the legs are of equal height and distance from the midline. The legs need to be gently secured with paper tape and padding.

For a thoracotomy (e.g. for tracheoesophageal fistula), consideration needs to be given to extra support for the overhead arm and padding between the legs. Tape with padding or table extensions to prevent the baby rolling sideways must also be carefully positioned.

The prone position (e.g. for excision of sacrococcygeal teratoma), requires support under the chest and pelvis allowing the abdomen to be unrestricted. If the abdomen is compressed this will compromise venous return and ventilation through diaphragmatic splinting.

The arms must lie rostrally, pronated along the sides of the head, symmetrically and padding must be applied under the knees and elbows. The head should be gently supported to one side with care taken over the positioning of the endotracheal tube. It is important to inspect the eyes and ears to ensure there is no pressure on them.

In any position it is crucial to inspect the whole patient after final positioning before the surgical drapes go on. Access to intravenous cannulae or invasive monitoring, position of urimeter, temperature monitoring, etc., needs to be easily manageable throughout the operation. It is also necessary to consider whether X-ray or image intensification will be required intraoperatively as that may affect the position on the table.

Anaesthesia

Regardless of which anaesthetic technique is used (general or regional anaesthesia or a combination of both), the aim is to reduce the humoral stress response, pain, and emotional distress. General anaesthesia aims to produce unconsciousness removing any perception of experience and amnesia. Neonates are extremely sensitive to painful stimuli, and preterm neonates even more so. Not surprisingly, decreased stress responses have been associated with improved clinical outcome in terms of morbidity and mortality postoperatively.[8] However, over-aggressive management of perioperative pain has its own morbidity (bradycardia, hypotension and respiratory depression side effects of opioids).

In the vast majority of cases neonates undergo general anaesthesia for surgery. (Exceptions to this may include inguinal herniotomy, which could be performed under combined caudal/spinal regional anaesthesia). However, to minimize the use of postoperative opioids, regional techniques are frequently used in addition to general anaesthesia. Perineal or lower abdominal surgery can be well covered by a caudal block and this is routinely carried out. Other blocks which can be used include transverse abdominis plane blocks, and paravertebral, rectus sheath, penile, axillary, and femoral nerve blocks. Ultrasound guidance has revolutionized our ability to visualize the structures and more accurately place small volumes of local anaesthetic close to the peripheral nerves.

In some parts of the world, especially where resources are scarce, the potential benefits of regional anaesthesia are even more important. Minimizing use of opioids can significantly reduce ventilator days and PICU stay.[9]

Induction of anaesthesia usually takes place within the operating theatre as minimum movement decreases the risk to the baby and preserves heat. Either an intravenous or inhalational technique is used, followed by administration of a muscle relaxant. Most neonates are intubated even for short procedures. The tube position should be checked by auscultation (ensuring equal air entry bilaterally) and capnography.

Anaesthesia is usually maintained with a mixture of oxygen, air, and inhalational agent, as well as with muscle relaxation and analgesia (often a combination of opioids, paracetamol and local anaesthesia). Ventilation is usually pressure controlled to minimize the risk of barotrauma, aiming for tidal volumes of 7–10 mL/kg.

Monitoring

All neonates should have continuous intraoperative monitoring of:

- ECG
- pulse oximetry
- non-invasive blood pressure
- core and peripheral temperature
- capnography
- inhalational agent
- inspired oxygen
- airway pressure.

In certain situations it may be necessary for invasive monitoring:

- central venous access for central venous pressure monitoring (if significant fluid losses are expected), inotrope infusions, poor peripheral access
- arterial line for accurate 'beat to beat' monitoring of blood pressure, sampling for estimations of blood gases, haemoglobin, blood glucose, etc.
- oesophageal Doppler for monitoring of cardiac output.

All neonates should be commenced on intravenous maintenance fluid preoperatively from the onset of fasting. However, in many situations one intravenous cannula may not be sufficient for all the fluids (maintenance, replacement of losses, blood and products) and drugs (antibiotics, anaesthetic agents, analgesia) that are required. Adjuncts such as local warming, transillumination, epidermal nitroglycerine, ultrasound guidance, and peripheral venous cut down are useful when intravenous access is difficult.[10] Alternative sites may need to be considered (e.g. inside wrist, scalp, dorsum of foot, etc.).

Central venous access may be required intraoperatively for the reasons indicated above, but also for long-term administration of drugs or parenteral nutrition.

In the event of intravenous access being very difficult to establish an intraosseous cannula should be considered.[11] These cannulae are:

- quick to insert
- landmarks are easily identified
- success rates are high (85% in babies)
- complications are infrequent
- variety of drugs and fluid can be administered.

Recommended sites of insertion are:

- proximal tibia: most common site in children
- distal tibia: just above centre of medial malleolus
- distal femur: approached from anterior aspect.

Complications are uncommon but include:

- dislodgement of the cannula (10%)
- extravasation around the needle
- failure to penetrate the cortex producing haematoma and severe tissue necrosis (particularly with hypertonic solutions e.g. bicarbonate, glucose, catecholamines or cytotoxic drugs) and compartment syndrome
- subcutaneous abscess
- osteomyelitis with prolonged infusion
- tibial fracture (babies).

Temperature control

The neutral thermal environment is defined as the ambient temperature range which leads to minimal O_2 consumption (so the body temperature remains normal with the minimum metabolic effort). The stress of allowing a neonate to cool may result in increased oxygen consumption and energy expenditure leading to hypoxia and acidosis, hypoglycaemia, pulmonary hypertension, increased capillary permeability, general impairment of enzyme activity, and a reduction in surfactant production.

Premature and sick neonates have a further reduced ability to control body temperature because of high surface area to mass ratio and little subcutaneous fat, significant transepidermal water losses, rapid depletion of brown fat stores, and immature temperature regulatory mechanisms by the hypothalamus.

The infant can increase heat production in response to cold stress by non-shivering thermogenesis. The release of catecholamines causes oxidative phosphorylation of brown fat (found around the scapulae, mediastinum, poles of kidneys, and adrenal glands) and release of energy in the form of heat. A newborn infant can double his rate of heat production by this mechanism.

In order to optimize the temperature of a neonate in the perioperative period the anaesthetist has to be meticulous about minimizing heat loss.

- The ambient temperature is maintained at 30C.
- Baby minimally exposed: covered in blankets where possible, bonnet, warm cotton wool.
- Warm intravenous fluids.
- Humidify inspiratory gases.
- Warm gel mattress to lie on.
- Warm air blankets.
- Warm irrigation fluids.
- Warm incubator for transfer back to ward.

Assessment of the injured child and Advanced Paediatric Life Support

Trauma is the most frequent cause of death in children over the age of 1 year, yet compared to adults, the absolute number of children involved in major trauma is low. Despite this, all clinicians who are responsible for the care of trauma patients must be familiar with the assessment and initial management of children. Assessment should follow Advanced Paediatric Life Support (APLS) [5] protocols that mirror adult Advanced Trauma Life Support using the mnemonic ABCDE, though consideration is given to the anatomical, physiological, and psychological differences between children and adults. This includes an awareness that the normal ranges of vital signs vary with age (see Table 7.1.2).

The majority of paediatric trauma is as a result of blunt trauma, with road traffic accidents and falls being the most common mechanisms of injury. Children suffer different injury patterns as compared to adults even when involved in similar accidents. The small size of the child leaves them susceptible to multiple injuries from a single impact, e.g. the bumper of a motor vehicle that causes lower limb injury in an adult can result in head, chest, and abdominal injuries in a child. Penetrating injury accounts for less than 10% of injuries; however, this is increasing in some urban areas. Although the majority of trauma is unintentional, non-accidental injury should always be considered, especially where there is an inconsistent history, or the suggested mechanism of injury and the injuries sustained do not correlate. When non-accidental injury is suspected, the patient must be referred to the local safeguarding team.

Effective paediatric trauma management requires a systematic team approach. A brief history should be obtained from the paramedics, though the initial priority is the primary survey: airway and cervical spine control, breathing, circulation and control of haemorrhage, disability, and exposure (ABCDE). Life-threatening problems should be treated as they are identified.

The paediatric airway is narrower, shorter, and softer than in the adult. A small amount of mucosal swelling results in a greater reduction in the diameter of the airway as compared to the adult and the risk of obstruction from small foreign bodies is increased. The large occiput in young children results in flexion of the neck which, in combination with a soft airway, results in collapse and obstruction. Hyperextension of the neck in young patients also results in obstruction of the airway, therefore a neutral position is required to maintain airway patency. Consideration should also be given to the effects of the large occiput on cervical spine alignment. During high-force trauma, the inherent elasticity of the ligaments of the paediatric vertebral column in combination with a large head renders the spinal cord susceptible to damage in the absence of bony injury: spinal cord injury without radiological abnormality (SCIWORA). This should be suspected in patients who have transient or permanent symptoms and or signs of neurological deficit.

Evaluation of breathing involves assessing for signs of respiratory distress including nasal flaring, tachypnoea, and intercostal/sternal recession, and by examination of the chest. Haemothorax and pneumothorax are relatively common, and if encountered, should be treated by immediate insertion of a chest drain. Incomplete ossification of the ribs results in increased thoracic compliance and transfer of energy to intrathoracic organs causing severe intrathoracic injuries even in the absence of rib fractures. When present, rib fractures indicate extreme force and are commonly associated with other injuries.

Circulation is assessed by heart rate, perfusion, and pulse volume. Hypotension is a late sign of hypovolaemia as children can remain normotensive until over 25% of blood volume is lost, therefore prolonged capillary refill time and tachycardia are more reliable signs of hypovolaemia. It is important to remember that small volumes of blood loss can represent a significant amount of the child's total blood volume. Insertion of two large bore cannulae is obligatory, but where intravenous access is impossible large volumes of fluid, including blood, can be administered through intraosseous needles. Currently, it is recommended that fluid be administered in aliquots of 10 mL/kg, with re-assessment after each bolus, up to a volume of 40 mL/kg when blood should be given and a surgical opinion sought.[1]

The relatively large head as compared to body size increases risk of head injury with neurological injury accounting for 80% of trauma deaths. Diffuse axonal injury and cerebral oedema are most common, with less than 10% of injuries having a surgically treatable haemorrhage. Neurological assessment can be challenging and must take into account the child's developmental age and an appreciation that a scared child is less cooperative. Where a head injury is suspected, a computed tomogram scan must be performed and a neurosurgical opinion sought.

High surface area to body mass ratio in children results in rapid heat loss so exposure of the child during the primary survey should be kept to a minimum.

Following the primary survey and emergency treatment, a secondary survey is performed and definitive management carried out.

References

1. Lloyd DA (ed.). *Paediatric Surgery: Standards of Care*. London: British Association of Paediatric Surgeons, 2002.
2. *National Service Framework for Children, Young People and Maternity Services*. London: Department of Health, Department for Education and Skills, 2004.
3. National Confidential Enquiry into Patient Outcomes and Death. *Surgery in Children: Are We There Yet? A Review of Organisational and Clinical Aspects of Children's Surgery*. London: National Confidential Enquiry into Patient Outcomes and Death, 2011.
4. National Institute for Health and Care Excellence. When to suspect child maltreatment, Clinical Guideline 89. Available from https://www.nice.org.uk/guidance/cg89 (accessed July 2015).
5. Advance Life Support Group. *Advanced Paediatric Life Support: The Practical Approach*, 5th edition. Oxford: John Wiley and Sons, 2011.
6. Boat AC, Sadhasivam S, Loepke AW, *et al*. Outcome for the extremely premature neonate: how far do we push the edge? *Pediatr Anesth* 2011; 21: 765–70.
7. Adewale L. Anatomy and assessment of the pediatric airway. *Pediatr Anesth* 2009; 19(suppl. 1): 1–8.
8. Weber F. Evidence for the need for anaesthesia in the neonate. *Best Prac Res Clin Anaesthesiol* 2010; 24: 475–84.
9. Bosenberg AT, Johr M, Wolf AR. Pro con debate: the use of regional vs systemic analgesia for neonatal surgery. *Pediatr Anesth* 2011; 21: 1247–58.
10. Simhi E, Kachko L, Bruckheimer E, *et al*. A vein entry indicator device for facilitating peripheral intravenous cannulation in children: a prospective, randomised, controlled trial. *Anesth Analg* 2008; 107(5): 1531–5.
11. Peutrell JM. Intraosseous cannulation. *Anaesth Intensive Care Medicine*. London: The Medical Publishing Company Ltd, 2002: 452–5.

CHAPTER 7.2

Principles of child protection and safeguarding

Alison Pike, Kalpesh Dixit, and Hilary Smith

Introduction to Child Protection

Safeguarding and promoting the welfare of children refers to the process of protecting children from abuse or neglect, preventing impairment of their health and development, and ensuring they are growing up in circumstances consistent with the provision of safe and effective care that enables children to have optimum life chances and enter adulthood successfully.[1]

Child protection is part of this safeguarding and is the process of protecting individual children identified as either suffering or likely to suffer significant harm as a result of abuse or neglect.[1] The Children Act 1989 introduced the concept of significant harm as the threshold that justifies compulsory intervention in family life in the best interests of children and gives the local authority a duty to make enquiries to decide whether they should take action to safeguard or promote the welfare of the child.

Arrangements for Safeguarding Children

These are set out in the document 'Working Together to Safeguard Children'.[1] This covers the legislative requirements and expectations on individual services to safeguard and promote the welfare of children, and provides a framework for Local Safeguarding Children Boards to monitor the effectiveness of local services. Similar documents are produced by departments of the devolved governments in Wales, Scotland, and Northern Ireland.

Local safeguarding children boards

Local safeguarding children boards (LSCBs) were established in every local authority area in England as a requirement of the Children Act 2004. Each board is responsible for agreeing how the relevant organizations in their area will cooperate to safeguard and promote the welfare of children, and for ensuring the effectiveness of what they do.

Representatives are drawn from all the local organizations that commission or provide services for children and young people. For the health service, this includes clinical commissioning groups, area teams, and provider trusts. Boards must also have access to expertise and advice from a designated doctor and nurse for safeguarding. The designated professionals are responsible for providing advice to commissioners of health services, and supporting and supervising those with lead safeguarding responsibilities in provider organizations. They also have a role in ensuring that appropriate training is available for all health staff.

Provider organizations

All organizations have a safeguarding team with a named doctor and nurse who have a key role in promoting good practice. They provide advice and expertise for fellow professionals on safeguarding matters and ensure appropriate safeguarding training is in place in the organization. They will work closely with the organization's safeguarding lead, the designated professional, and the LSCBs.

Serious Case Reviews

When a child dies and abuse or neglect are known or suspected to be a factor, the Local Safeguarding Children Board must undertake a serious case review to establish what lessons can be learned about the way in which the local professionals and organizations worked individually and together in order to safeguard future children. A serious case review may also be held when a child sustains potentially life-threatening injury or suffers serious harm through abuse (including sexual abuse) or neglect. Review panels have an independent chair and receive internal management review reports from all organizations involved with the child(ren) and family. The review report is published, with an emphasis on identification of areas for learning and improvement.

Child death overview panel (CDOP)

This panel is a statutory subcommittee of the LSCB and is responsible for reviewing all the available information relating to the deaths of children normally resident in their area. The collection and analysis of information is intended to identify matters of concern affecting the safety and welfare of children in the area, and any wider public health or safety concerns arising from a particular death or pattern of deaths. The CDOP may refer cases back to the LSCB for consideration of a serious case review.

In addition, when a child has died unexpectedly, the CDOP must ensure that there is a coordinated 'rapid response' that brings together relevant professionals to make immediate enquiries and evaluate the circumstances of the death, and ensure the family receive appropriate support and information.

Understanding child protection law and children's rights

Children's rights are enshrined in the Convention on the Rights of the Child that was adopted by the United Nations (UN) in 1989. The 54 Articles set out how children everywhere are entitled to special protection so that they can develop in conditions of freedom and dignity, and are protected from neglect, cruelty and exploitation. In addition, every child and young person has the right to the best possible health and health services, and for his or her views to be given due weight depending on age and maturity.

Children Act 1989 and Children Act 2004

In the United Kingdom, the principles of the UN convention on children's rights were incorporated into the Children Act 1989. The Act makes the welfare of the child paramount, and requires those working with children and young people to ensure that safeguarding and promoting their welfare forms an integral part of their care. Specific sections of the Act cover the duties of local authorities towards Children in Need (Section 17), and children for whom there is reasonable cause to suspect that a child has suffered or is likely to suffer significant harm (Section 47). There are also a range of powers that permit emergency action to safeguard children. These include emergency protection orders, which give authority for a child to be removed and placed under protection, and police protection orders, which allow the police to remove a child to a suitable accommodation or to prevent the removal of a child from hospital.

The Children Act 2004 builds on the 1989 Act and adds the requirement for organizations to cooperate with the local authority and to ensure that their services recognize the need to safeguard and promote the welfare of children. The 2004 Act also established the role of Children's Commissioner for England, and requires local authorities to appoint a Director of Children's services and identify an elected lead member for children's services who is ultimately accountable for delivery of services.

Messages from key reports

Lord Laming led the enquiry into the death of Victoria Climbie and reported in 2003, making wide-ranging recommendations that influenced the 2004 Children Act. Lord Laming produced a further report in 2009 following the death of Peter Connolly, leading to changes in the training and management of social workers. A 2011 report by Professor Eileen Munro called for a more child-focused system, and has heavily influenced the 2013 revision of Working Together.

Criminal law has also been amended following child deaths with a new offence of 'causing or allowing the death of a child', and a further amendment extending the offence to 'causing serious physical harm'.

Responsibilities of doctors in protecting children and young people

Good Medical Practice states that 'all Doctors must safeguard and protect the health and wellbeing of children and young people'.[2]

All Doctors need to be aware of the risk factors that have been linked to abuse and neglect and look out for signs that a child or young person may be at risk, whether they are dealing directly with children and their families or treating adult patients. Doctors working with children and young people must have the knowledge and skills to recognize signs and symptoms of abuse and neglect.[3]

All doctors have a duty to act on any child protection concerns; they must have a working knowledge of local policies and procedures for protecting children and young people in their area. A doctor's first concern must be the safety and care of the child: they must ensure the clinical needs of children and young people continue to be met and are not overshadowed by child protection concerns.[3]

The intercollegiate document 'Safeguarding Children and Young People: Roles and Competencies for all Healthcare Staff (2014 updated)[4] outlines a set of abilities that enable staff to effectively safeguard, protect, and promote the welfare of children and young people. Doctors must work within their competence to deal with child protection issues and keep up to date with best practice and undertake training appropriate to their role.

Parental responsibility

Parental responsibility is the rights and responsibilities that parents have in law for their child, including the right to consent to medical treatment for them until they reach 18 years in England, Wales, and Northern Ireland and 16 years in Scotland.

Mothers and married fathers automatically have parental responsibility as do unmarried fathers of children born after 15th April 2002 in Northern Ireland, after 1 December 2003 in England and Wales, and after 4th May 2006 in Scotland as long as the father is named on the birth certificate. Unmarried fathers before these times, or since if not named on the birth certificate, do not automatically have this responsibility; they can acquire it through a parental responsibility agreement with the mother or a parental responsibility order through the courts.

Parental responsibility is not lost unless a child is adopted. Parental responsibility is shared with the local authority when a child is 'looked after' and is subject to a care order. Adoptive parents gain parental responsibility with the adoption order; it can also be gained by carers through a special guardianship order or residence order awarded through the courts.

Consent

The General Medical Council states that treatment can be provided to a child and young person with their consent if they are competent to give it or with the consent of a parent or the court. Emergency treatment can be provided without consent, to save the life of or prevent serious deterioration in the health of a child or young person.[2] (see Chapter 4.4)

The capacity to consent is not age dependant, but for those under 16 years consideration should be given as to whether the young person is able to understand the nature, purpose, and possible consequences of investigations or treatment as well as the consequences of no treatment. If they can understand, retain, and use this information and communicate it to others, they can consent. At 16 years a young person is presumed to have this capacity and can legally give consent. Consent should be assessed on an individual basis considering the complexity and importance of the decision. If a young person cannot give consent, this is sought from the person with parental responsibility for the child.

If a young person has the capacity to consent, but refuses to do so, this cannot be overridden by either medical staff or the parents; similarly, if the person with parental responsibility withholds consent, legal advice should be sought if the view is that the treatment is in the best interests of the young person.

Box 7.2.1 Risk factors for abuse

◆ Parental factors: history of cruelty in their own childhood, physical or mental illness, learning difficulties, substance misuse, domestic violence

◆ Factors in the child: premature or demanding baby, any special needs

◆ Environmental factors: Overcrowding, poverty, poor support network

Recognizing the possibility of abuse or maltreatment

Child abuse can be seen in all sections of society, but there are recognized factors that are more commonly seen in children who are suffering abuse (see Box 7.2.1). The absence of these features should not deter from suspecting abuse if the presenting features suggest this.

Definitions and features of the different types of abuse

For full definitions please see 'Working Together to Safeguard Children'[1] and 'Alerting Features' from National Institute of Health and Care Excellence guidance.[5]

Physical abuse

Physical violence, punishment, and aggression directed towards children constitutes physical abuse and includes hitting, shaking, scalding, drowning, suffocating, poisoning, and fabrication or induction of illness in the child (see Figures 7.2.1 and 7.2.2; Table 7.2.1).

Neglect

Neglect is defined as the persistent failure to meet a child's basic physical and/or psychological/emotional needs, likely to result

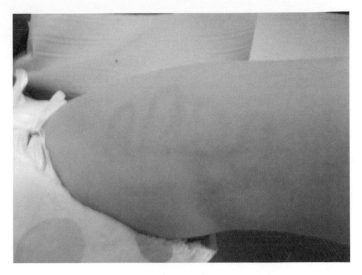

Fig. 7.2.2 Imprint from hand slap to the thigh.
Reproduced courtesy of Solent NHS Trust.

in the serious impairment of the child's health or development. Neglect includes inability to protect, supervise, or ensure access to appropriate medical care (see Table 7.2.2).

Table 7.2.1 Alerting features for consideration and suspicion of physical abuse

Alerting features to *consider* child maltreatment	Alerting features to *suspect* child maltreatment
Any serious or unusual injury	Bruising in shape of hand, ligature, stick, teeth mark, grip or implement
Cold injuries (swollen, red hands/feet) or Hypothermia	Bruising or petechiae, that are multiple (bruising) or in clusters, of similar shape and size,
Oral injury (e.g. torn frenulum)	Lacerations/abrasions/scars that are multiple or of symmetrical distribution
	Burns/scalds: shape of implement or pattern of forced immersion (e.g. glove and stocking)
	Fractures, especially of different ages
	Retinal haemorrhage or eye injury
	Intracranial haemorrhage without an explanation, especially if under 3 years, or associated with other injuries (or with multiple subdural haemorrhages)
	Spinal, intra-abdominal or intrathoracic injury without major accidental trauma
With an absent or unsuitable medical explanation	Without a suitable explanation or a discrepancy between account and injury
	In the absence of a medical disorder (e.g. coagulopathy or predisposition to fragile bones)
	On parts of the body that are not normally exposed or on non-bony parts
	Child who is not independently mobile

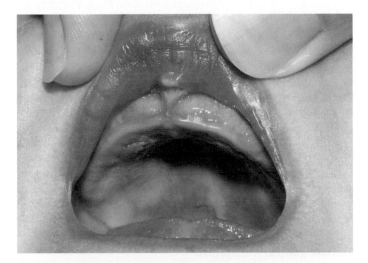

Fig. 7.2.1 This baby's mother took him to the general practitioner at aged 7 weeks with facial bruising and the torn frenulum was noted. Further investigation showed five rib fractures and a fractured metacarpal.
Reproduced courtesy of Solent NHS Trust.

Source: data from National Institute for Health and Care Excellence (NICE), *When to suspect child maltreatment*, NICE Clinical Guidelines 89, Copyright © NICE 2009, available from https://www.nice.org.uk/guidance/cg89/resources/guidance-when-to-suspect-child-maltreatment-pdf

Table 7.2.2 Alerting features for consideration and suspicion of neglect

Alerting features to *consider* child maltreatment	Alerting features to *suspect* child maltreatment
Severe persistent infestations	Not following medical advice compromising health
Delay in seeking treatment	Smelly and dirty
Failed appointments	Inadequate home environment (including hygiene, safety, food)
Missed child health surveillance	
Inappropriate clothes	
Poor growth and development	
Inadequate supervision causing injury	

Source: data from National Institute for Health and Care Excellence (NICE), *When to suspect child maltreatment*, NICE Clinical Guidelines 89, Copyright © NICE 2009, available from https://www.nice.org.uk/guidance/cg89/resources/guidance-when-to-suspect-child-maltreatment-pdf

Table 7.2.3 Alerting features for consideration and suspicion of emotional abuse

Alerting features to *consider* child maltreatment	Alerting features to *suspect* child maltreatment
Behaviour or emotional state inconsistent with age and development without medical explanation (e.g. withdrawn, clingy)	Scavenges or hoards food
Responsibilities interfere with activities	Indiscriminate, precocious or coercive sexualized behaviour
Marked behaviour change	
Extreme responses	
Self-harm/running away/deliberate soiling or wetting	

Source: data from National Institute for Health and Care Excellence (NICE), *When to suspect child maltreatment*, NICE Clinical Guidelines 89, Copyright © NICE 2009, available from https://www.nice.org.uk/guidance/cg89/resources/guidance-when-to-suspect-child-maltreatment-pdf

Emotional abuse

Persistent emotional maltreatment, so as to cause severe and persistent adverse effects on child's emotional development, constitutes emotional abuse. This includes conveying to the child their worthlessness, being unloved, imposing developmentally inappropriate expectations, overprotection, limitation of learning, bullying (including cyber bullying), and causing children to feel frightened, exploited or corrupted (see Table 7.2.3). This may occur alone although is involved in all types of abuse.

Sexual abuse

Sexual molestation of children, whether penetrative or non-penetrative, forced or coerced, involvement in looking at sexual activities or encouragement to behave in a sexually inappropriate way, constitutes sexual abuse (see Table 7.2.4).

Differential diagnosis

The main differential diagnosis is accidental trauma. Bruises which occur in mobile children are usually limited to extensor surfaces and bony prominences, and the explanation given is consistent with the injury seen. It is important to exclude conditions that may predispose to bruising (e.g. idiopathic thrombocytopenic purpura or haemolytic

Table 7.2.4 Alerting features for consideration and suspicion of sexual abuse

Alerting features to *consider* child maltreatment	Alerting features to *suspect* child maltreatment
Sexually transmitted infections including hepatitis B, anogenital warts	An allegation
Persistent anogenital discomfort or symptoms	Persistent recurrent anogenital symptoms with a change in behaviour
Pregnancy under 16 years	Anogenital injury without explanation
	Sexually transmitted Infection less than 13 years
	Unusual sexualized behaviour especially in a pre-pubertal child

Source: data from National Institute for Health and Care Excellence (NICE), *When to suspect child maltreatment*, NICE Clinical Guidelines 89, Copyright © NICE 2009, available from https://www.nice.org.uk/guidance/cg89/resources/guidance-when-to-suspect-child-maltreatment-pdf

uraemic syndrome) or fractures (e.g. osteogenesis imperfecta or rickets) or that may look similar (e.g. impetigo to burns).[6,7]

Investigations

A thorough history and examination are key to the determination of abuse.

Investigations are often not needed, but in unexplained bruising haematological investigations, including a blood count and coagulation tests, should be undertaken to rule out coagulopathy. In unexplained fractures, biochemical tests (bone profile, vitamin D levels) should be undertaken.[6]

All infants less than 2 years with abusive or inadequately explained intracranial trauma, or infants less than 1 year with signs of physical abuse should have neuroimaging (computed tomogram scan) and fundoscopic assessment. A full skeletal survey is indicated in all infants less than 1 year old with suspected physical abuse.[6,8]

Photographs of injuries need to be taken for documentation and future reference in case of legal proceedings.

Fabricated illness

Children with suspected fabricated or induced illness may present to the full range of medical specialists. Fabricated illness needs to be considered when the child's history, presentation, examination, or investigations are discrepant with a recognized clinical condition. There may be a poor response to treatment with the onset of new symptoms. The history of events may be unlikely and there is often frequent and varied medical consultations causing limitation of a child's activities and wellbeing.

When fabricated illness is suspected, health practitioners should not discuss their concerns with carers immediately. A senior clinician should be informed and the case discussed with the named doctor for safeguarding and local pathways should be followed.[9]

Female genital mutilation

Female genital mutilation (FGM) or female circumcision is considered child abuse in the UK and is illegal. It comprises all procedures involving the partial or total removal of the female external genitalia or other injury to the female genital organs for non-medical reasons. If a child is identified as being at risk of FGM or has had FGM, this information must be shared with social care and the police. It is then their responsibility to investigate and safeguard and protect any girls or women involved.[10]

Appropriate referral pathways

All doctors need to be familiar with their organization's local safeguarding pathway and know what actions to take when abuse is suspected. These include:

- Recording in writing concerns about a child's welfare, including whether or not further action is taken.

- Informing a senior colleague.

- Notifying the safeguarding team who may then carry out further assessments as necessary. If there is no dedicated safeguarding team, notification should be made directly to children's social care.

- The police should be informed immediately in the case of alleged or suspected sexual abuse or assault, presentation of a seriously injured child to a medical setting, or if there is a threatened removal of a child thought to be in danger.

- Children's social care and police also need to be informed if abuse or neglect are suspected, where the circumstances indicate that the child or siblings are unprotected or if serious abuse has been witnessed.

- Hospital admission is indicated for medical investigations, treatment of injuries, or if the family and social situation necessitates an emergency place of safety for the child and siblings until this is found by social care. If a child is admitted to the hospital, the decision to discharge the child is made by the consultant in discussion with the safeguarding team and with appropriate notification of other professionals prior to discharge.

Documentation relating to child protection

Record keeping

This is of paramount importance as records may be needed for legal purposes. All records should include:

- Documentation of accounts given verbatim.

- The examination findings in detail.

- A list of personnel present.

- Who the lead professional responsible for the care of the child is.

- Subsequent discussions, communications and any contact details relating to the assessment.

- Specific documentation about any discrepancies in the history and examination.

- Observations about any emotional accompaniments as well as limitations to the history.

- Any opinion formulated explained in detail giving reasons.

- All entries signed and dated with documentation of grade of the professional.

Reports

Care must be taken in the preparation of any report as it may be used as medical evidence in court.

Any report should follow a sequential pattern, starting with the doctor's details and qualification followed by detailed history and examination, clear professional opinion considering appropriate differential diagnosis and the reasons for the opinion. It is often a good idea to crosscheck the report with a colleague.

Police statements, if needed, are filled out on specific forms.

All reports need to be signed and dated with documentation of grade of the professional.

Communicating effectively

Effective communication between doctors and children and young people is essential to the provision of good care.[2]

- Involve the child and young person in discussions about their care.

- Give them time.

- Be open and honest with the child and their parents.

- Listen to them, respect their views and take them seriously.

- Give the opportunity to ask questions and respond to their concerns and questions.

- Explain in a way they understand.

- Give the child or young person the opportunity to be seen alone if they wish.

Good communication with parents is essential and doctors should be sensitive and responsive in providing information and support. When there are concerns about a child's welfare, the doctor should tell the parents of their concerns, explain their professional duty to act and explain how this will be done, and advise them where they can get support. If there is uncertainty about whether telling parents will cause further risks to the child, advice should be sought from a designated or named professional or a lead clinician first. Parents should be kept informed about what is happening and given opportunities to ask questions. Being open and honest with parents and avoiding judgemental comments, encourages families to cooperate.

Doctors must work with and communicate effectively with colleagues in their team and organization, and with other professionals and agencies.

Confidentiality and information sharing principles

Confidentiality is an essential part of good care. There are principles that apply when using, sharing or disclosing information about children and young people or adults and include:[7]

- Disclose information that identifies the patient only if necessary.

- Inform the patient about how this information will be used.

- Ask for consent before disclosing information that may identify them.

- Keep disclosures to a minimum.

The duty of confidentiality to children is the same as for adults and consent should be sought before sharing information. If consent is refused by either a competent child or adult with parental responsibility, then information should not be shared unless withholding the information puts the child at risk of harm. A disclosure is required by law or if there is an overriding public interest in the disclosure.

In safeguarding situations, information can be shared without explicit consent according to the following principles:[3]

+ Information sharing should be proportionate to the risk of harm.

+ If in doubt, seek further advice from a named or designated professional, lead clinician, experienced colleague, or the Caldicott guardian, or from a professional body, defence union, or the General Medical Council.

+ It is possible to justify raising a concern, even if it turns out to be groundless, if this has been done honestly and on the basis of reasonable belief through the appropriate channels.

+ Doctors have a duty to share their concerns if a child or young person is at risk of harm.

Sharing information with the right people can help protect children and young people from harm and ensure they get the help they need.

Conclusion

All professionals who come into contact with children and families have a responsibility to be alert and able to identify symptoms and triggers of abuse and neglect, share information appropriately, and work together to safeguard children.

Recommended reading

Department for Education. *Working Together to Safeguard Children: A Guide to Inter-Agency Working to Safeguard Children*. DFE-00130-2015, 2015.

Royal College Paediatrics and Child Health. Intercollegiate Document— Safeguarding Children and Young People: Roles and competencies for Healthcare Staff 3rd edition), 2014.

References

1. Department of Education. *Working Together to Safeguard Children*. London: HM Government, 2015.
2. General Medical Council. *0-18 years: Guidance for all Doctors*. London: General Medical Council, 2012.
3. General Medical Council. *Protecting Children and Young People: The responsibilities of all Doctors*. London: General Medical Council, 2012.
4. Royal College Paediatrics and Child Health *Intercollegiate Document— Safeguarding Children and Young People: Roles and competencies for Healthcare Staff* 3rd edn. London: Royal College Paediatrics and Child Health,2014.
5. National Institute for Health and Care Excellence. NICE Clinical Guidelines 89: When to suspect child maltreatment. Available from https://www.nice.org.uk/guidance/cg89/resources/guidance-when-to-suspect-child-maltreatment-pdf.
6. Royal College Paediatrics and Child Health. *Child Protection Companion* 2nd edn. London: Royal College Paediatrics and Child Health, 2013.
7. Barker J, Hodes D. *The Child in Mind: A Child protection Handbook* (3rd edn) New York, NY: Routledge, 2007).
8. Kemp A. Abusive head trauma: Recognition and the essential investigation. *Arch Dis Child Educ Pract Ed* 2011; 96: 202–8.
9. Department fo Education. *Safeguarding Children in whom Illness is Fabricated or Induced*. Supplementary guidance to working together to safeguard children. London: HM Government, 2013
10. Department of Education. *Female Genital Mutilation*. Supplementary guidance to working together to safeguard children. London: HM Government, 2013.

CHAPTER 7.3

Common paediatric surgical conditions

James A. Morecroft and Ross J. Craigie

Pyloric stenosis

Pyloric stenosis is defined as hypertrophy of the circular muscle layer of the pyloric sphincter that results in a narrowing of the gastric outlet. It is the most common cause of gastric obstruction in children and one of the most frequent reasons for surgical intervention in infants.

Incidence of pyloric stenosis

Pyloric stenosis occurs in 2-4 per 1000 live births. There is a 4:1 male to female ratio with infants of Caucasian descent being most commonly affected. It is uncommon in Asian and African populations.

Aetiology of pyloric stenosis

The cause of pyloric stenosis remains unknown but is thought to be multifactorial with proposed aetiologies including: increased gastric acidity causing pyloric spasm and muscle hypertrophy, abnormal innervation of the pylorus, and a reduction in pacemaker cells causing abnormal motility. A genetic component is suggested by the fact that 20% of males and 7% of females of an affected mother, and 5.5% of males and 2.5% of females of an affected father, develop pyloric stenosis.

Presentation of pyloric stenosis

Presentation is between 3 to 6 weeks of age, with either gradual or rapid onset of forceful projectile vomiting that occurs shortly after feeding. The vomit is always non-bilious but may be coffee ground as a result of gastritis or oesophagitis. The infant remains hungry and if the symptoms have been prolonged there will be significant dehydration, weight loss, and failure to thrive. This is now rare due to increased awareness of the condition and earlier referral. Differential diagnosis includes gastro-oesophageal reflux, over feeding, sepsis from any source, and rarely, intracranial pathology and other obstructive conditions such as duodenal web.

Diagnosis of pyloric stenosis

Following a thorough examination of the infant, a test feed should be performed. Once the infant is relaxed, visible peristalsis, and upper abdominal distension may be seen. Gentle and progressively deep palpation over the right upper quadrant and epigastrium reveals a palpable mobile firm olive-shaped mass. Where the mass is not felt but clinical suspicion remains, an ultrasound should be performed. Single-wall thickness of greater than 3 mm and length of greater than 15 mm is diagnostic of pyloric stenosis (Figure 7.3.1). Upper gastrointestinal contrast is rarely required but if performed, reveals a narrowed pyloric channel.

Other investigations include full blood count, biochemistry profile and capillary blood gas. Loss of hydrogen and chloride, and to a lesser extent potassium and sodium, from persistent vomiting results in the picture of hypochloraemic, hypokalaemic metabolic alkalosis. As the infant becomes more dehydrated, aldosterone acts to absorb sodium and water from the distal tubules and collecting ducts of the nephron. This is associated with further loss of potassium and hydrogen in the urine resulting in paradoxical aciduria. The low chloride level causes renal tubular absorption of bicarbonate with the sodium, worsening the metabolic alkalosis.

Management of pyloric stenosis

Prior to any surgical intervention it is imperative to correct the deranged metabolic picture as alkalosis prolongs the depression of the respiratory drive and may result in apnoeas and hypoventilation postoperatively.

The infant is placed nil by mouth and a nasogastric tube is inserted. Intravenous fluids of 0.45% saline and 5% dextrose with 10 mmol KCl per 500 mL should be commenced at 150 mL/kg/day.

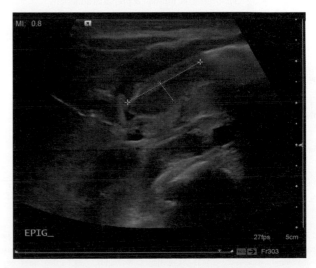

Fig. 7.3.1 Ultrasound image of pyloric stenosis indicating length of muscle hypertrophy.

KCl should not be added where there are concerns regarding poor urine output. Nasogastric losses are replaced with normal saline and 10 mmol KCl per 500 mL. Serum electrolyte levels and the metabolic status of the patient should be rechecked every 12 hours until corrected.

Ramstedt's pyloromyotomy is performed through either an open (periumbilical) or laparoscopic approach. A longitudinal incision is made in the serosa from the pyloroduodenal junction proximally on to the anterior wall of the stomach. The hypertrophic muscle fibres are then divided by blunt dissection to reveal the bulging mucosa. Adequate myotomy is confirmed when the muscle either side of the myotomy move independently. Leakage of bile or air indicates mucosal perforation necessitating repair with an omental patch. Postoperative feeding regimes vary; however, early introduction of feeds is associated with earlier discharge with no significant increase in vomiting.

Pyloromyotomy is associated with a low incidence of complications. Rates of infection and wound dehiscence are 1%. Mucosal perforation occurs in 1–4%, and, although postoperative vomiting affects up to 31% of patients, incomplete myotomy is exceedingly rare.

Non-operative management of pyloric stenosis with atropine is rarely used and is reserved for cases where surgical intervention is not possible.

There are no long-term sequelae and as such, routine follow-up is not required.

Phimosis

Introduction to phimosis

Phimosis is the normal physiological condition in which the foreskin covers the glans penis. During development the inner layer of the foreskin is adherent to the glans and separation of these two layers usually starts from the foreskin meatus and proceeds proximally towards the coronal sulcus allowing the foreskin to retract. The age at which retraction is possible is variable and Figure 7.3.2 shows the percentage of boys at a given age who still have a physiological phimosis or residual preputial adhesions.

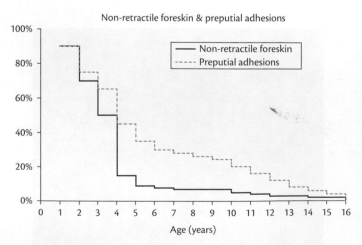

Fig. 7.3.2 Prevalence of non-retractile foreskin and preputial adhesions with age.
Source: data from Gairdner D., The Fate of the Foreskin: A Study of Circumcision, *British Medical Journal*, Volume 2, Issue 4642, pp. 1433–7, Copyright © 1949; and Oster J., Further fate of the foreskin: Incidence of preputial adhesions, phimosis, and smegma among Danish schoolboys, *Archives of Disease in Childhood*, Volume 43, Issue 228, pp. 200–3, Copyright © 1968.

Incidence of phimosis

There is a sharp drop in incidence up until about 6 years of age when 8% foreskins are not retractile, followed by a more shallow reduction up to 16 years of age when only 1% remain non-retractile.

If separation of the foreskin occurs proximally prior to distal separation, sebum accumulates in the coronal sulcus and forms a preputial pearl. This will discharge spontaneously once distal separation occurs. Pathological phimosis can occur because of scarring, either secondary to forcible retraction or ballanitis xerotica obliterans.

Management of phimosis

Circumcision involves removal of the foreskin and reattaching of the shaft skin to the coronal sulcus. Application of corticosteroids can be used to increase the suppleness of the foreskin as an alternative to circumcision.

Undescended testis

Introduction to the undescended testis

The testes develop on the posterior abdominal wall in relation to the developing kidneys and descend to the scrotum in two phases: an initial intra-abdominal phase results in the testis reaching the internal inguinal ring, and this is followed by an inguino-scrotal phase that takes the testis through the inguinal canal and into the scrotum. The gubernaculum 'steers' the testis by its main attachment to the scrotum, but also has other attachments that can result in the testis being drawn into an ectopic position such as the inner thigh or perineum. However, 95% testes are in the scrotum at birth increasing to 99% at 1 year of age.

Diagnosis of undescended testis

Clinical examination involves placing the thumb and forefinger of the non-dominant hand to cover both external rings, suppressing the cremasteric reflex and preventing escape of the testes from the scrotum; the examining hand can then assess the degree of tension upon the spermatic cord. If a testis cannot be felt, the examining hand sweeps down the inguinal canal while the non-dominant hand is removed and then reapplied. A normal testis can be brought to the bottom of the scrotum without any undue tension. Retraction due to the cremasteric reflex is normal and does not require treatment.

Management of undescended testis

An undescended testis cannot be brought to the bottom of the scrotum and orchidopexy should be performed to preserve testicular function. Eighty per cent of undescended testes are palpable along the line of descent from superficial inguinal ring towards the scrotum. A testis may be impalpable because it is within the abdomen or because it has undergone a neonatal catastrophe such as extravaginal torsion leading to atrophy of the testis. Laparoscopy is useful to differentiate these causes, and in performing a two-stage orchidopexy if the testis is intra-abdominal, as the vessels then are usually short preventing a standard type of orchidopexy.

Inguinal orchidopexy is performed similar to inguinal herniotomy by first separating the spermatic cord from the processus remnant, gently mobilizing the vessels and placing the testis well down in the scrotum within a subdartos pouch.

Prognosis of undescended testis

Unilateral undescended testis is associated with a reduced fertility but normal paternity rate, whereas if the condition is bilateral, paternity is also decreased. Undescended testes were associated with a higher malignant potential when orchidopexy was commonly performed later in childhood. Now that orchidopexy is performed around 1 year of age the increased risk has become negligible.

As an intra-abdominal testis rarely functions and has an increased malignant potential, orchidectomy rather than orchidopexy may be considered, particularly in an older boy with a normal contralateral testis.

Hernias

Introduction to hernias

The common sites for abdominal wall hernias in childhood are inguinal, umbilical, epigastric, and femoral.

Inguinal hernia and infantile hydrocoele

Aetiology of inguinal hernia and infantile hydrocoele

Inguinal hernia in children is related to persistence of the processus vaginalis that is involved in testicular descent. Normally this out-pouching of peritoneum around the descending testis closes at the internal inguinal ring once descent is complete. It is more common in boys, but can also occur in girls (male to female ratio is 3:1). A narrow processus allows small amounts of peritoneal fluid to collect around the testis causing a hydrocoele. There is a high rate (95%) of spontaneous resolution of such hydrocoeles and surgical intervention is usually reserved for persistence after 3 years of age.

Presentation of inguinal hernia and infantile hydrocoele

Enlargement of the processus can result in an indirect inguinal hernia. Both inguinal hernias and hydrocoeles transilluminate in childhood. With a hydrocoele, the swelling is usually confined to the scrotum, whereas an inguinal hernia can be reduced back through the inguinal canal. Encysted hydrocoeles can occur as a swelling separate from the testis in boys or in the labia majora of girls.

Incarceration of bowel in an inguinal hernia can lead to vascular compromise of the testicle in boys and in girls an ovary can herniate alongside the bowel and be at similar risk.

The risk of incarceration is inversely related to age, and inguinal hernias should be repaired as soon as possible. Thirty-three per cent of children with hernias present with incarceration and a further 5% develop incarceration between diagnosis and referral.

Management of inguinal hernia and infantile hydrocoele

Inguinal herniotomy rather than herniorraphy is performed in children. The indirect inguinal sac is separated from the vas and vessels in boys and transfixed at the level of the internal inguinal ring; in girls the sac should be opened to confirm that the ovary or fallopian tube is not within the sac before similar closure.

Umbilical hernia

Following separation of the umbilical stump the defect in the midline fascia around the umbilical vessels closes through cicatrization. It is common for this to result in an umbilical hernia in the first few months of life; however, 95% of these will resolve without any intervention. If the defect persists after 3 years of age, surgical closure can be considered although the risk of incarceration of such a hernia is very low in the UK. Umbilical hernia is more common in black African and black Caribbean children.

Epigastric hernia

An epigastric hernia is a small midline lump anywhere between the xiphoid process and the umbilicus caused by extraperitoneal fat herniating through a defect in the linear alba. In contrast to other abdominal wall hernias, these never have a peritoneal sac and incarceration of bowel cannot occur. The herniated fat may become strangulated, causing pain and swelling but if allowed to settle with analgesia, the swelling and defect will usually resolve. Surgical closure of the defect can be performed, but recurrence is common as the linea alba is thin around the defect reducing the chance of a sound surgical repair and the resulting scar is often more unsightly than the original lump.

Divarification of the recti is apparent in younger children in whom the rectus abdominus muscle has not yet developed the strength and size seen in adults, thus leading to a midline bulge between the sternum and umbilicus when the child attempts to sit from lying. No treatment is necessary.

Femoral hernia

Occasionally a groin swelling in a child turns out to be a femoral rather than inguinal hernia. The clinical features are less obvious than in the adult patient and the diagnosis is most often made when at operation an indirect inguinal sac is not found or the lump persists following inguinal herniotomy. Laparoscopy may be useful in both diagnosis and treatment. Care must be taken with regard to closure of the femoral canal, as this can risk vascular compromise in a growing child.

Further reading

Blumhagen JD, Maclin L, Krauter D, et al.Sonographic diagnosis of hypertrophic pyloric stenosis. *Am J Roentgenol* 1988; 150(6): 1367–70.
Gairdner D. Fate of the foreskin. *Br Med J* 1949; 2 (4642): 1433–7.
Oster J. Further fate of the foreskin. Incidence of preputial adhesions, phimosis, and smegma among Danish schoolboys. *Arch Dis Child* 1968; 43(228): 200–3.

Management of the dying patient

Section editor: Bill Noble

CHAPTER 8.1

Management of the dying patient in consultation with the palliative care team

Katharine Burke, Simon Noble, Bee Wee, and Bill Noble

Introduction

While the role of the hospice can be traced back to the time of the Roman Empire, the medical speciality of palliative medicine was only formally recognized in the United Kingdom by the Royal College of Physicians in 1987 and in the United States of America as a sub-specialty by the American Board of Medical Specialities in 2006. An understanding of how palliative care can integrate with surgical practice and familiarity with local team can greatly enhance the ward and outpatient care management of the patient. However, it should be acknowledged that unfamiliarity with other specialties can lead to poor appreciation of roles and consequently inappropriate use of each other's expertise. Since surgery is often the only definitive cure for many cancers, a close working relationship with the palliative care team may seem counterintuitive. However, palliative care services have developed in line with the medical and surgical innovations that have improved patient survival, and as such the role of a palliative care team extends far beyond that of providing terminal care. There are even data within the lung cancer population that suggest that lung cancer patients receiving early palliative care experience less depression, increased quality of life, and survive 2.7 months longer than those receiving standard oncologic care.[1] Patient referrals between surgical and palliative care services are rarely a one-way process in which a surgeon seeks assistance to manage the care of a dying patient or discharge a patient from an acute surgical ward; it is not uncommon for palliative care teams to request surgical colleagues to perform surgical procedures with the intent to alleviate complex symptoms.

Palliative care services

Since palliative care teams see patients throughout their disease, at varying stages of their illness, it is necessary that they offer a range of care within the acute hospital, community, and hospice setting. This may range from managing the physical symptoms in patients receiving treatment for cancer, to treating depression in patients with advanced disease, to the care of patients in their last days and hours. Much of the work involves helping patients with complex or severe physical, psychological, social, and spiritual problems. In the UK over half of patients are improved sufficiently to return home.

Palliative care hospital support teams

The surgical team is most likely to encounter palliative care services in the acute hospital setting. Within the UK, it is a minimum requirement that all new cancer diagnoses are discussed in a cancer multidisciplinary team meeting and that access to palliative care input at the point of diagnosis is available where necessary. Most multidisciplinary teams will have a palliative care team member present, especially for cancers that commonly present with severe symptoms (such as upper and lower gastrointestinal cancers) and those with poor prognosis (such as lung cancer).

The first UK hospital palliative care team was set up in St Thomas Hospital, London in 1976.[2] Over the following 30 years more than 300 services have been established, such that access to specialist palliative care is now a minimum requirement for all acute hospitals. The service includes providing supportive care and symptom control expertise alongside the current hospital treatment, assessment for transfer to hospice, advising on prognosis, and discharge support. However, since 1976, hospital teams have become involved at earlier stages in disease trajectories and have broadened referral case loads to include patients with non-malignant disease. For most services feature a multidisciplinary team consisting of physicians, pharmacists, registered nurses, nursing assistants, social workers, hospice chaplains, physiotherapists, occupational therapists, complementary therapists and volunteers.

Ongoing access and interaction with the hospital specialist palliative care team will ensure patients receive appropriate supportive and palliative care during their inpatient stay. For patients in the terminal stages of their illness, the team is able to provide support in managing end of life care as well as support for family members. For many, the main role for the palliative care team will be to provide ongoing advice as to the most appropriate symptom management and support of patients no longer requiring an acute hospital environment. While the promise of admission to a hospice may appear an easy way of planning a discharge with the patient and their family, it is not always available or the preferred place to continue management. An understanding of the other services available will allow teams to identify the best way to plan future patient care.

National Health Service palliative care units

While the majority of specialist palliative care inpatient units are owned and run by the voluntary sector as hospices, some hospices are wholly funded and run by the National Health Service (NHS). Several hospitals have inpatient palliative care units on site. Criteria for transfer or admission tend to be focused on management of complex symptoms that require intensive monitoring and intervention or ongoing access to support from the acute hospital service. Such examples would include the management of patients with epidural or intrathaecal pain delivery systems, those requiring frequent radiotherapy sessions, intensive rehabilitation, infusions, and those with specialist nursing needs such as tracheostomy management or the containment of severe delirium. They are rarely used for the provision of simple terminal care alone and the average bed stay of such units tends to be less than 14 days.

Hospice care

The first modern hospices was founded in London in 1960s and provided end of life care to patients with terminal cancer. While today's hospices are still concerned with the provision of end of life care, the scope of services has expanded. As the disease trajectory of malignant disease has changed, so to has hospice care. Patients are no longer solely admitted to die; many are admitted for control of symptoms that cannot be resolved at home or within the acute sector. As such the discharge rate of hospice admissions varies between 40–50% with an median length of bed stay around 13 days. The other difference in today's hospices is that their remit has expanded beyond cancer with advanced non-malignant diseases such as end-stage respiratory, cardiac, and neurological conditions being supported as well. Hospices rarely provide long-term care for patients, so transfers of patients with longer or uncertain prognoses should only be done with the expectation that they will be transferred or discharged.

Home care

The majority of patients when asked would prefer to have their end of life managed in their own home. Even those who would prefer to die in a hospice or hospital are likely to spend the most of their terminal illness in the community setting.

It follows that supporting patients and their families to remain in their own environment for as long as possible not only delivers patient-centred care, but also avoids unnecessary admissions to acute sector facilities. The level of community support will vary between regions but several components will be core to all services. General practitioners are key, often the clinician in overall charge of the patients care, usually supported by a palliative care clinical nurse specialist and district nurses. Depending upon the patient's needs, provision of allied health professional support, social services, and basic nursing care may also be available.

Integrated palliative care with a comprehensive range of specialist palliative care services delivered in the community is available in some centres. It is seen as a cost-effective alternative to hospice admission, but will require a radical reorganization of funding streams and coordination of palliative care within localities to become mainstream.

Palliative medicine clinics

Many palliative care services now offer outpatient clinics where patients can be referred for ongoing symptom management.

Various models have been established. Palliative care clinics within the NHS outpatient service may run in isolation, but the preferred model is to run the clinics in parallel with other services such as surgical and or oncology clinics. This allows optimum continuity of care with the opportunity for clinicians to refer patients quickly. In joint or parallel clinics the transition to supportive or palliative management is more seamless and less distressing for patients. It also allows for the provision of ongoing support by the clinic staff who may be involved with the patients care throughout the terminal illness.

Day hospice

Many hospices offer palliative care outpatient services within the environment of the hospice grounds. They are able to offer ongoing symptomatic support as well as access to the day hospice facilities that may include physiotherapy, occupational therapy, benefits advice, and advance care planning. For many patients, this outpatient model provides an introduction to the hospice service for those who may later need end of life care. The disadvantages of such a model are that many independent hospices are located off site and as such may not have access to diagnostic facilities such as blood tests and radiology access that a hospital outpatient service would provide. However, the provision of social care, rehabilitation, occupational and art therapy in a supportive environment go together to offer weekly day-respite to the carers of many hospice outpatients.

Education and training

Most palliative care organizations offer education and training for colleagues as part of their range of service. Surgical colleagues may find these study days and courses helpful in terms of formal knowledge and skills development as well as the opportunity to share experiences and learn from these. Since 2010, an e-learning programme has been available, covering assessment, symptom management, communication skills, and other areas relevant to end of life care. These are available free of charge to professionals working in the UK and with a subscription cost to those outside the UK (www.e-elca.org.uk). In the rest of this section, the relevant e-learning session numbers are listed for ease of reference.

The medical management of distressing symptoms

A variety of drugs are now used to control symptoms and those used at the end of life should be chosen with no less consideration for safety and avoidance of adverse reactions. Drug interactions, deteriorating renal function, drug interactions, metabolic abnormalities, poor hepatic function, poor cognition, and changing therapeutic priorities all play a part in the clinical decisions around prescribing in the dying patient.

Analgesics

e-ELCA sessions 04-07 (Assessment of pain), 04-08 (Principles of pain management), 04-09 (Drug management of pain – core knowledge)

Pain is a common symptom at the end of life, particularly in the context of cancer, and one which engenders fear. Patient's reporting of pain remains the gold standard of pain assessment, as pain is a subjective experience. Do not rely on single observations, or your own preconceptions about a patient's pain. Instead, conduct careful and regular assessments of your patient's symptoms and use these to form a management plan for pain control.

The oral route is usually preferable (unless there are significant problems with absorption, for example in severe dysphagia or bowel obstruction). Analgesics should be prescribed regularly in cases of constant pain, with additional 'breakthrough' analgesia as required. The World Health Organization analgesic ladder describes three classes of analgesics: non-opioids, weak opioids, and strong opioids, as well as adjuvant drugs. The the ladder may be useful when thinking about analgesia for patients at the end of life.[3] However, each person's response is unique, so an individual approach must be taken and referral to specialist palliative care teams must be made if the patient does not readily respond to straightforward analgesic regimes.

Non-opioids are drugs such as paracetamol and non-steroidal anti-inflammatory drugs (NSAIDs). The mechanism of action of paracetamol is still incompletely understood, but is probably active centrally to prevent the conversion of inactive cyclooxygenase (COX) to active oxidized COX.[4] It is an effective and safe drug, though caution should be taken in patients with extremely low body weight or pre-existing severe hepatic impairment. There have been case reports of death after unintentional overdose in patients with a body weight <30 kg and doses should be adjusted for patients' weight and circumstances.[5] There is conflicting evidence for the benefit of adding paracetamol to strong opioids, and given that full daily dose paracetamol is a considerable tablet load, it may be appropriate to consider a trial without paracetamol if patients are struggling with multiple medications.[6]

NSAIDs work predominantly by their action on COX. There are two COX isoforms: COX-1 is part of the body's normal physiology and COX-2 is generated by inflammation, dehydration, and trauma. NSAIDs are now generally classified by their relative action on these isoforms and this dictates their adverse effects (Table 8.1.1).

Patients at particular risk of gastrointestinal side effects are those older than 65 years, who have metastatic cancer, or who are already on medications that increase bleeding risk: aspirin, warfarin or selective serotonin reuptake inhibitors (SSRIs). A proton pump inhibitor (PPI) should be considered in these patients.

In palliative care patients it is probably reasonable to use a non-selective NSAID ± PPI for those with no cardiovascular risk and no gastrointestinal risk, and a COX-2 inhibitor ± PPI for those with no cardiovascular risk and significant gastrointestinal risk. Patients with pre-existing cardiovascular risk factors should have alternative analgesics first, then a non-selective NSAID ± PPI with caution.

Step 2 opioids ('weak' opioids) are drugs such as codeine phosphate or tramadol. Codeine is metabolized by CYP2D6 on the cytochrome P450 chain to morphine, which is the active metabolite and its mechanism of action. Ten per cent of the Caucasian population lack CYP2D6 activity and they have a poor analgesic effect from codeine. This is of particular relevance when converting from codeine to strong opioids, where you may inadvertently overdose a patient who has been taking codeine but has not been able to metabolize it. It is approximately one-tenth as strong as oral morphine.

Tramadol is a synthetic, centrally acting analgesic with both opioid and non-opioid (serotoninergic) properties. It is also metabolized by CYP2D6 to its active metabolite and has been shown to have particular benefit in neuropathic pain. Conversion ratios vary, but it is probably also approximately one-tenth as strong as oral morphine. Because of its effects on serotonin, it has the potential to cause serotonin toxicity when combined with SSRIs. It also lowers the seizure threshold and care should be taken in using tramadol in patients with a history of seizures.

Step 3 opioids are the mainstay of analgesia in palliative care and are safe and effective when prescribed carefully and correctly. Morphine is the first-line strong opioid for cancer pain, though other strong opioids can be used if morphine produces intolerable side effects. Its analgesic effect is via mu opioid receptors, but its dose-related side effects include nausea, constipation, cough suppression, and respiratory depression. The major metabolites are excreted by the kidneys and these can accumulate significantly in renal impairment. It can be used with caution in mild–moderate renal impairment (using lower than usual doses with increased dose intervals), but in renal impairment and renal failure it is generally sensible to seek specialist advice about using a strong opioid that is not excreted by the renal route.

Breakthrough doses of morphine should be prescribed as one-sixth of the total daily dose. When adjusting the dose of long-acting morphine, the PRN (*pro re nata*/prescribed-as-needed) usage should be taken into account and dosages should be increased by no more than one-third to one-half. Patients starting on regular strong opioids should also be prescribed a regular laxative unless there is a good reason not to (e.g. an ileostomy) and an antiemetic should be prescribed for PRN use.

The analgesic ladder described above is suitable for nociceptive pain. In other pain mechanisms, adjuvant drugs can be useful for enhancing pain relief. Steroids or non-steroidal anti-inflammatory drugs can be a helpful addition for visceral pain such as that caused by a swollen liver capsule. Pain caused by bone metastases often responds to non-steroidal anti-inflammatory drugs and localized radiotherapy. Both bone pain and peripheral vascular disease limb pain incorporate elements of neuropathic pain due to nerve rupture or ischaemia. Neuropathic pain often requires a combination of opioid, antidepressant and anticonvulsant drugs. These tend to be complex pain states and it is best to refer to specialist palliative care or pain teams early on. It is important to realize that if all these therapeutic measures fail to bring relief, palliative care teams will consider further treatments in refractory pain such as opioid switching, ketamine infusions and spinal analgesia or regional blocks.

Table 8.1.1 Action and adverse effects of non-steroidal anti-inflammatory drugs

COX isoform affinity	Drug	Relative adverse effects
Non-selective	Ibuprofen	Gastrointestinal ++
	Naproxen	Renal ++
		Cardiovascular +
COX-2 preferential	Diclofenac	Gastrointestinal ++
		Renal ++
		Cardiovascular ++
COX-2 selective	Celecoxib	Cardiovascular ++
	Etoricoxib	Gastrointestinal +
	Parecoxib	Renal ++
	Valdecoxib	

COX, cyclooxygenase.

Antiemetics

e-ELCA 04-15 (Causes of nausea and vomiting), 04-16 (Assessment of nausea and vomiting), 04-17 (Management of nausea and vomiting)

Nausea and vomiting are distressing symptoms in palliative care, and ongoing nausea is particularly difficult for patients to tolerate. There are many different antiemetics available and you should make an effort to determine the cause of the nausea and/or vomiting in order to choose the appropriate drug treatment. Remember that if patients are vomiting their oral absorption of medication will be unreliable and antiemetics should then be given subcutaneously or via continuous subcutaneous injection over 24 hours (in a syringe driver). Antiemetics for inoperable bowel obstruction should be given via continuous subcutaneous injection, except levomepromazine and haloperidol that have long half-lives and can be given once a day at bedtime to minimize sedating side effects. Table 8.1.2 outlines therapeutic approaches to a range of mechanisms that underlie vomiting in advanced disease.

Care should be taken when combining antiemetics and you should choose complementary drugs. For example, cyclizine may be combined effectively with haloperidol, hyoscine butylbromide, or levomepromazine, but the combination of cyclizine and metoclopramide is not recommended as the prokinetic activity of metoclopramide is via a final cholinergic pathway, antagonized by cyclizine.

Table 8.1.2 Common causes of nausea and vomiting in palliative care and their drug management

Cause	Example	Example drug treatment
Drug-induced or metabolic abnormality	Hypercalcaemia Uraemia Opioids	Haloperidol 0.5–1.5 mg tds po/sc prn
Delayed gastric emptying	Gastritis Gastric stasis Upper GI bowel obstruction without colic	Metoclopramide 10–20 mg po/sc qds
Intracranial	Raised intracranial pressure Motion sickness	Cyclizine 50 mg po/sc tds Dexamethasone 2–16 mg po od
Bowel obstruction with colic	Inoperable abdominal malignancy, inoperable peritoneal adhesions	Hyoscine butylbromide 60 mg sc in 24 hours Hyoscine hydrobromide 1200 micrograms sc in 24 hours Dexamethasone 4-8mg sc/po od
Vagal stimulation via 5HT3 gut wall receptors	Chemotherapy Radiotherapy	Ondansetron 8 mg bd for five days
Broad spectrum	Multiple causes or when other antiemetics are ineffective	Levomepromazine 6.25 mg nocte Cyclizine 50mg sc tds

bd, *bis die*, twice a day; nocte, at night; po, *per os*, by mouth; prn, *pro re nata*, as needed; sc, subcutaneous; qds, *quater die sumendus*, four times a day; tds, *ter die sumendum*, three times a day.

Laxatives

e-ELCA 04-18 (Assessment of constipation), 04-19 (Management of constipation)

Constipation is common in palliative care patients, due to immobility, reduced food intake, and routine use of opioids. Most patients prescribed a regular opioid will also need a regular laxative: opioids cause constipation by decreasing peristalsis and increasing the reabsorption of fluid, leading to harder stools that are more difficult to pass. Laxatives can be classified by their mode of action:

◆ stimulant (e.g. senna, bisacodyl, dantron)

◆ osmotic (e.g. lactulose, macrogols, magnesium hydroxide)

◆ softening (e.g. sodium docusate)

◆ bulk-forming (e.g. Fybogel®).

Stimulant laxatives are the usual first choice of laxative in opioid-induced constipation and act by stimulating secretion and peristalsis within the large intestine. The dose should be titrated according to the result and fluids should also be encouraged during this time.

If there is no effect from the maximum dose of a stimulant laxative or if it causes intestinal colic, osmotic laxatives may be used. Macrogols are more effective than lactulose,[7] but the volume required per dose is often not well tolerated by palliative care patients.

Softening laxatives such as sodium docusate act by lowering surface tension and allowing water and fat to penetrate faeces, and are useful as single agents in partial bowel obstruction. They are often used in combination with a stimulant laxative for opioid-induced constipation, though there is no evidence to support this regime.

Bulk-forming laxatives are not recommended for use in patients taking constipating drugs or with reduced food intake, so they are rarely prescribed in palliative care. They can be useful in patients with ileostomies/colostomies to make the stool more formed.

Psychotropics

e-ELCA 04-32 (Assessment of mood), 04-33 (Assessment and management of anxiety), 04-34 (Management of depression), 04-35 (Assessment and management of agitation)

Anxiety, depression, agitation, and delirium are common symptoms at the end of life and cause significant distress to patients, families, and staff. It is important to try to identify and treat potentially reversible causes. Pain, metabolic disturbance, infections, cerebral metastases, and medications can all alter patients' psychological and psychiatric state. Pre-existing cognitive impairment can progress more rapidly in patients with cancer and this can exacerbate delirium or agitation.

Benzodiazepines are used in palliative care to manage symptoms of insomnia, anxiety, and terminal agitation, as well as for antiepileptic management in some patients. They activate the alpha-subunit of the $GABA_A$ receptor (an inhibitory neurotransmitter). Tolerance and dependence may occur with benzodiazepines after long-term use and caution is required in severe hepatic impairment and severe renal impairment as they may accumulate. The choice of drug depends on the indication, route of administration, and familiarity, but typical doses include those shown in Table 8.1.3.

Antipsychotics are used in end of life care to treat agitation and delirium (for use in nausea and vomiting see Antiemetic section). They act via dopaminergic systems throughout the cerebral cortex

Table 8.1.3 Use of benzodiazepine and cyclopyrrolone sedatives

Drug	Half-life	Doses and indication
Midazolam	2–5 hours	2.5–5 mg sc every 2 to 4 hours for terminal agitation
		10 mg sc or iv stat for status epilepticus (repeat after 10 minutes if necessary)
Diazepam	24–120 hours	2–4 mg tds po for anxiety
Zopiclone	2–5 hours	7.5–15 mg po at bedtime for insomnia
Temazepam	8–15 hours	10–20 mg po at bedtime for insomnia

iv, intravenous; po, *per os*, by mouth; prn, *pro re nata*, as needed ; sc, subcutaneous; tds, *ter die sumendum*, three times a day.

to correct dopamine overactivity and improve symptoms of delusions and hallucinations. They also act via some systems to augment dopamine underactivity and exacerbate negative symptoms of apathy and cognitive blunting, and can cause extrapyramidal side effects of tremor, rigidity, and akathisia. Older 'typical' antipsychotics such as haloperidol and levomepromazine have a higher risk of extrapyramidal side effects, whereas newer, 'atypical' antipsychotics such as olanzapine and quetiapine reduce this risk.

All antipsychotics cause an increased risk of stroke, particularly in elderly patients. They also lower the seizure threshold and should be avoided in patients with Parkinson's disease and Lewy body dementia. Antipsychotics should therefore be used with caution, particularly in patients with co-existing cognitive impairment. Where they are needed for delirium (for example, where non-drug measures such as orientation and environmental modifications have failed), the lowest possible dose should be used for the shortest possible time[8] (e.g. haloperidol 0.5–1 mg tds). However, in terminal agitation (agitation in the last 48 hours of life), symptom control should be the priority.

The prevalence of depression in palliative care patients is estimated at around 25% (though some studies have identified up to 49%).[9] Depression is poorly managed in medically ill patients generally, possibly because it is harder to make a diagnosis in the presence of physical symptoms. It is also difficult to distinguish between the diagnoses of anxiety or depression and the emotional reactions of fear and sadness. However, the decision to prescribe antidepressants in palliative care may be made with regard to targeting particularly troublesome depressive symptoms as well as the need to avoid side effects that augment the symptoms of physical disease (Table 8.1.4). Drug treatment does not preclude other interventions and the effects of drugs and psychotherapy are complementary.

All classes of antidepressants have their own contraindications, interactions, and cautions, for example, renal impairment, hepatic disease, heart disease, gastrointestinal bleeding, epilepsy, nausea, glaucoma, delirium, sexual dysfunction, bladder neck obstruction, and analgesic therapy. Nevertheless, evidence indicates that antidepressants are effective in depressed patients with physical illness and benefits accrue from 4 to 5 weeks and persist after 18 weeks. In palliative care patients, the onset of response tends to be delayed and in a meta-analysis, significant benefits were first apparent after 4 weeks with tricyclics and after 16 weeks with SSRIs.[10] Therefore, antidepressants require careful selection and proper titration to achieve their desired effect and this should be done as quickly as possible.

It is worth becoming familiar with one or two antidepressants, such as mirtazepine (15 mg po on, titrating every week by 15 mg to a maximum of 45 mg) or sertraline (50 mg po od, titrating every 4 weeks by 50 mg to a maximum of 200 mg) Antidepressants should not be stopped abruptly in order to avoid discontinuation reactions. Seek specialist advice if there is no response to treatment after titration or if suicidal ideation ensues.

Surgical intervention in palliative care

In the tradition and heritage of surgery, the control of suffering is of equal importance to the cure of disease. Through closer collaborative working, it is inevitable that palliative care services will call upon their surgical colleagues for palliative surgery of some sort.

Table 8.1.4 Antidepressants in palliative care and considerations relating to their use

Indication	Management	Comments
For patients with anorexia, insomnia, anxiety or agitation	Mirtazepine 15–45 mg po at night	May improve appetite. May be sedative. Available as a 'melt' tablet
Alternative antidepressants when both sedation and stimulation need to be avoided	Sertraline 50–200 mg po once daily Citalopram 20 mg po once daily	May exacerbate anxiety, nausea, anorexia, and gastrointestinal bleeding. May potentiate the action of opioids
Alternative antidepressants when both sedation and stimulation need to be avoided and SSRIs are contraindicated	Lofepramine 70–210 mg po once daily	Less sedative and less toxic in overdose than older tricyclics
For patients with sleepiness or drowsiness	Fluoxetine 20–60 mg po once daily	May exacerbate anxiety, nausea, anorexia, seizures and gastro-intestinal bleeding
For patients with insomnia or a history of seizures	Trazodone 100–300 mg at night to a maximum of 300 mg twice a day	Thought to be less cardiotoxic than tricyclics. Commonly prescribed in patients with seizures. May cause dysphoria
May be prescribed for depression where analgesic for neuropathic pain is also required.	Amitriptyline 25–200 mg po at night Nortriptyline 25–150 mg po at night	Contraindicated in heart disease, epilepsy, glaucoma and bladder neck obstruction, but safe in renal failure. Dry mouth, sedation and QTc changes limit dose

po, *per os*, by mouth.

Studies have suggested that palliative procedures may account for 6–12% of surgical interventions.[11,12] Miner and colleagues (2004) concluded that when 'experienced clinicians' across a spectrum of surgical fields selected patients for palliative procedures, it resulted in improvement or resolution of specific symptoms 80% of the time.[12] A multidisciplinary approach is essential since comparable symptoms may demand different responses based upon the biology of each primary disease, and, often subtle, distinctions may need to be appreciated to provide the finest care. Factors such as symptom severity, the degree of symptom resolution, the timing and choice of procedure, the durability of the intervention, associated complications, and patient preferences all play major roles in determining the overall benefit of the palliative operation and the role of the surgeon.

While there are various definitions of palliative surgery, they generally refer to surgery performed with the intent of improving quality of life or relieving symptoms caused by advanced disease. Confusion sometimes arises when the concept of palliative surgery and non-curative surgery are used interchangeably. The key difference lies with the *intent* of the surgery; as such surgery that intends to relieve symptoms without consideration of oncological benefit is considered palliative, whereas surgery undertaken in asymptomatic patients with the intent of oncological cure but not curative in itself (i.e. debulking surgery) is deemed non-curative. The scope of palliative procedures that the surgeon may be requested to consider will vary according to the specialty of the team and not necessarily to primary cancer diagnosis. Examples of surgical procedures commonly provided to palliative patients are outlined in the following section.

Gastrointestinal symptoms

Upper and lower gastrointestinal surgery has much to offer the palliation of advanced cancer. Malignant bowel obstruction occurs in 3% of all cancer but is most common in cancers of the stomach, colon, and ovary. It is estimated that 25–40% of patients with ovarian cancer and 16% with colon cancer will develop malignant bowel obstruction.

Patients with malignant bowel obstruction who have failed to recover bowel function with conservative treatment may be considered for surgery if the clinical status of the patient permits and the patient is willing to undergo further surgery. Surgical options include:

◆ resection of the obstruction with re-anastomosis

◆ bypass procedures

◆ defunctioning colostomy/ileostomy formation

◆ division of adhesions.

The mortality rate from surgery in these patients is 20%. Survival rates of 43% have been reported at 60 days but recurrent symptoms are common. Survival is better after surgery in patients with the following characteristics:

◆ tumour has low grade/stage

◆ good performance status

◆ good nutritional status

◆ low metastatic disease burden

◆ age under 65

◆ benign cause for obstruction e.g. surgical adhesions or radiotherapy stricture.

Venting gastrostomy tubes are an acceptable way of decompressing the stomach and upper gastrointestinal tract in patients with intractable nausea and large volume vomiting or pain from gastric distension. They are arguably a preferable alternative to a nasogastric tube since it is less unsightly than a nasogastric tube and less likely to fall out requiring replacement. They can be introduced at laparotomy but are most commonly placed endoscopically or radiologically. The combination of a venting gastrostomy and feeding jejunostomy can successfully ameliorate symptoms of high outflow upper gastrointestinal obstruction while providing nutritional support.

Self-expanding metallic stents have been used for a long time in the palliation of malignant oesophageal symptoms strictures. Their use is becoming more commonplace to relieve obstruction in the stomach, jejunum, colon, and rectum. They are inserted under light sedation using radiological or endoscopic techniques but are contraindicated in patients with peritoneal carcinomatosis or multiple obstructions. Recognized complications include stent migration, pain and bowel perforation.

Cardiothoracic procedures

The two main interventions offered by cardiothoracic services will be with the intention of providing long-term relief from malignant pleural or pericardial effusions.

The management of malignant pleural effusions often falls between the respiratory physicians and the cardiothoracic surgeons. In general, the repeated aspiration of 1–1.5 L of fluid is a reasonable approach for patients with poor performance status and limited prognosis. However, recurrence rates are almost 100% at 1 month and attempts to prevent recurrence of the effusion should be considered with patients of better prognosis. The scope of available management options is likely to differ locally but may include:

◆ Thoracoscopy or video-assisted thoracic surgery (VATS): The lung is collapsed, giving a good view of the pleural cavity followed by introduction of 2–5 g of talc poudrage. Both techniques are considered equally effective. Recognized complications include empyema.

◆ Pleurectomy: While effective, open pleurectomy is associated with a 10–13% mortality rate and a significant morbidity. VATS pleurectomy is considered safer but dependant on availability and expertise.

◆ Pleuroperitoneal shunting: This option is most commonly used for patients with trapped lung and effusions refractory to other treatments. The shunt may be inserted with VATS or a limited thoracotomy. Complications include infection, shunt occlusion, and peritoneal seeding.

◆ Long-term indwelling catheter: This has become one of the most commonly offered procedures and tends to be well tolerated by patients. It is usually inserted as a day case and has been shown to reduce hospital admissions as well as improve overall quality of life.

◆ Management of pericardial effusions: The initial management of a pericardial effusion is likely to have been insertion of pericardial drain under ultrasound guidance. However, since most pericardial effusions accumulate, preventative methods have been developed. Subxiphoid percardiostomy (pericardial window) is the most widely used technique and can be performed under local anaesthesia. Following excision of a small piece of pericardium a draining chest tube is left *in situ* for 4 to 5 days to promote local inflammation and fusion of the visceral and parietal pericardium. A recurrence rate of 3% and complication rate lower than 2% makes this a preferable intervention.

◆ Percutaneous balloon pericardiostomy: Following pericardiocentesis a balloon catheter is inserted and inflated to tear open the needle tract, thus creating a window. While the success rate is 92%, the complication rate has been reported at 18% (mainly pleural effusions). As such it is a less favourable option to pericardiostomy.

◆ Thoracotomy with pericardiectomy: This approach was associated with a mortality rate of 13% and with the introduction of less invasive approaches is now largely obsolete.

Wound management and debridement

The management of complex wounds are considered the mainstay of palliative care services and aggressive management of severe wounds will often improve symptoms, quality of life, and prognosis. Extensive necrotic wounds are unlikely to heal until the excess dead tissue is removed and it is not uncommon for surgical colleagues to be asked to assist in debriding such wounds. While technically not a challenging surgical procedure for many, it must be remembered that such patients are likely to be of very poor performance and nutritional status. As such, anaesthetic risk is high.

For some patients the cause of the wound is not the cancer itself but the complications. The formation of feculent or urinary fistulae with the bladder or vagina will lead to progressive inflammation and skin breakdown unless the outflow of materials is reduced. Diversionary procedures in patients fit enough to undergo surgery offers a significant relief of symptoms.

Urinary tract surgery

Urostomy is usually performed after cystectomy for bladder cancer. It may be used for urinary diversion of presence of urinary leakage associated wounds. As the chemotherapeutic options available to patients increases, it has necessarily followed that surgeons are asked to help in aggressively managing the local compressive/obstructive consequences of advanced cancer. While the onset of renal failure secondary to obstructive bilateral hydronephrosis previously heralded the terminal phase of the malignant disease process, relief of ureteric obstruction and restoration of renal function may now allow patients ongoing palliative oncological treatments.

Although the radiological insertion of nephrostomies or cystoscopic approach to introduce stents may seem straightforward, the provision of such an intervention should be given due consideration to the long-term benefit afforded the patient. It is tempting for colleagues to promise further chemotherapy once the patient is fitter, rather than engage in the difficult conversation that confirms that disease has reached the terminal stages. The relief of hydronephrosis is appropriate if it provides symptomatic improvement or allows a suitable patient to receive disease-modifying therapy. However, poor selection of patients may result in prolonged hospital admissions with no impact on symptoms or clinical outcome. It is important that the patient understands that nephrostomy and urinary stent insertion is a life prolonging procedure as part of the conversation around consent. Some patients will regard a death by renal failure as preferable to the experience that follows it.

Orthopaedic procedures

Bone metastases are a common complication of many cancers including prostate, breast, lung, thyroid, renal, and gastrointestinal cancer as well as being a primary site of disease activity for myeloma. Metastatic bone disease usually presents with pain that can be usually be managed with analgesia and radiotherapy. Regular bisphosphonate therapy may also be given for prophylactic treatment to reduce the incidence of pain, fractures, and hypercalcaemia in patients with bone metastases due to breast cancer and myeloma. Evidence for their use in other cancers is less clear. Metastatic bone disease has a propensity to pathological fractures and it is not uncommon for patients with advanced cancer to present as part of the acute trauma service. For this reason, it is always important to obtain a bone biopsy during internal fixation of any fracture thought to be pathological. Frequently, such patients will have been symptomatic from the bone metastases for some while, and by the time they present with a fracture may be too unwell to withstand a general anaesthetic or surgical procedure. Prophylactic pinning of bones at high risk of fracture is preferred to fixation of actual pathological fracture since it will involve a shorter operating time, decreased morbidity, and quicker postoperative recovery. Several methods are available to help identify those at greatest risk of pathological fracture. These include evidence of more than 50% destruction of cortical bone and the presence of significant functional pain. Two formal staging systems (Harrington's criteria and Mirel's criteria) can also be used. However, it is beyond the scope of this chapter to cover these in detail.

Surgery is an option in the managing of metastatic spinal cord compression, although radiotherapy and steroids remains the mainstay treatment since the majority of patients will be unsuitable for surgery. The intention of surgery in this context is decompression of the spinal cord and mechanical stabilization. The type of surgery will depend upon the disease site; the most common site of metastatic disease is the vertebral body and an anterior approach will offer the most direct and accessible route. Resection of the vertebral body followed by methylmethacrylate cement and instrumentation used to attach to adjacent vertebral bodies will provide maximal stability. A surgical series has reported pain relief in 85–97% of patients, improvement or stabilization of motor function in 90% of patients, and reduction of incontinence in most patients.[13] Laminectomy in which the posterior arch of the vertebral body is removed to decompress the cord is reserved for posterior vertebral lesions.

Accepted indications for surgery include:

◆ spinal instability of bony neural compression
◆ good performance status prior to metastatic spinal cord compression
◆ neurological deterioration despite radiotherapy
◆ previous irradiation of spine to maximal tolerated dose
◆ intractable pain unrelieved by other measures
◆ unknown diagnosis.

Surgery is usually inappropriate if one or more of the following features are present:

◆ prognosis less than 3 months
◆ multiple levels of cord compression

* paraplegia present longer than 12 to 24 hours
* presence of serious co morbidities/poor performance status prior to diagnosis of metastatic spinal cord compression.

Further reading

Dunn G (ed.). *Surgical Palliative Care, An Issue of Surgical Clinics*. Philadelphia: Saunders, 2005.

Dunn G, Ganapathy S, Chan VWS (eds). *Surgical Palliative Care and Pain Management, An Issue of Anesthesiology Clinics* Philadelphia, 2012.

Wichmann M, Maddern G. *Palliative Surgery*. New York: Springer, 2014.

References

1. Temel JS, Greer JA, Muzikansky A, *et al.* Early palliative care for patients with metastatic non–small-cell lung cancer. *N Engl J Med* 2010; 363:733–42.
2. Bates T, Hoy AM, Clarke DG, *et al.* The St Thomas Hospital terminal care support team. A new concept of hospice care. *Lancet* 1981; 1: 1201–3.
3. World Health Organization. *Cancer Pain Relief*. Geneva: WHO, 1986.
4. Mattia A, Coluzzi F. What anesthesiologists should know about paracetamol (acetaminophen). *Minerva Anestesiol* 2009; 75: 644–53.
5. Claridge LC, Eksteen B, Smith A, *et al.* Acute liver failure after administration of paracetamol at the maximum recommended daily dose in adults. *BMJ* 2010; 341: c6764.
6. Axelsson B, Christensen S. Is there an additive analgesic effect of paracetamol at step 3? A double-blind randomised controlled study. *Palliat Med* 2003; 17: 724–5.
7. Lee-Robichaud H, Thomas K, Morgan J, *et al.* Lactulose versus polyethylene glycol for chronic constipation. *Cochrane Database of Syst Rev* 2010; 7: CD007570.
8. British Geriatrics Society and Royal College of Physicians. *The Prevention, Diagnosis and Management of Delirium in Older People*. National Guidelines. London: Royal College of Physicians; 2006.
9. Mitchell AJ, Chan M, Bhatti H, *et al.* Prevalence of depression, anxiety and adjustment disorder in oncological, haematological and palliative-care settings: a meta-analysis of 94 interview-based studies. *Lancet Oncol* 2011; 12(2): 160–74.
10. Rayner L, Price A, Evans A, *et al.* Antidepressants for the treatment of depression in palliative care: systematic review and meta-analysis. Palliative Med 2011; 25(1): 36-51.
11. Krouse RS, Nelson RA, Farell BR, *et al.* Surgical palliation at a cancer center: incidence and outcomes. Arch Surg 2001; 136: 773–8.
12. Miner TJ, Brennan MF, Jaques DP. A prospective, symptom related, outcomes analysis of 1022 palliative procedures for advanced cancer. *Ann Surg* 2004; 240: 719–26.
13. Levack P, Buchanan D, Dryden H, *et al.* Specialist palliative care provision in a major teaching hospital and cancer centre—an eight-year experience. *J R Coll Physic Edinb* 2008; 38: 112–9.

Terminal care of the dying patient, supporting their family and ethical considerations

Katharine Burke, Simon Noble, Bee Wee, and Bill Noble

Ethical issues and resuscitation

e-ELCA 03-30 (Discussing 'do not attempt CPR' decision), 03-31 (Discussing food and fluids)

Even when patients are dying, they should continue to be as involved as they can be, and wish to be, in decision-making about their care. Some find the prospect burdensome and prefer that this responsibility be taken by somebody else, but others wish to remain involved with decisions about medication, investigations, preferred place of care, and discharge planning. This should be supported by the healthcare team.[1] The Mental Capacity Act 2005 (England and Wales) governs this principle, and it is fundamental to the Act that adults should be assumed to have capacity to make decisions on their own behalf unless proven otherwise.[2] Equally, decision-making capacity should be maximized before deciding that an individual does not have the capacity to make a decision, for example by providing communication support or by assessing at a specific time of day around medication regimes. Mental capacity is decision-specific; for example, some patients at the end of life will retain the capacity to make decisions about their medications and some investigations or treatments, but may not have the capacity to make more complex decisions about discharge. An assessment of capacity should not be based on a patient's age, appearance, or any assumptions about their condition.

Where a patient does not have the capacity to make decisions about their treatment, any decision taken on their behalf should be made in their best interests. It may be appropriate to involve those close to the patient to establish what the patient may have wanted, but the best interest of the patient is paramount, not what others would themselves want for the patient.

The provision of food and drink by mouth is part of basic care, and you should make every effort to ensure that your dying patients are assisted to eat and drink as long as they wish to do so. The provision of clinically assisted nutrition and hydration (i.e. intravenous fluids, nasogastric or percutaneous endoscopic gastrostomy feeding or total parenteral nutrition) is classified in law as a medical treatment and should be treated in the same way as other medical interventions (i.e. a best-interest judgement). Such interventions may provide symptom relief but can also cause problems (e.g. nausea, peripheral oedema or infection) and the current evidence about the benefits and harms is not clear. In addition, for some patients and families the provision of

nutrition and hydration by any route is seen as a part of basic care and therefore the belief is that it should always be provided. For this reason, it is important to make individual clinical assessments of the benefits and harms of clinically assisted nutrition and hydration in patients and to discuss with patients and their families wherever possible.[3]

Decisions about whether or not to attempt cardiopulmonary resuscitation (CPR) or do not attempt cardiopulmonary resuscitation (DNACPR) orders can be difficult to undertake in clinical practice. The survival rate to discharge after an in-hospital cardiac arrest is, at best, approximately 15–20%[4] and the survival rate to discharge after an *unexpected* in-hospital cardiac arrest in patients with metastatic cancer is significantly lower than this (approximately 5%).[4] If the patient appears moribund due to the burden of disease, CPR is extremely unlikely to be successful and may prolong suffering or provide a distressing death. Wherever possible, decisions about CPR should be made by the most senior clinician responsible for the patient's care and should involve the whole healthcare team.[6]

When a decision is made not to attempt resuscitation because there is no prospect of it being successful and the patient has not expressed a wish to discuss CPR, very careful consideration should be given to informing the patient of the decision. Following the Tracey judgement, UK law dictates that the patient or their relative should be informed, unless the information is likely to cause harm.[7] For patients who know that they are in the last few days of life information about interventions that will not be offered because they will not be successful may cause more distress. However, for most patients and families it is more distressing either to find out by chance that a DNACPR order has been made without discussion, or that any decision is being made without explanation or communication and the Tracey judgement does not regard distress in receiving the information as harm.[7] It is good practice therefore to establish exactly what information patients and families want at the end of life and let this guide discussion. An example with the possible steps this might cover is shown in Box 8.2.1.

Family and carers

e-ELCA 02-10 (Carer assessment and support)

Cancer can also have an enormous impact on the whole family and close friends. This includes people in heterosexual and same-sex

Box 8.2.1 Some possible examples of ways to discuss decisions about cardiopulmonary resuscitation a do not attempt resuscitation decision

'I thought it might be useful if we talked a bit about what treatments we have used so far. Is that OK? What do you understand about what's been happening?'

'One of the things that can be useful to discuss is what might happen and what might be the right thing to do if things got worse. Have you had any thoughts about what might happen in the future?'

'One of the more difficult things to think about is what might happen if you were to deteriorate very suddenly, for example if your heart were to stop beating. If that were to happen, I don't think it would be the right thing to do lots of unpleasant things to try to start it again. This is sometimes called 'resuscitation'. Unfortunately I don't think that this would work, but I think the attempt would cause you and your family more distress and suffering. That doesn't mean that we will stop doing anything to try to improve things and we will certainly keep trying to treat your infection/control your bleeding/help control your symptoms. This might have been upsetting to hear—do you have any questions that you want to ask me?'

Box 8.2.2 Recognising dying

Communication and interaction

- Sleeping longer
- Drowsiness
- Reduced conversation
- Poor cooperation with nursing care
- Disorientation

Oral intake

- Decreased intake of fluids
- Poor appetite
- Difficulty swallowing
- Difficulty taking oral medication

Activity and appearance

- Requiring assistance with personal care
- Mostly bed-bound
- Profound fatigue
- Cachexia

relationships and others who have strong emotional or social bonds with a patient, for example step-families, older parents, or grandparents. They often provide crucial support and care, but professionals may not recognize their needs for emotional and practical support, particularly at times of increased stress such as severe illness, recurrence of cancer, or the end of life. You should ask family members and other carers about their own needs, for example asking them what information or explanation they require (which may well be different from what the patient is asking for), what help and support they may need to continue caring for the patient at home, or whether they would want further emotional support such as informal or formal counselling.[8] This may be available from their own general practitioner or alternatively through centres such as Maggie's Centres where these are available locally.

Terminal care

e-ELCA 04-23 (Recognising the dying phase, last days of life and verifying death), 04-24 (Managing death rattle), 04-25 (Managing agitation and restlessness in the dying phase), 04-26 (Managing distress during the dying phase)

Recognising dying and the end of life is one of the most difficult skills to develop as a doctor, particularly in the acute hospital setting where the primary intention is usually to preserve and prolong life. It is important to be aware of the signs and symptoms of dying in order to minimize unnecessary and burdensome treatments and investigations, and shift the focus of care towards the patient's wishes and concerns. These patients will show deterioration in their condition on a day-to-day basis: if a more sudden change is noticed on a background of previously relatively good function, attention should be paid to investigating and treating reversible causes such as infection, biochemical abnormalities, or possible side effects of medications. However, even when it is has been recognized that the patient is likely to be dying soon, decisions concerning treatment and investigation must be reviewed every few days in case the general condition changes and a recovery becomes a possible outcome. Box 8.2.2 highlights signs and symptoms to notice.

Patients and their carers will often be aware that things are deteriorating and it is important that this is discussed with them sensitively and carefully. However, some families may have less experience of somebody dying, so it is also important that your communication is very clear. A possible way to formulate a discussion with patients and/or carers about the diagnosis of dying is given in Box 8.2.3. It is only through training, experience, and reflection that one can develop the necessary skills to discuss such issues effectively. The following is an example that highlights the main issues that need to be covered. Individual clinicians will need to develop an approach with which they feel comfortable and modify it to be appropriate for the patient and/or carer. Always remember the basic rules of good communication apply here more than ever: find an appropriate place away from the busy ward, give your bleep to someone else, take another member of the healthcare team with you if possible, and allow plenty of time for questions or silence where appropriate. Above all, listen and pay attention to the concerns and what is being asked of you.

Box 8.2.3 A possible way to discuss the diagnosis of dying with patients and/or carers

'I wanted to talk to you about what's been happening with your mother's treatment. I'm afraid that things have not gone as well as we had hoped.'

'We have been trying to treat your mother's infection with antibiotics, but unfortunately despite these we as a team think that she has been deteriorating day-by-day. Was this something that you had been thinking about?'

'I think things have been changing very quickly recently, and although we have all been doing our best to treat the infection we have not been able to control it. I'm sorry to tell you that I don't think that she will survive this and I'm afraid she is dying.'

Symptom management in the terminal phase follows the same pattern as described previously. However, careful attention must be paid to assessment of symptoms in a patient who is less able to communicate or semiconscious. Medications should be prescribed by a parenteral (usually subcutaneous) route in anticipation of a patient's deterioration. It is not wise to attempt to convert transdermal patch medication to subcutaneous infusions, since the calculations are not reliable. It is best to continue patches as prescribed previously, unless a dose reduction is required, and add subcutaneous injections as required or a continuous infusion to substitute for oral regimes when the oral route is no longer viable. Daily review of these decisions is necessary to accommodate changes in the patient's condition that might presage an unexpected recovery.

There are at least five distressing sensations that appear to be capable of penetrating the terminal coma, producing signs of distress such as frowning, grimacing, vocalization or agitation. Pain, delirium, thirst, dyspnoea, and urinary retention may be the cause of distress in a comatose or semicomatose, moribund patient. Continuous nursing assessment and at least daily medical assessment to detect and treat these is a vital element of good terminal care. It is important that care of the dying person is individualized and shaped around that individual's needs and preferences. The report on One Chance to Get it Right sets out five priorities for care of the dying person which provides a framework for care.[3] Common dilemmas include the prescription by alternative route and the withdrawal or dose adjustment of anticoagulants, steroids, insulin, diuretics, and anticonvulsants. Dry mouth is treated by regular mouthcare, for example with oral sponges, ice cubes or saliva replacements. Intravenous hydration has not been shown to improve the symptoms of dry mouth at the end of life.[9] However, there is evidence that rehydration may be effective in the treatment of delirium[10] and previous poor oral intake or a prolonged terminal phase may produce dehydration before death supervenes, when artificial hydration by the subcutaneous or intravenous route is indicated.

Discharge and referral

When a patient is approaching the end of their life and there are no more secondary care interventions that are desirable or appropriate, it may be necessary to consider discharge. Every attempt should be made to explore with the patient where they would prefer to be cared for and what their wishes would be about further interventions or escalation of care. This should also include discussion with families and carers, who often bear huge responsibility for the care of the dying patient.

Points to consider and discuss with patients and families when planning discharge include:

◆ Where does the patient want to be cared for?

◆ Where do the patient's family/carers feel is the best place?

◆ What level of care and nursing support does the patient currently require? What level are they likely to need in the future?

◆ What might happen when the patient's condition deteriorates? Would it be appropriate to come back to hospital in the future if this happens?

◆ What plans could you put in place to manage problems if further hospital admission is not appropriate? This might

include anticipatory prescribing of subcutaneous end of life drugs, referral to district nursing, and/or a written advance care plan.

◆ Is it appropriate to discuss a DNACPR form at this time to go home with the patient?

◆ Who is going to follow-up the patient? This is likely to be the patient's general practitioner. Have you discussed with them directly what the plans are?

◆ Is a referral to specialist palliative care services appropriate?

Certification of death and the role of the coroner

Completion of the medical certificate of cause of death should be completed as soon as possible. The medical certificate of cause of death should have the immediate cause of death on line 1a and the underlying cause of death should be on the lowest completed line. The underlying cause of death will have caused all of the conditions on the lines above. Other diseases, injuries, or conditions that contributed to the death but were not part of the direct chain of events should be entered in part two of the certificate (see Box 8.2.4). Where death has occurred because of cancer, it is important that the histological site and anatomical location of the cancer is specified.[11]

In England and Wales there is a legal duty to report deaths to the coroner that may be due to accident, suicide, violence, neglect (by self or others), or if the death was thought to be due to industrial disease. Deaths in the perioperative period or before full recovery from surgery should also be reported, as should deaths occurring while in custody. In Scotland, deaths that may have been related to adverse effects of medical or surgical treatment, or to standards of care, or about which there has been any complaint, should be reported to the procurator fiscal.[12] If you are unsure about whether to report a death, contact the coroner's officer who will be able to advise you whether a formal report is appropriate.

When a death is referred to the coroner, it cannot be registered until the coroner's enquiries have been completed and a death certificate issued and provided to the Registrar of Births and Deaths. The coroner may request a post mortem to provide further information about the cause of death but this may not be necessary.

If the death is thought to be unnatural (including the result of an accident, industrial disease, or a surgical procedure), an inquest will be held. Normally the coroner will issue the authority for registration of death that permits a funeral to be held even though the inquest has not taken place. Inquests are generally opened soon after a death and adjourned until other investigations or inquiries are complete and this may take between three and nine months.

Box 8.2.4 Example of a completed medical certificate of cause of death

1a Massive lower gastrointestinal bleeding
1b Primary adenocarcinoma of the rectum with liver metastases
2 Non-insulin dependent diabetes mellitus, ischaemic heart disease

Further reading

Randall F, Downie R. *End of Life Choices: Consensus and Controversy.* Oxford: Oxford University Press, 2009.

References

1. General Medical Council. *Treatment and Care Towards the End of Life: Good Practice in Decision Making.* London: General Medical Council, 2010. Available from http://www.gmc-uk.org/guidance/ethical_guidance/end_of_life_care.asp (accessed 5 October 2015).

2. Great Britain. Mental Capacity Act. Chapter 9. [Act of Parliament online]. London: Stationery Office; 2005. Available from http://www.legislation.gov.uk/ukpga/2005/9/contents/enacted (accessed 5 October 2015).

3. Sandroni C, Nolan J, Cavallaro F, *et al.* In-hospital cardiac arrest: incidence, prognosis and possible measures to improve survival. *Intensive Care Med* 2007; 33: 237–45.

4. Reisfield GM, Wallace SK, Munsell MF, *et al.* Survival in cancer patients undergoing in-hospital cardiopulmonary resuscitation: a meta-analysis. *Resuscitation* 2006; 71(2): 152–60.

5. British Medical Association, Resuscitation Council (UK), Royal College of Nursing (Great Britain). *Decisions relating to cardiopulmonary resuscitation: guidance from the British Medical Association, the Resuscitation Council (UK) and the Royal College of Nursing.* Available from https://www.resus.org.uk/dnacpr/decisions-relating-to-cpr/ (accessed 5 October 2015).

6. National Institute for Clinical Excellence. Guidance on Cancer Services. *Improving Supportive and Palliative Care for Adults with Cancer: The Manual.* London: National Institute for Clinical Excellence, 2004.

7. Tracey v. Cambridge University Hospital NHS Foundation Trust and others. EWCA Civ2014. p. 822.

8. Leadership Alliance for the Care of Dying People (2014). *One Chance to Get it Right.* Available from https://www.gov.uk/government/uploads/system/uploads/attachment_data/file/323188/One_chance_to_get_it_right.pdf (accessed 18th May 2015).

9. Burge FI. Dehydration symptoms of palliative care cancer patients. *J Pain Symptom Manag* 1993; 8: 454–64.

10. Bruera E, Hui D, Dalal S, *et al.* Parenteral hydration in patients with advanced cancer: a multicenter, double-blind, placebo-controlled randomized trial. J Clin Oncol 2013; 31(1): 111–8.

11. Office for National Statistics Death Certification Advisory Group. *Guidance for doctors completing Medical Certificates of Cause of Death in England and Wales*, B0521 8/08. London: Stationery Office, 2010.

12. Ministry of Justice Coroners and Burials Division. *A guide to coroners and inquests.* London: Stationery Office; 2010.

Principles of organ and tissue transplantation

Section editor: J. Andrew Bradley

CHAPTER 9.1

Organ donation

Pankaj Chandak and Christopher J. Callaghan

Introduction

Overcoming the severe shortage in human donor organs is the major challenge facing transplantation. This chapter provides an overview of organ donation with an emphasis on UK practice; topics include donor types, the demand and supply of organs, and the organ donation pathway from assessment to organ procurement, storage, preservation, and allocation.

Deceased donor types and their implications

Death in deceased organ donors is declared using either standard criteria (i.e. donation after circulatory death [DCD]) or criteria for brain death (donation after brain death [DBD]). DCD donors can be further subdivided on the basis of the context of cardiac arrest and the timing of any failed cardiopulmonary resuscitation attempts (the modified Maastricht classification; Table 9.1.1).[1] Most DCD donors in the UK are currently Maastricht III donors.

Donor classification is important because it describes the physiological insult suffered by organs prior to preservation; this impacts on transplant outcome. Organs from DCD donors undergo a variable period of warm ischaemia (i.e. the absence of adequate oxygenated blood flow before the organ has been cooled). Organs from DBD donors do not incur significant warm ischaemia, but are subjected instead to the physiological disturbances associated with brain death. Organs from DCD donors are more susceptible to damage during cold storage.

Transplant outcomes for kidneys from controlled DCD and DBD donors are similar.[3,4] In contrast, graft survival after a DBD donor liver transplant is superior to that after transplantation with a DCD donor liver. DCD donor pancreas transplants are being carried out increasingly and the outcome is broadly similar to that for DBD pancreas transplants.

Donor organ supply and demand in the UK

In the UK, recent legal and organizational changes have led to an increase in transplantation activity with a decrease in the combined waiting list for all organ types (Figure 9.1.1) that is primarily due to an increase in kidney transplant activity.

The recent expansion in deceased donor numbers is largely attributable to an increase in the numbers of DCD donors (Figure 9.1.2). DBD donor numbers have plateaued because of improvements in road safety, better neurosurgical care, and more effective disease prevention. Although deceased donor numbers overall are increasing, the average age of donors is rising, as is the percentage of donors with co-morbidities that reduce organ quality.

Organization of organ retrieval in the UK

To address the shortage of deceased organ donors in the UK, an Organ Donation Taskforce was set up by the UK government in 2006.[5] The Taskforce focused on three major areas: effective donor identification and referral; improved donor coordination; and efficient organ retrieval processes. Changes implemented in response to the Taskforce findings include the introduction of a National Organ Retrieval Service and a comprehensive network of specialist nurses in organ donation (SN-ODs).

National Organ Retrieval Service

The National Organ Retrieval Service comprises 13 teams (seven abdominal and six cardiothoracic). Each team covers donor hospitals in a defined geographical location and comprises a lead surgeon, assistant surgeon, scrub nurse, and usually a perfusionist. National Health Service Blood and Transplant (NHSBT), a Special Health Authority, provides oversight and governance of the retrieval service.

Referral pathways

In the UK, SN-ODs are pivotal in the process of deceased organ donation. SN-ODs work in regional teams and take referrals of potential deceased organ donors from hospital clinicians based

Table 9.1.1 The modified Maastricht classification of DCD donors[1,2]

Category	Description	Donor subtype
I	Sudden death occurring outside hospital. No CPR	Uncontrolled
II	Unsuccessful CPR that started outside of hospital	Uncontrolled
III	Death expected after treatment withdrawal in a hospital environment	Controlled
IV	Cardiac arrest in a patient already confirmed dead by brain death criteria	Controlled
V	Unexpected cardiac arrest in a hospitalized patient	Uncontrolled

CPR, cardiopulmonary resuscitation.

Adapted from *Transplantation Proceedings*, Volume 27, Issue 5, Kootstra G. et al., Categories of non-heart-beating donors, pp. 2893–4, Copyright © 1995 Elsevier Inc. All rights reserved., with permission from Elsevier, http://www.sciencedirect.com/science/journal/00411345; with data from Sánchez-Fructuoso A.I. et al, Renal transplantation from non-heart beating donors: a promising alternative to enlarge the donor pool, *Journal of the American Society of Nephrology*, Volume 11, Issue 2, pp. 350–8, Copyright © 2000 by the American Society of Nephrology.

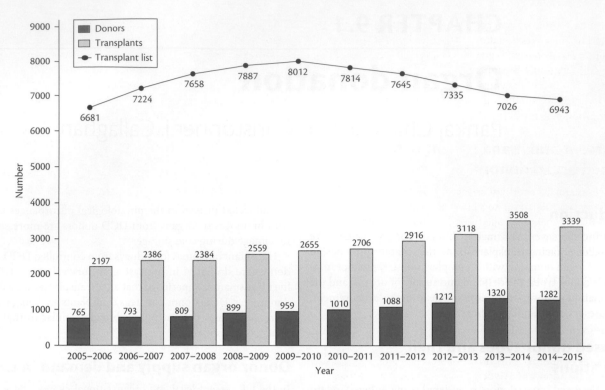

Fig. 9.1.1 The number of deceased donors, transplants in the UK, *1 April 2005–31 March 2015*, and patients on the active transplant list at 31 March 2015.
Reproduced with permission from *NHS Blood and Transplant Organ Donation and Transplantation Activity Report 2014/15*, Copyright © NHS Blood and Transplant, available from http://nhsbtmediaservices.blob.core.windows.net/organ-donationassets/pdfs/activity_report_2014_15.pdf

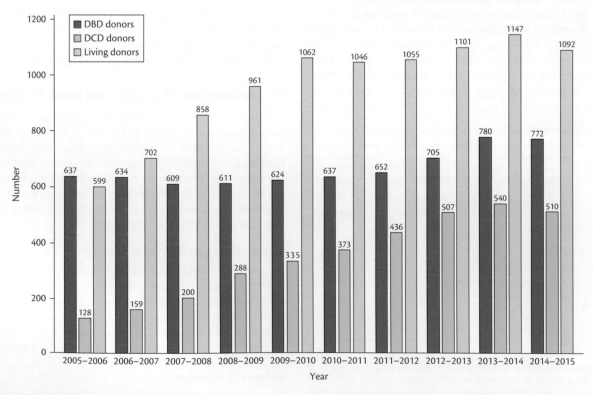

Fig. 9.1.2 Graph showing donor types in the UK 2005–2015.
Reproduced with permission from *NHS Blood and Transplant Organ Donation and Transplantation Activity Report 2014/15*, Copyright © NHS Blood and Transplant, available from http://nhsbtmediaservices.blob.core.windows.net/organ-donationassets/pdfs/activity_report_2014_15.pdf

in intensive care units or emergency departments. The SN-ODs are usually present when donation is discussed with the potential donor's family and if consent is given, notify NHSBT to enable them to mobilize the regional National Organ Retrieval Service team. Organ offers to implanting centres are made either by SN-ODs, or by NHSBT, depending on the organ type and allocation system (see Organ allocation systems in the UK section).

Assessment and management of potential deceased organ donors

The SN-OD performs an initial assessment of the potential donor to identify contraindications to donation (Box 9.1.1), and record core information including age, blood group, body mass index, history of the current admission, past medical history, current and previous medications, and relevant investigations.

Diagnosing death in potential deceased organ donors

The diagnosis of death can be complex as there are legal, religious, and ethical aspects that influence diagnostic criteria, making transplantation from deceased donors controversial in some cultures. Death can be defined as the irreversible loss of the capacity for consciousness combined with the irreversible loss of the capacity to breathe.[6] DBD donors have death diagnosed using neurological criteria, whereas combined neurological and circulatory criteria are used to diagnose death in DCD donors.

Diagnosis of death in DBD donors

Before testing for brain death, pre-conditions must be met and alternative diagnoses excluded. Pre-conditions require the patient

---

Box 9.1.1 Absolute contraindications to deceased organ donation

Absolute contraindications to organ donation

- Age > 85 years
- Acquired immunodeficiency syndrome (organs from well-controlled HIV infection may be suitable for HIV+ recipients)
- Any cancer with evidence of spread outside the affected organ within the last 3 years (excluding non-melanotic skin cancers)
- Definite, probable or possible human transmissible spongiform encephalopathy, including Creutzfeldt-Jakob disease and variant Creutzfeldt-Jakob disease, family history of familial Creutzfeldt-Jakob disease, other neurodegenerative diseases associated with infectious agents
- Malignant melanoma (other than completely excised stage I cancers)
- Choriocarcinoma
- Active haematological malignancy (myeloma, lymphoma, leukaemia)
- Tuberculosis (active or untreated)

Adapted with permission from Organ Donation and Transplantation, *Contraindications to Organ Donation—A Guide for SNODs*, Copyright © NHS Blood and Transplant, available from http://www.odt.nhs.uk/pdf/contraindications_to_organ_donation.pdf. The role of the list is to be a guide to non-approach for a potential donor family.

---

to be comatose and mechanically ventilated for apnoea. The cause of the coma must be known and irreversible. Non-neurological causes for coma must be excluded such as hypothermia, endocrine or metabolic disturbances, and the effects of drugs (e.g. barbiturates or neuromuscular blockade). Tests for absence of brainstem function and the afferent and efferent nerve pathways are shown in Table 9.1.2. Additional confirmatory investigations (e.g. electroencephalography, cerebral angiography) are not required in the UK.

The diagnosis of brain death must be made by two doctors (at least one Consultant), competent in the procedure, and registered for more than 5 years. The doctors should undertake testing together and neither should be a member of the transplant team. Tests must be performed twice.

Diagnosis of death in DCD donors

For DCD donors, death is diagnosed on circulatory and neurological criteria.[6] The patient must be unconscious with no capacity to breath, an absent pupillary response to light, an absent corneal reflex, and lack a motor response to supraorbital pressure. In addition, the potential donor must have lost the capacity to breathe as demonstrated by 5 minutes observation of maintained cardiorespiratory arrest (absence of respiratory effort and loss of cardiac output)—the 'stand-down' period.

For Maastricht III donors, withdrawal of life-sustaining treatment can occur in the intensive care unit, anaesthetic room adjacent to theatres, or in theatre itself. Death is diagnosed by an intensive care doctor or anaesthetist and organ procurement can begin immediately afterwards.

Consent for donation

The consent process for organ donation varies between countries, and may impact on organ donation rates. Broadly, consent systems may be 'opt in' (consent for donation is sought from the family or indicated by prior donor registration on an organ donation register) or 'opt out' (all potential deceased donors are considered to have agreed to donation unless they have indicated otherwise, i.e. 'presumed consent'). The UK (excluding Wales) has an 'opt in' system and approximately 40% of families of potential deceased donors refuse consent for donation.

Pre-donation management of the potential deceased donor

The medical management of potential deceased donors is complex due to the many physiological disturbances that occur around the time of death.

DBD donors

In patients with brain death, the presence of ischaemic cerebral tissue with failure of the neuroendocrine axis leads to changes in the cardiovascular, endocrine, haematological, and thermoregulatory systems. Cardiovascular disturbances include a hyperdynamic phase due to sympathetic over-activity ('catecholamine storm'), leading to tachycardia, hypertension, increased cardiac output, and raised systemic vascular resistance. Subsequent cardiovascular collapse and hypotension may result from loss of sympathetic tone, vasodilatation, and hypovolaemia secondary to diabetes insipidus. Endocrine changes originate from anterior and posterior pituitary failure leading to reduced thyroid hormone and anti-diuretic hormone secretion; lack of the latter causes diabetes insipidus). After the initial catecholamine storm, cortisol production decreases.

Table 9.1.2 Tests for absence of brainstem function and the afferent and efferent nerve pathways

Test	Findings in brainstem death	Afferent (sensory) nerve	Absent efferent (motor) nerve response
Pupillary reaction to light	Fixed and dilated pupils	Optic nerve (CN II)	Parasympathetic fibres carried on the oculomotor nerve (CN III)
Corneal reflexes	Absent corneal reflexes	Trigeminal nerve, ophthalmic division (CN V)	Facial nerve (CN VII)
Eye movement on caloric testing (vestibulo-ocular reflex)	Absent eye movements	Vestibulocochlear nerve (CN VIII)	Oculomotor, trochlear, and abducens nerves (CNs III, IV, and VI, respectively)
Motor responses in the cranial nerve distribution in response to stimulation of face, trunk or limbs	Absent motor responses in the cranial nerve distribution	Multiple	Facial nerve (VII)
Gag reflex	Absent gag reflex	Glossopharyngeal nerve (CN IX)-	Vagus nerve (CN X)
Cough reflex	Absent cough reflex	Vagus nerve (CN X)	Vagus (CN X) and phrenic nerves
Respiratory response to hypercarbia (P_aCO_2 >6 kPa) and ventilator disconnection for at least 5 minutes	Absent respiratory response	Central chemoreceptors (medulla) and peripheral chemoreceptors (carotid body—glossopharyngeal nerve [CN IX], and aortic body—vagus nerve [CN X])	Phrenic and intercostal nerves

CN, cranial nerve.

Disseminated intravascular coagulation is common due to the release of tissue thromboplastin from ischaemic brain tissue. Hypothermia can result from impaired hypothalamic function, loss of muscular activity, and peripheral vasodilatation.

If consent is given for organ donation, the emphasis of care changes from preservation of brain function to optimizing organ function for transplantation. Hypovolaemia should be corrected, but, if possible, inotropes should be avoided. Hormone replacement therapy may be needed to reduce inotrope requirements (e.g. vasopressin or desmopressin for diabetes insipidus, and triiodothyronine for hypothyroidism). Methylprednisolone is commonly given to reduce the inflammatory response. Insulin infusions are often needed to counteract hyperglycaemia associated with methylprednisolone and the 5% dextrose given intravenously to replace water loss from diabetes insipidus. Electrolyte imbalances should be corrected and hypothermia treated by active warming. Disseminated intravascular coagulation should be corrected with fresh frozen plasma and platelets at the time of organ procurement if haemostasis is problematic.

Potential controlled DCD donors

Management of a potential Maastricht III DCD organ donor on the intensive care unit is ethically complex, as the patient is still alive and any intervention that might potentially cause harm or distress must be avoided. The decision on withdrawal of life-sustaining treatments must be made independently of, and prior to, any consideration of organ donation. The intensive care team must make decisions on management before donation, with the patient's best interests in mind; the transplant team has no role in these decisions. In some countries, administration of heparin, phentolamine (a vasodilator), or placement of vascular cannulae prior to death, is allowed in potential Maastricht III DCD donors. These are not legal in the UK at present.

Withdrawal of life-sustaining treatment consists of stopping infusions and disconnecting respiratory support devices (extubation of or disconnection of the endotracheal tube).

Abdominal multiorgan retrieval surgery

The main objective in multiorgan retrieval is to remove organs safely, efficiently, and in an optimal condition. There are variations in the technique of abdominal organ retrieval.[7] A full laparotomy and thoracotomy is mandatory to detect any pathology. The techniques described here assume that cardiothoracic organ procurement is not taking place.

Operative procedure for DBD donors

A midline incision from the suprasternal notch to the pubic symphysis is made. Median sternotomy is performed and the pericardium opened. The right colon, small bowel mesentery, and duodenum are mobilized and the distal abdominal aorta isolated in preparation for arterial cannulation.

If the liver is to be procured, the portal triad is dissected, the common bile duct is ligated distally and divided proximally, and the origin of the gastroduodenal artery (GDA) from the common hepatic artery identified. The portal vein is identified and if portal perfusion is required, the inferior or superior mesenteric veins are identified near the pancreas, or in the root of the small bowel mesentery, respectively.

Once the anaesthetist, surgical team, and perfusionist are ready, high-dose intravenous heparin can be given to enable full anticoagulation. The distal abdominal aorta is ligated at the bifurcation, occluded proximally, and cannulated with a large (e.g. 20 Fr) cannula. The inferior mesenteric vein (or superior mesenteric vein) is then cannulated if needed. A cross-clamp is applied to the descending thoracic aorta to isolate the abdominal contents for cold perfusion. Cold preservation fluid is run through the aortic (± portal) cannula(e) and iced saline slush placed into the abdominal cavity to assist organ cooling. Venting of preservation fluid can be achieved by transecting the inferior vena cava (IVC) in the pericardium.

Organs are removed in the following order: liver, pancreas, kidneys. The gastroduodenal artery and splenic artery are cut off the common hepatic artery and the arterial blood supply to the liver via the coeliac artery is taken on a patch of abdominal aorta. The portal vein is divided, and the infrahepatic IVC transected above the right renal vein. The IVC is divided in the pericardium, and the liver removed with a cuff of diaphragm attached.

The pancreas is mobilized and the pylorus and proximal jejunum divided using a stapling device, as is the small bowel mesentery. The transverse mesocolon is transected, the superior mesenteric artery divided close to its origin, and the pancreas is removed with a 'C' of duodenum and spleen attached.

For donor nephrectomy, the left colon is mobilized and the ureters are transected distally. The left renal vein is divided at its confluence with the IVC and the distal abdominal aorta is transected at the bifurcation. The anterior aortic wall is opened in the midline and the orifices of the main renal arteries and any polar arteries visualized. The posterior wall of the abdominal aorta is divided in the midline and the IVC transected at the level of aortic bifurcation. Each kidney is then mobilized in turn, with wide dissection planes posterior to the aorta to avoid damaging renal vessels. The ureter is dissected with a wide cuff of peri-ureteric tissues.

Lymph nodes and splenic samples are removed for cross-matching. If the liver or pancreas are procured, iliac vessels are also excised to enable vascular reconstructions.

Operative procedure for controlled DCD donors

The surgical approach to DCD donors differs from that of DBD donors due to the requirement to minimize organ warm ischaemic damage. The 'super rapid' retrieval technique is described for controlled DCD donors. Uncontrolled DCD donors initially undergo organ perfusion via groin cannulae, prior to the consent process and subsequent organ removal (not described further here).

For Maastricht III DCD donors, the organ retrieval team prepare for surgery while treatment is withdrawn. The time between treatment withdrawal and death is highly variable, and a prolonged period of hypotension or hypoxia (warm ischaemic time) prior to death may render organs unusable. Acceptable warm ischaemic limits vary between organs. In general, systolic blood pressure <50 mmHg for more than 30 minutes, or time from withdrawal to death of more than 60 minutes, would be unacceptable for liver or pancreas donation. These limits are less restrictive for Maastricht III DCD kidney donors and kidneys have been successfully transplanted from donors dying up to 4 hours after withdrawal.

If the donor dies within an acceptable time frame, they are transferred rapidly to the operating theatre. A midline incision is made from the suprasternal notch to the symphysis pubis and the abdomen rapidly entered. The right common iliac artery or distal abdominal aorta is cannulated and perfusion with cooled, heparinized, organ preservation solution commenced. Iced saline slush is placed in the abdomen, and the chest opened through a median sternotomy. The descending thoracic aorta is cross-clamped and the IVC vented in the pericardium. This 'super rapid' approach minimizes the warm dissection phase (less than 10 minutes).

The right colon, duodenum, and small bowel mesentery are mobilized, and the liver hilum is dissected, as described in the Operative procedure for DBD donors section. If the liver is to be procured, cannulation of the superior mesenteric vein or portal vein may be required. Further dissection in the cold phase and organ removal proceeds as for the DBD donor.

Back-table surgery, packing, and closure

Removed organs are inspected noting possible damage, anatomical variation, quality of perfusion, pathology (e.g. tumours, cysts), and any other abnormalities (e.g. degree of steatosis or fibrosis of the liver and/or pancreas). Organs are often perfused further on the back-table with cold preservation solution before being packed and placed in ice. Donor incisions are carefully closed.

Organ preservation and storage

Aims and basic principles

The aim of organ preservation techniques is to minimize further deterioration prior to transplantation. Without adequate organ preservation, cells undergo progressive cellular damage due to metabolic acidosis, activation of autolysis, and loss of cell wall integrity due to ATP depletion and failure of the Na^+K^+- ATPase. Organ preservation techniques can be divided into static cold storage or machine perfusion.

Static cold storage

Cooling organs facilitates preservation by reducing enzyme activity. Static cold storage (i.e. cold perfused organs stored in an ice box) is the most common approach to organ preservation due to its low cost, simplicity, and proven efficacy. Cold (4°C) organ preservation solution is used to perfuse the organ as soon as possible after loss of circulation in the donor. Several different preservation solutions have been developed and choice is often based on cost and familiarity. Preservation solutions may contain an osmotic agent to reduce cellular swelling (e.g. mannitol, lactobionate), buffers to reduce intracellular acidosis (e.g. phosphate, bicarbonate), and electrolytes to maintain intracellular ionic homeostasis. Some solutions contain antioxidants (e.g. glutathione, allopurinol), metabolic energy substrates (e.g. adenosine, ketoglutarate), and amino acids.

In the UK, the most commonly used cold preservation solutions for abdominal organs are University of Wisconsin (UW) solution (e.g. ViaSpan, SPS-1, Belzer-UW), and Marshall's hypertonic citrate solution (e.g. Soltran). UW solution is widely regarded as the gold standard.[8] For DBD donor organs, acceptable cold ischaemic times are: liver, 10 to 12 hours; pancreas, 12 to 14 hours; kidney, 20 to 24 hours; and small bowel, 5 to 6 hours. Cold ischaemic limits for DCD donors are more stringent: liver, 9 hours: pancreas 10 hours; and kidney 12 to 15 hours.

Machine perfusion techniques

Machine perfusion involves connecting the deceased donor or organ to a machine through which preservation fluid or blood is cycled. The perceived advantages of machine perfusion include thorough washout of metabolic wastes, ongoing provision of nutrients, and assessment of organ viability. This may lead to better organ selection, prolonged preservation, and improved graft function.

Machine perfusion can take place at 4°C (hypothermic machine perfusion [HMP]) or body temperature (normothermic machine perfusion [NMP]). HMP is widely used for kidney storage although two recent randomized controlled trials comparing HMP to static cold storage[9,10] showed inconsistent findings with respect to its value. NMP restores metabolism and cold injury is reduced, but NMP technology is complex and expensive and its potential role is not yet clear.

Organ allocation schemes in the UK

Organ allocation schemes aim to balance the competing requirements of equity (equal access to organs) and utility (best use of organs). A system based solely on equity would give all patients on the waiting list an equal chance of receiving an organ, whereas one based solely on utility would only allocate organs to recipients who would derive greatest survival benefit from it.

In order to include an element of utility into a scheme, the factors that determine technical feasibility and outcome must be known. These include ABO blood group compatibility (all organs), donor–recipient size-matching (liver, small bowel), donor–recipient age matching, and the need to minimize cold ischaemic time. The importance of HLA matching between the donor and recipient varies widely between organs. For kidney transplantation it is helpful to minimize HLA mismatches between the donor and recipient, whereas in liver transplantation HLA matching is not important.

Liver

In the UK, livers are allocated on a regional basis. Livers from deceased donors dying in hospitals within the regional zone around a liver transplant unit are first offered locally. Clinicians at the transplant centre allocate the organ based on the donor-recipient ABO blood groups, donor-recipient size and age, and recipient clinical urgency. Patients with acute (fulminant) liver failure who meet specific criteria may be placed on the 'super-urgent' list that affords national priority. Livers from deceased donors aged <40 years may be suitable for splitting, for use in two recipients (usually an adult and a child).

Pancreas

Deceased donor pancreases are allocated nationally. Patients on the UK waiting list are awarded points based on seven clinically relevant factors: donor–recipient age matching, donor body mass index, waiting time, total HLA mismatch, degree of sensitization to HLA, travel time between the donor and recipient hospitals, and whether the recipient is currently requiring dialysis or not. For each ABO- and HLA-compatible pancreas, a ranking list is generated based on a computer algorithm that scores the above factors. The pancreas (along with a kidney if needed) is then offered to the transplant centre where the highest-scoring patient is registered, for implantation into that patient.

Kidney

DBD kidneys are allocated through a national sharing scheme that requires ABO blood group compatibility and favours HLA matching. For adult patients with similar degrees of HLA matching,

prioritization is determined by a points-based system that takes into account time on the waiting list, donor–recipient age difference, and several other factors. The kidney is offered to the transplant unit where the highest-scoring patient is registered. Kidneys from DCD donors are currently allocated regionally to minimize cold ischaemic times.

Further reading

Academy of Medical Royal Colleges. *UK guidelines on the diagnosis and confirmation of death* Available from: http://www.bts.org.uk/documents/a%20code%20of%20practice%20for%20the%2diagnosis%20and%20confirmation%20of%20death.pdf (accessed 20 July 2013).

National Health Service Blood and Transplant. *UK transplant activity report 2011–2012.* Available from https://nhsbtmediaservices.blob.core.windows.net/organ-donationassets/pdfs/activity_report_2011_12.pdf (accessed 20 July 2013).

Organ and Donar Transplantation. General information on UK transplant organisations, policies, and outcomes. Availabe from www.odt.nhs.uk (accessed 20 July 2013).

References

1. Kootstra G, Daemen JH, Oomen AP. Categories of non-heart-beating donors. *Transplant Proc* 1995; 27(5): 2893–4.
2. Sánchez-Fructuoso AI, Prats D, Torrente J, *et al.* Renal transplantation from non-heart beating donors: a promising alternative to enlarge the donor pool. *J Am Soc Nephrol* 2000; 11(2): 350–8.
3. Summers DM, Johnson RJ, Allen J, *et al.* Analysis of factors that affect outcome after transplantation of kidneys donated after cardiac death in the UK: a cohort study. *Lancet* 2010; 376(9749): 1303–11.
4. Summers DM, Johnson RJ, Hudson A, *et al.* Effect of donor age and cold storage time on outcome in recipients of kidneys donated after circulatory death in the UK: a cohort study. *Lancet* 2013; 381(9868): 727–34.
5. Department of Health (UK). *The Organ Donor Taskforce First Report, January 2008,* http://www.bts.org.uk/Documents/Publications/Organs%20for%20transplants%20-%20The%20Organ%20Donor%20Task%20Force%20201st%20report.pdf (accessed 20 July 2013).
6. Gardiner D, Shemie S, Manara A, *et al.* International perspective on the diagnosis of death. *Br J Anaesth* 2012; 108(Suppl 1): i14–28.
7. Brockmann JG, Vaidya A, Reddy S, *et al.* Retrieval of abdominal organs for transplantation. *Br J Surg* 2006; 93(2): 133–46.
8. O'Callaghan JM, Knight SR, Morgan RD, *et al.* Preservation solutions for static cold storage of kidney allografts: a systematic review and meta-analysis. *Am J Transplant* 2012; 12(4): 896–906.
9. Moers C, Pirenne J, Paul A, *et al.* Machine perfusion or cold storage in deceased-donor kidney transplantation. *N Engl J Med* 2012; 366(8): 770–1.
10. Watson CJ, Wells AC, Roberts RJ, *et al.* Cold machine perfusion versus static cold storage of kidneys donated after cardiac death: a UK multicenter randomized controlled trial. *Am J Transplant* 2010; 10(9): 1991–9.

Principles of transplant immunology and immunosuppressive therapy

Eleanor M. Bolton and J. Andrew Bradley

Introduction

All types of organ transplant stimulate a powerful immune response in the recipient that, in the absence of immunosuppressive therapy, leads to rapid graft rejection. A basic understanding of the immunological principles of graft rejection and knowledge about how best to overcome rejection using appropriate immunosuppressive agents are essential prerequisites for effective clinical management (Table 9.2.1).

Table 9.2.1 Immunosuppressive agents used in organ transplantation

Agent	Mode of action	Therapy
Prednisolone	Anti-inflammatory	Induction and maintenance, acute rejection
Azathioprine	Antiproliferative	Maintenance
Mycophenolate	Antiproliferative	Maintenance
Ciclosporin	Calcineurin inhibitor	Maintenance
Tacrolimus	Calcineurin inhibitor	Maintenance
Sirolimus and Everolimus	Mammalian target of rapamycin (mTOR) inhibitor	Maintenance when calcineurin inhibitors are to be avoided
Anti-thymocyte globulin, anti-lymphocyte serum	Depletion of lymphocytes	Induction therapy, acute rejection
Basiliximab	Anti-CD25: inhibition of activated T cells	Induction therapy
Alemtuzumab	Anti-CD52: depletion of lymphocytes and natural killer cells	Induction therapy
Rituximab	Anti-CD20: depletion of B lymphocytes	Induction therapy, acute rejection
Belatacept	CTLA4-Ig fusion protein: blockade of lymphocyte activation	Maintenance

Immunological barriers to transplantation

ABO blood groups

ABO blood group antigens are widely expressed in all organs and successful transplantation requires ABO blood group compatibility. Blood group O recipients develop both anti-A and anti-B antibodies in infancy and are therefore incompatible with both group A and B donors. Group A recipients have anti-B antibodies and group B recipients have anti-A antibodies and are incompatible with groups B and A donors, respectively. Group AB recipients have no antibodies and are 'universal recipients' whereas blood group O donors are 'universal donors'. Inadvertent transplantation of an ABO-incompatible organ risks causing hyperacute graft rejection. ABO-incompatible living donor kidney transplantation may be performed in recipients with levels of antibody to their ABO-incompatible living donor that are low enough to be removed by plasmapheresis or immunadsorption before transplantation.[1,2] (see Chapter 9.3, Kidney Transplantation, Allocation of deceased donor kidneys in the UK and Urological problems sections).

Human leukocyte antigens

Human leukocyte antigens (HLA) are the major immunological barrier to transplantation. They are widely expressed cell-surface glycoproteins whose normal physiological function is that of antigen-recognition elements, but in the context of transplantation they are highly antigenic. HLA molecules are coded for by the major histocompatibility complex on chromosome 6 and are highly polymorphic such that genetically unrelated individuals inevitably differ widely at numerous HLA alleles. The six HLA alleles that are most relevant to transplantation are the class I molecules HLA-A, HLA-B, and HLA-C, and the class II molecules HLA-DR, HLA-DP, and HLA-DQ. The HLA type of an individual is determined by DNA sequencing in the tissue-typing laboratory. Individuals express HLA genes from both the maternally derived and paternally derived chromosomes so that a total of 6 to 12 different HLA antigens are expressed, depending on the degree of homozygosity (shared antigens) at each of the 6 main HLA loci. Knowing the HLA type of the organ donor and recipient is necessary when attempting to achieve a degree of HLA match between donor and recipient as is done when allocating deceased donor kidneys and pancreases for transplantation. In the UK, only mismatches at HLA-A, HLA-B, and HLA-DR are taken into account when sharing deceased donor kidneys. Mismatches at each of the two loci for these three alleles are expressed as three digits where, for example, 1:2:1 is a four-antigen mismatched kidney with one mismatch at HLA-A, two mismatches at HLA-B, and one mismatch at HLA-DR. It is necessary to know the HLA type of the donor and recipient in order to determine the clinical significance of HLA antibodies in the recipient, both before and after transplantation.

Immunological basis of rejection

Transplant rejection is the result of recognition by the recipient's adaptive immune system (T and B lymphocytes) of non-self HLA molecules. A primary rejection response is initiated when CD4 T 'helper' lymphocytes recognize non-self HLA originating from the transplant. Following alloantigen recognition, CD4 T cells must be activated in order to coordinate the complex molecular and cellular interactions that result in rejection. This can only happen if CD4 T cells recognize alloantigen in the context of antigen-presenting cells (APC) that are able to provide the necessary 'second signal'. Both B lymphocytes and dendritic cells generally perform the function of APC; whereas the distribution of B cells is largely restricted to the haematopoietic system and lymphoid tissues, dendritic cells are present both in the blood and extensively in interstitial tissues throughout the body and are highly effective at processing and presenting antigen. Following reperfusion of an organ transplant, tissue dendritic cells migrate from the graft to draining lymph nodes and spleen where they encounter CD4 T cells. T-cell receptor engagement induces the APC to express co-stimulatory molecules that, in turn, activate the T cells.[3]

Mechanisms of graft rejection

Cytokines produced by activated CD4 T cells have inflammatory, chemotactic, and vasodilatory activity that facilitates activation and trafficking of immune effector cells. These include CD8 cytotoxic T lymphocytes, B lymphocytes (that differentiate into alloantibody-producing plasma cells), and inflammatory cells (including natural killer cells, polymorphonuclear leukocytes, granulocytes and macrophages)[4] (Figure 9.2.1). Inflammatory cells mediate cellular damage that is not antigen-specific and resembles a delayed-type hypersensitivity response; organ damage results from longer-term effects of inflammation that include capillary damage, cellular necrosis, and fibrosis. In contrast, the cell-mediated cytotoxicity characteristic of B cells and CD8 T cells is highly alloantigen specific; B cells produce HLA-specific antibody that binds to target cells and 'tags' them for clearance by phagocytosis or by natural killer cells, while CD8 cytotoxic cells bind directly to their target cells and kill them by release of perforins at the immune synapse (or point of contact) and by induction of apoptosis. Like CD4 T cells, B cells and CD8 T cells differentiate to become long-surviving memory cells that respond rapidly and specifically to a repeat challenge by proliferation and expansion of the effector cell pool.

Clinical patterns of rejection

The clinical pattern of rejection is defined by the nature of the immune effector mechanisms responsible and the timescale of the rejection process.

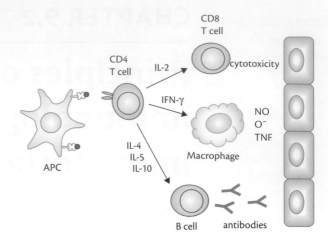

Fig. 9.2.1 Mechanisms of graft rejection. The CD4 T-helper cell is central to the effector mechanisms resulting in transplant rejection. CD4 T cells activated by recognition of mismatched donor HLA secrete cytokines that mediate activation and maturation of effector cell types including CD8 cytotoxic T cells that lyse target cells through release of granzymes and perforins, B lymphocytes that mature to form antibody-secreting plasma cells, and antigen non-specific cells such as macrophages and natural killer cells that have inflammatory activity and cause tissue damage through a range of pathways including release of free radicals, vasodilation, recruitment of granulocytes, and activation of the complement and coagulation cascades.

Hyperacute rejection

Hyperacute rejection occurs as a result of pre-existing circulating antibodies against ABO or HLA antigens. It occurs within minutes of re-establishing the transplant's blood supply, causing intravascular thrombosis, interstitial haemorrhage, and extensive tissue injury. Kidney allografts are particularly susceptible to hyperacute rejection and liver allografts are relatively resistant to such damage. Hyperacute rejection is rarely seen since it is avoided by ensuring ABO blood group compatibility and performing a pre-transplant cross-match test to exclude the presence of pre-existing donor-specific cytotoxic HLA antibodies before proceeding with transplantation. Such antibodies arise in response to past blood transfusion, pregnancy or a failed previous organ transplant.

Acute rejection

Acute rejection typically occurs within the first 6 months after transplantation and is a result of a *de novo* cellular and/or antibody-mediated immune response against HLA antigens expressed by the graft.[5] The rejection may be cellular or antibody-mediated or both. Acute cellular rejection is characterized by a lymphocytic infiltrate that is focal and perivascular initially and becomes heavier and diffuse, accompanied by an influx of macrophages, granulocytes, and plasma cells, together with associated parenchymal tissue damage and oedema. Antibody-mediated or humoral rejection is characterized by detection of complement components, particularly C4d, on the graft vasculature indicating the presence of antibodies binding to endothelial cells, and accompanied by graft oedema, interstitial haemorrhage, and accumulation of neutrophils. Acute rejection episodes are relatively common (occurring in up to 25% of transplant patients during the first year). They are usually reversible, although antibody-mediated rejection may be associated with inferior graft outcome.

Chronic rejection

Chronic rejection develops insidiously over months and years post-transplant and is the major cause of graft failure. The most characteristic pathological feature of chronic rejection is progressive occlusion of small arteries (graft vasculopathy), with concentric thickening of the intima caused by smooth muscle cell proliferation, and multilamellar or damaged elastic lamina, accompanied by graft fibrosis, and loss of parenchymal structures. Organ-specific features comprise glomerular sclerosis and tubular atrophy in the kidney, vanishing bile duct syndrome in the liver, and acinar cell loss and islet destruction in the pancreas. The likely causes of chronic rejection are an ongoing low-level cellular and particularly humoral immune response, compounded by other adverse factors including ischaemia/reperfusion injury, hyperlipidaemia and drug toxicity.[6]

Detection of human leukocyte antigen antibodies

The detection and characterization of pre-existing HLA antibodies in sensitized recipients before transplantation is important, so as to avoid inadvertently implanting an antibody incompatible donor organ, or to instigate desensitization if the levels are sufficiently low.[7] Detection of HLA antibodies following transplantation is also important to aid the diagnosis of antibody-mediated rejection. Historically, antibodies to HLA antigens were detected by their ability to mediate complement-dependent cytotoxicity against human cell lines expressing known HLA antigens. This test has now been supplemented by the more sensitive techniques of flow cytometric cross-match testing and Luminex technology that uses HLA coated beads to define HLA antibody specificities.[8]

Immunosuppression

General principles

Patients are treated with a range of immunosuppressive agents that aim to prevent rejection by targeting different arms of the immune response, while leaving adequate immune surveillance against infection and cancer. Immunosuppressive treatment is started at the time of transplant and continued indefinitely, with more intensive treatment given in the earliest stages. There is no consensus regarding the best combination of drugs and this depends on individual circumstances. Antibody induction therapy is widely used at the time of transplant and consists of antibodies to temporarily disable or deplete lymphocytes. Most transplant recipients receive a triple drug regimen for induction and maintenance therapy consisting of corticosteroids, a calcineurin inhibitor (ciclosporin or tacrolimus), and an antiproliferative agent (azathioprine or mycophenolic acid). Steroid withdrawal is often undertaken and sometimes steroids are omitted completely.

Episodes of acute rejection are relatively common and usually respond to treatment with steroids. Steroid-resistant rejection is treated with lymphocyte-depleting antibodies. Antibody-mediated acute rejection is treated by plasmapheresis and sometimes depleting therapeutic antibodies.

Induction agents

Basiliximab (anti-CD25) inhibits activated T lymphocytes by binding to their interleukin-2 receptor and is widely used as an induction agent to reduce the incidence of acute rejection. For recipients at high risk of acute rejection, antithymocyte globulin or alemtuzumab (anti-CD52) may be used to deplete circulating lymphocytes that might otherwise initiate an early acute rejection response.[9–11]

Corticosteroids

Corticosteroids have broad-spectrum anti-inflammatory effects and are widely used, although in relatively modest doses. Long-term use is associated with serious side effects including hyperlipidaemia, osteoporosis, insulin resistance, as well as the immediate side effects of skin thinning, fluid retention, and impaired wound healing.

Calcineurin inhibitors

Calcineurin inhibitors are the mainstay of most maintenance regimens.[12] Both ciclosporin and tacrolimus bind to immunophilins and inhibit translocation of the transcription factor (nuclear factor of activated T cells) across the nucleus thereby preventing secretion of a range of cytokines, particularly interleukin-2 that is critical for lymphocyte activation and clonal expansion. Tacrolimus is more commonly used than ciclosporin. Optimal drug dosing is based on monitoring whole blood concentration. Agent-specific side effects include nephrotoxicity, hypertension, glucose intolerance, and hyperlipidaemia. Ciclosporin may cause gum hypertrophy and hirsutism, and tacrolimus is more neurotoxic and diabetogenic than ciclosporin.

Antiproliferative agents

Azathioprine and mycophenolic acid inhibit the *de novo* synthesis of nucleotides thereby preventing lymphocyte proliferation.[13] Mycophenolic acid is more selective for lymphocytes than azathioprine, and some, though not all, studies have suggested mycophenolic acid is superior. It is also more expensive and in the UK azathioprine is still widely used. In contrast to calcineurin inhibitors, therapeutic monitoring of azathioprine and mycophenolic acid is not usually undertaken. Gastrointestinal effects and myelotoxicity are common side effects but usually respond to reduced dosing.

mTOR inhibitors

The mTOR inhibitors sirolimus and everolimus inhibit a serine/threonine protein kinase that regulates G1 to S phase cell cycling. They impair lymphocyte proliferation and are a possible alternative to calcineurin inhibitors for selected recipients, particularly those with calcineurin nephrotoxicity.[14,15] While mTOR inhibitors are not nephrotoxic, they impair wound healing, are sometimes poorly tolerated, and may cause interstitial pneumonitis. They may have a role in recipients with malignancy because of their antitumour activity.

Other agents

Rituximab is an anti-CD20 antibody that depletes B lymphocytes and may have a role in preventing and treating humoral rejection.[16] Belatacept is a fusion protein (CTLA4-Ig) that targets the co-stimulation requirement for lymphocyte activation.[17,18] Increasingly, the extended range of immunosuppressive agents with subtly different effects may be used in new combinations to address particular problems associated with current standard immunosuppression.

Complications of immunosuppression

Infection

All patients undergoing organ transplantation are at increased risk of infection because of the immunosuppression they receive, particularly during the early post-transplant period. The risk and type of infection vary according to the amount of immunosuppression given and the time after transplantation. Approaches to prophylaxis are governed by the type of organ transplanted and the individual patient circumstances.

Bacterial infections

In the first month following organ transplant, recipients are particularly prone to nosocomial (hospital acquired infection) that are mostly bacterial and related directly to transplant surgery. Wound infection, urinary tract infection, intra-abdominal, and chest infection are all relatively common. While many of these infections might have occurred in the absence of immunosuppression, they are more potentially more serious in immunosuppressed patients. A high index of suspicion and aggressive management are important.

Viral infections

Immunosuppressive therapy markedly impairs the protective effect of T-cell immunity against viral infection, and viral infection poses a serious threat particularly in the first 6 months after transplantation when levels of immunosupression are greatest. Of particular concern are members of the herpes virus family of DNA viruses (cytomegalovirus [CMV], Epstein–Bar virus [EBV] and herpes simplex and varicella zoster infection). In the normal population these rarely cause serious problems, but in immunosuppressed transplant recipients can cause major morbidity and life-threatening illness. In most cases infection arises through reactivation of latent virus infection rather than a primary infection. However, the transplanted organ is capable of transmitting infection from an organ donor who has a latent virus infection and primary infections can be particularly severe in immunosuppressed patients.

Cytomegalovirus infection

CMV infection is a particular concern after organ transplantation.[19] Infection may arise from reactivation of latent virus or as a primary infection most often acquired by transmission from the donor organ. CMV disease typically presents with pyrexia, lymphopaenia, and thrombocytopaenia, along with additional symptoms according to the predominant site of tissue invasion. Pneumonitis, hepatitis, or gastrointestinal inflammation are all common. CMV infection is also associated with an increased risk of acute rejection. Organ transplant recipients at high risk should be given CMV prophylaxis, including CMV-seronegative recipients of an organ from a CMV-seropositive donor and CMV-seropositive recipients receiving T-cell depleting antibody therapy. Prophylaxis with valganciclovir for 100 days is widely used. An alternative approach is to monitor recipients with weekly blood samples for CMV viraemia and start antiviral prophylaxis if CMV DNA levels exceed a predefined threshold. Established CMV disease is diagnosed by detection of CMV DNA in whole blood and when possible histological confirmation of disease in biopsy tissue. It is treated by oral valganciclovir or intravenous ganciclovir, a common side effect of which is neutropaenia.

BK virus infection

BK virus is a polyoma virus that is widespread in the general population where it is of little significance. However in immunosuppressed renal transplant recipients latent virus residing in the renal tract epithelium may become reactivated and cause infection to ascend into the renal tubules where it causes BK nephropathy.[20] This presents with graft dysfunction and the diagnosis is confirmed by identification of viral inclusions on graft biopsy. Treatment comprises careful reduction in immunosuppression to allow the immune system to regain control of the virus.

Fungal infections

Immunosuppressed patients are particularly vulnerable to fungal infections of which candida infection is the most common problem.[21] Nystatin or amphotericin prophylaxis is given routinely for 1 to 3 months to prevent oral and oesophageal candidiasis. The environmental fungi *Aspergillus* and *Cryptococcus* are a serious concern and may infect the lungs of transplant recipients and occasionally produce disseminated infection or localized disease elsewhere. Serology and antigen detection techniques aid the diagnosis of fungal infection but culture of infected fluid and histology of infected tissue allows a definitive diagnosis. Aggressive treatment with intravenous antifungals is required, but there is a high mortality rate for disseminated disease. *Pneumocystis jirovecii* is widespread in the environment and often colonizes the respiratory tract in healthy individuals. Prophylaxis with co-trimoxazole is commonly given.

Late infections

In the longer term, transplant recipients remain more susceptible than normal to community-acquired infections, but this should not limit their activities. Symptoms of infection should, however, be investigated promptly and consideration given to the possibility of infection by opportunistic pathogens, including CMV.

Malignancy

Long-term immunosuppression increases the risk of malignancy in recipients of organ transplants. There is a twofold to fivefold increase in most types of cancer in transplant recipients, but a much greater increase in the risk of certain types of cancer, most notably post-transplant lymphoproliferative disorder and squamous cell cancer of the skin.

Post-transplant lymphoproliferative disorder

This is the second most common type of malignancy in adult transplant recipients (2–5% recipients) and the most common malignancy in children after organ transplantation (5–10% recipients).[22,23] The term encompasses a range of malignancies arising in lymphoid cells, but most are B-cell lymphomas whose proliferation is driven by EBV. In children primary infection with EBV is usually the cause, whereas in most adults reactivation of EBV infection is responsible. Post-transplant lymphoproliferative disorder is more common after thoracic organ transplantation than after abdominal organ transplantation, because these patients receive more immunosuppression. Clinical presentation is highly variable and may occur at any time after transplantation, although half of cases present in the first year. The disease may be localized to lymph nodes, but more often is extranodal, often involving multiple sites, including the organ graft itself. Definitive diagnosis is based on tissue biopsy and histological evaluation. Initial treatment is reduction in immunosuppression to promote an anti-EBV immune response, but this risks triggering graft rejection. Many patients require additional treatment in the form of anti-CD20 antibody and systemic chemotherapy. The outcome is variable: patients with monomorphic disease have a poor prognosis but in patients with early (after transplantation) or polymorphic disease the prognosis is better with around 50% 5-year survival.

Cancer of the skin

Non-melanoma skin cancer (NMSC) is the most common malignancy in adult transplant recipients and affects around 50% of recipients.[24] Nearly all are either squamous cell carcinomas or basal cell carcinomas, with a predominance of squamous cell lesions. The risk of NMSC increases with the duration and amount of immunosuppression, and some cases may be related to infection by human papilloma virus, particularly those in the anogenital region. Exposure to ultraviolet radiation is a major risk factor and most NMSC are multi-focal and occur on sun-exposed areas. Transplant recipients should, therefore, be advised to avoid direct exposure to sunlight.

Most NMSCs are localized to the skin, although 5% of squamous cell carcinomas show lymph node metastasis; these can cause serious morbidity and are occasionally fatal. Early diagnosis and effective management by a specialist dermatologist is important. Regular (usually annual) skin surveillance after transplantation should be performed, preferably in a dedicated clinic, and new or suspicious lesions biopsied; if malignant they should be treated by excision or application of topical treatment. In patients with skin cancer, switching from calcineurin-based immunosuppression to mTOR may be helpful in preventing recurrence or managing aggressive lesions.[25]

Further reading

Danovitch GM (ed.). *Handbook of Kidney Transplantation*, 5th edition. Philadelphia: Lippincott Williams & Wilkins, 2009.

MacPhee I, Fronek F (eds). *Handbook of Renal and Pancreatic Transplantation*. Oxford: Wiley-Blackwell, 2012.

Morris PJ, Knechtle SJ (eds). *Kidney Transplantation: Principles and Practice*, 6th edition. Philadelphia: WB Saunders Elsevier, 2008.

Murphy K. *Janeway's Immunobiology*, 8th edition. New York: Garland Science, 2012.

References

1. Fehr T, Stussi G. ABO-incompatible kidney transplantation. *Curr Opin Organ Transplant* 2012; 17(4): 376–85.
2. Becker LE, Süsal C, Morath C. Kidney transplantation across HLA and ABO antibody barriers. *Curr Opin Organ Transplant* 2013; 18(4): 445–54.
3. Ali JM, Bolton EM, Bradley JA, *et al*. Allorecognition pathways in transplant rejection and tolerance. *Transplantation* 2013; 96(8): 681–8.
4. Wood KJ, Goto R. Mechanisms of rejection: current perspectives. *Transplantation* 2012; 93(1): 1–10.
5. Mengel M, Husain S, Hidalgo L, *et al*. Phenotypes of antibody-mediated rejection in organ transplants. *Transpl Int* 2012; 25(6): 611–22.
6. Renders L, Heemann U. Chronic renal allograft damage after transplantation: what are the reasons, what can we do? *Curr Opin Organ Transplant* 2012; 17(6): 634–9.
7. Montgomery RA, Warren DS, Segev DL, *et al*. HLA incompatible renal transplantation. *Curr Opin Organ Transplant* 2012; 17(4): 386–92.
8. Taylor CJ, Kosmoliaptsis V, Summers DM, *et al*. Back to the future: application of contemporary technology to long-standing questions about the clinical relevance of human leukocyte antigen-specific alloantibodies in renal transplantation. *Hum Immunol* 2009; 70(8): 563–8.
9. Rostaing L, Saliba F, Calmus Y, *et al*. Review article: use of induction therapy in liver transplantation. *Transplant Rev* 2012; 26(4): 246–60.
10. Morgan RD, O'Callaghan JM, Knight SR, *et al*. Alemtuzumab induction therapy in kidney transplantation: a systematic review and meta-analysis. *Transplantation* 2012; 93(12): 1179–88.
11. Wagner SJ, Brennan DC. Induction therapy in renal transplant recipients: how convincing is the current evidence? *Drugs* 2012; 72(5): 671–83.
12. Rush D. The impact of calcineurin inhibitors on graft survival. *Transplant Rev* 2013; 27(3): 93–5.
13. Villarroel MC, Hidalgo M, Jimeno A. Mycophenolate mofetil: An update. *Drugs Today* 2009; 45(7): 521–32.
14. Gurk-Turner C, Manitpisitkul W, Cooper M. A comprehensive review of everolimus clinical reports: a new mammalian target of rapamycin inhibitor. *Transplantation* 2012; 94(7): 659–68.
15. Halleck F, Duerr M, Waiser J, *et al*. An evaluation of sirolimus in renal transplantation. *Expert Opin Drug Metab Toxicol* 2012; 8(10): 1337–56.
16. Jordan SC, Kahwaji J, Toyoda M, *et al*. B-cell immunotherapeutics: emerging roles in solid organ transplantation. *Curr Opin Organ Transplant* 2011; 16(4): 416–24.
17. Grinyó JM, Budde K, Citterio F, *et al*. Belatacept utilization recommendations: an expert position. *Expert Opin Drug Saf* 2013; 12(1): 111–22.
18. Wojciechowski D, Vincenti F. Belatacept in kidney transplantation. *Curr Opin Organ Transplant* 2012; 17(6): 640–7.
19. Kotton CN. CMV: Prevention, diagnosis and therapy. *Am J Transplant* 2013; 13 Suppl 3: 24–40
20. Cannon RM, Ouseph R, Jones CM, *et al*. BK viral disease in renal transplantation. *Curr Opin Organ Transplant* 2011; 16(6): 576–9.
21. Shoham S, Marr KA. Invasive fungal infections in solid organ transplant recipients. *Future Microbiol* 2012; 7(5): 639–55.
22. Green M, Michaels MG. Epstein-Barr virus infection and posttransplant lymphoproliferative disorder. *Am J Transplant* 2013; 13(Suppl 3): 41–54
23. Taylor AL, Marcus R, Bradley JA. Post-transplant lymphoproliferative disorders (PTLD) after solid organ transplantation. *Crit Rev Oncol Hematol* 2005; 56(1): 155–67.
24. Euvrard S, Kanitakis J, Claudy A. Skin cancers after organ transplantation. *N Engl J Med* 2003; 348(17): 1681–91.
25. Euvrard S, Morelon E, Rostaing L, *et al*. Sirolimus and secondary skin-cancer prevention in kidney transplantation. *N Engl J Med* 2012; 367(4): 329–39.

CHAPTER 9.3

Kidney transplantation

J. Andrew Bradley and Michael Nicholson

Introduction

The incidence of end-stage renal failure in the UK is fairly steady at around 108 pmp.[1] The common causes of end-stage renal disease are shown in Table 9.3.1, with diabetes being the most common. All ages are affected, although elderly patients predominate, and the mean age of adult patients accepted for renal replacement therapy is 65 years.[1] Renal replacement therapy comprises haemodialysis, peritoneal dialysis, and kidney transplantation. Around one-third of patients with end-stage renal disease are suitable candidates for renal transplantation. Over 2500 kidney transplants were performed during 2012 in the UK: two-thirds were deceased donor and one third are living donor transplants. Transplant numbers are increasing gradually but remain two to three fold short of the number needed.

Vascular and peritoneal access for dialysis

Patients with end-stage renal disease require dialysis to keep them alive. This most often comprises haemodialysis requiring vascular access but in a minority dialysis is delivered in the form of peritoneal dialysis.

Vascular access for dialysis

Vascular access for haemodialysis should, whenever possible, be planned well in advance. An arteriovenous (AV) fistula is the preferred type of vascular access for patients starting haemodialysis. If this is not possible, an AV graft or, failing this, a venous catheter may be used (tunnelled rather than non-tunnelled is preferred). Venous catheters are usually only employed as a last resort for long-term dialysis because of the associated risk of infection and increased mortality. It is important to avoid, whenever possible, venepuncture or insertion of a cannula into the forearm and the upper arm cephalic vein at a site where an arteriovenous fistula may be needed. When choosing where to site an AV fistula, the approach should be

Table 9.3.1 Causes of chronic renal failure in UK adults starting dialysis[1]

Diabetic nephropathy	25%
Hypertension/renovascular disease	14%
Glomerulonephritis	13%
Adult polycystic kidney disease (APKD)	7%
Pyelonephritis	7%
Unknown or other	34%

Source: data from Feest TG et al., *15th Annual Report of the Renal Association*, UK Renal Registry, Bristol, UK Copyright © UK Renal Registry 2012, available from www.renalreg.com/Reports/2012.html

to start distally in the non-dominant arm. In pre-dialysis patients with declining kidney function, a fistula should be created at least 3 months before it is likely to be required, allowing adequate time for it to mature. It is standard practice to give all patients undergoing creation of an AV fistula antiplatelet therapy, at least until it matures, to prevent early failure.

The radiocephalic fistula (Brescia–Cimino fistula) is the preferred first option. An end-to-side anastomosis is fashioned between the cephalic vein and the radial artery. In the UK, this is most commonly performed at the wrist but may also be sited more distally in the 'anatomical snuffbox' or proximal to the wrist. The expected primary patency rate for a standard radiocephalic fistula is approximately 60% at 5 years. If a radiocephalic fistula is not possible, then a brachiocephalic fistula at the elbow is usually the second choice, and failing this a brachio-basilic fistula at the elbow with transposition of the basilic vein (as a single-stage or two-stage procedure) so that it lies more superficially in the upper arm and is more readily accessible for cannulation. Other options are increasingly described, including an ulnar artery–basilic vein fistula at the wrist. Preoperative vascular mapping with the aid of Doppler ultrasound examination is used increasingly to assist the planning of fistula formation. If the opportunities for a standard AV fistula have been exhausted, then a graft of either autologous saphenous vein or synthetic graft may need to be used to create a functional fistula. This is usually placed in the forearm with anastomosis to the vessels in the ante-cubital fossa. Insertion of such grafts in the thigh is a last resort because of the risks of infection.

Complications of AV fistula include:

- failure of fistula to mature
- thrombosis
- aneurysm formation (single or multiple)
- haemorrhage
- steal syndrome
- fistula-related high-output cardiac failure (rare).

Aneurysm formation may lead to sudden rupture or thrombosis and its occurrence can be reduced by good needling technique. If a stenosis is suspected, it should be confirmed by duplex ultrasound (or angiography) and treated by percutaneous transluminal angioplasty or surgical revision of the fistula. Thrombosis may, if recognized early, be amenable to treatment by balloon angioplasty, but is often associated with stenosis that also requires correction. It is often possible to salvage a failing but patent radiocephalic fistula by performing a new anastomosis to the proximal cephalic vein obviating the need to progress to a fistula at the elbow.

Vascular access induced ischaemia is seen more commonly in the elderly and those with diabetes, and often results in 'steal syndrome'. For elbow fistulas, the incidence of steal syndrome is 10–20%. If severe it results in rest pain and atrophic changes. Intervention to reduce the blood flow through the fistula or ligation of the graft may be needed.

Peritoneal dialysis

A long-term indwelling silicone peritoneal dialysis catheter is used to deliver dialysis solutions into the peritoneal cavity, providing either continuous ambulatory dialysis or overnight machine exchanges. The dialysis catheter (Tenckhoff catheter) is made of silicon with one or more Dacron cuffs, which serve to anchor the catheter in the abdominal wall and provide a seal against infection. The most commonly used type is curled distally and has both end and side holes. The tip should be situated in the pelvis. The catheter can either be inserted via a small open sub-umbilical incision, tunnelling the proximal catheter laterally, or laparoscopically.

Potential contraindications to peritoneal dialysis include:

- intra-abdominal adhesions
- abdominal wall hernia
- obesity
- respiratory disease
- encapsulating (sclerosing) peritonitis.

The complications of peritoneal dialysis are:

- peritonitis
- exit site infection
- catheter obstruction (by omentum)
- fluid leak
- catheter tip migration
- hernia (at the site of incision or port site)
- encapsulating (sclerosing) peritonitis.

Advantages of transplantation over dialysis

For those able to withstand the challenges of transplant surgery and long-term immunosuppressive therapy, kidney transplantation offers improved longevity and superior quality of life. The complications of dialysis are avoided and uraemic symptoms are corrected, with no need for dietary and fluid restriction. Exercise capacity is increased and pregnancy is possible. Transplantation is also more cost-effective than dialysis.

Selection of patients for transplantation

Selection for renal transplantation should focus on the identification and evaluation of major co-morbid disease that precludes transplantation. Old age per se is not a contraindication to transplantation, but older patients have more co-morbid conditions that make transplantation inadvisable. Conditions with a life expectancy of less than 5 years are a contraindication to transplantation, as are uncontrolled infection and malignancy.[2] Patients with end-stage renal failure have a greatly increased risk of cardiovascular disease and it is important to perform a thorough cardiovascular risk assessment. High-risk patients should undergo a cardiac stress test (e.g. a stress echocardiogram), and those with symptoms of coronary artery disease should be referred for coronary angiography. Smokers should be strongly encouraged to stop before listing for transplantation. Morbid obesity (body mass index > 35) is a contraindication to transplantation because of the high risk of surgical complications and poorer patient and graft survival.

It is important to ensure that transplantation is technically feasible. If there are concerns about the anatomy or patency of the iliac and more distal blood vessels, this should be evaluated by duplex ultrasound and, if necessary, angiography. Patients with small poorly compliant bladders may need bladder augmentation or creation of an ileal conduit prior to transplantation. Pre-transplant native nephrectomy may be necessary in patients with very large polycystic kidneys to make room for a transplant or in patients with intractable renal tract infection. For patients who have had a malignant disease (excluding non-melanoma cancers of the skin), transplantation should only be considered when at least two years have elapsed since successful treatment.

Assessment should be performed in a timely manner and, where possible, patients should be listed for transplantation pre-emptively (within 6 months of the anticipated initiation of dialysis). Patients on the waiting list for transplantation should be formally re-evaluated annually (6 monthly if high risk) to confirm that they remain suitable candidates for renal transplantation.

Allocation of deceased donor kidneys in the UK

There is a national waiting list for deceased donor kidney transplantation in the UK and all kidneys from donation after brain death (DBD) donors are allocated according to an algorithm that aims to ensure equity of access and minimize the number of patients waiting many years.[3] Absolute priority is given to 0.0.0 human leukocyte antigen (HLA)-A, HLA-B, and HLA-DR mismatched patients and well-matched paediatric patients. Thereafter, kidneys are assigned according to a points-based system where length of time on the waiting list is the most influential factor but HLA mismatch is also taken into account, especially in younger recipients who may in the future require re-transplantation. The allocation algorithm also avoids allocating old kidneys to young recipients and vice versa. The average wait for a deceased donor transplant in the UK is around 3 years. Kidneys from younger donation after circulatory death (DCD) donors are also shared using similar criteria to those for DBD donor kidneys, but on a supra-regional rather than national basis to reduce the cold ischaemic time involved with shipping.

Living donor transplantation

For the recipient, a pre-emptive living donor kidney transplant offers the best chance of rehabilitation. All living donor transplants performed in the UK must first be approved by the Human Tissue Authority, a regulatory body established to oversee the working of the Human Tissue Act 2004 (or the Human Tissue Act (Scotland) 2006). Approval requires that an independent assessor authorized by the Human Tissue Authority has conducted separate interviews with the prospective donor and recipient and is satisfied that the donor is not rewarded, appropriate consent has been given, and that the donor and recipient are fully informed.

Assessment of the living donor

Prospective living donors must undergo a rigorous workup to confirm their medical suitability to donate, with a particular emphasis on excluding cardiovascular, respiratory, and kidney disease.[4] In addition to a full history and clinical examination, this includes extensive blood tests (including coagulation screen and serological testing to exclude viral infection), cardiovascular stress test, repeated urine dipstick testing, renal ultrasound, measurement of glomerular filtration rate, and either magnetic resonance angiogram or computed tomography angiogram to delineate the anatomy of the renal vasculature. Twenty-five per cent of individuals have two or more arteries to one or both kidneys. If both kidneys have single vessels, left donor nephrectomy is preferred since the longer renal vein facilitates implantation.

If hypertension (blood pressure > 140/90) is detected, ambulatory blood pressure monitoring should be performed. Mild to moderate hypertension that is readily controlled by no more than two antihypertensive agents and is not associated with end-organ damage need not necessarily exclude kidney donation. Similarly, microscopic haematuria on dipstix testing need not necessarily exclude donation, but requires cystoscopy and possible renal biopsy before donation can proceed.

All prospective donors should be counselled that nephrectomy might increase their risk of developing hypertension or making pre-existing hypertension more difficult to control. Prospective donors with obesity (body mass index 30–35) should be counselled about the long-term risk of kidney disease, the likely increased risk of perioperative complications, and be advised to reduce their body mass index to less than 30 prior to nephrectomy. Potential donors should also be told that if they sustain major trauma or develop a carcinoma of their remaining kidney then life-saving nephrectomy may be required, leaving them dialysis dependent.

Live donor nephrectomy

Nephrectomy is undertaken by a minimally invasive approach (total laparoscopic donor nephrectomy or hand-assisted laparoscopic donor nephrectomy). It is a relatively safe procedure (perioperative mortality rate 1 in 2000). Major perioperative complications occur in 5% of donors.[5] These include the need for blood transfusion, deep vein thrombosis, wound and chest infection, re-operation, and damage to an intra-abdominal viscus. After nephrectomy, a compensatory increase in glomerular filtration rate occurs (60–70% of pre-donation glomerular filtration at 1 year). Apart from increasing the risk of hypertension, nephrectomy appears to have no long-term detrimental effect. Donors should undergo annual screening with measurement of blood pressure, serum creatinine and urine dipstix testing.

Types of living donor

Transplants may be genetically related (most often between siblings or from parent to child) or genetically unrelated (most often between spouses or partners). Transplant outcome is similar in both groups and HLA mismatching is not associated with poorer graft survival.[6] A third of all potential recipients are antibody incompatible with their prospective living donor either because of ABO blood group incompatibility (ABOi) or because of antibodies directed against donor HLA antigens (HLAi). Historically, ABOi- and HLAi-incompatible transplants were not performed because of

the high risk of hyperacute rejection. Patients whose antibody levels are not too high can be desensitized by a combination of antibody removal (plasma exchange or immunoabsorption) and inhibition of new antibodies (using intravenous immunoglobulin or anti-CD20 antibody). For ABOi and HLAi pairs whose antibody levels are too high for desensitization, the UK paired/pooled scheme offers a possible route to transplantation.[7] Incompatible donor recipient pairs are entered into a national pool that seeks to identify two or three way exchanges that enable antibody-compatible live donor transplants to proceed. Unfortunately, less than half of recipients entered into the scheme find a suitable antibody-compatible donor.

Healthy individuals in the UK can volunteer to donate a kidney altruistically to a stranger recipient, subject to strict criteria that include a favourable psychiatric assessment. Kidneys are allocated via the national kidney allocation scheme or are entered into the paired/pooled exchange scheme, where they are often able to facilitate additional pooled exchanges.

Renal transplant surgery

Preparation for surgery

Before surgery, it should be confirmed that the cross-match test is negative and that the donor kidney is blood group compatible with the recipient (unless a deliberate plan to carry out ABOi transplantation has been made). Prior to starting the implant procedure, the donor kidney should be inspected to confirm its suitability for transplantation and any necessary preparatory surgery should be carried out. This includes ligation of any divided branches of the renal vessels. The renal arteries are end-arteries, so it important whenever possible to preserve all branches and, if there are multiple renal arteries, to plan how best to implant these, carrying out reconstructive bench surgery as appropriate. Very small upper polar arteries can be safely ligated, but lower polar vessels should be preserved if possible since they may help supply the ureter. Smaller renal veins can be safely ligated, as there is overlap of venous drainage.

After induction of anaesthesia, a urinary catheter is inserted along with any central venous lines necessary for haemodynamic monitoring. Prophylaxis for deep vein thrombosis and renal vessel thrombosis is given (usually low-molecular-weight heparin) together with a broad spectrum antibiotic as prophylaxis for wound infection.

Implantation

The donor kidney is placed extraperitoneally in one or other iliac fossa with anastomosis of the renal vessels to the iliac vessels, and the donor ureter to the bladder (Figure 9.3.1). The donor kidney can be implanted in either iliac fossa, although some surgeons have a preference for the right iliac fossa because the iliac vein is more accessible, and others prefer to place the kidney in the contralateral iliac fossa because the renal pelvis is more accessible should urological complications occur. If peripheral vascular disease is present, the side with less disease should be used to avoid worsening distal ischaemia. A curvilinear incision is made in the iliac fossa, dividing the muscles displacing the intact peritoneum medially to expose the iliac vessels.

Typically, the donor renal vein is anastomosed to the external iliac vein and the donor renal artery (on a Carrel patch of donor aorta when available) to the external iliac artery. In the case of

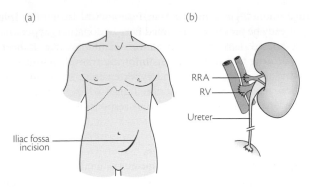

Fig. 9.3.1 Technique for kidney transplantation. (a) Curved incision in iliac fossa. (b) Deceased donor kidney implanted to external iliac vessels. RA, renal artery on patch of aorta; RV, renal vein.

a living donor kidney some surgeons prefer, when possible, to anastomose the renal artery end-to-end to the divided internal iliac artery rather than to the side of the external iliac artery. After the kidney has been re-vascularized, the ureter is shortened, spatulated, and anastomosed to the bladder with absorbable sutures. A double J ureteric stent is used to reduce the incidence of urine leak and obstruction. It is removed by cystoscopy at around 6 weeks. Care should be taken to ensure the transplanted kidney lies in a position that allows satisfactory orientation of the renal vessels, typically positioning the graft in a sub-rectus 'pocket'.

Dual kidney transplantation

Deceased donor kidneys considered very marginal in quality because of donor adverse characteristics or the features of a pre-implantation biopsy (Remuzzi score[8]) may be implanted as a dual transplant into the same recipient to provide adequate nephron mass. There is, however, little evidence on which to base the decision as to whether marginal donor kidneys should be implanted singly or as a dual transplant.

En-bloc transplantation of paediatric donor kidneys

Kidneys from young paediatric donors (aged 2–5 years) may be implanted into selected adults *en-bloc*. The donor aortic conduit is anastomosed to the recipient iliac artery and the donor vena cava to the iliac vein. Such kidneys rapidly hypertrophy and usually provide excellent long-term renal function for the recipient.

Renal transplantation in children

End-stage renal failure in children is rare (annual incidence of 2 per million population). Kidney transplantation enables growth and development to occur and markedly improves quality of life. In very young children where there is a size mismatch between recipient and donor kidney (which may be an adult organ), the kidney may be placed intraperitoneally, with anastomosis of the renal artery to the distal aorta or common iliac artery and anastomosis of the renal vein to the inferior vena cava or common iliac vein.

Immunosupression

The immunosuppressive agents used and their agent-specific and generic side effects (infection and malignancy) are described in Chapter 9.2. In the UK, immunosuppression for renal transplantation typically comprises induction therapy with the anti-CD25 antibody, followed by calcineurin-based therapy (most often tacrolimus) given with steroids and an antiproliferative agent (azathioprine or mycophenolic acid). Alemtuzumab induction therapy is often used for patients at high risk of graft rejection. Some centres favour early steroid withdrawal or steroid avoidance. Sirolimus is sometimes substituted for a calcineurin inhibitor in patients who are more than 1 year post-transplant to reduce nephrotoxicity or if a malignancy develops.

Early postoperative management

Careful monitoring of haemodynamic status is important during and following implantation to ensure appropriate maintenance of the intravascular volume and electrolyte balance. Central venous pressure monitoring (target 8–10 mmHg) is routine for 24 hours. Blood pressure should be maintained. Hypertension, if persistent, should be treated by cautious reduction of fluid intake and use of antihypertensive agents if necessary. Hyperkalaemia is a common and potentially serious problem in the early post-transplant period, particularly if graft function is delayed. Serum potassium levels should be monitored sequentially and hyperkalaemia managed by intravenous glucose and insulin or by haemodialysis. If there is concern about vascularity of the graft in the early post-transplant period a Doppler ultrasound examination should be performed.

Delayed graft function

Delayed graft function (defined as the need for dialysis) is usually due to acute tubular necrosis resulting from ischaemia reperfusion injury. It occurs in up to 5% of living donor recipients, 30% of recipients of kidneys from DBD donors, and 60% of kidneys from DCD donors. Other causes of oliguria (e.g. vascular thrombosis, urinary catheter blockage, and ureteric obstruction) should be excluded. Supportive management (haemodialysis, maintenance of intravascular volume, and avoidance of calcineurin blocker nephrotoxicity) allows graft function to recover within a few days but it may take several weeks. Kidney transplants that never function are classified as having primary non-function and this may be due to vascular thrombosis or irreversible ischaemic injury of the donor kidney.

Early postoperative complications

Vascular thrombosis

Renal vein or arterial thrombosis occurs in the first few days and is seen in <5% of transplants. It is often related to surgical technique and effective prophylaxis with low-dose heparin or aspirin is important. Vascular thrombosis is confirmed by Doppler ultrasound, but salvage of the graft is rarely possible.

Lymphocoele

Lymphocoeles adjacent to the graft occur in up to 20% recipients. Most are small and resolve spontaneously. Large lymphocoeles may cause compression of the transplant ureter, or of the iliac vessels leading to a deep vein thrombosis. Symptomatic lymphocoeles are treated initially by percutaneous aspiration or drainage, but if they fail to resolve may require open or laparoscopic fenestration.

Urological problems

Urine leak is uncommon (<2%) when a ureteric stent is used.[9] It may be associated with ischaemia or necrosis of the distal ureter and initial management is by inserting a percutaneous nephrostomy. Surgery is sometimes required with re-implantation of the donor ureter into the bladder or joining it to the native ureter. Ureteric obstruction is usually due to distal ischaemia and stenosis and may occur at any stage after removal of the ureteric stent. Hydronephrosis is readily detectable by ultrasound and the diagnosis confirmed by an antegrade nephrostogram. Ureteric strictures may be amenable to balloon dilatation or stenting but surgical intervention is often required.

Causes of early graft dysfunction

Deterioration in graft function in the early post-transplant period is diagnosed by increasing serum creatinine, possible accompanied by oliguria. Possible causes are:

- hypovolaemia
- sepsis
- renal vein or renal artery thrombosis
- ureteric obstruction or urine leak
- obstructed urinary catheter
- calcineurin inhibitor toxicity
- pyelonephritis
- acute rejection.

Unless the cause is obvious, urgent investigation is required and should include Doppler ultrasound examination to exclude vascular thrombosis or urological causes. Acute rejection should be suspected unless another obvious cause is found, and transplant biopsy should be performed unless there is a good response to empirical treatment with steroids. If acute rejection is suspected, serum should be tested for the presence of donor-specific HLA antibodies to help determine if acute antibody-mediated rejection is likely.

Longer-term decline in graft function

Causes of declining graft function

Progressive decline in renal allograft function in the months and years after transplantation may be due to:

- acute cell-mediated or antibody-mediated rejection
- chronic antibody-mediated rejection
- ureteric or bladder outflow obstruction
- recurrent pyelonephritis
- BK virus nephropathy
- calcineurin toxicity
- recurrent glomerulonephritis
- renal artery stenosis
- hypertension.

The term 'chronic allograft nephropathy' is used to describe a kidney allograft showing interstitial fibrosis and tubular atrophy which is the stereotypical response to injury. There are multiple causes,

both immunological and non-immunological in nature. Injury may already be present at the time of organ donation (hypertensive or age-related damage), occur at transplantation (e.g. ischaemic injury or drug toxicity) or occur following transplantation (rejection, infection, drug toxicity, and hypertension). The term 'chronic rejection' may be used to describe a graft where alloantibody or cell-mediated rejection is shown to be responsible for chronic graft injury.

BK virus nephropathy

Management usually comprises cautious reduction in immunosuppression and leads to recovery in most cases, but graft loss through progressive nephropathy or acute rejection triggered by reducing immunosuppression may occur (see Chapter 9.2, Principles of transplant immunology and immunosuppressive therapy section).

Recurrent renal disease

Glomerulonephritis commonly recurs in a kidney transplant. Some types recur more often than others and are more likely to cause graft failure. Recurrent glomerulonephritis is a relatively common cause of long-term graft loss and is largely refractory to treatment. Most cases of recurrence are relatively benign in nature and progress over many years, and concern about recurrence should not usually be a contraindication to transplantation. However, if early loss of a first graft has been attributed to recurrent glomerulonephritis, a repeat transplant is likely to suffer the same fate.

Renal artery stenosis

This occurs in 1–5% of grafts and usually presents with increasingly difficult to control hypertension and progressive graft dysfunction.[10] It may be a consequence of arterial injury incurred at the time of organ donation or during the transplant procedure and typically occurs at or just distal to the arterial anastomosis.

Colour Doppler ultrasound is a useful first investigation for diagnosing haemodynamically significant stenosis. Definitive diagnosis is made by angiography and if hypertension remains refractory and/or graft function declines, interventional treatment is either by angioplasty (with or without stenting) or, as a last resort, surgical revascularization.

Transplant nephrectomy

Kidney transplants with primary non-function are usually excised. Most grafts that fail after months or years become smaller and fibrosed and do not require excision unless causing symptoms or as a preparatory procedure to make room for a further renal transplant. In such cases, the kidney is densely adherent to surrounding tissues and necessitates intracapsular dissection and ligation of the renal vascular pedicle.

Long-term outcome after transplantation

The early results after kidney transplantation have improved markedly as a result of better assessment of immune compatibility, and improved prophylaxis and treatment of acute rejection and early infection. In contrast, longer-term graft outcome has improved relatively little and graft failure attributable to chronic allograft nephropathy or premature death with a functioning transplant remain a major problem. While transplantation provides a survival advantage, it only partly offsets the high risk of cardiovascular events associated with chronic renal failure. Recipient death accounts for half of all graft failures after the first year and the majority of deaths are due to cardiovascular events.

Living donor kidney transplantation gives superior outcomes to deceased donor transplantation with five-year patient and graft survival of more than 95% and 90%, respectively.[6,11] Patient and graft survival is similar for DBD and DCD kidneys, with 5-year patient and graft survival rates of >85%.[11,12] Long cold ischaemia (>12 hours for DCD kidneys and >24 hours for DBD kidneys) is associated with reduced graft survival.[12] For all types of kidney, increasing donor age is associated with poorer graft survival.[6,12] In the USA, the term extended or expanded criteria donor kidneys is used to describe kidneys from sub-optimal donors.[13] They are defined as kidney donors aged older than 60 years or 50–59 years with two of: history of donor hypertension, donor death from cerebrovascular accident, and serum creatinine of >133 μmol/L. Longer-term graft survival is around 10% worse for kidneys from expanded criteria donors than those from a non-expanded criteria donor. The impact of HLA matching on kidney transplant outcome has diminished as immunosuppressive therapy has improved. Most large registry analyses still show an incremental decrease in graft survival with increasing HLA-A, HLA-B and HLA-DR mismatch.[3] A recent UK analysis of living donor kidney transplants, however, showed no apparent benefit of HLA matching on transplant survival. This does not exclude the possibility that recipients of poorly HLA-matched grafts may require a greater burden of immunosuppression and hence suffer more side effects. In addition, recipients of poorly HLA-matched grafts who may subsequently require a further renal transplant are more likely to develop HLA alloantibodies that limits their access to an HLA antibody-compatible kidney.[6]

Further reading

Bradley JA. Transplantation. In: Williams NS, Bulstrode CJK, O'Connell PR (eds) *Bailey and Love's Short Practice of Surgery*, 25th edition, London: Hodder Arnold, 2008, pp 1407–30.

Morris PJ (ed.). *Kidney Transplantation: Principles and Practice*, 5th edition. Philadelphia: Saunders Company, 2001.

Torpey N, Moghal NE, Watson E, et al. (eds). *Renal Transplantation*. Oxford: Oxford University Press, 2010.

References

1. The UK Renal Registry, 15th Annual report, 2012. https://www.renal-reg.org/reports/2012-the-fifteenth-annual-report/ (accessed 27 March 2016).
2. British Transplantation Society. *Guideline Development Policy, revised version 25th November 2011*. http://www.bts.org.uk/documents/guidelines/active Assessment_of_the_Potential_Kidney_Transplant_Recipient_-_Final_Version_12_January_2011%20endorsed%20by%20BTS.pdf (accessed 27 March 2016).
3. Johnson RJ, Fuggle SV, Mumford L, et al. A New UK 2006 National Kidney Allocation Scheme for deceased heart-beating donor kidneys. *Transplantation* 2010; 89(4): 387–94.
4. British Transplant Society. *UK Guidelines for living donor kidney transplantation*. http://www.bts.org.uk/Documents/Guidelines/Active/UK%20Guidelines%20for%20Living%20Donor%20Kidney%20July%202011.pdf (accessed 27 March 2016).
5. Hadjianastassiou VG, Johnson RJ, Rudge CJ, et al. 2509 living donor nephrectomies, morbidity and mortality, including the UK introduction of laparoscopic donor surgery. *Am J Transplant* 2007; 7(11): 2532–7.
6. Fuggle SV, Allen JE, Johnson RJ, et al. Factors affecting graft and patient survival after live donor kidney transplantation in the UK. *Transplantation* 2010; 89(6): 694–701.
7. Johnson RJ, Allen JE, Fuggle SV, et al. Early experience of paired living kidney donation in the United Kingdom. *Transplantation* 2008; 86(12): 1672–7.
8. Remuzzi G, Cravedi P, Perna A, et al. Long-term outcome of renal transplantation from older donors. *N Engl J Med* 2006; 354(4): 343–52.
9. Saeb-Parsy K, Kosmoliaptsis V, Sharples LD, et al. Donor type does not influence the incidence of major urologic complications after kidney transplantation. *Transplantation* 2010; 90(10): 1085–90.
10. Seratnahaei A, Shah A, Bodiwala K, et al. Management of transplant renal artery stenosis. *Angiology* 2011; 62(3): 219–24.
11. National Health Service Blood and Transplantation. http://www.odt.nhs.uk/pdf/organ_specific_report_kidney_2015.pdf (accessed 27 March 2016).
12. Summers DM, Johnson RJ, Hudson A, et al. Effect of donor age and cold storage time on outcome in recipients of kidneys donated after circulatory death in the UK: a cohort study. *Lancet* 2013; 381(9868): 727–34.
13. Metzger R A, Delmonico F L, Feng S, et al. Expanded criteria donors for kidney transplantation. *Am J Transplant* 2003: 3(Suppl); 114–25.

CHAPTER 9.4

Pancreas and islet transplantation

John J. Casey

Pancreas transplantation

Indications

The aim of pancreas transplantation is to render diabetic patients free of exogenous insulin and modify the secondary effects of diabetes. The pancreas is most commonly transplanted simultaneously along with a kidney in patients with type I diabetes and end-stage renal disease due to diabetic nephropathy (SPK). The pancreas can be also transplanted at a later date after a renal transplant (PAK), often after a live donor kidney has been transplanted. A pancreas transplant alone (PTA) can be carried out for patients with diabetes without renal impairment, usually for impaired awareness of hypoglycaemia and glycaemic lability. Although pancreas transplantation is normally offered to patients with confirmed type I diabetes, evidence is emerging that some patients with type II diabetes may also benefit.[1]

Assessment

The majority of patients referred for SPK transplantation have multiple co-morbidities associated with diabetes such as retinopathy, neuropathy, microvascular disease, and macrovascular disease. As a result many units have an arbitrary upper age limit of 50–55 years. Cardiovascular disease is the most common cause of mortality after pancreas transplantation. The best way in which to undertake cardiovascular assessment is, however, controversial. Some centres routinely perform coronary angiography, whereas others rely on functional assessments such as treadmill testing (Bruce protocol), myocardial perfusion scanning, stress echo or, more recently, cardiopulmonary exercise testing.

Procedure

Back table preparation of the pancreas

Meticulous back table preparation of the pancreas is essential for successful implantation. Haemorrhage from multiple points at reperfusion is a particular problem in pancreas transplantation, but this can be avoided by carefully ligating all potential bleeding points. The duodenal loop is then trimmed to an appropriate length and the stapled end of the mesenteric vessels under run. The pancreas derives its blood supply from both the superior mesenteric artery and the splenic artery and these two vessels are reconstructed on the back table to form a single arterial conduit using donor iliac vessels (Figure 9.4.1). The venous drainage is via the portal vein, and this is dissected to provide adequate length for implantation. If necessary it may be extended using donor iliac vein.

Vascular implantation

The pancreas is most commonly implanted intraperitoneally in the right iliac fossa. The kidney can also be implanted onto the left side using this approach, although a separate left iliac fossa retroperitoneal approach as for a standard kidney transplant is commonly used. The portal vein of the donor pancreas is implanted onto the lower inferior vena cava or common iliac vein and the arterial conduit is anastomosed to the common iliac artery (Figure 9.4.2). Pancreas transplant recipients typically have significant atheroma affecting the aorto-iliac segment and so alternative sites for implantation may be required, such as the external or internal iliac vessels.

Exocrine drainage

The exocrine secretions of the pancreas must be internally drained either into the bladder or small bowel. The bladder was initially chosen because of the lower risk of anastomotic leakage (compared to enteric drainage) and because amylase levels could be measured in the urine as a surrogate marker of rejection. Enteric drainage (either onto proximal jejunum or a roux loop) is now most commonly used as urinary amylase is a very unreliable marker of pancreas rejection and patients with bladder drainage suffer from severe chemical cystitis, dehydration and electrolyte loss.

Outcomes

Graft and patient survival

Since the first description of pancreas transplantation in 1966, pancreas graft and patient survival have improved year on year. The best outcomes are seen with SPK transplantation, with a 1-year pancreas graft survival of 89% and a 5-year graft survival of

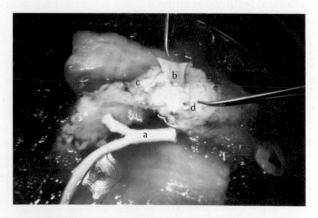

Fig. 9.4.1 Back table preparation of the pancreas for transplantation. a, Donor iliac vessels (Y-graft); b, portal vein; c, splenic artery; d, superior mesenteric artery.

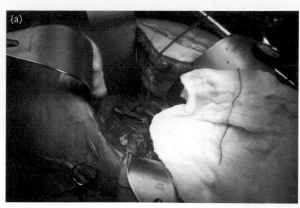
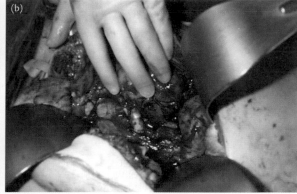

Fig. 9.4.2   (a) Exposure of donor right common iliac artery and lower inferior vena cava for pancreas implantation. (b) Reperfusion of the pancreas.

71%. Graft survival after PAK transplantation is similar at 85% at 1 year and 65% at 5 years. The outcome after PTA transplantation is inferior at both 1 and 3 years (82%% and 58%, respectively).[2] This is probably due to the difficulty in detecting early acute rejection in PTA grafts. It is very common for pancreas and renal graft rejection to occur simultaneously and so renal transplant rejection can be used as a surrogate marker. The diagnosis of pancreas rejection can be confirmed by computed tomogram or ultrasound-guided biopsy. Patient survival at 1 and 3 years is excellent at 95% and 92% for SPK, 97% and 90% for PAK, and 96% and 92% for PTA, respectively. It should be noted that type I diabetic patients who remain on dialysis will have an expected 5-year survival of only 50%.[3]

Secondary complications of diabetes

The Diabetes Control and Complications Trial Research Group's trial of intensive insulin therapy against standard therapy demonstrated that maintaining tight glycaemic control results in a significantly reduced incidence of secondary complications of diabetes, and pancreas transplantation to a large extent reflects this.[4,5] Pancreas transplantation can reverse the histological changes of diabetes on both the renal graft and native kidneys, so preserving long-term kidney function.[6] Chronic rejection and drug toxicity are more common causes of renal graft loss than recurrent diabetic nephropathy in SPK transplantation. The progression of retinopathy can be slowed after pancreas transplantation, but it is important that proliferative retinopathy is treated prior to pancreas transplantation as this can rapidly progress post transplant. The symptoms of diabetic nephropathy are expected to improve after pancreas transplantation, though this may take months or years.[7] Reversal of microvascular and macrovascular disease is not seen after pancreas transplantation, but progression may be slowed and pancreas transplantation appears to modify the cardiovascular risk of diabetic patients.[8]

Complications

Approximately 10% of pancreas grafts fail due to early complications. Vascular thrombosis is the most common cause occurring in 5% of transplants.[9] Other complications include haemorrhage, sepsis due to intra-abdominal collections, enteric leak or pancreatic fistula, and graft pancreatitis. Bladder drainage results in specific complications as previously discussed.

Islet transplantation

The islets of Langerhans account for only 1% of the mass of the pancreas, but contain the beta and alpha cells responsible for insulin and glucagon production necessary for glycaemic control. Although the first successful human islet transplant was carried out in the late 1970s, islet transplantation was only considered a viable clinical option in 2000 when the Edmonton group demonstrated that long-term insulin independence was possible in a small series of patients.[10]

There are two principal indications for islet transplantation:

1. *Severely impaired awareness of hypoglycaemia despite optimum insulin therapy* occurs in 20–25% of patients with type I diabetes and is potentially life threatening. Defective recognition of hypoglycaemia increases the risk of severe hypoglycaemic episodes that can result in coma and death. The impact on quality of life for these patients is substantial and social activities and employment can be severely restricted. In the UK, patents with impaired awareness of hypoglycaemia cannot hold a driving license.

2. *Patients with type I diabetes and a functioning kidney allograft who are unable to maintain their HbA1^C below 7%*. In this patient group, it has been shown that the improved glycaemic control after islet transplantation in this setting is associated with a reduction in long-term diabetic complications.

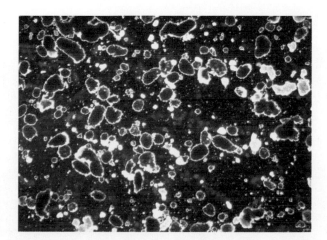

Fig. 9.4.3   Human islets of Langerhans stained red with dithizone.

Islets are extracted from a human cadaveric pancreas in a good manufacturing practice standard laboratory using collagenase digestion (see Figure 9.4.3).[11,12] The islets are then infused into the recipient patient's portal vein under fluoroscopic guidance. Complications of the procedure are rare but haemorrhage, bile leak, and portal vein thrombosis have been described.[13]

Over 1000 patients have now undergone islet transplantation and reversal of impaired awareness of hypoglycaemia is seen in nearly all patients. Insulin independence is reported in 50–90% of patients.[14]

References

1. Gruessner AC, Sutherland DER, Gruessner RWG. Pancreas transplantation in the United States: a review. *Curr Opin Organ Transplant* 2010; 15: 93–101.
2. Gruessner RWG, Gruessner AC. The current state of pancreas transplantation. *Nat Rev Endocrinol* 2013; 9(9): 555–62.
3. McMillan MA, Briggs JD, Junor BJ. Outcome of renal replacement treatment in patients with diabetes mellitus. *BMJ* 1990; 301: 540–4.
4. The Diabetes Control and Complications Trial Research Group. The effect of intensive treatment of diabetes on the development and progression of long-term complications in insulin dependent diabetes mellitus. *N Engl J Med* 1993; 329: 977–86.
5. DCCT/EDIC Research Group, de Boer IH, *et al.* Intensive diabetes therapy and glomerular filtration rate in type 1 diabetes. *N Engl J Med* 2011; 365(25): 2366–76.
6. Fioretto P, Steffes MW, Sutherland DER, *et al.* Reversal of lesions of diabetic nephropathy after pancreas transplantation. *N Eng J Med* 1998; 339: 69–75.
7. Navarro X, Sutherland DER, Kennedy WR. Long term effects of pancreatic transplantation on diabetic neuropathy. *Ann Neurol* 1997; 42: 727–36.
8. Fiorina P, La Rocca E, Venturini M, *et al.* Effects of kidney-pancreas transplantation on atherosclerotic risk factors and endothelial function in patients with uremia and type 1 diabetes. *Diabetes* 2001; 50(3): 496–501.
9. Farney AC, Rogers J, Stratta RJ. Pancreas graft thrombosis: causes, prevention, diagnosis, and intervention. *Current Opinion Organ Transplant* 2012; 17: 87–92.
10. Shapiro AM, Lakey JR, Ryan EA, *et al.* Islet transplantation in seven patients with type 1 diabetes mellitus using a glucocorticoid-free immunosuppressive regimen. *N Engl J Med* 2000; 343: 230–8.
11. Ricordi C, Lacy PE, Scharp DW. Automated islet isolation from human pancreas. *Diabetes* 1989; 38(Suppl 1): 140–2.
12. Lake SP, Bassett PD, Larkins A, *et al.* Large-scale purification of human islets utilizing discontinuous albumin gradient on IBM 2991 cell separator. *Diabetes* 1989; 38(Suppl 1): 143–5.
13. Takita M, Matsumoto S, Noguchi H, *et al.* Adverse events in clinical islet transplantation: one institutional experience. *Cell Transplant* 2012; 21: 547–51.
14. Barton FB, Rickels MR, Alejandro R, *et al.* Improvement in outcomes of clinical islet transplantation: 1999-2010. *Diabetes Care* 2012; 35: 1436–45.

CHAPTER 9.5

Liver transplantation

Simon J. F. Harper and Raaj K. Praseedom

Introduction

Liver transplantation remains the only effective treatment option for patients with end-stage or fulminant liver disease. Outcomes have continued to improve since the first liver transplant by Starzl in 1963,[1] but liver transplantation remains a huge challenge for all involved. The most common indications for liver transplantation in adults are alcoholic liver disease, viral hepatitis, autoimmune liver disease, metabolic liver disease, hepatocellular carcinoma, and increasingly non-alcoholic steato hepatitis related to obesity. In children, the leading indications are biliary atresia, α1-antitrypsin deficiency, non-cirrhotic metabolic diseases (e.g. Crigler–Najjar), autoimmune hepatitis, and acute viral hepatitis.

Indications and assessment for liver transplantation

End-stage chronic liver disease

Allocation of organs for transplantation is underpinned by the ethical principles of justice (prioritization according to the need of individual patients) and utility (ensuring fair access to a scarce resource). In liver transplantation this is particularly difficult, as the sickest patients tend to be those most in need of a transplant but also the least likely to survive the procedure. In the UK, the United Kingdom Model for End-Stage Liver Disease score incorporates international normalized ratio, serum bilirubin, creatinine, and sodium in an algorithm that predicts mortality on the waiting list.[2] Patients are eligible for transplantation when their score is more than 49 as this correlates with a predicted 1-year mortality of more than 9%, thereby exceeding the mortality at 1-year after transplantation. In addition, to ensure maximum gain from each organ, a detailed patient assessment is performed to ascertain that the estimated 5-year survival after transplantation is at least 50%. Allowance is also made for 'variant syndromes' that carry particular morbidity (e.g. hepatopulmonary syndrome).[3]

Hepatocellular carcinoma

Hepatocellular carcinoma on a background of decompensated cirrhosis is an indication for liver transplantation. Candidate selection for patients with HCC is currently based on the Milan criteria, which require a single lesion <5 cm in diameter or up to five lesions each £3 cm in the absence of vascular invasion or extrahepatic disease.[4]

Acute liver failure

Acute liver failure patients are given highest priority for organ allocation, but strict criteria must be met to differentiate between patients that are likely to deteriorate beyond effective intervention and those likely to recover without needing a liver transplant. In the UK, specific physiological parameters (e.g. acidosis, prolonged prothombin time) are applied to causes of acute liver failure, such as paracetamol overdose, acute viral hepatitis, idiosyncratic drug reactions, acute Wilson's disease, Budd-Chiari syndrome, early allograft failure, or hepatic artery thrombosis and acute liver failure after live liver donation.[5]

The liver transplant procedure

Severe liver disease leads to profound pathophysiological changes that affect most organ systems. Liver failure is associated with coagulopathy, malnutrition, portal hypertension, pulmonary and systemic microvascular shunting, renal impairment, and encephalopathy. In addition, patients invariably have other co-morbidities, many related to the underlying liver disease (e.g. obstructive airways disease in α1-antitrypsin deficiency). The perioperative management for liver transplantation, as such, represents a huge challenge and requires a dedicated multidisciplinary team at a specialist centre.

The liver transplant procedure comprises four components: donor hepatectomy, graft preservation and bench preparation, recipient hepatectomy, and implantation of the donor liver. Liver transplants are performed successfully using organs from donation after brainstem death, donation after circulatory death and living donation. In deceased donors, the liver is perfused with cold preservation solution via the hepatic artery (HA) and portal vein (PV). The main HA is preserved along with any accessory hepatic arteries. The PV, suprahepatic vena cava, and infrahepatic vena cava and bile duct are transected precisely. In live donation, three main types of graft are used: left lateral segment (adult to child) and full right or full left hemi-livers (adult to adult).

At the recipient centre, the liver is assessed in terms of suitability for transplantation and prepared on the bench for implantation. Vascular reconstruction may be required and high-quality livers may be split to allow transplantation into two recipients.

The recipient hepatectomy is often started while the liver is in transit to minimize the cold ischaemic time to less than 12 hours. The recipient hepatectomy is frequently the most difficult part of the procedure as a result of distorted liver anatomy, intra-abdominal varices, and coagulopathy. The 'classical' technique involves resection of the diseased liver with the retrohepatic portion of the inferior vena cava (IVC) and replacement with the new liver and IVC (Figure 9.5.1). The main disadvantage of this approach is the need to cross-clamp the IVC, which may lead to haemodynamic instability requiring temporary extracorporal venovenous bypass (femoral to jugular) to provide adequate cardiac venous return. A commonly

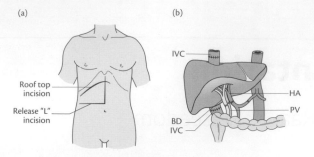

Fig. 9.5.1 Liver transplantation. (a) Incision, either 'roof top' or 'reverse L'. (b) Completed implantation of donor liver. BD, bile duct; IVC, inferior vena cava; HA, hepatic artery; PV, portal vein.

used alternative is preservation of the IVC during recipient hepatectomy and anastomosis of the donor IVC directly onto recipient IVC ('piggyback' or cavo-cavoplasty).[6,7]

The donor PV is usually anastomosed directly to recipient PV, although jump grafts to mesenteric veins may be required in PV thrombosis. The donor HA is anastomosed either directly to recipient HA or via a conduit from the aorta created using donor blood vessels (e.g. iliac artery). Reperfusion of the liver is particularly dangerous; significant instability and even cardiac arrest may occur due to the combination of a marked systemic ischaemia-reperfusion response, significant blood loss, and 'washing out' of potassium-rich preservation fluid. The transplant is completed by anastomosis of the donor bile duct directly to the recipient bile duct or onto a Roux-en-Y loop of jejunum.

Early postoperative course after liver transplantation

Liver transplant recipients are transferred to the intensive care unit for immediate postoperative care, although most do not require prolonged ventilation. Immunosuppression regimens usually include tacrolimus, azathioprine or mycophenolate mofetil and variably steroids although these are often stopped. The major complications observed in the first 24 to 48 hours are bleeding, primary non-function, and hepatic artery thrombosis (HAT). Primary non-function is essentially an immediate, irreversible graft failure and is often apparent intraoperatively with progressive features of multiorgan failure following graft reperfusion. Donation after circulatory death, prolonged preservation, increased donor age and graft steatosis are recognized risk factors and the only effective management is re-transplantation.[8]

The risk of HAT increases with complexity of arterial reconstruction and re-transplantation.[9] Surveillance imaging with Doppler ultrasound may facilitate timely diagnosis of HAT allowing emergency thrombectomy. However, most cases require re-transplantation, as even in the absence of immediate graft infarction, severe cholangiopathy will rapidly develop. Bile leaks often require re-exploration and formation of hepaticojejunostomy. Graft dysfunction in the first few postoperative weeks is common. The differential diagnosis is sepsis, biliary and vascular complications, or rejection. Rejection is treated with adjustment of immunosuppression and/or pulsed intravenous methylprednisolone.

Long-term care after liver transplantation

The results after liver transplantation are good overall, with recipient survival rates after elective liver transplantation in adults of >85% at 1 year and >70% at 5 years. The leading causes of death in liver transplant recipients after the first postoperative year are malignancy, recurrent liver disease, cardiovascular disease, infection, and chronic rejection.[10] Deaths from cancer occur as a result of the underlying liver disease (e.g. colorectal cancer in primary sclerosing cholangitis PSC), virus-related, (e.g. lymphoma), or direct recurrence of hepatocellular carcinoma. Recurrent liver disease arising in the graft is a particular problem in viral hepatitis, autoimmune disease and, of course, recidivism in alcoholism. There is a disproportionately high incidence of obesity, diabetes, hypertension, and hyperlipidaemia leading to significant cardiovascular morbidity in the post-transplant population.[11] The effect of immunosuppression underlies all of these morbidities, including a significant incidence of renal impairment. The liver is notably less prone to rejection than other allografts and as such immunosuppression with a single agent (usually tacrolimus) or conversion to a less nephrotoxic agent (e.g. sirolimus) can often be achieved with an aim to mitigate side effects. However, a proportion of patients will develop late acute rejection and/or chronic ductopenic rejection requiring increased immunosuppression and in some cases re-transplantation. Re-transplantation is the only option for patients with a failing graft and patients are assessed on a case-by-case basis, as each subsequent transplant is associated with an escalating risk of mortality.

Multivisceral transplantation

Multivisceral transplantation, including intestinal transplantation, is currently only indicated in patients with life-threatening complications (e.g. liver injury) or unacceptable quality of life on total parenteral nutrition, or following evisceration for extensive intra-abdominal tumours. The most common underlying pathologies in children are gastroschisis, volvulus, necrotizing enterocolitis, and pseudo-obstruction; the most common underlying pathologies in adults are mesenteric vascular disease, Crohn's disease, trauma, dysmotility disorders, and desmoid tumours. Intestinal failure patients in the absence of significant irreversible liver disease are best served with an isolated intestinal graft. A combined liver and intestinal transplant is indicated in patients with significant liver disease, almost always as a result of long-term total parenteral nutrition and in patients requiring a liver transplant where there is extensive portomesenteric thrombosis. Pathology affecting the foregut may require more extensive grafts including the stomach, duodenum and pancreas.

Multivisceral transplantation is technically demanding. The transplant recipient has frequently undergone multiple previous laparotomies resulting in profoundly distorted intra-abdominal anatomy, portal hypertension, vascularized adhesions, and lack of space for the incoming graft. The multivisceral allograft is generally retrieved and implanted *en bloc* to allow rapid implantation. The most important early complications are acute rejection and sepsis, which frequently occur together. Long-term survival remains a major challenge, with chronic rejection and malignancy being the leading causes of graft loss and mortality.

Further reading

NHS Blood and Transplant Liver Advisory Groups Protocols and Guidelines https://www.organdonation.nhs.uk/about_transplants/organ_allocation/pdf/adult_protocols_guidelines.pdf (accessed April 2013).

References

1. Starzl TE, Marchioro TL, Vonkaulla KN, *et al*. Homotransplantation of the liver in humans. *Surg Gynecol Obstet* 1963; 117: 659–76.
2. Barber K, Madden S, Allen J, *et al*. Elective liver transplant list mortality: Development of a united kingdom end-stage liver disease score. *Transplantation* 2011; 92: 469–76.
3. Wiesner R, Lake JR, Freeman RB, *et al*. Model for end-stage liver disease (meld. exception guidelines. *Liver Transpl* 2006; 12: S85–7.
4. Mazzaferro V, Regalia E, Doci R, *et al*. Liver transplantation for the treatment of small hepatocellular carcinomas in patients with cirrhosis. *N Engl J Med* 1996; 334: 693–9.
5. O'Grady JG, Schalm SW, Williams R. Acute liver failure: Redefining the syndromes. *Lancet* 1993; 342: 273–5.
6. Calne RY, Williams R. Liver transplantation in man. I. Observations on technique and organization in five cases. *BMJ* 1968; 4: 535–40.
7. Tzakis A, Todo S, Starzl TE. Orthotopic liver transplantation with preservation of the inferior vena cava. *Ann Surg* 1989; 210: 649–52.
8. Strasberg SM, Howard TK, Molmenti EP, *et al*. Selecting the donor liver: Risk factors for poor function after orthotopic liver transplantation. *Hepatology* 1994; 20: 829–38.
9. Bekker J, Ploem S, de Jong KP. Early hepatic artery thrombosis after liver transplantation: A systematic review of the incidence, outcome and risk factors. *Am J Transplant* 2009; 9: 746–57.
10. Watt KD, Pedersen RA, Kremers WK, *et al*. Evolution of causes and risk factors for mortality post-liver transplant: Results of the niddk long-term follow-up study. *Am J Transplant* 2010; 10: 1420–7.
11. Desai S, Hong JC, Saab S. Cardiovascular risk factors following orthotopic liver transplantation: Predisposing factors, incidence and management. *Liver Int* 2010; 30: 948–57.

SECTION 10

Evidence-based surgery, research, and audit

Section editor: Jane M. Blazeby

CHAPTER 10.1

Research in surgery

Alan A. Montgomery and Jane M. Blazeby

Introduction

Surgical innovation is an important part of surgical practice. Assessment of standard and new interventions provides evidence to inform health policy and individual clinician and patient decision making. Historically, research in surgery was often poorly conducted and the majority of published papers in surgical journals consisted of reports of single-centre and single-surgeon case series. This generated poor-quality evidence resulting in little uniformity in the standard of care and surgery became dependent upon individual surgeon or patient preferences. The past two decades, however, have seen increasing investment and leadership in scientific evaluation of surgery and a subsequent rise in the quality and number of surgical research studies. The increased funding opportunities available in the UK to support surgical research and to develop and evaluate surgical interventions has been mirrored by investment in the clinical academic career pathway through the National Institute of Health Research and the creation of academic posts at all levels of surgical training. The combined opportunities for surgical research provide surgeons with time and resources to work together with methodologists to design studies to evaluate surgery and to create high-quality evidence.

There are several different study designs available to evaluate surgery and these create different levels of evidence. Meta-analyses and systematic reviews of well-designed and well-conducted trials, with concealment of allocation, form the highest level of evidence, whereas expert opinion and conventional wisdom form the lowest level of evidence. One of the best methods for evaluating healthcare interventions is the randomized controlled trial and while this is possible in surgery, there are particular methodological and practical challenges that need to be considered. These include problems related to ensuring surgeons can recruit into trials and explain clinical equipoise to patients, methods related to selection and measurement of outcomes that are relevant to patients as well as surgeons, and there are issues associated with the complexity of interventions in surgery that need special attention in trial design. This chapter covers these challenging areas as well as the basic methodological features that are important to the design, conduct, and reporting of trials. The need to understand the importance of methodology in the evaluation of surgery needs to be supplemented with a cultural shift in surgical research to become multidisciplinary and collaborative. Well-designed large pragmatic randomized controlled trials in surgery require that surgeons work together to answer important questions for patients and the health service. Increased collaboration and participation in trials is required to achieve this. Efforts to conduct high-quality studies in surgery will mean that future patient care will be informed by evidence of the effectiveness and cost-effectiveness of surgical interventions.

Trial design

Planning and study design

While many of the 'rules' to follow in planning a research study depend on the research question and the optimum study design, perhaps one that is universal is the need to plan early and often. Successful studies require multidisciplinary teams comprising personnel with clinical, scientific, and methodological expertise, and establishing good working relationships between surgeons and other team members is essential. Major statistical input is required at the design stage, since leaving this until the end of the study is likely to lead to difficulties that cannot be resolved. Once it has been determined that a randomized study is feasible and ethical, there is the question of trial design. The two-arm parallel design, where participants are individually randomized to receive either a new type of intervention or a comparator, is the most familiar and widely used. However, a question may be better addressed using an alternative design, such as crossover (participants receive first one treatment and then the other, with the order randomly allocated and usually with a washout period in-between), factorial (where more than one intervention is tested, and in its simplest 2×2 design, participants receive either both, one or the other, or no intervention), or cluster (where groups, or *clusters*, of participants are randomized rather than individuals). Further details of these trial designs can be found in other texts.[1,2] The issues discussed in this chapter generally apply regardless of the trial design employed.

Minimizing risk of bias

A well-planned and well-conducted randomized study minimizes the risk of bias and provides the best evidence about the effects of healthcare interventions. Selection bias occurs when individuals allocated to each trial arm differ in some important characteristic(s) associated with the primary outcome. This can be minimized by generating a random allocation sequence and ensuring that the sequence is concealed from those enrolling patients into the study. Performance bias occurs when there is unequal provision of care between trial arms apart from the treatment under evaluation. Detection bias refers to biased assessment of outcomes, where the outcome assessor's (including the patient) reporting of outcomes in the treatment and control groups is different and is influenced by preferences or beliefs about the effectiveness of the treatment. Risk of bias is also greater for more subjective outcomes. These biases can be minimized by blinding study participants, personnel, and anyone else involved in participants' care to allocated treatment. Attrition bias refers to the exclusion from analysis of any randomized participants. As described in the Trial analysis section, this can be minimized by analysing data using an 'intention to treat' (ITT) approach combined with appropriate sensitivity analyses exploring various assumptions about treatment adherence and missing outcome data. A tool developed by the Cochrane Collaboration makes the process of assessing risk of bias in published trials clearer and more accurate.[3]

Eligibility criteria

Eligibility criteria for patients who will be included in, or excluded from, the trial must be clearly defined. Studies of patients who are representative of the population normally treated for a given problem have greater external validity, or generalizability, than studies with more restricted eligibility criteria. There may be good reasons to exclude some patients from a trial, for example, contraindications to a new treatment or inability to follow study requirements. A well-planned and well-executed trial has high internal validity, regardless of the type of patients who make it into the study. However, the applicability of trial results to normal healthcare practice is likely to be reduced when a greater number of exclusion criteria are applied. Therefore, when reporting the results of trials it is important to be clear about which patients were included and excluded, the numbers excluded, and the reasons why any eligible patients were not randomized.

Intervention and comparison

The intervention must be defined in sufficient detail such that it can be delivered consistently during the study, and reliably reproduced afterwards if it is to be implemented in practice. For drug interventions this may describe the formulation, dosing instructions, and duration of treatment. For more complex interventions, such as surgery, it may require a lengthy and detailed treatment manual, with supplemental material such as video if appropriate. Consideration should also be given to training those who will deliver the intervention, and whether a 'run-in' period is necessary to allow learning effects to stabilize.

The comparison group must also be clearly defined. For a drug trial, this may be an identically matched placebo if there is no valid current treatment of proven efficacy. In trials of complex interventions, this group often receives whatever treatment is currently used in typical care, which may not be the same in different countries, or in different parts of the same country, or even among clinicians working in the same healthcare centre. There may be no desire or possibility to standardize usual care for the purposes of the trial, but this makes it vital that usual care during the trial is carefully documented so that the effects of the new intervention can be properly interpreted.

Outcomes

Selection of the most appropriate outcomes is dependent on the nature of the study. Before describing the different categories of outcome it is necessary to define the concepts of primary and secondary outcomes in the context of randomized trials. Primary outcomes are of central interest to the investigators. If the trial results are to lead to changes in practice then it will be on the basis of these outcomes. Secondary outcomes relate to other relevant questions in the same study but are not the main focus. They receive less emphasis in reports of trial results and may be used to generate new hypotheses. Decision making about which outcomes are defined as primary or secondary is essential at the planning stage as

it has implications for sample size estimation and analytical strategy. By forcing investigators to define in advance which outcomes are of main interest, it guards against later selective reporting only of outcomes for which a treatment effect was observed.

Rather than be too prescriptive about how many primary outcomes there can be in a particular trial, it is better to consider the nature of the intervention and the number of independent domains considered to be relevant to the decision making process once the trial is completed. In practice though, there will usually be between one and three primary outcomes, which may be chosen to represent the different perspective of, for example, clinicians, patients, regulatory bodies, or healthcare purchasers. The concept of core outcome sets is a growing area of research to develop consensus about which outcomes should always be collected in trials of a specific condition, making it easier for the results of trials to be compared and combined.[4] Clinical outcomes may be binary, indicating whether an event—such as death from any cause or from a disease-specific cause—has occurred within a specified time period following randomization. Alternatively the same outcome might be analysed according to the time taken for the event to occur. Other clinical outcomes may reflect the occurrence, or relief from, particular symptoms, or may be a surrogate outcome that is a good predictor of the clinical outcome of 'real' interest but that can be measured sooner, potentially allowing a trial of fewer participants and shorter duration. One should be cautious about converting continuous outcomes into binary or categorical outcomes. The usual argument for doing this is to ease clinical interpretation, with a score on one side of a threshold value indicating that the outcome was present, and a score on the other side indicating absence. Statistically this results in reduced power since useful information is discarded, and hence requires more participants in the study in order to detect an equivalent effect size. But it does not always make good clinical sense either, since outcomes such as mortality or presence of disease aside, most variables that can be measured in humans are naturally continuous and the choice of number of categories and their respective cut-points may be rather arbitrary.

Whatever the view among clinicians of the main outcomes of interest in a trial, it is often the case that rather different outcomes matter more to patients (for example, pain). Patient-reported outcomes, as the name suggests, are outcomes that are collected directly from participants, usually via questionnaires that either the participant completes them self or by responding to questions from an interviewer. These outcomes often reflect aspects of function or quality of life not captured in more clinical outcomes, and the questionnaires may be generic such as the SF-36[5] or EQ5D,[6] or condition-specific such as the EORTC QLQ-C30[7] designed for patients with cancer. It is worth noting here the importance of collecting adverse outcomes in trials, since these too may form an important part of deciding whether an intervention should be adopted into routine practice. This is particularly true of unanticipated adverse outcomes that may not be apparent until large-scale randomized trials are conducted.

The final category of outcomes to consider is those relating to health economics. It seems reasonable to assume that a new intervention that is more clinically effective, produces fewer adverse events, is well-tolerated by patients, and is cheaper than the current best available treatment should become the new standard treatment in practice. But what if the new intervention is both more effective and more expensive than the current treatment? Is it worth spending the extra for the expected gains in health? The costs of the intervention itself plus any indirect costs or savings on other aspects of healthcare can be combined with the effects of an intervention, usually in terms of quality-adjusted life-years, into a cost-effectiveness ratio. This describes the additional cost of gaining an extra year of life or a benefit in quality of life for the patient, and can be used when making decisions about which treatments a healthcare system can provide.

Sample size estimation

All studies that involve an element of quantitative data analysis should be subject to a sample size calculation at the planning stage. There are many formal equations, commands in statistical packages, and freely available internet tools to assist in this process, details of which will not be given here. Rather, the emphasis for this section is on the concepts involved and the information required for the calculations to proceed. First, though, it is worth noting that in practice the determination of required sample size is not an exact science. Many of the decisions about design and analysis are interrelated with the specifications for the sample size, and the process is not one with a single solution. This of course is no reason to abandon the exercise, but reinforces the need for the determination of sample size to be one element of discussions among members of the research team, including someone with appropriate statistical expertise.

There are three fundamental approaches: one based on the required precision of an estimate; another on requiring the study to have adequate probability (power) of detecting a certain effect size; and a third where the aim is to demonstrate equivalence between treatment groups. The second of these is the most commonly used in randomized trials, and is the one that we describe here in more detail in order to demonstrate the concepts involved. We also assume a simple trial design (i.e. a two-arm parallel design). Other designs may require additional statistical considerations.

All studies involving human participants include random noise in the outcomes assessed, in the shape of sampling, and measurement errors. When planning a clinical trial, we want to be reasonably confident that the study includes enough participants to be able to distinguish a true treatment effect, if it exists, from random noise. Estimating a sample size requires four components (Box 10.1.1).

Keeping all else constant, smaller values of alpha, beta, and target difference will require a larger sample size, as will greater variability of the primary outcome and a proportion of patients in the control arm with the outcome closer to 50%. The specified target difference arguably requires greatest consideration. Investigators should seek clinical, patient, and healthcare provider opinion of how small a difference would need to be before it was no longer considered worthwhile, and should avoid basing the target difference solely on effects observed in previous studies. A common error is to overestimate the likely effects of a new treatment or the minimum clinically important difference. This requires a smaller study, but it also reduces precision of the estimated treatment effect, and may yield an inconclusive trial, with a confidence interval for the between-group comparison for the primary outcome that is consistent with benefit, harm, and with no effect at all. It is stressed again that there is no single answer, and agreeing the final target sample size may involve several iterations and take into account other factors such as the availability of eligible participants, the amount of funding

available, and the time horizon within which an answer to the research question is required.

Trial registration

Registering a trial means publishing key details of the study in the public domain prior to commencing recruitment of participants.[8] Registration helps researchers and funding agencies avoid unnecessary duplication, can make it easier to identify gaps in clinical research, and may facilitate more effective collaboration including prospective meta-analysis. Decisions about healthcare should be made on the basis of all the available evidence, and trial registration allows identification of studies for which the main results were never published. Publishing the study protocol is similarly useful and provides greater detail than is possible in a trial registration database.

Research governance

For studies conducted in the UK National Health Service, ethical approval must be obtained from a Research Ethics Committee. The research and development departments in the NHS Trust(s) where the study will be conducted must also give their approval. Trials of medicines may require authorization from the Medicines and Healthcare products Regulatory Agency. Applications for all of these approvals and others are managed through a single online system, the Integrated Research Application System.

Trial conduct

Informed consent

Patients must give informed consent to participate in research before randomization. For consent to be ethically valid the researchers must provide potential participants with full information about what taking part in the study involves, including disclosure of all the potential risks and benefits of the study treatments. The patient must be competent to understand this information and must give consent voluntarily. Research without consent is possible, for example in emergency medicine, although justification must be given in the application for ethical approval.

Box 10.1.1 Elements required when estimating sample size

1. *Alpha*: The probability of a false positive result (i.e. erroneously concluding that the intervention is effective). Conventionally set at 5% but may be set lower if investigators wish to reduce the risk of this type I error.

2. *Beta*: The probability of a false negative result (i.e. erroneously concluding that the intervention is not effective). Conventionally set at 20% but again may be set lower. Power derives from this type II error, and is equal to $1-\beta$.

3. (a) *Binary outcomes*: estimated proportion of participants in the control arm who will experience the outcome.

   (b) *Continuous outcomes*: estimated variability of the outcome, expressed as a standard deviation.

4. *Target difference*: Often called the minimum clinically important difference (i.e. the smallest difference between the trial arms that would need to be observed in order to change clinical practice).

Randomization

The single feature that distinguishes randomized trials from other study designs is that participants have an equal probability of being allocated to any of the groups being compared. Thus we expect to end up with groups that are, on average, similar to each other in all respects other than the treatment(s) under investigation. Randomization does not ensure that groups are the same, rather it ensures, when conducted properly, that any differences between the groups in their measured or unmeasured characteristics at baseline are due to chance. Randomization itself involves two key stages. The first is generation of an unpredictable random allocation sequence. This is usually done using computer-generated random numbers. The second is concealment of the allocation sequence from the investigators enrolling patients into the study. This is usually achieved using an automated telephone or web-based randomization service, although sometimes it is only practical to use sequentially numbered, sealed opaque envelopes or drug containers prepared by an independent supplier and numbered in advance. This is known as adequate concealment and means that it is impossible for the investigator to have any influence over who is allocated to which trial arm—it should not be confused with blinding or masking of treatment after randomization has occurred. Any knowledge of the allocation sequence in advance could possibly result in investigators allocating certain patients to receive either the new or control treatment based on their age, sex, disease severity, or any other prognostic variable. In the context of a randomized study, this is called selection bias.

Allocation may be based on a simple random number sequence, equivalent to flipping an unbiased coin each time a patient is recruited. Although any differences between the trial arms in number or characteristics of patients is by definition due to chance, for smaller studies in particular this can lead to statistical inefficiency. Refinements of simple randomization, known collectively as 'restricted randomization', include stratification, blocking, and minimization, and these methods can help encourage greater balance between the trial arms in both the number and characteristics of patients in each.

Blinding

Blinding is when the various parties involved in a trial (i.e. patients, carers, those providing the study treatment, other healthcare providers, outcome assessors, and data analysts) are kept unaware of the treatment allocation following the act of randomization itself, and before, during, and after administration of the trial treatment. Blinding of patients and practitioners can be highly dependent on the type of treatment and control being compared. For example, consider a placebo-controlled drug trial, a study comparing different types of surgery that leave the same wound, a study of surgical versus medical management, and a trial of a complex behavioural intervention such as an exercise and diet programme. The potential to blind the different parties involved in such trials would vary significantly in each of these examples. Blinding of outcome assessors is more important for subjective than objective outcomes. Blinding is employed in order to prevent some of the biases that can make interpretation of the trial results more difficult, as discussed in Minimizing risk of bias section. Reports of trials often use the terms 'single' or 'double blind' but these are used inconsistently and it is unclear who was blinded. It is better to explicitly report the blinding status of study participants and investigators.

Deviations from protocol

The perfect randomized trial is one where all eligible patients are randomized, everyone fully adheres to their allocated treatment, and complete outcome data for the entire duration of the follow up period are collected. Of course this rarely happens in practice, and the way in which deviations from the protocol after randomization are handled during study conduct, analysis, and reporting can impact on interpretation of the results. Deviations from protocol can take many forms. Recruiters can fail to properly apply the inclusion and exclusion criteria. The patient may receive none or some of the allocated treatment, they may stop and start the treatment periodically, or take it in some other way than that directed by the investigators. Patients may receive the comparator treatment in addition to or instead of the treatment they were allocated to receive, or may seek further treatments not under investigation in the study. And finally they may provide incomplete outcome data. Dealing with these deviations in the analysis is dealt with in the Trial analysis section; suffice to say here that investigators should do everything possible to try and minimize them, and certainly document them as fully as possible when they occur.

Trial analysis

This section does not contain any technical details of statistical methods, some of which are described in Chapter 10.3, while more details are available in standard texts.[9,10] Rather, a general approach to analysing randomized trials is described. The key elements of the statistical analysis should be planned in advance and specified in the protocol and any deviations from or additions to this should be clearly identified in trial reports.

Representativeness and baseline comparability

The first stage is to compare the representativeness of those randomized with the target population of eligible patients. The numbers of eligible patients who were and were not randomized should be presented, with reasons for the latter. Descriptive statistics can be used to compare important characteristics such as age, sex, and the disease severity of participants and those declining. The second stage is to compare the treatment groups at the point of randomization (baseline). Again this should done using descriptive statistics such as means and standard deviations or numbers and percentages of demographic and prognostic variables, including baseline values of the outcomes. A common error at this stage is to conduct statistical tests for differences between groups. This should be avoided, since by definition any differences are due to chance if randomization was performed correctly. Furthermore the study is not designed (powered) to test for these differences, and the importance of the magnitude of any difference should be judged in the context of any variable's strength of relationship with the primary outcome.

Primary analyses

The primary approach to analysing data from randomized trials is that of ITT, that is, analysis of participants according to what the investigators intended their treatment to be, regardless of the type or amount of treatment actually received. This approach is not always intuitive when first encountered, but is used for reasons of avoiding bias. Since the deviations from protocol described previously are rarely at random, other approaches to analysis (e.g. according to treatment received) may result in comparing groups of participants that are different from each other in many respects and not just by the treatment received. Strictly speaking, the term 'intention to treat' means inclusion in the analysis of all randomized participants, whether or not outcome data were actually collected. For many trials, collection of outcome data is incomplete, and therefore missing outcome data must be imputed for an ITT analysis. Methods for imputing missing data in health research have developed rapidly in recent years and a detailed discussion is beyond the scope of this chapter.[11]

Results of the between-group analysis of the primary outcome should comprise an appropriate measure of effect dependent on the variable type, such as a difference in means or a risk ratio, some measure of uncertainty around this estimate, usually a 95% confidence interval, and a p-value from the appropriate hypothesis test. These can be obtained from linear or logistic regression models, which can also be used to adjust for the outcome at baseline if it was measured, as well as any stratification or minimization variables. It is emphasized that exact p-values should be presented and interpreted as a measure of strength of evidence against the null hypothesis rather than simply whether or not it is below some arbitrary threshold. The main focus for interpretation should be on the magnitude and direction of the between-group difference, and the clinical importance, whether benefit or harm, of the confidence limits.

Other analyses

Analysis of secondary outcomes can proceed in the same way as for primary outcomes. For all outcomes, approaches other than ITT may be explored, depending on the extent of deviations from protocol. Of course the ideal is to produce a treatment that is both highly effective and that patients are prepared to take. Where this occurs, both ITT and other types of analyses will give a reasonable estimate of a treatment's *efficacy* (i.e. the effect of treatment if actually taken as intended). However, where treatment adherence is sub-optimal, an ITT analysis tends to underestimate true efficacy and instead give an estimate of the treatment's *effectiveness* (i.e. the average effect that might be expected if introduced into practice). A 'per-protocol' analysis excludes treatment non-compliers and poor compliers, the falsely included, and those not providing outcome data. The justification is that this gives a better estimate of the true treatment effect, but the analyst should be aware of the reasons why participants do not comply with their allocated treatment or drop out of the study and the potential for bias in this kind of analysis. Advances in statistical methodology in this area seek to estimate causal effects of treatments if actually taken as intended while also minimizing risk of bias.[12,13] Other secondary analyses may investigate whether the intervention is more or less effective in certain types of patients. This is done by introducing appropriate interaction terms into regression models. These subgroup analyses should be specified in advance and reported in full.

Trial reporting

Consolidated Standards of Reporting Trials guidance

The Consolidated Standards of Reporting Trials (CONSORT) statement is an evidence-based minimum set of recommendations of reporting randomized trials. By requesting that authors prepare trial reports in a complete and transparent way, aids their critical appraisal and interpretation. The statement comprises a checklist and flow diagram, is endorsed by many medical journals, and is always evolving with further updates and extensions encompassing alternative trial designs and interventions.[14]

References

1. Senn SS. *Cross-over Trials in Clinical Research*, second edition. Chichester: John Wiley and Sons Ltd, 2002.
2. Eldridge S, Kerry S. *A Practical Guide to Cluster Randomised Trials in Health Services Research*. Chichester: John Wiley and Sons Ltd, 2012.
3. Higgins JPT, Altman DG, Gøtzsche PC, *et al.* The Cochrane Collaboration's tool for assessing risk of bias in randomised trials. *BMJ* 2011; 343: d5928.
4. COMET Initiative. *Core Outcome Measures in Effectiveness Trials*. http://www.comet-initiative.org/ (accessed 1 April 2013).
5. Ware JE, Kosinski M, Bjorner JB, *et al. User's Manual for the SF36v2 Health Survey*. Lincoln, RI: Quality Metric Inc., 2007.
6. The EuroQol Group. EuroQol-a new facility for the measurement of health related quality of life. *Health Policy* 1990: 16(3); 199–208.
7. Aaronson NK, Ahmedzai S, Bergman B, *et al.* The European Organization for Research and Treatment of Cancer QLQ-C30: A Quality-of-Life Instrument for Use in International Clinical Trials in Oncology. *J Natl Cancer Inst* 1993; 85(5): 365–76.
8. World Medical Association. *Declaration of Helsinki*, sixth revision, 2008. http://www.wma.net/en/30publications/10policies/b3/ (accessed 1 April 2013).
9. Altman DG. *Practical Statistics for Medical Research*. London: Chapman & Hall, 1991.
10. Kirkwood BR, Sterne JAC. *Essential Medical Statistics*, second edition. Oxford: Blackwell Science Ltd, 2003.
11. Carpenter JR, Kenward MG. *Multiple Imputation and its Application*. Chichester: John Wiley and Sons Ltd, 2013.
12. Dunn G, Maracy M, Tomenson B. Estimating treatment effects from randomized clinical trials with noncompliance and loss to follow-up: the role of instrumental variable methods. *Stat Methods Med Res* 2005; 14(4): 369–95.
13. Emsley R, Dunn G, White IR. Mediation and moderation of treatment effects in randomised controlled trials of complex interventions. *Stat Methods Med Res* 2010; 19(3): 237–70.
14. Schulz KF, Altman DG, Moher D. CONSORT 2010 Statement: updated guidelines for reporting parallel group randomised trials. *BMJ* 2010; 340: c332.

CHAPTER 10.2

Quality improvement

Rob Bethune and Jane M. Blazeby

Introduction

Healthcare and all aspects of surgery are dependent upon practices, pathways, teams, and individuals acting within and between systems in a complex organization. Improvements in the quality of healthcare, therefore, are reliant upon improving the systems within which teams and individuals work. Changing complex systems, that have dependent and interdependent components, is not easy and requires an understanding of the systems as well as the use of tried and tested methodologies for improvement. During the process of improvement there is a need for an iterative approach with careful attention and continuous measurements of performance. This topic area has expanded over the last few years and it is designed to complement research and training to establish real and sustainable changes and improvements in surgery. In this chapter a basic understanding of the terms and concepts that underpin quality improvement are provided and the key methodologies are described, and illustrated with real life examples and case studies relevant to surgical care.

Quality improvement

Definitions of quality

Over the last few years, terms such as 'quality', 'safety', and 'human factors' have become common parlance in medical practice. The official definitions of these are listed in Box 10.2.1. In essence, quality is simply how good we are at healthcare and it encompasses several domains: safety (avoiding harm), effectiveness (treating medical conditions), patient experience, efficiency (reducing cost and waste), and equity. These terms may also be worded from the patients' perspective, and then quality becomes 'making me better' (effectiveness), 'not harming me while you make me better' (safety), 'making it as pleasant as it can be for me' (patient experience), 'doing it for the least cost in terms of money and resources' (efficiency), and 'treating me the same regardless of my race, wealth, religion or any other personal or social factors' (equity). Historically, medicine has focused primarily on effectiveness using evidence-based medicine to find treatments that improve outcome from disease, but this is only part of the picture.

Quality improvement and clinical audit

Knowing what quality really is, clarifies the definition of quality improvement. In its broadest sense quality is improving all aspects of care. Improving care does not happen by chance; it needs not only dedication, but crucially also a methodology that works. Clinical audit is an example of a quality improvement methodology and involves data collection of performance against an established standard, performing an intervention to improve performance,

and then re-auditing the data to assess the effect of the intervention. While clinical audit has led to some important developments over the past two decades, there are also areas of healthcare where audit has not been sufficient to lead to real and sustained changes. More recently developed methods of quality improvement, including 'the model of improvement', have been used successfully to transform healthcare systems and other industries. The three stages

---

Box 10.2.1 Definitions of key terms in quality improvement

Quality is achieving the highest standard of care in four main areas; safety, effectiveness, efficiency and patient experience.[1]

Patient safety is concerned with harm done to patients during treatment. This harm can either be from omission (a patient getting a pulmonary embolus from not receiving venous thrombo-embolism prophylaxis) or commission (development of a central line related infection).

Effectiveness is providing services based on scientific knowledge to all who could benefit, and refraining from providing services to those not likely to benefit.[2]

Efficiency is avoiding waste, including waste of equipment, supplies, ideas, and energy.[2]

Patient experience is providing care that is respectful of and responsive to individual patient preferences, needs, and values, and ensuring that patient values guide all clinical decisions. Care must also be delivered in a timely fashion.

Quality improvement is the process of improving all aspects of care given to patients. The three main areas are; education and training, research, and service improvement.

Service improvement (which may be used synonymously with quality improvement) is the process of systematically improving the standard of healthcare, within the four domains (patient experience, effectiveness, efficiency, and safety).

Clinical audit is the systematic and critical analysis of the quality of clinical care, including the procedures for the diagnosis, treatment and care, the associated use of resources and the resulting outcome and quality of life for the patient.[3] Practically, this has been simplified to the audit cycle (see Figure 10.2.3).

Human factors refers to errors relating to non-technical skills. Technical skills are knowledge and practical skills. Non-technical skills are categorized as; communication, leadership, team work, decision making, situational awareness and coping with stress and fatigue.[4]

of 'the model for improvement' will be discussed in the model for improvement section, illustrating these with clinical examples.

Patient safety

The chasm between the best possible healthcare in the National Health Service (NHS) (which may be defined in the hypothetical setting as the application of the best available evidence, by the perfectly trained clinical team functioning within a seamless system for 100% of the time) and what actually happens in practice in hospitals and within the NHS is enormous.[2] This gap is well recognized and although hospitals and clinical teams are attempting to reduce it, closing the chasm and increasing safety is critical. One method, initiated in 2001, was the creation of the NHS National Patient Safety Agency, which is a body that investigates safety incidents within healthcare and proposes solutions to improve safety. This is essential as repeated studies show that 10–20% of patients admitted to hospital experience errors in their care that can result in harm (i.e. an adverse event), and of those, up to a further 10% may die from such errors.[5] In this setting, an adverse event is defined as an unintended injury that results in temporary or permanent disability, death, or prolonged hospital stay that was caused by the system of healthcare rather than the patient's disease.[5] This statistic holds true for surgery as well. A study of ten surgical units in The Netherlands documented some 881 unintended events over a 3 month period.[5] The consequences of the events were analysed and these included suboptimal care, inconveniences to patients, extra interventions, prolonged hospital stays, and physical and mental injury.

The surgical safety checklist

The translation of the risk of experiencing an adverse event while in hospital to population data demonstrates the scale of the problem. In the UK, there are 3 million hospital admissions per year, meaning that approximately 300 000 patients may suffer unintended events each year as a result of error, leading to significant morbidity and mortality. The challenge to staff within the health service, therefore, is to consider how these adverse events can be prevented and to take action to change systems to improve safety.[6] One of the best examples of a system change that can reduce adverse events in surgery is the introduction of the surgical safety checklist.[7] This demonstrated a 36% reduction in mortality following its introduction (Box 10.2.2).

Human factors

Adverse events

When surgical adverse events are analysed in detail, the factors contributing to them are overwhelmingly related to human error (72.7%), followed by systematic organizational failings (16.1%); technical errors are the smallest group (5.7%).[5] The terms used to encompass human error within an organizational setting are nowadays referred to as 'human factors' or 'non-technical skills', and these include communication, leadership, team work, decision making, situational awareness, and coping with stress and fatigue.[4] Recognition of the need for excellence in human (non-technical) factors among surgeons, who traditionally focus on the acquisition of technical skills, is a significant advance in healthcare and in the attempt to reduce human error and improve healthcare systems. The widespread use of methods that mitigate human factors error

---

Box 10.2.2 The surgical safety checklist

In a landmark study, Atul Gawande and colleagues trialled a simple 20-point checklist to be used perioperatively as well as preoperative briefings and training for staff on the use of these tools.[7] The study was conducted in eight hospitals in eight cities, four in the developed world and four in the developing world. Over 7000 operations were observed, half using the checklist and the other half as a control. In the group where the checklist was being used the reduction in mortality was 46% and in morbidity was 36%. Both of these were highly statistically significant results. As the authors point out in their discussion, the exact impact of the checklist is difficult to untangle as there were almost certainly other factors that influenced the outcome. First, the use of preoperative and postoperative briefings have been shown to improve communication and improve efficiency[8] and, in addition, the findings may have been subject to the Hawthorne effect, an improvement in performance due to subject's knowledge of being observed. Despite these potential pitfalls the magnitude of the effect cannot be ignored.

Source: data from *The Institute for Medicine, Crossing the Quality Chasm: A New Health System for the 21st Century*, National Academy Press, Washington, D.C., USA, Copyright © 2001; Flin R. et al. (Eds.), *Safety at the Sharp End: A guide to non-technical skills*, Ashgate Publishing Limited, Copyright © 2008; Working for patients: NHS White Paper, New diagnosis—new prescription, *Health Service Journal*, Volume 99, Issue 5136, pp. 134–7, Copyright © 1989; and Darzi A., *High Quality Care For All: NHS Next Stage Review Final Report*, ©Crown Copyright 2008, licensed under the Open Government Licence v3.0.

(such as the surgical checklist) have huge potential for reducing adverse events in surgery.

Communication

Effective communication underpins the other human factor domains and is fundamental to workplace safety and efficiency.[4] There are checklists or *aide-mémoires* designed to improve and formalize communication within clinical teams with the aim of maximizing the accuracy of information transfer.[9] An example of this is the situation, background, assessment, and recommendation (SBAR) communication tool (Box 10.2.3).[10] While this tool was developed in the aviation industry, and used within the military, it has now been adapted for healthcare where the effective (or ineffective) use of a structured communication can be a matter of life and death.

Situational awareness and decision making

Situational awareness refers to the human facet of simply being aware and knowing what is going on around you. While this may seem very obvious, without situational awareness in surgery, serious mistakes may occur. One such example is the loss of situational awareness in theatre in a unilateral operation leading to wrong-side surgery.[13] Decision making refers to the ability to process the available information and make an informed choice based on this. In reality, decision making is a continuous process of monitoring the environment, re-evaluating, and then making the appropriate decision.[4] A classic medical example of where decision making goes

Box 10.2.3 Situation, background, assessment, and recommendation—the communication tool recommended to improve hand over in clinical teams

The SBAR (situation, background, assessment, and recommendation) tool was developed to formalize communications and help both the sender and the receiver to transmit meaning accurately.[9–12] It consists of four parts.

S—Situation: A brief outline of the current state of the patient ('Mrs X is hypotensive and tachycardic')

B—Background: What has happened running up to this moment ('Mrs X is previously fit and well and had a laparoscopic cholecystectomy this morning')

A—Assessment: The state of play now. ('Her respiratory rate is 35, blood pressure 90/70 and heart rate is 130. I think she is in class III hypovolaemic shock, she has received 2 litres of crystalloid')

R—Recommendation: What the sender wants the receiver to do. ('Can you please come to ward 31 immediately as I think she needs to go back to theatre')

(N.B In Australia it is called, i-SBAR, the first i standing for *intro-ducing yourself*.)

Adapted from the SBAR Toolkit, available from the Institute for Healthcare Improvement at: http://www.ihi.org/knowledge/Pages/Tools/SBARToolkit.aspx. The SBAR Toolkit was originally developed by Michael Leonard, Doug Bonacum, and Suzanne Graham at Kaiser Permanente of Colorado.

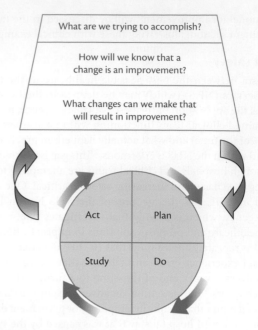

Fig. 10.2.1 The model for improvement.

Reproduced with permission from Langley GL, *et al.*, *The Improvement Guide: A Practical Approach to Enhancing Organizational Performance*, Second Edition, Wiley-Blackwell, Chichester UK, Copyright © 2009 Gerald J Langley, Ronald D Moen, Kevin M Nolan, Thomas W Nolan, Clifford I Norman, Lloyd P Provost. All rights reserved.

wrong is 'tunnel vision'. A clinician makes a diagnosis and sticks to that diagnosis, despite evidence (from tests and investigations) to the contrary. This can lead to major error, and yet if iterative processes and team working were in place, it is possible that such problems could be avoided.

Stress and fatigue

Coping with stress at work involves understanding that emergency situations affect our ability to function and take appropriate decisions. The development and use of systems such as the surgical safety checklist may mitigate against flawed thinking when under pressure by ensuring that basic standards of care are adhered to and that the whole team is involved in achieving the standards. As healthcare operates 24/7, all healthcare workers will at some point experience fatigue at work. This needs to be recognized and minimized as much as possible and, in addition to using safe systems, the use of safe and 'humane' shift patterns of work are essential to reduce the potential for harm that fatigue inevitably produces in individuals and teams.

The model for improvement

The aim

One of the most widely used methods for implementing change in healthcare, is the 'model for improvement'.[14,15] This consists of three simple steps that are applied to achieve change in a system. The first is to be clear about the aim of the project, the second is to measure the process and outcomes, and finally there is the need to test for change (Figure 10.2.1).[15] Ensuring that the aim of any project is clear is critical for it to be achieved. An aim should be specific

in content and nature and also it should be realistic. For example, a clear aim will ask exactly what and where is the target of the project, for example, 'what' (how many patients have documented venous thrombo-embolism risk assessments) and 'where' (on the surgical ward 7B).

Measurement

Measurement is crucial to quality improvement and it is essential to measure the effects of implemented changes. The main measurements that can be made include measures of process, outcomes and of balance.

Process measures

Process measures (like the quality of weekend handovers or discharge summaries) may be used to assess part of the overall system that delivers care and, as such, they are not measures of clinical outcomes. Process measures, however, will be linked to and often associated with clinical outcomes, and by improving them it would be expected that a clinical outcome would improve. Although it may be hard to prove the association between an improvement in a process measure and clinical outcome, the links will usually be very plausible. For example, a better communicated handover between clinical teams will result in better patient care and, therefore, a reduced number of adverse events (clinical outcomes). This is plausible and may be explained because of accurate and timely exchange of information between key personnel at the hand over.

Outcome measures

There are many different outcomes that can be measured in healthcare, including clinical outcomes (e.g. rates of wound infection), patient-reported outcomes (outcomes described by patients themselves such as walking distance after a total knee replacement or patient experience and satisfaction with healthcare), cost-related outcomes (e.g. cost of improved life year gained), and observer-assessed outcomes (e.g. symptoms assessed by doctors). Selection of the right measures to assess any changes is often difficult and it is likely that a combination of outcome measures will be used to complement measures of process and balance. The chapter on research includes a detailed summary of each of these types of outcomes. Careful and accurate measurement will reveal the underlying complexity of a system and allow a deeper understanding of it and further the goal of improving it. As Peter Drucker said 'if you can't measure it, you can't manage it'.[16]

Balancing measures

Balancing measures attempt to quantify the undesired or the side effects of any change. They are a crucial, but often forgotten, part of the programmes that implement change. Measures of the undesired effects provide data to understand the balance of the overall impact of the intervention. In the handover example (Box 10.2.4) between doctors using weekend handover stickers, a measure of balance would be time lost completing the handover, which may erode into time to complete technical tasks. An often cited example of a major change in the NHS that did not fully balance the impact of the change was the introduction of the 4-hour wait target in emergency departments in 2003.[17]Although within 4 years the target was met successfully (98.5% of patients in the UK were seen within 4 hours in 2007), there was a lack of consideration of some of the unintended consequences and side effects of achieving this. For example, sick patients were removed from the safe environment of the emergency department to wards that were unable to provide the acute care.[18,19] As balancing measures were not collected it is difficult to truthfully comment on the success of the programme.

Measurement also acts to provide continuity to the project. In the example (Figure 10.2.2), data regarding improving the handover between F1 doctors was collected weekly and, although it did not take long to collect the data, the very action of data collection brought the project back to the attention of the F1s. During periods when no changes were being made, the project's drumbeat was the data collection.

The plan–do–study–act cycle

The plan–do–study–act (PDSA) is the 'doing' bit of the model for improvement. It is as simple and intuitive as it sounds. Once

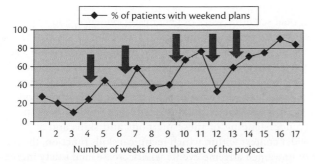

Fig. 10.2.2 Run chart showing % of weekend plans documented in the notes. The red arrows refer to the plan–do–study–act cycles. The x-axis is the time period. Data was collected on a weekly basis for the 4 months the project was run.

Box 10.2.4 Improving weekend handover: a junior doctor-led quality improvement project

The aim: what are we trying to accomplish

A group of F1 doctors realized that the weekend handover at their trust was not as good as it could be. When they were doing the weekend on call they were frustrated that the key information regarding patients had not been passed to them, which meant they were often reacting to events rather than preventing them. At the same time as they were conceiving their plan, a significant amount of media attention was being paid to a Dr Foster report that highlighted a significantly higher mortality of patients at weekends and specifically highlighted poor handover as one of the causes.

They decided to try and improve weekend handover, and they used the model for improvement to help them. The aim was to ensure that 95% of surgical inpatients on two wards had a documented and adequate weekend handover plan in the patient's notes.

Measurement: how do we know if our changes are an improvement?

Often this is one of the harder stages of an improvement project. The area being measured (the 'metric') can sometimes be hard to define, but in this case it was simple. On a Monday morning, the group would check the notes of all the patients on the ward. Clear definitions are important to allow the data to be consistent. In this case, the only patients included were ones that had been admitted before 5pm on the Friday and had stayed in until Monday. The notes were quickly reviewed to see if an adequate weekend handover had been documented (adequate was defined as a clear diagnosis and management plan as well as whether the patient needed daily review). This allowed one metric per week to be collected and plotted on a run chart (Figure 10.2.2). Six data points were collected before any changes were implemented.

Tests of change: the plan–do–act–study (PDSA) cycle

Once measurement was securely in place, the F1 doctors started devising their first test of change. They knew of a group in another hospital who had done a similar project successfully using a sticker that was filled in and then placed in the notes. They contacted the other team and their first PDSA used the sticker from the other hospital. As a result of local variations in practice, several modifications were made to the sticker (PDSA cycles), before the final one was agreed. Further PDSA cycles had to be conducted to work out how to get the stickers to the F1s, so they had them on Friday. For example, one PDSA was to give the stickers out during the F1 teaching at lunchtime. This sounded like a good idea, but in fact several teams wanted to fill most of the stickers out on the morning ward round, so other plans had to be made. The results in the run chart speak for themselves. After a series of PDSAs (marked with red arrows but in practice there were many more), the percentage of adequate weekend plans in the notes went from the baseline of 30% up to 95%. When analysed using a statistical process chart the change was significant.

measurement is in place and a suitable number of baseline points have been collected and examined, then it is possible to make system changes to improve practice. The PDSA cycle is initially done on a very small scale. For example, in the weekend handover project the initial test of change was to try out one sticker before a weekend with just one F1 (plan and do), then this F1 could feedback on the sticker (study) that would allow change and modification (act). The updated sticker was then re-tested on the same scale again by the F1 until s/he was happy with it. The next step was to try it on three F1s using the same feedback processes until they all agreed it was working, and then finally it was tested on a larger group of five F1s on two wards. This iterative process is crucial to quality improvement and an essential ingredient to develop and modify a solution to a problem before examining its impact on a large scale (i.e. start the tests small and scale them up when they are working). Multiple PDSA cycles are often needed to generate improvement (Figure 10.2.2).

The model for improvement is a tried and tested method for improving frontline care.[20–22] The iterative approach with multiple small tests of change and continuous data collection contrasts starkly to clinical audit where data is collected only twice and only one intervention is attempted.

Clinical audit

In 1989, the Department of Health highlighted the need for clinical audit in the white paper 'Working for Patients'.[3] It defined clinical audit as the 'systematic and critical analysis of the quality of clinical care, including the procedures for the diagnosis, treatment and care, the associated use of resources and the resulting outcome and quality of life for the patient.' This relatively sophisticated and complicated description has been simplified to the idea of the audit cycle (Figure 10.2.3). In practice, this means identifying a problem for which standards exist, collecting a large amount of data associated with it, performing an intervention, and then re-collecting the data at a later date (to close the audit loop).

Although the use of the audit process has had some major impact and successes over the past two decades, particularly with nationally led projects, many aspects of it have also had a chequered history, particularly small-scale projects that are led by junior doctors. Retrospective analysis of audit (an audit of audits) has shown that only 5% resulted in any significant and lasting improvement.[23] In addition, audit is not popular with junior doctors; 25% feel a negative personnel benefit of performing audit and a further 27% felt it was a waste of time. Also, it is rarely carried out properly, which is probably a major contributing factor to the lack of belief by junior staff in the process.[24–26] There is also evidence to show that the audit loop is only ever completed in 20% of cases.

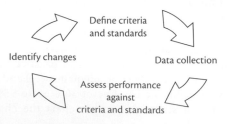

Fig. 10.2.3 The audit cycle.

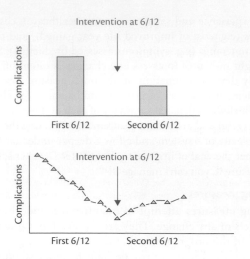

Fig. 10.2.4 The danger of isolated interval data.
Reproduced with permission from O'Brien T, *et al.*, Why don't Mercedes Benz publish randomized trials?, *BJU International*, Volume 105, Issue 3, pp. 293–5, Copyright © 2010 The Authors. Journal Compilation © 2010 BJU International.

There are a variety of reasons why clinical audit may fail. Many clinical audits are done as a 'tick box' exercise, with little understanding of why the audit is being carried out. Large amounts of time are needed to extract meaningful data from notes and written records; this makes completion of the audit cycle difficult. However, the most significant problem is the lack of structure and support the clinicians running the audit have which limits their ability to do it properly and to use the data afterwards to make meaningful changes.[23] Further to the above procedural problems, with audit there is a methodological flaw when looking at performance that only collects data on two occasions. This method is occasionally used in research as well where it is called an interrupted time series analysis. The two graphs in Figure 10.2.4 describe the potential inaccuracy associated with this method.[27] Large grouped collections of data can hide real trends that can go against the conclusion drawn from looking at pooled data. Although the example shown is extreme, it would seem sensible to always display data over time to avoid this potential error.

Conclusion

Recent recognition of the number and type of avoidable errors and unwanted events within healthcare has highlighted the need to better understand healthcare systems and how care is delivered. Methods to improve the quality of health systems differ from the traditional scientific ways of generating evidence, and require the consideration of non-technical skills as well as technical factors. The whole process of quality improvement, however, is not a separate part of healthcare and it runs through every aspect and involves every member of the healthcare team. Indeed, both undergraduate and postgraduate curricula require training in these methods and factors. It is anticipated that as healthcare professionals increase their understanding of these methods and skills and appreciate the wider context within which technical skills function, the number of unwanted adverse events will decrease, and safety increase. Clinical audit has played a part in understanding variation within clinical practice, but it seems the newer methodologies such as the model for improvement will become increasingly important in the transformation of healthcare. The chasm between the best possible care and what is currently provided to patients will be bridged by frontline clinicians working to improve the systems in which they work.

References

1. Darzi A. High quality care for all: NHS Next Stage Review final report, 2008. Available from https://www.gov.uk/government/uploads/system/uploads/attachment_data/file/228836/7432.pdf (accessed 6 October 2015).
2. The Institute for Medicine. *Crossing the Quality Chasm: A New Health System for the 21st Century*. Washington DC: National Academy of Medicine, 2001.
3. Working for Patients. NHS White Paper. New diagnosis—new prescription. *Health Serv J* 1989; 99(5136): 134–7.
4. Flin R, O'Connor P, Crichton M. *Safety at the Sharp End: a guide to non-techincal skills*. Farnham: Ashgate Publishing Limited, 2008.
5. van Wagtendonk I, Smits M, Merten H, *et al*. Nature, causes and consequences of unintended events in surgical units. *Br J Surg* 2010; 97(11): 1730–40.
6. Kable AK, Gibberd RW, Spigelman AD. Adverse events in surgical patients in Australia. *Int J Qual Health Care* 2002; 14(4): 269–76.
7. Haynes AB, Weiser TG, Berry WR, *et al*. A surgical safety checklist to reduce morbidity and mortality in a global population. *N Engl J Med* 2009; 360(5): 491–9.
8. Bethune R, Sasirckha G, Sahu A, *et al*. Use of briefings and debriefings as a tool in improving team work, efficiency, and communication in the operating theatre. *Postgrad Med J* 2011; 87(1027): 331–4.
9. Telem DA, Buch KE, Ellis S, *et al*. Integration of a formalized handoff system into the surgical curriculum: resident perspectives and early results. *Arch Surg* 2011; 146(1): 89–93.
10. Marshall S, Harrison J, Flanagan B. The teaching of a structured tool improves the clarity and content of interprofessional clinical communication. *Qual Saf Health Care* 2009; 18(2): 137–40.
11. Haig KM, Sutton S, Whittington J. SBAR: a shared mental model for improving communication between clinicians. *Jt Comm J Qual Patient Saf* 2006; 32(3): 167–75.
12. Mitchell EL, Lee DY, Arora S, *et al*. SBAR M&M: a feasible, reliable, and valid tool to assess the quality of, surgical morbidity and mortality conference presentations. *Am J Surg* 2012; 203(1): 26–31.
13. Neily J, Mills PD, Paull DE, *et al*. Sharing lessons learned to prevent incorrect surgery. *Am Surg* 2012; 78(11): 1276–80.
14. Courtlandt CD, Noonan L, Feld LG. Model for improvement—Part 1: A framework for health care quality. *Pediatr Clin North Am* 2009; 56(4): 757–78.
15. Langley GJ, Moen RD, Nolan KM, et al. *The Improvement Guide: A Practical Approach to Enhancing Organizational Performance*. San Francisco: Jossey-Bass, 2009.
16. Drucker P. *On Knowledge Management*. Boston: Harvard Business School Press, 1987.
17. Locker TE, Mason MM. Analysis of the distribution of time that patients spend in emergency departments. *BMJ* 2005; 330: 1188–89.
18. Mortimore A, Cooper S. The '4-hour target': emergency nurses' views. *Emerg Med J* 2007; 24(6): 402–4.
19. Weber EJ, Mason S, Carter A, *et al*. Emptying the corridors of shame: organizational lessons from England's 4-hour emergency throughput target. *Ann Emerg Med* 2011; 57(2): 79–88.e1.
20. Vogel P, Vassilev G, Kruse B, *et al*. Morbidity and Mortality conference as part of PDCA cycle to decrease anastomotic failure in colorectal surgery. *Langenbecks Arch Surg* 2011; 396(7): 1009–15.
21. Batalden PB, Davidoff F. What is 'quality improvement' and how can it transform healthcare? *Qual Saf Health Care* 2007; 16(1): 2–3.
22. Pronovost P. Interventions to decrease catheter-related bloodstream infections in the ICU: the Keystone Intensive Care Unit Project. *Am J Infect Control* 2008; 36(10):S171: e1–5.
23. Hillman T, Roueche A. Clincal audit is dead, long live quality improvement. *BMJ Careers* 2011. Available from http://careers.bmj.com/careers/advice/view-article.html?id=20002524 (accessed 6 October 2015).
24. Greenwood JP, Lindsay SJ, Batin PD, *et al*. Junior doctors and clinical audit. *J R Coll Physicians Lond* 1997; 31(6): 648–51.
25. Guryel E, Acton K, Patel S. Auditing orthopaedic audit. *Ann R Coll Surg Engl* 2008; 90(8): 675–8.
26. John CM, Mathew DE, Gnanalingham MG. An audit of paediatric audits. *Arch Dis Child* 2004; 89(12): 1128–9.
27. O'Brien T, Viney R, Doherty A, Thomas K. Why don't mercedes benz publish randomized trials? *BJU Int* 2010; 105(3): 293–5.

CHAPTER 10.3

Statistics for surgeons

Vimal J. Gokani and Matthew J. Bown

Describing data

Types of data

When reading a paper or analysing data it is important to understand the type of data (Figure 10.3.1). Usually it will be either *categorical* (e.g. blood group, where patients can be categorized into groups A, B, AB, and O) or *numerical* (e.g. height, where patients are measured and height is expressed as an absolute measure on a scale). If analysing numerical data, it is usual to examine it first by plotting a histogram. This gives information about the spread and uniformity of the data in the sample and considering these histograms helps to understand some of the language of statistics. If the data conforms to a classic bell-shaped normal distribution it can be summarized using the *parameters* mean and standard deviation, leading to the classification that this is *parametric* data (and can be analysed using parametric statistical techniques). If data is skewed and concentrated around the more positive values (compared to the average value), the dataset is positively skewed. If the data are concentrated around a less positive value (compared with the average), the dataset is negatively skewed. Non-normally distributed (skewed) datasets are *non-parametric*. By looking at the distribution of the data it is possible to make a decision about whether to use parametric or non-parametric statistical techniques.

The average

When describing data it is usual to summarize the data (but when presenting data graphically it is preferable to show every data point wherever possible). The most commonly used summary measure is the 'average' (i.e. the value around which observations are spread). The three commonly used averages are the mean, median, and mode.

The (arithmetic) *mean* is defined as the sum of all values divided by the number of values. The mean takes into account all values; however, it is distorted by skewed data and outliers. For normally distributed data the standard deviation (σ) can be used to describe the spread of the data around the mean. It is important to note that if data is skewed, or not normal, the mean and the standard deviation do not accurately summarize the data. The *median* is the central value of the set of data when ordered from smallest to largest. If n is odd, the median is simple to calculate. If it is even, it is calculated as the arithmetic mean of the two middle values. Although the median ignores much of the data, it is little affected by the skew of the data or the presence of outliers. Therefore when data appears non-parametric or an assessment cannot be made (i.e. due to small sample sizes, skewed data or outliers), then it is preferable to use the median to describe the data. The *mode*, which represents the most common observation, is appropriately used when describing categorical data.

The spread of data

When discussing continuous data, the spread (or variability) can be described. For parametric data this can easily be achieved using the standard deviation. The *standard deviation* (σ), is the square-root of the *variance*, describes the spread of the data around the mean: the larger the standard deviation, the larger the variability. For non-parametric data it is usual to use the *range*, defined as the difference between the largest and smallest values. This is unaffected by skew but it is affected by outliers. The *interquartile range* has the advantage that it is unaffected by both of these. This is the range between the 25th percentile value and the 75th percentile value and contains the middle 50% of the values in the dataset. As the interquartile range simply excludes the bottom and top 25% of values, another measure of dispersion of data may be required.

Confidence intervals

Scientific studies are performed on a sample taken from an entire population. When a sample is studied, conclusions are made and the sample is described using measures such as mean and standard deviation. However, it is often more useful to think of what the result may represent for the population from which it is drawn. Confidence intervals allow us to estimate the range in which the true population value for a measurement or outcome is likely to lie. Using the mean, standard deviation, and size of the sample, a range in which the true population value lies can be estimated. It is common to use a *95% confidence interval*. This means that for a given outcome one can be 95% certain that the true population value for this outcome is within the quoted 95% confidence interval.

Displaying data

Data can usually be described using appropriate figures or tables. Parametric data or categorical data can easily be summarized in tables. Often authors use bar charts with error bars for parametric data. For non-parametric continuous data boxplots (Figure 10.3.2) are usually used. Figures for more specialized data are considered later. Wherever possible it is ideal to display the actual measures for individuals/experimental units in a study.

Measurement of risk

Comparisons between groups in clinical and epidemiological studies are often assessed using *odds ratio* (OR), *relative risk* (RR), relative risk reduction (RRR), and *absolute risk reduction* (ARR), but these

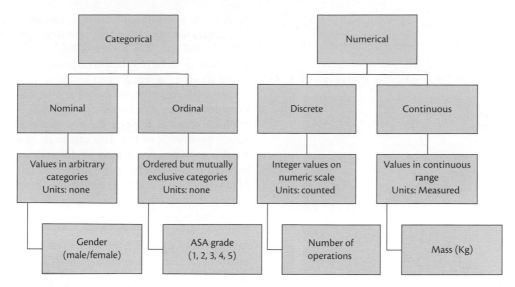

Fig. 10.3.1 Types of data. ASA, American Society of Anesthesiologists.

are not interchangeable. RR is usually applied to prospective cohort studies that assess the exposure of groups to some risk factor of interest. OR are commonly used for analysis of case-control studies. The difference between OR and RR becomes smaller when the prevalence (the number of instances of an event per unit time in a specified population) of the disease in question becomes low (<10%). RRR is usually reserved for interpretation of interventional trials. However, it is possible to calculate all of these measures in many instances, but it is not necessarily correct to do so. It is important therefore to seek advice on what measure to use in each particular circumstance.

The *odds* is simply the proportion of adverse events to non-adverse events and the OR is the ratio of the odds in one group

compared to another. The RR is the change in incidence of adverse events between two groups (e.g. intervention and no intervention). The RRR is the proportion of RR between two groups. The RR is more intuitive, and therefore often easier to understand; however, there are certain instances where RR cannot be calculated. The *absolute risk* is the incidence of an event (the number of events in a defined population at a given time). The ARR is the difference between the proportion of adverse outcomes in the population undergoing an intervention and the proportion of adverse outcomes in the population undergoing no intervention or another intervention. The *number needed to treat*, defined as the number of patients who need to be treated to prevent one defined event (e.g. death), is calculated by taking the reciprocal of the ARR.

To illustrate this, consider a study that has tested two treatments (treatment A and treatment B) to manage a disease (see Figure 10.3.3). At the end of the study, the numbers of people who have died from the disease and those who are alive are recorded.

Hypothesis testing

The null hypothesis

Clinical research must begin with a question (e.g. is endovascular abdominal aortic aneurysm (AAA) repair (EVAR) better than open repair, in terms of mortality rate?), which is converted to a hypothesis (EVAR is associated with lower mortality than open repair). The *null hypothesis* (H_0) is the theory that there is no difference (in our example, there is no difference between mortality for EVAR and open repair). Hypothesis tests will allow the null hypothesis to be either accepted or rejected. If rejected, the *alternative hypothesis*, (H_1) must be true (i.e. there is a difference in the mortality between open repair and EVAR).

Type 1 and type 2 error

In hypothesis testing, there are two types of error (i.e. incorrectly accepting or rejecting the null hypothesis). A *type 1 error* is when the null hypothesis is incorrectly rejected. A *type 2 error* occurs when the null hypothesis is incorrectly accepted. When performing power calculations for research design the proposed type 1 error

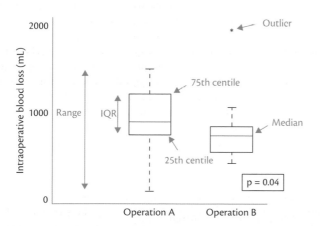

Fig. 10.3.2 A box-and-whisker plot of two operations (A and B), and their associated blood loss. In this example, range is demonstrated by the whiskers (dotted lines) and interquartile range (IQR) is demonstrated by the box. The upper limit of the box represents the 75th percentile, and the lower limit of the box represents the 25th centile. In operation A, the median (represented by the red line) is lower than the 50th centile, therefore the data exhibit a negative skew. In operation B, the median is larger than the 50th centile, therefore these data exhibit a positive skew. As $p=0.04$, there is a 4% chance that this finding occurred by chance. This is accepted as statistically significant. Although this may be statistically significant, it may not be clinically significant as the blood loss, although statistically different, is very similar for both operations (900 mL versus 950 mL). The asterisk marks outliers.

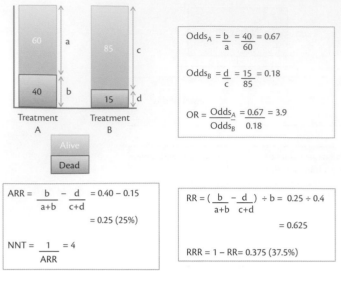

$$\text{Odds}_A = \frac{b}{a} = \frac{40}{60} = 0.67$$

$$\text{Odds}_B = \frac{d}{c} = \frac{15}{85} = 0.18$$

$$\text{OR} = \frac{\text{Odds}_A}{\text{Odds}_B} = \frac{0.67}{0.18} = 3.9$$

$$\text{ARR} = \frac{b}{a+b} - \frac{d}{c+d} = 0.40 - 0.15$$
$$= 0.25\ (25\%)$$

$$\text{NNT} = \frac{1}{\text{ARR}} = 4$$

$$\text{RR} = \left(\frac{b}{a+b} - \frac{d}{c+d}\right) \div b = 0.25 \div 0.4$$
$$= 0.625$$

$$\text{RRR} = 1 - \text{RR} = 0.375\ (37.5\%)$$

Fig. 10.3.3 The odds of dying if undergoing treatment A (O_A) is (40/60 =) 0.67. The odds of dying if a patient undergoes treatment B (O_B) is (15/85 =) 0.18. The odds ratio (OR) therefore, is (0.67/0.18 =) 3.9x. Patients have 3.9 the odds of dying if they have treatment B instead of A. If undergoing treatment A, the probability of death is (40/100 =) 0.4. For treatment B, the probability of death is (15/100 =) 0.15. The absolute risk reduction (ARR) of dying with treatment A over treatment B is (40/100–15/100 =) 0.25 (25%). The number needed to treat (NNT) is (1/0.25 =) 4, indicating that four people need to undergo treatment A as opposed to treatment B to prevent one death. The relative risk (RR) of dying if undergoing treatment A compared to treatment B is ((0.4–0.15)/0.4 =) 0.625 (62.5%). There is a 62.5% increased risk of dying if undergoing treatment B, compared to undergoing treatment A. The relative risk reduction (RRR) is 1–RR (1–0.625 =) 0.375. Relative risk therefore, does not indicate the size of the actual risk.

rate (alpha) and power (one minus the type 2 error rate (beta)) are used (see Chapter 10.1, Research in Surgery).

The *p*-value

The *p-value* is the probability that the observed outcome of the study occurs due to chance alone. Conventionally a probability of less than 5% is accepted as being statistically significant ($p < 0.05$). It is important to remember that statistical significance does not equate to clinical significance. The lower the *p*-value, the stronger the evidence is that the null hypothesis can be rejected.

Choosing the correct statistical test

Hypothesis testing is based on choosing the correct statistical test for the dataset being tested. For basic approaches, the choice of test depends on the *type of data* (numerical or categorical), the *distribution* (parametric or non-parametric), the *number of groups* being compared (one, two, or more than two), and whether the measurements are *paired* or *unpaired* (e.g. weight measurements on the same person before and after an intervention are paired). Figure 10.3.4 shows an algorithm for choosing statistical tests for simple datasets.

Chi-squared tests are used for categorical data if the sample size is large enough (arbitrarily greater than 20 observations with no counts of under 5). Fisher's exact test can be used for 2×2 tables with small numbers; however, there is no alternative for tables larger than 2×2 with small numbers. In this case, providing it can

be done in a meaningful manner, categories can be combined. McNemar's test can be used for paired categorical data.

Numerical data can be considered as those datasets where a numerical outcome (e.g. height) is being compared in a small number of groups (e.g. females and males) or those where a numerical outcome is being compared with another numerical explanatory variable (e.g. height and weight).

Where data are grouped the first step is to assess whether the data is parametric or not. This can be done using statistical tools, but it is good practice to start off doing this manually. Differences between two groups for non-parametric data can be tested using Mann-Whitney U test (e.g. comparing the number of monocytes in tissue biopsies from patients with either tumour type X or Y). For paired non-parametric data, such as a randomized controlled trial comparing two chemotherapeutic agents A or B on patient weight before and after treatment (i.e. repeat (paired) measurements in the same individual), the Wilcoxon signed rank test is used. Where there are more than two groups to be tested either a Mann-Whitney U test (non-paired data) or a Friedman test (paired data) can be used.

For unpaired parametric data, the Student's *t*-test is used to compare two groups, such as evaluating the effect of a two different operations on postoperative pain scores. For paired data there is a corresponding paired *t*-test. For datasets where there are more than two groups, such as comparing C-reactive protein levels in patients with pancreatitis on three different anti-inflammatory agents an Analysis Of Variance (ANOVA) is used.

Correlation

Correlation is used to determine whether there is any association between numerical variables. A scatter plot can demonstrate any association graphically and usually the presence/absence of a linear relationship between the two variables is determined (although other mathematical relationships can exist). The strength and direction of the relationship can be described using a correlation coefficient. *Pearson's correlation* (r) coefficient is such an example, and ranges from +1 to –1. This is used when testing associations between at least one normally distributed variable to another. The size of r delineates how close the association between the variables is, and the positive or negative sign denotes the direction of the association: negative correlation is where as one variable increases, the other decreases. When $r = 0$, there is no linear correlation between the variables. When $r = 1$, there is a very strong positive linear relationship between the variables. A very strong negative linear relationship is indicated by $r = -1$. Of note, a strong correlation between x and y does not suggest a causal relationship. *p*-Values from correlation analyses are the probability that the observed relationship occurred by random chance.

Associations of non-parametric data series can be tested using *Spearman's rank correlation*. This test should be used if sample sizes are too small to assess the data for normality, if both x and y are non-parametric or in a few other special situations.

Regression

Correlation can determine whether two variables are associated but often we need to determine the degree of *association* (i.e. how much one variable changes with a given change in another). Regression

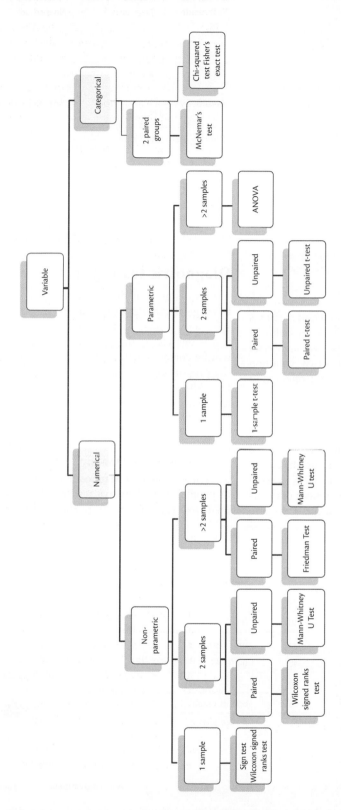

Fig. 10.3.4 Hypothesis testing: a suggested flow diagram of which statistical test to use when testing hypotheses.

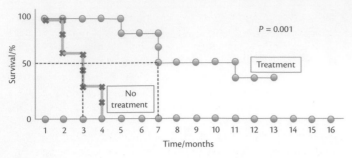

Fig. 10.3.5 A Kaplan-Meier survival curve. When reading this chart, note the *y*-axis. Not all curves are presented with a percentage scale, and the *y*-axis may be presented as mortality instead of survival. The graph shows the survival curves of a disease with treatment (blue line) and without treatment (green line). In the treatment arm, the first death occurred at 5 months, and between months 6 and 7 there were two deaths. Between months 10 and 11 no further death occurred, and no patients were followed up after 13 months. The median survival is measured by drawing a line across from the 50% survival, and down to the *x*-axis. The median survival of patients who do not receive treatment is 3 months, and 7 months for those who receive this treatment. If the follow-up is long enough, the 5-year survival can also be reported. The survival curves are statistically significantly different as P = 0.001 (i.e. *p* < 0.05).

tests the *relationship* between variables which exhibit and measures it. Regression can also examine the effect of multiple variables on one outcome variable (multivariate analyses). This is very powerful but often over-used. Incorrect use of regression is easy, common and can lead to erroneous conclusions. Expert help is required to perform such analyses.

Survival analysis

When dealing with outcomes after surgery we are often interested in how long it takes for a certain event to occur (death, cancer recurrence, etc.). These time-to-event data are usually assessed using Kaplan-Meier curves that demonstrate the number of events of interest occurring over time, and when they occur. The curve

Table 10.3.1 Sensitivity and specificity

Test result	Disease	No disease	Total
Positive	a	b	a + b
Negative	c	d	c + d
Total	a + c	b + d	n = a + b + c + d

$$\text{Sensitivity} = \frac{a}{(a+c)} \qquad \text{Specificity} = \frac{d}{(b+d)}$$

$$\text{Positive predictive value} = \frac{a}{(a+b)} \qquad \text{Negative predictive value} = \frac{d}{(c+d)}$$

of survival against time looks like a series of steps, with each step down representing an individual reaching an end point (see Figure 10.3.5). When two or more individuals reach an end point in a given time period, the step down is proportionately larger.

Diagnostic testing accuracy

The assessment of diagnostic accuracy is a common question in surgical examinations and is measured using sensitivity and specificity primarily. The *sensitivity* of a diagnostic or screening test is defined as the proportion of people with a disease who will be correctly detected by that test. The *specificity* of a test is the proportion of people without a disease who have a negative test. Although it would be ideal if all tests had a sensitivity and specificity of 100%, this is often not the case. Whether a test aims for a high sensitivity depends on the disease being detected. In cases of diseases which are easily treated, a high specificity may be acceptable. In cases of severe untreatable disease, a test with high specificity would protect against false positives. The *positive predictive value* of a diagnostic test is defined as the proportion of people with a positive test that has the disease. The *negative predictive value* is the proportion of people that has a negative

	Intervention		Control			Odds Ratio [95% CI]
Study	Events	n	Events	n	Weight (%)	
1	20	50	4	50	10	0.3 [−1–1.2]
2	60	100	20	100	15	0.8 [0.1–1.4]
3	225	450	85	450	40	0.7 [0.35–1.5]
4	5	50	0	50	10	−0.2 [−1.2–0.9]
5	130	150	20	150	25	0.95 [0.4–1.7]
Total	420	800	129	800		0.75 [0.2–1.1]

Test for overall effect: Z = 5.89 (P=0.003)

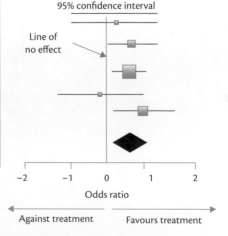

Fig. 10.3.6 An example of results from a meta-analysis. In the table each study is represented (1 to 5). Each study is weighted by the inverse of the variance, a measure of study accuracy. In the forest plot, each blue box represents the point estimate in a study and the size of the box its weight in the analysis. The grey lines at each end of the boxes represent the 95% confidence interval of each study. The black diamond represents the overall combined result, with the overall 95% confidence interval represented by its width. If the diamond is to the right of the line of no effect, the study shows that the treatment is of benefit. In this example, this is numerically confirmed by the *p*-value for the test for the overall effect (0.003).

result and does not have the disease. Table 10.3.1 demonstrates this. Sensitivity and specificity relate to the test, however, positive predictive values explain how likely it is that individuals do or do not have a disease.

Graphs of specificity (false positive rate) against sensitivity (true positive rate) for a given diagnostic test can be drawn to produce receiver operating characteristic curves. This allows comparison of diagnostic tests across a range of diagnostic thresholds. The area under the curve is transformed to a value between zero and one, with one representing the perfect test. The larger the area under the curve, the 'better' the test (i.e. the fewer false positives and the fewer false negatives).

Systematic reviews and meta-analyses

It is common for junior (and senior) surgeons to embark upon these types of projects. A systematic review is a *comprehensive assimilation* of all data (published and unpublished) relevant to a particular question. When data from individual studies in a systematic review are *weighted* and *combined* statistically, this is termed a meta-analysis and special statistical techniques have been developed to do this. There are published guidelines for the conduct and preparation of systematic reviews and meta-analyses. Meta-analysis results are displayed as a forest plot (see Figure 10.3.6). Meta-analyses can be a very valuable tool in clinical decision making. However, care must be made in their interpretation: a number of biases can flaw the data, for example publication bias, where negative results are not published, and therefore not accounted for in the combination of the data.

Further reading

Kirkwood B. Sterne J. *Essential Medical Statistics*, 2nd edition. Oxford: Wiley-Blackwell, 2003.
Peacock J, Peacock P. *Oxford Handbook of Medical Statistics*. Oxford: Oxford University Press, 2010.
Petrie A, Sabin C. *Medical Statistics at a Glance*, 3rd edition. Oxford: Wiley-Blackwell, 2009.

Index